The
Bethesda Handbook
of Clinical
Oncology

FIFTH EDITION

The
Bethesda Handbook
of Clinical
Oncology

FIFTH EDITION

EDITORS

JAME ABRAHAM, MD, FACP

Director, Breast Oncology Program Taussig Cancer Institute,
Professor of Medicine, Lerner College of Medicine,
Cleveland Clinic, Cleveland, Ohio

JAMES L. GULLEY, MD, PHD, FACP
Director, Medical Oncology Service
Center for Cancer Research; National Cancer Institute
National Institutes of Health; Bethesda, Maryland
Formerly of Emory University School of Medicine, and
Loma Linda University School of Medicine

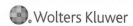

. Wolters Kluwer

Philadelphia • Baltimore • New York • London
Buenos Aires • Hong Kong • Sydney • Tokyo

Senior Acquisitions Editor: Ryan Shaw
Editorial Coordinator: John Larkin
Marketing Manager: Rachel Mante Leung
Production Project Manager: Kim Cox
Design Coordinator: Holly McLaughlin
Manufacturing Coordinator: Beth Welsh
Prepress Vendor: Newgen Knowledge Works Pvt. Ltd., Chennai, India

Fifth Edition
Copyright © 2019 Wolters Kluwer.

2001 Market Street, Philadelphia, PA 19103 USA

Printed in China

Library of Congress Cataloging-in-Publication Data
Names: Abraham, Jame, editor. | Gulley, James L. (James Leonard), 1964– editor.
Title: The Bethesda handbook of clinical oncology / editors, Jame Abraham, James L. Gulley.
Other titles: Handbook of clinical oncology
Description: Fifth edition. | Philadelphia, PA : Wolters Kluwer, [2019] |
Includes bibliographical references and index.
Identifiers: LCCN 2017056079 | ISBN 9781496344182 (Hardback : alk. paper)
Subjects: | MESH: Neoplasms–therapy | Handbooks
Classification: LCC RC262.5 | NLM QZ 39 | DDC 616.99/4–dc23
LC record available at https://lccn.loc.gov/2017056079

*We dedicate this book to those lives that are touched by cancer and
to their caregivers who spend endless hours taking care of them.*

"May I never forget that the patient is a fellow creature in pain.
May I never consider him merely a vessel of disease."
—Maimonides *(Twelfth-century philosopher and physician)*

Contributors

Jame Abraham, MD, FACP Director, Breast Oncology Program, Taussig Cancer Institute, Professor of Medicine, Lerner College of Medicine, Cleveland Clinic, Cleveland, Ohio

David J. Adelstein, MD Professor, Department of Medicine, Cleveland Clinic, Lerner College of Medicine of Case Western Reserve University, Cleveland, Ohio; Staff, Department of Hematology and Medical Oncology, Cleveland Clinic, Taussig Cancer Institute, Cleveland, Ohio

Piyush K. Agarwal, MD Head, Bladder Cancer Section, Urologic Oncology Branch, Center for Cancer Research, National Cancer Institute, National Institutes of Health, Bethesda, Maryland; Tenure-Track Investigator, Urologic Oncology Branch, Center for Cancer Research, National Cancer Institute, National Institutes of Health, Bethesda, Maryland

Sanjiv S. Agarwala, MD Professor, Temple University School of Medicine, Philadelphia, Pennsylvania; Chief of Medical Oncology and Hematology; Director, Melanoma and Immunology Program, St. Luke's Cancer Center, Easton, Pennsylvania

Christina M. Annunziata, MD, PhD Investigator, Women's Malignancies Branch, National Cancer Institute, Bethesda, Maryland

Andrea B. Apolo, MD Chief, Bladder Cancer Section, Investigator and Lasker Scholar, Center for Cancer Research, Genitourinary Malignancies Branch, National Cancer Institute, National Institutes of Health, Bethesda, Maryland

Ananth K. Arjunan, MD Fellow, Division of Hematology and Oncology, University of Pittsburgh, Pittsburgh, Pennsylvania

Philip M. Arlen, MD Attending Physician, National Cancer Institute, National Institutes of Health, Bethesda, Maryland

Ann Berger MSN MD Chief of Pain and Palliative Care, National Institutes of Health, Clinical Center, Bethesda, Maryland

Christina Brzezniak, DO Chief of Thoracic Oncology, John P. Murtha Cancer Center, Walter Reed National Military Medical Center, Bethesda, Maryland

Brian Burkey, MD Professor, Otolaryngology—Head and Neck Surgery, Vice-Chairman, Head and Neck Institute, Cleveland Clinic and Foundation, Cleveland, Ohio

George Carter, MMS PA-C National Institutes of Health, NCL, Medical Oncology Branch, Bethesda, Maryland

Julia Cheringal, MD Medical Oncology Fellow, John P. Murtha Cancer Center, Walter Reed National Military Medical Center, Bethesda, Maryland

Michael Craig, MD Professor, Department of Medicine, Section Chief, West Virginia University Cancer Institute, Morgantown, West Virginia

William L. Dahut, MD Senior Investigator, Genitourinary Malignancies Branch, National Institutes of Health, Bethesda, Maryland

Erin F. Damery, PharmD, BCOP Clinical Oncology Pharmacist, Pharmacy Department, University of Kansas Health System, Kansas City, Kansas

Robert Dean, MD Department of Hematology/Oncology, Taussig Cancer Institute, Cleveland Clinic, Cleveland, Ohio

Jaydira Del Rivero, MD Staff Clinician, Medical Oncology Service, Center for Cancer Research, National Cancer Institutes, National Institutes of Health, North Bethesda, Maryland

Marnie Grant Dobbin, MS, RDN, CNSC Clinical Research Dietitian, Nutrition Department, National Institutes of Health, Bethesda, Maryland

Daniel E. Elswick, MD, FAPM Clinical Associate Professor, Behavioral Medicine and Psychiatry, West Virginia University School of Medicine, Morgantown, West Virginia

Bassam Estfan, MD Assistant Professor of Medicine, Taussig Cancer Institute, Cleveland Clinic, Lerner College of Medicine, Case Western Reserve University, Cleveland, Ohio; Staff, Hematology/Oncology, Cleveland Clinic, Cleveland, Ohio

Sheryl B. Fleisch, MD Assistant Professor, Psychiatry and Behavioral Sciences, Vanderbilt University Medical Center, Nashville, Tennessee

Juan C. Gea-Banacloche, MD Senior Clinician, Experimental Transplantation and Immunology Branch, National Cancer Institute, National Institutes of Health, Bethesda, Maryland; Chief, Infectious Diseases Consultation Service, NIAID/NCI, NIH Clinical Center, Bethesda, Maryland

Thomas J. George, Jr., MD, FACP Associate Professor, Department of Medicine, University of Florida, Gainesville, Florida; Director, GI Oncology Program, Department of Medicine, University of Florida Health Cancer Center, Gainesville, Florida

Aaron T. Gerds, MD, MS Assistant Professor of Medicine, Hematology and Medical Oncology, Cleveland Clinic, Cleveland, Ohio; Staff, Leukemia Program, Cleveland Clinic, Cleveland, Ohio

Azam Ghafoor, MD Oncology Fellow, Medical Oncology Branch, National Cancer Institute, Bethesda, Maryland

Mark R. Gilbert, MD Senior Investigator and Chief, Neuro-Oncology Branch, National Institutes of Health/National Institute of Neurologic Disorders and Stroke, National Institutes of Health, Bethesda, Maryland

Ann W. Gramza, MD Medical Oncologist, Division of Hematology and Oncology, Lombardi Comprehensive Cancer Center, Georgetown University, Washington, DC

Megan Greally MB, BCh, BAO Advanced Oncology Fellow, Gastrointestinal Oncology, Memorial Sloan Kettering Cancer Center, New York

F. Anthony Greco, MD Director Sarah Cannon Cancer Center, Centennial Medical Center Sarah Cannon Cancer Center, Nashville, Tennessee

James L. Gulley, MD, PhD, FACP Director, Medical Oncology Service, Center for Cancer Research, National Cancer Institute, National Institutes of Health, Bethesda, Maryland; Formerly of Emory University School of Medicine, and Loma Linda University School of Medicine

Mehdi Hamadani, MD Associate Professor of Medicine, Hematology/Oncology, CIBMTR & Medical College of Wisconsin, Milwaukee, Wisconsin; Director, Blood and Marrow Transplant Program, Hematology/Oncology, Froedtert Hosptial, Milwaukee, Wisconsin

Hannah W. Hazard-Jenkins, MD, FACS Associate Professor, Department of Surgery, Director of Clinical Services, WVU Cancer Institute, West Virginia University Hospital, Morgantown, West Virginia

Brandie Heald, MS, LGC Licensed Genetic Counselor, Genomic Medicine Institute, Cleveland Clinic, Cleveland, Ohio

Upendra P. Hegde, MD Associate Professor, Department of Medicine, University of Connecticut, Farmington, Connecticut; Associate Director, Melanoma and Cutaneous Oncology Program, Neag Comprehensive Cancer Center, John Dempsey Hospital, Farmington, Connecticut

Thomas E. Hughes, PharmD, BCOP Clinical Pharmacy Specialist, Pharmacy Department, National Institutes of Health, Clinical Research Center, Bethesda, Maryland

Nikhil P. Joshi, MD Assistant Professor of Medicine, Cleveland Clinic, Lerner College of Medicine, Cleveland, Ohio; Staff Physician, College of Medicine, California; Staff Physician, Department of Radiation Oncology, Cleveland Clinic Foundation, California

Matt Kalaycio, MD Department of Hematology/Oncology, Taussig Cancer Institute, Cleveland Clinic, Cleveland, Ohio

Abraham S. Kanate, MD Assistant Professor of Internal Medicine, Osborn Hematopoietic Malignancy and Transplantation Program, West Virginia University, Morgantown, West Virginia

Alok A. Khorana, MD, FACP Professor of Medicine, Taussig Cancer Institute, Cleveland Clinic Lerner College of Medicine, Case Western Reserve University, Cleveland, Ohio; Staff, Hematology/Oncology, Cleveland Clinic, Cleveland, Ohio

David R. Kohler, PharmD Oncology Clinical Pharmacy Specialist, Pharmacy Department, National Institutes of Health Clinical Center, Bethesda, Maryland

Elise C. Kohn, MD, CAPT (ret), USPHS Head, Gynecologic Cancer Therapeutics, Clinical Investigations Branch, Cancer Therapy Evaluation Program, National Cancer Institute, Bethesda, Maryland

Megan Kruse, MD Department of Hematology-Oncology, Cleveland Clinic, Cleveland, Ohio

Chaoyuan Kuang, MD, PhD Fellow, Division of Hematology and Oncology, University of Pittsburgh, Pittsburgh, Pennsylvania; Fellow, Division of Hematology and Oncology, University of Pittsburgh Medical Center, Pittsburgh, Pennsylvania

Shaji K. Kumar, MD. Professor of Medicine, Consultant, Division of Hematology, Chair, Dysproteinemia Group; Medical Director, Cancer Clinical Research Office, Rochester, Minnesota

Charles A. Kunos, MD, PhD Medical Officer and Coordinator, Investigational Therapeutics & Radiation, Investigational Drug Branch, Cancer Therapy Evaluation Program, Division of Cancer Treatment and Diagnosis, National Cancer Institute, National Institutes of Health, Rockville, Maryland

Arjun Lakshman, MD, MRCP Post-doctoral Research Fellow, Division of Hematology, Mayo Clinic, Rochester, Minnesota; Post-doctoral Research Fellow, Division of Hematology, Mayo Clinic, Rochester, Minnesota

Paulette Lebda, MD Department of Radiology, Cleveland Clinic, Cleveland, Ohio

James J. Lee, MD, PhD Associate Professor of Medicine, Division of Hematology-Oncology, Department of Medicine, University of Pittsburgh School of Medicine, Pittsburgh, Pennsylvania

Jung-min Lee, MD Investigator and Lasker Clinical Research Scholar, Women's Malignancies Branch, Center for Cancer Research, National Cancer Institute, Bethesda, Maryland

Gregory D. Leonard University Hospital Galway, Galway, Ireland

Ravi A. Madan, MD Clinical Director of the Genitourinary Malignancies Branch at the National Cancer Institute, National Institutes of Health, Bethesda, Maryland

Bindu Manyam, MD Department of Radiation Oncology, Cleveland Clinic, Cleveland, Ohio

Christopher Melani, MD Staff Clinician, Lymphoid Malignancies Branch, National Cancer Institute, National Institutes of Health, Bethesda, Maryland; Staff Clinician, Lymphoid Malignancies Branch, National Cancer Institute, National Institutes of Health, Bethesda, Maryland

Lekha Mikkilineni, MD, MA Fellow in Hematology/
Oncology, National Cancer Institute, National Institutes
of Health, Bethesda, Maryland; Clinical Fellow, National
Cancer Institute, Clinical Center - NIH, Bethesda,
Maryland

Emanuela Molinari Neurology Department, Neuroscience
Division, The Queen Elizabeth University Hospital,
Glasgow, United Kingdom; Consultant Neurologist,
Neurology, The Queen Elizabeth University Hospital,
Glasgow, United Kingom

Andreas Niethammer, MD, PhD Associate Professor
of Experimental Oncology, Department of Radiation
Oncology, Ruprecht-Karls-Universitaet Heidelberg,
Heidelberg, Germany

Michelle A. Ojemuyiwa, MD Assistant Professor,
Department of Medicine, Hematology Oncology
Uniformed Services, University of Health Sciences Walter
Reed National Military Medical Center, Bethesda, Maryland

Maryland Pao, MD Clinical Professor, Department of
Psychiatry, Georgetown University School of Medicine,
Washington, DC; Clinical & Deputy Scientific Director,
National Institute of Mental Health, National Institutes of
Health, Bethesda, Maryland

Hiral Parekh, MD, MPH Assistant Professor, Department
of Medicine, University of Florida, Gainesville, Florida;
Oncologist, Department of Medicine, University of Florida
Health Cancer Center, Gainesville, Florida

Holly Jane Pederson, MD Associate Professor, Medicine,
Cleveland Clinic, Lerner College of Medicine, Cleveland,
Ohio; Director, Medical Breast Services, Breast Services,
Department of General Surgery, Cleveland Clinic,
Cleveland, Ohio

Jean-Paul Pinzon, DO Medical Director, Palliative Care,
Inova Schar Cancer Institute, Fairfax, Virginia

Muzaffar H. Qazilbash, MD Professor of Medicine, Stem
Cell Transplantation and Cellular Therapy, University of
Texas, MD Anderson Cancer Center, Houston, Texas

Jason M. Redman, MD Medical Oncology Fellow, Medical
Oncology Service, National Cancer Institute, National
Institutes of Health, Bethesda, Maryland

Kevin R. Rice, MD Associate Professor of Surgery,
Urology Service Uniformed Services, University of Health
Sciences, Walter Reed National Military Medical Center,
Bethesda, Maryland

Mark Roschewski, MD Staff Clinician, Lymphoid
Malignancies Branch, National Cancer Institute, National
Institutes of Health, Bethesda, Maryland; Staff Clinician,
Lymphoid Malignancies Branch, National Cancer Institute,
National Institutes of Health, Bethesda, Maryland

Donald L. Rosenstein, MD Professor and Vice Chair for
Hospital Psychiatry, Psychiatry and Medicine, University
of North Carolina at Chapel Hill, Chapel Hill, North
Carolina; Director, Comprehensive Cancer Support
Program, North Carolina Cancer Hospital, Chapel Hill,
North Carolina

Inger L. Rosner, MD Associate Professor, Department of
Surgery, Uniformed Services University, Bethesda, Maryland;
Director, Urologic Oncology, Department of Surgery, Walter
Reed National Military Medical Center, Bethesda, Maryland

Kerry Ryan, MPH, MS PA-C National Institutes of Health,
NHLBI, Pulmonary Branch, Bethesda, Maryland.

Meena Sadaps, MD Medical Resident, Department
of Internal Medicine, Cleveland Clinic Foundation,
Cleveland, Ohio

Yogen Saunthararajah, MD Professor of Medicine,
Hematology and Oncology, Case Western Reserve
University, Cleveland, Ohio; Staff, Hematology and
Oncology, Cleveland Clinic, Cleveland, Ohio

Mikkael A. Sekeres, MD, MS Professor of Medicine,
Director, Leukemia Program, Cleveland Clinic, Cleveland,
Ohio; Director, Leukemia Program, Cleveland Clinic,
Cleveland, Ohio

Chirag Shah, MD Associate Professor, Department of
Radiation Oncology, Cleveland Clinic Lerner College of
Medicine, Cleveland, Ohio; Staff Physician, Director of
Clinical Research, Department of Radiation Oncology,
Cleveland Clinic, Cleveland, Ohio

Dale R. Shepard, MD, PhD Director, Taussig Cancer
Institute Phase I and Sarcoma Programs; Staff, Hematology
and Medical Oncology and Center for Geriatric Medicine,
Cleveland Clinic, Cleveland, Ohio; Assistant Professor
of Medicine, Internal Medicine, Cleveland Clinic, Lerner
College of Medicine, Cleveland, Ohio; Director, Taussig
Institute Phase I and Sarcoma Programs, Hematology and
Medical Oncology, Cleveland Clinic, Cleveland, Ohio

Davendra P. S. Sohal, MD, MPH Assistant Professor of
Medicine, Taussig Cancer Institute, Cleveland Clinic, Lerner
College of Medicine, Case Western Reserve University,
Cleveland, Ohio; Staff, Hematology/Oncology, Cleveland
Clinic, Cleveland, Ohio

Ramaprasad Srinivasan, MD, PhD Investigator and Head,
Molecular Cancer Section, Urologic Oncology Branch,
Center for Cancer Research, National Cancer Institute,
Bethesda, Maryland

Samer A. Srour, MB ChB, MS Assistant Professor of
Medicine, Department of Medicine, Dan L. Duncan
Comprehensive Cancer Center, Hematology and Oncology
Section, Baylor College of Medicine, Houston, Texas

Jason S. Starr, DO Assistant Professor, Department
of Medicine, University of Florida, Gainesville, Florida;
Oncologist, Department of Medicine, University of Florida
Health Cancer Center, Gainesville, Florida

James P. Stevenson, MD Vice-Chairman, Department
of Hematology and Medical Oncology, Cleveland Clinic,
Taussig Cancer Institute, Cleveland, Ohio

Julius Strauss, MD Staff Clinician, Laboratory of Tumor
Immunology and Biology, Center for Cancer Research,
National Cancer Institute, National Institutes of Health,
Bethesda, Maryland

Christina Tafe, MSN, ACNP-BC, ACHPN Nurse Practitioner, Advanced Disease Management, Heartland Care Partners, Fairfax, Virginia

Sarah M. Temkin, MD Professor, Massey Cancer Center, Virginia Commonwealth University, Richmond, Virginia; Division Director, Gynecologic Oncology, Virginia Commonwealth University, Richmond, Virginia

Anish Thomas, MBBS, MD Investigator, Developmental Therapeutics Branch, National Cancer Institute, Bethesda, Maryland

Neel Trivedi, MD Hematology/Oncology Fellow, Division of Hematology/Oncology, Lombardi Comprehensive Cancer Center, Washington, DC

Chaitra Ujjani, MD Associate Professor, Division of Hematology/Oncology, Lombardi Comprehensive Cancer Center, Washington, DC

Stephanie Valente, DO Department of Surgery, Cleveland Clinic, Cleveland, Ohio

Leticia Varella, MD Assistant Professor, Department of Medicine, Division of Hematology & Oncology, Weill Cornell Medicine, Cornell University, New York, New York

Andrew Vassil, MD Department of Radiation Oncology, Cleveland Clinic, Cleveland, Ohio

Christopher E. Wee, MD Chief Medical Resident, Department of Internal Medicine, Cleveland Clinic Foundation, Cleveland, Ohio

Kristen P. Zeligs, MD Gynecologic Oncologist, Department of Obstetrics and Gynecology, Walter Reed National Military Medical Center, Bethesda, Maryland

Peter A. Zmijewski, MD Chief Resident, West Virginia University General Surgery Residency, West Virginia University School of Medicine, Morgantown, West Virginia

Preface

The Bethesda Handbook of Clinical Oncology is a clear, concise, and comprehensive reference book for the busy clinician to use in his or her daily patient encounters. The book has been compiled by clinicians who are working at the National Cancer Institute, National Institutes of Health, Cleveland Clinic, M.D. Anderson, Mayo Clinic as well as scholars from other academic institutions. To limit the size of the book, less space is dedicated to etiology, pathophysiology, and epidemiology and greater emphasis is placed on practical clinical information. For easy accessibility to the pertinent information, long descriptions are avoided, and more tables, pictures, algorithms, and phrases are included.

The Bethesda Handbook of Clinical Oncology is not intended as a substitute for the many excellent oncology reference textbooks available that are essential for a more complete understanding of the pathophysiology and management of complicated oncology patients. We hope that the reader-friendly format with its comprehensive review of the management of each disease with treatment regimens, including dosing and schedule, makes this book unique and useful for oncologists, oncology fellows, residents, students, oncology nurses, and allied health professionals.

The landscape of oncology has changed substantially since we published the first edition of this book more than 16 years ago. For the fifth edition, we have updated all chapters and added two new chapters, "Clinical Genetics" and "Diagnosis-Driven Individualization of Cancer Care." Since we are publishing a companion Board Review Book *The Bethesda Review of Clinical Oncology,* in this edition we have eliminated the questions at the end of each chapters.

As always, we have attempted to capture the advances in the field and listened to the feedback from readers to improve this edition. We hope that anyone needing a comprehensive review of oncology will find *The Bethesda Handbook of Clinical Oncology* to be an indispensable resource.

Jame Abraham and James L. Gulley

Acknowledgments

Our sincere thanks to all our esteemed colleagues and friends who contributed to this book.

We thank our publisher, Wolters Kluwer, and dedicated staff members at the company who have been supporting this book for more than 13 years. We would like to thank Ms. Grace Caputo for carefully editing many chapters and offering suggestions.

We thank our wives, Shyla, and Trenise, for their encouragement and support in this endeavor.

Above all, we thank you for your support and feedback.

Contents

Head and Neck 1

Nikhil P. Joshi, David J. Adelstein, and Brian Burkey

EPIDEMIOLOGY AND RISK FACTORS

The overwhelming majority of head and neck cancers are squamous cell cancers (HNSCC). More than 500,000 cases of HNSCC are diagnosed worldwide, and 40,000 to 60,000 cases occur in the United States. HNSCC comprise approximately 3% to 5% of all new cancers and 2% of all cancer deaths in the United States. Most patients are older than 50 years, incidence increases with age, and the male-to-female ratio is 2:1 to 5:1. The age-adjusted incidence is higher among black men, and, stage-for-stage, survival among African Americans is lower overall than in whites. Death rates have been decreasing since at least 1975, with rates declining more rapidly in the past decade. Human papillomavirus (HPV)–related oropharyngeal cancer is a subset of head and neck cancers that is increasing in number and is associated with a better prognosis, in part due to better response to treatment. The most common sites of head and neck cancer are the oral cavity, pharynx, larynx, and hypopharynx in the United States. Nasal cavity, buccal, paranasal sinus cancers, salivary gland malignancies, and various sarcomas, lymphomas, and melanoma are less common. This chapter will limit its discussion to the more common tumors found in the head and neck region, namely squamous cell carcinomas and related histologies. Lymphomas, sarcomas, cutaneous malignancies including melanoma and thyroid gland cancer will not be discussed.

Common risk factors include tobacco (smoking tobacco and other forms) and alcohol intake. Heavy alcohol consumption increases the risk of developing squamous head and neck cancer 2- to 6-fold, whereas smoking increases the risk 5- to 25-fold, depending on gender, race, and the amount of smoking. Both factors together increase the risk 15- to 40-fold. Smokeless/chewing tobacco and snuff are associated with oral cavity cancers. Use of smokeless tobacco, or chewing betel with or without tobacco, and slaked lime (common in many parts of Asia and some parts of Africa), is associated with premalignant lesions and oral squamous cancers. Chronic dental irritation due to ill-fitting dentures, sharp teeth, or inflammatory lesions like oral lichen planus also predispose to oral cavity cancers.

Multifocal mucosal abnormalities have been described in patients with head and neck cancer ("field cancerization"). There is a 2% to 6% risk per year for a second head and neck, lung, or esophageal cancer in patients with a history of a tobacco-related cancer in this area. Those who continue to smoke have the highest risk. Second primary cancers represent a major risk factor for death among survivors of an initial squamous carcinoma of the head and neck.

Epstein-Barr virus (EBV) has been detected in almost all nonkeratinizing and undifferentiated nasopharyngeal cancers in North America but less consistently in keratinizing squamous nasopharyngeal cancers. HPV infection is associated with up to 70% of cancers of the oropharynx (base of tongue and tonsil), and some squamous nasopharyngeal cancers. The incidence of HPV-related oropharyngeal cancers is increasing in several countries, and HPV positivity is more common in cancers of nonsmokers. Disorders of DNA repair (e.g., Fanconi anemia and dyskeratosis congenita) as well as organ transplantation with immunosuppression are also associated with increased risk of squamous head and neck cancer.

ANATOMY AND PATHOLOGY

A simplified depiction of extracranial head and neck anatomy is presented in Figure 1.1. The major regions and subsites of the upper aerodigestive tract are divided into the nose and paranasal sinuses; nasopharynx (NP); oral cavity (OC; lips, gingiva, buccal areas, floor of mouth, hard palate, and tongue anterior to the circumvallate papillae); oropharynx (OP; soft palate, tonsils, base of tongue and lingual tonsils, and pharyngeal wall between palate and vallecula); hypopharynx (HP; posterior pharyngeal wall between vallecula and esophageal inlet, piriform sinuses, and postcricoid space); and larynx (supraglottis, glottis, and subglottis). The supraglottic larynx comprises the epiglottis, aryepiglottic folds, false vocal cords, and ventricles. The glottis comprises the true vocal cords, anterior commissure, and posterior commissure. The subglottis extends under the glottis to the cricoid cartilage and continues as the trachea.

Knowledge of the lymphatic drainage of the neck assists in identification of the site of a primary tumor when a palpable lymph node is the initial presentation, and in staging metastatic spread, enabling the surgeon or radiation oncologist to plan appropriate treatment of both primary and neck disease. The patterns of lymphatic drainage divide the neck into several levels (Fig. 1.2): Level I includes the submental or submandibular nodes, which are most often involved with lesions of the oral cavity, nasal cavity, or submandibular salivary gland. Level II (upper jugular lymph nodes) extends from the skull base to the hyoid bone, and is frequently the site of metastatic presentation of naso- or oropharyngeal primaries. Level III (middle jugular lymph nodes between the hyoid bone and the lower border of the cricoid cartilage) and level IV (lower jugular lymph nodes between the cricoid cartilage and the clavicle) are most often involved by metastases from the hypopharynx, larynx, or above. Level V is the posterior triangle, including cervical nodes along cranial nerve XI, frequently involved along with level II sites in cancers of the naso- and oropharynx. Level VI is the anterior compartment from the hyoid bone to the

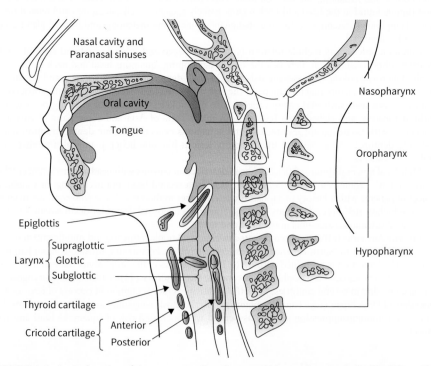

FIGURE 1.1 Sagittal section of the upper aerodigestive tract. (Adapted from Oatis CA. *Kinesiology: The Mechanics and Pathomechanics of Human Movement*. Baltimore, MD: Lippincott Williams & Wilkins; 2004.)

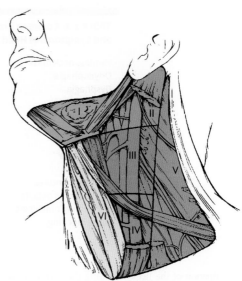

FIGURE 1.2 Diagram of the neck showing levels of lymph nodes. Level I, submandibular; level II, high jugular; level III, midjugular; level IV, low jugular; level V, posterior triangle; level VI, tracheoesophageal; level VII, superior mediastinal, is not shown. (From Robbins KT, Samant S, Ronen O. Neck dissection. In: Flint PW, Haughey BH, Lund VJ, et al., eds. *Cumming's Otolaryngology Head and Neck Surgery*. 5th ed. Copyright Elsevier, 2010. Used with permission.)

suprasternal notch bounded on each side by the medial carotid sheath, and is an important region for the spread of laryngeal and thyroid carcinomas. Level VII is the area of the superior mediastinum, and mostly portends distant metastasis except for thyroid cancers.

PRESENTATION, EVALUATION, DIAGNOSIS, AND STAGING

Signs and symptoms most often include pain and/or mass effects of tumor, involving adjacent structures, nerves, or regional lymph nodes (Table 1.1). This is common for oral cavity cancers. Adult patients with any of these symptoms for more than 2 weeks should be referred to an otolaryngologist. Delay in diagnosis is common due to patient delay, repeated courses of antibiotics for otitis media or sore throat, or lack of follow-up. A persistent lateralized symptom or firm cervical mass is highly suggestive of malignancy, and may represent a squamous cell carcinoma (Fig. 1.3). For nasopharyngeal and oropharyngeal cancers, a common presenting symptom is a neck mass, often in a node in the jugulodigastric area and/or the posterior triangle. In advanced lesions, cranial nerve abnormalities may be present. Symptoms like hoarseness, hemoptysis, and odynophagia or dysphagia may indicate a laryngeal or hypopharyngeal primary. Distant metastases are uncommon at presentation, but may occur with nasopharyngeal, oropharyngeal, and hypopharyngeal cancers. The most common sites of distant metastases are lung and bone; liver and central nervous system involvement is less common.

The history should include the following:

1. Signs and symptoms as listed in Table 1.1 and above
2. Tobacco exposure (pack-years; amount chewed; and duration of habit, current or former)
3. Alcohol exposure (number of drinks per day and duration of habit)
4. Other risk factors (chewing betel nut, chronic dental irritation, oral lichen planus, oral submucous fibrosis, leukoplakia, or erythroplakia)
5. Cancer history of patient and family; history of immunosuppression or congenital disorder
6. Thorough review of systems

The head and neck physical examination should include the following:

1. Careful inspection of the scalp, ears, nose, and mouth.

**TABLE 1.1 Common Presenting Signs
and Symptoms of Head and Neck Cancer**

Painless neck mass
Odynophagia
Dysphagia
Hoarseness
Hemoptysis
Trismus
Otalgia
Otitis media
Loose teeth
Ill-fitting dentures
Cranial nerve deficits
Nonhealing oral ulcers
Nasal bleeding

2. Palpation of the neck including the thyroid gland and oral cavity, assessment of tongue mobility, determination of restrictions in the ability to open the mouth (trismus), and bimanual palpation of the base of the tongue and floor of the mouth.
3. During examination of the nasal passages, NP, oropharynx, hypopharynx, and larynx, flexible endoscopes or mirrors as appropriate should be strongly considered for symptoms of hoarseness, sore throat, or enlarged lymph nodes not cured by a single course of antibiotics. When a neck mass with occult primary is the first presentation, the primary site can be located by clinical or flexible endoscopic examination in approximately 80% of cases.
4. Special attention to the examination of cranial nerves.
5. Look for possible skin cancers.

For abnormalities identified by history, physical examination, and/or endoscopy, the following evaluations should be performed. Superficial cutaneous or oral mucosal lesions, with irregular shape, erythema, induration, ulceration, and/or friability (easy bleeding) of greater than 2-week duration warrant biopsy, as these frequently are early indicators of severe dysplasia, carcinoma in situ, or invasive malignant process. For findings or lesions involving the nose, NP, oropharynx, hypopharynx and larynx, or neck with unknown primary, computed tomography (CT), and/or magnetic resonance imaging (MRI) with contrast should first be performed to identify origin, extent, and potential vascularity of lesions. Surgical biopsy of a neck mass before endoscopy is generally not advisable if a squamous cell carcinoma is suspected. Open biopsy may complicate regional control although an open biopsy may provide additional information to that obtained from fine needle aspiration (FNA) or a core needle biopsy. A direct laryngoscopy is still necessary for staging and treatment planning. Tissue diagnosis obtained by FNA biopsy of the node has a sensitivity and specificity approaching 99%. However, a nondiagnostic FNA or negative flexible endoscopy does not rule out the presence of tumor. Positron emission tomography (PET) scans combined with CT (PET/CT) or MRI can often localize smaller or submucosal primaries of the naso- and oropharynx that present with level II or V cervical adenopathy. Intraoperative endoscopic biopsy is then done with a secure airway under anesthesia. Bilateral tonsillectomy will sometimes reveal the source of an occult cancer, especially for HPV+ cancers. Esophagoscopy and bronchoscopy may be indicated for symptoms such as dysphagia, hoarseness, cough, or to search for occult primary. Transoral robotic surgery (TORS) can also be used to diagnose otherwise occult oropharyngeal cancers.

After a diagnosis of cancer is established, the patient should be staged using physical examination, endoscopic studies, and radiologic studies, which usually include CT scan and/or MRI of the primary tumor, neck, and chest. CT scan is considered the primary imaging study for evaluation of bone involvement, regional, mediastinal, and pulmonary metastasis. MRI may complement the CT scan with

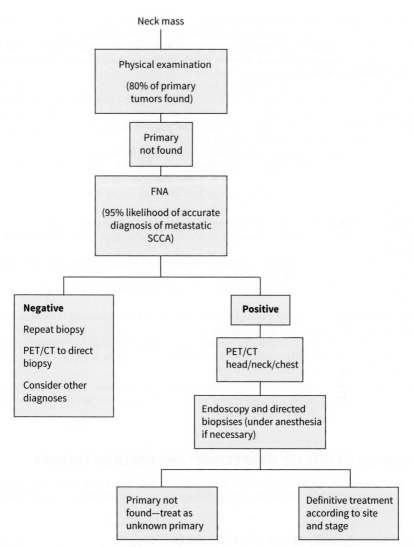

FIGURE 1.3 Evaluation of cervical adenopathy when a primary cancer of the head and neck is suspected.

greater resolution of soft tissue for primary tumor staging, and evaluation of skull base and intracranial involvement. PET/CT scans are being used more frequently to detect tumors or nodes that are not obvious on other scans and for monitoring for disease recurrence in patients with advanced locoregional disease treated with concurrent chemotherapy and radiotherapy. PET/CT scanning is also indicated for staging patients with unknown primaries and for advanced head and neck cancers. A chest CT (or PET/CT) may also be useful for patients with locally advanced disease because of the risk of metastasis or a second lung malignancy.

Specialized tests include tissue p16 immunostaining for oropharyngeal cancers, and tissue Epstein-Barr encoded RNA (EBER) and plasma EBV DNA copy number for nasopharyngeal carcinoma. Laboratory tests typically obtained prior to initiating therapy include complete blood counts, renal and liver function tests, serum calcium and magnesium (if platinum-based chemotherapy is to be given), baseline thyroid function tests, and pregnancy testing in females of child-bearing age. Baseline and post treatment EBV DNA levels are recommended in EBV-related nasopharyngeal cancers.

Dental evaluation should be performed and any necessary extractions should be carried out at least 2 weeks prior to any planned radiation. Baseline speech, swallow, and audiometry evaluation may be indicated depending on the primary site involved and the treatment anticipated.

Clinical staging is based on physical and endoscopic examinations and imaging tests. The staging systems of the American Joint Committee for Cancer (AJCC) or the Union Internationale Contre le Cancer (UICC) (tumor, node, metastasis [TNM], stages I to IV) are used. The AJCC classification has further subdivided the most advanced disease stages into stage IVA (moderately advanced), stage IVB (very advanced), and stage IVC (distant metastatic).

The staging of primary tumors is different for each site within the head and neck, although some common themes exist. The *AJCC Cancer Staging Manual*, which entered its eighth edition in 2017, has made several significant changes in the previous T, N, and staging definition.

Below is a summary of the pertinent changes for head and neck cancer staging detailed in the *AJCC* eighth edition:

(1) Oral cavity cancer staging now reflects the depth of invasion as an important factor.
(2) p16-positive and p16-negative oropharynx cancers have separate staging systems for their T and N stage.
(3) The nodal staging for p16-positive oropharynx cancer is more akin to nasopharynx nodal staging; the stage grouping is different from other head and neck subsites as well.
(4) The tumor staging for nasopharynx cancer has been revised to more accurately reflect anatomic involvement.
(5) The nodal staging for nasopharynx cancer has been revised to reflect involvement above and below the cricoid cartilage; stage IVC has been eliminated.
(6) Nonoropharyngeal/nasopharyngeal cancer nodal staging has been revised to reflect the importance of extranodal extension (ENE)—clinical and pathologic nodal staging is different on the basis of node size and presence of ENE.

Discussion regarding staging in this chapter refers to the seventh edition of the *AJCC staging manual*. The eighth edition of the *AJCC Staging Manual* will be used to stage head and neck cancers starting January 2018 and should be consulted for details.

PRINCIPLES OF DISEASE MANAGEMENT AND GOALS OF THERAPY

Since head and neck cancer involves multiple individual sites of disease, it is useful to think of disease management principles according to the extent of disease. Certain common themes of management are evident as described below.

Early Disease (Usually Stages I, II, and Selected Stage III)

Early disease is optimally managed with single modality treatment. This could include surgery or radiation. The objective is to achieve high rates of locoregional control and cure while limiting morbidity of treatment and preserving functional outcomes. Organ conservation is central to management of early cancers. The choice of modality is dependent on how best these goals are achieved along with availability of expertise and patient choice.

Locoregionally Advanced Disease (Usually Stages III, IVA, IVB)

This is a heterogeneous group of patients spanning the spectrum of resectable and unresectable disease. Two or more treatment modalities are often combined to achieve optimal disease control. The primary modality of treatment depends on the site of disease. For example, while primary surgery is considered standard for oral cavity cases, radiation with chemotherapy might be considered for laryngeal cancer cases. Nasopharyngeal cases are treated with definitive chemoradiation in most cases. Trimodality treatment is necessary on occasion. Examples include surgery followed by adjuvant chemoradiation for locally advanced oral cavity cancers or surgical salvage after definitive chemoradiation for oropharynx/larynx/hypopharynx cancers. While organ preservation remains an important goal for larynx and hypopharynx cancers, disease control is the primary objective. Multimodality therapy including surgical resection is often required to reduce the risk of locoregional recurrence and/or distant metastases and improve survival when organ preservation is not possible.

Recurrent/Metastatic Disease (Stage IVC)

Recurrent and metastatic diseases often have equally poor prognoses. Exceptions may include "oligo-metastatic" disease, second cancers after a long disease-free interval and metastatic disease from HPV-associated oropharyngeal cancers. These categories may have a long natural history and a comparatively long disease course with therapy. Long term cures though uncommon are seen, especially with second cancers. This is discussed separately below. The large bulk of recurrent/metastatic cancers are best treated with palliative therapy. Palliative radiation, palliative chemotherapy, or a combination of the two is often used. Occasionally surgery might be used to debulk the cancer and offer quick relief of symptoms. A tracheostomy may be necessary for airway compromise and a feeding tube procedure may be required for alimentation. High-dose radiation with stereotactic techniques may be used to achieve durable palliation with lower toxicity rates. Early intervention with hospice care and palliative medicine may be appropriate during the course of disease.

PRINCIPLES OF SURGERY

Surgery plays a central role in the management of head and neck cancers. This includes management of the primary and the neck in most cases. For the primary cancer, surgical goals include resection of the tumor with an adequate margin (usually 0.5 cm microscopic margin) while preserving function (for early cancers), often with an en-block resection. Piece-meal resection is usually not favored. Exceptions include resection of sinus tumors via an endoscopic approach as opposed to an open surgical approach. The extent of primary oncologic cancer surgery depends on the subsite involved and is variably described as such. For example, oral tongue cancer surgery can span the spectrum of wide local excision to hemi-glossectomy to total glossectomy depending on the extent of the disease. Early oropharynx and larynx cancers are amenable to transoral robotic resection or transoral microsurgery using laser. These modern procedures are far less morbid than open procedures like a transcervical approach or mandibular swing done in the past. On occasion however, an open procedure might be necessary and the morbidity of this approach has to be balanced against the alternative of nonoperative therapy. While transoral procedures are becoming more popular, appropriate case selection is crucial to optimize outcomes.

Management of the neck includes removal of all fibrofatty tissue in the neck levels at risk for disease spread for early disease or removal of all grossly involved nodes along with structures involved by the nodes for locoregionally advanced disease. The extent of neck dissection depends on the amount of neck disease. More aggressive neck dissections are needed for more extensive neck disease. For example, a selective neck dissection or modified radical neck dissection (type III) is adequate for elective nodal dissection/limited neck disease but a more extensive neck dissection might be needed if various structures in the neck are involved by disease (type I). A radical neck dissection might be needed in the salvage setting or if extensive neck disease is present, which involves the sternoclei-domastoid muscle (SCM) and/or internal jugular vein. On occasion, multimodality surgical expertise is needed—cardiovascular surgery for reconstructing the carotid and subclavian artery or neurosurgery to assist with skull base resections or intracranial disease.

Surgical resection, as described, inevitably results in tissue deficits, which can significantly affect function and cosmesis or both. This has led to a separate practice of surgery dedicated to reconstructive surgery. This entails various grafts involving the transfer of skin and muscle/bone to reconstruct or cover tissue defects. This is especially of value for salvage of recurrent disease after initial surgery or definitive radiation/chemoradiation. A detailed discussion is beyond the scope of this chapter, but suffice it to say that modern day head and neck surgery requires the ability to do elaborate reconstruction simultaneously with tumor extirpation.

PRINCIPLES OF RADIATION

Radiation, like surgery, also plays an important role in the treatment of HNSCC. It involves the precise delivery of radiation using x-rays or electrons to tumor targets while sparing as much normal tissue as reasonably possible. The intent of radiation therapy may be definitive (with or without concurrent chemotherapy), adjuvant after surgery (for microscopic disease), or palliative. Definitive doses of radiation (70 Gy equivalent) are generally used to treat gross disease, while lower doses (60 to 66 Gy equivalent) are used to treat microscopic disease in the postoperative setting. Certain recurrent cases may be treated with definitive reirradiation or with postoperative reirradiation. Reirradiation may be delivered once daily or twice daily as hyperfractionated radiation. Occasionally, induction radiation (with or without chemotherapy) may be used. In general, definitive doses of radiation are used for single modality treatment or when combined with chemotherapy for nonsurgical treatment of locally advanced disease. The dose is usually 70 Gy delivered at 2 Gy per fraction over 7 weeks. This is considered standard fractionation in the United States. However, other definitive dose fractionation schedules have been used around the world. Examples include 60 Gy in 25 fractions over 5 weeks, 64 Gy in 40 fractions over 4 weeks, and 55 Gy in 20 fractions over 4 weeks. Altered fractionation schemes include acceleration (same dose given over shorter periods of time), hyperfractionation (2 or more smaller fractions per day, higher total dose, and same overall treatment period), and hypofractionation (larger doses per fraction with a lower total dose). Hyperfractionation has shown an overall survival benefit and locoregional control benefit compared with standard fractionation. Toxicity profiles are different as well. In general, acute toxicities are worse but late toxicities are similar with hyperfractionation compared with standard fractionation. Adjuvant radiation after surgery is used to reduce the risk of locoregional recurrence. This is combined with chemotherapy for high-risk disease (positive margins or extracapsular nodal disease) based on a combined analysis of two studies (RTOG 9501 and EORTC 22931). The doses of adjuvant radiation are 60 to 66 Gy in 2 Gy fractions given over 6 to 6½ weeks. General indications for adjuvant radiation include T3, T4 disease, close margins (<0.5 cm), positive margins, lymphovascular space invasion, perineural disease, and node positive disease.

The technique of radiation delivery has improved dramatically over the years, and intensity modulated radiation therapy (IMRT) is considered standard for HNSCC. This involves using multiple beams of radiation to target the disease with variable radiation beam intensity in order to optimally spare normal tissue. Many centers have graduated to volumetric modulated arc therapy (VMAT). This is a special form of IMRT using radiation arcs to generate more degrees of freedom and modulate the radiation intensity better. Moreover, this technique is now usually combined with image guidance (IGRT). This involves the use of daily cone-beam CT scanning while the patient is on the treatment machine to ensure precise and reproducible patient positioning, thereby reducing the amount of normal tissue in the radiation field.

Palliative radiation involves the delivery of a quick and limited volume of radiation often to the gross disease for rapid relief of symptoms. Different fractionation schemes include 20 Gy in 5 fractions, 30 Gy in 10 fractions, 8 Gy in one fraction, or 14 Gy in 4 fractions (2 fractions a day, 6 hours apart). The response is often short-lived but serves the goal for patients with 4 to 6 months life expectancy. Apart from HPV/EBV positive disease involving the oropharynx or nasopharynx, HNSCC remains a locoregionally recurrent problem. Recognition of this pattern of recurrence combined with the short-lived response to conventional palliative radiation has led to the development of stereotactic body radiotherapy (SBRT). SBRT is a high-precision radiation delivery technique used to deliver a very high-dose of radiation over a few treatments (usually 5) in the recurrent/metastatic disease setting. This technique is associated with durable response rates with acceptable morbidity and is favored when life expectancy is more than 6 months.

Proton therapy is a special form of radiation which enables the deposition of dose in the target while sparing the structures beyond the target. It is most often used for pediatric tumors, skull base tumors, and tumors close to optic structures and spinal cord, especially in the recurrent setting. Proton therapy is only recently being used for HNSCC and has yet to establish a role for routine cases. There remain several challenges with Proton therapy for HNSCC. Some of these are technique specific (range uncertainty, radiobiologic effectiveness values near the end of range, need for intensity modulation, lack of image guidance, etc.). Perhaps, the most important challenge remains the cost of proton therapy, which is several fold higher than standard photon therapy. More evidence for proton therapy in HNSCC is warranted before considering this therapy as a standard option especially when compared with techniques like VMAT IGRT using photons. Lastly, all these sophisticated techniques have a long learning curve, and there is evidence of better outcomes for patients treated at high-volume centers.

PRINCIPLES OF SYSTEMIC THERAPY

The use of systemic therapy in head and neck cancer is based on the assumption that squamous cell malignancies of the head and neck share a common sensitivity to chemotherapy. Thus most clinical trials of systemic chemotherapy have included patients with multiple and varied disease subsites. As for most solid tumors, initial exploration of the role of systemic chemotherapy began with the use of these agents as palliation for patients with recurrent or metastatic cancers deemed incurable by other treatment modalities. Despite the fact that these patients were often heavily pre-treated with surgery and radiation therapy, and often had a poor or suboptimal performance status, multiple single chemotherapeutic agents were found to have modest activity. Drugs such as methotrexate, bleomycin, fluorouracil, the platins (cisplatin and carboplatin), the taxanes (docetaxel and paclitaxel), and gemcitabine have all demonstrated modest efficacy as single agents prompting further study of their use in combination. The best studied of these combinations has been the fluorouracil and cisplatin regimen, which has produced consistent responses in approximately one third of patients with advanced disease. Other drug combinations have been similarly effective. Although these responses can have important palliative benefit, overall survival was not meaningfully impacted by this treatment.

The epidermal growth factor receptor inhibitors, including both the monoclonal antibodies like cetuximab, and the tyrosine kinase inhibitors like gefitinib, erlotinib, and afatinib have resulted in very marginal response rates in recurrent disease patients progressing after conventional chemotherapy, although temporary disease stability has been frequently possible. When cetuximab was added to the fluorouracil and cisplatin (or carboplatin) combination, however, for the first time, a modest survival improvement was identified in the European EXTREME clinical trial reported in 2008.

Recent success using the immune checkpoint inhibitors in other diseases has led to their study in patients with recurrent head and neck cancer. Phase III data have now been generated demonstrating a survival benefit for the anti-PD-1 monoclonal antibodies when used after failure of first line platinum containing therapeutic regimens, and these drugs have now been approved for use in this setting. Although response rates are quite modest, the responses seen can be durable and active study of these agents is ongoing. Table 1.2 depicts selected chemotherapy regimens used for palliation.

TABLE 1.2 Selected Palliative Systemic Therapy Regimens for Metastatic Head and Neck Cancer

Regimens	Common Toxicities
Cisplatin 100 mg/m² IV (or Carboplatin AUC 5) on day 1 every 3 wk for six cycles plus 5-FU 1,000 mg/m²/day by continuous IV infusion on days 1–4 every 3 wk for six cycles plus cetuximab 400 mg/m² IV loading dose on day 1, then 250 mg/m² IV weekly (EXTREME regimen)	Nephrotoxicity, ototoxicity, myelosuppresion, mucositis, diarrhea, hand foot syndrome, allergic reaction, and acneiform rash
Carboplatin AUC 6 IV on day 1 plus paclitaxel 175–200 mg/m² IV on day 1 every 3 wk	Neuropathy, myelosuppresion, alopecia
Methotrexate 40 mg/m² IV weekly	Mucositis, myelosuppresion
Docetaxel 30–40 mg/m² weekly	Neuropathy, alopecia, diarrhea

The activity of systemic chemotherapy in poor performance status patients with advanced disease suggested that there might be better ways to utilize this treatment modality. As for other malignancies, the previously untreated patients given systemic chemotherapy experience a considerably higher response rate than that seen in patients with recurrent tumors. In head and neck cancer, the fluorouracil and cisplatin combination results in only a 30% response rate in the previously treated recurrent disease patient, but has been reported to produce response rates of up to 90% in the previously untreated. When patients continue to receive multiple course of chemotherapy, however, they invariably progress, and single modality chemotherapy cannot be considered a curative treatment when given alone. The obvious suggestion, instead, would be to exploit this biologic activity as part of definitive management, rather than limiting its use to the recurrent and metastatic disease setting. This has led to a number of multimodality treatment schedules.

The first approach considered was the use of induction chemotherapy. This is based on the high response rates in previously untreated patients and the hope that tumor shrinkage induced by chemotherapy might result in more successful definitive locoregional management. Multiple phase II clinical trials of induction chemotherapy were successfully completed suggesting a high but transient response rate to systemic chemotherapy, with good tolerance of subsequent locoregional definitive management. Phase III trials, however, comparing induction followed by definitive radiation or surgery, to definitive treatment alone, were unsuccessful, and failed to produce any meaningful survival improvement. As such this treatment schedule has not been adopted.

The alternative of adding systemic chemotherapy after definitive surgery and/or radiation has also been tested. Phase III trials of this approach have similarly failed to demonstrate an improvement in overall survival. It should be noted however that with both the induction and the adjuvant schedules the use of systemic chemotherapy was successful in reducing the risk of distant metastatic disease. The lack of impact on overall survival likely reflected the limited importance of distant metastases in disease natural history.

It is only when the chemotherapy is given concurrently with radiation that any benefit can be consistently identified. Concurrent treatment appears to be effective due to the ability of chemotherapy to potentiate the impact of radiation, coupled with its demonstrated success in reducing the risk of distant micrometastatic disease. The approach has several potential disadvantages however, including the additive toxicity from the concurrent use of two treatment modalities, which then results in a tendency to compromise dose intensity of either radiation or chemotherapy. Nonetheless, phase III trials comparing concurrent chemotherapy and radiation with radiation alone have now reproducibly demonstrated a clear survival benefit for the concomitant regimens. The best studied of these concurrent regimens has employed high-dose single-agent cisplatin given every three weeks in conjunction with the radiation. Alternative single agent and multiagent concurrent chemoradiotherapy regimens have also proven successful, but have been less well studied. Meta-analysis data from more than 17,000 patients and 93 clinical trials have confirmed the lack of a survival benefit from either induction or adjuvant chemotherapy, compared to a clear improvement in survival when chemotherapy is used concurrently. As a result, this treatment approach has become the standard of care in the definitive nonsurgical management of patients with locoregionally advanced disease. Table 1.3 includes induction and concurrent chemotherapy regimens used most often.

The monoclonal anti-EGFR antibody cetuximab has also been studied in conjunction with radiation and compared to radiation therapy alone. Again, a survival benefit was demonstrated for the combination. This approach has thus become another potential treatment option for the nonoperative management of locoregionally advanced disease. It remains unknown however whether radiation and concurrent cetuximab is equivalent to radiation and concurrent chemotherapy. Clinical trials are addressing this question but the results are not yet available.

The marked improvement in locoregional control achieved with concurrent chemoradiotherapy has, not surprisingly, been accompanied by an increase in the relative frequency of distant metastatic disease. Given the reproducible benefit of induction chemotherapy on the incidence of distant metastases, the suggestion has emerged that the use of induction chemotherapy followed by concurrent chemoradiotherapy, or "sequential treatment" might further improve treatment results. In addition, the incorporation of a taxane into the fluorouracil and cisplatin induction combination has proven successful in increasing the response rates after induction chemotherapy suggesting additional potential benefit from a three-drug regimen in this sequential schedule. Although a theoretically attractive approach, this

TABLE 1.3 Concurrent and Induction Therapy Systemic Agents in Head and Neck Cancer

Regimens	Common Toxicities
Concurrent: Cisplatin 100 mg/m² IV every 21 days during radiation or cisplatin 40 mg/m² every week	Nephrotoxicity, severe nausea/delayed vomiting, dehydration, mucositis, ototoxicity, neuropathy, myelosuppresion
Concurrent: Carboplatin 70 mg/m²/day IV on days 1–4, 22–25, and 43–46 plus 5-FU 600 mg/m²/day by continuous IV infusion on days 1–4, 22–25, and 43–46	Thrombocytopenia, mucositis, diarrhea, hand foot syndrome, neuropathy
Concurrent: Cetuximab loading dose 400 mg/m² IV followed by 250 mg/m²/week IV	Acneiform rash, mucositis, allergic reaction
Induction: Docetaxel 75 mg/m² IV day 1, Cisplatin 100 mg/m² IV day 1, 5-FU 1,000 mg/m² per day (continuous 24-hour infusion) for 4 days (Days 1–4)	Nephrotoxicity, severe nausea/delayed vomiting, dehydration, mucositis, ototoxicity, neuropathy, myelosuppresion, diarrhea
Induction: Cisplatin 80–100 mg/m² IV day 1, 5-FU 1,000 mg/m² per day (continuous 24-hour infusion) for 4–5 days	Nephrotoxicity, severe nausea/delayed vomiting, dehydration, mucositis, ototoxicity, neuropathy, myelosuppresion, diarrhea

treatment paradigm is accompanied by an increase in treatment duration, an increase in treatment toxicity, and a significant increase in expense. To date, three phase III trials comparing concurrent chemoradiotherapy to sequential induction followed by concurrent chemoradiotherapy have been completed. None of these three trials have demonstrated a survival benefit for the sequential treatment, and all have resulted in increased toxicity. Thus the current standard of care for the nonoperative management of locoregionally advanced disease is the use of concurrent chemoradiotherapy, and the sequential treatment schedules have no defined role.

Many patients however will first undergo surgical resection but are then found to have pathologic features suggesting a high risk of disease recurrence. The standard approach for these high risk patients has been the use of postoperative adjuvant radiation. Two phase III cooperative group clinical trials from the RTOG and the EORTC have explored the role of postoperative radiation and concurrent high-dose cisplatin, compared to radiation alone in patients with high-risk features after surgical resection. These trials both reported a clear improvement in local disease control and disease-free survival in the concurrently treated patients. When an unplanned subgroup analysis was conducted of pooled data from both trials, it appeared that this benefit was limited to those patients with extracapsular nodal spread or margin positivity. As such, the use of concurrent high dose cisplatin with radiation has become a treatment standard for this subgroup of postoperative patients.

SPECIAL CONSIDERATIONS

Oral Cavity

The oral cavity includes the lip, anterior two-thirds of the tongue, floor of the mouth, buccal mucosa, gingiva, hard palate, and retromolar trigone. Approximately 20,000 new cases are diagnosed annually in the United States. The epidemiology, natural history, common presenting symptoms, risk of nodal involvement, and prognosis for specific subsites are shown in Table 1.4

Early oral cavity cancers are treated with surgery alone. This usually involves a wide local excision of the primary with surgical management of the neck. Elective nodal dissection is considered standard except for very small, superficial primaries (tumors less than 4 mm thick). Small primaries of the oral cavity resected with a wide margin, without adverse pathologic features and with negative nodes may be

TABLE 1.4 Head and Neck Cancer: Oral Cavity

Site	Epidemiology	Natural History and Common Presenting Symptoms	Nodal Involvement
Lip	Risk factors are sun exposure and tobacco; 3,600 new cases a year; 10–40 times more common in white men than in black men or women (black or white)	Exophytic mass or ulcerative lesion; more common in lower lip (92%); slow-growing tumors; pain and bleeding	5%–10% Midline tumors spread bilaterally Level I more common (submandibular and submental); upper lip lesions metastasize earlier: Level I and also preauricular
Alveolar ridge and retromolar trigone	10% of all oral cancers; M:F, 4:1	Exophytic mass or infiltrating tumor, may invade bone; bleeding, pain exacerbated by chewing, loose teeth, and ill-fitting dentures	30% (70% if T4) Levels I and II more common
Floor of mouth	10%–15% of oral cancers, (occurrence 0.6/100,000); M:F, 3:1; median age, 60 y	Painful infiltrative lesions, may invade bone, muscles of floor of mouth and tongue	T1, 12%; T2, 30%; T3, 47%; and T4, 53% Levels I and II more common
Hard palate	0.4 cases/100,000 (5% of oral cavity); M:F, 8:1; 50% cases squamous, 50% salivary glands	Deeply infiltrating or superficially spreading pain	Less frequently: 6%–29%
Buccal mucosa	8% of oral cavity cancers in United States; women > men	Exophytic more often, silent presentation; pain, bleeding, difficulty in chewing, trismus	10% at diagnosis

M:F, male-to-female ratio.

followed without adjuvant management. An alternative approach to manage the primary is with definitive radiation, usually using brachytherapy. This approach remains dependent on local practice patterns and availability of expertise and is generally not a standard of care in the United States.

Locoregionally advanced cases including T2 oral tongue cancers with more than 4 mm thickness are usually treated with wide local excision and neck dissection. The extent of primary site excision depends on the size of the primary and its extent. For example, an oral tongue resection might range from a wide local excision to a near total or total glossectomy. Similarly, the extent of neck dissection varies by the extent of disease in the neck. A recent phase III trial of elective nodal dissection versus therapeutic nodal dissection at relapse for early-stage lateralized oral squamous cell carcinoma has shown a survival advantage to elective nodal dissection. A selective neck dissection (levels I to IV) or modified radical neck dissection is done in most cases for node negative necks and those with minimal neck disease. Patients with more extensive neck disease and salvage cases may require a more extensive surgery like a radical neck dissection. Of late, sentinel lymph node biopsy is gaining popularity especially for oral cavity cancers. Head and neck cancers have complex lymph node drainage patterns, and oral tongue cancers have traditionally been known to drain directly to the lower neck while skipping intervening lymph nodal stations. Sentinel lymph node biopsy is not considered standard and is not recommended outside of a clinical trial. Tumor thickness, especially for oral tongue cancers, has traditionally been a prognostic factor for disease outcomes and also correlates with neck nodal disease. It is generally agreed that increasing thickness of the tumor correlates with outcome. The actual thickness however is variable across studies. Most cases require reconstruction with the help of a surgeon trained in head and neck reconstruction techniques. Definitive radiation or chemoradiation is an inferior alternative to initial surgical management of locally advanced oral cavity cancers and is not favored unless the patient is medically inoperable or unresectable.

Radiation plays an important role in the adjuvant management of locoregionally advanced oral cavity cancers and has been shown to improve locoregional control. Chemotherapy is generally added for positive margin or extracapsular extension of nodal disease. This approach has been shown to provide a locoregional control benefit over radiation alone. Several intermediate risk factors are recognized including close margins (<5 mm), lymphovascular space invasion, perineural invasion, T3/T4 disease, T2 oral cancer with >5 mm thickness of primary and node positive disease without extracapsular extension. Adjuvant radiation with cetuximab is being explored in a phase III trial to improve outcomes for intermediate risk disease where surgery and radiation remain the current standard but locoregional control still remains far from optimal. Similarly, even with adjuvant chemoradiation after surgery for high-risk disease (extracapsular extension from a node, positive margin), locoregional control and overall survival remain poor. RTOG 0234 was a phase II study exploring the safety and efficacy of docetaxel and cetuximab to further intensify treatment for high-risk disease. Encouraging results from this study have resulted in the ongoing RTOG 1216 study comparing radiation with cisplatin to radiation with docetaxel or radiation with docetaxel and cetuximab for the management of high-risk cancers.

Oropharynx

The oropharynx includes the base of the tongue, vallecula, tonsils, posterior pharyngeal wall, and the soft palate. The epidemiology, natural history, common presenting symptoms, and risk of nodal involvement are shown in Table 1.5.

Oropharyngeal cancers can be divided into two large prognostic groups by their etiology, namely HPV-induced or HPV-unrelated, usually tobacco-induced cancers and the most recent AJCC staging system now recognizes these as two different diseases with two separate staging systems. The overwhelming majority of oropharyngeal cancers are HPV positive in the western world. Positive immunohistochemistry for p16 is a surrogate for the presence of HPV as a causative factor. A large RTOG experience has validated the prognostic value of HPV and divided oropharyngeal cancers in low, intermediate, and high-risk groups. Data from the Princess Margaret Hospital in Canada have further categorized HPV positive disease into low- and high-risk groups. Age and smoking have stood out as prognostic factors as well. Based on these data, it is clear that the HPV positive disease has a far better prognosis than HPV negative tumors. Although, at present, treatment algorithms are the same for HPV-induced and carcinogen-induced oropharynx cancer, active investigation is currently underway in an effort to identify whether these treatments can be altered based on disease etiology.

Early stage oropharynx cancers are usually managed with single modality treatment, namely surgery or definitive radiation (T1/T2, N0/N1). Locoregional control and overall survival remain high for these stages. More locally advanced disease is traditionally managed with definitive chemoradiation or bioradiation (with cetuximab) with surgery reserved for salvage (especially for advanced neck disease). A select subset of patients can be managed with surgery followed by adjuvant treatment. Surgical options include transoral resection (less commonly open surgery) and appropriate neck dissection. Case selection is often tailored to achieve optimal outcomes and avoid multiple modalities of therapy thereby minimizing morbidity. For example, a T2N2bM0, tonsil primary amenable to TORS may undergo this procedure and neck dissection in the absence of clinical extracapsular extension of disease in the nodes, thereby avoiding the addition of concurrent chemotherapy with adjuvant radiation.

It must again be emphasized that the current standard of care treatment does not differ by HPV status. However, for low risk, HPV positive disease (T1-T3, N1-2b, </= 10 pack-years smoking history), locoregional control and distant control are excellent and have encouraged treatment de-escalation trials

TABLE 1.5 Head and Neck Cancer: Oropharynx

Site	Epidemiology	Natural History and Common Presenting Symptoms	Nodal Involvement
Base of tongue	4,000 new cases annually in the United States; M:F ratio, 3–5:1. May be HPV-associated	Advanced at presentation (silent location, aggressive behavior); pain, dysphagia, weight loss, and otalgia (from cranial nerve involvement); neck mass is a frequent presentation	All stages: 70% (T1) to 80% (T4) Levels II and III more commonly involved
Tonsil, tonsillar pillar, and soft palate	Tobacco and alcohol; HPV common	Tonsillar fossa: more advanced at presentation: 75% stage III or IV, pain, dysphagia, weight loss, and neck mass Soft palate: more indolent, may present as erythroplakia	Tonsillar pillar T2, 38% Tonsillar fossa T2, 68% (55% present with N2 or N3 disease)
Posterior pharyngeal wall		Advanced at diagnosis (silent location); pain, bleeding, and weight loss; neck mass is common initial symptom	Clinically palpable nodes T1, 25% T2, 30% T3, 66% T4, 75% Bilateral involvement is common

in order to maintain good outcomes and reduce the morbidity of treatment. This includes the recently concluded RTOG 1016 study comparing chemoradiation with cisplatin to bioradiation with cetuximab. Other studies like the ECOG 3311 are exploring the role of TORS to choose patients for radiation dose de-escalation while the HN 002 study is exploring the role of radiation dose de-escalation and elimination of chemotherapy. These and other studies being conducted will help to establish the role of treatment de-escalation for low risk HPV-related disease.

High risk HPV positive oropharyngeal cancer (T4, N2c-N3 disease) is still associated with a high locoregional control rate but distant failure occurs in up to a quarter of cases. Therefore, this group may not benefit from treatment de-escalation (particularly elimination of systemic therapy) and strategies to improve systemic control are warranted. High risk HPV negative cancer (T3, T4, N2c-N3 disease) is associated with equally poor distant failure. Locoregional control is also inferior with about 40% failure at 3 years. Fortunately, this group of patients is becoming less common. Aggressive therapy is warranted for these patients and usually takes the form of definitive chemoradiation followed by surgical salvage as needed.

Larynx

Laryngeal cancers can be supraglottic, glottic, and/or subglottic. The epidemiology, natural history, common presenting symptoms, risk of nodal involvement, and prognosis for specific subsites of the larynx are shown in Table 1.6.

Larynx cancer mainly comprises cancers of the glottis and supraglottis and less commonly of the subglottis. This distinction is important considering the glottis is devoid of lymphatics while the supraglottis and subglottis are rich in lymphatics.

Early T1 glottic cancers can be managed with voice conserving transoral laryngeal microsurgery. The local control with this technique is excellent often with superior voice quality. In general, superficial lesions affecting one vocal cord and not extending to the anterior commissure are best treated with this technique. Local recurrences can be managed with further surgery so long as they are superficial.

TABLE 1.6 Head and Neck Cancer: Larynx

Site	Epidemiology	Natural History and Common Presenting Symptoms	Nodal Involvement
Supraglottis	35% of laryngeal cancers	Most arise in epiglottis; early lymph node involvement due to extensive lymphatic drainage; two-thirds of patients have nodal metastases at diagnosis	Overall rate: T1, 63%; T2, 70%; T3, 79%; T4, 73% Levels II, III, and IV more common
Glottis	Most common laryngeal cancer	Most favorable prognosis; late lymph node involvement; usually well differentiated, but with infiltrative growth pattern; hoarseness is an early symptom; 70% have localized disease at diagnosis	Sparse lymphatic drainage, early lesions rarely metastasize to lymph nodes. Clinically positive: T1, T2 Levels II, III, and IV more common T3, T4, 20%–25%
Subglottis	Rare, 1%–8% of laryngeal cancers	Poorly differentiated, infiltrative growth pattern unrestricted by tissue barriers; rarely causes hoarseness, may cause dyspnea from airway involvement; two-thirds of patients have metastatic disease at presentation	20%–30% overall pretracheal and paratracheal nodes more commonly involved

M:F, male-to-female ratio.

Deeply invasive lesions require more extensive surgery. While these lesions are technically resectable, more extensive surgery or multiple surgeries can lead to deterioration in the voice quality. Such procedures are thus avoided.

Definitive radiation is considered an alternative for early glottic cancers especially when the lesion is more extensive and not suitable for microsurgical excision. Voice quality is often superior with radiation but depends on the baseline voice quality. Early glottic cancers can be treated with definitive radiation with excellent outcomes. The radiation field is usually a small laryngeal parallel-opposed field. Mild hypofractionation to 2.25 Gy has shown improved local control versus 2 Gy fractions.

T1 cancers of the supraglottis can be treated with transoral voice preserving surgery. An open or endoscopic supraglottic laryngectomy is often done and some form of bilateral neck management is usually advocated given the high risk of lymph node spread. Definitive radiation is an alternative management option and usually includes both necks in the treatment field.

T2 tumors of the glottis and supraglottis can be managed with either surgery or definitive radiation. Various forms of voice preserving laryngectomy procedures are utilized based on the extent of the tumor. Some of these options include a supraglottic laryngectomy, supracricoid laryngectomy, and a vertical partial laryngectomy. Bilateral neck dissections are also advised for supraglottic disease. Alternatively the primary and both necks can be treated with definitive radiation. The dose is usually slightly higher than for T1 tumors. Though not a part of formal AJCC staging, T2 glottic cancers have been divided into T2a and T2b based on true vocal cord mobility restriction. T2b glottic cancers have a worse outcome with standard-dose radiation alone. It is believed that these cases represent early paraglottic space involvement, and these may require more intensive treatment. Hyperfractionation and chemoradiation are some strategies utilized to achieve better local control.

The management of T3N0M0 laryngeal cancer is controversial. In certain cases, a voice preserving surgical approach may be warranted. A fixed cord is usually a contraindication for such a procedure like a vertical partial laryngectomy. If no adverse postoperative pathologic factors are identified, the patient may be observed without further adjuvant treatment. Total laryngectomy is usually avoided but remains an oncologically acceptable option. Definitive chemoradiation remains an alternative voice preserving treatment strategy.

The management of locally advanced laryngeal cancer takes into account the baseline function of the larynx, baseline swallowing function, and disease extent. The standard surgical procedure remains a total laryngectomy with bilateral node dissection. This may be followed by adjuvant radiation or chemoradiation based on the pathologic risk factors. This surgical management approach is best used for patient with severely compromised laryngeal and/or swallowing function. Select cases might undergo a voice-preserving surgery for the primary with neck dissections followed by adjuvant treatment as indicated. Perioperative speech rehabilitation is critically important for patients with advanced laryngeal cancer who are undergoing total laryngectomy. Phonation options include tracheoesophageal puncture at the time of total laryngectomy, esophageal speech, or a mechanical electrolarynx. Most patients can obtain satisfactory communication through one of these techniques.

Nonetheless, because of the significant resulting functional compromise, a total laryngectomy is not a surgical procedure that is readily embraced by patients. Larynx-preserving, nonoperative approaches have emerged as reasonable options, and are most appropriate for those patients without significant pre-existing laryngeal and/or swallowing dysfunction. The nonoperative management of locally advanced larynx cancer with radiation/chemoradiation has evolved in a systematic fashion. The VA larynx study compared induction chemotherapy with cisplatin/5-FU followed by radiation with total laryngectomy followed by radiation for locally advanced larynx cancers. The rate of larynx preservation was 64% and overall survival was not compromised. The RTOG 91-11 study compared induction chemotherapy followed by radiation to either definitive concurrent chemoradiation or to radiation alone. Large volume T4 lesions (with destruction of larynx or massive extension of supraglottic laryngeal cancer to the base of tongue) were excluded as these are felt to be best treated with a primary surgical approach. The larynx preservation rate at 10 years was 82% for the concurrent chemoradiation arm and this approach has become a treatment standard in North America. Although the overall survival was statistically similar between all three treatment arms, likely reflecting the success of salvage surgery, a concerning trend toward an inferior survival was noted in the concurrent arm for reasons that are not entirely clear. As a result, induction chemotherapy followed by radiation, or even radiation alone remain acceptable treatment standards despite the reduced likelihood of larynx preservation.

Hypopharynx

The epidemiology, natural history, common presenting symptoms, risk of nodal involvement, and prognosis for specific subsites of the hypopharynx are shown in Table 1.7.

The large majority of hypopharynx cancers present at an advanced stage. The hypopharynx has a rich lymphatic network and nodal metastases are common at presentation. The retropharyngeal nodes may be involved as well. Early stage primary cancers may be addressed with transoral or open voice conserving procedures with neck dissections as indicated. Adjuvant therapy can then be administered if required.

The standard surgical approach for locally advanced hypopharynx cancer is a total laryngectomy with a partial pharyngectomy and bilateral node dissections. Microvascular free flap reconstruction of the surgical defect is common in the modern era. Adjuvant treatment is based on the adverse factors noted on pathology and usually includes adjuvant radiation. Similar to the trials conducted in larynx cancer, voice conserving nonoperative treatment has been studied for hypopharygeal cancers as well. The EORTC 24891 study compared induction cisplatin/5-FU followed by radiation with surgery followed by radiation. Larynx preservation at 5 years was 22% (in surviving patients). Overall survival was similar in both arms. Several recent retrospective institutional series have shown high larynx preservation rates (around 90% at 3 years) with better overall survival (around 50% at 3 years) with modern radiation/chemoradiation techniques. Overall, similar to larynx cancer, patients with significant laryngeal/swallowing dysfunction are best treated with initial surgery and adjuvant therapy. Patients with retained laryngeal and swallowing function may be best served by definitive nonoperative chemoradiation. General medical fitness for either approach is of paramount importance since these patients are often medically compromised.

TABLE 1.7 Head and Neck Cancer: Hypopharynx, Nasal Cavity, Paranasal Sinuses, and Nasopharynx

Site	Epidemiology	Natural History and Common Presenting Symptoms	Nodal Involvement
Hypopharynx	2,500 new cases yearly in United States; etiology: tobacco, alcohol, and nutritional abnormalities	Aggressive, diffuse local spread, early lymph node involvement; occult metastases to thyroid and paratracheal node chain; pain, neck stiffness (retropharyngeal nodes), otalgia (cranial nerve X), irritation, and mucus retention 50% present as neck mass; high risk of distant metastases	Abundant lymphatic drainage Up to 60% have clinically positive lymph nodes at diagnosis
Nasal cavity and paranasal sinuses	Rare 0.75/100,000 occurrence in United States Nasal cavity and maxillary sinus, four-fifths of all cases M:F, 2:1 Increased risk with exposure to furniture, shoe, textile industries; nickel, chromium, mustard gas, isopropyl alcohol, and radium	Nonhealing ulcer, occasional bleeding, unilateral nasal obstruction, dental pain, loose teeth, ill-fitting dentures, trismus, diplopia, proptosis, epiphora, anosmia, and headache, depending on the site of invasion Usually advanced at presentation	10%–20% clinically positive nodes Levels I and II more common
Nasopharynx	Rare (1/100,000) except in North Africa, Southeast Asia, and China, far northern hemisphere Associated with EBV, diet, genetic factors	Most common initial presentation: neck mass Other presentations: otitis media, nasal obstruction, tinnitus, pain, and cranial nerve involvement	Clinically positive: WHO I, 60% WHO II and III, 80%–90%

M:F, male-to-female ratio; EBV, Epstein-Barr virus.

Nasopharynx

The epidemiology, natural history, common presenting symptoms, risk of nodal involvement, and prognosis for nasopharyngeal cancer are shown in Table 1.7.

Nasopharyngeal cancers span a spectrum from more endemic EBV-associated undifferentiated carcinoma (WHO type III) to keratinizing squamous cell carcinoma (WHO type I). More recently, a p16-positive, EBV-negative subset has also been identified. The nasopharynx is very rich in lymphatics and nodal metastases are commonly found with nasopharyngeal cancer. The anatomy of the nasopharynx generally precludes a primary surgical approach especially since both necks are at risk from disease spread. As such, radiation plays a major role in the management of this cancer. Early node negative primaries of the nasopharynx are treated with radiation alone. This includes the primary and both necks. Appropriate elective skull base coverage is necessary. Locally advanced nasopharyngeal cancers are often treated with definitive chemoradiation followed by three cycles of adjuvant chemotherapy, based on the INT 0099 study, which demonstrated a large survival benefit with concurrent and adjuvant chemotherapy versus radiation alone. Despite several criticisms to this approach and the demographic differences noted with nasopharyngeal SCC in the west versus the east, this approach remains standard. The ongoing NRG HN 001 study is a randomized trial exploring the importance of this adjuvant chemotherapy based on clinical response and plasma EBV DNA levels. Patients with undetectable plasma EBV DNA after concurrent chemoradiation will be randomized to standard adjuvant CDDP/5-FU versus observation. Patients with detectable plasma EBV DNA after concurrent chemoradiation will be randomized to standard adjuvant CDDP/5-FU versus an alternative combination of paclitaxel/gemcitabine. Locally recurrent nasopharyngeal cancer that is nonmetastatic can be treated with surgical and nonsurgical approaches. Re-irradiation is usually advocated especially when the patient is not a surgical candidate.

Nasal Cavity and Paranasal Sinuses

The epidemiology, natural history, common presenting symptoms, risk of nodal involvement, and prognosis for carcinomas of the nasal cavity and paranasal sinuses are shown in Table 1.7. Nasal cavity and the paranasal sinus tumors comprise a broad variety of tumors. Some of these include squamous cell carcinomas, various types of adenocarcinomas, transitional cell carcinomas, minor salivary gland carcinomas, small cell carcinomas, esthesioneuroblastomas, and sinonasal undifferentiated carcinomas. Rare benign tumors like hemangiomas and angiofibromas may be seen.

There is no consensus on the management of these tumors. In general, these tumors are resected surgically, optimally using an endoscopic approach, or if necessary a combined open and endoscopic approach. Tumor resection often proceeds in a piecemeal rather than en-bloc fashion, and negative margins are often difficult to obtain. A combined team approach with neurosurgery may be needed especially for tumors involving the skull base. Certain cases where the tumor approaches the orbit might necessitate an orbital exenteration. Exceptions include radiosensitive and chemosensitive tumors like small cell carcinoma, which may be treated with definitive chemoradiation. Adjuvant radiation/chemoradiation usually follows surgical management. Locally advanced unresectable tumors may be treated with definitive chemoradiation provided the patient has adequate performance status and is medically fit to receive aggressive chemoradiation therapy. The remaining patients are best treated with palliative radiation and chemotherapy.

Salivary Glands

Salivary gland cancers are a rare subset of head and neck cancers. They comprise a variety of histologies and are found in various locations throughout the head and neck region, including the major and minor salivary glands. Salivary gland cancers may be both benign and malignant. Benign lesions are more commonly found in major salivary glands while lesions of the minor salivary glands are more likely to be malignant. Although the current pathologic classification of salivary gland cancers is currently under revision, the WHO 2005 system is still most commonly used. The benign salivary gland tumors are listed in Table 1.8.1 and malignant salivary gland tumors are listed in Table 1.8.2.

The clinical characteristics and prognosis of specific malignant salivary gland tumors are shown in Table 1.8.3.

While major salivary gland cancers are clinically obvious as to site of origin, minor salivary gland tumors are often mistaken for more common mucosal lesions. Pretreatment imaging and tissue diagnosis are important for optimal management. Inadvertent partial excision of a lesion can compromise further oncological surgical excision. FNA biopsy is usually the first diagnostic step although definitive classification of salivary gland cancers can be difficult using this approach. Definitive surgical management is considered the standard initial treatment. In the absence of clear diagnosis, major salivary gland lesions are often resected with intraoperative frozen section for diagnosis. An oncological resection is attempted after establishing the diagnosis. Benign lesions like pleomorphic adenomas are also resected keeping oncological principles in mind (no tumor spillage) since these tumors show preponderance for local recurrence. Obviously malignant lesions (fast preoperative growth, facial nerve paralysis) are resected with a wide local margin. Negative resection margins are desired but may be difficult to obtain

TABLE 1.8.1 Salivary Gland Benign Tumors

Pleomorphic adenoma (benign mixed tumor)
Warthin tumor (papillary cystadenoma lymphomatosum)
Monomorphic adenoma
Benign lymphoepithelial lesion
Oncocytoma
Ductal papilloma
Sebaceous lymphadenoma

TABLE 1.8.2 Salivary Gland Malignant Tumors

Acinic cell carcinoma
Mucoepidermoid carcinoma
Adenoid cystic carcinoma
Polymorphous low-grade adenocarcinoma
Epithelial-myoepithelial carcinoma
Basal cell adenocarcinoma
Sebaceous carcinoma
Papillary cystadenocarcinoma
Mucinous adenocarcinoma
Oncocytic carcinoma
Salivary duct carcinoma
Adenocarcinoma
Myoepithelial carcinoma
Carcinoma ex pleomorphic adenoma
Squamous cell carcinoma
Small cell carcinoma

in proximity to the facial nerve. The facial nerve is usually preserved if it is functioning preoperatively and grossly uninvolved intraoperatively. A paralyzed facial nerve is sacrificed and an attempt is made to obtain a negative proximal margin. Meticulous skull base dissection may be required. The facial nerve should be reconstructed (grafted) during the primary surgery, and other adjunct procedures considered for facial reanimation, for example, temporalis tendon transfer. Management of the neck is controversial. In general, patients with T3/T4, high grade, or node positive diseases are usually managed with ipsilateral neck dissection.

The adjuvant management of salivary gland cancers is based on retrospective data. Adjuvant radiation appears to play an important role in improving locoregional control. General indications for postoperative radiation include T3/T4 primary lesions, high grade, lymphovascular space invasion, perineural invasion, close/positive margins, node positive disease, or recurrent disease. The principles of adjuvant radiation including doses required are similar to more common mucosal tumors discussed previously. Adjuvant radiation also plays a role in improving locoregional control for benign tumors like multiply recurrent pleomorphic adenomas. The role of chemotherapy is controversial and far less established for salivary gland tumors. The RTOG 1008 trial is a phase III trial exploring the role of concurrent cisplatin with radiation for high-risk salivary gland tumors. Some histologic subtypes may express potential hormonal or other therapeutic targets, such as HER2 and androgen receptors in salivary duct carcinomas. The role of targeted therapies for these diseases is being explored. Like other head and neck cancers, single modality adjuvant chemotherapy currently does not have a defined role in the current management of salivary gland cancers.

TABLE 1.8.3 Selected Salivary Gland Malignant Tumors: Clinical Characteristics and Prognosis

Histology	Clinical Characteristics
Mucoepidermoid carcinoma	Most common malignant tumor in major salivary glands; most common in parotid glands (32%)
	Low grade: local symptoms, long history, cure with aggressive resection; rarely metastasizes
	t(11;19)(q21;p13) in 50%–70%
	High grade: locally aggressive, invades nerves and vessels, and metastasizes early
Adenocarcinoma	16% of parotid and 9% of submandibular malignant tumors
	Grade correlates with survival
Squamous cell carcinoma	Very rare
	Grade correlates with survival
	Squamous cell carcinoma of temple, auricular, and facial skin can metastasize to parotid nodes and can be confused with primary parotid tumor
Acinic cell carcinoma	<10% of all salivary gland malignant tumors
	Low grade with slow growth, infrequent facial nerve involvement, infrequent and late metastases (lungs)
	Regional metastasis in 5%–10% of patients
Adenoid cystic carcinoma	Most common malignant tumor in submandibular gland (41%), 11% of parotid gland
	High incidence of nerve invasion, which compromises local control
	t(6;9)(q22–23;p23–24) in 50%
	40% of patients develop metastases; most common site of metastases is the lung. Patients may live many years with lung metastasis, but visceral or bone metastases indicate poor prognosis

Unknown Primary of the Head and Neck

Unknown primary of the head and neck region comprises about 3% of all head and neck cancers. While squamous cell carcinomas are thought to originate from mucosal sites, other histologies are also seen and may indicate the source of their primary origin. For example, adenocarcinomas might arise from the salivary glands or the thyroid/parathyroid gland. The site of lymph node presentation is often linked to the potential site of the primary and this knowledge helps in evaluation and management. For example, a level III node might arise from the larynx, hypopharynx, or upper cervical esophagus. A level IA node is likely to arise from an oral cavity primary, while a level IB node might indicate a primary in the oral cavity, maxillary sinus, or nasal cavity. A level II node might indicate a primary in the oropharynx although several sites primarily drain to level II. A level V node raises the possibility of a nasopharynx or skin cancer. A parotid gland node usually indicates a cutaneous primary squamous cell carcinoma. An isolated supraclavicular node is very unlikely to indicate a head and neck primary. The primary in this case is almost always below the clavicle (lung, thoracic esophagus, breast, etc.). Evaluation follows the usual workup of head and neck cancers. A core needle biopsy of the node is preferred especially to obtain p16 and EBER evaluation, which may point to an HPV-related oropharyngeal primary or nasopharyngeal primary, respectively. However, caution is advised while doing so and the primary drainage pattern of the involved node should be taken into account before interpreting the immunohistochemistry results. For example, an isolated level V node might be p16+ but is more likely to indicate a cutaneous primary/nasopharynx primary rather an oropharyngeal primary. A PET CT should be considered before surgical diagnostic procedures are performed since this information might aid in finding the primary. A tonsillectomy, tongue base, and nasopharynx biopsy are considered standard although the yield is low for blind biopsies. Transoral lingual tonsillectomy (tongue base resection) is being increasingly utilized to detect a tongue base primary and is usually found in a high number of cases with a level II node presentation.

When no primary is found after surgical biopsies, management usually follows the purported site of the primary. For example, a level I node is subjected to a neck dissection assuming the oral cavity as the primary site. N1 disease may be resected and in the absence of adverse pathologic features, the patient may be observed without further treatment. This is based on the fact that data regarding emergence rates of the primary, although inconsistent in the literature, appear low. When radiation is used for treatment, however, it is considered standard to prophylactically radiate potential primary sites. For example, a p16+ level II node is treated with definitive neck radiation and prophylactic coverage of the oropharynx. A p16– level II node is treated similarly but prophylactic coverage often includes the nasopharynx and hypopharynx as well. An EBV+ node is treated along the lines of nasopharynx cancer. In general, the oral cavity, larynx, and hypopharynx are excluded in the prophylactic radiation volume since this approach is considered excessively morbid with low yield. More advanced disease may be treated with surgery followed by radiation with or without chemotherapy based on pathologic risk factors. When treating N2/N3 disease nonoperatively, concurrent chemotherapy is usually added to the radiation although the benefit of this is unclear. Salvage surgery may be needed for more advanced neck disease. Patients with distant metastases presenting with a neck node and no primary are treated with palliation (radiation and chemotherapy). The results of treatment usually follow similarly staged head and neck cancers with a known primary site. Therefore, in nonmetastatic cases, a cure is possible despite not knowing where the primary originated.

Recurrent Nonmetastatic Disease

Local recurrence is the most frequent pattern of disease failure in patients with locally advanced head and neck cancer. Distant failure however is being recognized more frequently, particularly in patients with HPV-induced oropharyngeal tumors. Locoregionally recurrent disease remains a major challenge in clinical oncology. These cancers could either be true recurrent disease or second primaries, a distinction that is often difficult, especially if disease is identified within 2 to 3 years of the primary disease. Management is based on the intent of treatment, which may be either palliative or definitive. Recurrent cancer within a short time span (usually 6 months), advanced age, poor performance status, and large burden of unresectable disease are factors associated with particularly poor outcomes and are best treated with palliative radiation and/or systemic palliative therapy. SBRT may be an option for some cases with an estimated survival of more than 6 months. This strategy is employed to quickly deliver reasonably durable palliative treatment with acceptable morbidity.

More favorable disease features include second primaries, or recurrent disease occurring more than 3 years after treatment of the initial tumor, young age, good performance status, low volume disease, resectable disease, and low morbidity from previous treatment. When possible, these patients should be treated with surgery followed by adjuvant chemoradiation. The GORTEC trial demonstrated a disease-free survival, but not overall survival advantage to adjuvant chemoradiation versus observation after surgery in this group of patients. The adjuvant radiation may be hyperfractionated or once daily radiation aimed at minimizing the side effects of therapy. The volume of radiation is usually minimized to include the recurrent disease bed while maximally sparing normal tissue thereby sparing morbidity. Case selection is crucial since the morbidity of this approach is not trivial. More modern and technologically advanced radiation delivery may offset the morbidity noted historically.

TOXICITY MANAGEMENT AND FOLLOW-UP

Acute Toxicities of Treatment

Patients treated with radiation therapy or concomitant chemoradiation therapy require frequent clinical assessment and prompt institution of supportive care to avoid severe or fatal consequences during the acute phase of treatment (during treatment and for the first several months after treatment).

Nutrition

Careful assessment of the need for a feeding tube should be done. In general, reactive feeding tube placement is preferred to prophylactic placement before therapy begins. These devices have been shown to be beneficial for patients who are thin, or have lost significant weight. They are not necessary for all patients, but if not placed, such patients must be assessed every 1 to 2 weeks for toxicity and weight loss.

Hydration

Radiation and chemoradiation leads to increased fluid loss, especially with severe mucositis, and/or with loss of normal taste or appetite. Patients should be assessed every 1 to 2 weeks for skin turgor, orthostatic blood pressure changes, lightheadedness on standing, or renal dysfunction (especially when platinum-based chemotherapy is used).

Mucositis

A significant number of patients receiving chemoradiation therapy will develop severe mucositis that impairs nutrition and causes severe pain. Candida infection of the affected mucosal surfaces is fairly common. At the first sign of candidiasis, antifungal therapy should be instituted, topically and/or orally. A preparation containing an antifungal, anesthetic, and calcium carbonate suspension is useful. Narcotic pain control should be aggressive and patients should be taught to track pain severity and self-administer their narcotics before the peak of pain occurs. It is useful to use a transdermal administration route, using careful dose calculation based on the total use of short acting narcotic, plus a short-acting (liquid) narcotic to control pain.

Radiation Dermatitis and Rash

Mild radiation dermatitis is managed with a moisturizer during and after radiation. Moist desquamation may be managed with vinegar soaks and saline dressings. These reactions will often heal after radiation is concluded. Superficial infections should be managed with antibiotics.

Cetuximab may cause an acneiform rash in the upper torso and face, which may become infected if not treated. Patients should be started prophylactically on moisturizers as topical therapy. Steroid-containing topical creams and minocycline are also helpful for a more severe rash (confluent in more than one body area). The rash often improves after the first few weeks, and may not be present in the radiation fields.

Allergic Reactions

Severe and life-threatening allergic reactions have occurred with cisplatin, taxanes, carboplatin, and antiepidermal growth factor receptor (EGFR) antibodies. Infusion of these agents should only be done when appropriate emergency equipment and trained personnel are available.

Late Toxicities of Treatment

Xerostomia

Risk of dry mouth due to incidental radiation to the salivary glands is present but has been lessened by more accurate treatment planning and delivery with intensity-modulated radiation therapy (IMRT) methods. Initial management typically includes saliva substitutes, oral mucosal lubricants, and frequent sips of water. Systemic cholinergic agonists can be considered for xerostomia that persists for more than 1 year after treatment completion. There is growing evidence supporting a role for acupuncture or acupuncture-like transcutaneous electrical nerve stimulation (ALTENS) in palliation of xerostomia as well.

Late Dysphagia

A minority of patients will have swallowing difficulties for several years or permanently, with attendant risk of aspiration and pneumonia. Swallowing therapy and potentially continued enteral nutrition with a percutaneous tube may be necessary for these patients. Serial dilatations of the oropharyngeal inlet and esophagus might be needed to deal with radiation- /surgery-related strictures.

Dental Caries

An increased risk of developing dental caries accompanies any change in salivary flow or composition. For this reason, any patient who has had head and neck radiation should have regular, frequent dental evaluations. Long-term, daily use of fluoride trays is often recommended. Meticulous oral hygiene can reduce the likelihood of other late effects, such as osteoradionecrosis (ORN).

Osteoradionecrosis

Bone exposure following radiation may lead to progressive ORN, which occurs in 5% to 7% of patients treated with radiation. To prevent ORN, extractions should be performed in patients with poor dentition and allowed adequate time for healing prior to therapy (at least 2 weeks). If ORN develops, patients with dead sequestra (necrotic bone) should be referred to an oral maxillofacial surgeon for sequestrectomy. Culture may provide sensitivities for IV antibiotic therapy. Sequestrectomy coupled with long-term pentoxifylline has been reported to result in healing in most patients within 1 year. Hyperbaric oxygen has been used for many years, but was not found to be of benefit in a randomized clinical trial. Nonresponsive or advanced ORN requires open surgical resection (e.g., segmental mandibulectomy) and reconstruction with vascularized tissue, for example, Fibula free flap reconstruction for segmental mandibulectomy.

Mobility Impairment

Both surgery and radiation can cause fibrosis of soft tissues of the neck, impacting cosmesis and/ or neck mobility. Treatment often includes physical therapy for neck stretching and strengthening and massage. Greater regression is generally achieved with earlier initiation of therapy.

Hypothyroidism

Up to 75% of patients may have increased thyroid stimulating hormone levels (TSH) after radiation therapy. Following radiation treatment to the neck, TSH should be monitored regularly and appropriate replacement therapy instituted.

Follow-Up

Curative treatment of patients with head and neck cancer should be followed by a comprehensive head and neck physical examination every 1 to 3 months during the first year after treatment, every 2 to 4 months during the second year, every 3 to 6 months from years 3 to 5, and every 6 to 12 months after year 5. In patients treated nonoperatively, restaging imaging studies should be done approximately 12 weeks after completion of radiation therapy and then as needed for any symptoms or signs suggesting recurrence or second primary cancer. A recent study established the role of PET CT obtained 12 weeks after definitive chemoradiation for disease surveillance. Neck dissection is warranted for incomplete response and equivocal findings on imaging. This approach resulted in equally good survival and was cost effective compared with planned neck dissections. The highest risk of relapse is during the first 3 years after treatment. After 3 years, a second primary tumor in the lung or head and neck is the most important cause of morbidity or mortality. Because of this risk, annual chest imaging, particularly in smokers, is recommended.

PREVENTION

The most important recommendation for prevention of head and neck cancer is to encourage smoking cessation and to limit alcohol intake. HPV vaccination should be given to all adolescents. It is currently approved by the U.S. Food and Drug administration for prevention of cervical cancer (bivalent or quad-rivalent vaccines) in females and genital warts in males (quadrivalent vaccine), as well as for prevention of anal precancers (quadrivalent vaccine). Data are currently being gathered on the effect of vaccination on incidence of HPV-related head and neck cancer.

Premalignant lesions occurring in the oral cavity, pharynx, and larynx may manifest as leukoplakia (a white patch that does not scrape off and that has no other obvious cause) or erythroplakia (friable reddish or speckled lesions). These lesions require biopsy and potentially excision. The risk of leuko-plakias without dysplasia progressing to cancer is about 4%. However, up to 40% of severe dysplasias or erythroplasias progress to cancer.

Presently, there is no effective chemoprevention for patients at risk for head and neck squamous cancer and chemoprevention outside a clinical trial is not recommended.

Suggested Readings

1. Al-Sarraf M, LeBlanc M, Giri PG, et al. Chemoradiotherapy versus radiotherapy in patients with advanced nasopharyn-geal cancer: phase III randomized Intergroup study 0099. *J Clin Oncol.* 1998;16:1310–1317.
2. Ang KK, Harris J, Wheeler R, et al. Human papillomavirus and survival of patients with oropharyngeal cancer. *N Engl J Med.* 2010;363:24–35.
3. Bernier J, Domenge C, Ozsahin M, et al. Postoperative irradiation with or without concomitant chemotherapy for locally advanced head and neck cancer. *N Engl J Med.* 2004;350:1945–1952.
4. Blanchard P, Baujat B, Holostenco V, et al. Meta-analysis of chemotherapy in head and neck cancer (MACH-NC): a com-prehensive analysis by tumour site. *Radiother Oncol.* 2011;100:33–40.
5. Bonner JA, Harari PM, Giralt J, et al. Radiotherapy plus cetuximab for squamous-cell carcinoma of the head and neck. *N Engl J Med.* 2006;354:567–578.
6. Byers RM, Weber RS, Andrews T, et al. Frequency and therapeutic implications of "skip metastases" in the neck from squamous carcinoma of the oral tongue. *Head Neck.* 1997;19:14–19.
7. Cooper JS, Zhang Q, Pajak TF, et al. Long-term follow-up of the RTOG 9501/intergroup phase III trial: postoperative concurrent radiation therapy and chemotherapy in high-risk squamous cell carcinoma of the head and neck. *Int J Radiat Oncol Biol Phys.* 2012;84:1198–1205.
8. D'Cruz AK, Vaish R, Kapre N, et al. Elective versus therapeutic neck dissection in node-negative oral cancer. *N Engl J Med.* 2015;373:521–529.
9. Daly ME, Le QT, Jain AK, et al. Intensity-modulated radiotherapy for locally advanced cancers of the larynx and hypo-pharynx. *Head Neck.* 2011;33:103–111.
10. Davis KS, Byrd JK, Mehta V, et al. Occult primary head and neck squamous cell carcinoma: utility of discovering primary lesions. *Otolaryngol Head Neck Surg.* 2014;151:272–278.
11. Forastiere AA, Zhang Q, Weber RS, et al. Long-term results of RTOG 91-11: a comparison of three nonsurgical treatment strategies to preserve the larynx in patients with locally advanced larynx cancer. *J Clin Oncol.* 2013;31:845–852.
12. Gillison ML, D'Souza G, Westra W, et al. Distinct risk factor profiles for human papillomavirus type 16-positive and human papillomavirus type 16-negative head and neck cancers. *J Natl Cancer Inst.* 2008;100:407–420.
13. Janot F, de Raucourt D, Benhamou E, et al. Randomized trial of postoperative reirradiation combined with chemotherapy after salvage surgery compared with salvage surgery alone in head and neck carcinoma. *J Clin Oncol.* 2008;26:5518–5523.
14. Jemal A, Bray F, Center MM, et al. Global cancer statistics. *CA Cancer J Clin.* 2011;61:69–90.
15. Lefebvre JL, Chevalier D, Luboinski B, et al. Larynx preservation in pyriform sinus cancer: preliminary results of a European Organization for Research and Treatment of Cancer phase III trial. EORTC head and neck cancer cooperative group. *J Natl Cancer Inst.* 1996;88:890–899.
16. Mehanna H, Wong WL, McConkey CC, et al. PET-CT surveillance versus neck dissection in advanced head and neck cancer. *N Engl J Med.* 2016;374:1444–1454.
17. Mok G, Gauthier I, Jiang H, et al. Outcomes of intensity-modulated radiotherapy versus conventional radiotherapy for hypopharyngeal cancer. *Head Neck.* 2015;37:655–661.
18. Moore KA, Mehta V. The growing epidemic of HPV-positive oropharyngeal carcinoma: a clinical review for primary care providers. *J Am Board Fam Med.* 2015;28:498–503.
19. O'Sullivan B, Huang SH, Siu LL, et al. Deintensification candidate subgroups in human papillomavirus-related oropha-ryngeal cancer according to minimal risk of distant metastasis. *J Clin Oncol.* 2013;31:543–550.
20. Terhaard CH, Lubsen H, Rasch CR, et al. The role of radiotherapy in the treatment of malignant salivary gland tumors. *Int J Radiat Oncol Biol Phys.* 2005;61:103–111.
21. The Department of Veterans Affairs Laryngeal Cancer Study Group. Induction chemotherapy plus radiation compared with surgery plus radiation in patients with advanced laryngeal cancer. *N Engl J Med.* 1991;324:1685–1690.
22. Trotti A, Zhang Q, Bentzen SM, et al. Randomized trial of hyperfractionation versus conventional fractionation in T2 squamous cell carcinoma of the vocal cord (RTOG 9512). *Int J Radiat Oncol Biol Phys.* 2014;89:958–963.

23. Vargo JA, Ferris RL, Ohr J, et al. A prospective phase 2 trial of reirradiation with stereotactic body radiation therapy plus cetuximab in patients with previously irradiated recurrent squamous cell carcinoma of the head and neck. *Int J Radiat Oncol Biol Phys.* 2015;91:480–488.
24. Wuthrick EJ, Zhang Q, Machtay M, et al. Institutional clinical trial accrual volume and survival of patients with head and neck cancer. *J Clin Oncol.* 2015;33:156–164.
25. Yamazaki H, Nishiyama K, Tanaka E, et al. Radiotherapy for early glottic carcinoma (T1N0M0): results of prospective randomized study of radiation fraction size and overall treatment time. *Int J Radiat Oncol Biol Phys.* 2006;64:77–82.

2 Non–Small Cell Lung Cancer

Christina Brzezniak, Julia Cheringal, and Anish Thomas

EPIDEMIOLOGY

- Lung cancer, broadly divided into small cell lung cancer (SCLC) and non–small cell lung cancer (NSCLC), is the leading cause of cancer death in both men and women in the United States and worldwide.
- An estimated 224,390 new cases of lung and bronchus cancer (117,920 in men and 106,470 in women) will be diagnosed in 2016 in the United States, resulting in 158,080 deaths (85,920 in men, 72,160 in women).
- More than 70% of patients are diagnosed with advanced disease that is not amenable to curative therapy.
- The 5-year relative survival rate for lung cancer is approximately 18%, reflecting a slow but steady improvement from 13.7% in the 1970s.
- Stage at diagnosis accounts for the most marked variation in prognosis. Patient characteristics associated with poorer prognosis include older age, male gender, and African-American heritage.
- In the United States, it is estimated that as many women now die from lung cancer as die from breast, uterine, and ovarian cancers combined. The increase in lung cancer risk among women reflects changes in smoking habits during the 20th century. By 1987, lung cancer had surpassed breast cancer as the leading cause of cancer death in women as a result of an increase in the prevalence of female smokers.
- Rates of cigarette smoking have declined in the United States in the past 10 years, but developing nations are now seeing an alarming increase in smoking rates.

ETIOLOGY AND RISK FACTORS

- The vast majority of lung cancer deaths are directly attributable to cigarette smoking.
- Tobacco smoke contains a highly complex mixture of carcinogens that have the potential to damage DNA. Polycyclic aromatic hydrocarbons, aromatic amines, and tobacco-specific nitrosamines have been implicated as the major mutagenic carcinogens responsible for DNA adduct formation. The number of DNA adducts formed is directly related to the number of cigarettes consumed; in heavy smokers they can be responsible for as many as 100 mutations per cell genome.
- Compared to those who have never smoked, smokers have an approximate 20-fold increase in lung cancer risk. The likelihood of developing lung cancer decreases among those who quit smoking compared to those who continue to smoke.
- Estimates indicate that passive smoking accounts for approximately 3,000 lung cancer deaths per year in the United States.
- Radon, a radioactive gas produced by the decay of radium 226, is the second leading cause of lung cancer in the United States, accounting for 6,000 to 36,000 cases of lung cancer each year. The decay of radium 226 produces substances that emit alpha particles, which may cause cell damage. Residential exposure has been associated with an increased risk of developing lung cancer.
- Occupational exposure to carcinogens such as asbestos, arsenic, chromates, chloromethyl ethers, nickel, polycyclic aromatic hydrocarbons, and other agents is estimated to cause approximately 9%

to 15% of lung cancers. Asbestos exposure in smokers is associated with a synergistic risk of developing lung cancer. Cigarette smoking impairs bronchial clearance and thereby prolongs the presence of asbestos in the pulmonary epithelium.
- The contribution of hereditary factors to the development of lung cancer is less well understood than for any other of the common forms of solid tumors in human. Proof that the familial occurrence of lung cancer has a genetic basis is complicated by the central role of cigarette smoking in the etiology of lung cancer.
- Although hereditary lung cancer syndromes are rare, T790M germline mutations of the epidermal growth factor receptor (EGFR) gene have been reported to predispose to the development of lung cancer.
- Large randomized, double-blind, placebo-controlled chemoprevention trials reported in the 1990s provided no evidence that specific dietary constituents confer protection against lung cancer.

PATHOLOGY

- NSCLC can be divided into three major subtypes:
  - Adenocarcinoma
  - Squamous cell carcinoma
  - Large cell carcinoma
- Adenocarcinoma is the most frequently diagnosed form of NSCLC in both men and women in the United States. Tumors are classically peripheral and arise from surface epithelium or bronchial mucosal glands. Histologic examination reveals gland formation, papillary structures, or mucin production. The histologic characteristics of lung cancer in several developed countries, including the United States, have changed in the past few decades, demonstrating that the frequency of adenocarcinoma has risen while the frequency of squamous cell carcinoma has declined.
- A revised multidisciplinary classification of lung adenocarcinoma recommends discontinuing the use of the term bronchioloalveolar carcinoma (BAC) and instead has introduced new categories to better categorize tumors based on histo-pathologic subtypes.
  - Preinvasive lesions include: atypical adenomatous hyperplasia (AAH) and adenocarcinoma in situ (AIS) ≤3 cm (formerly BAC)
  - Minimally invasive adenocarcinoma (MIA) ≤3 cm of lepidic tumor with ≤5 mm of invasion.
  - Invasive adenocarcinoma including lepidic predominant with >5 mm of invasion (formerly nonmucinous BAC), and variants such as invasive mucinous adenocarcinoma (formerly mucinous BAC).
- Squamous cell carcinoma accounts for approximately 25% of NSCLC and has the strongest association with cigarette smoking. This tumor arises most frequently in the central proximal bronchi and can lead to bronchial obstruction, with resultant atelectasis or pneumonia. Histologic examination reveals visible keratinization, with prominent desmosomes and intercellular bridges.
- Large cell carcinoma is the least common subtype of lung cancer, accounting for approximately 10% of all NSCLCs.

BIOLOGY

- Lung cancer evolves through a multistep process from normal bronchial epithelium to dysplasia to carcinoma in situ and finally to invasive cancer. These changes include activation of oncogenes, inactivation of tumor suppressor genes, and loss of genomic stability. Changes can be both genetic (via deletions or mutations) or epigenetic (methylation), leading to altered cell proliferation, differentiation, and apoptosis. Mutations in multiple tumor suppressor genes and oncogenes have been associated with the development of NSCLC (Table 2.1). A small subset of somatic mutations ("driver mutations") are essential for lung carcinogenesis and tumor progression and confer a selective growth

TABLE 2.1 Frequency of Common Molecular Alterations in NSCLC

Description	Percentage
KRAS mutations	15–25
EGFR mutations	10–35
PTEN mutations	4–8
ALK rearrangement	3–7
HER2 mutations	2–4
PIK3CA mutations	1–3
AKT mutations	1–3
BRAF mutations	1–3
NRAS mutations	1
MEK1 mutations	1
RET rearrangement	1
ROS rearrangement	1

advantage to the cancer cell. Cancer cells are often "addicted to" the continued activity of these somatically mutated genes for maintenance of their malignant phenotype.

- p53 is involved in DNA repair, cell division, apoptosis, and growth regulation. In normal conditions, p53 production increases when DNA damage occurs. Increased amounts of p53 induce cell cycle arrest in the G1 phase, allowing DNA repair. If a p53 deletion or mutation exists, G1 arrest is not achieved and the abnormal cell proceeds to S phase, further dividing and propagating genetic damage. Mutations in p53 are found in 50% of NSCLC.
- The RB gene also regulates G1 growth arrest. Hypermethylation of the CpG-rich island at the 5' end of the RB gene is thought to lead to the silencing of the RB gene and tumor progression. RB gene mutations occur in 15% of NSCLC.
- The human epidermal growth factor receptor (HER) family is a group of four trans-membrane tyrosine kinase receptors: EGFR, ErbB1, or HER1; ErbB2 (HER2/nu or HER2); ErbB3 (HER3), and ErbB4 (HER4). Following binding of a ligand to its extracellular receptor, dimerization occurs, leading to activation of tyrosine kinases and a subsequent increase in downstream signaling pathways, including RAS-RAF and AKT protein kinases. These pathways regulate angiogenesis, cell proliferation, and survival. Point mutations within EGFR exons 18 to 21 which encode a portion of the EGFR tyrosine kinase domain predict tumor sensitivity to EGFR tyrosine kinase inhibitors (TKIs). Common EGFR sensitizing mutations include exon 19 deletions and exon 21 L858R point mutations These mutations are more frequently found in female patients with adenocarcinoma histology, patients of Asian origin, or never or light smokers. They occur in up to 10% of US or European populations and 30% to 50% of Asian patients with NSCLC.

■ KRAS is a member of the RAS family of oncogenes and codes for a 21-kDa guanine-binding protein that mediates signal transduction pathways from cell surface receptors to intracellular molecules. The RAS-RAF pathway produces signaling downstream of the EGFR trans-membrane tyrosine kinase and promotes survival and proliferation. Mutations in EGFR and KRAS are, in general, mutually exclusive, and KRAS mutations confer primary resistance to EGFR TKIs. The RAS oncogene can be activated either by a point mutation or by overexpression. KRAS mutations are found with greater frequency in patients with adenocarcinomas (~15% to 30%), Caucasians, and smokers and are less frequent in Asians.

■ The anaplastic lymphoma kinase (ALK) is a receptor tyrosine kinase that is aberrant in a variety of malignancies. ALK rearrangements occur because of a chromosomal inversion within the short arm of chromosome 2, which results in the formation of the echinoderm microtubule-associated protein-like 4 (EML4)-ALK fusion oncogene. ALK fusion—with its most frequent fusion partner EML4 and less frequently with a variety of other partner genes—results in its dimerization and constitutive kinase activity, which leads to activation of pathways involved in cell growth and pro-liferation. Approximately 3% to 7% of NSCLC harbor ALK fusions. ALK fusions are more common in younger patients, never or light-smokers, and patients with adenocarcinoma with signet ring or acinar histology and in most cases are mutually exclusive of EGFR and KRAS mutations. ALK fusions predict sensitivity to ALK/MET tyrosine kinase inhibitors.

■ ROS1 is a receptor tyrosine kinase of the insulin receptor family. Chromosomal rearrangements involving the ROS1 gene lead to constitutive kinase activity and are found in approximately 2% of NSCLC. The clinical characteristics of ROS1-rearranged NSCLC is similar to that of ALK-rearranged NSCLC; more common in younger patients, never-smokers, and those with adenocarcinomas. Although there are no ROS1-specific agents in clinical practice, rearrangements predict sensitivity to the ALK inhibitor crizotinib.

■ In addition to the above genes, alterations in several other oncogenes including DDR2, FGFR1, MET, and RET are important for lung cancer pathogenesis.

■ Both cellular (T lymphocyte mediated) and humoral (antibody mediated) immune antitumor responses are known to occur in patients with advanced lung cancer. Despite this, spontaneous tumor regressions rarely occur, indicating that the tumor cells are able to escape an immune response.

■ NSCLC is increasingly being recognized to employ a number of mechanisms to escape the host immune response and promote immune tolerance. These include suppression of antigen-presenting machinery (e.g., altered human leukocyte antigen expression that prevents antigen presenta-tion and an effective immune response), release of immune inhibitory cytokines (e.g., interleukin 10 and transforming growth factor-β), immunosuppressive cells in the tumor microenvironment (e.g., tumor-infiltrating T lymphocytes and myeloid-derived suppressor cells), and expression of immune checkpoints. Immune checkpoints are molecules expressed on the surface of T lymphocytes that modulate the immune response to antigens via inhibitory or stimulatory signaling to T cells. Cytotoxic T-lymphocyte antigen-4 (CTLA-4) and programmed death 1 (PD-1) are among the most extensively studied immune checkpoints. Activation of immune checkpoints causes downregulation and inhibition of immune responses.

LUNG CANCER SCREENING

■ Randomized trials of screening with chest radiography with or without sputum cytology have shown no reduction in lung-cancer mortality.

■ Low-dose computed tomography screening may benefit individuals at an increased risk for lung cancer.
  ● The National Lung Screening Trial (NLST), a randomized trial compared annual screening by low-dose chest CT (LDCT) with chest x-ray for three years in high risk individuals (age between 55 and 74 years with at least 30 pack-year cigarette smoking, and former smokers who had quit within the previous 15 years), enrolling 53,454 individuals.
  ● There were 247 deaths from lung cancer per 100,000 person-years in the LDCT group and 309 deaths per 100,000 person-years in the radiography group, representing a relative reduction in mortality from lung cancer with LDCT screening of 20.0% (95% CI, 6.8 to 26.7; $P = 0.004$).
  ● The rate of death from any cause was reduced in the LDCT group, as compared with the radiog-raphy group by 6.7% (95% CI, 1.2 to 13.6; $P = 0.02$).
  ● This significant mortality risk reduction changed the approach to lung cancer surveillance and provided a validated means to screen high risk patients for lung cancer.

CLINICAL PRESENTATION

■ A minority of patients present with an asymptomatic lesion discovered incidentally on chest radio-graph. No set of signs or symptoms are pathognomonic of lung cancer, so diagnosis is usually delayed.

■ Clinical signs and symptoms of lung cancer are outlined in Table 2.2.

TABLE 2.2 Clinical Signs and Symptoms of Lung Cancer

Primary disease
  Central or endobronchial tumor growth
    Cough
    Sputum production
    Hemoptysis
    Dyspnea
    Wheeze (usually unilateral)
    Stridor
    Pneumonitis with fever and productive cough (secondary to obstruction)
  Peripheral tumor growth
    Pain from pleural or chest wall involvement
    Cough
    Dyspnea
    Pneumonitis
Regional involvement (either direct or metastatic spread)
  Hoarseness (recurrent laryngeal nerve paralysis)
  Dysphagia (esophageal compression)
  Dyspnea (pleural effusion, tracheal/bronchial obstruction, pericardial effusion, phrenic nerve palsy,
    lymphatic infiltration, superior vena cava obstruction)
  Horner's syndrome (sympathetic nerve palsy)
Metastatic involvement (common sites)
  Bone (pain exacerbated by movement or weight bearing, often worse at night; fracture)
  Liver (right hypochondrial pain, icterus, altered mental status)
  Brain (altered mental status, seizures, motor and sensory deficits)
Paraneoplastic syndromes
  Hypertrophic pulmonary osteoarthropathy
  Hypercalcemia
  Dermatomyositis (Eaton-Lambert syndrome)
  Hypercoagulable state
  Gynecomastia

CLINICAL EVALUATION

Single Pulmonary Nodule (SPN)

- Definition: solitary mass, often found incidentally, surrounded by lung tissue, well circumscribed, measures <3 cm without mediastinal or hilar adenopathy.
- Benign inflammatory vascular abnormalities or infectious lesions can mimic more sinister lesions. Review of previous chest imaging is a crucial first step. A stable lesion over a 2-year period suggests a benign condition.
- Computed tomography (CT) of the chest is required to assess for other nodules, adenopathy, or chest wall invasion.
- FDG-PET (^{18}F-fluorodeoxyglucose-positron emission tomography) is used to evaluate SPNs. False-positive PET scans may occur in conditions such as tuberculosis or histoplasmosis. False-negative results have been reported for small lesions (<1 cm) and neoplasms with low metabolic activity, such as in some cases of preinvasive or minimally invasive disease. Mean sensitivity of FDG-PET is 96%; mean specificity is 75%. The negative and positive predictive value of PET for pulmonary nodules is approximately 90%.
- A growing SPN needs a pathologic diagnosis. Tissue can be obtained by fine needle aspiration (FNA), transbronchial biopsy, or surgical resection. Flexible fiber optic bronchoscopy is appropriate for central lesions and can lead to a diagnosis in 97% of cases via biopsies, bronchial washings, and brushings.

- Invasive carcinomas can present with a spectrum of nodular patterns including ground glass opacities (GGO), mixed GGO/solid nodules, or consolidations.
- Observation may be reasonable in a low-risk individual (<40 years old and has never smoked) with a negative FDG-PET and a stable lesion measuring <2 cm. Reimaging with regular CT scans and follow-up clinic appointments are recommended.

Suspected Lung Cancer

- Full history and physical examination are recommended, followed by complete blood count and chemistry tests, chest x-ray, and CT of the chest and abdomen (including adrenal glands).
- Sputum analysis may be helpful in cases of central lesions.
- Bone scans and plain films of affected areas are warranted where bone pain exists. Routine imaging of the brain in asymptomatic patients is controversial.
- Peripheral lesions may require percutaneous transthoracic FNA, which can be performed under CT or fluoroscopic guidance.
- Mediastinoscopy, a more invasive method, may be needed to obtain a histologic diagnosis in difficult-to-reach primary tumors. Mediastinoscopy can reveal unsuspected tumors in mediastinal lymph nodes—a negative implication for survival. Evaluation of the mediastinum is recommended before surgery in suspected mediastinal disease and intraoperatively prior to any planned resections.
- An accurate pathologic diagnosis and staging of disease is essential in the management of lung cancer. Stage of disease determines whether surgical resection is warranted. Clinical staging often underestimates the true extent of the disease. The combination of PET evaluation and mediastinoscopy is routinely used to complete staging.
- Preresection forced expiratory volume/1 second (FEV1) should be ≥2 L for pneumonectomy, 1 L for lobectomy, or 0.6 L for segmentectomy.
- Preresection forced vital capacity should be ≥1.7 L.
- In patients who undergo surgical resection, surgical/pathologic staging should be used to predict recurrence and to evaluate the need for adjuvant therapy.

STAGING

- The tumor-node-metastasis (TNM) staging system bases patient prognoses on tumor size, lymph node involvement, and metastasis. Median overall survival for patients with pathologic stage IA, IB, IIA, IIB, IIIA, IIIB, and IV are 119, 81, 49, 31, 22, 13, and 17 months, respectively.
- The seventh edition of the *TNM Classification of Malignant Tumours* (UICC) was adopted by the American Joint Committee on Cancer (AJCC) in 2010. A summary of the TNM classification, stage grouping, and anatomical drawing can be found at http://www.cancerstaging.org/staging/posters/lung12x15.pdf. In stages I and II, disease is limited to one lung and does not involve the mediastinum or more distant sites. Involvement in stage III is heterogeneous, and ranges from tumor ≤2 cm with metastasis in ipsilateral mediastinal and/or subcarinal lymph node (T1a, N2-stage IIIA) to a tumor of any size with local invasion or a separate nodule in a different ipsilateral lobe with metastasis in contralateral mediastinal or hilar nodes (T4, N3-stage IIIB). Stage IV includes tumor involvement in a contralateral lobe, presence of malignant pleural (or pericardial) effusions, or distant metastases.

TREATMENT

Stages I and II

- Stages I and II NSCLC are considered early-stage disease. These two stages combined account for 25% to 30% of all lung cancers.
- Five-year survival rates are 58% to 73% for stage I and 36% to 46% for stage II.

- Surgical resection is the recommended treatment for patients with stage I and stage II NSCLC. In patients who are medically fit for surgical resection, lobectomy or greater resection is recommended rather than sublobar resections (wedge or segmentectomy).
  - A study of the Surveillance, Epidemiology, and End Results database evaluating wedge resection versus lobectomy found that OS and lung cancer specific survival (LCSS) favored lobectomy when compared with segmentectomy or wedge resection in patients with tumors ≤1 cm and >1 to 2 cm. With sublobar resection, lower OS and LCSS was demonstrated for NSCLC >1 to 2 cm after wedge resection, whereas similar survivals were observed for NSCLC ≤1 cm.
- Video-assisted thorascopic surgery (VATS) is an acceptable alternative to open thoracotomy.
- Intraoperative systematic mediastinal lymph node sampling or dissection is recommended for accurate pathologic staging.
- Even with complete resection, approximately half of the patients eventually experience relapse, with a 2- to 3-fold higher proportion of distant metastases over local recurrences.
  - In selected patients who undergo complete surgical resection, several large trials have demonstrated a statistically significant survival benefit from cisplatin-based adjuvant chemotherapy (IALT, ANITA, JBR 10).
  - The lung adjuvant cisplatin evaluation (LACE) meta-analysis which used individual patient data (n = 4,584) from five trials with a median follow-up of 5.2 years found that adjuvant cisplatin-based chemotherapy was associated with a decrease in absolute risk of death of 5.4 % at five years compared with no chemotherapy (hazard ratio [HR] 0.89; 95% CI, 0.82 to 0.96).
- Among completely resected early-stage NSCLC, adjuvant chemotherapy is not recommended for stage IA, is standard for stage II, and may be useful in a subset of patients with stage IB.
  - In the LACE meta-analysis, the overall survival benefit varied considerably by stage of disease, with potential harm seen in stage IA (HR 1.40; 95% CI, 0.95 to 2.06), a trend toward benefit in stage IB (HR 0.93; 95% CI, 0.78 to 1.10), and clear benefit in stage II (HR 0.83; 95% CI, 0.73 to 0.95) patients.
- Since there is no reliable way to identify which stage IB patients may derive benefit from adjuvant chemotherapy, current guidelines recommend chemotherapy in stage IB high risk patients, defined by large size (more than 4 cm), poor differentiation, vascular invasion, visceral involvement, and suboptimal resection.
- Cisplatin-based doublet is the usual adjuvant chemotherapy of choice. Vinorelbine, docetaxel, or gemcitabine and pemetrexed (the latter for nonsquamous histology) can be combined with cisplatin. Although OS and DFS have been shown to be similar with these combinations, adverse event profiles vary. Cisplatin is preferred over carboplatin in the adjuvant setting unless the patient has comorbidities such as pre-existing hearing loss or neuropathy that might be worsened with cisplatin.
- Current evidence suggests that postoperative radiotherapy is associated with decreased survival for patients with stage I (N0) and stage II (N1) NSCLC. However, most meta-analyses included several older studies that used radiotherapy methods that are inferior to current methods.
- If surgery is contraindicated in early-stage NSCLC, radiotherapy can be an effective means of local control. In clinical studies, accelerated radiotherapy (54 Gy in 12 days) was associated with better 4-year survival than conventional radiotherapy (60 Gy in 6 weeks). Stereotactic body radiation therapy (SBRT), which delivers a high-dose to a target volume and spares surrounding normal tissues, may be an option for patients with primary tumors <5 cm and in whom surgery is contraindicated.
- The role of targeted therapies and immunotherapy in the adjuvant setting is under investigation. The Adjuvant Lung Cancer Enrichment Marker Identification and Sequencing Trial (ALCHEMIST) is evaluating the benefit of erlotinib or crizotinib as adjuvant therapy in molecularly selected patients with stage IB to IIIA NSCLC. Several trials are evaluating the role of immune checkpoint inhibitors in the adjuvant setting.

Stage IIIA

- Stage IIIA (N2) NSCLC is a therapeutically challenging and controversial subset of lung cancer, with a 5-year survival rate of only 24%.

▪ Randomized trials strongly suggest a combined modality approach in stage IIIA disease. Conflicting data, however, have led to difficulties in proposing specific management guidelines. This, in part, is secondary to the heterogenous nature of stage IIIA disease.

▪ Clinically N0 or N1 patients are often taken for upfront surgical resection with cure achievable in 25% to 50% of these patients. However, should incidentally discovered N2 disease be found at surgery, complete tumor resection and mediastinal lymphadenectomy is recommended. With the high rate of recurrence in this patient population adjuvant chemotherapy to address micrometastatic disease is recommended.

  • The International Adjuvant Lung Cancer Trial of 1,867 patients with stages IB to IIIA (39% stage IIIA) randomized patients to three to four cycles of postoperative cisplatin-based chemotherapy versus surgery alone, with adjuvant 60 Gy radiotherapy given to both arms of stage IIIA patients (the use of radiotherapy was left to investigator's choice). After a median 56-month follow-up, the overall survival rate was significantly higher in the chemotherapy group (HR 0.86), with a 5-year survival rate of 44.5% in the chemotherapy group versus 40.4% in the control arm, with the strongest benefit in patients with stage III disease.

  • The ANITA study randomized 840 completely resected patients with stages I to IIIA (35% stage IIIA) to four postoperative cycles of cisplatin and navelbine versus observation (radiotherapy as per preference of participating center). After a median follow-up of >70 months, long-term 5-year survival of stage IIIA patients in the chemotherapy arm was significantly greater at 42% versus 26% in the observation arm ($P = 0.013$).

▪ Postoperative radiation therapy (PORT) while reducing local recurrence, does not improve survival, may be detrimental and is not recommended as standard of care. Advocates of radiotherapy have emphasized that there are several differences between the treatment administered in several trials included in this meta-analysis and current practices in the United States.

  • The PORT meta-analysis (Meta-Analysis Trialist Group) of 2,128 patients treated in nine randomized trials with a median follow-up of 3.9 years found a significant increase in risk of death with PORT (overall risk ratio 1:21; $P = 0.001$).

▪ Evidence has yet to be established substantiating the benefit of adding adjuvant radiotherapy to adjuvant chemotherapy in fully resected stage IIIA patients.

▪ Postoperative radiotherapy is recommended for patients with a positive surgical margin following surgical resection of stage III disease.

▪ Individuals with clinically apparent (bulky) N2 disease or N2 disease found at mediastinoscopy prior to thoracotomy should not undergo upfront surgery based on the poor results of primary resection for bulky stage IIIA disease. Selected patients with nonbulky N2 disease, defined as a single N2 positive node less than 2 cm, may be considered for surgical resection followed by adjuvant therapy. However, thorough discussion regarding lack of data illustrating optimal treatment in this setting is needed.

▪ Poor survival rates with surgery alone in N2 disease, even with postoperative chemotherapy or radiotherapy, have led to the use of radiotherapy and/or chemotherapy in the neoadjuvant setting, with the aim of making an unresectable tumor resectable and improving long-term survival. Theoretically, advantages include shrinking the tumor to allow for easier resection and nodal clearance, decreased surgical seeding, in vivo chemosensitivity testing of the chemotherapy regimen, and increased patient acceptance and compliance. Disadvantages of neoadjuvant therapy may include delayed tumor resection and increased surgical morbidity and mortality. While high rates of pathologic complete response and negative mediastinal nodes result from neoadjuvant chemoradiotherapy, it is also associated with substantial toxicity.

  • A meta-analysis evaluating neoadjuvant chemotherapy found a nonstatistically significant trend in favor of neoadjuvant chemotherapy (HR 0.65; 95% CI, 0.41 to 1.04).

  • Two clinical trials (European Organization for Research and Treatment of Cancer 08941 and North American Intergroup 0196) showed no significant difference in overall survival between patients with bulky stage IIIA NSCLC treated with neoadjuvant chemotherapy then surgery versus definitive chemoradiation alone (no surgery).

▪ The use of concurrent chemotherapy/radiotherapy versus sequential treatment has been addressed in numerous trials. At present, for patients with bulky N2 disease treatment with concurrent over sequential chemotherapy/radiotherapy is recommended.

- Concurrent chemotherapy/radiotherapy followed by consolidation chemotherapy is currently not recommended as standard of care.

Stage IIIB

- All patients with N3 (metastasis in contralateral mediastinal, contralateral hilar, ipsilateral or contralateral scalene, or supraclavicular node) involvement or T4 N2 disease are stage IIIB. Anticipated 5-year survival for most patients with stage IIIB disease is 3% to 7%.
- Optimal treatment depends on extent of disease, age of patient, co-morbidities, performance status (PS), and weight loss.
- Stage IIIB lung cancers are not amenable to curative surgical resection unless they are highly selected.
- For patients with stage IIIB disease with PS of 0 to 1, and minimal weight loss (<5%), platinum-based combination chemoradiotherapy followed by chemotherapy is recommended.
- The standard dose-fractionation of radiation is 60 Gy given in 2-Gy once-daily fractions over 6 weeks.
- The most common chemotherapeutic agents used concurrently with radiotherapy are etoposide, vinblastine, pemetrexed, and paclitaxel in conjunction with cisplatin or carboplatin. No randomized phase III trials of concurrent chemoradiotherapy have shown the superiority of one chemotherapy regimen over another.
- Studies have shown that induction chemotherapy followed by concurrent chemoradiotherapy is not superior to initial treatment with concurrent therapy.
- The role of additional cycles of chemotherapy following concurrent chemoradiotherapy is uncertain; however, this is usually administered to manage potential micrometastatic disease, especially if full doses of systemic chemotherapy were not delivered during radiotherapy.

Stage IV or Recurrent Disease

- Prognosis for patients with advanced-stage NSCLC is poor. Best supportive care produces median survival rates of 16 to 17 weeks and 1-year survival rates of 10% to 15%. Addition of chemotherapy improves 1-year survival to >35%.
- Subsets of patients with stage IIIB disease who are treated as though they have stage IV disease include those with advanced ipsilateral supraclavicular adenopathy, and those whose intrathoracic disease is not amenable to combined treatment modalities.
- Therapy options for patients with advanced or metastatic disease includes chemotherapy or targeted therapy as these are shown to improve quality of life and reduce symptoms from disease burden. However, systemic therapy is only palliative in nature, and not curative, therefore supportive therapy alone may be chosen if the patient is unable to tolerate systemic treatments due to poor PS or other comorbidities.
- Chemotherapeutic regimens can be divided into first-line, maintenance, second-line, and beyond second line or subsequent treatment strategies.
- In the era of personalized oncology—where therapy is tailored toward each patients individual tumor molecular profile—it is important to understand the concept of targeted therapies.

Driver Mutations and Targeted Therapy

- Classically, a lung cancer diagnosis was based on histology, but now it incorporates molecular profile of tumors. Improved sequencing technologies have had a major impact on the identification of specific molecular alterations that drive each tumor enabling widespread use of targeted therapies.
- KRAS.
  - The prognostic value of KRAS mutations in NSCLC has been controversial. It is thought to vary depending on the specific KRAS codon that is mutated as well as the disease stage at the time of diagnosis. For resectable disease, the prognostic value of KRAS appears to be minimal whereas in stage IV NSCLC, KRAS mutation is associated with poor prognosis. KRAS mutation is highly associated with smoking and generally portends a lack of response to targeted therapy. There has been limited success in directly inhibiting the KRAS protein.

- EGFR
  - Point mutations within EGFR exons 18 to 21, which encode a portion of the EGFR tyrosine kinase domain, predict tumor sensitivity to EGFR TKIs, including erlotinib, gefitinib, and afatinib.
  - The Iressa Pan-Asia Study (IPASS) randomized 1,217 patients with untreated Stage IIIB or IV lung adenocarcinoma to gefitinib or carboplatin and paclitaxel. In addition to adenocarcinoma histology, patients were nonsmokers or former light smokers and therefore were more likely to have EGFR mutated tumors. IPASS met its primary end point of 12-month PFS of 24.9% in gefitinib group versus 6.7% in the chemotherapy arm. Several additional trials for gefitinib, erlotinib, and afatinib versus chemotherapy confirmed improved ORR and PFS and quality of life in previously untreated patients with EGFR mutated NSCLC.
  - EGFR TKIs yield response rates of 55% to 80% and PFS of 9 to 14 months in patients with EGFR-mutated NSCLC. The activity of EGFR-TKIs differs among various types of EGFR mutations with deletion mutations in exon 19 responding more favorably than exon 21 L858R mutations.
  - The eventual development of acquired resistance generally limits the duration of response to EGFR TKIs. Almost 50% of patients whose disease progresses on an EGFR TKI develop an EGFR T790M "gatekeeper mutation." Less common resistance mechanisms include MET amplification, PIK3CA mutation, epithelial-to-mesenchymal transition, and SCLC transformation among others.
  - Multiple treatment strategies are now available for patients whose disease has progressed on initial EGFR TKI, including therapies targeting both T790M, and non-T790M-mediated resistance. Third-generation EGFR TKIs that block activating EGFR mutations as well as the T790M resistance mutation yield marked responses among patients with EGFR-mutated NSCLC and acquired resistance to initial TKIs. Osimertinib was the first of these drugs to receive US Food and Drug Administration (FDA) approval. Osimertinib yielded a response rate of 61% in patients who had progressed on an EGFR TKI and had confirmed EGFR T790M resistance. Response rate was 21% among patients with EGFR T790M-negative tumors. The median PFS was 9.6 months in EGFR T790M-positive patients and 2.8 months in EGFR T790M-negative patients.
  - EGFR TKIs, in general, have a favorable toxicity profile, with diarrhea, cutaneous eruption, nausea, and anorexia reported as the most common adverse effects.
- ALK
  - Crizotinib is an oral small molecule inhibitor of the ALK, MET, and ROS tyrosine kinases. It was granted FDA approval based on response rates of 57% and median PFS 9.7 months. Crizotinib is approved for first-line therapy in patients with ALK-rearranged nonsquamous NSCLC.
  - Two additional ALK inhibitors, ceritinib and alectenib, can be used to treat patients with progressive disease after crizotinib treatment or patients who are intolerant of this agent.
  - Ceritinib is a second-generation ALK TKI that is more potent than crizotinib. It received FDA accelerated approval based on a response rate of 56% in patients who had received prior ALK inhibitor and 72% in ALK inhibitor-naïve patients. The median duration of response was 8.3 months in patients with prior crizotinib and 17.0 months in ALK inhibitor-naïve patients.
  - Alectinib is another second-generation ALK TKI that received FDA-accelerated approval based on response rates of about 50% in patients with ALK-translocated locally advanced or metastatic NSCLC who had progressed on crizotinib. Alectinib is the preferred ALK TKI in patients with ALK-translocated NSCLC and brain metastases given its better CNS penetration and activity in CNS disease. Common adverse events from crizotinib include visual disorders, gastrointestinal effects (nausea, diarrhea, vomiting, constipation), edema, and fatigue. The second generation ALK TKIs have a similar adverse event profile, but visual disorders are uncommon.
- ROS1
  - Crizotinib has antitumor activity in patients with advanced ROS1-rearranged NSCLC and is approved for use in such patients. In a single-arm trial of 50 patients with ROS1-rearranged NSCLC, crizotinib yielded response rate of 72%, and median PFS of 19.2 months.
- In general, tumor tissue is obtained using a biopsy and is tested for a panel of genes to assess for the presence of targetable driver mutation. In the setting of known oncogenic driver mutations, serial

tumor biopsies at the time of progression is important to detect resistance mechanisms. Given the difficulties in obtaining reliable biopsies especially in patients who are ill, there is growing interest in detecting actionable mutations in plasma specimens so-called liquid biopsy. An approved liquid biopsy test is now available to detect exon 19 deletions or L858R substitution mutations in the EGFR gene to identify patients with metastatic NSCLC eligible for treatment with erlotinib.

Immunotherapy and Checkpoint Inhibition

- Research on immune checkpoint inhibitors has shown promising results for the treatment of NSCLC. These inhibitors alter the tumor microenvironment and block the evasion of the immune system thereby disrupting the tumor ability to grow and proliferate.
- New evidence has pointed to the utility of harnessing the adaptive immune system, one of the most important regulators in the elimination of malignant cells from the human body through the formation of cancer-specific T lymphocytes.
- The adaptive immune system utilizes NK cells, macrophages, and additional inflammatory cells to penetrate the microenvironment as antigen-presenting cells, which subsequently activate T cells leading to the formation of CD4 and CD8 cells. The goal of this pathway is the destruction of cancer cells. However, two normal immune pathways, or checkpoints, have been found to suppress this T cell response. These include the checkpoint proteins cytotoxic T-lymphocyte-associated protein 4 (CTLA-4) and programmed dealth-1 (PD-1).
- PD-1 activation primarily affects the later stages of T-cell immune response, thus affecting the effector T cells and cytotoxic T lymphocytes in the lymph node and tissue microenvironment, such as that seen in and around tumor cells. PD-1 and PD-L1 pathway inhibition can, therefore, reactivate tumor-specific T lymphocytes, leading to a prolonged antitumor response. This research has led to the approval of two anti–PD-1 antibodies, nivolumab and pembrolizumab, now in clinical use. PD-L1 antibodies such as atezolizumab and MEDI-4736 are in clinical development.
- In a phase I expansion trial of nivolumab, 129 patients with advanced NSCLC who were heavily pretreated were treated with three different doses of nivolumab (1, 3, or 10 mg/kg) every 2 weeks. Median OS was 9.9 months, and patients receiving the dose of 3 mg/kg (the eventual FDA approved dose) had impressive OS rates of 56%, 42%, and 27% at 1, 2, and 3 years, respectively. Treatment was well tolerated, with 14% of patients experiencing grade 3/4 adverse events. Three deaths from presumed treatment-related pneumonitis occurred. Responses were seen in patients with both squamous and nonsquamous histology.
- Two subsequent phase III trials confirmed the benefit of nivolumab over docetaxel as second-line treatment in patients with advanced NSCLC.
  - In the CheckMate 017 trial of 272 patients with squamous NSCLC, median OS was 9.2 months with nivolumab versus 6.0 months with docetaxel. Hazard ratio (HR) for death was 0.59 with nivolumab ($P < 0.001$), and the 1-year OS rate was 42% with nivolumab versus 24% with docetaxel.
  - The CheckMate 057 trial evaluated nivolumab versus docetaxel in patients with advanced nonsquamous NSCLC. Median OS was 12.2 in patients treated with nivolumab versus 9.4 months in patients treated with docetaxel. HR for death was 0.73 with nivolumab ($P = 0.002$), and 1-year OS rate was 51% with nivolumab versus 39% with docetaxel. Subgroup analysis from this trial showed higher efficacy for all end points in patients with PD-L1–positive tumors.
- It is important to note that response to nivolumab was independent of PD-L1 tumor expression.
- The KEYNOTE-010 trial evaluated the role of pembrolizumab in patients with previously treated advanced NSCLC. Patients enrolled on this trial had at least 1% of tumor cells with PD-L1 expression. A total of 1,034 patients received either pembrolizumab 2 mg/kg or 10 mg/kg versus docetaxel 75 mg/m^2 every 3 weeks. With pembrolizumab, median OS was 10.4 months at the 2 mg/kg dose and 12.7 months on 10 mg/kg versus 8.5 months with docetaxel. OS was improved with both the doses of pembrolizumab compared with docetaxel. In patients with at least 50% of tumor cells expressing PD-L1, OS was 14.9 months with pembrolizumab 2 mg/kg and 17.3 months with pembrolizumab 10 mg/kg versus 8.2 months with docetaxel.

- Based on these trials, the FDA has approved both nivolumab and pembrolizumab as single agents for the second-line therapy of patients with advanced NSCLC. Nivolumab use does not require testing for PD-L1 expression. Pembrolizumab is currently approved for patients with PD-L1 overexpression. Immunotherapy has emerged as the standard second line treatment in advanced NSCLC based on these data.
- Toxicities of both of these antibodies can include immune-related adverse side effects, with 10% to 14% of patients experiencing grade 3 or higher side effects. The most common side effects with PD-1 antibodies are rash and pruritus. Grade 3/4 diarrhea or colitis is seen in about 1% of patients, and grade 3/4 pneumonitis is seen in about 2% of patients. Other less-common immune-mediated side effects include transaminitis, nephritis, thyroiditis, hypophysitis, iritis, uveitis or conjunctivitis, and pericarditis.

First-Line Therapy

- Several factors have to be considered in choice of first-line treatment for metastatic or recurrent NSCLC: age, PS and co-morbidities of the patient, molecular abnormalities, and histology of the tumor (Figure 2.1).
- Patients with tumors harboring EGFR sensitizing mutations should receive an EGFR tyrosine kinase inhibitor. The relevant clinical trial data are discussed above under "Driver mutations and targeted therapy."
- Patients with tumors harboring ALK translocations should receive therapy targeting this translocation for which there are now three FDA-approved options—crizotinib, ceritinib, and alectinib. The relevant clinical trial data are discussed above under "Driver Mutations and Targeted Therapy."
- Patients with ROS1-translocated NSCLC should receive crizotinib.
- The optimal sequencing of these targeted therapies is not fully clear, but it is reasonable to consider repeat biopsy after progression on a targeted therapy to maximize their use and evaluate for the presence of resistance mutations.
- Patients with tumors harboring neither EGFR mutations, ALK translocation or ROS1 translocation nor who have exhausted all targeted therapy options should receive standard chemotherapy. Four to six cycles of platinum-based doublets prolong survival and improve symptom control and is the standard of care for patients with recurrent or metastatic NSCLC and good PS. However, no single regimen has demonstrated superiority, and treatment decisions should be based on individual patient and tumor characteristics.
  - An ECOG study which randomized 1,207 patients to a reference regimen of cisplatin and paclitaxel or to one of three experimental regimens: cisplatin and gemcitabine, cisplatin and docetaxel, or carboplatin and paclitaxel found comparable efficacy for all four regimens. This trial yielded an objective response rate of 19%, with a median survival of 7.9 months, a 1-year survival rate of 33% and a 2-year survival rate of 11%.
- Histology is an important determinant of the choice of chemotherapy agent. A phase III trial comparing pemetrexed/cisplatin to cisplatin/gemcitabine in 1,700 advanced/metastatic patients in the first-line setting found OS between both treatment arms to be the same. However, subset analysis for histology revealed significant differences.
  - In patients with adenocarcinoma histology, combination of pemetrexed with cisplatin demonstrated improved survival and reduced toxicity compared with gemcitabine/cisplatin. OS was 12.6 months in the pemetrexed arm versus 10.9 months in the gemcitabine arm.
  - Conversely those with squamous histology showed improved survival with cisplatin/gemcitabine (10.8 months) as initial chemotherapy treatment versus pemetrexed/cisplatin (9.4 months).
- Bevacizumab, a recombinant humanized monoclonal antibody that is directed against VEGF, (thereby preventing its interaction with the VEGF receptor) is approved for treatment of nonsquamous histology advanced/metastatic disease in combination with chemotherapy as first-line treatment.
  - ECOG 4599 which randomized selected patients with nonsquamous NSCLC ($n = 878$) to chemotherapy (carboplatin/paclitaxel) alone or with bevacizumab found significant improvements in OS (median 12.3 vs. 10.3 months), PFS (median 6.2 vs. 4.5 months), and response rates (35% vs. 15%). The risk of treatment-related deaths was higher in patients who received bevacizumab.
  - The AVAiL trial further evaluated bevacizumab in nonsquamous histology tumors randomizing patients to cisplatin/gemcitabine with or without two different doses of bevacizumab. Although

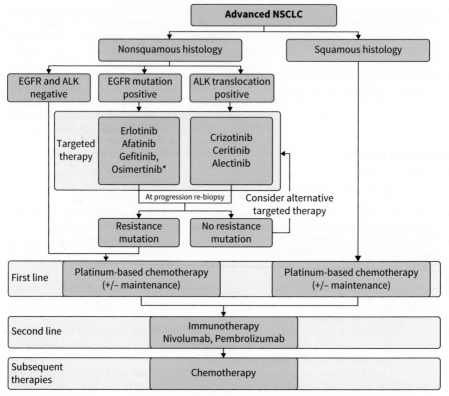

FIGURE 2.1 Treatment algorithm for non–small cell lung cancer patients; Repeat biopsy after progression on targeted therapy should be considered to determine if a resistance mutation has developed. If no resistance mutation is present, consider alternative targeted therapies based on patient characteristics, CNS disease, and T790M mutations; First-line treatment with combination of platinum agent plus gemcitabine is recommended for squamous histology; Treatment with bevacizumab or pemetrexed is not indicated in patients with squamous histology; Immunotherapy is considered the standard second-line treatment option for patients without a contraindication to this treatment; Subsequent therapies include any cytotoxic therapy not previously utilized including docetaxel, docetaxel/ramucirumab, gemcitabine, or pemetrexed.

*T790M only

addition of bevacizumab significantly prolonged PFS, the improvement was modest (median 6.7 and 6.5 months, respectively for bevacizumab 7.5 mg/kg and 15 mg/kg, respectively; 6.1 months for placebo), and there was no OS benefit with addition of bevacizumab. It is unclear if the lack of OS benefit is secondary to differences in chemotherapy between the two trials.
- The PointBreak trial compared carboplatin and bevacizumab with either pemetrexed or paclitaxel in the first-line setting for nonsquamous NSCLC patients with PS 0 to 1. After four cycles, patients in the pemetrexed arm received maintenance bevacizumab plus pemetrexed whereas those in the paclitaxel arm received maintenance with bevacizumab alone. OS did not improve in the pemetrexed arm compared with the paclitaxel arm (12.6 vs. 13.4 months).
■ Cetuximab is a monoclonal antibody that binds to the EGFR. Given the significantly increased toxicity seen in the phase III FLEX trial, the combination of cisplatin/vinorelbine/cetuximab is not generally used despite a small yet significant OS benefit (OS of 11.3 months for cetuximab arm vs. 10.1 months in the control arm).

▪ Addition of a third chemotherapeutic agent to platinum-based doublets has failed to show a superior survival benefit; response rates improved only at the cost of substantially increased toxicity.

Maintenance Chemotherapy

▪ Maintenance therapy is the use of systemic therapy in patients with a response or stable disease after first-line therapy until disease progression or unacceptable toxicity with goals of delaying disease progression and to extend survival, without adversely affecting quality of life.

▪ One of the drugs used in first-line therapy (continuation maintenance) or a new agent (switch maintenance) may be used for maintenance.

▪ Pemetrexed, bevacizumab, gemcitabine, or pemetrexed plus bevacizumab may all be chosen as continuation maintenance options.

- The PARAMOUNT trial, double-blind, placebo-controlled trial, which investigated continuation pemetrexed maintenance therapy in patients with nonsquamous histology, found that pemetrexed maintenance resulted in a 36% reduction in risk of progression (HR 0.64; 95% CI, 0.51 to 0.81; $P = 0.00025$).

- The phase III, IFCT-GFPC 0502 trial randomized patients to maintenance gemcitabine, erlotinib, or observation after lack of progression on cisplatin/gemitabine as upfront therapy. A significant improvement in PFS was observed for the gemcitabine maintenance (HR 0.51; 95% CI, 0.39 to 0.66). Gemcitabine may be used in patients with squamous histology for continuation maintenance.

- The Pointbreak trial discussed previously showed a very small PFS improvement (6 vs. 5.6 months) with pemetrexed/bevacizumab maintenance at the expense of increased toxicity in the form of neurotoxicity, neutropenia, and alopecia.

▪ Pemetrexed, docetaxel, and erlotinib are options for switch maintenance therapy.

- A phase III study evaluated the use of pemetrexed maintenance following nonprogression with nonpemetrexed-containing platinum-based chemotherapy versus best supportive care. Pemetrexed significantly improved not only PFS (4.3 vs. 2.6 months; HR 0.5; 95% CI, 0.42 to 0.61; $P < 0.0001$) but also OS (13.4 vs. 10.6 months; HR 0.79; 95% CI, 0.65 to 0.95; $P = 0.012$) compared to placebo, respectively.

- Erlotinib switch maintenance has been studied after nonprogression on platinum-based chemotherapy. PFS was significantly longer for the erlotinib arm compared to placebo, regardless of EGFR mutational status (12.3 vs. 11.1 weeks; $P < 0.0001$). However patients with EGFR mutations were the ones who benefited the most from maintenance erlotinib.

- In patients with squamous histology docetaxel maintenance may be considered.

▪ Maintenance chemotherapy may be ideal in patients where close monitoring for disease progression is not feasible and for whom rapid disease progression after the completion of first-line treatment may preclude administration of active second-line agents.

Second Line and Subsequent Therapies (Beyond Second Line)

▪ Most patients who undergo first-line therapy will eventually develop disease progression, and second-line therapy is administered in this setting.

▪ Second-line therapy has an impact on survival and quality of life in advanced NSCLC; therefore, patients with a PS of 0 to 2 should be offered further treatment following progression.

▪ Immunotherapy is considered the preferred second-line treatment option. Based on data discussed above, nivolumab or pembrolizumab should be considered in patients without a contraindication to this treatment after progression on platinum doublet +/– maintenance therapy.

▪ If no targeted treatment options remain or patients have progressed on or cannot be treated with immunotherapy, and continue to have a good PS (0 to 2), then cytotoxic chemotherapies not previously utilized remain viable options including: docetaxel, docetaxel/ramucirumab, gemcitabine, or pemetrexed.

- The TAX 317, a phase III trial which randomized patients with advanced NSCLC and prior platinum-based chemotherapy ($n = 104$) to docetaxel (75 mg/m² IV every 21 days) or best supportive care, found longer overall survival with docetaxel (median 7.5 vs. 4.6 months).

- In an open-label randomized phase III trial of patients with advanced NSCLC after failure of one chemotherapy regimen ($n = 571$), pemetrexed (500 mg/m² IV every 21 days) resulted in equivalent efficacy outcomes with docetaxel (median OS 8.3 vs. 7.9 months for docetaxel) but with significantly fewer side effects.

- BR 21, a randomized (2:1), double blind, placebo-controlled trial of unselected advanced NSCLC patients after failure of one or two chemotherapy regimens ($n = 731$), demonstrated improved OS with erlotinib (150 mg PO qday) (6.7 vs. 4.3 months for placebo). The phase III REVEL trial ($n = 1,253$) enrolled patients with squamous or nonsquamous NSCLC who had progressed during or after a first-line platinum-based chemotherapy to receive docetaxel and either ramucirumab or placebo. A slight increase in median OS was seen with the combination versus docetaxel alone (10.5 vs. 9.1 months, respectively). This came at the expense of increased rates of gastrointestinal bleeding, perforation, or fistula as well as hypertension in the combination arm.

- If disease progression occurs on subsequent chemotherapy or all therapeutic options are exhausted, it is recommended that patients with a PS of 0 to 2 be enrolled in a clinical trial or treated with best supportive care.

Suggested Readings

1. Arriagada R, Bergman B, Dunant A, et al. Cisplatin-based adjuvant chemotherapy in patients with completely resected non-small cell lung cancer. *N Engl J Med*. 2004;350:351–360.
2. Azzoli CG, Baker S Jr, Temin S, et al. American Society of Clinical Oncology Clinical Practice Guideline update on chemotherapy for stage IV non-small-cell lung cancer. *J Clin Oncol*. 2009;27(36):6251–6266.
3. Baumgart M. New molecular targets on the horizon in non-small cell lung cancer. *Am J Hematol/Oncol*. 2014;11(6):10–12.
4. Bergethon K, Shaw A, Ou S, et al. ROS1 rearrangements define a unique molecular class of lung cancers. *J Clin Oncol*. 2012;30(8):863–870.
5. Berghmans T, Paesmans M, Meert AP, et al. Survival improvement in resectable non-small cell lung cancer with (neo) adjuvant chemotherapy: results of a meta-analysis of the literature. *Lung Cancer*. 2005;49:13–23.
6. Borghaei H, Paz-Ares L, Horn L, et al. Nivolumab versus decetaxel in advanced nonsquamous non-small-cell lung cancer. *N Engl J Med*. 2015;373:1627–1639.
7. Brahmer J, Reckamp KL, Baas P, et al. Nivolumab vs. docetaxel in advanced squamous non-small-cell lung cancer. *N Engl J Med*. 2015;373:123–135.
8. Burdett S, Stewart L. Postoperative radiotherapy in non-small cell lung cancer: update of an individual patient data meta-analysis. *Lung Cancer*. 2005;47:81–83.
9. Camidge DR, Bang YJ, Kwak EL, et al. Activity and safety of crizotinib in patients with ALK-positive non-small-cell lung cancer: updated results from a phase 1 study. *Lancet Oncol*. 2012;13:1011–1109.
10. Cappuzzo F, Ciuleanu T, Stelmakh L, et al. Erlotinib as maintenance treatment in advanced non-small-cell lung cancer: a multicentre, randomised, placebo-controlled phase 3 study. *Lancet Oncol*. 2010;11:521–529.
11. Chan BA, Hughes B. Targeted therapy for non-small-cell lung cancer: current standards and the promise of the future. *Transl Lung Cancer Res*. 2015;4(1):36–54.
12. Ciuleanu T, Brodowicz T, Zielinski C, et al. Maintenance pemetrexed plus best supportive care versus placebo plus best supportive care for non-small-cell lung cancer: a randomised, double-blind, phase 3 study. *Lancet*. 2009;374: 1432–1440.
13. Cui JJ, Tran-Dube M, Shen H, et al. Structure based drug designed of crizotinib (PF-02341066), a potent and selective dual inhibitor of mesenchymal-epithelial transition factor (c-MET) kinase and anaplastic lymphoma kinase (ALK). *J Med Chem*. 2011;54:6342–6363.
14. Dai C, Shen J, Ren Y, et al. Choice of surgical procedure for patients with NSCLC ≤ 1 cm or > 1 to 2 cm among lobectomy, segmentectomy, and wedge resection: a population-based study. *J Clin Oncol*. 2016 (epub ahead of print).
15. Douillard J, Rosell R, Delena M, et al. Adjuvant vinorelbine plus cisplatin versus observation in patients with completely resected stage IB-IIIA non-small-cell lung cancer (Adjuvant Navelbine International Trialist Association [ANITA]): a randomised controlled trial. *Lancet Oncol*. 2006 Sep;7(9):719–727.
16. Fischer BM, Mortensen J, Hojgaard L. Positron emission tomography in the diagnosis and staging of lung cancer: a systematic, quantitative review. *Lancet Oncol*. 2001;2:659–666.
17. Garon EB, Ciuleanu TE, Arrieta O, et al. Ramucirumab plus docetaxel versus placebo plus docetaxel for second-line treatment of stage IV non-small-cell lung cacner after disease progression on platinum-based therapy (REVEL): a multicenter, double-blind, randomized phase 3 trial. *Lancet*. 2014;384:665–673.
18. Gazdar A1, Robinson L, Oliver D, et al. Hereditary lung cancer syndrome targets never smokers with germline EGFR gene T790M mutations. *J Thorac Oncol*. 2014;9(4):456–463.
19. Gettinger SN, Horn L, Gandhi L, et al. Overall survival and long-term safety of nivolumab (anti-programmed death 1 antibody, BMS-936558, ONO-4538) in patients with previously treated advanced non-small-cell lung cancer. *J Clin Oncol*. 2015;33:2004–2012.

20. Goldstraw P, Crowley J, Chansky K The IASLC Lung Cancer Staging Project: proposals for the revision of the TNM stage groupings in the forthcoming (seventh) edition of the TNM Classification of malignant tumours. *J Thorac Oncol.* 2007;2:706–714.

21. Gould MK, Maclean CC, Kuschner WG, Rydzak CE, Owens DK. Accuracy of positron emission tomography for diagnosis of pulmonary nodules and mass lesions: a meta-analysis. *JAMA.* 2001; 285:914–924.

22. Hamilton M, Wolf JL, Rusk J, et al. Effects of smoking on the pharmacokinetics of erlotinib. *Clin Cancer Res.* 2006;12:2166–2171.

23. Hanna N, Shepherd FA, Fossella FV, et al. Randomized phase III trial of pemetrexed versus docetaxel in patients with non-small-cell lung cancer previously treated with chemotherapy. *J Clin Oncol.* 2004;22:1589–1597.

24. Herbst RS, Baas P, Kim DW, et al. Pembrolizumab versus docetaxel for previously treated, PD-L1-positive, advanced non-small-cell lung cancer (KEYNOTE-010): a randomised controlled trial. *Lancet.* 2016;387(10027):1540–1550.

25. Keedy VL, Temin S, Somerfield MR, et al. American Society of Clinical Oncology provisional clinical opinion: epidermal growth factor receptor (EGFR) Mutation testing for patients with advanced non-small-cell lung cancer considering first-line EGFR tyrosine kinase inhibitor therapy. *J Clin Oncol.* 2011;29:2121–2127.

26. Kilgoz HO, Bender G, Scandura JM, Viale A, Taneri B. KRAS and the Reality of Personalized Medicine in Non-Small-Cell Lung Cancer. *Mol Med.* 2016;22:380–387.

27. Kwak EL, Bang YJ, Camidge DR, et al. Anaplastic lymphoma kinase inhibition in non-small-cell lung cancer. *N Engl J Med.* 2010;363:1693–1703.

28. Lubin JH, Boice JD Jr. Lung cancer risk from residential radon: meta-analysis of eight epidemiologic studies. *J Natl Cancer Inst.* 1997;89:49–57.

29. Lynch TJ, Bell DW, Sordella R, et al. Activating mutations in the epidermal growth factor receptor underlying responsiveness of non-small-cell lung cancer to gefitinib. *N Engl J Med.* 2004; 350:2129–2139.

30. Maemondo M, Inoue A, Kobayashi K, et al. Gefitinib or chemotherapy for non-small-cell lung cancer with mutated EGFR. *N Engl J Med* 2010;362:2380–2388.

31. Masters G and Shah D. Immunotherapy in lung cancer treatment: current treatment and future directions. June 3, 2016. https://am.asco.org/immunotherapy-lung-cancer-treatment-current-status-and-future-directions. Accessed September 22, 2016.

32. Mitsudomi T, Morita S, Yatabe Y, et al. Gefitinib versus cisplatin plus docetaxel in patients with non-small-cell lung cancer harbouring mutations of the epidermal growth factor receptor (WJTOG3405): an open labe, randomized phase 3 trial. *Lancet Oncol.* 2010;11:121–128.

33. Mok TS, Wu YL, Thongprasert S, et al. Gefitinib or carboplatin-paclitaxel in pulmonary adenocarcinoma. *N Engl J Med.* 2009;361:947.

34. NationalComprehensive Cancer Network. *Practice Guidelines in Oncology Version 3*; 2017. Available at: https://www.nccn.org/professionals/physician_gls/default.aspx.

35. Okawara G, Ung YC, Markman BR, et al. Postoperative radiotherapy in stage II or IIIA completely resected non-small cell lung cancer: a systematic review and practice guideline. *Lung Cancer.* 2004;44:1–11.

36. Patel JD, Socinski MA, Garon EB, et al. Pointbreak: a randomized phase III study of pemetrexed plus carboplatin and bevacizumab followed by maintenance pemetrexed and bevacizumab versus paclitaxel plus carboplatin and bevacizumab followed by maintenance bevacizumab in patients with stage IIIB or IV nonsquamous non-small cell lung cancer. *J Clin Oncol.* 2013;31:4349–4357.

37. Perez-Soler R, Chachoua A, Hammond LA, et al. Determinants of tumor response and survival with erlotinib in patients with non-small-cell lung cancer. *J Clin Oncol.* 2004;22:3238–3247.

38. Pignon JP, Tribodet H, Scagliotti GV, et al. Lung Adjuvant Cisplatin Evaluation (LACE): a pooled analysis of five randomized clinical trials including 4,584 patients. *J Clin Oncol.* 2006;24(18S):7008.

39. Postoperative radiotherapy in non-small-cell lung cancer: systematic review and meta-analysis of individual patient data from nine randomized controlled trials. PORT Meta-analysis Trialist Group. *Lancet.* 1998;353:257–263.

40. Sandler A, Gray R, Perry MC, et al. Paclitaxel-carboplatin alone or with bevacizumab for non-small-cell lung cancer. *N Engl J Med.* 2006;355:2542.

41. Saunders M, Dische S, Barrett A, Harvey A, Gibson D, Parmar M. Continuous hyperfractionated accelerated radiotherapy (CHART) versus conventional radiotherapy in non-small cell lung cancer: a randomised, multicentre trial: CHART Steering Committee. *Lancet.* 1997;350:161–165.

42. Scagliotti GV, Parikh P, von Pawel J, et al. Phase III study comparing cisplatin plus gemcitabine with cisplatin plus pemetrexed in chemotherapy-naive patients with advanced-stage non-small-cell lung cancer. *J Clin Oncol.* 26;3543–3551.

43. Schiller JH, Harrington D, Belani CP, et al. Comparison of four chemotherapy regimens for advanced non-small-cell lung cancer. *N Engl J Med.* 2002;346:92.

44. Senan S, Brade A, Wang LH, et al. PROCLAIM: randomized phase III trial of pemetrexed-cisplatin or etoposide-cisplatin plus thoracic radiation therapy followed by consolidation chemotherapy in locally advanced nonsquamous non-small-cell lung cancer. *J Clin Oncol.* 2016;34(9):953–962.

45. Sequist LV, Waltman BA, Dias-Santagata D, et al. Genotypic and histological evolution of lung cancers acquiring resistance to EGFR inhibitors. *Science Transl Med.* 2011;3:75ra26.

46. Shaw AT, Yeap BY, Mino-Kenudson M, et al. Clinical features and outcome of patients with non-small-cell lung cancer who harbor EML4-ALK. *J Clin Oncol.* 2009;27:4247–4253.
47. Shaw AT, Yeap BY, Solomon BJ, et al. Effect of crizotinib on overall survival in patients with advanced non-small lung cancer harbouring ALK gene rearrangement: a retrospective analysis. *Lancet Oncol.* 2011;12:1004–1012.
48. Shepherd FA, Pereira J, Ciuleanu TE, et al. Erlotinib in previously treated non-small-cell lung cancer. *N Engl J Med.* 2005;353:123–132.
49. Shepherd FA, Dancey J, Ramlau R, et al. Prospective randomized trial of docetaxel versus best supportive care in patients with non-small-cell lung cancer previously treated with platinum-based chemotherapy. *J Clin Oncol.* 2000;18:2095–2103.
50. Siegel R, Naishadham D, Jemal A. Cancer statistics, 2012. *CA Cancer J Clin.* 2012;62:10–29.
51. Travis WD, Brambilla E, Noguchi M, et al. International association for the study of lung cancer/american thoracic society/european respiratory society international multidisciplinary classification of lung adenocarcinoma. *J Thorac Oncol.* 2011;6:244–285.
52. Van Meerbeeck JP, Kramer G, Van Schil PE, et al. A randomized trial of radical surgery versus thoracic radiotherapy in patients with stage IIIA-N2 non-small cell lung cancer after response to induction chemotherapy (EORTC 08941) [abstract]. *J Clin Oncol.* 2005;23(Suppl):7015.
53. Winton T, Livingston R, Johnson D, et al. Vinorelbine plus cisplatin vs. observation in resected non–small-cell lung cancer. *N Engl J Med.* 2005;352:2589–2597.
54. Wood K, Hensing T, Malik R, et al. Prognostic and predictive value in KRAS in non–small-cell lung cancer. *JAMA Oncol.* 2016;2(6):805–812.
55. Zhou C, Wu YL, Chen G, et al. Erlotinib versus chemotherapy as first-line treatment for patients with advanced EGFR mutation-positive non-small-cell lung cancer (OPTIMAL, CTONG-0802): a multicenter, open-label, randomized, phase 3 study. *Lancet Oncol.* 2011;12:735–742.

Small Cell Lung Cancer 3

Christopher E. Wee and James P. Stevenson

EPIDEMIOLOGY

Small cell lung cancer (SCLC) makes up approximately 13% of all new lung malignancies and is primarily a disease of the smoking population. SCLC is a biologically aggressive disease, but multimodality therapy in early-stage SCLC can lead to prolonged survival and potential cure in subsets of patients. However, while SCLC is highly responsive to chemotherapy, it often relapses, and thus generally has a poor prognosis.

PATHOLOGY

Small cell lung cancer (SCLC) is classified into three groups: classical small cell carcinoma, large cell neuroendocrine tumor, and a combination of small cell carcinoma with areas of non–small cell lung carcinoma (NSCLC). SCLC is often poorly differentiated with high mitotic rate and proliferation index. Immunohistochemical stains consistent with small cell characteristics include keratin, tissue transcription factor-1 (TTF-1), and epithelial membrane antigen. Neuroendocrine markers such as chromogranin and synaptophysin are often present, but their absence does not rule out small cell histology. Thirty percent of SCLC biopsies can contain NSCLC, thus leading to the hypothesis that lung carcinoma originates from a pluripotent stem cell. Even expert pathologists can have difficulty differentiating NSCLC from SCLC approximately 5% of the time, and thus review by multiple pathologists may be necessary.

CLINICAL PRESENTATION

SCLC is typically symptomatic at presentation, as a result of bulky locoregional disease and/or the presence of distant metastases. Because SCLC is often located centrally, patients are commonly susceptible to pulmonary complications, including dyspnea and postobstructive infection. Common metastatic sites include the brain, liver, bones, and adrenal glands. Classically, SCLC is associated with a number of paraneoplastic syndromes, which are typically associated with poor prognosis:

- Lambert-Eaton syndrome
- Syndrome of inappropriate antidiuretic hormone (SIADH)
- Ectopic ACTH production (Cushing's syndrome)
- Ectopic parathyroid hormone production
- Sensory neuropathy
- Paraneoplastic encephalomyelitis

STAGING

The AJCC staging system defines the TNM subsets used to stage SCLC.

- This staging classification can be helpful in prognostication and selection of patients who might benefit from multimodality treatment approaches, including surgical resection in select cases.

Traditionally, however, SCLC has been divided into limited-stage (LS) and extensive-stage (ES) disease.

- LS SCLC is disease that is encompassed safely into one radiation field, and thus is amenable to definitive chemoradiation.
- ES SCLC is tumor burden that extends beyond one radiation field, and therefore treatment is primarily systemic chemotherapy with palliative intent.

This simplified approach to staging has practical utility, given that the majority of patients present with bulky lymphadenopathy and/or distant metastases at time of diagnosis. However, as the role of surgical resection has increased and become more well-defined, the classic division of cases as LS and ES has become less relevant. The AJCC TNM staging system definitions are more precise and allow for better selection for patients who may be candidates for multimodality therapy.

IMAGING

Routine testing generally consists of a CT of the chest and abdomen, and brain imaging. Once extensive stage has been established, further staging workup is optional, except brain imaging, which should occur in all patients.

Brain imaging is important because 10% to 15% of SCLCs have brain metastases at presentation, and early detection and treatment have been shown to improve both patient morbidity and mortality, and will guide therapeutic decisions. MRI is preferred over CT, unless there is a contraindication, due to its greater sensitivity in detecting parenchymal brain metastases.

Positron emission tomography (PET) is recommended if limited-stage disease is suspected after initial imaging. Fischer et al. demonstrated that PET/CT had a sensitivity and specificity of 93% and 100% compared to 79% and 100% with standard staging. PET/CT is not recommended for assessment of treatment response. Additional imaging is recommended only if it will impact treatment approach. For patients who appear to have T1-2N0 disease after initial imaging, invasive mediastinal staging should be performed if the patient is a surgical candidate.

SURVIVAL

Median overall survival (OS) for treated LS SCLC is 15 to 20 months, and treated ES SCLC is 8 to 12 months. If untreated, median OS for ES SCLC is 6 to 12 weeks. The 2-year survival for LS SCLC is 20% to 40% and <5% for ES SCLC.

TREATMENT

Limited-Stage Small Cell Lung Cancer (Stages I to III)

General Concepts

Multimodal approaches are recommended in early-stage disease. While surgical resection has not classically been considered a primary treatment approach in SCLC, recent data has indicated surgical intervention may benefit a subset of patients, specifically, those with clinical T1-2N0 disease (about 5% of patients with SCLC) that has been subsequently confirmed by pathologic mediastinal lymph node staging. The optimal adjuvant approach for surgical patients has not been well defined, but generally includes adjuvant chemotherapy or chemoradiation.

Stages I to III disease that is not amenable to surgery (due to nodal involvement or medical contraindications), but can be encompassed within one radiation portal, should be treated with definitive concurrent chemoradiation. Patients treated with chemotherapy alone for LS SCLC have an 80% rate of local recurrence, and the addition of thoracic radiotherapy improves OS and reduces the rate of local recurrence. A meta-analysis of thoracic radiotherapy and chemotherapy in LS SCLC showed an increase

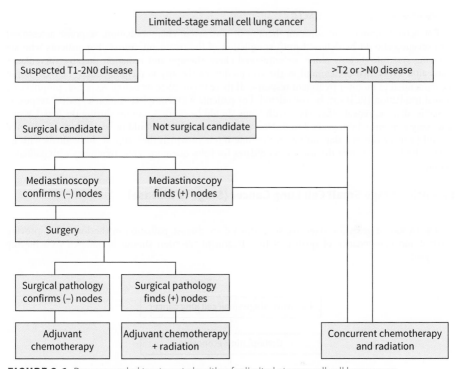

FIGURE 3.1 Recommended treatment algorithm for limited-stage small cell lung cancer.

in the rate of local control by 25% to 30%, with a 5% to 7% improvement in 2-year overall survival when compared to chemotherapy alone.

Chemotherapy in LS SCLC

The most commonly used chemotherapy regimen for LS SCLC is cisplatin and etoposide, and is the preferred regimen. Carboplatin may be substituted in patients who are not candidates for cisplatin (e.g., renal insufficiency, neuropathy) or unable to tolerate fluid load. Myeloid growth factors are not recommended for use during concurrent chemoradiation; a randomized controlled trial of patients with LS SCLC undergoing chemotherapy and radiation with and without granulocyte-macrophage colony-stimulating factors (GM-CSF) found that while the cohort randomized to receive GM-CSF had higher WBC and neutrophil nadirs, there was no significant difference in grade 4 neutropenia or leukopenia. Paradoxically, those randomized to the GM-CSF group had significantly more life-threatening thrombocytopenia, toxic deaths, nonhematologic toxicities, days in hospital, and transfusions.

Radiation Therapy in LS SCLC

Concurrent chemoradiation produces superior outcomes compared to sequential therapy. Candidates for concurrent therapy must be carefully selected, as this approach produces increased toxicity compared to either modality alone. Early thoracic radiotherapy delivered concurrently with cycle 1 or 2 of the standard 3-weekly cisplatin and etoposide (EP) combination is the current standard of care as it is associated with significantly increased survival.

Thoracic radiotherapy may be delivered in single daily fractions over 6 weeks for a total dose of 60 Gy, or a hyperfractionated schedule of 45 Gy over 3 weeks, twice daily. The efficacy of these two treatment schedules is currently being investigated in the CALGB 30610 trial.

Monitoring Response in LS SCLC

For patients undergoing adjuvant therapy, or concurrent chemoradiation, response assessment with imaging should be deferred until completion of the treatment course. For patients who are receiving systemic therapy alone, or sequential chemotherapy and radiation therapy, surveillance scans after every two cycles, and at the completion of therapy is recommended. PET/CT is not recommended to monitor treatment response. If there is complete or partial response, prophylactic cranial irradiation (PCI) can be considered. For patients with complete response, partial response, or stable disease, repeat office visits with scans should be every 3 months during the first 2 years, and every 6 months from years 3 to 5. New pulmonary nodules should be worked up as potential second primary tumors, depending on the time frame in which they appear. Individuals with LS SCLC who have recurrent disease are candidates for subsequent systemic treatment with palliative intent.

Extensive-Stage Small Cell Lung Cancer (Stage IV Disease)

General Concepts

The treatment goals for extensive-stage disease are disease palliation in the form of improving survival and maintenance of quality of life. Treatment selection should be tailored to achieving these goals.

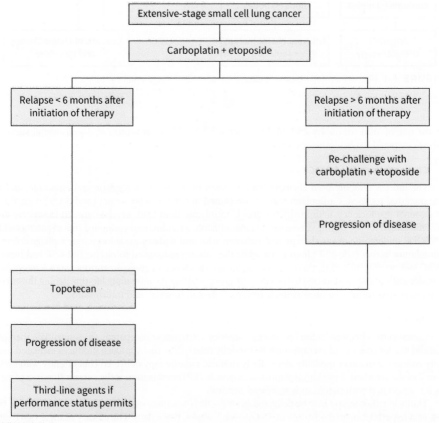

FIGURE 3.2 Recommended treatment algorithm for extensive-stage small cell lung cancer.

Chemotherapy in ES SCLC

Platinum and etoposide regimens also remain the standard of care for extensive-stage disease. Carboplatin is often used in extensive-stage disease because of its more favorable side-effect profile. A meta-analysis of four trials comparing cisplatin and carboplatin in front-line treatment of SCLC demonstrated similar outcomes; of the 663 patients included in the analysis, 68.3% had extensive-stage disease. For cisplatin and carboplatin, median OS was 9.6 months versus 9.4 months, respectively, and median PFS was 5.5 months versus 5.3 months. These outcomes and baseline characteristics (e.g., sex, stage, performance status, age) were not significantly different.

Multiple trials have explored the possible substitution of the topoisomerase I inhibitor irinotecan for etoposide in ES SCLC. While an initial phase III Japanese trial demonstrated longer median OS (12.8 vs. 9.4 months) and higher two-year survival (19.5% vs. 5.2%) when cisplatin and irinotecan were compared with cisplatin and etoposide, this result was not reproduced in two US trials, and therefore irinotecan is not recommended for front-line use.

Relapsed/Refractory SCLC

Eighty percent of patients with SCLC and nearly all with ES SCLC will relapse within the first 12 months after first-line therapy. If the cancer relapses within 3 months of initial therapy, it is defined as refractory/resistant disease and is associated with a poor prognosis. Sensitive disease applies to patients who exhibit disease progression more than 3 months after completion of front-line platinum-based chemotherapy. A systematic analysis of 21 trials reported that patients with sensitive SCLC had higher response rates (27.7% vs. 14.8%) and longer median OS (7.73 vs. 5.45 months) when compared with resistant/refractory SCLC.

Patients who relapse greater than 6 months after completion of front-line chemotherapy represent a group with more favorable prognosis and may be retreated with carboplatin + etoposide as this regimen is associated with a greater response rate than single agents. Topotecan is the current therapy of choice for patients who have refractory disease or relapse within the first 6 months of completion of front-line chemotherapy. Oral or intravenous topotecan may be used since efficacy and toxicity are similar. When compared to best supportive care in a randomized trial, topotecan was found to improve both quality of life and survival. A phase III trial comparing topotecan to combination CAV (cyclophosphamide, doxorubicin, vincristine) demonstrated similar response rate and overall survival, but improved tolerability. Single agent irinotecan, docetaxel, paclitaxel may also be considered. Phase I/II immunotherapy trials have shown responses with nivolumab, or combination of ipilimumab and nivolumab, and these treatments are under further investigation in randomized trials.

Radiation Therapy in ES SCLC

In a phase III randomized controlled trial, patients with ES SCLC who responded to chemotherapy were randomized to receive thoracic radiotherapy or no thoracic radiotherapy. All patients received PCI. While the primary endpoint of one-year survival did not differ between the groups, secondary analysis did demonstrate a significant two-year survival difference of 13% in the radiotherapy group versus 3% in the control. Thus in patients who respond to initial cytotoxic therapy, the addition of thoracic radiotherapy may be considered in selected patients.

Monitoring Response in ES SCLC

During systemic therapy for ES SCLC, CT scans should be obtained after every two to three cycles of systemic therapy. Responding patients should continue therapy for at least six cycles in the front-line setting, and until disease progression for subsequent lines of therapy, if tolerated.

Prophylactic Cranial Irradiation

Intracranial metastases occur in more than half of patients with SCLC. Brain metastases represent an area of significant morbidity and mortality in SCLC. Prophylactic cranial irradiation (PCI) consists of five to ten fractions of whole-brain radiotherapy delivered to prevent the onset of symptomatic brain metastases. Each treatment consists of 1.5 to 2.0 Gy per fraction. Higher doses (>3.0 Gy), concurrent chemotherapy, and high total radiotherapy doses have been associated with late neurologic toxicity. In LS SCLC, a meta-analysis demonstrated a 25% reduction in the cumulative incidence of brain metastases at 3 years (33% to 58%) and an improvement in 3-year OS with PCI (20.7% vs. 15.3%). There are conflicting data regarding the use of PCI in ES SCLC. An EORTC trial of PCI versus observation in patients who exhibited either a partial or complete response to combination chemotherapy showed decreased incidence of brain metastases and improved one-year OS from 13.3% to 27.1%. However, a recent Japanese phase III trial demonstrated no survival benefit for those with ES SCLC when administered PCI versus no PCI.

Thus, PCI is recommended for LS SCLC who achieve a PR or CR and may be considered for ES SCLC after weighing risks and benefits. Its use in patients with ES SCLC can be considered on an individual basis, but is not routinely recommended given the poor OS for these patients. PCI is not recommended for patients with a poor ECOG PS (3 to 4), multiple comorbidities, or impaired cognitive function. PCI is not given concurrently with chemotherapy due to potentially cumulative neurotoxicity.

New Therapeutic Directions

Many chemotherapeutic combinations have been evaluated against platinum plus etoposide in the front-line setting, but none have clearly demonstrated superior outcomes. A phase III trial demonstrated no benefit with the addition of paclitaxel to cisplatin and etoposide in ES SCLC, with an increase in treatment-related mortality in the experimental arm (6.5% vs. 2.4%).The addition of the antiangiogenic agent bevacizumab showed promise in phase II studies in combination with platinum-based chemotherapy; however, a randomized trial failed to demonstrate survival benefit of the addition of bevacizumab to chemotherapy alone.

Breakthroughs in immunotherapy have already changed the standards of care in many common malignancies, including NSCLC, melanoma, and renal cell carcinoma. Two agents, ipilimumab (CTLA-4 inhibitor) and nivolumab (PD-1 inhibitor), upregulate T-cell antitumor activity, and produce significant responses in these malignancies, as well as others. An open-label phase I/II trial including 216 SCLC patients who had disease progression following a platinum-containing regimen demonstrated objective disease response in 10% to 33% of patients receiving differing doses of nivolumab monotherapy or combination nivolumab plus ipilimumab. Randomized controlled trials of nivolumab +/– ipilimumab are currently underway to further determine efficacy.

Another agent, rovalpituzumab tesirine (Rova-T), targets delta-like protein 3 (DLL-3), which is present on nearly two-thirds of SCLC tumor cells. This is an antibody-drug conjugate, delivering the toxin pyrrolobenzodiazepine to the DLL-3 expressing tumor cell. A phase I trial of rovalpituzumab in recurrent small cell lung cancer included 74 patients who had progressed on at least one prior therapy. Nine of the 74 patients were not assessable for analysis (e.g., patient died prior to scan, adverse event, withdrew consent). Of the 65 that were analyzed, 11 (17%) had objective response, 35 (54%) had stable disease; therefore, disease control was achieved in 47 (71%) of patients. Moreover, responses were greater in those who were over-expressed DLL-3, signaling that rovalpituzumab may be the first molecular-targeted agent in patients with SCLC.

Suggested Readings

1. Antonia SJ, López-Martin JA, Bendell J, et al. Nivolumab alone and nivolumab plus ipilimumab in recurrent small-cell lung cancer (CheckMate 032): a multicentre, open-label, phase 1/2 trial. *Lancet Oncol.* 2016;17(July):883–895. doi:10.1016/S1470-2045(16)30098-5.
2. Auperin A, Arriagada R, Pignon J. Prophylactic cranial irradiation for patients with small-cell lung cancer in complete remission. *N Engl J Med.* 1999;341:476–484.
3. Bunn Jr. PA, Crowley J, Kelly K, et al. Chemoradiotherapy with or without granulocyte-macrophage colony-stimulating factor in the treatment of limited-stage small-cell lung cancer: a prospective phase III randomized study of the Southwest Oncology Group. *J Clin Oncol.* 1995;13(0732-183X):1632–1641.
4. Fischer BM, Mortensen J, Langer SW, et al. A prospective study of PET/CT in initial staging of small-cell lung cancer: comparison with CT, bone scintigraphy and bone marrow analysis. *Ann Oncol.* 2007;18:338–345. doi:10.1093/annonc/mdl374.

5. Fischer BM, Mortensen J, Langer SW, et al. PET/CT imaging in response evaluation of patients with small cell lung cancer. *Lung Cancer*. 2006;54. doi:10.1016/j.lungcan.2006.06.012.

6. Govindan R, Page N, Morgensztern D, et al. Changing epidemiology of small-cell lung cancer in the United States over the last 30 years: analysis of the surveillance, epidemiologic, and end results database. *J Clin Oncol*. 2006;24:4539–4544. doi:10.1200/JCO.2005.04.4859.

7. Hanna N, Bunn PA, Langer C, et al. Randomized phase III trial comparing irinotecan/cisplatin with etoposide/cisplatin in patients with previously untreated extensive-stage disease small-cell lime cancer. *J Clin Oncol*. 2006;24(13):2038–2043. doi:10.1200/JCO.2005.04.8595.

8. Lara PN, Natale R, Crowley J, et al. Phase III trial of irinotecan/cisplatin compared with etoposide/cisplatin in extensive-stage small-cell lung cancer: clinical and pharmacogenomic results from SWOG S0124. *J Clin Oncol*. 2009;27(15):2530–2535. doi:10.1200/JCO.2008.20.1061.

9. Niell HB, Herndon JE, Miller AA, et al. Randomized phase III intergroup trial of etoposide and cisplatin with or without paclitaxel and granulocyte colony-stimulating factor in patients with extensive-stage small-cell lung cancer: cancer and Leukemia Group B trial 9732. *J Clin Oncol*. 2005;23(16):3752–3759. doi:10.1200/JCO.2005.09.071.

10. Noda K, Nishiwaki Y, Kawahara M, et al. Irinotecan plus cisplatin compared with etoposide plus cisplatin for extensive small-cell lung cancer. *N Engl J Med*. 2002;346(2):85–91. doi:10.1056/NEJMoa003034.

11. O'Brien MER, Ciuleanu TE, Tsekov H, et al. Phase III trial comparing supportive care alone with supportive care with oral topotecan in patients with relapsed small-cell lung cancer. *J Clin Oncol*. 2006;24(34):5441–5447. doi:10.1200/JCO.2006.06.5821.

12. Owonikoko TK, Behera MM, Chen Z, et al. A systematic analysis of efficacy of second-line chemotherapy in sensitive and refractory small-cell lung cancer. *JTO Acquis*. 2012;7(5):866–872. doi:10.1097/JTO.0b013e31824c7f4b.

13. Pawel BJ Von, Schiller JH, Shepherd FA, et al. Topotecan versus cyclophosphamide, doxorubicin, and vincristine for the treatment of recurrent small-cell lung cancer. 2016;17(2):658–667.

14. Pignon J-P, Arriagada R, Ihde DC. A meta-analysis of thoracic radiotherapy for small-cell lung cancer. *N Engl J Med*. 1992;327(23):1618–1624.

15. Pijls-Johannesma M, De Ruysscher D, Vansteenkiste J, Kester A, Rutten I, Lambin P. Timing of chest radiotherapy in patients with limited stage small cell lung cancer: a systematic review and meta-analysis of randomised controlled trials. *Cancer Treat Rev*. 2007;33(5):461–473. doi:10.1016/j.ctrv.2007.03.002.

16. Pujol JL, Lavole A, Quoix E, èt al. Randomized phase II-III study of bevacizumab in combination with chemotherapy in previously untreated extensive small-cell lung cancer: Results from the IFCT-0802 trial. *Ann Oncol*. 2015;26(5):908–914. doi:10.1093/annonc/mdv065.

17. Rossi A, Di Maio M, Chiodini P, et al. Carboplatin- or cisplatin-based chemotherapy in first-line treatment of small-cell lung cancer: The COCIS meta-analysis of individual patient data. *J Clin Oncol*. 2012;30:1692–1698. doi:10.1200/JCO.2011.40.4905.

18. Rudin CM, Pietanza MC, Bauer TM, et al. Rovalpituzumab tesirine, a DLL3-targeted antibody-drug conjugate, in recurrent small-cell lung cancer: a first-in-human, first-in-class, open-label, phase 1 study. *Lancet Oncol*. 2016;2045(16):1–10. doi:10.1016/S1470-2045(16)30565-4.

19. Slotman B, Faivre-Finn C, Kramer G, et al. Prophylactic cranial irradiation in extensive small-cell lung cancer. *N Eng J Med*. 2007;357:664–672.

20. Slotman BJ, Van Tinteren H, Praag JO, et al. Use of thoracic radiotherapy for extensive stage small-cell lung cancer: a phase 3 randomised controlled trial. *Lancet*. 2015;385(9962):36–42. doi:10.1016/S0140-6736(14)61085-0.

21. Takada M, Fukuoka M, Kawahara M, et al. Phase III study of concurrent versus sequential thoracic radiotherapy in combination with cisplatin and etoposide for limited-stage small-cell lung cancer: results of the Japan Clinical Oncology Group Study 9104. *J Clin Oncol*. 2002;20:3054–3060. doi:10.1200/JCO.2002.12.071.

22. Takahashi T, Yamanaka T, Seto T, et al. Prophylactic cranial irradiation versus observation in patients with extensive-disease small-cell lung cancer: A multicentre, randomised, open-label, phase 3 trial. *Lancet Oncol*. 2017;18(5):663–671. doi:10.1016/S1470-2045(17)30230-9.

23. Travis WD. Advances in neuroendocrine lung tumors. *Annals of Oncology*. Vol. 21.; 2010. doi:10.1093/annonc/mdq380.

24. Warde P, Payne D. Does Thoracic irradiation improve survival and local control in limited-stage small-cell carcinoma of the lung? A meta-analysis. *J Clin Oncol*. 1992;10:890–895.

4 Esophageal Cancer

Megan Greally and Gregory D. Leonard

Worldwide, esophageal cancer is the eighth most commonly occurring cancer and the sixth most common cause of cancer-related mortality. Approximately 50% to 60% of patients present with incurable locally advanced or metastatic disease. Recent years have seen advances in the management of esophageal cancer resulting in meaningful improvements in outcomes.

EPIDEMIOLOGY

United States

Esophageal cancer occurs less frequently in the United States than in other geographic regions. It is estimated that there will be 16,910 cases and 15,690 deaths in 2016, 2.6% of all cancer deaths in the United States. The age-adjusted incidence from 2009 to 2013 was 4.3 per 100,000 per year. The median age at diagnosis is 67 years.

Esophageal cancer is approximately four times more common in men than women. The incidence is higher in lower socioeconomic groups and in urban areas, particularly in black men. Overall the incidence is similar among black people and white people. Squamous cell carcinoma (SCC) is more common in black people than adenocarcinoma (ADC). Incidence of ADC has increased significantly, and ADC now account for over half of all cases in Western countries. After a steep increase from 1973 to 2001, there has been a plateau in incidence in recent years. In contrast, rates for SCC have been decreasing because of reduced tobacco and alcohol consumption. Five-year relative survival rates were 5% from 1975 to 1977, 10% from 1987 to 1989, and 20% from 2005 to 2011.

Worldwide

About 80% of cases of esophageal cancer occur in less developed regions. The highest incidence occurs in Asia (Northern China, India, and Iran) followed by Southern and Eastern Africa. In the high risk areas of Asia, 90% of cases are SCC, which may be related to low intake of fruits and vegetables and drinking beverages at high temperatures.

ETIOLOGY

Recognized causes of esophageal cancer are described in Table 4.1 above. Smoking has a synergistic effect with alcohol consumption and together they are responsible for 90% of all SCC cases in Western countries. Barretts esophagus is the greatest risk factor for ADC. It increases the risk of ADC 30-fold over the general population. Management recommendations are as follows:

- Nondysplastic Barrett's esophagus: endoscopy every 3 to 5 years.
- Low-grade dysplasia: endoscopic ablation or surveillance every 6 to 12 months.

TABLE 4.1 Causes of Esophageal Adenocarcinoma and Squamous Cell Carcinoma

Adenocarcinoma	Squamous Cell Carcinoma
Barrett's esophagus	Tobacco smoking
Induced by chronic GERD	Alcohol
GERD	Achalasia
Obesity	Plummer–Vinson syndrome
Due to risk of GERD	Tylosis
Smoking	Human papillomavirus (HPV)
	Celiac disease
	Esophageal diverticula and webs
	Dietary factors

TABLE 4.2 Clinical Presentation of Esophageal Cancer

Local Tumor Effects	
Dysphagia (solids then liquids)	Odynophagia
Weight loss and anorexia	Regurgitation of undigested food
Iron-deficiency anemia secondary to chronic gastrointestinal blood loss	
Invasion of Surrounding Structures	
Hoarseness secondary to recurrent laryngeal nerve involvement	
Tracheo- or bronchio-esophageal fistula	Hiccups (phrenic nerve invasion)
Distant Metastases	
Cachexia	Pain
Hypercalcemia	Dyspnoea/Jaundice/ascites (metastatic sites)

▪ High-grade dysplasia: endoscopic eradication therapy (resection of visible irregularities followed by radiofrequency ablation) preferred over esophagectomy or intensive three monthly endoscopy.

CLINICAL PRESENTATION

Both ADC and SCC have similar presentations. Early symptoms are subtle and nonspecific. Later symptoms are described in Table 4.2. Physical signs, usually only seen at late presentation, include Horner syndrome, left supraclavicular lymphadenopathy (Virchow's node), hepatomegaly, and those related to a pleural effusion.

DIAGNOSIS

Endoscopy is the gold standard investigation and allows for histological confirmation with biopsy. It has been shown that several biopsies improve diagnostic accuracy and six to eight biopsies are recommended to allow sufficient tissue for histological interpretation and yield a diagnostic accuracy close to 100%.

PATHOLOGY

The common histologic subtypes are ADC and SCC, which account for approximately 90% of esophageal cancers. Rarely, small cell carcinoma, melanoma, sarcoma, lymphoma, or carcinosarcoma may arise in the esophagus. Fifty percent of tumors arise in the lower one-third, 40% in the middle one-third, and 10% in the upper one-third of the esophagus. Most SCCs occur in the upper and mid esophagus while ADC generally arises in the distal esophagus and esophagogastric junction (EGJ). Metastases to locoregional lymph nodes occur early because the lymphatics are located in the lamina propria. Involvement of celiac and perihepatic nodes is more common in ADC due to distal tumor location.

STAGING

Adequate staging is required in order to determine the appropriate therapeutic approach. Patients should be assigned a clinical stage according to the American Joint Committee on Cancer (AJCC) tumor-node-metastasis (TNM) classification. The advent of modern staging modalities has resulted in more accurate clinical TNM staging. The Siewert classification subclassifies EGJ tumors into three types according to their anatomic location and may be useful for selecting the surgical approach. Type I are distal esophagus tumors, type II are cardia tumors, and type III are subcardia gastric tumors.

Standard staging includes computed tomography (CT) and endoscopic ultrasonography (EUS). CT evaluates for the presence of metastatic disease, with an accuracy of over 90%, and for direct invasion of local structures, which may preclude surgical intervention. EUS allows assessment of the relationship of an esophageal mass to the five-layered esophageal wall and is superior to CT in evaluating the histologic depth of the tumor and determining nodal burden (accuracy of ~80% and 75%, respectively). EUS can facilitate fine-needle aspiration of suspicious lymph nodes to allow confirmation of disease involvement. The accuracy of EUS is operator dependent and interobserver variability is significant.

Positron emission tomography (PET)/CT is more sensitive than CT for detecting distant disease, and guidelines recommend its use in patients who are surgical candidates after routine staging. Several studies have suggested a change in management in up to 20% of patients with the use of PET/CT in preoperative assessment. The role of laparoscopy in outruling peritoneal disease is uncertain. It is an optional staging investigation for those with no evidence of distant metastatic disease who have distally located tumors.

TREATMENT

An overview of management strategies for localized and advanced disease is shown in Figure 4.1.

Surgical Management

- Esophageal cancer is confined to the esophagus in about 22% and regional nodal disease accounts for a further 30% of cases. Therefore, approximately 50% of patients are potential surgical candidates.
- In recent years, the improved survival seen with combined modality treatment has meant that surgery alone is generally only considered for patients with T1-2N0M0 disease.
- Endomucosal resection (EMR) is a treatment option for select patients with T1a disease as similar cure rates to esophagectomy have been reported in specialized centers. EMR is not recommended for T1b cancers as submucosal involvement is associated with a 30% rate of nodal metastases.
- Advances in staging techniques and patient selection have improved surgical morbidity and mortality. Surgical expertise, multidisciplinary management, and audit of outcomes in high volume centers all contribute to operative mortality rates of less than 5%.
- Surgical principles include a wide resection of the primary tumor and regional lymphadenectomy. Intraoperative frozen section can assess for the presence of residual disease, which may be R1 (microscopic tumor) or R2 (macroscopic tumor). The resection status is one of the strongest prognostic

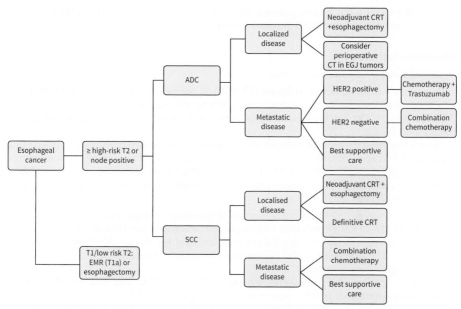

FIGURE 4.1 Algorithm for management of esophageal cancers, localized and metastatic.

factors in esophageal cancer. The probability of achieving an R0 resection (no residual tumor) is associated with the depth of tumor infiltration into the esophageal wall.

▪ Definitive chemoradiotherapy (CRT) is favored for patients with cervical carcinoma of the esophagus (above the aortic arch) as they are usually not surgical candidates, and is standard in those with unresectable disease (T4 or extensive nodal burden) or poor performance status.

▪ The transhiatal, transthoracic (Ivor-Lewis), and tri-incisional esophagectomy procedures are the usual approaches employed in the United States while esophagectomy with an extended (three-field) lymphadenectomy is commonly utilized in Asia.

▪ A total thoracic esophagectomy (TTE) is recommended for patients with thoracic esophageal cancer. This involves a cervical esophagogastrostomy, radical two-field lymph node dissection (mediastinum and upper abdomen nodes), and jejunostomy feeding.

▪ A tri-incisional approach involving laparotomy, thoracotomy and a left neck incision for cervical anastomosis is generally advocated over an Ivor-Lewis transthoracic procedure as tri-incisional surgery allows for more extensive proximal resection margins and a reduced risk of reflux.

▪ A transhiatal (TH) esophagectomy is utilized in patients with Siewert II and III EGJ tumors. This involves laparotomy and cervical esophagogastrostomy after resection of the distal esophagus and partial or extended gastrectomy with a two-field lymphadenectomy. TH esophagectomy can also be used for Siewert I EGJ tumors, but a TTE and partrial gastrectomy with two-field lymphadenectomy is an option based on a randomized study which showed a nonsignificant improvement in overall survival (OS) for this approach compared to TH esophagectomy.

▪ Minimally invasive laparoscopic and thoracoscopic techniques aim to reduce complication rates and enhance recovery times. One randomized trial showed a 3-fold decrease in postoperative pulmonary infection rate after minimally invasive surgery compared with open transthoracic surgery. This is significant as pulmonary complications, including pneumonia, are the most frequent complications following esophageal surgery. However, more data are required regarding this approach and open surgery remains standard of care.

▪ The minimum number of lymph nodes that should be removed has not been established. Some data suggest that a more extensive lymphadenectomy is associated with a better survival. Three-field lymphadenectomy is standard for proximal tumors in Asia but it is unclear if this approach improves outcomes and it is associated with increased toxicity.

Chemoradiotherapy

Neoadjuvant (Trimodality Approach)

In patients with locally advanced disease (T3-4, N0-3), preoperative therapy is standard. With surgery alone, an R0 resection is not possible in about 30% to 50% and long-term survival rarely exceeds 20%. Preoperative CRT has been shown to result in higher rates of complete resection, better local control, and OS.

Several randomised trials have evaluated preoperative CRT versus surgery alone. Neoadjuvant CRT is standard for T3 and resectable T4 esophageal cancers based on two of these studies demonstrating a statistically significant OS benefit for CRT. Three studies did not show a benefit, however, two of these were underpowered and debate continues regarding their interpretation. The two most important studies are the CROSS and CALGB 9781 studies:

- CALGB 9781 was a randomized Intergroup trial of trimodality therapy versus surgery alone in 56 patients (42 ADC, 14 SCC) with stage I–III esophageal cancer. Five-year OS was 39% versus 16% in favor of trimodality therapy but this did not reach statistical significance. A pathological complete response (pCR) was achieved in 40% of assessable patients in the trimodality arm, and there was no increase in perioperative mortality.
- The CROSS trial included 363 patients, a majority (75%) had ADC, over 80% had T3/4 tumors, and over 60% were node positive. Preoperative radiation, at a dose of 41.4 Gy, concurrent with carboplatin and paclitaxel weekly for 5 weeks was compared to surgery alone. A significant 5-year OS advantage of 47% versus 33% in favor of the CRT arm was observed, HR 0.67. The benefit appeared greater in patients with SCC. There was also a higher rate of R0 resections (92% vs. 69%) and a 29% complete response rate observed with the use of CRT. Treatment was well tolerated and there was no increased postoperative mortality associated with the use of CRT.

A meta-analyses in 2011 reported a benefit for trimodality therapy over surgery alone. This included 12 randomized trials of concurrent or sequential neoadjuvant CRT versus surgery alone. The above studies were included. There was an absolute OS benefit of 8.7% at 2 years and benefit was observed across histologic subtypes.

Management of patients with clinical T2N0 disease is less well defined. These patients were included in three trials including the CROSS trial that showed survival benefit for neoadjuvant CRT but currently there is no clear consensus as to the best approach. An RTOG phase III study is currently ongoing evaluating the addition of trastuzumab to trimodality therapy in patients with HER2 positive disease based on the survival advantage seen in the ToGA trial in patients with advanced disease.

Neoadjuvant CRT has been compared with neoadjuvant chemotherapy in three trials, which reported similar results. There was no difference in OS between groups but higher rates of pathologic complete response and R0 resections were observed in the CRT groups in all three studies. Of note, two of these trials were underpowered to show a survival advantage.

Definitive Chemoradiotherapy in Resectable Disease

Direct comparisons of CRT versus surgery in resectable esophageal cancer are limited. Definitive CRT is reasonable in patients who are not surgical candidates and in those with SCC and an endoscopic complete response. The benefit of nonoperative management (avoidance of morbidity and mortality) must be weighed against the lower rates of local control. Patients with ADC have lower rates of pCR after CRT and there is limited data on nonsurgical management in this group. Some retrospective studies have reported inferior survival with a nonsurgical approach and it is recommended that definitive CRT is reserved for ADC patients with major operative risk.

Two randomized trials have compared CRT with CRT followed by surgery and have provided evidence to support a nonsurgical approach in select patients. Despite better local control neither showed improved survival with trimodality therapy. The patient populations were predominantly SCC.

- A German study evaluated 172 patients with locally advanced resectable SCC. Patients received three cycles of induction 5-FU, leucovorin, etoposide, and cisplatin followed by concurrent CRT (cisplatin/ etoposide with 40 Gy radiotherapy) and patients with at least a partial response were randomized to continued CRT (chemotherapy with 20 Gy radiotherapy) or surgery. There was an improvement in local control rates with surgery (64% vs. 41% at 2 years), but no difference in OS, and early mortality was less in the CRT arm (12.8% vs. 3.5%; $P = 0.03$).

- FFCD 9102 randomized 444 patients with T3, N0-1, M0 disease to definitive CRT with cisplatin and 5-FU or CRT (lower dose of radiation) and surgery (patients with at least a partial response were randomly assigned to continue CRT or undergo surgery). The majority (89%) had SCC. There was no significant difference in 2-year OS (34% vs. 40% for surgery and CRT, respectively) between the groups. Surgically resected patients had lower rates of local recurrence and were less likely to require palliative procedures.

- A Cochrane analysis published in 2016 explored this question further, including these two trials, two others comparing CRT alone versus surgery alone and one comparing CRT with surgery and chemotherapy. Again, most patients had SCC. There was no difference in long-term mortality in the CRT group compared with the surgery group (HR 0.88; 95% CI, 0.76 to 1.03). However, the evidence was considered low-quality and included trials had a high risk of bias.

Experienced multidisciplinary teamwork is required for appropriate use of definitive CRT and decision making around surgery versus CRT should be taken together with the informed patient.

Definitive Chemoradiotherapy in Inoperable Disease

Locally advanced unresectable esophageal cancer is generally incurable but combined modality therapy does offer a small chance of lasting disease control and long-term survival as well as improving quality of life through relief of dysphagia.

The optimal combination, doses and schedule of drugs, that should be used during CRT is not definitively established. Based on the RTOG 85-01 study, cisplatin and 5-FU with radiotherapy is recommended for patients with SCC. This study demonstrated an OS advantage (14 vs. 9 months median survival and 27% vs. 0% 5-year survival) in favor of CRT over radiotherapy alone. The majority of patients had SCC but eligibility for this study did not require surgical unresectability and patients with T4 disease and high nodal burden were not included. Therefore, this cohort likely represents a prognostically more favorable population. A number of randomized trials of CRT versus radiotherapy alone have failed to duplicate these results; however, a Cochrane review has confirmed the superiority of CRT over radiotherapy in patients with a good performance status. Combination cisplatin/5-FU is associated with significant toxicity and weekly carboplatin plus paclitaxel and oxaliplatin/5-FU based chemotherapy have been shown in phase II and phase III trials, respectively, to be appropriate alternative options.

Adjuvant Chemoradiotherapy

There are few data available on the use of postoperative CRT in esophageal cancer. It is generally recommended in patients with resected node-positive or T3-4 disease who did not undergo preoperative therapy.

- An influential Intergroup trial compared postoperative CRT with 5-FU/calcium leucovorin, to surgery alone in resected stage ≥ IB esophagogastric (20% of patients) and gastric ADC. The 3-year OS (50% vs. 41%) was significantly better with CRT. While EGJ tumors are usually treated with neoadjuvant therapy, postoperative CRT remains a standard option based on this data when required. However, there may be significant toxicity associated with this approach.

- The CALGB 80101 investigated the use of more intensive chemotherapy (ECF) given before and after the INT-0116 protocol regimen, but found no improvement in survival compared with the 5-FU regimen used in the Intergroup trial.

- The CRITICS trial compared postoperative epirubicin, cisplatin/oxaliplatin and capecitabine (ECC or EOC) to postoperative cisplatin/capecitabine-based CRT in patients with gastric ADCs. Patients received three cycles of preoperative ECC or EOC. In a preliminary report at the American Society of

Clinical Oncology (ASCO) 2016 meeting there was no significant difference in 5-year OS (40.8% vs. 40.9%). Seventeen percent of patients had EGJ tumors.

- Only one half to two thirds of patients in INT-0116 and CRITICS completed planned postoperative therapy, providing further rationale for the use of preoperative therapy in this patient group.

Chemotherapy

Neoadjuvant and Perioperative Chemotherapy

Several trials have evaluated the benefit of preoperative and perioperative chemotherapy with the rational that haematogenous relapses remain a significant issue and early systemic therapy might eradicate micrometastatic disease. To date, trials have focused on distal esophagus and EGJ disease and mixed results have been observed:

- INT-0113 randomized 440 patients to preoperative chemotherapy with three cycles of cisplatin and 5-FU or immediate surgery. There was no significant difference in survival in either the overall population or between the SCC and ADC groups.
- The Medical Research Council (MRC) OE2 trial of surgery with or without preoperative cisplatin/ 5-FU demonstrated a survival benefit for this approach.
- MRC MAGIC evaluated perioperative ECF versus surgery alone in gastric and EGJ ADC. Of 503 patients, 15% and 11% had EGJ and lower esophageal tumors, respectively. Patients who received chemotherapy in addition to surgery had better 5-year OS (23% vs. 36%). Only 42% of patients completed all planned treatment, again highlighting the difficulty administering postoperative therapy.
- Preliminary results of the MRC OEO5 study were presented at the ASCO 2015 annual meeting. This study examined the optimal duration of preoperative chemotherapy and compared four cycles of epirubicin, cisplatin, and capecitabine (ECX) to two cycles of cisplatin/5-FU, both followed by surgery, in patients with T3N0-1 lower esophageal and EGJ ADC. There was no significant difference in disease-free survival (DFS) or OS despite use of ECX being associated with higher R0 resection and pCR rates. There was less toxicity associated with CF but surgical morbidity was similar between the groups.
- The FLOT trial composed the combination of docetaxel, oxaliplatin and fluorouracil to a "MAGIC" regimen and improved the median survival from 35 months to 50 months. This is likely to be a new standard of case.
- A 2015 meta-analysis that included nine randomized comparisons of preoperative chemotherapy versus surgery alone for esophageal or EGJ cancers showed a survival benefit for neoadjuvant chemotherapy with a hazard ratio of 0.88. No significant difference in the rate of R0 resections or risk of distant recurrence was observed.

With the above data in mind, perioperative chemotherapy is considered a rational approach in patients unable to tolerate trimodality therapy.

Adjuvant Chemotherapy

In patients who have not received preoperative chemotherapy or CRT, postoperative chemotherapy may be beneficial but data is limited. One study evaluating adjuvant chemotherapy have been completed in Asian patients. The JCOG 9204 is a Japanese trial that compared surgery alone to surgery followed by two cycles of cisplatin and 5-FU in 242 patients with esophageal SCC. The 5-year DFS was significantly better with chemotherapy (55% vs. 45%) but there was no significant difference in OS (61% vs. 52%). The JCOG 9907 study showed superiority of neoadjuvant cisplatin/5-FU over adjuvant cisplatin/5-FU. With regards to EGJ ADC, data for the use of adjuvant chemotherapy may be extrapolated from gastric cancer where a benefit has been seen. For example, one such trial, the CLASSIC trial demonstrated a benefit for postoperative capecitabine/oxaliplatin in gastric cancer and a small proportion of EGJ tumors were included (2.3%).

Palliative Therapy

The goals of therapy in the metastatic setting include improvement in disease-related symptoms and quality of life as well as prolongation of survival. When deciding on the most appropriate treatment strategy, performance status, histologic subtype, symptom burden, and patient preference should be considered.

There is limited data for chemotherapy in the setting of advanced disease and most evidence is extrapolated from gastric cancer trials that include EGJ tumors. In the first instance therefore, clinical trial enrolment should be considered as there remains a lack of consensus as to the best regimen in the first line setting. Combination chemotherapy regimens provide higher response rates, in the range of 25% to 45% versus 15% to 25% for single agent therapies, but this has been shown to translate into only limited improvements in duration of disease control and survival. Patients with ADC should have their tumors evaluated for HER2 overexpression using immmunohistochemical (IHC) or fluorescence in situ hybridization (FISH) analysis. Approximately 7% to 22% of EGJ adenocarcinomas overexpress HER2.

There are a number of first-line chemotherapy options:

- Cisplatin and 5-FU (CF) is a well-established regimen although, despite higher response rates, the combination did not show a statistically significant survival benefit over cisplatin alone in a randomized trial of patients with advanced esophageal SCC.
- 5-FU/calcium leucovorin with either oxaliplatin or irinotecan (FOLFOX or FOLFIRI) has shown equivalence to cisplatin and 5-FU in advanced EGJ studies and is potentially less toxic.
- Docetaxel, cisplatin, and 5-FU (DCF) have been compared to CF and demonstrated an improvement in response rates (37% vs. 25%), time to progression (5.6 vs. 3.7 months) and 2-year OS (18% vs. 9%). However, DCF was associated with significant toxicity in this study and doses have been modified in other trials evaluating this regimen.
- The REAL-2 trial published in 2008 was a landmark trial, which evaluated oxaliplatin and capecitabine as alternatives to cisplatin and 5-FU. It randomized 1,002 patients to ECF, ECX (epirubicin/cisplatin/capecitabine), EOF (epirubicin/oxaliplatin/5-fluorouracil), or EOX (epirubicin/oxaliplatin/capecitabine). The median survival was 9.9, 9.9, 9.3, and 11.2 months, respectively. As OS was highest with EOX ($P = 0.02$) EOX subsequently became a standard of care in the first-line setting in many institutions.
- Increasingly, in many institutions, doublet regimens are preferred over triplet regimens as the latter are not felt to offer a significant advantage and result in more toxicity.
- S1 in combination with cisplatin or docetaxel showed superiority compared to S1 in Asian studies. The FLAGS study was subsequently conducted in a global population and showed equivalence of cisplatin/S1 and cisplatin/5-FU in the first-line setting. Cisplatin/S1 was associated with a favorable toxicity profile.
- In elderly patients and those with poor performance status single agent chemotherapy with 5-FU/leucovorin, capecitabine, weekly taxanes, or irinotecan is appropriate.

Targeted therapies have been evaluated in the first-line setting:

- The addition of Trastuzumab to combination chemotherapy is recommended in patients with HER2 positive esophageal ADC. The ToGA trial demonstrated an improvement in response rate (47% vs. 35%) and OS (13.8 vs. 11.1 months) for patients treated with trastuzumab in combination with cisplatin/5-FU compared with cisplatin/5-FU alone. In a post-hoc subgroup analysis, patients whose tumors were IHC 2+ and FISH positive or IHC 3+ benefitted substantially from addition of Trastzumab with an OS benefit of 16 versus 11 months, HR 0.65. In contrast, patients whose tumors were IHC 0/1+ and FISH positive did not demonstrate a significant improvement in OS (10 vs. 8.7 months; HR 1.07). National Comprehensive Cancer Network (NCCN) guidelines (www.nccn.org) suggest that Trastuzumab can be used with most active first-line regimens except those containing anthracyclines.
- Other anti-HER2 agents have also been evaluated. The LOGiC study assessed the addition of lapatinib to first-line chemotherapy (capecitabine/oxaliplatin) and found no benefit while the JACOB study evaluating addition of Pertuzumab to first-line chemotherapy (cisplatin/5-FU) with Trastuzumab and also showed no benefit.
- The benefit of bevacizumab in combination with capecitabine and cisplatin in EGJ ADC in the first-line treatment was evaluated in the phase III AVAGAST trial and found no improvement in OS (12.1 vs. 10.1 months) despite improvements in response rates and progression free survival. Subgroup analysis suggests a potential benefit for patients in the Americas and while biomarkers may prove useful in identifying patients who might gain from addition of Bevacizumab to standard therapy, its role remains poorly defined.
- EGFR is expressed in the majority of esophageal SCC but addition of Panitumumab or Cetuximab to chemotherapy in the first-line setting showed no benefit in two phase III trials.

Decision-making around second-line therapy upon progression should also take performance status, patient preference, and histological subtype into account and clinical trials should be considered where available.

- Phase III data has shown benefit for docetaxel, irinotecan, or weekly paclitaxel with or without ramicirumab. Best supportive care is recommended for patients with poor performance status or significant comorbidities.
- Vascular endothelial growth factor receptor-2 (VEGFR-2) was evaluated as a therapeutic target in the second-line setting in the REGARD and RAINBOW phase III trials. REGARD demonstrated a modest but significant OS benefit with the use of the VEGFR-2 inhibitor ramucirumab compared to placebo after progression on first-line therapy and RAINBOW reported an improvement in OS with the addition of ramucirumab to weekly paclitaxel.
- Anti-HER2 therapy has also been evaluated in the second-line setting. Lapatinib did not show benefit when added to a taxane in the TyTAN study and T-DM1 demonstrated no benefit when compared to a taxane in the GATSBY study.

In the third-line setting, apatinib was shown to modestly improve OS when compared to placebo in a Chinese population and regorafenib has demonstrated modest activity in the second- and third-line settings in a randomized phase II study. However, neither of these agents is considered standard.

Finally, immunotherapy is also being evaluated in esophageal cancer. KEYNOTE-059 demonstrated the benefit of pembrolizumab in third line and was given FDA approval for this indication.

Nivolumab showed a similar benefit over placebo in an Asian study published in the Lancent in 2017. Studies are also ongoing evaluating the role for immunotherapy in early-stage disease.

Radiotherapy alone may be used in the palliative setting for control of dysphagia. Endoscopic laser or balloon dilatation or stenting are alternative options and placement of a gastrostomy or jejunostomy may improve a patient's nutritional status.

Surveillance of Patients with Locoregional Disease

The majority of recurrences develop within one year and over 90% develop within 2 to 3 years.

Isolated local recurrences occur more frequently after definitive CRT where salvage surgery may have a role and more vigilant surveillance is recommended in the first 2 years.

There is currently no data that demonstrate improved survival from earlier detection of recurrences or to guide the optimal surveillance strategy. The European Society of Medical Oncology (ESMO) guidelines suggest surveillance with clinical review and multidisciplinary input, however, NCCN do advocate imaging and endoscopy in selected patients.

Suggested Readings

1. Ajani JA, Rodriguez W, Bodoky G, et al. Multicenter phase III comparison of cisplatin/S-1 with cisplatin/infusional fluorouracil in advanced gastric or gastroesophageal adenocarcinoma study: the FLAGS trial. *J Clin Oncol.* 2010;28:1547–1553.
2. Al-Batran SE, Homann N, Schmalenberg H, et al. Perioperative chemotherapy with docetaxel, oxaliplatin, and fluorouracil/leucovorin (FLOT) versus epirubicin, cisplatin, and fluorouracil or capecitabine (ECF/ECX) for resectable gastric or gastroesophageal junction (GEJ) adenocarcinoma (FLOT4-AIO): A multicenter, randomized phase 3 trial. *J Clin Oncol.* 2017;35(15_suppl):Abstract 4004.
3. Alderson D, Langley RE, Nankivell MG, et al. Neoadjuvant chemotherapy for resectable oesophageal and junctional adenocarcinoma: results from the UK Medical Research Council randomised OEO5 trial. *J Clin Oncol.* 2015;33(suppl):Abstract 4002.
4. Allum WH, Stenning SP, Bancewicz J, et al. Long-term results of a randomized trial of surgery with or without preoperative chemotherapy in esophageal cancer. *J Clin Oncol.* 2009;27:5062–5067.
5. Best LM, Mughal M, Gurusamy KS. Non-surgical versus surgical treatment for esophageal cancer. *Cochrane Database Syst Rev.* 2016;3:CD011498.
6. Conroy T, Galais MP, Raoul JL, et al. Definitive chemoradiotherapy with FOLFOX versus fluorouracil and cisplatin in patients with oesophageal cancer (PRODIGE5/ACCORD17): final results of a randomised, phase 2/3 trial. *Lancet Oncol.* 2014;15:305–314.
7. Cooper JS, Guo MD, Herskovic A, et al. Chemoradiotherapy of locally advanced esophageal cancer: long-term follow-up of a prospective randomized trial (RTOG 85-01). Radiation Therapy Oncology Group. *JAMA.* 1999;281(17):1623–1627.

8. Cunningham D, Allum WH, Stenning SP, et al. Perioperative chemotherapy versus surgery alone for resectable gastro-esophageal cancer. *N Engl J Med.* 2006;355:11–20.

9. Cunningham D, Starling N, Rao S, et al. Capecitabine and oxaliplatin for advanced esophagogastric cancer. *N Engl J Med.* 2008;358:36–46.

10. Fuchs CS, Doi T, Jang RW, et al. KEYNOTE-059 cohort 1: Efficacy and safety of pembrolizumab (pembro) monotherapy in patients with previously treated advanced gastric cancer. *J Clin Oncol.* 2017;35(15_suppl):Abstract 4003.

11. Fuchs CS, Niedzwiecki D, Mamon HJ, et al. Adjuvant chemoradiotherapy with epirubicin, cisplatin, and fluorouracil compared with adjuvant chemoradiotherapy with fluorouracil and leucovorin after curative resection of gastric cancer: results from CALGB 80101 (Alliance). *J Clin Oncol.* 2017;35(32):3671–3677.

12. Fuchs CS, Tomasek J, Yong CJ, et al. Ramucirumab monotherapy for previously treated advanced gastric or gastro-oesophageal junction adenocarcinoma (REGARD): an international, randomized, multicentre, placebo-controlled, phase 3 trial. *Lancet.* 2014;383:31–39.

13. Hecht JR, Bang YJ, Qin SK, et al. Lapatinib in combination with capecitabine plus oxaliplatin in human epidermal growth factor receptor 2-positive advanced or metastatic gastric, esophageal or gastroesophageal adenocarcinoma: TRIO-013/LOGIC—a randomized phase III trial. *J Clin Oncol.* 2016;34(5):443–451.

14. Kang YK, Boku N, Satoh T, et al. Nivolumab in patients with advanced gastric or gastro-oesophageal junction cancer refractory to, or intolerant of, at least two previous chemotherapy regimens (ONO-4538-12, ATTRACTION-2): a randomised, double-blind, placebo-controlled, phase 3 trial. *Lancet.* 2017;390:2461–2471.

15. Kelsen DP, Ginsberg R, Pajak TF, et al. Chemotherapy followed by surgery compared with surgery alone for localized esophageal cancer. *N Engl J Med.* 1998;339(27):1979–1984.

16. Kidane B, Coughlin S, Vogt K, et al. Preoperative chemotherapy for resectable thoracic esophageal cancer. *Cochrane Database Syst Rev.* 2015;(5):CD001556.

17. MacDonald JS, Smalley SR, Benedetti J, et al. Chemoradiotherapy after surgery compared with surgery alone for adeno-carcinoma of the stomach or gastroesophageal junction. *N Engl J Med.* 2001;345:725–730.

18. Njei B, McCarty TR, Birk JW, et al. Trends in esophageal cancer survival in United States adults from 1973-2009: A SEER database analysis. *J Gastroenterol Hepatol.* 2016;31(6):1141–1146.

19. Ohtsu A, Shah MA, Van Cutsem E, et al. Bevacizumab in combination with chemotherapy as first-line therapy in advanced gastric cancer: a randomized, double-blind, placebo-controlled phase III study. *J Clin Oncol.* 2011;29:3968–3976.

20. Omloo JM, Lagarde SM, Hulscher JB et al. Extended transthoracic resection compared with limited transhiatal resection for adenocarcinoma of the mid/distal esophagus. Five-year survival of a randomized clinical trial. *Ann Surg.* 2007;246:992–1000.

21. Satoh T, Xu RH, Chung HC, et al. Lapatinib plus paclitaxel versus paclitaxel alone in the second-line treatment of HER2-amplified advanced gastric cancer in Asian populations: TyTAN—a randomized, phase III study. *J Clin Oncol.* 2014;32:2039–2049.

22. Siegel RL, Miller KD, Jemal A, et al. Cancer statistics, 2016. *CA Cancer J Clin.* 2016;66:7–30.

23. Sjoquist KM, Burmeister BH, Smithers BM, et al. Survival after neoadjuvant chemotherapy or chemoradiotherapy for resectable esophageal carcinoma: an updated meta-analysis. *Lancet Oncol.* 2011;12(7):681–692.

24. Stahl M, Stuschke M, Lehmann N, et al. Chemoradiation with and without surgery in patients with locally advanced squamous cell carcinoma of the esophagus. *J Clin Oncol.* 2005;23(10):2310–2317.

25. Tepper J, Krasna MJ, Niedzwiecki D, et al. Phase III trial of trimodality therapy with cisplatin, fluorouracil, radiotherapy, and surgery compared with surgery alone for esophageal cancer: CALGB 9781. *J Clin Oncol.* 2008;26(7):1086–1092.

26. Tougeron D, Scotté M, Hamidou H, et al. Definitive chemoradiotherapy in patients with esophageal adenocarcinoma: an alternative to surgery? *J Surg Oncol.* 2012;105(8):761–766.

27. Van Cutsem E, Moiseyenko VM, Tjulandin S, et al. Phase III study of docetaxol and cisplatin plus fluorouracil compared with cisplatin and fluorouracil as first-line therapy for advanced gastric cancer: a report of the V325 Study Group. *J Clin Oncol.* 2006;24:4991–4997.

28. Van Hagen P, Hulshof MC, van der Gaast A, et al. Preoperative chemoradiotherapy for esophageal or junctional cancer: Results from a multicentre randomized phase III trial. *N Engl J Med.* 2012;366:2074–2084.

29. Verheij M, Jansen EPM, Cats A, et al. A multicenter randomized phase III trial of neo-adjuvant chemotherapy followed by surgery and chemotherapy or by surgery and chemoradiotherapy in resectable gastric cancer: first results from the CRITICS study (abstract). *J Clin Oncol.* 2016;34(suppl): abstr 4000.

30. Wong R, Malthaner R. Combined chemotherapy and radiotherapy (without surgery) compared with radiotherapy alone in localized carcinoma of the esophagus. *Cochrane Database Syst Rev.* 2006;(1):CD002092.

5 Gastric Cancers

Hiral Parekh and Thomas J. George, Jr.

EPIDEMIOLOGY

Worldwide, gastric carcinoma represents the fifth most common malignancy. The frequency of gastric carcinoma at different sites within the stomach has changed in the United States over recent decades. Cancer of the distal half of the stomach has been decreasing in the United States since the 1930s. However, over the past two decades, the incidence of cancer of the cardia and gastroesophageal junction has been rapidly rising, particularly in patients younger than 40 years. There are expected to be 28,000 new cases and 10,960 deaths from gastric carcinoma in the United States in 2017.

RISK FACTORS

- Average age at onset is fifth decade.
- Male-to-female ratio is 1.7:1.
- African-American-to-white ratio is 1.8:1.
- Precursor conditions include chronic atrophic gastritis and intestinal metaplasia, pernicious anemia (10% to 20% incidence), partial gastrectomy for benign disease, *Helicobacter pylori* infection (especially childhood exposure—3- to 5-fold increase), Ménétrier's disease, and gastric adenomatous polyps. These precursor lesions are largely linked to distal (intestinal type) gastric carcinoma.
- Family history: first degree (2- to 3-fold); the family of Napoléon Bonaparte is an example; familial clustering; patients with hereditary nonpolyposis colorectal cancer (Lynch syndrome II) are at increased risk; germline mutations of E-cadherin (*CDH1* gene) have been linked to familial diffuse gastric cancer and associated lobular breast cancer. Gastric adenocarcinoma and proximal polyposis of the stomach (GAPPS) is an autosomal dominant syndrome characterized by fundic gland polyposis and intestinal type adenocarcinoma.
- Tobacco use results in a 1.5- to 3-fold increased risk for cancer.
- High salt and nitrosamine food content from fermenting and smoking process.
- Deficiencies of vitamins A, C, and E; β-carotene; selenium; and fiber.
- Blood type A.
- Alcohol.
- The marked rise in the incidence of gastroesophageal and proximal gastric adenocarcinoma appears to be strongly correlated to the rising incidence of Barrett's esophagus.

SCREENING

In most countries, screening of the general populations is not practical because of a low incidence of gastric cancer. However, screening is justified in countries where the incidence of gastric cancer is high. Japanese screening guidelines include initial upper endoscopy at age 50, with follow-up endoscopy for abnormalities. Routine screening is not recommended in the United States.

PATHOPHYSIOLOGY

Most gastric cancers are adenocarcinomas (more than 90%) of two distinct histologic types: intestinal and diffuse. In general, the term "gastric cancer" is commonly used to refer to adenocarcinoma of the stomach. Other cancers of the stomach include non-Hodgkin's lymphomas (NHL), leiomyosarcomas, carcinoids, and gastrointestinal stromal tumors (GIST). Differentiating between adenocarcinoma and lymphoma is critical because the prognosis and treatment for these two entities differ considerably. Although less common, metastases to the stomach include melanoma, breast, and ovarian cancers.

Intestinal Type

The *epidemic* form of cancer is further differentiated by gland formation and is associated with precancerous lesions, gastric atrophy, and intestinal metaplasia. The intestinal form accounts for most distal cancers with a stable or declining incidence. These cancers in particular are associated with *H. pylori* infection. In this carcinogenesis model, the interplay of environmental factors leads to glandular atrophy, relative achlorhydria, and increased gastric pH. The resulting bacterial overgrowth leads to production of nitrites and nitroso compounds causing further gastric atrophy and intestinal metaplasia, thereby increasing the risk of cancer.

The recent decline in gastric carcinoma in the United States is likely the result of a decline in the incidence of intestinal-type lesions but remains a common cause of gastric carcinoma worldwide. Intestinal-type lesions are associated with an increased frequency of overexpression of epidermal growth factor receptor *erbB-2* and *erbB-3*.

Diffuse Type

The *endemic* form of carcinoma is more common in younger patients and exhibits undifferentiated signet-ring histology. There is a predilection for diffuse submucosal spread because of lack of cell cohesion, leading to linitis plastica. Contiguous spread of the carcinoma to the peritoneum is common. Precancerous lesions have not been identified. Although a carcinogenesis model has not been proposed, it is associated with *H. pylori* infection. Genetic predispositions to endemic forms of carcinoma have been reported, as have associations between carcinoma and individuals with type A blood. These cancers occur in the proximal stomach where increased incidence has been observed worldwide. Stage for stage, these cancers have a worse prognosis than do distal cancers.

Diffuse lesions have been linked to abnormalities of fibroblast growth factor systems, including the *K-sam* oncogene as well as E-cadherin mutations. The latter results in loss of cell–cell adhesions.

Molecular Analysis

- Loss of heterozygosity of chromosome 5q or APC gene (deleted in 34% of gastric cancers), 17p, and 18q (*DCC* gene).
- Microsatellite instability, particularly of transforming growth factor-β type II receptor, with subsequent growth-inhibition deregulation.
- p53 is mutated in approximately 40% to 60% caused by allelic loss and base transition mutations.
- Mutations of E-cadherin expression (*CDH1* gene on 16q), a cell adhesion mediator, is observed in diffuse-type undifferentiated cancers and is associated with an increased incidence of lobular breast cancer.
- Epidermal growth factor receptor overexpression, specifically *Her2/neu* and *erbB-2/erbB-3* especially in intestinal forms.
- Epstein-Barr viral genomes are detected.
- *Ras* mutations are rarely reported (less than 10%) in contrast to other gastrointestinal cancers.

DIAGNOSIS

Gastric carcinoma, when superficial and surgically curable, typically produces no symptoms. Among 18,365 patients analyzed by the American College of Surgeons, patients presented with the following symptoms: weight loss (62%), abdominal pain (52%), nausea (34%), anorexia (32%), dysphagia (26%), melena (20%), early satiety (18%), ulcer-type pain (17%), and lower-extremity edema (6%).

Clinical findings at presentation may include anemia (42%), hypoproteinemia (26%), abnormal liver functions (26%), and fecal occult blood (40%). Medically refractory or persistent peptic ulcer should prompt endoscopic evaluation.

Gastric carcinomas primarily spread by direct extension, invading adjacent structures with resultant peritoneal carcinomatosis and malignant ascites. The liver, followed by the lung, is the most common site of hematogenous dissemination. The disease may also spread as follows:

- To intra-abdominal nodes and left supraclavicular nodes (Virchow's node).
- Along peritoneal surfaces, resulting in a periumbilical lymph node (Sister Mary Joseph node, named after an operating room nurse at the Mayo Clinic, which form as tumor spreads along the falciform ligament to subcutaneous sites).
- To a left anterior axillary lymph node resulting from the spread of proximal primary cancer to lower esophageal and intrathoracic lymphatics (Irish node).
- To enlarged ovary (Krukenberg tumor; ovarian metastases).
- To a mass in the cul-de-sac (Blumer shelf), which is palpable on rectal or bimanual examination.

Paraneoplastic Syndromes

- Skin syndromes: acanthosis nigricans, dermatomyositis, circinate erythemas, pemphigoid, and acute onset of seborrheic keratoses (Leser-Trélat sign).
- Central nervous system syndromes: dementia and cerebellar ataxia.
- Miscellaneous: thrombophlebitis, microangiopathic hemolytic anemia, membranous nephropathy.

Tumor Markers

Carcinoembryonic antigen (CEA) is elevated in 40% to 50% of cases. It is useful in follow-up and monitoring response to therapy, but not for screening. α-Fetoprotein and CA 19-9 are elevated in 30% of patients with gastric cancer, but are of limited clinical use.

STAGING

The American Joint Committee on Cancer (AJCC) has designated staging by TNM classification. In the 2017 AJCC eighth edition, tumors arising at the gastroesophageal junction (GEJ) or in the cardia of the stomach within 5 cm of the GEJ that extend into the GEJ or esophagus are termed esophageal rather than gastric cancers. Gastric tumors involving muscolaris propria (T2), subserosa (T3), and serosa (T4a) are considered resectable whereas tumors with invasion of adjacent structures (T4b) are not. Nodal stage relates to number of involved regional nodes: N1, 1 to 2 involved nodes; N2, 3 to 6 involved nodes; N3a, 7 to 15 involved nodes; and N3b, 16 or more involved nodes. The presence of positive peritoneal cytology is considered M1 as are distant metastases. Many of these staging classifiers represent changes from previous AJCC staging system editions but continue to refine prognostic groups based on the best available outcomes data (Table 5.1). Of note, alternative staging systems are used in Japan.

- Initial upper gastrointestinal endoscopy and double-contrast barium swallow identify suggestive lesions and have diagnostic accuracy of 95% and 75%, respectively, but add little to preoperative staging otherwise.
- Endoscopic ultrasonography assesses the depth of tumor invasion (T staging) and nodal involvement (N staging) with accuracies up to 90% and 75%, respectively.
- Computerized tomographic scanning is useful for assessing local extension, lymph node involvement, and presence of metastasis, although understaging occurs in most cases.
- Although whole-body 2-[18F]fluoro-2-deoxyglucose (FDG)–positron emission tomography (PET) may be useful in detecting metastasis as part of preoperative staging in some gastric cancer patients, the sensitivity in detecting early stage gastric cancer is only about 20% and overall appears less reliable than in esophageal cancer.

TABLE 5.1 Observed Survival Rates for Surgically Resected Gastric Adenocarcinomas in a Representative Western Population

Stage	Survival Rates		
	5 year (%)	10 year (%)	Median (mo)
IA	82	68	ND
IB	69	60	151
IIA	60	43	102
IIB	42	32	48
IIIA	28	18	28
IIIB	18	11	19
IIIC	11	6	12
IV	6	5	9

ND, not determined.

Modified from Reim D, Loos M, Vogl F, et al. Prognostic implications of the seventh edition of the international union against cancer classification for patients with gastric cancer: the Western experience of patients treated in a single-center European institution. *J Clin Oncol.* 2013 Jan 10;31(2):263–271.

PROGNOSIS

Pathologic staging remains the most important determinant of prognosis (Table 5.1). Other prognostic variables that have been proposed to be associated with an unfavorable outcome include the following:

- Older age
- Male gender
- Weight loss greater than 10%
- Location of tumor
- Tumor histology: Diffuse versus intestinal (5-year survival after resection, 16% vs. 26%, respectively); high grade or undifferentiated tumors
- Four or more lymph nodes involved
- Aneuploid tumors
- Elevations in epidermal growth factor or P-glycoprotein level
- Overexpression of ERCC1 and p53; loss of p21 and p27

MANAGEMENT OF GASTRIC CANCER

Standard of Care

Although surgical resection remains the cornerstone of gastric cancer treatment, the optimal extent of nodal resection remains controversial. The high rate of recurrence and poor survival of patients following surgery provide a rationale for the use of adjuvant or perioperative treatment. Adjuvant radiotherapy alone does not improve survival following resection. In addition to complete surgical resection, either postoperative adjuvant chemoradiotherapy (chemoRT) or perioperative polychemotherapy appear to confer survival advantages. The results of the Intergroup 0116 study show that the combination of 5-fluorouracil (5-FU)–based chemoRT significantly prolongs disease-free (DFS) and overall survival (OS) when compared to no adjuvant treatment. Similarly, the use of polychemotherapy pre- and postoperatively can increase DFS and OS compared to observation.

In advanced gastric cancer, chemotherapy enhances quality of life and prolongs survival when compared with the best supportive care. Human epidermal growth factor receptor 2 (HER2), a key driver of tumorigenesis, is overexpressed in 7% to 34% of esophagogastric tumors. The standard of care for HER2 overexpressing advanced or metastatic gastric cancer is trastuzumab in combination with cytotoxic chemotherapy. Of the commonly used regimens, triple combination chemotherapy with either docetaxel, cisplatin, and 5-FU (DCF) or epirubicin, oxaliplatin, and capecitabine (EOX) probably has the strongest claims to this role for the majority of fit patients, with modified FOLFOX (5-FU, leucovorin, and oxaliplatin) also frequently used in the United States. However, there is a pressing need for assessing new agents, both cytotoxic and molecularly targeted, in the advanced and adjuvant settings and enrollment in clinical trial is highly encouraged.

Resectable Disease

Surgery

Complete surgical resection of the tumor and adjacent lymph nodes remains the only chance for cure. Unfortunately, only 20% of U.S. patients with gastric cancer have disease at presentation amenable to such therapy. Resection of gastric cancer is indicated in patients with stage I to III disease. Tumor size and location dictate the type of surgical procedure to be used. An exploration to exclude carcinomatosis just prior to the definitive resection is justified in this disease. Current surgical issues include subtotal versus total gastrectomy, extent of lymph node dissection, and palliative surgery.

Subtotal versus Total Gastrectomy

Subtotal gastrectomy (SG) may be performed for proximal cardia or distal lesions, provided that the fundus or cardioesophageal junction is not involved (Fig. 5.1). Total gastrectomy (TG) is more appropriate if tumor involvement is diffuse and arises in the body of the stomach, with extension to within 6 cm of the cardia. TG is associated with increased postoperative complications, mortality, and quality-of-life decrement, necessitating thorough consideration of complete gastric resection (Fig. 5.2).

Extent of Lymph Node Dissection

Regional lymph node dissection is important for accurate staging and may have therapeutic benefit as well. The extent of lymphadenectomy is categorized by the regional nodal groups removed (Table 5.2). At least 16 lymph nodes must be reported for accurate AJCC staging. D2 lymphadenectomy is reported to improve survival in patients with T1, T2, T3, and some serosa-involved (currently T4a) lesions as compared to D1. However, factors such as operative time, hospitalization length, transfusion requirements, and morbidity are all increased. The routine inclusion of splenectomy in D2 resections is no longer advocated given higher postoperative complications. The greatest benefit of more extensive lymph node dissection may occur in early gastric cancer lesions with small tumors and superficial mucosal involvement as up to 20% of such lesions have occult lymph node involvement.

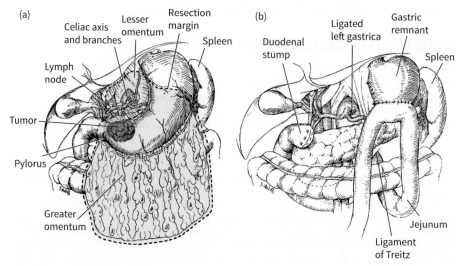

FIGURE 5.1 (a) and (b): Subtotal gastrectomy.

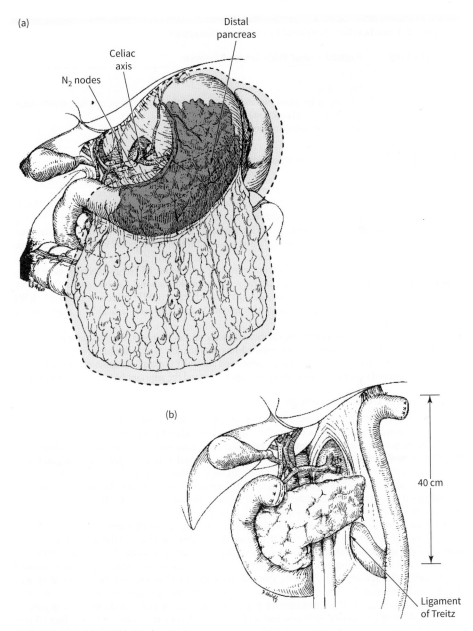

FIGURE 5.2 (a) and (b): Total gastrectomy.

Radiation Therapy

- For patients with locally advanced or metastatic disease, moderate doses of external-beam radiation can be used to palliate symptoms of pain, obstruction, and bleeding but do not routinely improve survival.
- Local or regional recurrence in the gastric or tumor bed, the anastomosis, or regional lymph nodes occurs in 40% to 65% of patients after gastric resection with curative intent. The high frequency of such relapses has generated interest in perioperative therapy. Radiotherapy (RT) in this setting is

TABLE 5.2 Classification of Regional Lymph Node Dissection

Dissection (D)	Regional Lymph Node Groups Removed
D0	None
D1	Perigastric
D2	D1 plus nodes along hepatic, left gastric, celiac, and splenic arteries; splenic hilar nodes; +/– splenectomy
D3[a]	D2 plus periaortic and portahepatis

[a] Periaortic and portahepatis nodes are typically considered distant metastatic disease.

limited by the technical challenges inherent in abdominal irradiation, optimal definition of fields, diminished performance status, and nutritional state of many patients with gastric cancer.

- A prospective randomized trial from the British Stomach Cancer Group failed to demonstrate a survival benefit for postoperative adjuvant radiation alone, although locoregional failures had decreased from 27% to 10.6%.
- Attempts to improve the efficacy and minimize toxicity with newer RT techniques have been investigated. Sixty patients who underwent curative resection at the National Cancer Institute were randomized to receive either adjuvant intraoperative radiotherapy (IORT) or conventional RT. IORT failed to afford a benefit over conventional therapy in OS and remains unavailable to many outside of a clinical trial or specialized center.
- In patients with locally unresectable pancreatic and gastric adenocarcinoma, the Gastrointestinal Tumor Study Group (GITSG) has shown that combined-modality therapy is superior to either RT or chemotherapy alone. On the basis of this concept, combined chemoRT (typically in combination with 5-FU) has been evaluated in both the neoadjuvant (preoperative) and the adjuvant (postoperative) settings.

Perioperative Chemoradiotherapy

Aside from GEJ and high gastric cardia tumors, the available data on the role of neoadjuvant chemoRT for gastric cancer are not conclusive. Although neoadjuvant therapy may reduce the tumor mass in many patients, several randomized controlled trials have shown that compared with primary resection, a multimodal approach does not result in a survival benefit in patients with potentially resectable tumors. In contrast, for some patients with locally advanced tumors (i.e., patients in whom complete tumor removal with upfront surgery seems unlikely), neoadjuvant chemoRT may increase the likelihood of complete tumor resection on subsequent surgery. However, predicting those likely to benefit from this approach remains an ongoing research question.

Adjuvant chemoRT has been evaluated in the United States. In a phase III Intergroup trial (INT-0116), 556 patients with completely resected stage IB to stage IV M0 adenocarcinoma of the stomach and gastroesophageal junction were randomized to receive best supportive care or adjuvant chemotherapy (5-FU and leucovorin) and concurrent radiation therapy (45 Gy). With >6-year median follow-up, median survival was 35 months for the adjuvant chemoRT group as compared to 27 months for the surgery-alone arm ($P = 0.006$). Both 3-year OS (50% vs. 41%; $P = 0.006$) and relapse-free survival (48% vs. 31%; $P < 0.0001$) favored adjuvant chemoRT. Although treatment-related mortality was 1% in this study, only 65% of patients completed all therapy as planned and many had inadequate lymph node resections (54% D0). After 10-year median follow-up, persistent benefit in OS (HR 1.32; 95% CI, 1.10 to 1.60; $P = 0.0046$) and relapse-free survival (HR 1.51; 95% CI, 1.25 to 1.83; $P = 0.001$) were observed without excess treatment related late toxicities. This study established adjuvant chemoRT as a standard of care for gastric cancer in the United States.

Perioperative Chemotherapy

In Japan, patients who underwent complete surgical resection for stage II or III gastric cancer with D2 lymphadenectomy appeared to benefit from adjuvant S-1, a novel oral fluoropyrimidine. In a randomized controlled trial, patients were randomized to 1 year of monotherapy or surveillance alone.

The study was closed early after interim analysis confirmed a 3-year OS (80% vs. 70%; $P = 0.002$) and relapse-free survival (72% vs. 60%; $P = 0.002$) advantage in favor of adjuvant chemotherapy. At 5-year follow up, the improved OS rate (72% vs. 61%) and relapse-free survival rate (65% vs. 53%) persisted. S-1 is approved for adjuvant therapy for gastric cancer in Japan and for advanced gastric cancer in Europe, but it is not commercially available in the United States.

In Europe, focus has been on the role of more potent polychemotherapy regimens in the perioperative setting without RT. The UK Medical Research Council conducted a randomized controlled trial (MAGIC trial) comparing three cycles of pre- and postoperative epirubicin, cisplatin, and 5-FU (ECF) to surgery alone in patients with resectable stage II to IV nonmetastatic gastric cancer; 503 patients were stratified according to surgeon, tumor site, and performance status. Perioperative chemotherapy improved 5-year OS (36% vs. 23%; $P = 0.009$) and reduced local and distant recurrence. There appeared to be significant downstaging by chemotherapy treatment, with more patients deemed by the operating surgeon to have had a "curative" resection (79% vs. 70%; $P = 0.03$), smaller tumors (median 3 vs. 5 cm; $P < 0.001$), T1/T2 stage tumors (52% vs. 37%; $P = 0.002$), and N1/N2 stage disease (84% vs. 71%; $P = 0.01$). Toxicity was feasible with postoperative complications comparable; however, nearly one-third of patients who began with preoperative chemotherapy did not receive postoperative chemotherapy owing to progressive disease, complications, or patient request.

A French multicenter trial also showed a survival benefit for perioperative chemotherapy. Patients with potentially resectable stage II or higher adenocarcinoma of the stomach, GEJ or distal esophagus (total 224) were randomly assigned to two or three preoperative cycles of cisplatin/5-FU infusion and three or four postoperative cycles of the same regimen versus surgery alone. At a median follow-up of 5.7 years, 5-year OS (38% vs. 24%; HR 0.69; 95% CI, 0.50 to 0.95; $P = 0.02$) and DFS (34% vs. 19%; HR 0.65; 95% CI, 0.48 to 0.89; $P = 0.003$) were improved in the polychemotherapy arm. Curative resection rate was significantly improved with perioperative polychemotherapy (84% vs. 73%; $P = 0.04$) with similar postoperative morbidity in the two groups. The phase II/III FLOT4-AIO trial compared four preoperative and four postoperative courses of the docetaxel-based triplet FLOT regimen (docetaxel, oxaliplatin, and 5FU) versus epirubicin-based triplet therapy in patients with resectable adenocarcinoma of the stomach or EGJ. In the 716 enrolled patients, FLOT was associated with a median OS improvement (50 vs. 35 months; HR 0.77; $P = 0.012$). In Europe, perioperative polychemotherapy is considered a standard of care.

Postoperative Chemoradiotherapy versus Perioperative Chemotherapy

There are no randomized controlled trials directly comparing these two standards of care. The ARTIST randomized phase III trial did not show a survival improvement with adjuvant chemoRT compared to adjuvant chemotherapy alone in patients with D2 resected gastric cancer. Patients ($n = 458$, stage IB-IV M0) were randomly assigned to chemotherapy (capecitabine and cisplatin) or chemoRT (cisplatin/capecitabine followed by capecitabine/radiation [45 Gy] followed by cisplatin/capecitabine). After >4 years follow-up, no significant difference in locoregional recurrences (8.3% in chemo alone vs. 4.8% in chemoRT; $P = 0.3533$) or distant metastases (24.6% in chemo vs. 20.4% in chemoRT; $P = 0.5568$) was observed. Treatment completion rate was better than the INT-0116 trial with 75% of patients having completed the planned chemotherapy and 82% the chemoRT. Given that a multivariate analysis showed that chemoRT improved 3-year DFS in those with node-positive disease (HR 0.68; 95% CI, 0.47 to 0.99; $P = 0.047$), a subsequent phase III trial (ARTIST-II) study to evaluate the benefit of chemoRT in patients who have undergone D2 lymph node dissection with positive lymph nodes is currently enrolling.

CALGB 80101, a US Intergroup study, compared the INT-0116 adjuvant chemoRT versus postoperative ECF before and after chemoRT. Patients ($n = 546$) with completely resected gastric or GEJ tumors that were ≥T2 or node positive were included. Through a preliminary report, patients receiving ECF had lower rates of diarrhea, mucositis, and grade ≥4 neutropenia. However, the primary endpoint of OS was not significantly better with ECF at 3 years (52% vs. 50%). The primary tumor location did not affect treatment outcome.

With the goal of assessing the role of postoperative intensification of treatment with chemoRT, the phase III CRITICS study recently completed. Patients with stage Ib-IVa gastric cancer ($n = 788$) were treated with preoperative epirubicin, capecitabine, and a platinum compound (cisplatin or oxaliplatin) followed by surgery. After surgery, patients were randomized to an additional three cycles of the same chemotherapy versus chemoRT (45 Gy with weekly cisplatin and daily capecitabine). There was no difference in the 5-year survival between two arms. (40.8% vs. 40.9%).

Unresectable or Metastatic Disease

Primary goals of therapy should focus on improvement in symptoms, delay of disease progression, pain control, nutritional support, and quality of life. Although a role for palliative surgery and radiotherapy exists (see previous sections), chemotherapy remains the primary means of palliative treatment in this setting. The most commonly administered chemotherapeutic agents with objective response rates in advanced gastric cancer include mitomycin, antifolates, anthracyclines, fluoropyrimidines, platinums, taxanes, and topoisomerase inhibitors. Monotherapy with a single agent results in a 10% to 30% response rate with mild toxicities (Table 5.3). 5-FU is the most extensively studied, producing a 20% response rate. Complete responses with single agents are rare and disease control is relatively brief. Combination chemotherapy provides a better response rate with survival advantage over best supportive care in randomized studies. Molecularly targeted therapies against the HER2 and vascular endothelial growth factor (VEGF) pathways now have an active role in the treatment of metastatic gastric cancer.

Palliative Surgery and Stents

Palliative surgery and stents should be considered in patients with obstruction, bleeding, or pain, despite operative mortalities of 25% to 50%. Gastrojejunostomy bypass surgery alone may provide a 2-fold increase in mean survival. The selection of patients most likely to benefit from this or other palliative surgical interventions require further evaluation with prospective studies and multidisciplinary conference discussion.

Plastic and expansile metal stents are associated with successful palliation of obstructive symptoms in more than 85% of patients with tumors in the GEJ and in the cardia.

Palliative Chemotherapy

Various combinations of active agents have been reported to improve the response rate (20% to 50%) among patients with advanced gastric carcinoma (Table 5.4). While utilizing 5-FU as a backbone, FAMTX (5-FU, doxorubicin, methotrexate) became an international standard after direct comparison to FAM (5-FU, doxorubicin, mitomycin) supported a superiority with a survival advantage for FAMTX. The addition of cisplatin into combination regimens was supported by subsequent studies in both Europe and the United States.

Historically, the most commonly used combination regimens include FAMTX, FAM, FAP, ECF, ELF, FLAP (5-FU, leucovorin, doxorubicin, cisplatin), PELF (cisplatin, epidoxorubicin, leucovorin, 5-FU with glutathione and filgrastim), and FUP or CF (5-FU, cisplatin). The combination of a fluoropyrimidine and platinum is most commonly used in the United States.

Cytotoxic Chemotherapy Agents

Chemotherapeutic agents, including irinotecan, docetaxel, paclitaxel, and alternative platinums and fluoropyrimidines, have shown promising activity as single agents and have been actively incorporated into combination therapy (see Tables 5.3 and 5.4). A complete review of all agents is beyond the scope of this chapter.

Docetaxel is Federal Drug Administration approved in combination with cisplatin and 5-FU (DCF) in patients with advanced or metastatic gastric cancer, based on the results of a large phase III international

TABLE 5.3 Antineoplastic Therapy with Activity in Advanced Gastric Cancer

Class	Examples
Antifolates	Methotrexate
Anthracyclines	Doxorubicin, epirubicin
Fluoropyrimidines	5-FU, capecitabine, S-1, UFT
Platinums	Cisplatin, carboplatin, oxaliplatin
Taxanes	Docetaxel, paclitaxel
Topoisomerase inhibitors	Etoposide, irinotecan
Targeted therapies	Trastuzumab, ramucirumab, apatinib

TABLE 5.4 Randomized Studies of Combination Antineoplastic Therapy in Advanced Gastric Cancer

Treatment Arms	Patients (n)	RR (%)	Median Survival (mo)
FAMTX vs. FAM	213	41 vs. 9[a]	10.5 vs. 7.3[a]
PELF vs. FAM	147	43 vs. 15[a]	8.8 vs. 5.8
FAMTX vs. EAP	60	33 vs. 20	7.3 vs. 6.1
ECF vs. FAMTX	274	45 vs. 21[a]	8.9 vs. 5.7[a]
DCF vs. CF	445	37 vs. 25[a]	9.2 vs. 8.6[a]
EOX vs. ECF	488	48 vs. 40	11.2 vs. 9.9[a]
Cis/S-1 vs. Cis/5-FU	1,053	29 vs. 32	8.6 vs. 7.9
CF + Trastuzumab vs. CF	298	47 vs. 35	13.8 vs. 11.1
PAC + Ram vs. PAC	655	28 vs. 16	9.6 vs. 7.4
Ram vs. BSC	355	8 vs. 3	5.2 vs. 3.8
Apatinib vs. BSC	270	3 vs. 0	6.5 vs. 3.7

[a] Difference is statistically significant ($P < 0.05$).

RR, response rate; FAMTX, 5-FU, doxorubicin, and methotrexate; FAM, 5-FU, doxorubicin, mitomycin-C; PELF, cisplatin, epidoxorubicin, leucovorin, 5-FU with glutathione and filgrastim; EAP, etoposide, doxorubicin, cisplatin; ECF, epirubicin, cisplatin and 5-FU; EOX, epirubicin, oxaliplatin, capecitabine; DCF, docetaxel, cisplatin, 5-FU; CF, cisplatin, 5-FU; S-1, oral fluoropyrimidine; Ram, ramucirumab; PAC, paclitaxel; BSC, best supportive care.

trial; 445 patients were randomized to receive cisplatin and 5-FU with or without docetaxel. The addition of docetaxel resulted in an improvement in tumor response (37% vs. 25%; $P = 0.01$), time to progression (5.6 vs. 3.7 months; $P < 0.001$), and median survival (9.2 vs. 8.6 months; $P = 0.02$) with a doubling of 2-year survival (18% vs. 9%). These findings were at the cost of anticipated increased toxicity; however, maintenance of quality of life and performance status indices were longer for DCF. In a Japanese study, 20% of patients who showed no response to previous chemotherapy had a partial response to monotherapy with docetaxel.

S-1 is an oral fluoropyrimidine derivative composed of tegafur (5-FU prodrug), 5-chloro-2, 4-dihydroxypyridine (inhibitor of 5-FU degradation), and potassium oxonate (inhibitor of gastrointestinal toxicities). Because of the favorable safety profile of S-1 compared to infusional 5-FU, a multicenter prospective randomized phase III trial was conducted in 24 Western countries including the United States. Previously untreated patients ($n = 1,053$) with advanced gastric or GEJ adenocarcinoma were randomized to either cisplatin/S-1 or cisplatin/infusional 5-FU. The median OS (8.6 vs. 7.9 months; $P = 0.20$), overall response rate (29.1% vs. 31.9%; $P = 0.40$), median duration of response (6.5 vs. 5.8 months; $P = 0.08$), and treatment-related deaths (2.5% vs. 4.9%; $P < 0.05$) favored the cisplatin/S-1 arm. The cisplatin/S-1 arm had significant favorable toxicities as well. The lack of survival benefit but improved toxicity profile could have been due to the lower dose of cisplatin used in the cisplatin/S-1 arm.

Capecitabine is another oral fluoropyrimidine that has been substituted for infusional 5-FU in a variety of settings. It was formally evaluated with encouraging results in combination with a platinum alternative.

Oxaliplatin is a third-generation platinum with less nephrotoxicity, nausea, and bone marrow suppression than cisplatin. In a two-by-two designed study in patients with advanced gastric cancer, standard ECF chemotherapy was modified with oxaliplatin substituted for cisplatin and capecitabine substituted for 5-FU; 1,002 patients were randomly allocated between the four arms (ECF, EOF, ECX, and EOX). Capecitabine and oxaliplatin appeared as effective as 5-FU and cisplatin, respectively. Response rates and progression-free survival were nearly identical between the groups, with the EOX regimen showing superiority in OS over ECF (11.2 vs. 9.9 months; $P = 0.02$).

Biologic/Targeted Agents/Immunotherapy

New biologic therapies designed to inhibit or modulate targets of aberrant signal transduction in gastric cancer have been actively investigated. Inhibition of angiogenesis, vascular endothelial growth factor (VEGF), and epidermal growth factor (EGF) pathways are undergoing clinical testing and have shown early promising activity (see Tables 5.3 and 5.4). Immunotherapy (IO) treatments are active in advanced disease and represent a relatively new option for some patients. Predictors of durable response remain elusive to date.

Epidermal Growth Factor Receptor-2 (HER2)

Overexpression of EGF receptor (EGFR)-2 (HER2) is seen in approximately 7% to 22% of esophageogastric cancers. The prognostic significance of HER2 overexpression in esophagogastric adenocarcinoma is unclear. Similar to breast cancer, HER2 overexpression is predictive for response to anti-HER2 therapies. HER2 protein expression is assessed by immunohistochemical (IHC) staining and gene amplification by fluorescence in situ hybridization (FISH). HER2 overexpression in esophagogastric cancer is different from that in breast cancer because it tends to spare the digestive luminal membrane. Thus, an esophagogastric cancer with only partially circumferential (i.e., "basolateral" or "lateral") membrane staining can still be categorized as 2+ or 3+. In contrast, a breast tumor must demonstrate complete circumferential membrane staining to be designated as 2+ or 3+. Using breast cancer HER2 interpretation criteria may underestimate expression in esophagogastric cancers. Modified criteria for interpreting HER2 by IHC in esophagogastric cancers were developed and validated with a high concordance rate of HER2 gene amplification and HER2 protein overexpression for IHC 0-1+ and 3+ cases. For an equivocal IHC 2+ expression, FISH analysis is recommended for confirmation.

Therapeutic targeting of HER2 overexpressing esophagogastric adenocarcinoma by a monoclonal antibody, trastuzumab, was studied in combination with chemotherapy. Patients (n = 592) with HER2-overexpressed advanced gastric and GEJ adenocarcinoma (ToGA trial) were randomized to standard chemotherapy (cisplatin/5-FU) with or without trastuzumab. The study demonstrated improved median OS (13.8 vs. 11.1 months; HR 0·74; 95% CI 0·60 to 0·91; P = 0.0046) in those receiving trastuzumab. The toxicities between the two arms were comparable. Subgroup analysis demonstrated patients with HER2 IHC 3+ scores derived the greatest benefit from targeted therapy (HR 0.66; 95% CI 0.50 to 0.87). This trial established a new standard of care for advanced HER2 overexpressing esophagogastric tumors. Lapatinib, an orally active small molecule targeting EGFR1 and EGFR2 (HER2), failed to show a survival benefit when added to chemotherapy with capecitabine and oxalaplatin. Lapatinib also failed to improve OS when combined with paclitaxel in second-line therapy but demonstrated a trend toward improvement in the median OS (11 vs. 8.9 months; P = 0.1044). It is noteworthy that few patients had received prior trastuzumab (only 7% in lapatinib arm and 15% in combination). Thus, testing for and targeting HER2 overexpressing tumors with trastuzumab represents a clinically meaningful treatment option.

Epidermal Growth Factor Receptor (EGFR)

Overexpression of EGFR is seen in 27% to 64% of gastric cancers with some studies suggesting it as a poor prognostic variable. Cetuximab is a partially humanized murine anti-EGFR monoclonal antibody that has been most extensively studied in gastric cancer. This agent has minimal activity as a single agent while in combination with doublet or triplet chemotherapy regimens it showed variable overall response rates (Table 5.4). The EXPAND trial randomized 904 patients with metastatic or locally advanced gastric cancer to chemotherapy (cisplatin and capecitabine) with or without cetuximab. The addition of cetuximab provided no benefit in progression-free survival but added toxicity. A fully humanized anti-EGFR monoclonal antibody (panitumumab) in combination with EOC (epirubicin, oxaliplatin, and capecitabine) was investigated in a randomized phase III (REAL-3) study. The addition of panitumumab to chemotherapy significantly reduced survival from 11.3 to 8.8 months. Of note, small molecule tyrosine kinase inhibitors of the EGFR (i.e., erlotinib and gefitinib) showed very limited activity in multiple phase II trials. Based upon currently available evidence, anti-EGFR therapy should not be used outside the context of a clinical trial.

Targeting Angiogenesis

A high tumor and circulating serum level of vascular endothelial growth factor (VEGF) in gastric cancer is associated with a poor prognosis. Ramucirumab, a recombinant monoclonal antibody of the IgG1 class targeting VEGFR-2, has demonstrated a survival advantage for palliative patients with previously treated gastric cancer. In the phase III REGARD trial, 355 previously treated patients with advanced or metastatic esophagogastric adenocarcinoma were randomly assigned to ramucirumab versus best supportive care. Ramucirumab was associated with significantly improved median progression free (2.1

vs. 1.3 months) and OS (5.2 vs. 3.8 months; HR 0.78; 95% CI 0.60 to 0.998; $P = 0.047$). The phase III RAINBOW trial added ramucirumab or placebo to weekly paclitaxel in 665 patients with metastatic esophagogastric adenocarcinoma who had disease progression on or within four months after first-line platinum and fluoropyrimidine-based combination therapy. The combination treatment was also associated with an improved median progression free (4.4 vs. 2.9 months) and OS (9.6 vs. 7.4 months; HR 0.807; 95% CI 0.678 to 0.962; $P = 0.017$). Ramucirumab, either alone or in combination with paclitaxel, is considered a standard targeted therapy for previously treated patients with metastatic gastric adenocarcinoma. Clinical trials are ongoing to determine any benefit in the first-line setting.

Of note, another monoclonal antibody against VEGF, bevacizumab, has already been tested in combination with first line chemotherapy (cisplatin/capecitabine or 5-FU) in advanced gastric cancer. Although the initial phase II study showed promising OS, the benefit was not sustained in the global, phase III AVAGAST study. This study randomized 774 patients to cisplatin/fluoropyrimidine combination chemotherapy with or without bevacizumab. Response rate (46% vs. 37%; $P = 0.0315$) and progression-free survival (6.7 vs. 5.3 months; $P = 0.0037$) were both improved with bevacizumab; however, there was no improvement in OS (12.2 vs. 10.1 months; $P = 0.1002$). Bevacizumab is currently under investigation in the perioperative setting.

Another orally active VEGFR 2 inhibitor is currently approved for use in China based on a multicenter randomized, double-blind trial in which 270 patients with advanced gastric cancer were randomly assigned in a 2:1 ratio to apatinib (850 mg daily) or placebo. Apatinib was associated with prolonged median progression free (2.6 vs. 1.8 months) and OS (6.5 vs. 4.7 months; HR 0.709; 95% CI, 0.537 to 0.937; $P = 0.0156$).

Immunotherapy

Immunotherapy targeting programmed cell death receptor and ligand (PD-1 or PD-L1) has shown activity in early phase clinical trials using single or combination checkpoint inhibitors. The anti PD-1 antibody, nivolumab, was compared to placebo in a phase 3 study enrolling patients with refractory gastric cancer. Compared to placebo, nivolumab was associated with modest improvement in median OS. (5.26 months vs 4.14 months; HR 0·63; 95% CI 0·51 to 0·78; $P < 0·0001$). Based on this study, nivolumab obtained approval for the treatment of advanced gastric cancer that has progressed after conventional chemotherapy in Japan. Pembrolizumab, another anti PD-1 antibody, was similarly studied in 259 patients with recurrent or advanced gastric or gastroesophageal junction (GEJ) adenocarcinoma who have received 2 or more lines of chemotherapy. In this study, 143 of 259 patients had PD-L1 positive tumor and the ORR was 13.3%. PD-L1 positivity was assessed by PD-L1 IHC 22C3 pharmDx Kit (Dako) with PD-L1 positivity based on a combined positive score (CPS) ≥ 1. CPS was determined by the number of PD-L1 staining cells (tumor cells, lymphocytes, macrophages) divided by total number of tumor cells evaluated, multiplied by 100. The duration of response among the 19 responding patients ranged from 2.8 to 19.4 months with responses being 6 months or longer in 11 (58%) patients and 12 months or longer in 5 (26%) patients. Based on these results, pembrolizumab obtained FDA-approval for the treatment of PD-L1 positive recurrent or advanced gastric or gastroesophageal junction (GEJ) adenocarcinoma who have received 2 or more lines of chemotherapy.

As described earlier, a small percentage of patients harbor microsatellite instability-high (MSI-H) or mismatch repair deficient (dMMR) gastroesophageal tumors. The safety and efficacy of pembrolizumab was studied in 149 patients with 15 different tumor types (5 patients with gastric ca) across five single arm clinical trials. In this patient population, the ORR was 39.6% and for 78% of responders, response lasted more than 6 months. Based on this data, pembrolizumab obtained FDA-approval for MSI-H or dMMR cancers (including gastroesophageal cancers) after progression of standard treatments.

TREATMENT OF GASTRIC CANCER ACCORDING TO STAGE

Stage 0 Gastric Cancer

Stage 0 indicates gastric cancer confined to the mucosa. Based on the experience in Japan, where stage 0 is diagnosed more frequently, it has been found that more than 90% of patients treated by gastrectomy with lymphadenectomy will survive beyond 5 years. An American series has confirmed these findings. No additional perioperative therapy is necessary.

Stage I and II Gastric Cancer

1. One of the following surgical procedures is recommended for stage I and II gastric cancer:
   - Distal SG (if the lesion is not in the fundus or at the cardioesophageal junction)
   - Proximal SG or TG, with distal esophagectomy (if the lesion involves the cardia)
   - TG (if the tumor involves the stomach diffusely or arises in the body of the stomach and extends to within 6 cm of the cardia or distal antrum)
   - Regional lymphadenectomy is recommended with all of the previously noted procedures
   - Splenectomy is not routinely performed
2. Postoperative chemoRT is recommended for patients with at least stage IB disease.
3. Perioperative polychemotherapy could also be considered for patients who present with at least a T2 lesion preoperatively.

Stage III Gastric Cancer

1. Radical surgery: Curative resection procedures are confined to patients who do not have extensive nodal involvement at the time of surgical exploration.
2. Postoperative chemoRT or perioperative polychemotherapy is recommended. The latter should be considered particularly for bulky tumors or with significant nodal burden.

Stage IV Gastric Cancer

Patients with Distant Metastases (M1)

All newly diagnosed patients with hematogenous or peritoneal metastases should be considered as candidates for clinical trials. For many patients, chemotherapy may provide substantial palliative benefit and occasional durable remission, although the disease remains incurable. Patients with HER2 overexpression should be treated with trastuzumab in combination with chemotherapy. Balancing the risks to benefits of therapy in any individual patient is recommended.

Peritoneal Carcinomatosis

In approximately 50% of patients with advanced gastric cancer, the disease recurs locally or at an intraperitoneal site, and this recurrence has a negative effect on quality of life and survival. Intraperitoneal (IP) 5-FU, cisplatin, and/or mitomycin have been used at select centers. IP chemotherapy administration does not routinely alter survival and should be reserved only for clinical trial at an experienced center.

POSTSURGICAL FOLLOW-UP

- Follow-up in patients after complete surgical resection should include routine history and physical, with liver function tests and CEA measurements being performed.
- Evaluation intervals of every 3 to 6 months for the first 3 years, then annually thereafter have been suggested.
- Symptom-directed imaging and laboratory workup is indicated, without routine recommendations otherwise.
- If TG is not performed, annual upper endoscopy is recommended due to a 1% to 2% incidence of second primary gastric tumors.
- Vitamin B_{12} deficiency develops in most TG patients and 20% of SG patients, typically within 4 to 10 years. Replacement must be administered at 1,000 mcg subcutaneously or intramuscularly every month indefinitely.

PRIMARY GASTRIC LYMPHOMA

Gastric lymphomas are uncommon malignancies representing 3% of gastric neoplasms and 10% of lymphomas.

Classification and Histopathology

Gastric lymphomas can be generally classified as primary or secondary:

- Primary gastric lymphoma (PGL) is defined as a lymphoma arising in the stomach, typically originating from mucosa-associated lymphoid tissue (MALT). PGL can spread to regional lymph nodes and can become disseminated. Most are of B-cell NHL origin, with occasional cases of T-cell and Hodgkin's lymphoma seen. Examples of PGLs include extranodal marginal zone B-cell lymphoma of MALT type previously called low-grade MALT lymphoma, diffuse large B-cell lymphoma (DLBCL) previously called high-grade MALT lymphoma, and Burkitt's and Burkitt's-like lymphoma. This section will primarily address PGLs.
- Secondary gastric lymphoma indicates involvement of the stomach associated with lymphoma arising elsewhere. The stomach is the most common extranodal site of lymphoma. In an autopsy series, patients who died from disseminated NHL showed involvement of the gastrointestinal tract in 50% to 60% of cases. Examples of secondary gastric lymphoma include several common advanced-stage systemic NHLs, particularly mantle cell lymphoma.

Epidemiology

- The prevalence of PGL has been increasing over the past 20 years without a clear explanation.
- PGL incidence rises with age, with a peak in the sixth to seventh decades with a slight male predominance.
- Risk factors include *H. pylori*-associated chronic gastritis (particularly low-grade MALT lymphoma), autoimmune diseases, and immunodeficiency syndromes including AIDS and chronic immunosuppression.

Diagnosis

Clinical symptoms that are most common at presentation include abdominal pain, weight loss, nausea, vomiting, and early satiety. Frank bleeding is uncommon and patients rarely present with perforation. Findings on upper endoscopy are diverse and may be identical to typical adenocarcinoma.

Since PGL can infiltrate the submucosa without overlying mucosal changes, conventional punch biopsies may miss the diagnosis. Deeper biopsy techniques should be employed. If an ulcer is present, the biopsy should be at multiple sites along the edge of the ulcer crater. Specimens should be pathologically evaluated by both standard techniques to determine histology and *H. pylori* positivity as well as flow cytometry to determine clonality and characteristics of any infiltrating lymphocytes. The latter requires fresh tissue placed in saline, not preservative. In addition, fluorescence in situ hybridization (FISH) or polymerase chain reaction (PCR) are used to test for $t(11;18)$. This cytogenetic finding is associated with more advanced disease and relative resistance to *H. pylori* therapy.

Staging

Lugano staging system is commonly used for gastric lymphoma because the Ann Arbor stating system is considered to be inadequate as it does not incorporate depth of tumor invasion, which is known to affect the prognosis. Early (stage IE/IIE) disease includes a single primary lesion or multiple, noncontiguous lesions confined to the GI tract that may have local or distant nodal involvement. There is no stage III in the Lugano system. Advanced (stage IV) has disseminated nodal involvement or concomitant supradiaphragmatic involvement. Patients present with stage IE and stage IIE PGL with an equal prevalence ranging between 28% and 72%.

Presentation with high-grade and low-grade disease is also equal, with 34% to 65% of disease presenting as high-grade lymphoma and 35% to 65% presenting as low-grade lymphoma. CT scanning of the chest and abdomen is important to determine the lymphoma nodal involvement. FDG-PET scanning and bone marrow biopsy may be useful in high-grade PGL staging.

Treatment

Treatment of PGL is dependent primarily by stage and histologic grade of the lymphoma. However, given the rarity of the disease and lack of clinical trial data, treatment recommendations are based primarily on retrospective studies.

Extranodal marginal zone B-cell lymphoma of MALT type is usually of low-grade histology (40% to 50%) and confined to the stomach (70% to 80% stage IE). Very good epidemiologic data support *H. pylori*-induced chronic gastritis as a major etiology for this tumor. Eradication of *H. pylori* infection with antibiotics should be the initial standard treatment. Complete histologic regression of the lymphoma has been demonstrated in 50% to 80% of patients treated in this manner with good long-term DFS. Radiation therapy (RT) can provide durable remission for cases that relapse or are *H. pylori*-negative. One third of PGL is associated with the *t*(11;18) translocation, which has a low response to *H. pylori* therapy and should warrant consideration of RT as a primary treatment. More advanced stage or aggressive histologies at presentation should be treated like DLBCL.

Previously called high-grade MALT lymphoma, DLBCL is a more aggressive PGL. Eradication of *H. pylori* provides less reliable and durable disease control. Gastrectomy was the traditional treatment of choice; however, this appears to be no longer necessary. Five hundred eighty-nine patients with stage IE and IIE DLBCL PGL were randomized to receive surgery, surgery plus radiotherapy, surgery plus chemotherapy, or chemotherapy alone. Chemotherapy was six cycles of cyclophosphamide, doxorubicin, vincristine, and prednisone (CHOP). Overall survivals at 10 years were 54%, 53%, 91%, and 96%, respectively. Late toxicity and complications were more frequent and severe in those receiving surgery. Gastric perforation or bleeding as a result of initial chemotherapy was not evident. Organ preservation has been a major advance for this disease with the use of chemotherapy.

Highly aggressive PGLs including Burkitt's and Burkitt's-like lymphoma have seen dramatic improvement in survival over the past decade as a result of potent chemotherapy combinations for systemic disease as well as better treatment of underlying immunodeficiency states (i.e., highly effective antiretroviral therapy for AIDS).

Suggested Readings

1. A comparison of combination chemotherapy and combined modality therapy for locally advanced gastric carcinoma. *Gastrointestinal Tumor Study Group. Cancer.* 1982;49:1771–1777.
2. Adachi Y, Yasuda K, Inomata M, Sato K, Shiraishi N, Kitano S. Pathology and prognosis of gastric carcinoma: well versus poorly differentiated type. *Cancer.* 2000;89:1418–1424.
3. Ajani JA, Rodriguez W, Bodoky G, et al. Multicenter phase III comparison of cisplatin/S-1 with cisplatin/infusional fluorouracil in advanced gastric or gastroesophageal adenocarcinoma study: the FLAGS trial. *J Clin Oncol.* 2010;28:1547–1553.
4. Al Batran S-E, Homann N, Schmalenberg H, et al. Perioperative chemotherapy with docetaxel, oxaliplatin, and fluorouracil/leucovorin (FLOT) versus epirubicin, cisplatin, and fluorouracil or capecitabine (ECF/ECX) for resectable gastric or gastroesophageal junction (GEJ) adenocarcinoma (FLOT4-AIO): A multicenter, randomized phase 3 trial (abstract). *J Clin Oncol.* 2017;35 (suppl; abstr 4004).
5. Amin M, Edge S, Greene F, et al. AJCC Cancer Staging Manual. 8th ed. Chicago, IL: Springer; 2018.
6. Avilés A, Nambo MJ, Neri N, et al. The role of surgery in primary gastric lymphoma: results of a controlled clinical trial. *Ann Surg.* 2004;240:44–50.
7. Bang YJ, Van Cutsem E, Feyereislova A, et al. Trastuzumab in combination with chemotherapy versus chemotherapy alone for treatment of HER2-positive advanced gastric or gastro-oesophageal junction cancer (ToGA): a phase 3, open-label, randomised controlled trial. *Lancet.* 2010;376:687–697.
8. Bonenkamp JJ, Hermans J, Sasako M, et al. Extended lymph-node dissection for gastric cancer. *N Engl J Med.* 1999;340:908–914.
9. Cocconi G, Bella M, Zironi S, et al. Fluorouracil, doxorubicin, and mitomycin combination versus PELF chemotherapy in advanced gastric cancer: a prospective randomized trial of the Italian Oncology Group for Clinical Research. *J Clin Oncol.* 1994;12:2687–2693.
10. Cunningham D, Allum WH, Stenning SP, et al. Perioperative chemotherapy versus surgery alone for resectable gastroesophageal cancer. *N Engl J Med.* 2006;355:11–20.
11. Cunningham D, Starling N, Rao S, et al. Capecitabine and oxaliplatin for advanced esophagogastric cancer. *N Engl J Med.* 2008;358:36–46.
12. Fuchs CS DT, Jang RW-J, et al. KEYNOTE-059 cohort 1: Efficacy and safety of pembrolizumab (pembro) monotherapy in patients with previously treated advanced gastric cancer (abstract). *J Clin Oncol.* 2017;35 (suppl; abstr 4003).
13. Fuchs CS, Tomasek J, Yong CJ, et al. Ramucirumab monotherapy for previously treated advanced gastric or gastro-oesophageal junction adenocarcinoma (REGARD): an international, randomised, multicentre, placebo-controlled, phase 3 trial. *Lancet.* 2014;383:31–39.
14. Fuchs CS,TJ, Niedzwiecke D, et al. Postoperative adjuvant chemoradiation for gastric or gastroesophageal junction (GEJ) adenocarcinoma using epirubicin, cisplatin, and infusional (CI) 5-FU (ECF) before and after CI 5-FU and radiotherapy (CRT) compared with bolus 5-FU/LV before and after CRT: intergroup trial CALGB 80101. *J Clin Oncol.* 2011;29:256s (abstract 4003).
15. Hallissey MT, Dunn JA, Ward LC, Allum WH. The second British Stomach Cancer Group trial of adjuvant radiotherapy or chemotherapy in resectable gastric cancer: five-year follow-up. *Lancet.* 1994;343:1309–1312.
16. Hecht JR, Bang YJ, Qin SK, et al. Lapatinib in combination with capecitabine plus oxaliplatin in human epidermal growth factor receptor 2-positive advanced or metastatic gastric, esophageal, or gastroesophageal adenocarcinoma: TRIO-013/LOGiC—a randomized phase III trial. *J Clin Oncol.* 2016;34:443–451.

17. Jemal A, Bray F, Center MM, et al. Global Cancer Statistics. *CA Cancer J Clin.* 2011;61(2):69–90.
18. Kang YK, Boku N, Satoh T, et al. Nivolumab in patients with advanced gastric or gastro-oesophageal junction cancer refractory to, or intolerant of, at least two previous chemotherapy regimens (ONO-4538-12, ATTRACTION-2): a randomised, double-blind, placebo-controlled, phase 3 trial. *Lancet.* 2017.
19. Kattan MW, Karpeh MS, Mazumdar M, Brennan MF. Postoperative nomogram for disease-specific survival after an R0 resection for gastric carcinoma. *J Clin Oncol.* 2003;21:3647–3650.
20. Kelsen D, Atiq OT, Saltz L, et al. FAMTX versus etoposide, doxorubicin, and cisplatin: a random assignment trial in gastric cancer. *J Clin Oncol.* 1992;10:541–548.
21. Le DT, Durham JN, Smith KN, et al. Mismatch repair deficiency predicts response of solid tumors to PD-1 blockade. *Science.* 2017;357:409–413.
22. Lee J, Lim DH, Kim S, et al. Phase III trial comparing capecitabine plus cisplatin versus capecitabine plus cisplatin with concurrent capecitabine radiotherapy in completely resected gastric cancer with D2 lymph node dissection: the ARTIST trial. *J Clin Oncol.* 2012;30:268–273.
23. Li J, Qin S, Xu J, et al. Randomized, double-blind, placebo-controlled phase III trial of apatinib in patients with chemotherapy-refractory advanced or metastatic adenocarcinoma of the stomach or gastroesophageal junction. *J Clin Oncol.* 2016;34:1448–1454.
24. Lordick F, Kang YK, Chung HC, et al. Capecitabine and cisplatin with or without cetuximab for patients with previously untreated advanced gastric cancer (EXPAND): a randomised, open-label phase 3 trial. *Lancet Oncol.* 2013;14:490–499.
25. Macdonald JS, Smalley SR, Benedetti J, et al. Chemoradiotherapy after surgery compared with surgery alone for adenocarcinoma of the stomach or gastroesophageal junction. *N Engl J Med.* 2001;345:725–730.
26. Marrelli D, Morgagni P, de Manzoni G, et al. Prognostic value of the 7th AJCC/UICC TNM classification of noncardia gastric cancer: analysis of a large series from specialized Western centers. *Ann Surg.* 2012;255:486–491.
27. Ohtsu A, Shah MA, Van Cutsem E, et al. Bevacizumab in combination with chemotherapy as first-line therapy in advanced gastric cancer: a randomized, double-blind, placebo-controlled phase III study. *J Clin Oncol.* 2011;29:3968–3976.
28. Sakuramoto S, Sasako M, Yamaguchi T, et al. Adjuvant chemotherapy for gastric cancer with S-1, an oral fluoropyrimidine. *N Engl J Med.* 2007;357:1810–1820.
29. Sasako M, Sakuramoto S, Katai H, et al. Five-year outcomes of a randomized phase III trial comparing adjuvant chemotherapy with S-1 versus surgery alone in stage II or III gastric cancer. *J Clin Oncol.* 2011;29:4387–4393.
30. Satoh T, Xu RH, Chung HC, et al. Lapatinib plus paclitaxel versus paclitaxel alone in the second-line treatment of HER2-amplified advanced gastric cancer in Asian populations: TyTAN—a randomized, phase III study. *J Clin Oncol.* 2014;32:2039–2049.
31. Smalley SR, Benedetti JK, Haller DG, et al. Updated analysis of SWOG-directed intergroup study 0116: a phase III trial of adjuvant radiochemotherapy versus observation after curative gastric cancer resection. *J Clin Oncol.* 2012;30:2327–2333.
32. Songun I, Putter H, Kranenbarg EM, Sasako M, van de Velde CJ. Surgical treatment of gastric cancer: 15-year follow-up results of the randomised nationwide Dutch D1D2 trial. *Lancet Oncol.* 2010;11:439–449.
33. Stephens J, Smith J. Treatment of primary gastric lymphoma and gastric mucosa-associated lymphoid tissue lymphoma. *J Am Coll Surg.* 1998;187:312–320.
34. Van Cutsem E, Bang YJ, Feng-Yi F, et al. HER2 screening data from ToGA: targeting HER2 in gastric and gastroesophageal junction cancer. *Gastric Cancer.* 2015;18:476–484.
35. Van Cutsem E, Moiseyenko VM, Tjulandin S, et al. Phase III study of docetaxel and cisplatin plus fluorouracil compared with cisplatin and fluorouracil as first-line therapy for advanced gastric cancer: a report of the V325 Study Group. *J Clin Oncol.* 2006;24:4991–4997.
36. Verheij MJE, Cats A, et al. A multicenter randomized phase III trial of neo-adjuvant chemotherapy followed by surgery and chemotherapy or by surgery and chemoradiotherapy in resectable gastric cancer: first results from the CRITICS study. *J Clin Oncol.* 2016;34(suppl): abstr 4000.
37. Waddell T, Chau I, Cunningham D, et al. Epirubicin, oxaliplatin, and capecitabine with or without panitumumab for patients with previously untreated advanced oesophagogastric cancer (REAL3): a randomised, open-label phase 3 trial. *Lancet Oncol.* 2013;14:481–489.
38. Webb A, Cunningham D, Scarffe JH, et al. Randomized trial comparing epirubicin, cisplatin, and fluorouracil versus fluorouracil, doxorubicin, and methotrexate in advanced esophagogastric cancer. *J Clin Oncol.* 1997;15:261–267.
39. Wilke H, Muro K, Van Cutsem E, et al. Ramucirumab plus paclitaxel versus placebo plus paclitaxel in patients with previously treated advanced gastric or gastro-oesophageal junction adenocarcinoma (RAINBOW): a double-blind, randomised phase 3 trial. *Lancet Oncol.* 2014;15:1224–1235.
40. Wils JA, Klein HO, Wagener DJ, et al. Sequential high-dose methotrexate and fluorouracil combined with doxorubicin—a step ahead in the treatment of advanced gastric cancer: a trial of the European Organization for Research and Treatment of Cancer Gastrointestinal Tract Cooperative Group. *J Clin Oncol.* 1991;9:827–831.
41. Worthley DL, Phillips KD, Wayte N, et al. Gastric adenocarcinoma and proximal polyposis of the stomach (GAPPS): a new autosomal dominant syndrome. *Gut.* 2012;61:774–779.
42. Ychou M, Boige V, Pignon JP, et al. Perioperative chemotherapy compared with surgery alone for resectable gastroesophageal adenocarcinoma: an FNCLCC and FFCD multicenter phase III trial. *J Clin Oncol.* 2011;29:1715–1721.

6 Biliary Tract Cancer

Davendra P. S. Sohal and Alok A. Khorana

INTRODUCTION

Carcinomas of the biliary tract include cancers arising in either the gallbladder or the bile duct system—the latter usually referred to as cholangiocarcinomas and further categorized as intra- or extrahepatic. There will be an estimated 11,420 new cases of gallbladder and biliary tract cancers (excluding intrahepatic biliary tract cancer) in 2016 in the United States with 3,710 expected deaths. Worldwide, 186,000 cases and 140,000 deaths were reported in 2013. Gallbladder cancer is the most common biliary tract cancer, occurring nearly twice as often as cholangiocarcinomas. The epidemiology, clinical features, staging, and surgical treatment are distinct for carcinomas arising in the gallbladder and bile duct, therefore, these are described separately. The systemic therapy options are similar and are discussed together later in the chapter.

CARCINOMA OF THE GALLBLADDER

Epidemiology

- Women have a 2- to 6-fold higher incidence of gallbladder cancer.
- There is a prominent geographic variation in the incidence of gallbladder cancer. Higher rates are seen among Native Americans, in South American countries (particularly Chile), and in countries such as India, Pakistan, Japan, and Korea. These populations share a high prevalence of cholelithiasis, which is a common risk factor.
- The United States is considered a low-incidence area. The age-adjusted incidence of carcinoma of the gallbladder is 1.2 per 100,000 population in the United States.

Etiology

- Cholelithiasis (gallstones): A history of gallstones appears to be one of the strongest risk factors for gallbladder cancer. Most (70% to 90%) patients have gallstones. The risk increases with an increase in the size and duration of the stones.
- Porcelain gallbladder: Extensive calcium deposition in the gallbladder wall was associated with cholecystitis in nearly all cases. Previously, the incidence of gallbladder cancer in patients with this condition was thought to range from 12.5% to 60%, although more recent data suggest the incidence is closer to 2% to 3%. Stippled, mucosal calcifications appear to be associated with a higher risk than diffuse intramural calcifications.
- Chronic infection: Carriers or those colonized with *Salmonella typhi* and *Helicobacter pylori* may be at increased risk of developing gallbladder cancer.
- Gallbladder polyps: Polyps >1 cm have the greatest malignant potential and therefore are an indication for cholecystectomy.
- An anomalous pancreatobiliary duct junction may contribute to the development of gallbladder cancer.

▪ Miscellaneous: Obesity, diabetes, medications (methyldopa, estrogens, isoniazid), and carcinogen exposure (radon, chemicals from the rubber industry, cigarettes) have also been associated with this disease.

Clinical Features

Early-stage disease may be asymptomatic or present with very nonspecific symptoms, including the following:

▪ Often, it is noted as an incidental finding on cholecystectomy for cholelithiasis or cholecystitis
▪ Pain
▪ Weight loss
▪ Anorexia
▪ Nausea or vomiting
▪ Mass in the right upper quadrant
▪ Jaundice
▪ Abdominal distension
▪ Pruritus

Diagnosis

Three clinical scenarios exist in patients presenting with gallbladder cancer: final pathology after a routine laparoscopic cholecystectomy incidentally discovers gallbladder cancer; gallbladder cancer is suspected/diagnosed intraoperatively; or gallbladder cancer is suspected preoperatively.

▪ An incidental surgical or pathologic finding is the most common clinical scenario. It is estimated that 1% to 2% of patients undergoing exploration for presumed benign disease will be found to have gallbladder cancer.
▪ Ultrasound is a useful modality in the preoperative workup for gallbladder pathology. In the case of gallbladder cancer, the ultrasonographic findings may include a thickened or calcified wall, a protruding mass, or a loss of gallbladder to liver interface; however, these may not be specific for gallbladder cancer.
▪ Triple-phase computed tomography (CT) scan (liver protocol), which includes a noncontrast phase, a hepatic arterial phase, and a portal venous phase, allows visualization of the extent of tumor growth, can aid in determining the nodal status as well as identifying distant metastases, and is particularly useful in determining the relationship of the tumor mass to the major hilar inflow structures, which is an important preoperative determinant. This modality is less helpful in distinguishing benign from malignant polyps.
▪ Cholangiography: Magnetic resonance cholangiopancreatography (MRCP) can provide further information regarding the extent of disease.
▪ Laboratory studies are generally not diagnostic. Elevated serum bilirubin or alkaline phosphatase can indicate biliary obstruction. CA19.9, a tumor marker, is often checked, but is neither sensitive nor specific for a diagnosis.

Pathology

▪ Adenocarcinoma accounts for close to 85% of cases. It is further classified into papillary, tubular, mucinous, or signet cell type. Other histologies include anaplastic, squamous cell, small-cell neuroendocrine tumors, sarcoma, and lymphoma.

Staging

There are several staging systems available for gallbladder cancer. The original staging system was developed by Nevin in 1976; the preferred classification scheme in the United States is the TNM staging system of the American Joint Committee on Cancer (AJCC) (Table 6.1).

▪ The AJCC TNM staging classification was updated in 2010.
▪ The updated stage groupings were realigned to better correlate with resectability and prognosis.

TABLE 6.1 AJCC Staging System for Gallbladder Cancer

Primary Tumor (T)	
TX	Primary tumor cannot be assessed
T0	No evidence of primary tumor
Tis	Carcinoma in situ
T1	Tumor invades lamina propria or muscular layer
T1a	Tumor invades lamina propria
T1b	Tumor invades muscular layer
T2	Tumor invades perimuscular connective tissue; no extension beyond serosa or into liver
T3	Tumor perforates the serosa (visceral peritoneum) and/or directly invades the liver and/or one other adjacent organ or structure, such as the stomach, duodenum, colon, pancreas, omentum, or extrahepatic bile ducts
T4	Tumor invades main portal vein or hepatic artery or invades two or more extrahepatic organs or structures

Regional Lymph Nodes (N)	
NX	Regional lymph nodes cannot be assessed
N0	No regional lymph node metastasis
N1	Metastases to nodes along the cystic duct, common bile duct, hepatic artery, and/or portal vein
N2	Metastases to periaortic, pericaval, superior mesenteric artery, and/or celiac artery lymph nodes

Distant Metastasis (M)	
M0	No distant metastasis
M1	Distant metastasis

Anatomic Stage/Prognostic Groups			
Stage 0	Tis	N0	M0
Stage I	T1	N0	M0
Stage II	T2	N0	M0
Stage IIIA	T3	N0	M0
Stage IIIB	T1-3	N1	M0
Stage IVA	T4	N0-1	M0
Stage IVB	Any T	N2	M0
	Any T	Any N	M1

Treatment

Surgery

- Surgical resection remains the only potentially curative therapy.
- The lack of a peritoneal lining on the side of the gallbladder that is attached to the liver represents an important anatomic consideration in the surgical management of gallbladder cancer. In a simple cholecystectomy, the surgeon dissects the plane between the muscularis of the gallbladder and the cystic plate, which is a fibrous lining that occupies the space between the gallbladder and the liver. For this reason, simple cholecystectomy is considered inadequate surgical therapy for all but the earliest stages of the disease.
- Factors determining resectability include the stage of the tumor as well as the location. T0-2 tumors are potentially resectable with curative intent. T3 tumors are difficult to resect.

▪ For incidentally detected gallbladder cancer after simple cholecystectomy, careful clinical, laboratory, radiologic, and pathologic evaluation should be conducted to assess the extent of disease.

▪ For completely resected (margin-negative) nonperforated T1a tumors with no evidence of nodal or metastatic disease, observation alone is usually sufficient as 5-year overall survival is over 90%.

▪ Patients with T1b or greater lesions should undergo extended cholecystectomy after metastatic disease has been ruled out. Optimal resection (extended cholecystectomy) includes a cholecystectomy with en bloc hepatic resection and regional lymphadenectomy with or without bile duct excision. Achievement of R0 resection margins correlates strongly with long-term survival.

▪ The type of resection that is ultimately required to achieve an R0 resection can at times depend on the location of the tumor within the gallbladder. Tumors of the body and fundus may be manageable with a localized segment IV/V resection while those of the infundibulum may require division of inflow structures and consequently major hepatic resection with or without bile duct resection/reconstruction.

▪ Contraindications to surgery include distant metastases, extensive involvement of the porta hepatis causing jaundice, significant ascites, and encasement or occlusion of major vessels. Direct involvement of adjacent organs is not an absolute contraindication.

▪ If cancer is suspected, perforation of the gallbladder (such as during percutaneous biopsy) during surgery should be avoided to prevent seeding of the peritoneal cavity.

Radiation

▪ A number of reports have documented improvements in survival rates in cases of intraoperative or postoperative adjuvant radiotherapy. No prospective randomized controlled trials have been performed to address this issue. In 2003, however, Jarnigan and colleagues found that only 15% of patients had locoregional recurrence as their only site of recurrent disease, which highlights the importance of effective, adjuvant systemic strategies.

Systemic Therapy and Palliation

The benefits and options available for systemic therapy and palliation of carcinoma of the gallbladder are the same as those for cholangiocarcinoma, which is discussed in the next section.

Survival

The various aspects of survival following treatment of gallbladder cancers according to stage are given in Table 6.2.

TABLE 6.2 Treatment and 5-Year Survival of Gallbladder Cancers According to Stage

TNM Stage	Treatment	Median Survival (mo)	5-Y Survival (%)
I	Simple cholecystectomy	19	60–100
	Radical cholecystectomy		
II	Radical cholecystectomy	7	10–20
	+/– Radiation therapy (not standard)		
III	Radical cholecystectomy	4	5
	+/– Radiation therapy (not standard)		
IV	Palliation with stent placement	2	0
	Surgery or radiation or chemotherapy or combination of these		

CARCINOMA OF THE BILE DUCTS (CHOLANGIOCARCINOMA)

Epidemiology

- Cholangiocarcinomas arise from the epithelial cells of either intrahepatic or extrahepatic bile ducts.
- The reported incidence within the United States is 1 to 2 cases per 100,000 persons.
- Median age at diagnosis is between 50 and 70 years. However patients with primary sclerosing cholangitis (PSC) and those with choledochal cysts tend to present at younger ages.
- In contrast to gallbladder cancer, cholangiocarcinomas are more common in males.
- Cholangiocarcinomas are categorized into proximal extrahepatic (perihilar or Klatskin tumor; 50% to 60%), distal extrahepatic (20% to 25%), intrahepatic (peripheral tumor; 20% to 25%), and multifocal (5%) tumors.
- Extrahepatic cholangiocarcinomas are more common than intrahepatic cholangiocarcinomas, and perihilar cholangiocarcinoma is the most common type.

Etiology

A number of risk factors have been associated with the disease in some patients; however, no specific predisposing factors have been identified.

- Inflammatory conditions: PSC is associated with an annual risk of 0.6% to 1.5% per year and a 10% to 15% lifetime risk of developing cholangiocarcinoma. Ulcerative colitis and chronic intraductal gallstone disease also increase risk. Nearly 30% of cholangiocarcinomas are diagnosed in patients with coexistent ulcerative colitis and PSC.
- Bile duct abnormalities: Caroli disease (cystic dilatation of intrahepatic ducts), bile duct adenoma, biliary papillomatosis, and choledochal cysts increase risk. The overall incidence of cholangiocarcinoma in these patients can be as high as 28%.
- Infection: In Southeast Asia, the risk can be increased 25- to 50-fold by parasitic infestation from *Opisthorchis viverrini* and *Clonorchis sinensis*. These parasitic infections are more commonly associated with intrahepatic cholangiocarcinoma. An association with viral hepatitis has also been seen. A higher than expected rate of hepatitis C-associated cirrhosis was noted in patients with cholangiocarcinoma. An association with hepatitis B has also been suggested.
- Genetic: Lynch syndrome II and multiple biliary papillomatosis are associated with an increased risk of developing cholangiocarcinoma. Biliary papillomatosis should be considered a premalignant condition as one study noted that up to 83% will undergo malignant transformation. More recently, certain genetic polymorphisms (NKG2D) have been determined to be possible risk factors for developing cholangiocarcinoma.
- Miscellaneous: Smoking, toxic exposures, such as thorotrast (a radiologic contrast agent used in the 1960s), asbestos, radon, and nitrosamines are also known to increase the risk. Recently, patients with diabetes or a metabolic syndrome have been noted to have an increased risk of developing a cholangiocarcinoma as well.

Clinical Features

Cholangiocarcinomas usually become symptomatic when the biliary system becomes obstructed.

- Extrahepatic cholangiocarcinoma usually presents with symptoms and signs of cholestasis (icterus, pale stools, dark urine, pruritus, or cholangitis, which includes pain, icterus, and fever). Laboratory studies will typically suggest biliary obstruction with elevated direct bilirubin and alkaline phosphatase.
- Intrahepatic cholangiocarcinoma may present as a mass, be asymptomatic, or produce vague symptoms such as pain, anorexia, weight loss, night sweats, and malaise. These patients are less likely to be jaundiced.

Diagnosis

- A cholestatic picture may be seen as described previously. Liver function tests may be elevated, particularly with intrahepatic cholangiocarcinoma. Tumor markers such as CEA and CA-19-9 by themselves are neither sensitive nor specific enough to make a diagnosis. Ultrasonography is the first-line investigation for suspected cholangiocarcinoma, usually to confirm biliary duct dilatation, localize the site of obstruction, and rule out cholelithiasis. This technique can often overlook masses and is poor at delineating anatomy.

- CT/MRI is recommended as part of the diagnostic workup of cholangiocarcinoma, intrahepatic tumors in particular. These imaging modalities can help determine tumor resectability by evaluating the tumor and the surrounding structures (major vessels, lymph nodes, presence of metastases).
- Cholangiography: MRCP is noninvasive and can provide excellent imaging of the intrahepatic and extrahepatic bile ducts. This provides valuable information about disease extent and surgical options. Due to their ability to obtain brushings from as well as stent across strictures within the biliary tree, ERCP, and/or PTC offer both diagnostic and therapeutic value in the workup and management of biliary obstruction; however, the diagnostic yield on cytology obtained from biliary brushings can be low.
- EUS may be useful in visualizing the extent of tumor and lymph node involvement of distal bile duct lesions. Its role in proximal bile duct lesions is less clear.

Pathology

- Adenocarcinomas account for 90% to 95% of tumors. The remainder are squamous cell carcinomas. Adenocarcinomas are graded as well, moderately and poorly differentiated, and are further classified as sclerosing, nodular, and papillary subtypes. Patients with papillary tumors present with earlier disease and have the highest resectability and cure rates; however, they are the least common subtype.

Staging

- The AJCC TNM staging system is primarily based on the extent of ductal involvement by the tumor.
- The seventh edition staging system for extrahepatic cholangiocarcinomas separates perihilar and distal bile duct tumors. These changes have improved the prognostic stratification of the TNM staging system. Please refer to the seventh edition AJCC Staging Manual for details.
- Cancers arising in the perihilar region have been also further classified according to their patterns of involvement of the hepatic ducts, the Bismuth-Corlette classification.

Treatment

Surgery

Except in the case of distal common bile duct cancer, cholangiocarcinoma is a disease that, when managed surgically, often requires major hepatic resection (segmentectomy, anatomic lobectomy, and trisegmentectomy) with or without bile duct resection/reconstruction. Therefore, the general principles of such resection(s) should be reviewed.

From the standpoint of major hepatic resection, the surgical principles are simple and revolve primarily around leaving the patient with an adequate volume of a functioning liver remnant to sustain them postoperatively. This requires executing an operation that ensures both adequate inflow to (hepatic artery and portal vein) and outflow from (hepatic vein and bile duct) the remnant liver.

Generally speaking, roughly 75% of a patient's liver volume can safely be resected; however, consideration must be given to the health of the background liver. Such consideration includes underlying chronic liver disease (hepatitis, prior alcohol use, and steatosis/steatohepatitis) as well as any acute insults, which in the case of cholangiocarcinoma often involves cholestasis. The former issues can limit the extent of resection that can safely be performed, while the latter often necessitates preoperative delays while the cholestatic picture resolves.

If there is any concern about the adequacy of the planned future liver remnant, portal vein embolization on the side of the liver that is anticipated to be resected can be performed in an attempt to allow the contralateral side to hypertrophy preoperatively.

Intrahepatic Cholangiocarcinoma

- Surgery is the only potentially curative therapy for patients with intrahepatic cholangiocarcinoma; however, most patients present with advanced disease and are not surgical candidates.
- Multiple hepatic tumors, regional lymph node involvement, large tumor size, and vascular invasion predict poor recurrence-free survival postresection.
- The extent of surgery is dictated by what is necessary to obtain clear margins. R0 resection with adequate margins is the aim and is ultimately associated with significantly longer survival rates that can range from 30% to 67%.
- If microscopic positive tumor margins (R1) or residual local disease (R2) is noted after resection, patients should be evaluated for possible re-resection versus chemoradiation options.
- The role of routine nodal dissection in the management of intrahepatic cholangiocarcinoma is controversial.
- During laparotomy, thorough assessment of the intra-abdominal lymph node basins should be undertaken prior to hepatic resection, suspicious nodes should be biopsied, and attempts at resection should be aborted if nodal metastases are confirmed intraoperatively.

Distal Cholangiocarcinoma

- Primarily treated with a Whipple procedure (pancreaticoduodenectomy).

Perihilar Cholangiocarcinoma

- The main curative therapy for patients with extrahepatic perihilar cholangiocarcinoma is complete surgical resection.
- Surgery for extrahepatic hilar cholangiocarcinomas is based on the stage of disease, and the goal of surgical intervention is to obtain a tumor-free margin (Table 6.3).
- For patients with hilar cholangiocarcinoma, bile duct resection leads to high local recurrence rates. Hilar resection with lymphadenectomy and en bloc liver resection and biliary reconstruction are recommended for lesions in the extrahepatic biliary tree. Caudate resection is often required to achieve an R0 resection, particularly for tumors involving the left hepatic duct.
- Five-year survival rates range from 20% to 40% in patients treated with surgical resection for hilar cholangiocarcinoma.

TABLE 6.3 Treatment and Survival of Cholangiocarcinomas According to Location

Location	Treatment	Median Survival (mo)	5-Y Survival (%)
Extrahepatic (hilar)	Type I + II: en bloc resection of extrahepatic bile ducts, gallbladder, regional lymphadenectomy, and roux-en-Y hepaticojejunostomy Type III: as above plus right/left hepatectomy Type IV: as above plus extended right/left hepatectomy	12–24	9–18
Extrahepatic (distal)	Pancreaticoduodenectomy	12–24	20–30
Intrahepatic	Resect involved segments or lobe of liver	18–30	10–45

Adjuvant Chemotherapy and Chemoradiation

▪ Adjuvant chemotherapy with capecitabine is being recognized as a new standard of care for resected biliary tract cancers. This is based on presentation of results from the BILCAP study, which showed that adjuvant capecitabine for 6 months improved median overall survival from 36 months with placebo to 51 months (HR 0.80; $P = 0.097$). While not statistically significantly different, the results were encouraging, and parsing further, most improvement was seen for patients with positive nodes and higher grade of disease.

Chemotherapy in Advanced-Stage Disease

▪ For metastatic biliary tract cancer, the standard of care is combination chemotherapy with gemcitabine and cisplatin, based on a large randomized controlled trial (ABC-02 study) that showed improved overall survival with the combination, compared with gemcitabine alone (11.7 vs. 8.1 months; HR 0.64; 95% CI, 0.52 to 0.80).

▪ Oxaliplatin can be considered instead of cisplatin, in combination with gemcitabine, to minimize toxicities from therapy, based on extrapolation of data from phase II studies.

Targeted Therapy

▪ Several targeted agents (cetuximab, panitumumab, erlotinib, bevacizumab, etc.) have been tested in advanced biliary tract cancers but have failed to show improvement in survival. Currently, therefore, there are no data to support the use of targeted therapies in this setting.

Palliation

▪ Patients with unresectable or metastatic disease may benefit from palliative surgery, radiation, chemotherapy, or a combination of these.

▪ Biliary drainage can be achieved by Roux-en-Y choledojejunostomy, bypass of the site of obstruction to left or right hepatic duct, or endoscopic or percutaneously placed stents (metal-wall stents have a larger diameter and are less prone to occlusion or migration and are preferably used in patients with a life expectancy of greater than 6 months and/or in those who have unresectable disease).

▪ Celiac plexus blockade may also ameliorate symptoms of pain in the patient with inoperable disease.

Suggested Readings

1. DeOliveira ML, Cunningham SC, Cameron JL, et al. Cholangiocarcinoma: thirty-one-year experience with 564 patients at a single institution. *Ann Surg.* 2007;245:755–762.
2. Eckel F, Schmid RM. Chemotherapy in advanced biliary tract carcinoma: a pooled analysis of clinical trials. *Br J Cancer.* 2007;96:896–902.
3. Edge SB, Byrd DR, Compton CC, et al., eds. *American Joint Committee on Cancer Staging Manual.* 7th ed. New York: Springer; 2010:211pp.
4. Endo I, Gonen M, Yopp AC, et al. Intrahepatic cholangiocarcinoma: rising frequency, improved survival, and determinants of outcome after resection. *Ann Surg.* 2008;248:84–96.
5. Farges O, Fuks D, Le Treut Y-P, et al. The AJCC 7th edition of TNM staging accurately discriminates outcomes of patients with resectable intrahepatic cholangiocarcinoma. *Cancer.* 2011;117:2170–2177.
6. Gruenberger B, Schueller J, Heubrandtner U, et al. Cetuximab, gemcitabine, and oxaliplatin in patients with unresectable advanced or metastatic biliary tract cancer: a phase 2 study. *Lancet Oncol.* 2010;11(12):1142–1148.
7. Hsing AW, Gao YT, Han TQ, et al. Gallstones and the risk of biliary tract cancer: a population-based study in China. *Br J Cancer.* 2007;97(11):1577–1582.
8. Hueman MT, Vollmer CM, Pawlik TM. Evolving treatment strategies for gallbladder cancer. *Ann Surg Oncol.* 2009;16:2101–2115.
9. Ito F, Agni R, Rettammel RJ, et al. Resection of hilar cholangiocarcinoma: concomitant liver resection decreases hepatic recurrence. *Ann Surg.* 2008;248:273–279.
10. Jarnagin W, Belghiti J, Blumgart L, et al. *Blumgart's Surgery of the Liver, Biliary Tract and Pancreas.* 5th ed., Vol. 1. Chapters 49–50B. Philadelphia, PA: Elsevier Saunders; 2012.

11. Jarnagin WR, Bowne W, Klimstra DS, et al. Papillary phenotype confers improved survival after resection of hilar cholangiocarcinoma. *Ann Surg.* 2005;241(5):703–712.

12. Jarnagin WR, Ruo L, Little SA, et al. Patterns of initial disease recurrence after resection of gallbladder carcinoma and hilar cholangiocarcinoma: implications for adjuvant therapeutic strategies. *Cancer.* 2003;98:1689–1700.

13. Jensen EH, Abraham A, Habermann EB, et al. A critical analysis of the surgical management of early stage gallbladder cancer in the United States. *J Gastrointest.* 2009;13:722–727.

14. Khan SA, Thomas HC, Davidson BR, Taylor-Robinson SD. Cholangiocarcinoma. *Lancet.* 2005;366(9493):1303–1314.

15. Kim JH, Won HJ, Shin YM, et al. Radiofrequency ablation for the treatment of primary intrahepatic cholangiocarcinoma. *Am J Roentgenol.* 2011;196:W205–W209.

16. Kim TW, Chang HM, Kang HJ, et al. Phase II study of capecitabine plus cisplatin as first-line chemotherapy in advanced biliary cancer. *Ann Oncol.* 2003;14:1115–1120.

17. Kobayashi K, Tsuji A, Morita S, et al. A phase II study of LFP therapy (5-FU (5-fluorourasil) continuous infusion (CVI) and low dose consecutive (cisplatin) CDDP) in advanced biliary tract carcinoma. *BMC Cancer.* 2006;6:121.

18. Koeberle D, Saletti P, Borner M, et al. Patient-reported outcomes of patients with advanced biliary tract cancers receiving gemcitabine plus capecitabine: a multicenter, phase II trial of the Swiss Group for Clinical Cancer Research. *J Clin Oncol.* 2008;26:3702–3708.

19. Lee J, Park SH, Chang HM, et al. Gemcitabine and oxaliplatin with or without erlotinib in advanced biliary-tract cancer: a multicentre, open-label, randomised, phase 3 study. *Lancet Oncol.* 2012;13(2):181–188.

20. Lee SS, Kim MH, Lee SK, et al. Clinicopathologic review of 58 patients with biliary papillomatosis. *Cancer.* 2004;100(4):783–793.

21. Lee SW, Kim HJ, Park JH, et al. Clinical usefulness of 18F-FDG PET-CT for patients with gallbladder cancer and cholangiocarcinoma. *J Gastroenterol.* 2010;45(5):560–566.

22. Lubner SJ, Mahoney MR, Kolesar JL, et al. Report of a multicenter phase II trial testing a combination of biweekly bevacizumab and daily erlotinib in patients with unresectable biliary cancer: a phase II Consortium study. *J Clin Oncol.* 2010;28(21):3491–3497.

23. Malka D, Trarbach T, Fartoux L, et al. A multicenter, randomized phase II trial of gemcitabine and oxaliplatin (GEMOX) alone or in combination with biweekly cetuximab in the first-line treatment of advanced biliary cancer: interim analysis of the BINGO trial. *J Clin Oncol.* 2009;27(15 suppl):Abstract 4520.

24. Melum E, Karlsen TH, Schrumpf E, et al. Cholangiocarcinoma in primary sclerosing cholangitis is associated with NKG2D polymorphisms. *Hepatology.* 2008;47(1):90–96.

25. Miller G, Schwartz LH, D'Angelica M. The use of imaging in the diagnosing and staging of hepatobiliary malignancies. *Surg Oncol Clin N Am.* 2007;16:343–368.

26. Misra S, Chaturvedi A, Misra NC, et al. Carcinoma of the gallbladder. *Lancet Oncol.* 2003;4(3):167–176.

27. Murakami Y, Uemura K, Sudo T, et al. Prognostic factors after surgical resection for intrahepatic, hilar, and distal cholangiocarcinoma. *Ann Surg Oncol.* 2011;18:651–658.

28. Nathan H, Aloia TA, Vauthey J-N, et al. A proposed staging system for intrahepatic cholangiocarcinoma. *Ann Surg Oncol.* 2009;16:14–22.

29. Nehls O, Oettle H, Hartmann JT, et al. Capecitabine plus oxaliplatin as first-line treatment in patients with advanced biliary system adenocarcinoma: a prospective multicenter phase II trial. *Br J Cancer.* 2008;98:309–315.

30. Nevin JE, Moran TJ, Kay S, et al. Carcinoma of the gallbladder, staging, treatment and prognosis. *Cancer.* 1976; 37:141–148.

31. Pawlik TM, Gleisner AL, Vigano L, et al. Incidence of finding residual disease for incidental gallbladder carcinoma: implications for re-resection. *J Gastrointest Surg.* 2007;11:1478–1486.

32. Philip P, Mahoney M, Allmer C, et al. Phase II Study of Erlotinib in patients with advanced biliary cancer. *J Clin Oncol.* 2006;24:3069–3074.

33. Randi G, Malvezzi M, Levi F, et al. Epidemiology of biliary tract cancers: an update. *Ann Oncol.* 2009;20:146–159.

34. Ries LAG, Melbert D, Krapcho M, et al. *SEER Cancer Statistics Review, 1975–2005.* Bethesda, MD: National Cancer Institute.

35. Rullier A, Le Bail B, Fawaz R, et al. Cytokeratin 7 and 20 expression in cholangiocarcinoma varies along the biliary tract but still differs from that in colorectal carcinoma metastasis. *Am J Surg Pathol.* 2000;24:870–876.

36. Sadamoto Y, Kubo H, Harada N, Tanaka M, Eguchi T, Nawata H. Preoperative diagnosis and staging of gallbladder carcinoma by EUS. *Gastrointest Endosc.* 2003;58:536–541.

37. Siegal R, Naishadham D, Jemal A. Cancer statistics, 2013. *CA Cancer J Clin.* 2013;63:11–30.

38. Thongprasert S, Napapan S, Charoentum C, Moonpraken S. Phase II study of gemcitabine and cisplatin as first-line chemotherapy in inoperable biliary tract carcinoma. *Ann Oncol.* 2005;16:279–281.

39. Primrose JN, Fox R, Palmer DH, et al. Adjuvant capecitabine for biliary tract cancer: The BILCAP randomized study. *J Clin Oncol.* 2017;35:15_suppl; 4006.

40. Valle J, Wasan H, Palmer DH, et al. Cisplatin plus gemcitabine versus gemcitabine for biliary tract cancer. *N Engl J Med.* 2010;362:1273–1281.

41. Welzel TM, Graubard BI, El-Serag HB, et al. Risk factors for intrahepatic and extrahepatic cholangiocarcinoma in the United States: a population-based case–control study. *Clin Gastroenterol Hepatol.* 2007;5(10):1221–1228.
42. Yee K, Sheppard BC, Domreis J, et al. Cancers of the gallbladder and biliary ducts. *Oncology.* 2002;16:939–957.
43. Zhu AX, Meyerhardt JA, Blaszkowsky LS, et al. Efficacy and safety of gemcitabine, oxaliplatin, and bevacizumab in advanced biliary-tract cancers and correlation of changes in 18-fluorodeoxyglucose PET with clinical outcome: a phase 2 study. *Lancet Oncol.* 2010;11(1):48–54.

7 Primary Cancers of the Liver

Bassam Estfan and Alok A. Khorana

INTRODUCTION

Hepatocellular carcinoma (HCC) arises from hepatocytes and is the most common type of primary liver cancer, generally occurring in the setting of cirrhosis. It is a leading cause of global cancer death. Intrahepatic cholangiocarcinoma arises from hepatic biliary epithelium. Secondary or metastatic cancer to the liver is the most common type of malignancy discovered in the liver. This section will focus on HCC.

EPIDEMIOLOGY

- Hepatocellular carcinoma is the sixth most common cancer, and second leading cause of death from cancer around the world. In the United States it is the thirteenth most common cancer but the fourth leading cause of cancer death.
- The highest incidence is in Asia and Africa, correlating with prevalence of Hepatitis B virus (HBV) infection. China accounts for more than 50% of global cases.
- In the United States the incidence has risen steadily since early 1980s but appears to have plateaued after 2010.
    - Incidence of HCC in the United States between 2008 and 2013 is 13 per 100,000 for men and 4.4 per 100,000 for women (http://seer.cancer.gov/statfacts/html/livibd.html).
    - Black, Hispanics, Pacific Islanders, and American Indians have higher incidence rates than White and non-Hispanics.
- Thirty-six percent of new cases are diagnosed between the ages of 55 and 65.
- In 2016, 39,230 new primary liver cancer cases and 27,170 deaths are expected in the United States.
- The 5-year overall survival (OS) for all stages is 17%.

ETIOLOGY

- In high incidence global regions, chronic HBV infection is the major risk factor for HCC. The risk increases with cirrhosis and higher serum levels of HBV DNA.
- HBV can lead to HCC through cirrhosis or integration into host DNA.
- In lower incidence regions such as the United States, cirrhosis due to chronic hepatitis C virus (HCV) infection, alcohol abuse, and non-alcoholic fatty liver disease plays a major role in hepatocellular carcinoma development.
    - HCV infection accounts for up to 50% of HCC cases in the United States.
    - Alcoholic cirrhosis accounts for 15% of HCC cases and commonly coexists with chronic HCV infection.
- Other less common etiologies include hemochromatosis, α1-antitrypsin deficiency, and aflatoxin exposure.
- Five-year cumulative risk of developing HCC in cirrhotic patients ranges from 5% to 30% depending on region, cause of cirrhosis, and degree of liver inflammation/cirrhosis.

CLINICAL FEATURES

▪ Hepatocellular carcinoma is commonly asymptomatic and is either incidentally found, or discovered during screening in cirrhotic patients.
▪ Symptoms are usually a sign of advanced disease (pain, constitutional symptoms), and most accompanying symptoms are due to cirrhosis or co-existing hepatic disease.
▪ HCC is usually confined to liver, but the risk of metastases increases with larger tumor size and vascular involvement.
  ◦ Common metastatic sites are regional lymph nodes, lung, and bone.
  ◦ There is a very small risk (<3%) of needle track seeding in abdominal wall following percutaneous biopsy.
▪ Acute pain with large and/or superficial tumors in the liver may indicate rupture.

DIAGNOSIS

▪ Diagnosis is usually suspected in patients with known cirrhosis with abnormal routine screening ultrasound of the liver and/or alpha-fetoprotein (AFP) serum levels.
▪ The American Association for the Study of Liver Disease has issued guidelines outlining the diagnosis, staging, and management of HCC.
▪ **Screening**
  ◦ At-risk population should be screened with liver ultrasound every 6 months.
  ◦ Abnormal liver ultrasound should be followed by dedicated liver sectional imaging such as computed tomography scan (CT), or magnetic resonance imaging (MRI).
  ◦ Alpha-fetoprotein (AFP) use for screening is controversial but commonly used; AFP has ineffective sensitivity and specificity for screening.
▪ **Liver Imaging**
  ◦ A multiphasic CT scan or MRI is indicated when HCC is suspected (arterial, venous, delayed phases).
  ◦ Organ Procurement and Transplantation Network (OPTN) has devised new imaging classification system for transplant listing approval.
    ◦ HCC compatible lesions are referred to as OPTN5 lesions.
  ◦ Characteristic HCC lesions show arterial phase enhancement and venous or delayed phase washout at risk population in lesions larger than 2 cm.
    ◦ Lesions less than 1 cm should be followed every 3 months.
    ◦ Lesions between 1 and 2 cm should have a pseudo-capsule in addition to meet diagnostic criteria.
  ◦ If first imaging modality was not confirmatory (CT or MRI) and suspicion was high, a diagnosis can be made if the other imaging modality shows characteristic OPTN5 lesions.
  ◦ The United Network for Organ Sharing allows only biopsy proven or OPTN5 lesions for orthotopic liver transplantation (OLT) approval.
▪ **Liver Biopsy**
  ◦ Liver biopsy is indicated for suspicious lesions when diagnosis cannot be confirmed radiologically, or if alternative diagnoses are suspected.
  ◦ Percutaneous biopsies should be avoided as much as possible especially in those who may be candidate for OLT due to risk of needle track seeding and abdominal wall recurrence.
▪ **AFP**
  ◦ The presence of a liver mass with cirrhosis and an AFP >400 ng/mL is usually indicative of HCC. This is not acceptable for OLT listing. Liver disease and cholangiocarcinoma can also elevate AFP.
  ◦ AFP is neither sensitive nor specific for diagnosis.
  ◦ AFP can be normal in up to 40% of cases.

PATHOLOGY

- Hepatocellular carcinoma is the most common primary liver cancer accounting for 80% to 90%, followed by intrahepatic cholangiocarcinoma (10% to 20%).
- Other rare primary liver malignancies include fibrolamellar carcinoma (a subtype of HCC), hepatoblastoma, angiosarcoma, hemangiosarcoma, and epithelioid hemangioendothelioma.
- Although rare, liver metastases should be suspected in cirrhotic patients with liver lesions not meeting radiological characteristics of HCC.
- HCCs are vascular tumors and are frequently associated with micro- or macrovascular invasion.

STAGING

- Multiple staging systems have been developed for HCC.
- Although the American Joint Committee on Cancer (AJCC) TNM staging system is prognostic, it lacks incorporation of liver function and functional status.
- Other staging systems such as Okuda, Cancer of the Liver Italian Program (CLIP), and Barcelona Clinic Liver Cancer (BCLC) have incorporated elements pertaining to liver function.
- The BCLC staging system is the most widely used and incorporates elements of cancer size, number, Child-Pugh score, and performance status with implications in regards to treatment options (Fig. 7.1).
- Child Pugh scoring system is key in assessment of liver health and determining management options (Table 7.1).
  - Child Pugh class corresponds to expected 1- and 2-year survival.

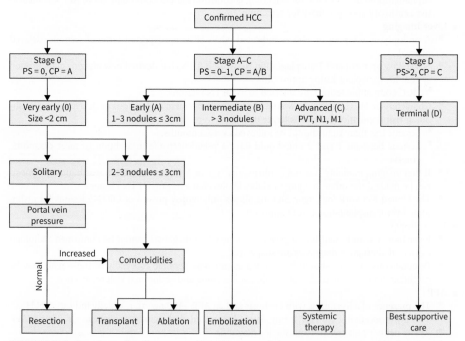

FIGURE 7.1 Barcelona clinic liver cancer (BCLC) hepatocellular carcinoma staging classification. The BCLC algorithm incorporates liver function, tumor characteristics, performance status and comorbidities in staging and treatment assignment. (Adapted from Bruix J, Sherman M. Management of hepatocellular carcinoma: an update. *Hepatology*. 2011;53:1020–1022.)

TABLE 7.1 Child Pugh Classification

Score Attribution	1	2	3
Bilirubin (mg/dL)	<2	2–3	>3
Albumin (g/dL)	>3.5	2.8–3.5	<2.8
INR (or PT)	<1.7 (<4)	1.7–2.3 (4–6)	>2.3 (>6)
Ascites	None	Mild (or medically suppressed)	Moderate to severe (or refractory)
Encephalopathy grade	None	1–2	3–4

Class A: score 5–6, Class B: score 7–9, Class C: score 10–15.

One and two year survival are 100% and 85% for Class A, 81% and 57% for Class B, and 45% and 35% for Class C, respectively.

INR, international normalization ratio; PT, prothrombin time.

TREATMENT

Surgery

- Surgery is the main curative option for HCC whether through resection or transplantation.
- Candidacy for surgery is determined by liver function, presence of portal hypertension, tumor burden (see Fig. 7.1), and to a certain extent anatomical location of lesions.
- Those who undergo surgery should have liver confined disease, no macrovascular invasion, and no regional lymph node involvement. Except in highly select situations, metastatic disease is a contraindication to surgery.
- **Hepatic resection**
  - Resection can be curative for those with liver-confined disease without underlying cirrhosis or fibrosis.
  - Cirrhotic patients without portal hypertension may be eligible for resection, but are still at risk of de novo HCC.
  - Five-year survival is 50% to 70%. Factors affecting survival include size and number of lesions.
  - Risk of recurrence at 5 years can be as high as 70% (60% intrahepatic metastases, 40% de novo HCC).
- **Liver transplantation**
  - Liver transplantation is the mainstay of curative management for patients with both HCC and cirrhosis.
  - Candidates for transplantation should meet Milan selection criteria:
    - One lesion ≤5 cm, or up to three lesions each ≤3 cm
    - No macrovascular invasion or portal vein thrombosis
    - No regional lymph node involvement or metastatic disease
  - Liver transplantation is dependent on available cadaveric livers. Living donor transplantation is another viable option.
  - For HCC within Milan criteria, OLT is associated with 4-year OS of 70% and recurrence free survival of 80%.
  - In the United States, eligible patients should have OPTN5 lesions, and can only be given exception points for enlisting after a period of 6 months of controlled or stable disease.
  - Locoregional control with chemoembolization is frequently used as "bridging" therapy awaiting transplantation.
  - Patients with chronic viral hepatitis infections should be treated with goal of sustained viral response prior to transplantation.

- **Postsurgical surveillance**
  - Imaging of chest, liver, and pelvis every 3 to 6 months for 2 years, then annually.
  - AFP ever 3 to 6 months for 2 years then every 6 months

Locoregional treatment

- Locoregional therapies for HCC can be employed with curative (ablation) or palliative intent for local control (embolization). They can also be used to maintain local control awaiting OLT.
- **Ablative therapy**
  - These include percutaneous ethanol injection (PEI), radiofrequency ablation (RFA), and microwave ablation (MWA).
  - RFA and MWA can be done percutaneously or laparascopically.
  - PEI is less commonly used in recent years.
  - RFA or MWA are very effective for local control in lesions <2 cm.
  - Local recurrence can be as high as 50% to 70%.
  - Factors influencing recurrence include larger size, proximity to major vessels, subcapsular lesions, percutaneous approach, and ablation margin <1 cm.
  - Best candidates are those with very early or early BCLC stage who are not candidate for resection.
  - Needle tract seeding recurrence can occur in up to 3% after RFA, especially with repeat intervention and treatment of subcapsular lesions.
- **Hepatic artery embolization**
  - Transarterial chemoembolization (TACE) and bland embolization are effective means of locoregional control of liver confined HCC, but are not considered curative interventions.
  - Eighty percent of HCC vascular supply is derived from hepatic artery branches; in contrast, normal liver parenchyma receives its main vascular supply from the portal vein.
  - TACE has been shown to improve survival compared to best supportive care with 2-year survival rate of 63% versus 27%, respectively.
  - TACE is commonly done using drug-eluting beads (DEBs) laden with doxorubicin.
    - A randomized trial of conventional TACE compared to DEBs in unresectable HCC showed better local control (44% vs. 52% at 6 months, respectively) and lower rate of toxicity in favor of DEB/TACE.
  - There is continued controversy in regards to the added benefit of chemotherapy to bead therapy.
  - Suitable patients are those with relatively preserved liver function (Child Pugh Class A-B), unresectable disease, "bridging" therapy prior to transplantation. Chemoembolization often requires more than one treatment for optimal local control.
  - TACE may be used with the intent of "down-staging" to meet Milan criteria.
  - There is no role for systemic therapy in conjunction with TACE per the SPACE phase II trial.
- **Radioembolization**
  - Hepatocellular carcinoma is radiosensitive but is also located in a radiosensitive organ. Normal liver can tolerate radiation up to about 20 Gy.
  - Radioembolization utilizes Yttrium-90 microspheres. Resin and glass microspheres are commercially available.
  - Glass microspheres have an FDA humanitarian device exemption approval for unresectable HCC.
  - A mapping hepatic artery angiogram is an important first step to rule out vascular shunting prior to therapy. Radiation pneumonitis is a major complication with large pulmonary radiation shunting.
  - It is generally contraindicated in decompensated hepatic function, and if bilirubin is >2 mg/dL.
  - Radiation segmentectomy is a method whereby the radiation dose is selectively delivered to one or two segments instead of the whole lobe. This allows higher radiation dose exposure leading to better tumor necrosis and local control.
  - There is indication overlap with chemoembolization. Larger lesions, significant lobar involvement, or diffuse disease are usually indications for radioembolization. Deciding the best locoregional therapeutic intervention should be done in a multidisciplinary tumor board setting.

Radiation

■ Stereotactic body radiation therapy (SBRT) is a precise and conformal way of delivering external radiation in high dosage to a specific area. In radiosensitive tumors SBRT has a high success rate of achieving local control.

■ SBRT for hepatocellular carcinoma is a plausible option in small (preferably less than 5 cm) lesions not amenable to locoregional therapy or ablation. Anatomically challenging location for ablation such as liver dome can be treated with SBRT.

■ Tumor thrombus (especially symptomatic) can also be treated with SBRT in combination with other locoregional treatment.

■ In one series, local control rate with or without TACE was 96% with an overall survival rate of 67% at 3 years.

Systemic Therapy

■ Systemic therapy for HCC is indicated in advanced disease not amenable to locoregional treatment, or metastatic disease. The goal of therapy is palliation with the main benefit being increase in life expectancy.

■ Patients with advanced HCC should be considered for clinical trials when possible.

■ While chemotherapy has been associated with low rates of partial response in certain series, it has not been shown to improve survival.

■ Sorafenib is a multikinase inhibitor with antiangiogenic properties. It targets RAF-1, BRAF, VGEFR1, 2, and 3, and PDGFR-β. It is the only FDA-approved drug for treatment of advanced HCC in the United States. It has mainly been studied in Child Pugh Class A cirrhosis.

■ In the SHARP trial, patients with advanced HCC and Child Pugh Class A cirrhosis where randomized to placebo or sorafenib at 400 mg twice daily. Survival was significantly improved with placebo (10.7 vs. 7.9 months). The Asia-Pacific trial used a similar design in Asian population and a statistically significant improvement in survival was also noted in favor of sorafenib (6.5 vs. 4.2 months).

■ Response rates are 2% to 3%; about 70% will have stable disease at follow-up.

■ Side effects of sorafenib include fatigue, diarrhea, hypertension, mouth sores, bone marrow, and hepatic toxicity. Palmar plantar erythema (hand-foot syndrome) can occur in up to 45% of patients. At least 30% will require dose reduction due to side effects.

■ Sorafenib should be used with caution in patient with Child Pugh Class B cirrhosis.

■ Other targeted therapies have been tried in HCC including sunitinib, brivanib, erlotinib, everolimus, linifanib, and ramucirumab. None have proven to be more effective or tolerable than sorafenib. Sunitinib was actually associated with worse survival.

■ There is no adjuvant role for sorafenib after curative intent resection or ablation. The STROM trial showed no difference in recurrence-free survival between adjuvant sorafenib and placebo given up to 4 years.

■ Sorafenib was studied in conjunction with TACE in locally advanced HCC in the phase II SPACE trial. There was no difference in time to progression between sorafenib and placebo.

■ In a randomized clinical trial of regorafenib versus placebo in patients with preserved liver function who had progressive hepatocellular carcinoma on sorafenib, regorafenib was associated with statistically significant improvement in survival (10.6 vs. 7.8 months, respectively). Nivolumab is a PD-1 monoclonal antibody, which has shown activity in HCC after progression on sorafenib. It was well tolerated and was associated with response rate of 20% and a 9 months survival rate of 74%. It has been approved for advanced HCC in the second-line setting.

Suggested Readings

1. Brown KT, Do RK, Gonen M, et al. Randomized trial of hepatic artery embolization for hepatocellular carcinoma using doxorubicin-eluting microspheres compared with embolization with microspheres alone. *J Clin Oncol.* 2016;34(17):2046–2053.

2. Bruix J, Qin S, Merle P, et al. Regorafenib for patients with hepatocellular carcinoma who progressed on sorafenib treatment (RESORCE): a randomised, double-blind, placebo-controlled, phase 3 trial. *Lancet.* 2017;389(10064):56–66.

3. Bruix J, Sherman M. Management of hepatocellular carcinoma: an update. *Hepatology.* 2011;53:1020–1022.

4. Bruix J, Takayama T, Mazzaferro V, et al. Adjuvant sorafenib for hepatocellular carcinoma after resection or ablation (STORM): a phase 3, randomised, double-blind, placebo-controlled trial. *Lancet Oncol.* 2015;16(13):1344–1354.
5. El-Khoueiry AB, Sangro B, Yau T, et al. Nivolumab in patients with advanced hepatocellular carcinoma (CheckMate 040): an open-label, non-comparative, phase 1/2 dose escalation and expansion trial. *Lancet.* 2017;389(10088):2492–2502.
6. El-Serag HB. Hepatocellular carcinoma. *N Engl J Med.* 2011;365:1118–1127.
7. Hickey RM, Lewandowski RJ, Salem R. Yttrium-90 radioembolization for hepatocellular carcinoma. *Semin Nucl Med.* 2016;46(2):105–108.
8. Lencioni R, Llovett JM, Han G, et al. Sorafenib or placebo plus TACE with doxorubicin-eluting beads for intermediate stage HCC: the SPACE trial. *J Hepatol.* 2016;64(5):1090–1098.
9. Llovet JM, Ricci S, Mazzaferro V, et al. Sorafenib in advanced hepatocellular carcinoma. *N Engl J Med.* 2008;359(4)378–390.
10. Llovet JM, Schwartz M, Mazzaferro V. Resection and liver transplantation for hepatocellular carcinoma. *Semin Liver Dis.* 2005;25(2); 181–200.
11. Lovet JM, Real MI, Montana X, et al. Arterial embolisation or chemoembolisation versus symptomatic treatment in patients with unresectable hepatocellular carcinoma: a randomised controlled trial. *Lancet.* 2002;359(9319):1734–1739.
12. Mazzaferro V, Regalia E, Doci R, et al. Liver transplantation for the treatment of small hepatocellular carcinomas in patients with cirrhosis. *N Engl J Med.* 1996;334(11):693–699.
13. McGlynn KA, Petrick JL, London WT. Global epidemiology of hepatocellular carcinoma: an emphasis on demographic and regional variability. *Clin Liver Dis.* 2015 May;19(2):223–238.
14. Riaz A, Gate VL, Atassi B, et al. Radiation segmentectomy: a novel approach to increase safety and efficacy of radioembolization. *Int J Radiat Oncol Biol Phys.* 2011;79(1):163–171.
15. Takeda A, Sanuki N, Tsurugai Y, et al. Phase 2 study of stereotactic body radiotherapy and optional transarterial chemoembolization for solitary hepatocellular carcinoma not amenable to resection and radiofrequency ablation. *Cancer.* 2016;122(13):2041–2049.
16. Wald C, Russo MW, Heimbach JK, et al. New OPTN/UNOS policy for liver transplant allocation: standardization of liver imaging, diagnosis, classification, and reporting of hepatocellular carcinoma. *Radiology.* 2013;266(2):376–382.

Gastrointestinal Stromal Tumors (GIST) 8

Dale R. Shepard and Alok A. Khorana

Gastrointestinal stromal tumors (GIST) are the most common mesenchymal tumors in the gastrointestinal tract. Most GIST tumors have a mutation in the proto-oncogene *KIT* or platelet-derived growth factor receptor alpha (*PDGFRA*) genes. Ideally, these tumors are resected, which is curative for many patients. The development of targeted therapies that inhibit *KIT* and *PDGFRA* has revolutionized recurrence after surgery and the treatment of metastatic disease.

EPIDEMIOLOGY

The incidence of GIST in the United States is approximately 7 to 20 per 1,000,000 people leading to 4000 to 6000 new cases annually. The majority of cases are sporadic with patients having no family history of GIST. In a SEER registry, the median age at diagnosis was 63 years of age. There are no established risk factors for the development of most GIST, although some conditions, including neurofibromatosis-1 (NF-1), are associated with the development of GIST.

PATHOLOGY

GIST originate from interstitial cells of Cajal. It is important to differentiate GIST from other subepithelial tumors of the GI tract, including leiomyosarcoma, leiomyoma, and desmoid tumors. GIST can be identified by the presence of KIT overexpression, present in 95% of GIST, or *KIT* mutations that are present in 80% of GISTs. DOG-1 is another sensitive and specific marker for diagnosis of GIST. Among *KIT* mutations, 70% are found on exon 11 and 10% on exon 9; exons 13 and 17 are rarely involved. Alterations in KIT, a transmembrane receptor tyrosine kinase, lead to activation of the transmembrane receptor and abnormal cell signaling. These KIT alterations can be detected by immunohistochemistry with anti-CD117 antibodies. GIST tumors may also have mutations in *PDGFRA*. *PDGFRA* mutations are homologous to those responsible for KIT- and Flt-3L-independent kinase activation in other malignancies, including acute myeloid leukemia, mast cell disorders, and seminomas. KIT and PDGFRA mutations and overexpression are usually mutually exclusive in GIST. Thirty-five percent of KIT wild-type GISTs have PDGFRA mutations. Mutations in both KIT and PDGFRA lead to dysregulation of downstream intracellular signaling processes involving protein kinases and transcription factors such as AKT, MAPK, and STATs (STAT1 and STAT3), which play a critical role in the development and progression of cancer.

Morphologically, GIST are characterized as spindle cell type (70%), epithelioid (20%) or mixed (10%). GIST are most common in the stomach or duodenum, followed by the remainder of the small intestine, rectum, and esophagus. GIST may also be found in the colon, mesentery, or retroperitoneum, but this is much less common. About 10% to 20% of patients present with metastatic disease at the time of diagnosis, predominantly with involvement of the liver, omentum, or peritoneum.

CLINICAL PRESENTATION

Small GIST may be asymptomatic and are usually found incidentally during imaging or endoscopy studies. Larger tumors may cause symptoms related to their location.

- Pain
- Bloating
- Early satiety
- Bleeding

PROGNOSTIC FACTORS

Factors associated with an increased risk for recurrence of GIST include tumor size, mitotic index, tumor location, and presence of rupture of the tumor (Table 8.1). Based on these tumor characteristics, patients can be stratified into very low, low, intermediate, or high risk of recurrence. Tumors less than 2 cm have very low risk while tumors greater than 10 cm are associated with high risk. A mitotic index of ≤5 per 50 high power fields is associated with a very low or low risk for recurrence. A mitotic index of greater than 10 leads to a high risk. Tumor rupture is prognostic for a high risk of recurrence regardless of tumor size or mitotic index. Gastric GISTs are associated with a better outcome than GISTs in other locations.

DIAGNOSIS

Computerized tomography (CT) scans of the abdomen and pelvis with contrast or MRI are recommended for initial staging to determine the resectability of the tumor and to evaluate for metastatic disease. Endoscopy with ultrasound may be used to further characterize submucosal GI lesions and a fine needle aspiration during this procedure may be used to collect tissue for cytology and immunohistochemistry to establish a diagnosis. These biopsies are not required for patients who have a resectable tumor with a high degree of suspicion for GIST. A biopsy should be obtained in patients with clearly unresectable tumors or with tumors that may become resectable if treated with preoperative imatinib. Positron emission tomography (PET) scans are not routinely used for the diagnosis or monitoring of patients with GIST.

TABLE 8.1 Modified NIH Risk Stratification for Recurrence of GIST

Risk	Size (cm)	Mitotic Index (per 50 HPFs)	Primary Tumor Site
Very low	<2	≤5	Any
Low	2.1 to 5	≤5	Any
Intermediate	2.1 to 5	>5	Gastric
	<5	6 to 10	Any
	5.1 to 10	≤5	Gastric
High	Any	Any	Tumor rupture
	>10	Any	Any
	Any	>10	Any
	>5	>5	Any
	2.1 to 5	>5	Any
	2.1 to 5	>5	Nongastric
	5.1 to 10	≤5	Nongastric

HPFs, high-power fields. Adapted from Joensuu H. *Hum Pathol.* 2008;39:1411.

TREATMENT

Upfront resection is generally the standard for resectable disease in patients with no contraindications to surgery. Preoperative imatinib may impact the assessment of the risk of recurrence and should be reserved for patients in whom a decrease in the size of the tumor will minimize the morbidity of the surgery. Following resection of the tumor, patients with an intermediate or high risk of recurrence (Table 8.1) should start adjuvant therapy with imatinib for at least 3 years. Patients who received neoadjuvant imatinib followed by a complete resection and patients who have residual disease after surgery should receive postoperative imatinib. During treatment, patients should be seen in clinic with a CT of the abdomen and pelvis every 3 to 6 months for 3 to 5 years, with surveillance annually afterward. Approximately 60% of patients with resected GIST will be cured with surgery alone. The median time to recurrence after resection of a primary high-risk GIST is about 2 years; however, metastatic disease can develop several years after initial resection of the primary tumor necessitating long-term clinical follow-up.

Patients with unresectable or metastatic disease at the time of their diagnosis should start treatment with imatinib and have repeat imaging with CT scans after 3 months to assess treatment response. Patients with initially unresectable disease who have a response to imatinib should be assessed again for possible resection although downstaging with neoadjuvant therapy generally requires several months of treatment. Patients who continue to have unresectable tumors or who have metastatic disease with stable disease or a response to therapy should remain on imatinib indefinitely.

Patients with recurrent GIST should be treated with imatinib, if not given previously. Treatment options for patients with recurrence who have received prior imatinib or progression of their GIST while receiving imatinib include resection, embolization, radiofrequency ablation, or palliative radiation, escalation of the dose of imatinib, or alternative agents such as sunitinib and regorafenib. Mutational testing of the tumor may help with therapeutic decisions. Tumors with a KIT exon 9 mutation may be more likely to benefit from an increase in the dose of imatinib from 400 mg daily to 800 mg daily. GIST tumors with a PDGFRA D842V mutation or without a mutation in KIT or PDGFRA have a decreased likelihood of response to imatinib.

Patients with GIST tumors in the stomach measuring less than 2 cm without high risk EUS features, such as irregular borders, cystic spaces, ulceration, foci of echogenicity, and heterogeneity, may be managed by surveillance with endoscopy and may not require surgery.

ADJUVANT THERAPY

Imatinib is approved as adjuvant therapy for patients with GIST based on the results of the American College of Surgeons Oncology Group (ACOSOG) Intergroup Adjuvant GIST Study Z9001 study. In this phase III trial, 713 patients were randomized to 1 year of imatinib 400 mg daily or placebo following complete gross resection of a primary GIST expressing KIT measuring at least 3 cm. Upon recurrence, patients were allowed to crossover to from placebo to imatinib or increase the dose of imatinib to 800 mg daily. Recurrence-free survival (RFS) at 1 year, the primary endpoint of the trial, was 98% in the imatinib arm versus 83% in the placebo arm (P < 0.0001). Overall survival (OS) was not statistically significant between the two arms, likely due to the short-term follow-up and the crossover from placebo to imatinib. A subsequent study in patients with a high risk for recurrence showed an improvement in both 5-year RFS (65.6% vs. 47.9% (P<0001)) for patients receiving 3 years versus 1 year of imatinib, respectively. There was also an improvement in OS (92.0% vs. 81.7% in the 3-year and 1-year arms, respectively (P = 0.02)).

NEOADJUVANT THERAPY

A prospective phase II trial, RTOG 0132/ACRIN 6665, evaluated the safety and efficacy of neoadjuvant treatment with imatinib for 8 to 12 weeks before surgery with continuation of imatinib for at least 2 years after surgery or disease progression. Patients had a resectable KIT positive GIST measuring at least 5 cm. In patients with a primary GIST, there was a partial response in 7% of patients and stable disease in 83%. There was 5% partial response and stable disease in 91% of patients with resectable metastatic disease. With a median follow-up of 5 years, the PFS rate for patients with a primary tumor was 57% and OS rate was 77%. Complications of surgery and toxicity from the imatinib were minimal.

DRUGS USED FOR TREATING PATIENTS WITH GIST

Imatinib

Imatinib is a tyrosine kinase inhibitor of c-KIT and PDGFRA receptors. Imatinib is approved for patients with unresectable or metastatic KIT (CD117) positive GIST or for adjuvant treatment after resection of KIT positive GIST. Two large randomized phase III trials confirmed the efficacy of imatinib in patients with advanced GIST. In the S0033 trial, patients were randomized to receive either 400 mg of imatinib once daily (with crossover to 800 mg per day with disease progression) or 400 mg twice daily. The median OS was 55 months and 51 months for patients receiving 400 mg and 800 mg imatinib daily, respectively. There were no significant differences in response rates, PFS, or OS between the two groups. In a subgroup analysis of a retrospective analysis, patients with KIT exon 9 mutations receiving 800 mg imatinib daily had an improvement in PFS, but not in OS. Approximately 80% of patients eventually develop secondary mutations in KIT exons resulting in progressive disease. Patients should start therapy at 400 mg daily, and increase to 800 mg daily for patients with progression of disease or have the presence of an exon 9 KIT mutation. Treatment with imatinib is generally well tolerated with nausea, diarrhea, periorbital edema, muscle cramps, fatigue, headache, and dermatitis as the most common toxicities.

Sunitinib

Sunitinib is an oral inhibitor of several tyrosine kinase receptors approved for the patients with GIST after disease progression on or intolerance to imatinib. In a double-blind placebo-controlled, multicenter, randomized phase III trial, patients with GIST with disease progression on or intolerance to imatinib were randomized to receive sunitinib 50 mg daily for 4 weeks, with 2 weeks off ($n = 207$) or placebo ($n = 105$). Objective response rates in the sunitinib and placebo arms were 8% and 0%, respectively, and the median time to progression was significantly longer in the sunitinib arm (6.3 vs. 1.5 months).

Regorafenib

Regorafenib, an inhibitor of multiple tyrosine kinases including KIT and PDGFRA is approved for patients who have progressed after imatinib and sunitinib. In a randomized phase III trial, the median PFS was 4.8 months for patients receiving regorafenib and 0.9 months for patients receiving placebo (HR 0.27; $P < 0.0001$).

Suggested Readings

1. Blanke CD, Rankin C, Demetri GD, et al. Phase III randomized, intergroup trial assessing imatinib mesylate at two dose levels in patients with or metastatic gastrointestinal stromal tumors expressing the kit receptor tyrosine kinase: S0033. *J Clin Oncol.* 2008;26(4):626–632.
2. Choi H, Charnsangavej C, Faria SC, et al. Correlation of computed tomography and positron emission tomography in patients with metastatic gastrointestinal stromal tumor treated at a single institution with imatinib mesylate: proposal of new computed tomography response criteria. *J Clin Oncol.* 2007;25(13):1753–1759.
3. Dematteo RP, Ballman KV, Antonescu CR, et al. Adjuvant imatinib mesylate after resection of localised, primary gastrointestinal stromal tumour: a randomised, double-blind, placebo-controlled trial. *Lancet.* 2009;373(9669):1097–1104.
4. Demetri GD, Reichardt P, Kang YK, et al. Efficacy and safety of regorafenib for advanced gastrointestinal stromal tumours after failure of imatinib and sunitinib (GRID): an international, multicentre, randomised, placebo-controlled, phase 3 trial. *Lancet.* 2013;381(9863):295–302.
5. Demetri GD, van Oosterom AT, Garrett CR, et al. Efficacy and safety of sunitinib in patients with advanced gastrointestinal stromal tumour after failure of imatinib: a randomised controlled trial. *Lancet.* 2006;368(9544):1329–1338.

6. Demetri GD, von Mehren M, Blanke CD, et al. Efficacy and safety of imatinib mesylate in advanced gastrointestinal stromal tumors. *N Engl J Med.* 2002;347(7):472–480.
7. Eisenberg BL, Harris J, Blanke CD, et al. Phase II trial of neoadjuvant/adjuvant imatinib mesylate (IM) for advanced primary and metastatic/recurrent operable gastrointestinal stromal tumor (GIST): early results of RTOG 0132/ACRIN 6665. *J Surg Oncol.* 2009;99(1):42–47.
8. Fletcher CD, Berman JJ, Corless C, et al. Diagnosis of gastrointestinal stromal tumors: a consensus approach. *Int J Surg Pathol.* 2002;10(2): 81–89.
9. Heinrich MC, Corless CL, Duensing A. et al. PDGFRA activating mutations in gastrointestinal stromal tumors. *Science.* 2003;299:708–710.
10. Heinrich MC, Owzar K, Corless CL, et al. Correlation of kinase genotype and clinical outcome in the North American Intergroup Phase III Trial of imatinib mesylate for treatment of advanced gastrointestinal stromal tumor: CALGB 150105 Study by Cancer and Leukemia Group B and Southwest Oncology Group. *J Clin Oncol.* 2008;26(33):5360–5367.
11. Joensuu H, Eriksson M, Sundby Hall K, et al. One vs three years of adjuvant imatinib for operable gastrointestinal stromal tumor: a randomized trial. *JAMA.* 2012;307(12):1265–1272.
12. Joensuu H, Roberts PJ, Sarlomo-Rikala M, et al. Effect of the tyrosine kinase inhibitor STI571 in a patient with a metastatic gastrointestinal stromal tumor. *N Engl J Med.* 2001;344(14):1052–1056.
13. Joensuu H, Vehtari A, Riihimäki J, et al. Risk of gastrointestinal stromal tumour recurrence after surgery: an analysis based on pooled population-based cohorts. *Lancet Oncol.* 2012;13(3):265–274.
14. Medeiros F, Corless CL, Duensing A, et al. KIT-negative gastrointestinal stromal tumors: proof of concept and therapeutic implications. *Am J Surg Path.* 2004;28:889–894.
15. Rubin BP, Fletcher JA, Fletcher CD. Molecular insights into the histiogenesis and pathogenesis of gastrointestinal stromal tumors. *Int J Surg Pathol* 2000;8:5–10.
16. Rubin BP, Singer S, Tsao C, et al. KIT activation is a ubiquitous feature of gastrointestinal stromal tumors. *Cancer Res.* 2001;61:8118–8121.
17. Tran T, Davila JA, El-Serag HH. The epidemiology of malignant gastrointestinal stromal tumors: an analysis of 1,458 case from 1992 to 2000. *Am J Gastroenterol.* 2005;100:162–168.
18. Verweij J, Casali PG, Zalcberg J, et al. Progression-free survival in gastrointestinal stromal tumours with high-dose imatinib: randomised trial. *Lancet.* 2004;364(9440):1127–1134.
19. Von Mehren M, Randall RL, Benjamin RS, et al. Gastrointestinal stromal tumors, version 2.2014. *J Natl Compr Canc Netw.* 2014;12:853–862.

9 Colorectal Cancer

Jason S. Starr and Thomas J. George, Jr.

EPIDEMIOLOGY

- Colorectal cancer (CRC) is the second leading cause of cancer deaths among men and women combined in the United States and is the third most common cause of cancer, separately, in men and in women.
- An estimated 135,430 cases of CRC (70% colon; 30% rectal) will be diagnosed in 2017, and over one-third will die as a result of the disease.
- The lifetime risk of developing CRC for both men and women is 5%.
- Surgery will cure almost 50% of all diagnosed patients; however, 40% to 50% of newly diagnosed CRC cases will eventually develop metastatic disease.
- The incidence of colon cancer is higher in the more economically developed regions, such as the United States or Western Europe, than in Asia, Africa, or South America.
- US incidence and mortality rates from CRC continue to decline among patients 50 years of age or older (4.5% decrease per year from 2008 to 2012). On the contrary, incidence rates have increased among patients younger than age 50 (1.8% increase per year from 2008 to 2012). The reason for this increase in younger adults is unclear.

RISK FACTORS

Although certain conditions predispose patients to develop colon cancer, up to 70% of patients have no identifiable risk factors:

- Age: More than 90% of colon cancers occur in patients older than 50 years.
- Gender: The incidence of colon cancer is similar in men and women, but rectal cancer is more prominent in men.
- Ethnicity: The occurrence of CRC is more common in African Americans than in whites, and mortality is nearly 45% higher in African Americans compared to whites.
- Personal history of CRC or adenomatous polyps:
  - Tubular adenomas (lowest risk)
  - Tubulovillous adenomas (intermediate risk)
  - Villous adenomas (highest risk)
- Tobacco use is associated with increased incidence and mortality from CRC compared to never smokers. The association is stronger for rectal cancers.
- Obesity: Two prospective cohort studies show a 1.5-fold increased risk of CRC in people that have a high body mass index (BMI) compared to that in normal.
- Dietary factors: High-fiber, low caloric intake, and low animal fat diets may reduce the risk of cancer.
- Calcium deficiency: Daily intake of 1.25 to 2.0 g of calcium was associated with a reduced risk of recurrent adenomas in a randomized placebo-controlled trial. Oral bisphosphonate therapy for at least 1 year's duration may also reduce CRC risk.

- Vitamin D: There is no prospective evidence that vitamin D supplementation reduces risk of colorectal adenomas or cancer although a meta-analysis of five studies showed that patients with CRC and higher levels of vitamin D had improved overall survival and disease-specific mortality.
- Micronutrient deficiency: Selenium and vitamins E and D deficiency may increase the risk of cancer. The role of folate remains unclear.
- Inflammatory bowel disease (IBD): IBD is associated with a 2.9-fold increase risk of CRC. The risk of CRC is associated with duration of IBD.
- Nonsteroidal anti-inflammatory drugs: An American Cancer Society study reported 40% lower mortality in regular aspirin users, and similar reductions in mortality were seen in prolonged nonsteroidal anti-inflammatory drug use in patients with rheumatologic disorders. The cyclooxygenase-2 (COX-2) inhibitor celecoxib is approved by the U.S. Food and Drug Administration (FDA) for adjunctive treatment of patients with familial adenomatous polyposis (FAP). Chemoprevention with selective COX-2 inhibitors must be balanced against increased cardiovascular risks.
- Family history: 80% of colon cancer cases are diagnosed in the absence of a positive family history. In the general population, if one first-degree relative develops cancer, it increases the relative risk for other family members to 1.72, and if two relatives are affected, the relative risk increases to 2.75. Increased risk is also observed when a first-degree relative develops an adenomatous polyp before age 60. True hereditary forms of cancer account for only 6% of CRCs.

FAMILIAL CANCER SYNDROMES

Familial Adenomatous Polyposis

FAP is an autosomal-dominant inherited syndrome with more than 90% penetrance, manifested by hundreds of polyps developing by late adolescence. The risk of developing invasive cancer over time is virtually 100%. Germline mutations in the adenomatous polyposis coli (APC) gene on chromosome 5q21 have been identified. The loss of the APC gene results in altered signal transduction with increased transcriptional activity of β-catenin. Several FAP variants with extraintestinal manifestations also exist:

- Attenuated FAP: This variant generates flat adenomas that arise at an older age. Mutations tend to occur in the proximal and distal portions of the APC gene.
- Gardner's syndrome: Associated with desmoid tumors, osteomas, lipomas, and fibromas of the mesentery or abdominal wall.
- Turcot's syndrome: Involves tumors (esp. medulloblastoma) of the central nervous system.
- Peutz–Jeghers syndrome: Includes non-neoplastic hamartomatous polyps throughout the gastrointestinal tract and perioral melanin pigmentation.
- Juvenile polyposis: Associated with hamartomas in colon, small bowel, and stomach.

Hereditary Nonpolyposis Colorectal Cancer (Lynch Syndrome)

The Lynch syndromes, named after Henry T. Lynch, include Lynch I or the colonic syndrome, which is an autosomal-dominant trait characterized by distinct clinical features, including proximal colon involvement, mucinous or poorly differentiated histology, pseudodiploidy, and the presence of synchronous or metachronous tumors. Patients develop colon cancer before 50 years, with a lifetime risk of cancer approximating 75%. In Lynch II or the extracolonic syndrome, individuals are susceptible to malignancies in the endometrium, ovary, stomach, hepatobiliary tract, small intestine, and genitourinary tract.

The Amsterdam criteria (3-2-1 rule) were established to identify potential kindreds and include the following:

- Histologically verified CRC in at least three family members, one being a first-degree relative of the other two members
- CRC involving at least two successive generations
- At least one family member being diagnosed by 50 years

Inclusion of extracolonic tumors and clinicopathologic and age modifications was introduced by the Bethesda criteria in 1997 and subsequently revised to account for microsatellite instability (MSI). Lynch syndrome is characterized by germline defects in DNA mismatch–repair genes (e.g., *hMLH1*, *hMSH2*, *hMSH6*, and *hPMS2*). These defects result in alterations to the length of microsatellites, segments of DNA with repeating nucleotide sequences, thus making them unstable and detectable in diagnostic assays. This MSI can be identified in virtually all Lynch syndrome kindred and in approximately 15% of sporadic CRCs.

SCREENING

Several professional societies have developed screening guidelines for the early detection of colon cancer. There are a number of early detection tests for colon cancer in average-risk asymptomatic patients. The American Cancer Society and US Preventative Service Task Force (USPSTF) screening guidelines (Table 9.1) are the most widely cited. The USPSTF does not endorse one test over the other, only that some form of recommended screening be done. Beginning at age 50, both men and women should discuss the full range of testing options with their physician. Any positive or abnormal screening test should be followed up with colonoscopy. Individuals with a family or personal history of colon cancer or polyps, or a history of chronic IBD, should be tested earlier and possibly more often.

PATHOPHYSIOLOGY

More than 90% of CRCs are adenocarcinomas, the focus of this chapter. Other primary cancers of the colon and rectum include Kaposi's sarcoma, non-Hodgkin lymphomas, small cell carcinoma, and carcinoid tumors. Metastases to the large bowel can rarely occur with melanoma, ovarian, and gastric cancer.

Colon carcinogenesis involves progression from hyperproliferative mucosa to polyp formation, with dysplasia, and transformation to noninvasive lesions and subsequent tumor cells, with invasive and metastatic capabilities. CRC is a unique model of multistep carcinogenesis resulting from the accumulation of multiple genetic alterations. Stage-by-stage molecular analysis has revealed that this progression involves several types of genetic instability, including loss of heterozygosity, with chromosomes 8p, 17p, and 18q representing the most common chromosomal losses. The 17p deletion accounts for loss of p53 function, and 18q contains the tumor-suppressor genes deleted in colon cancer (i.e., DCC) and the gene deleted in pancreatic 4 (i.e., DPC4).

TABLE 9.1 Recommended Colorectal Cancer Screening Guidelines for Asymptomatic Average-Risk Individuals Beginning at Age 50, All Patients at Average Risk of Colorectal Cancer Should Have *One* of the Screening Options Listed Below.[a]

Test	Frequency
Guaiac-based fecal occult blood test (gFOBT) or fecal immunochemical test (FIT)	Every year
Multitarget stool DNA	Every 3 y
Colonoscopy[b]	Every 10 y
Flexible sigmoidoscopy	Every 5 y
Flexible sigmoidoscopy with FIT	Flex sigmoidoscopy every 10 y, FIT every year
CT colonography (virtual colonoscopy)	Every 5 y

[a] 2016 USPSTF Recommendations did not specify which screening approach is preferred.

[b] Colonoscopy should be done if the fecal blood test shows blood in the stool or if sigmoidoscopy shows a polyp. This colonoscopy is considered a screening completion colonoscopy.

Colon carcinogenesis also occurs as a consequence of defects in the DNA mismatch–repair system (dMMR). The loss of *hMLH1* and *hMSH2*, predominantly, in sporadic cancers leads to accelerated accumulation of additions or deletions in DNA. This MSI contributes to the loss of growth inhibition mediated by transforming growth factor-β due to a mutation in the type II receptor. Mutations in the APC gene on chromosome 5q21 are responsible for FAP and are involved in cell signaling and in cellular adhesion, with binding of β-catenin. Alterations in the APC gene occur early in tumor progression. Mutations in the proto-oncogene *ras* family, including K-*ras* and N-*ras*, are important for transformation and also are common in early tumor development.

DIAGNOSIS

Signs and Symptoms

The presentation of CRC can include abdominal pain, which is typically intermittent and vague, weight loss, early satiety, and/or fatigue. Bowel changes may be noted for left-sided colon and rectal cancers, including constipation, decreased stool caliber (pencil stools), and tenesmus. Bowel obstruction or perforation is less common. Unusual presentations include deep venous thrombosis, nephrotic-range proteinuria, and *Streptococcus bovis* bacteremia with or without endocarditis. The clinical finding of iron deficiency in the absence of an overt source should prompt a diagnostic endoscopic workup.

Diagnostic Evaluation

- Endoscopic studies provide histologic information, potential therapeutic intervention, and overall greater sensitivity and specificity.
- CEA elevations occur in non–cancer-related conditions, reducing the specificity of CEA measurements alone in the initial detection of colon cancer.
- Basic laboratory studies including complete blood count, electrolytes, liver and renal function tests, and CT scan of the chest, abdomen, and pelvis with IV contrast are useful in initial cancer diagnosis and staging.
- In colon cancers, CT scan sensitivity for detecting distant metastasis is higher (75% to 87%) than for detecting nodal involvement (45% to 73%) or the extent of local invasion (~50%).
- FDG-PET scanning adds little over conventional imaging in the initial staging and diagnosis of CRC in the absence of abnormalities seen on CT scan.
- Contrast-enhanced magnetic resonance imaging (MRI) can help determine the status of suspicious lesions in the liver as well as the characteristics (not just size) of rectal cancers.
- For rectal cancers, endoscopic rectal ultrasound (ERUS) is a valuable tool in the preoperative evaluation, with high accuracy of determining the extent of the primary tumor (sensitivity 63% to 95%) and perirectal nodal status (sensitivity 63% to 82%). However, as compared to ERUS, MRI can better visualize proximal tumors and allow for noninvasive evaluation of circumferential (i.e., obstructing) tumors. Additionally, MRI can better characterize the perirectal lymph nodes and approximate the tumor to the pelvic side wall.

STAGING

The eighth edition of the American Joint Committee on Cancer Staging for CRC uses the TNM classification system. The Dukes or MAC staging systems are only of historic interest. The tumor designation, or T stage, defines the extent of bowel wall penetration including invasion into the submucosa (T1), muscularis propria (T2), pericolic tissue (T3), visceral peritoneal surface (T4a), or an adjacent organ or other structure (T4b). At least 12 lymph nodes must be sampled for accurate staging and represents an important quality control metric. The number of regional nodes involved varies from 1 to 3 (N1a/b) to 4 or more (N2a/b). N1c includes direct tumor deposits in the subserosa, mesentery, or nonperitonealized pericolic or perirectal tissues without regional nodal metastasis. Metastases confined to one organ or site (M1a) have a better prognosis than metastases confined to the peritoneum or multiple sites (M1b).

TABLE 9.2 Prognosis by Stage for Colorectal Cancers

Stage	5-Y Observed Survival Rate (%)
I	74
IIA	65
IIB	58
IIC	37
IIIA	73
IIIB	45
IIIC	28
IV	6

Adapted from Gunderson LL, Jessup JM, Sargent DJ, et al. Revised TN categorization for colon cancer based on national survival outcomes data. *J Clin Oncol.* 2010;28(2):264–271.

PROGNOSIS

Pathologic stage remains the most important determinant of prognosis (Table 9.2) with similar outcomes for both colon and rectal cancers in the modern era. Other prognostic variables proposed to be associated with an unfavorable outcome include advanced age of the patient, high tumor grade, perineural or lymphovascular invasion, high serum CEA level, and bowel obstruction or perforation at the time of presentation.

- Biochemical and molecular markers such as elevated thymidylate synthase, p53 mutations, loss of heterozygosity of chromosome 18q (DCC gene), and lack of CDX2 expression are also proposed as prognostic. The latter appears to portend for a worse 5-year disease-free survival (DFS) in patients with stage II and III colon cancers, yet adjuvant chemotherapy was associated with a significant DFS improvement upon retrospective analysis. However, a defective DNA mismatch–repair system (e.g., altered *MLH1*, *MSH2*; associated with Lynch syndrome) is associated with an improved outcome for patients with early stage, node-negative disease. Regardless of stage, the presence of a B-*raf* (V600E) mutation has been associated with a worse prognosis. The presence of a somatic B-*raf* mutation in the setting of *MLH1* absence precludes the germline diagnosis of Lynch syndrome. There are multiple commercially available multigene assays that have been developed to help define the risk of recurrence and prognosis for stage II CRC (see "Adjuvant Chemotherapy Regimens for Colon Cancer").

MANAGEMENT ALGORITHM

Surgery

- For colon cancers, the primary curative intervention requires en bloc resection of the involved bowel segment and mesentery, with pericolic and intermediate lymphadenectomy for both staging and therapeutic intent. Negative proximal, distal, and lateral surgical margins are of paramount importance. Laparoscopic techniques adhering to these surgical principles are an acceptable option.
- For rectal cancers, en bloc resection of the primary tumor with negative proximal, distal, and radial margins is critical as well as a sharp dissection of the mesorectum (total mesorectal excision) to optimally reduce local recurrence. The location of the tumor in relation to the anal sphincter is the primary determinant in a low anterior resection (LAR) versus an abdominoperineal resection (APR).

The latter generates a permanent colostomy. For highly selected early-stage rectal cancer cases, trans-anal endoscopic microsurgery may be considered.

■ Surgical intervention is indicated if polypectomy pathology reveals muscularis mucosa involvement or penetration.

■ Surgical palliation may include colostomy or even resection of metastatic disease for symptoms of acute obstruction or persistent bleeding.

Radiation Therapy

■ Routine administration of abdominal radiotherapy (RT) is limited by bowel-segment mobility, adjacent small bowel toxicity, previous surgery with adhesion formation, and other medical comorbidities.

■ Local control and improved DFS have been reported in retrospective series of patients with T4 lesions or perforations, nodal disease, and subtotal resections, who have been treated with 5,000 to 5,400 cGy directed at the primary tumor bed and draining lymph nodes. However, there are no randomized data to support the routine use of RT in the management of colon cancer.

■ In contrast, RT is routinely utilized in rectal cancers to reduce local recurrence and improve resectability. RT can also be useful for palliation of pain and bleeding in rectal cancer.

Pivotal Adjuvant Chemotherapy Studies for Colon Cancer

Establishing Benefit and Duration of Adjuvant Fluoropyrimidine Therapy

The Intergroup 0035 trial is of historic importance because it demonstrated that the use of 5-fluorouracil (5-FU) and levamisole (Lev) reduced the relapse rate by 41% and overall cancer mortality by 33%. This study resulted in the National Institutes of Health consensus panel recommending that 5-FU-based adjuvant therapy be administered to all patients with resected stage III colon cancer.

The subsequent Intergroup 0089 trial randomized 3,759 patients with stage II or III disease to one of four therapeutic arms. The results demonstrated that the 5-FU- and leucovorin (LV)-containing schedules (Mayo Clinic and Roswell Park regimens) were equivalent without the need for Lev. A 6-month schedule of the 5-FU and LV was similar to a protracted 12 months of therapy.

Utilization of an oral fluoropyrimidine (capecitabine) was evaluated in patients with stage III disease. Capecitabine (1,250 mg/m^2 b.i.d. for 14 days, every 3 weeks) was compared with the Mayo Clinic bolus of 5-FU and LV. The study was designed to demonstrate equivalency, with a primary endpoint of 3-year DFS. The capecitabine (cape) arm was non-inferior and demonstrated a trend toward DFS superiority (64% vs. 60%; HR 0.87; 95% CI, 0.75 to 1.00; P = 0.0526). Toxicity was improved in cape arm in all categories except hand–foot syndrome (HFS). A 3-year DFS endpoint was chosen because a retrospective analysis of more than 20,000 patients treated with 5-FU demonstrated equivalency to the conventional 5-year OS benchmark.

Intensifying Adjuvant Chemotherapy

With adjuvant fluoropyrimidine monotherapy well established, studies began testing the potential benefit of polychemotherapy. In Europe, 2,246 patients with stage II (40%) and III disease were treated with infusional 5-FU with LV modulation versus the same combination with oxaliplatin (FOLFOX4) every 2 weeks for 6 months, demonstrated a 3-year DFS benefit favoring the FOLFOX4 combination over standard 5-FU with LV (78.2% vs. 72.9%; HR 0.77; 95% CI, 0.65 to 0.92; P = 0.002). With a median 6-year follow-up, the OS advantage was confirmed in the patients with stage III disease (72.9% vs. 68.7%; HR 0.80; 95% CI, 0.65 to 0.97; P = 0.023). No difference in OS was seen in the stage II population. Treatment with FOLFOX4 was well tolerated, with 41% patients having grade 3 and 4 neutropenia, only 0.7% being associated with fever. Anticipated grade 3 peripheral neuropathy or paresthesias were observed (12%), which almost entirely resolved two years later (persisted in only 0.7% of patients).

The addition of oxaliplatin to three cycles of adjuvant Roswell Park 5-FU with LV (FLOX) was evaluated in 2,407 stage II (30%) and III patients. The combination improved 3-year DFS (76.1% vs. 71.8%; HR 0.80; 95% CI, 0.69 to 0.93; P = 0.003). Grade 3 diarrhea (38%) and peripheral neuropathy (8%) were significantly worse with FLOX without any difference in treatment-related mortality.

MOSAIC and C-07 established doublet adjuvant chemotherapy with fluoropyrimidine and oxaliplatin as a standard of care.

While 6 months of adjuvant therapy is currently the standard of care for adjuvant therapy, an ongoing global study (IDEA Study) is assessing the benefit of 3 versus 6 months of FOLFOX or CAPOX (capecitabine and oxaliplatin) chemotherapy in completely resected stage III patients. This potential practice changing study should have early results available in 2017.

Adjuvant Irinotecan

Unlike oxaliplatin, at least three studies failed to confirm a benefit for the use of adjuvant irinotecan. CALGB 89803 was a study of irinotecan with bolus 5-FU and LV (IFL) versus weekly 5-FU in patients with stage III disease. Increased grade 3 and 4 neutropenia and early deaths were observed in the experimental arm, and a higher number of patients withdrew from the study. Overall, IFL was not better than the 5-FU and LV arm. The two European studies (PETACC-3 and ACCORD) together randomized over 3,500 patients to infusional 5-FU with or without irinotecan. Both studies failed to reach their primary endpoint of 3-year DFS, although toxicities were less than in the IFL study. The use of irinotecan is thus not recommended in the adjuvant setting.

Adjuvant Biologics

Both cetuximab (cmab) and bevacizumab (bev) are biologic-targeted agents (see the metastatic CRC section) that have been shown to improve outcomes when combined with chemotherapy in metastatic CRC and have been definitively tested in the adjuvant setting.

Intergroup 0147 tested whether the addition of cmab to standard mFOLFOX6 adjuvant chemotherapy for resected stage III colon cancer improved outcomes. The protocol was amended to allow only patients with wild-type K-*ras* tumors to be eligible. The study terminated early after a second interim analysis demonstrated no benefit when adding cmab. Three-year DFS for patients with wild-type K-*ras* was 71.5% with mFOLFOX plus cmab and 74.6% with mFOLFOX alone (HR 1.21; 95% CI, 0.98 to 1.49; $P = 0.08$), suggesting a trend toward harm. There were no subgroups that benefitted from cmab, with increased toxicity and greater detrimental differences in all outcomes in patients aged greater than 70.

The addition of bev to mFOLFOX6 was tested in NSABP C-08. This randomized phase III trial assessed DFS in stage II (25%) and III patients. Bev was administered for 6 months concurrently with chemotherapy and then continued for an additional 6 months beyond (total of 1 year of biologic therapy). mFOLFOX6 plus bev did not significantly improve 3-year DFS compared to mFOLFOX6 (77.4% vs. 75.5%; HR 0.89; 95% CI, 0.76 to 1.04; $P = 0.15$). However, survival curve analysis suggested a time-dependent improvement in DFS with maximal separation of the curves occurring at 15 months, which correlated with 1 year of bev treatment followed by 3 months off drug. This benefit disappeared with time. No OS benefit, unexpected toxicity, or difference in patterns of relapse was seen. A study testing the benefit of expanded duration suppression of vascular endothelial growth factor (VEGF) in high risk stage III colon cancer patients using regorafenib or placebo after completion of standard adjuvant therapy is ongoing.

The AVANT trial also tested bev in a three-arm study that randomized 3,451 patients with high-risk stage II (17%) or stage III colon cancer to either FOLFOX4, FOLFOX4 plus bev, or CAPOX plus bev. The 3-year DFS was not significantly different between the groups with 5-year OS hazard ratio for FOLFOX 4 plus bev versus FOLFOX4 (HR 1.27; 95% CI, 1.03 to 1.57; $P = 0.02$), and CAPOX plus bev versus FOLFOX4 (HR 1.15; 95% CI 0.93 to 1.42; $P = 0.21$) suggesting a potential detriment.

Adjuvant Chemotherapy Regimens for Stage III Colon Cancer

Based on these studies, 6 months of adjuvant chemotherapy is recommended for all patients with stage III colon cancer. Several acceptable options exist (Table 9.3), with combination regimens offering increased efficacy and modest toxicity. Ongoing studies are assessing whether shorter duration adjuvant therapy is just as beneficial. The use of irinotecan or biologic-targeted therapies in the adjuvant setting is not recommended outside of a clinical trial. Adjuvant chemotherapy should be started within 8 weeks of surgery with data supporting that a delay beyond 2 months may compromise the effectiveness of adjuvant treatment.

TABLE 9.3 Acceptable Adjuvant Chemotherapy Regimens for Stage III Colon Cancer

Name	Regimen and Dose	Repeated (d)	Total Cycles
Mayo Clinic	LV 20 mg/m^2/d IV followed by 5-FU 425 mg/m^2/d IV days 1–5	28	6
Roswell Park	LV 500 mg/m^2 IV followed by 5-FU 500 mg/m^2 IV weekly × 6	8 wk	3–4
Capecitabine	1,250 mg/m^2 PO twice daily × 14 d	21	8
FOLFOX4	Oxaliplatin 85 mg/m^2 IV on day 1 followed by LV 200 mg/m^2/d IV on days 1 and 2 followed by 5-FU 400 mg/m^2/d IV on days 1 and 2 followed by 5-FU 600 mg/m^2/d CIVI for 22 h on days 1 and 2	14	12
FOLFOX6	Oxaliplatin 85–100 mg/m^2 IV on day 1 followed by LV 400 mg/m^2/d IV on day 1 followed by 5-FU 400 mg/m^2/d IV on day 1 followed by 5-FU 2,400 mg/m^2 CIVI for 46 h	14	12
FLOX	LV 500 mg/m^2 IV followed by 5-FU 500 mg/m^2 IV on days 1, 8, 15, 22, 29, 36 and Oxaliplatin 85 mg/m^2 IV on days 1, 15, and 29	8 wk	3
CAPOX	Oxaliplatin 100–130 mg/m^2 IV on day 1 Capecitabine 1,000 mg/m^2 PO twice daily on days 1–14	21	8

There is no role for biologic-targeted therapy or irinotecan-containing regimens in the adjuvant setting at this time.

LV, leucovorin; IV, intravenous; 5-FU, 5-fluorouracil; CIVI, continuous intravenous infusion.

Adjuvant Chemotherapy for Stage II Colon Cancer

Despite the 75% 5-year survival with surgery alone, some patients with stage II disease have a higher risk of relapse, with outcomes being similar to those of node-positive patients. Adjuvant chemotherapy provides up to 33% relative risk reduction in mortality, resulting in an absolute treatment benefit of approximately 5%.

Several analyses have reported varying outcomes in patients with stage II disease who received adjuvant treatment:

▪ The National Surgical Adjuvant Breast and Bowel Project (NSABP) summary of protocols (C-01 to C-04) of 1,565 patients with stage II disease reported a 32% relative reduction in mortality (cumulative odds, 0.68; 95% CI, 0.50 to 0.92; P = 0.01). This reduction in mortality translated into an absolute survival advantage of 5%.

▪ A meta-analysis by Erlichman et al. detected a nonsignificant 2% benefit (82% vs. 80%; P = 0.217) in 1,020 patients with high-risk T3 and T4 cancer treated with 5-FU and LV for 5 consecutive days.

▪ Schrag et al. reviewed Medicare claims for chemotherapy within the Surveillance, Epidemiology, and End Results (SEER) database and identified 3,700 patients with resected stage II disease among whom 31% received adjuvant treatment. No survival benefit was detected with 5-FU compared to surgery alone (74% vs. 72%) even with patients considered to be at high risk because of obstruction, perforation, or T4 lesions.

▪ The Quasar Collaborative Group study reported an OS benefit of 3.6% in 3,239 patients (91% Dukes B colon cancer) prospectively randomized to chemotherapy versus surgery alone. With a median follow-up of 5.5 years, the risk of recurrence (HR 0.78; 95% CI, 0.67 to 0.91; P = 0.001) and death (HR 0.82; 95% CI, 0.70 to 0.95; P = 0.008) favored 5-FU and LV chemotherapy.

- In the MOSAIC study, FOLFOX4 chemotherapy showed nonsignificant benefits in DFS over 5-FU and LV in patients with stage II disease (86.6% vs. 83.9%; HR 0.82; 95% CI, 0.57 to 1.17).
- The American Society of Clinical Oncology Panel concluded that the routine use of adjuvant chemotherapy for patients with stage II disease could not be recommended. A review of 37 randomized controlled trials and 11 meta-analyses found no evidence of a statistically significant survival benefit with postoperative treatment of stage II patients. However, treatment should be considered for specific subsets of patients (e.g., T4 lesions, perforation, poorly differentiated histology, or inadequately sampled nodes), and patient input is critical.
- For stage II patients without high-risk features, molecular analysis can provide improved recurrence risk determination.
- MSI is a surrogate marker for functional defects in the DNA mismatch–repair system. When these occur at a high frequency (MSI-high) in node-negative colon cancer, it portends a very favorable prognosis. There is controversy as to whether MSI-high tumors benefit from adjuvant fluoropyrimidine chemotherapy. Given the more favorable outcome and questionable response to adjuvant chemotherapy, it is recommended to test this molecular marker in all stage II patients to aid in personalized treatment decisions.
- Commercially available microarray gene expression profile assays may aid in determining the risk of recurrence of stage II CRC. An example is Oncotype Dx (Genomic Health, Inc), which uses a 12-gene signature and excludes patients with MSI-high tumors. A recurrence score can be generated for an individual patient with stage II disease that classifies them as low, intermediate, or high risk. Given these tests only offer prognostic and not predictive value, the National Comprehensive Cancer Network (NCCN) states there is insufficient evidence to recommend use of the multigene assays to determine adjuvant therapy.

Treatment for Rectal Cancer

In contrast to colon cancer, local treatment failures after potentially curative resections represent a major clinical problem. Combined-modality chemotherapy with RT (chemoRT) is the standard therapy for patients with stage II and III rectal cancer (T3, T4, and nodal involvement).

Establishing Combined Modality Neoadjuvant Therapy as Standard of Care

A four-arm study of 1,695 post-operative patients compared 5-FU alone, 5-FU and LV combination, 5-FU and Lev combination, and 5-FU and LV and Lev combination. Two cycles of chemotherapy were administered before and after chemoRT using 5,040 cGy of external beam RT (4,500 cGy with 540 cGy boost). The chemotherapy during the RT was given as a bolus with or without LV. The DFS and OS were similar in all treatment arms, leading to the conclusion that 5-FU alone was as effective as other combinations. Subsequent studies sponsored by the North Central Cancer Treatment Group (NCCTG) demonstrated improvements in both DFS and OS when continuous infusion of 5-FU was provided during RT compared with those receiving bolus 5-FU. This survival benefit has led to continuous infusion of 5-FU during RT being considered as a standard.

The benefit of delivering chemoRT in a preoperative (neoadjuvant) fashion was evaluated by the German Rectal Study Group in 421 patients compared to 401 similar patients randomized to receive postoperative chemoRT. In both groups, 5-FU was administered in a continuous fashion during the first and fifth weeks of RT. All patients received an additional four cycles of adjuvant 5-FU after chemoRT and surgery. Results of neoadjuvant treatment provided improvement in local recurrence (6% vs. 13%; $P = 0.006$), but no difference in 5-year OS. Both acute toxic effects (27% vs. 40%; $P = 0.001$) and long-term toxicities (14% vs. 24%; $P = 0.01$) were less common with neoadjuvant treatment. Preoperative chemoRT followed by surgical resection with postoperative 5-FU-based chemotherapy represents a standard for patients with stage II and III rectal cancer.

Intensifying Therapy

NSABP R-04 was a phase III, 2×2 non-inferiority trial, which evaluated the substitution of oral capecitabine (cape) for infusional 5-FU (CVI 5-FU) as well as the intensification of radiosensitization by adding oxaliplatin in stage II and III rectal carcinoma. Over 1,500 patients were randomized into one of four neoadjuvant chemoRT arms. The primary endpoint for this study was local regional tumor control. The 3-year local regional tumor event rates were similar in both the cape and CVI 5-FU arms, 11.2% versus 11.8%, respectively. There was also equivalence for cape and CVI 5-FU in terms of rates of pathologic complete response (pCR) and surgical downstaging. Rates of grade 3 diarrhea were equal in both arms (11.7%). However, the addition of oxaliplatin failed to improve DFS, OS, pCR rates, surgical downstaging, or sphincter-sparing surgery. The addition of oxaliplatin did increase (16.5% vs. 6.9%) grade 3 and 4 diarrhea. This and other studies confirmed that cape is an acceptable replacement for CVI 5-FU, and that adding oxaliplatin to chemoRT offers no benefit in the neoadjuvant treatment of rectal cancer.

Sequencing of Therapy and Future Directions

Most patients with rectal cancer who recur succumb to metastatic disease yet contemporary randomized controlled trials show that 25% to 70% of the patients never receive or complete their intended adjuvant systemic chemotherapy. Thus, a "total neoadjuvant therapy" (TNT) approach to care has been developed, which provides systemic chemotherapy and chemoRT preoperatively. This has proven to be safe and feasible in early studies and has the benefit of determining therapeutic response, which can guide potential delay or elimination of certain portions of traditional treatment in an attempt to reduce morbidity. For example, a multicenter randomized phase II trial (OPRA; ClinicalTrials.gov identifier: NCT02008656) is looking at the TNT approach whereby patients with a clinical complete response (cCR) will be managed nonoperatively. This trial is based on a Brazilian report of 265 patients with resectable rectal cancers who were treated with standard neoadjuvant chemoRT, and those with a cCR were observed while all others were taken to surgery. A provocative 27% of patients maintained a cCR at one year and were spared from TME. Another important phase II/III trial (PROSPECT; ClinicalTrials.gov #NCT01515787) is randomizing low risk patients with stage II and III rectal cancer to standard of care chemoRT versus induction chemotherapy (FOLFOX for 12 weeks) followed by MRI and/or ERUS. If the tumor decreases by >20% with neoadjuvant chemotherapy alone, patients proceed to surgery without chemoRT. Post-op chemoRT is allowable should pathology support that need, but avoidance of pelvic radiotherapy for those patients with highly chemo-sensitive disease is the goal of the study design. Lastly, of interest is the randomized phase II platform TNT study (NRG GI002; ClinicalTrials.gov #NCT02921256) that has parallel, noncomparative experimental arms with a single comparative control arm of neoadjuvant chemotherapy and chemoRT. The TNT experimental arms are testing new systemic therapies and/or radiation sensitizers to improve pathologic endpoints. The first two experimental arms are assessing the potential radiosensitizing activity of the poly [ADP-ribose] polymerase (PARP) inhibitor, veliparib and the potential immunogenic capability of chemoRT with pembrolizumab, a programmed cell death-1 (PD-1) inhibitor.

Combined-Modality Options for Rectal Cancer

1. Neoadjuvant therapy (chemoRT):
   - Continuous infusion 5-FU (1,000 mg/m²/day) given daily for 5 days during the first and fifth week of radiation therapy OR 225 mg/m²/day given Monday through Friday continuously throughout RT .
   - Oral capecitabine 825 mg/m² twice daily given Monday through Friday on days of RT.
   - All concurrent with external beam RT given in 180 cGy fractions to a total dose of 5,040 cGy.
2. Complete surgical resection adhering to total mesorectal excision standards.
3. Systemic therapy for 4 months (before or after from surgery):
   - 5-FU bolus (500 mg/m²/day) on days 1 to 5 repeated every 28 days for four cycles. Given the previously discussed data for adjuvant chemotherapy regimens in colon cancer, several different regimens (see Table 9.3) may also be considered as components of the systemic chemotherapy phase of therapy in rectal cancer (e.g., fluoropyrimidine and oxaliplatin).

FOLLOW-UP AFTER CURATIVE TREATMENT

Eighty percent of recurrences are seen within 2 years of initial therapy. The American Cancer Society recommends total colonic evaluation with either colonoscopy or double-contrast barium enema within 1 year of resection, followed every 3 to 5 years if findings remain normal. Synchronous cancers must be excluded during initial surgical resection, and metachronous malignancies in the form of polyps must be detected and excised before more malignant behavior develops.

History and physical evaluations with serum CEA measurements should be performed every 3 to 6 months for the first few years after therapy. These evaluations can be further reduced during subsequent years. Surveillance imaging should be reserved for those individuals who would be considered operable candidates if localized metastases were to be identified. Elevations of CEA postoperatively may suggest residual tumor or early metastasis. Patients with initially negative levels of CEA can subsequently exhibit positive levels; therefore, serial CEA measurements after completion of treatment may identify patients who are eligible for a curative surgery, in particular, patients with oligometastatic liver or lung recurrence.

TREATMENT FOR ADVANCED COLORECTAL CANCER

Unprecedented improvements in OS have been recognized during the past decade with systemic chemotherapy in advanced or metastatic disease. Median survival has improved from 6 months with best supportive care to approximately 30 months with incorporation of all active agents. Based upon clinical practice and supported by total cancer genomic analyses, there are no differences in the molecular characteristics or systemic management of metastatic colon or rectal cancers. Data also support proceeding with systemic therapy without surgical intervention on the primary tumor, as long as the intact primary tumor is asymptomatic. Determination of molecular profiling for *RAS*, *BRAF*, and MMR/MSI status at the time of diagnosis is now critical for optimal treatment selection.

Fluoropyrimidine-Based Chemotherapy

5-FU inhibits thymidylate synthase, an enzyme critical in thymidine generation. LV potentiates this inhibition. 5-FU and LV chemotherapy regimens in advanced CRC have objective response rates of 15% to 20%, with median survival of 8 to 12 months. Toxicity is predictable and manageable. The activity of continuous infusion of 5-FU may be equivalent to or slightly better than that of bolus 5-FU and LV and is generally well tolerated despite the inconvenience of a prolonged intravenous ambulatory infusion apparatus. Toxicities include mucositis and palmar–plantar erythrodysesthesia (HFS); however, myelosuppression is less common. Continuous infusions of 5-FU may have activity in patients who have progressed with bolus 5-FU.

Capecitabine, an oral fluoropyrimidine prodrug, undergoes a series of three enzymatic steps in its conversion to 5-FU. The final enzymatic step is catalyzed by thymidine phosphorylase, which is overexpressed in tumor tissues and upregulated by RT. Two phase III studies have compared single-agent capecitabine to the Mayo Clinic 5-FU and LV regimen and demonstrated higher response rates for the former but equivalent time to progression and median survival. Capecitabine was associated with decreased gastrointestinal and hematologic toxicities and fewer hospitalizations, but with an increased frequency of HFS and hyperbilirubinemia.

Trifluridine and tipiracil is an FDA-approved oral therapy for the treatment of metastatic CRC who have been previously treated with all other standard therapies. Trifluridine is a thymidine-based nucleoside analog while tipiracil is a thymidine phosphorylase inhibitor and in effect increases trifluridine activity. Once trifluridine is taken up in the cancer cell it is incorporated into the DNA and inhibits cell proliferation and interferes with DNA synthesis. The phase III, randomized placebo-controlled registration trial (RECOURSE) studied trifluridine and tipiracil in patients with previously treated (at least two prior lines) metastatic CRC. Results showed an improvement in median PFS (2 vs. 1.7 months; $P < 0.001$) and OS (7.1 vs. 5.3 months; $P < 0.001$) for trifluridine/tipiracil versus placebo, respectively. The main side effects of trifluridine/tipiracil were grade 3 to 4 asthenia/fatigue (7%), grade 3 anemia (18%), grade 3 to 4 neutropenia (38%), and grade 3 to 4 thrombocytopenia (5%).

Oxaliplatin

Oxaliplatin is an agent that differs structurally from other platinums in its 1,2-diaminocyclohexane (DACH) moiety, but acts similarly by generating DNA adducts. Oxaliplatin exhibits synergy with 5-FU with response rates as high as 66% even in patients who are refractory to 5-FU. Despite its unique toxicities (i.e., peripheral neuropathy, laryngopharyngeal dysesthesias, and cold hypersensitivities), oxaliplatin lacks the emetogenic and nephrogenic toxicities of cisplatin.

The North Central Cancer Treatment Group (NCCTG-9741) conducted a trial comparing first-line FOLFOX4 versus IFL versus IROX (irinotecan in combination with oxaliplatin). Higher 60-day mortality was detected in the IFL arm, resulting in a dose reduction in the protocol. The response rate, time to progression, and OS were significantly better in the FOLFOX4 arm than in the modified IFL arm. However, imbalances in the second-line chemotherapy administered to patients in this study may confound the survival differences. Approximately 60% of the oxaliplatin failures were treated with irinotecan, whereas only 24% of patients who were refractory to irinotecan received oxaliplatin. In addition, the study was not designed to address the effect of infusional 5-FU. The observed toxicities in the study were reflective of the specific drug combinations and included grade 3 or higher paresthesias (18%) in the FOLFOX arm and a 28% incidence of diarrhea in the IFL arm. Despite a higher degree of neutropenia (60% in FOLFOX vs. 40% in IFL) with FOLFOX, febrile neutropenia was significantly greater in the IFL arm. IROX also exhibited significant toxicities. Oxaliplatin was approved by the FDA for use in the first-line treatment of patients with metastatic CRC largely based on this study.

Although FOLFOX is clearly a superior regimen compared to IFL, the use of infusional 5-FU with irinotecan (FOLFIRI) may produce results similar to those seen using FOLFOX. Tournigand et al. reported an equivalent median survival of 21.5 months with FOLFIRI followed by FOLFOX and a median survival of 20.6 months with the opposite sequence ($P = 0.99$). Similar survival is observed in patients receiving either sequence, and both are acceptable first-line therapies for advanced disease.

Irinotecan

Irinotecan is a topoisomerase I inhibitor, with activity in advanced CRC deemed refractory to 5-FU. As a single agent, response rates as high as 20% are observed, and an additional 45% of patients achieve disease stabilization. Significant survival advantages have been shown for irinotecan as second-line therapy after 5-FU compared with supportive care or with continuous-infusion 5-FU regimens. Several schedules are typically administered with and without 5-FU; however, the cumulative data suggest that irinotecan should not be utilized with bolus 5-FU (i.e., IFL) due to excessive treatment-related mortality. Irinotecan obtained initial FDA approval based on a study comparing IFL to the 5-FU bolus Mayo Clinic regimen. A higher response rate (39% vs. 21%; $P = 0.0001$) and OS (14.8 vs. 12.6 months; $P = 0.042$) were observed favoring IFL.

Delayed-onset diarrhea is common and requires close monitoring and aggressive management (high-dose loperamide, 4 mg initially and then 2 mg every 2 hours until diarrhea stops for at least 12 hours). Neutropenia, mild nausea, and vomiting are common. This combination of toxicities can be severe and life-threatening, which was evident in NCCTG 9741 (see previous oxaliplatin section). A higher 60-day mortality was observed (4.5% vs. 1.8%), and the dose of irinotecan required reduction.

Anti-VEGF Therapies

Bevacizumab (bev) is a recombinant humanized monoclonal antibody targeting the VEGF, which blocks VEGF-induced angiogenesis by preventing it from binding to VEGF receptors. When added to IFL, bev increased the response rate (45% vs. 35%; $P = 0.004$) and had a longer median survival (20.3 vs. 15.6 months; $P < 0.001$). When added to FOLFOX in the second-line setting, response rates are again increased (23% vs. 9%; $P < 0.001$) along with an improvement in OS (12.9 vs. 10.8 months; $P = 0.0011$). Bev has been approved by the FDA for the treatment of patients with advanced CRC in combination with any intravenous 5-FU-based regimen. Two trials (ML18147, BRiTE) looked at bev beyond progression following first-line chemotherapy. Both studies showed PFS and OS advantage with continuation of bev with second line chemotherapy. This approach was further explored as a maintenance strategy. The CAIRO-3 study was a European study that enrolled 558 patients to receive "induction" chemotherapy with CAPOX plus bev for six cycles. Patients were then randomized to observation versus maintenance treatment with cape and bev. Upon progression (PFS1) patients on either observation or cape and bev were restarted on CAPOX plus bev, and the next progression (PFS2) was the primary endpoint. The maintenance group had a significantly improved PFS2 compared to observation, 11.7 versus 8.5 months, respectively (HR 0.67; 95% CI 0.56 to 0.81; $P < 0.0001$).

Ziv-aflibercept is a fully humanized recombinant fusion protein that blocks angiogenesis by binding to VEGF-A, VEGF-B, and placental growth factor and preventing their interaction with endogenous receptors. It is FDA approved for use in combination with FOLFIRI for second-line treatment in metastatic CRC based on results from the VELOUR study. This phase III, placebo-controlled trial randomized 1,226 meta-static patients with CRC after an oxaliplatin-based regimen to second-line therapy with FOLFIRI plus ziv-aflibercept or placebo. Median OS of FOLFIRI plus ziv-aflibercept was statistically superior to FOLFIRI (13.5 vs. 12 months; HR 0.87; 95% CI 0.713 to 0.937; $P = 0.0032$) as was PFS (6.9 vs. 4.7 months; $P < 0.0001$).

Ramucirumab is another humanized monoclonal antibody that blocks activation of VEGF recep-tor 2, effectively blocking the binding of VEGF-A, VEGF-C, and VEGF-D. It is FDA approved for use in combination with FOLFIRI for second-line treatment in metastatic CRC based on results from the RAISE study. This phase III, placebo-controlled trial randomized 1,072 patients with previously oxali-platin treated metastatic CRC to FOLFIRI plus ramucirumab or placebo. The addition of ramucirumab demonstrated a median PFS improvement of 1.2 months (5.7 vs. 4.5 months; $P < 0.001$) and median OS improvement of 1.6 months (13.3 vs. 11.7 months; $P = 0.023$).

The first and currently only approved oral multikinase inhibitor for metastatic CRC is regorafenib. This agent blocks several kinases involved in angiogenic and oncogenic survival pathways including VEGFR1, VEGFR2, VEGFR3, TIE2, KIT, RET, RAF1, BRAF, PDGFR, and FGFR. The CORRECT trial randomized heavily pretreated metastatic CRC patients who progressed within 3 months after treat-ment with all currently available standard therapies to oral regorafenib versus placebo. Median OS was found to be improved with regorafenib compared to placebo (6.4 vs. 5 months; HR 0.77; $P = 0.0052$). Studies which incorporate this treatment in earlier lines of therapy are ongoing.

Anti-Epidermal Growth Factor Therapies

The epidermal growth factor receptor (EGFR) and pathway represent another targeted approach in advanced CRC therapy. Two monoclonal antibodies are FDA approved for use in patients with metastatic CRC. Importantly, tumor EGFR positivity by IHC staining does not correlate with treatment response; however, K-ras, N-ras, and B-raf mutational status does. Both intracellular signal transduction proteins exist in either a wild-type (normal functional) or mutated (via activating mutation resulting in continuous over-activity) state. Mutations in K- and N-ras (~50% together) and B-raf (5% to 10%) have high concordance between primary and metastatic CRC tumors (in excess of 90%), with recommendations for testing these at the time of metastatic diagnosis. Of note, B-raf V600E mutations have become increasingly important in identifying a subset of CRC patients with a particularly aggressive disease associated with short PFS (4 to 6 months) and OS (9 to 14 months). Attempts to directly target this pathway with the B-raf inhibitor vemurafenib failed given unanticipated feedback through the EGFR accessory pathways. Treatments aimed at combining dual pathway targets or maximizing first-line cytotoxic regimens are under active investiga-tion. Testing for extended ras and raf mutations is recommended and widely commercially available.

Cetuximab (cmab) is a chimerized IgG1 antibody that prevents ligand binding to the EGFR and its heterodimers through competitive displacement. Panitumumab (pmab) is a fully humanized IgG2 antibody also targeting EGFR in a similar manner. These agents both block receptor dimerization, tyrosine kinase phosphorylation, and subsequent downstream signal transduction. Both can cause a skin rash, diarrhea, hypomagnesemia, and infusion reactions, but to a less degree with pmab for the latter two toxicities. A correlation between the intensity of the skin rash and improved survival has been consistently noted with agents in this class.

Cmab was initially FDA approved based on a study in irinotecan-refractory advanced disease. Patients were randomized to the combination of cmab and irinotecan versus cmab alone with improvements in the response rate (22.9% vs. 10.8%; $P = 0.0074$) and time to progression (4.1 vs. 1.5 months; $P < 0.0001$) favoring the combination. Despite manageable toxicity, no improvements in survival outcomes were observed, but tumor resensitization to irinotecan was clearly demonstrated. Cmab is also approved for use as first-line metastatic treatment for patients with wild-type K-ras tumors. The CRYSTAL phase III trial randomized 1,217 patients to FOLFIRI with or without cmab. FOLFIRI plus cmab demonstrated a 15% relative reduction in the risk of recurrence (HR 0.85; 95% CI 0.72 to 0.99; $P = 0.048$) with an improvement in the median PFS (8.9 vs. 8 months). The addition of cmab produced significantly more skin reactions, diarrhea, and infusional reactions. Median progression-free survival directly correlated with increased grade of skin rash. K-ras status was available on a subgroup analysis of 540 tissue samples. Patients with wild-type K-ras had a favorable outcome on response rate, OS, and PFS (HR 0.68). However, mutated K-ras tumors were associated with a decrease in OS and response rates, particularly with cmab addition, confirming that ras mutations are a negative predictor of response to EGFR inhibition.

Panitumumab is FDA approved as monotherapy given improvement in progression-free survival over best supportive care in heavily pretreated patients (HR 0.54; 95% CI 0.44 to 0.66; $P < 0.0001$), although no OS advantage was noted. This agent also has data supporting improvements in PFS when combined with FOLFIRI in the second-line treatment.

PD-1 Antibody

Programmed cell death protein 1 (PD-1) is expressed on activated T-cells and is a negative regulator of T-cell activity when it interacts with its ligand PD-L1. As a mechanism of immune evasion, tumor cells overexpress PD-L1. Antibodies to block this interaction have been developed with varying success in a multitude of malignancies. In CRC, anti-PD-1 therapy has been most notable in tumors harboring mismatch-repair deficiency (dMMR/MSI-High). This represents about 5% of patients with metastatic CRC.

The PD-1 checkpoint inhibitor, pembrolizumab, received accelerated approval from the FDA (May 2017) for dMMR and/or MSI-H metastatic CRC who have progressed on fluoropyrimidine, oxaliplatin, or irinotecan. Approval was based on aggregate data from 149 patients (90 with CRC) with dMMR/MSI-H status. For the CRC subset, ORR was 36% with median duration of response not reached. Shortly thereafter, the FDA granted an accelerated approval (August 2017) to nivolumab with the same indication. This approval was based on preliminary results of the Checkmate-142 trial that randomized dMMR/MSI-H metastatic CRC patients to nivolumab or nivolumab and ipilimumab, an anti CTLA-4 antibody. In the 74 patients who received single agent nivolumab the ORR was 31% with median duration of response was not reached. Current clinical trials are determining the impact of moving such agents earlier in treatment paradigms and stage. It remains critical to determine the MMR/MSI status of all patients with metastatic CRC at the time of diagnosis.

CHEMOTHERAPY REGIMENS FOR METASTATIC CRC

See Tables 9.3 and 9.4 and Figure 9.1. Investigations into the optimal timing and sequence of treatment combinations both with and without EGFR and VEGF inhibition continue.

Optimal Therapy Selection and Sequencing

CALGB 80405 was an important international phase III trial, which tested the optimal first line treatment in 1,137 patients with metastatic K-*ras* wild-type (WT) CRC. Patients were treated with FOLFOX (or FOLFIRI at provider discretion) and randomized to the addition of either cmab or bev. Median OS (the primary endpoint) was essentially the same (32 vs. 31.2 months; $P = 0.40$) between treatment with chemo and cmab versus bev, respectively. PFS was also similar between the arms. Retrospective analysis identified that left-sided tumors were associated with a longer median compared to those from the right colon (OS 33.3 vs. 19.4 months; $P < 0.0001$). Results suggested that bev may also benefit right sided tumors more than cmab-based chemotherapy (OS 24.2 vs. 16.7 months; $P < 0.0001$). The opposite was true for left-sided cancers suggesting cmab was more effective than bev-based chemotherapy (OS 36 vs. 31.4 months; $P < 0.0001$). This suggests distinct molecular variability of colon cancers depending on their "sidedness."

The FIRE-3 study was the European equivalent of the CALGB 80405 study. It enrolled 592 similar patients and randomized them to FOLFIRI plus either bev or cmab. In contrast to the prior study, the median OS favored treatment with cmab (33.1 vs. 25.6 months; $P = 0.011$). Importantly, there was no difference in PFS between the groups suggesting subsequent therapy may have accounted for the improvement in OS. It should be noted that neither trial prospectively tested for N-*ras* or B-*raf* mutations, as either predictive or prognostic biomarkers.

OLIGOMETASTATIC DISEASE

The liver is the most common site for metastasis, with one-third of cases involving only the liver. Approximately 25% of liver metastases are resectable, with certain patient subsets showing 30% to 40%

TABLE 9.4 Select Chemotherapy Regimens for Advanced Colorectal Cancer[a]

Name	Regimen and Dose	Repeated (d)
CAPOX	Oxaliplatin 100–130 mg/m² IV on day 1	21
	Capecitabine 850–1,000 mg/m² PO twice daily on days 1–14	
Irinotecan	300–350 mg/m² IV	21
Irinotecan	125 mg/m² IV on days 1, 8, 15, and 22	6 wk
FOLFIRI	Irinotecan 180 mg/m² IV on day 1 followed by	14
	LV 400 mg/m²/d IV on day 1 followed by	
	5-FU 400 mg/m²/d IV on day 1 followed by	
	5-FU 2,400 mg/m² CIVI for 46 h	
Bevacizumab[b]	5 mg/kg IV on day 1	14
Ziv-aflibercept	4 mg/kg IV on day 1	14
Ramucirumab	8 mg/kg IV on day 1	14
Cetuximab[c]	400 mg/m² IV on day 1 followed by	weekly
	250 mg/m² IV weekly thereafter	
Panitumumab[c]	6 mg/kg IV on day 1	14
Regorafenib	160 mg PO once daily for 21 d	28
Trifluridine and tipiracil	35 mg/m²/dose PO twice daily on days 1–5 and 8–12	28
Pembrolizumab[d]	200 mg IV on day 1	21
Nivolumab[d]	240 mg IV on day 1	14

[a] These are in addition to those presented in Table 9.3.

[b] In combination with any 5-FU–containing regimen.

[c] Only indicated for patients with *RAS* and/or *RAF* wild-type tumors.

[d] Only indicated for patients with dMMR or MSI-H tumors.

LV, leucovorin; IV, intravenous; 5-FU, 5-fluorouracil; CIVI, continuous intravenous infusion.

5-year survival after resection and 3% to 5% operative morbidity and mortality. Nonoperative ablative techniques (i.e., cryoablation, radiofrequency ablation, stereotactic RT, and hepatic artery embolization with or without chemotherapy) have not shown consistent durable prospective survival benefits. Intraoperative ultrasound is the most sensitive test for initial detection, followed by CT scan or MRI. PET scanning can help identify occult extrahepatic disease in select patients being considered for resection.

Patients with unresectable disease limited to the liver can be treated with locoregional hepatic artery infusion (HAI) or systemic chemotherapy. Kemeny et al. reported a 4-year DFS and hepatic disease-free benefit in patients with resected liver metastases who had received intra-arterial floxuridine with systemic 5-FU compared to those who did not receive any postoperative therapy, although there was no statistically significant difference in OS (62% vs. 53%; $P = 0.06$). Such an approach has typically been reserved for select centers and its utility has been challenged by the advent of more effective systemic chemotherapy.

The feasibility of converting initially unresectable disease to a potentially curative disease has been investigated by Bismuth and colleagues. Resection was possible in 99 patients with either downstaged or stable disease, and the 3-year survival was encouraging (58% for responders, 45% for patients with stable disease). Similar observations have been reported by Alberts using preoperative FOLFOX4 on 41% of patients undergoing resection with an observed median survival of 31.4 months (95% CI 20.4 to 34.8) for the entire cohort. Given objective response rates of 60% to 70% in RAS WT tumors treated initially with cmab-based chemotherapy, this could provide rationale for personalizing treatment selection to optimize response and improve chances of conversion of borderline or unresectable disease. Alternatively, for those with RAS mutations where anti-EGFR therapies are contraindicated, FOLFOXIRI (5-FU/LV, irinotecan, oxaliplatin) with bev demonstrated a 65% objective response rate, however the rate of hepatic R0 surgical resections was not improved over FOLFIRI with bev.

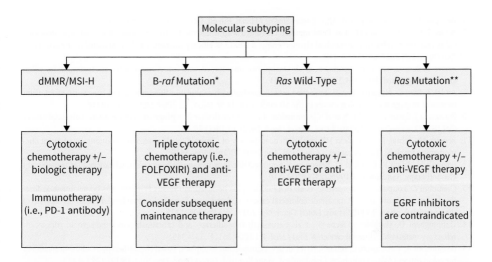

*B-*raf* mutation denotes exon 15, V600E.

**K-*ras*/N-*ras* mutations denote exons 2 (codons 12, 13), 3 (codons 59, 61) and 4 (codons 117, 146).

dMMR, defective mismatch-repair system; MSI-H, microsatellite instability high; PD-1, programmed cell death protein 1; EGFR, epidermal growth factor receptor; VEGF, vascular endothelial growth factor.

FIGURE 9.1 Palliative treatment considerations for metastatic colorectal cancer as defined by molecular subtypes. *Note: Consideration of clinical trial enrollment for each patient in these categories for each line of therapy is prudent.*

Indeed, current management of resectable liver disease typically includes appropriate patient selection, adequate imaging to confirm isolated and limited disease burden, multidisciplinary clinical collaboration, and consideration of perioperative systemic chemotherapy. The latter recommendation is based, in part, on the results of a European study showing a progression-free survival advantage to the use of 3 months of FOLFOX4 chemotherapy pre- and post-resection compared to surgery alone. However, attention must be paid to the potential hepatotoxicity and surgical complications from prolonged perioperative chemotherapy. The maximum radiographic response from chemotherapy is typically seen at 12 weeks. Importantly, systemic chemotherapy fails to sterilize hepatic metastases, even if radiographic complete response is noted. Patients with B-*raf* mutations appear to have limited benefit from oligometastatic management given the aggressive and refractory nature of metastatic disease.

Suggested Readings

1. Alberts SR, Donohue JH, Mahoney MR. Liver resection after 5-fluorouracil, leucovorin and oxaliplatin for patients with metastatic colorectal cancer (MCRC) limited to the liver: a North Central Cancer Treatment Group (NCCTG) Phase II Study. *Proc Am Soc Clin Oncol.* 2003; 22:268(abstr 1053).
2. Alberts SR, Sargent DJ, Nair S, et al. Effect of oxaliplatin, fluorouracil, and leucovorin with or without cetuximab on survival among patients with resected stage III colon cancer: a randomized trial. *JAMA.* Apr 2012;307(13):1383–1393.
3. Allegra CJ, Yothers G, O'Connell MJ, et al. Phase III trial assessing bevacizumab in stages II and III carcinoma of the colon: results of NSABP protocol C-08. *J Clin Oncol.* Jan 2011;29(1):11–16.
4. Allegra CJ, Yothers G, O'Connell MJ. Final results from NSABP protocol R-04: neoadjuvant chemoradiation comparing continuous infusion 5-FU with capecitabine with or without oxaliplatin in patients with stage II and III rectal cancer. *J Clin Oncol.* 2014; 32(5): 3603(abstr).
5. American Cancer Society. Cancer facts and figures 2016. http://www.cancer.org/acs/groups/content/@research/documents/document/acspc-047079.pdf. Accessed September 1, 2016.

6. Amin M, Edge S, Greene F, et al. *AJCC Cancer Staging Manual*. 8th ed. Chicago, IL: Springer; 2017.
7. André T, Blons H, Mabro M, et al. Panitumumab combined with irinotecan for patients with KRAS wild-type metastatic colorectal cancer refractory to standard chemotherapy: a GERCOR efficacy, tolerance, and translational molecular study. *Ann Oncol*. Feb 2013;24(2):412–419.
8. André T, Boni C, Mounedji-Boudiaf L, et al. Oxaliplatin, fluorouracil, and leucovorin as adjuvant treatment for colon cancer. *N Engl J Med*. Jun 2004;350(23):2343–2351.
9. André T, Boni C, Navarro M, et al. Improved overall survival with oxaliplatin, fluorouracil, and leucovorin as adjuvant treatment in stage II or III colon cancer in the MOSAIC trial. *J Clin Oncol*. Jul 2009;27(19):3109–3116.
10. Bennouna J, Sastre J, Arnold D, et al. Continuation of bevacizumab after first progression in metastatic colorectal cancer (ML18147): a randomised phase 3 trial. *Lancet Oncol*. Jan 2013;14(1):29–37.
11. Benson AB, Schrag D, Somerfield MR, et al. American Society of Clinical Oncology recommendations on adjuvant chemotherapy for stage II colon cancer. *J Clin Oncol*. Aug 2004;22(16):3408–3419.
12. Bismuth H, Adam R, Lévi F, et al. Resection of nonresectable liver metastases from colorectal cancer after neoadjuvant chemotherapy. *Ann Surg*. Oct 1996;224(4):509–520.
13. Cremolini C, Loupakis F, Antoniotti C, et al. FOLFOXIRI plus bevacizumab versus FOLFIRI plus bevacizumab as first-line treatment of patients with metastatic colorectal cancer: updated overall survival and molecular subgroup analyses of the open-label, phase 3 TRIBE study. *Lancet Oncol*. Oct 2015;16(13):1306–1315.
14. Cunningham D, Humblet Y, Siena S, et al. Cetuximab monotherapy and cetuximab plus irinotecan in irinotecan-refractory metastatic colorectal cancer. *N Engl J Med*. Jul 2004;351(4):337–345.
15. de Gramont A, Van Cutsem E, Schmoll HJ, et al. Bevacizumab plus oxaliplatin-based chemotherapy as adjuvant treatment for colon cancer (AVANT): a phase 3 randomised controlled trial. *Lancet Oncol*. Dec 2012;13(12):1225–1233.
16. Efficacy of adjuvant fluorouracil and folinic acid in B2 colon cancer. International Multicentre Pooled Analysis of B2 Colon Cancer Trials (IMPACT B2) Investigators. *J Clin Oncol*. May 1999;17(5):1356–1363.
17. Fearon ER, Vogelstein B. A genetic model for colorectal tumorigenesis. *Cell*. Jun 1990;61(5):759–767.
18. George TJ, Laplant KD, Walden EO, et al. Managing cetuximab hypersensitivity-infusion reactions: incidence, risk factors, prevention, and retreatment. *J Support Oncol*. 2010 Mar–Apr 2010;8(2):72–77.
19. Goldberg RM. N9741: a phase III study comparing irinotecan to oxaliplatin-containing regimens in advanced colorectal cancer. *Clin Colorectal Cancer*. Aug 2002;2(2):81.
20. Gray R, Barnwell J, McConkey C, et al. Adjuvant chemotherapy versus observation in patients with colorectal cancer: a randomised study. *Lancet*. Dec 2007;370(9604):2020–2029.
21. Grothey A, Sugrue MM, Purdie DM, et al. Bevacizumab beyond first progression is associated with prolonged overall survival in metastatic colorectal cancer: results from a large observational cohort study (BRiTE). *J Clin Oncol*. Nov 2008;26(33):5326–5334.
22. Grothey A, Van Cutsem E, Sobrero A, et al. Regorafenib monotherapy for previously treated metastatic colorectal cancer (CORRECT): an international, multicentre, randomised, placebo-controlled, phase 3 trial. *Lancet*. Jan 2013;381(9863):303–312.
23. Habr-Gama A, Perez RO, Nadalin W, et al. Operative versus nonoperative treatment for stage 0 distal rectal cancer following chemoradiation therapy: long-term results. *Ann Surg*. Oct 2004;240(4):711–717.
24. Haller DG, Catalano PJ, Macdonald JS. Fluorouracil (FU), leucovorin (LV) and levamisole (LEV) adjuvant therapy for colon cancer: five-year final report of INT-0089. *Proc Am Soc Clin Oncol*. 1998;15:211.
25. Heinemann V, von Weikersthal LF, Decker T, et al. FOLFIRI plus cetuximab versus FOLFIRI plus bevacizumab as first-line treatment for patients with metastatic colorectal cancer (FIRE-3): a randomised, open-label, phase 3 trial. *Lancet Oncol*. Sep 2014;15(10):1065–1075.
26. Hurwitz H, Fehrenbacher L, Novotny W, et al. Bevacizumab plus irinotecan, fluorouracil, and leucovorin for metastatic colorectal cancer. *N Engl J Med*. Jun 2004;350(23):2335–2342.
27. Johnson CM, Wei C, Ensor JE, et al. Meta-analyses of colorectal cancer risk factors. *Cancer Causes Control*. Jun 2013;24(6):1207–1222.
28. Kemeny MM, Adak S, Gray B, et al. Combined-modality treatment for resectable metastatic colorectal carcinoma to the liver: surgical resection of hepatic metastases in combination with continuous infusion of chemotherapy—an intergroup study. *J Clin Oncol*. Mar 2002;20(6):1499–1505.
29. Kim NK, Kim MJ, Yun SH, Sohn SK, Min JS. Comparative study of transrectal ultrasonography, pelvic computerized tomography, and magnetic resonance imaging in preoperative staging of rectal cancer. *Dis Colon Rectum*. Jun 1999;42(6):770–775.
30. Krook JE, Moertel CG, Gunderson LL, et al. Effective surgical adjuvant therapy for high-risk rectal carcinoma. *N Engl J Med*. Mar 1991;324(11):709–715.
31. Kuebler JP, Wieand HS, O'Connell MJ, et al. Oxaliplatin combined with weekly bolus fluorouracil and leucovorin as surgical adjuvant chemotherapy for stage II and III colon cancer: results from NSABP C-07. *J Clin Oncol*. Jun 2007;25(16):2198–2204.
32. Le DT, Uram JN, Wang H, et al. PD-1 blockade in tumors with mismatch-repair deficiency. *N Engl J Med*. Jun 2015;372(26):2509–2520.

33. Maalmi H, Ordóñez-Mena JM, Schöttker B, Brenner H. Serum 25-hydroxyvitamin D levels and survival in colorectal and breast cancer patients: systematic review and meta-analysis of prospective cohort studies. *Eur J Cancer*. May 2014;50(8):1510–1521.

34. Mamounas E, Wieand S, Wolmark N, et al. Comparative efficacy of adjuvant chemotherapy in patients with Dukes' B versus Dukes' C colon cancer: results from four National Surgical Adjuvant Breast and Bowel Project adjuvant studies (C-01, C-02, C-03, and C-04). *J Clin Oncol*. May 1999;17(5):1349–1355.

35. Mayer RJ, Van Cutsem E, Falcone A, et al. Randomized trial of TAS-102 for refractory metastatic colorectal cancer. *N Engl J Med*. May 2015;372(20):1909–1919.

36. McAndrew MR, Saba AK. Efficacy of routine preoperative computed tomography scans in colon cancer. *Am Surg*. Mar 1999;65(3):205–208.

37. Moertel CG, Fleming TR, Macdonald JS, et al. Levamisole and fluorouracil for adjuvant therapy of resected colon carcinoma. *N Engl J Med*. Feb 1990;322(6):352–358.

38. Saltz LB, Cox JV, Blanke C, et al. Irinotecan plus fluorouracil and leucovorin for metastatic colorectal cancer. Irinotecan Study Group. *N Engl J Med*. Sep 2000;343(13):905–914.

39. Saltz LB, Niedzwiecki D, Hollis D, et al. Irinotecan fluorouracil plus leucovorin is not superior to fluorouracil plus leucovorin alone as adjuvant treatment for stage III colon cancer: results of CALGB 89803. *J Clin Oncol*. Aug 2007;25(23):3456–3461.

40. Samowitz WS, Sweeney C, Herrick J, et al. Poor survival associated with the BRAF V600E mutation in microsatellite-stable colon cancers. *Cancer Res*. Jul 2005;65(14):6063–6069.

41. Sauer R, Becker H, Hohenberger W, et al. Preoperative versus postoperative chemoradiotherapy for rectal cancer. *N Engl J Med*. Oct 2004;351(17):1731–1740.

42. Schrag D, Rifas-Shiman S, Saltz L, Bach PB, Begg CB. Adjuvant chemotherapy use for Medicare beneficiaries with stage II colon cancer. *J Clin Oncol*. Oct 2002;20(19):3999–4005.

43. Simkens LH, van Tinteren H, May A, et al. Maintenance treatment with capecitabine and bevacizumab in metastatic colorectal cancer (CAIRO3): a phase 3 randomised controlled trial of the Dutch Colorectal Cancer Group. *Lancet*. May 2015;385(9980):1843–1852.

44. Tabernero J, Yoshino T, Cohn AL, et al. Ramucirumab versus placebo in combination with second-line FOLFIRI in patients with metastatic colorectal carcinoma that progressed during or after first-line therapy with bevacizumab, oxaliplatin, and a fluoropyrimidine (RAISE): a randomised, double-blind, multicentre, phase 3 study. *Lancet Oncol*. May 2015;16(5):499–508.

45. Tepper JE, O'Connell MJ, Petroni GR, et al. Adjuvant postoperative fluorouracil-modulated chemotherapy combined with pelvic radiation therapy for rectal cancer: initial results of intergroup 0114. *J Clin Oncol*. May 1997;15(5):2030–2039.

46. Thompson PA, Ashbeck EL, Roe DJ, et al. Celecoxib for the prevention of colorectal adenomas: results of a suspended randomized controlled trial. *J Natl Cancer Inst*. Dec 2016;108(12).

47. Tournigand C, André T, Achille E, et al. FOLFIRI followed by FOLFOX6 or the reverse sequence in advanced colorectal cancer: a randomized GERCOR study. *J Clin Oncol*. Jan 2004;22(2):229–237.

48. Twelves C, Wong A, Nowacki MP, et al. Capecitabine as adjuvant treatment for stage III colon cancer. *N Engl J Med*. Jun 2005;352(26):2696–2704.

49. Van Cutsem E, Hoff PM, Harper P, et al. Oral capecitabine vs intravenous 5-fluorouracil and leucovorin: integrated efficacy data and novel analyses from two large, randomised, phase III trials. *Br J Cancer*. Mar 2004;90(6):1190–1197.

50. Van Cutsem E, Köhne CH, Hitre E, et al. Cetuximab and chemotherapy as initial treatment for metastatic colorectal cancer. *N Engl J Med*. Apr 2009;360(14):1408–1417.

51. Van Cutsem E, Labianca R, Bodoky G, et al. Randomized phase III trial comparing biweekly infusional fluorouracil/leucovorin alone or with irinotecan in the adjuvant treatment of stage III colon cancer: PETACC-3. *J Clin Oncol*. Jul 2009;27(19):3117–3125.

52. Van Cutsem E, Peeters M, Siena S, et al. Open-label phase III trial of panitumumab plus best supportive care compared with best supportive care alone in patients with chemotherapy-refractory metastatic colorectal cancer. *J Clin Oncol*. May 2007;25(13):1658–1664.

53. Van Cutsem E, Tabernero J, Lakomy R, et al. Addition of aflibercept to fluorouracil, leucovorin, and irinotecan improves survival in a phase III randomized trial in patients with metastatic colorectal cancer previously treated with an oxaliplatin-based regimen. *J Clin Oncol*. Oct 2012;30(28):3499–3506.

54. Venook A, Niedzwiecki D, Lenz HJ. CALGB/SWOG 80405: phase III trial of FOLFIRI or mFOLFOX6 with bevacizumab or cetuximab for patients with KRAS wild-type untreated metastatic adenocarcinoma of the colon or rectum. *J Clin Oncol*. 2014;32(5s):LBA(abstr).

55. Venook A, Niewzwiecki D, Innocenti F. Impact of primary tumor location on overall survival and progression-free survival in patients with metastatic colorectal cancer: analysis of CALBG/SWOG 80405 (Alliance). *J Clin Oncol*. 2016;34:3504a.

56. Ychou M, Raoul RJ, Douillard JY, et al. A phase III randomized trial of LV5FU2+CPT-11 vs LV5FU2 alone in adjuvant high risk colon cancer (FNCLCC Accord02/FFCD9802). *J Clin Oncol*. 2005;23(suppl):3502a.

10 Pancreatic Cancer

Ananth K. Arjunan and James J. Lee

INTRODUCTION

The majority of pancreatic cancers arise from the exocrine pancreas and are of the pancreatic ductal adenocarcinoma (PDAC) subtype. PDAC comprises 90% of all primary pancreatic cancers. Other subtypes of exocrine pancreatic cancer such as acinar cell carcinoma are rare. The pancreatic neuroendocrine tumors that arise from the endocrine islet cells form a small minority of primary pancreatic cancers. The focus of this chapter is PDAC, which will hereafter be treated as synonymous with the term pancreatic cancer.

EPIDEMIOLOGY

In 2017, there will be 53,670 patients with newly diagnosed pancreatic cancer and 43,090 deaths due to pancreatic cancer in the United States. It only comprises 3.1% of all new cancer diagnoses, yet is the fourth leading cause of cancer-related death. About 88.3% of patients are diagnosed after age 55 and the median age of diagnosis is 70 years. Males have a slightly increased incidence compared to females. In comparison to all races, African Americans have a higher incidence (15.5 vs. 12.4 per 100,000) and higher mortality rate (13.5 vs. 10.9 per 100,000). Only a modest improvement in 5-year overall survival (OS) has been noted over several decades, from 3% for patients diagnosed in 1975 to 7.6% for patients diagnosed in 2008.

Risk Factors

- *Family history and hereditary syndromes.* There is clear association of family history with a lifetime risk of pancreatic cancer—6% with 1 affected first-degree relative (FDR), 40% with ≥3 affected FDRs. Approximately 10% of pancreatic cancer is attributable to a hereditary component. Table 10.1 summarizes inherited syndromes associated with pancreatic cancer.
- *Smoking.* Two-fold increased risk in active smokers. Risk correlates with smoking intensity and is less in former smokers. Twenty-five percent of pancreatic cancer is attributable to smoking.
- *Chronic pancreatitis.* Confers a five-fold increased risk. Patients with an underlying hereditary pancreatitis or tropical pancreatitis have at least 70-fold increased risk.
- *Alcohol.* There is strong evidence that heavy use (≥30 g or >3 drinks per day) is associated with a 20% increased risk.
- *Increased weight.* Risk is increased by 10% and 20% in overweight and obese patients, respectively. This association is not seen in the Asian population.
- *Insulin resistance.* There is at least a 50% increased risk with long-standing diabetes. Similar risk increase is seen in patients with metabolic syndrome.
- *Dietary intake and nutrition.* Meta-analyses of retrospective studies support an association with consumption of processed meat and red meat. There is conflicting evidence on risk reduction with fruit and vegetable intake. No clear association is noted with tea or coffee consumption. Vitamin D level has no clear association.

TABLE 10.1 Inherited Syndromes Associated with Pancreatic Cancer

	Affected Gene	Relative Risk	Comments
Hereditary pancreatitis	PRSS1 (cationic trypsinogen)	20–75	Present in youth with recurrent acute pancreatitis leading to chronic pancreatitis. Pancreatic cancer occurs 2–3 decades after onset of chronic pancreatitis.
Peutz-Jeghers syndrome	STK11/LKB1 (serine threonine kinase 11)	132	Tumor suppressor gene. Presents with benign GI polyps, melanosis of mouth/hands/feet. Also associated with breast, lung, endometrial, gonadal cancers.
Familial atypical multiple mole melanoma (FAMMM)	CDKN2A (p16)	13–22	Tumor suppressor gene. Also associated with melanoma, breast, endometrial, lung cancers.
Hereditary breast/ ovarian cancers (HBOC)	BRCA1 BRCA2 PALB2	2.3–3.6 3–10 Unknown	Tumor suppressor genes. BRCA2 is the most common hereditary risk factor for pancreatic cancer.
Familial adenomatous polyposis (FAP)	APC	5	Tumor suppressor gene. Associated with numerous colon polyps beginning in adolescence and colon cancer in young adulthood.
Hereditary non-polyposis colon cancer (HNPCC)	MSH2, MLH1	Unknown	Mismatch repair proteins. Less frequently from MSH6, PMS1, and PMS2 mutations. Associated with cancers of colon (especially right-sided), endometrium, ovary, stomach, small intestine, biliary tract, upper GU tract, brain, skin.

■ *Chronic infections.* Evidence supports a strong association with *Helicobacter pylori* and there is evidence of slight increased risk with Hepatitis B and Hepatitis C.
■ *ABO blood type.* Non-O blood groups have a 30% to 40% increased risk.

PATHOPHYSIOLOGY

The pancreas is anatomically divided into the *head* which lies within the duodenal curvature, the *neck*, the *body* which crosses midline posterior to the stomach pylorus, and finally tapers into the *tail* which terminates near the splenic hilum. About 70% of pancreatic cancer arises from the pancreatic head. The pancreas abuts major vascular structures including the aorta, celiac artery, gastroduodenal artery, splenic artery/vein, superior mesenteric artery/vein (SMA/SMV), and inferior vena cava (IVC). The pancreatic duct courses from the tail to the head and joins the common bile duct to exit in union at the ampulla into the second part of the duodenum. PDAC arises from the pancreatic ductal epithelium.

About 95% of invasive PDAC is preceded by pancreatic intraepithelial neoplasia (PanIN), a flat or papillary duct cell proliferation that is <0.5 cm in size. Other preinvasive changes such as intraductal papillary mucinous neoplasia (IPMN) and mucinous cystic neoplasia (MCN) are less common. IPMN lesions are frequently found on imaging, occurring in 2% of adults, and have a 25% chance of becoming invasive cancer.

Several driver gene mutations are implicated in PDAC—*KRAS, CDKN2A, SMAD4, TP53*. Activation of the *KRAS* oncogene and telomere shortening is observed in early PanIN lesions and is followed by inactivation of the tumor suppressor genes *CDKN2A*, *TP53*, and *SMAD4* as they progress toward a more invasive phenotype. When pancreatic cancer metastasizes, it typically involves the liver, peritoneum, or lung. *SMAD4* loss has been shown to correlate with presence of widely metastatic disease.

CLINICAL PRESENTATION

The most common symptoms of pancreatic cancer are fatigue, weight loss, anorexia, abdominal pain, jaundice, and dark urine. Loss of exocrine tissue or pancreatic duct obstruction leads to malabsorption and steatorrhea, which can necessitate the use of pancreatic enzyme supplementation. An atypical presentation of diabetes can occur from the loss of functioning islet cells with 40% of patients being diagnosed with diabetes in 36 months prior to a pancreatic cancer diagnosis. Pain in the abdomen and back occurs due to involvement of celiac and mesenteric nerve plexi. Symptoms from metastatic disease, such as ascites from peritoneal deposits may occur.

SCREENING AND DIAGNOSIS

There is no role for screening of the general population for pancreatic cancer. The Cancer of the Pancreas Screening (CAPS) consortium produced consensus guidelines in 2011 recommending screening by endoscopic ultrasound (EUS) or MRI of select individuals (FDRs of patients with pancreatic cancer from a familial kindred with ≥2 affected FDRs; patients with Peutz-Jeghers syndrome; and carriers of p16, BRCA2, HNPCC mutations with ≥1 affected FDR). No consensus was achieved on screening frequency or at what ages to implement screening.

Initial diagnostic evaluation in patients with suspected pancreatic cancer includes laboratories and abdominal imaging. The primary tumor marker associated with PDAC is carbohydrate antigen 19-9 (CA 19-9). It is useful for monitoring disease response with treatment, but remains a poor diagnostic test with a median sensitivity and specificity of 79% and 82%, respectively. CA 19-9 is a sialylated Lewis[a] blood group antigen and thus is not a useful marker in the 10% of Caucasians and 22% of African Americans who do not express the Lewis antigen.

The imaging study of choice is a "pancreatic protocol" CT scan, which involves triple-phase contrast enhancement on multidetector CT. The late arterial phase helps to distinguish the hypoattenuating tumor from normal parenchyma and the portal phase allows visualization of interface between the tumor and adjacent venous structures and detection of liver metastases. Abdominal ultrasound can identify pancreatic cancer as a solid, hypoechoic mass and show associated biliary ductal dilatation from tumor obstruction. However, it is subject to variability based on operator skill, may miss tumors <3 cm, and incompletely evaluates the pancreas when overlying bowel gas is present.

Endoscopic retrograde cholangiopancreatography (ERCP) is of limited diagnostic utility as the sensitivity of ERCP biopsy or brushing for cytology is low and classically described finding of the "double duct sign" (pancreatic and biliary duct dilatation) are not specific to pancreatic tumors. ERCP is likely more useful as a therapeutic intervention in relieving malignant biliary obstructions. EUS with fine-needle aspiration (FNA) has a sensitivity of 92% and specificity of 96% in diagnosing pancreatic cancer, and it is the preferred method of obtaining a histopathologic diagnosis. Percutaneous biopsy is avoided due to a theoretical concern for seeding of tumor in the biopsy needle tract or peritoneal cavity.

STAGING

The staging of pancreatic cancer is based upon the TNM system of the American Joint Committee on Cancer (AJCC). The AJCC designates T4 (tumor involving celiac axis or SMA) as unresectable disease, but studies have shown some T4 tumors can achieve R0 resection after neoadjuvant therapy. Practically speaking, the goal of staging evaluation in pancreatic cancer is to evaluate local disease for resectability and rule out distant metastases.

Triple-phase "pancreatic protocol" CT scan of the abdomen is the mainstay of staging. MRI scan and PET/CT scan can be done but provide no additional benefit in comparison to CT. EUS is good at local tumor and nodal staging, may evaluate for some distant metastases in liver, and can sample ascites fluid. However, it is invasive and evaluation of primary tumor can be confounded by parenchymal inflammation. Staging laparoscopy is considered in those at risk of occult peritoneal involvement (body/tail tumors, primary tumor >3 cm, very high initial CA 19-9, and imaging suggestive of occult disease).

TREATMENT

Pancreatic cancer can be split into treatment categories: (1) resectable, (2) borderline resectable, (3) locally advanced, unresectable, or (4) metastatic. Pancreatic cancer portends a high burden of morbidity and mortality, so palliative/supportive care should be implemented early. Patients are best evaluated by multidisciplinary teams at high-volume centers. Efforts should always be made to offer clinical trial enrollment to eligible patients.

Resectable Disease

Fifteen percent of patients present with resectable disease, which means there is no arterial tumor contact and no SMV or portal vein contact (or ≤180° contact without vein contour irregularity). Treatment involves surgical resection followed by 6 months of adjuvant chemotherapy with gemcitabine (GEM) or GEM plus capecitabine. There is no proven role for chemoradiotherapy (CRT) as of yet.

Surgical Resection. Resection offers a potentially curative treatment, but recurrences are common even with R0 resections. Patients must have good functional status to tolerate a major abdominal surgery. Resection is underutilized in the United States among early stage pancreatic cancer patients with 38.2% of appropriate candidates not undergoing resection. Pancreatic head tumors undergo conventional or pylorus-preserving pancreaticoduodenectomy (Whipple procedure), whereas pancreatic body/tail tumors undergo a distal pancreatectomy, often with splenectomy. Staging laparoscopy should be considered prior to resection with head/tail tumors given possibility of occult peritoneal metastases. Total pancreatectomy is done only if entire gland involved by tumor, but has a high attendant morbidity. Extended pancreatectomy and extended lymphadenectomy do not improve survival. Vein resection with reconstruction is performed when tumor focally involves the portal vein or SMV.

Adjuvant Chemotherapy. All patients who have had resection should receive 6 months of adjuvant chemotherapy with either GEM alone or GEM/Capecitabine. Chemotherapy is typically initiated 4 to 6 weeks after resection, though benefit is conferred even when initiation is delayed to 12 weeks. Completion of all planned cycles tends to be the more important factor in terms of outcomes. Relevant clinical trials involving adjuvant chemotherapy are summarized below:

- **ESPAC-1** used a 2 × 2 factorial design to randomize 289 patients after resection into four treatment arms: (1) chemoradiotherapy alone; (2) chemotherapy alone; (3) both chemoradiotherapy and chemotherapy; and (4) observation. Five-year OS was 21% in those who received chemotherapy versus 8% in those who did not ($P = 0.009$).
- **CONKO-001** randomized 368 patients after resection to 6 months of adjuvant chemotherapy with GEM versus observation. Median DFS was 13.4 and 6.7 months in the GEM and observation groups, respectively, with HR 0.55 ($P < 0.001$). Five-year OS was 20.7% and 10.4% with GEM and observation, respectively, with HR 0.76 ($P = 0.01$).
- **ESPAC-3 (v2)** randomized 1,088 patients after resection to 6 months of adjuvant chemotherapy with GEM versus 5-fluorouracil/folinic acid (5FU/FA). There was no significant difference in median survival of about 23 months in each group. More adverse events were noted with 5FU/FA.
- **RTOG 9704** randomized 451 patients with gross resection to receive chemotherapy with either GEM or 5FU/FA at 3 weeks prior and 12 weeks after planned chemoradiotherapy. No significant difference in OS was noted. The subset with pancreatic head tumors trended toward improved median survival and 5-year OS but did not reach statistical significance.
- **JASPAC 01** randomized 385 Japanese patients to receive adjuvant chemotherapy with GEM versus S-1 (an oral prodrug of 5FU). Five-year OS in the S-1 group was 44.1% versus 24.4% in the GEM group with HR 0.57 ($P < 0.0001$). S-1 is not currently approved in the United States and studies are needed to show validity in non-Asian populations.

- **ESPAC-4** randomized 732 patients to gemcitabine alone (N = 366) or gemcitabine plus capecitabine (N = 364). Enrolled patients received six cycles of either 1,000 mg/m^2 gemcitabine alone administered once a week for three of every 4 weeks (one cycle) or with 1,660 mg/m^2 oral capecitabine administered for 21 days followed by 7 days' rest (one cycle). The median OS was 28.0 months in the gemcitabine plus capecitabine group and 25.5 months in the gemcitabine monotherapy group (HR 0.82; 95% CI, 0.68 to 0.98; P = 0.032). There was increased incidence of grade 3 to 4 toxicities in the combination arm.
- Other ongoing trials of intensified chemotherapy in the adjuvant setting include **APACT** (GEM/nab-paclitaxel) and **PRODIGE/ACCORD24** (GEM/modified FOLFIRINOX).

Adjuvant Chemoradiotherapy (CRT). There is no recommendation for CRT in the adjuvant setting. Relevant clinical trials involving adjuvant CRT are summarized below:

- **ESPAC-1** (see above for trial design) showed trend toward harm with CRT with a 5-year OS of 10% versus 20% in those who did not receive CRT.
- **EORTC 40891** compared 218 patients receiving CRT versus observation alone. Median survival and 2-year survival rates had no significant differences.
- **GITSG** compared CRT to observation alone and showed 2-year survival rates of 43% with CRT versus 18% with observation (P < 0.03). Several criticisms of the trial include the poor patient accrual (only 43 patients) and atypical treatment schedule with a split course of radiation given and the 5FU component being given during the first week of radiation and continued for up to 2 years after.
- **RTOG 0848** is an ongoing phase III trial, which hopes to further investigate the role of adjuvant CRT by evaluating outcomes when it is added after 6 months of GEM in comparison to GEM chemotherapy alone.

Neoadjuvant Therapy. Theoretical advantages of neoadjuvant therapy in resectable disease include upfront treatment of micrometastases, higher likelihood of negative resection margins, and ability to give treatment before post-resection complications. Although there are no reliable data from randomized studies in this setting yet, neoadjuvant therapy is gaining more support at major centers, especially for patients with borderline resectable disease.

Borderline Resectable Disease

Borderline resectable disease is localized disease which is not likely to achieve negative resection margins. While there is no universal definition of borderline resectability, it typically means that tumor focally involves the visceral arteries (≤180°) or has short-segment encasement or occlusion of major veins. Treatment involves use of chemotherapy for 2 to 3 months to downstage the tumor before attempted resection. There is a paucity of evidence to guide which exact regimen to use but multi-agent chemotherapy is typically given (e.g., FOLFIRINOX or GEM/nab-paclitaxel). The **Alliance Trial A021101 (NCT01821612)** is an ongoing study in borderline resectable disease using mFOLFIRINOX and subsequent capecitabine-based chemoradiation before resection and adjuvant GEM. Initial results have shown 68% underwent surgery with 93% of those achieving R0 resection.

Locally Advanced, Unresectable Disease

About 35% of patients present with locally advanced, unresectable disease. Typically, it is treated with multi-agent chemotherapy (GEM/nab-paclitaxel or FOLFIRINOX based on extrapolation of data in the metastatic setting) for at least 3 months. CRT is then considered in those who have not progressed systemically. Upfront CRT is reserved for patients with poorly controlled pain or bleeding from local invasion. Repeat imaging to evaluate for response or progression is recommended every 2 to 3 months. Relevant clinical trials are summarized below:

- **ECOG 4201** compared CRT followed by GEM versus GEM alone with median OS of 11.1 and 9.2 months, respectively (one-sided P = 0.017). However, grade 4 or higher toxicity was more in CRT arm (41% vs. 9%). It was limited by poor accrual (only 74 patients).
- **FFCD-SFRO** enrolled 119 patients and compared CRT followed by GEM versus GEM alone. OS was shorter in the CRT group than in the GEM-alone group (8.6 vs. 13 months; P =0.03) and more grade 3 to 4 toxicity was seen in the CRT arm.

▪ **LAP 07** studied CRT versus GEM maintenance in patients who had already received induction chemotherapy for 4 months without progression. No difference in median OS was noted at 16.5 versus 15.3 months (HR 1.03; P = 0.83). However, CRT was associated with decreased local progression. There was no increased grade 3 to 4 toxicity in the CRT group except for nausea.

Metastatic Disease

At least 50% of patients present with metastatic disease. The first-line treatment of metastatic disease remains combination cytotoxic chemotherapy. Performance status is the major determinant of which regimen is used.

In 1997, GEM was proven to be superior to 5-FU/FA with regards to clinical benefit response and survival. Subsequently, several phase III studies of GEM combined with other cytotoxic or targeted agents were conducted but showed no significant improvement in survival. However, pooled analysis showed modest improvement in survival when GEM was combined with cytotoxic therapy in patients with good functional status. In recent years, use of the combination cytotoxic regimens FOLFIRINOX and GEM/nab-paclitaxel have shown benefit and are the main first-line regimens. Single-agent chemotherapy is recommended in those with poor performance status. Clinical trials should be encouraged in eligible patients.

▪ **PRODIGE4/ACCORD11** randomized 342 patients to receive FOLFIRINOX or GEM and showed superiority of FOLFIRINOX with HR for death of 0.57 (P < 0.01) and median survival improved by 4.3 months. Quality of life was preserved for a longer period despite more grade 3 to 4 toxicities in the FOLFIRINOX group.
▪ **MPACT** randomized 861 patients to receive GEM/nab-paclitaxel versus GEM alone with median OS of 8.5 versus 6.7 months (HR 0.72; P < 0.01).

Second-line therapy involves use of GEM-containing chemotherapy in those initially treated with 5FU/FA-containing regimen, and vice-versa. Recent data suggests benefit with addition of liposomal irinotecan.

▪ **NAPOLI-1** evaluated the use of nanoliposomal irinotecan with 5-FU/FA versus each agent alone in patients previously treated with GEM. Median survival improved in the combined treatment group compared to 5-FU/FA alone (6.1 vs. 4.2 months; HR 0.6; P = 0.012).
▪ **PANCREOX** showed no difference in PFS, worse OS, and more toxicity in patients receiving modified FOLFOX6 compared to 5FU/FA alone in the second-line setting after receiving GEM.

Immunotherapy of Pancreatic Cancer

Pancreatic cancer is generally considered to be a nonimmunogenic tumor. Trials with immune checkpoint inhibitors against CTLA-4 and PD-1 have not shown the same promising results seen in other solid tumors. Current efforts have focused on the PD-1 blockade +/– anti-CTLA-4 in combination with various immune-potentiating modalities including radiation or chemotherapy.

Suggested Readings

1. Aggarwal G, Kamada P, Chari ST. Prevalence of diabetes mellitus in pancreatic cancer compared to common cancers. *Pancreas.* 2013;42(2):198–201.
2. Bilimoria KY, Bentrem DJ, Ko CY, Stewart AK, Winchester DP, Talamonti MS. National failure to operate on early stage pancreatic cancer. *Ann Surg.* 2007;246(2):173–180.
3. Canto MI, Harinck F, Hruban RH, et al. International Cancer of the Pancreas Screening (CAPS) Consortium summit on the management of patients with increased risk for familial pancreatic cancer. *Gut.* 2013;62(3):339–347.
4. Chauffert B, Mornex F, Bonnetain F, et al. Phase III trial comparing intensive induction chemoradiotherapy (60 Gy, infusional 5-FU and intermittent cisplatin) followed by maintenance gemcitabine with gemcitabine alone for locally advanced unresectable pancreatic cancer. Definitive results of the 2000-01 FFCD/SFRO study. *Ann Oncol.* 2008;19(9):1592–1599.
5. Chen J, Yang R, Lu Y, Xia Y, Zhou H. Diagnostic accuracy of endoscopic ultrasound-guided fine-needle aspiration for solid pancreatic lesion: a systematic review. *J Cancer Res Clin Oncol.* 2012;138(9):1433–1441.
6. Conroy T, Desseigne F, Ychou M, et al. FOLFIRINOX versus gemcitabine for metastatic pancreatic cancer. *N Engl J Med.* 2011;364(19):1817–1825.
7. Edge SB, Byrd DR, Compton CC, Fritz AG, Greene FL, Trotti A, eds. Cancer survival analysis. In: *AJCC Cancer Staging Manual.* New York: Springer; 2010:15–20.
8. Esposito I, Segler A, Steiger K, Kloppel G. Pathology, genetics and precursors of human and experimental pancreatic neoplasms: an update. *Pancreatology.* 2015;15(6):598–610.

9. Gastrointestinal Tumor Study Group. Radiation therapy combined with Adriamycin or 5-fluorouracil for the treatment of locally unresectable pancreatic carcinoma. *Cancer.* 1985;56(11):2563–2568.

10. Gill S, Ko YJ, Cripps C, et al. PANCREOX: a randomized phase III study of 5-fluorouracil/leucovorin with or without oxaliplatin for second-line advanced pancreatic cancer in patients who have received gemcitabine-based chemotherapy. *J Clin Oncol.* 2016;34(32):3914–3920.

11. Goonetilleke KS, Siriwardena AK. Systematic review of carbohydrate antigen (CA 19-9) as a biochemical marker in the diagnosis of pancreatic cancer. *Eur J Surg Oncol.* 2007;33(3):266–270.

12. Greer JB, Lynch HT, Brand RE. Hereditary pancreatic cancer: a clinical perspective. *Best Pract Res Clin Gastroenterol.* 2009;23(2):159–170.

13. Hammel P, Huguet F, van Laethem JL, et al. Effect of chemoradiotherapy vs chemotherapy on survival in patients with locally advanced pancreatic cancer controlled after 4 months of gemcitabine with or without erlotinib: the LAP07 randomized clinical trial. *JAMA.* 2016;315(17):1844–1853.

14. Howlader N, Noone AM, Krapcho M, et al. *SEER Cancer Statistics Review, 1975–2013 [Internet].* Bethesda, MD: National Cancer Institute; 2016 [cited February 20, 2017].

15. Iacobuzio-Donahue CA, Fu B, Yachida S, et al. DPC4 gene status of the primary carcinoma correlates with patterns of failure in patients with pancreatic cancer. *J Clin Oncol.* 2009;27(11):1806–1813.

16. Katz MHG, Shi Q, Ahmad SA, et al. Preoperative modified FOLFIRINOX treatment followed by capecitabine-based chemoradiation for borderline resectable pancreatic cancer: alliance for clinical trials in oncology trial A021101. *JAMA Surg.* 2016;151(8):e161137.

17. Khorana AA, Mangu PB, Berlin J, et al. Potentially curable pancreatic cancer: American Society of Clinical Oncology Clinical Practice Guideline. *J Clin Oncol.* 2016;34(21):2541–2556.

18. Klinkenbijl JH, Jeekel J, Sahmoud T, et al. Adjuvant radiotherapy and 5-fluorouracil after curative resection of cancer of the pancreas and periampullary region: phase III trial of the EORTC gastrointestinal tract cancer cooperative group. *Ann Surg.* 1999;230(6):776–782; discussion 782–784.

19. Loehrer PJ, Feng Y, Cardenes H, et al. Gemcitabine alone versus gemcitabine plus radiotherapy in patients with locally advanced pancreatic cancer: an Eastern Cooperative Oncology Group trial. *J Clin Oncol.* 2011;29(31):4105–4112.

20. Maisonneuve P, Lowenfels AB. Risk factors for pancreatic cancer: a summary review of meta-analytical studies. *Int J Epidemiol.* 2015;44(1):186–198.

21. Neoptolemos JP, Palmer DH, Ghaneh P, et al. Comparison of adjuvant gemcitabine and capecitabine with gemcitabine monotherapy in patients with resected pancreatic cancer (ESPAC-4): a multicentre, open-label, randomised, phase 3 trial. *Lancet* 2017;389(10073):1011–1024.

22. Neoptolemos JP, Stocken DD, Bassi C, et al. Adjuvant chemotherapy with fluorouracil plus folinic acid vs gemcitabine following pancreatic cancer resection: a randomized controlled trial. *JAMA.* 2010;304(10):1073–1081.

23. Neoptolemos JP, Stocken DD, Friess H, et al. A randomized trial of chemoradiotherapy and chemotherapy after resection of pancreatic cancer. *N Engl J Med.* 2004;350(12):1200–1210.

24. Oettle H, Neuhaus P, Hochhaus A, et al. Adjuvant chemotherapy with gemcitabine and long-term outcomes among patients with resected pancreatic cancer: the CONKO-001 randomized trial. *JAMA.* 2013;310(14):1473–1481.

25. Porta M, Fabregat X, Malats N, et al. Exocrine pancreatic cancer: symptoms at presentation and their relation to tumour site and stage. *Clin Transl Oncol.* 2005;7(5):189–197.

26. Regine WF, Winter KA, Abrams R, et al. Fluorouracil-based chemoradiation with either gemcitabine or fluorouracil chemotherapy after resection of pancreatic adenocarcinoma: 5-year analysis of the U.S. Intergroup/RTOG 9704 phase III trial. *Ann Surg Oncol.* 2011;18(5):1319–1326.

27. Seufferlein T, Bachet JB, Van Cutsem E, Rouger P. Pancreatic adenocarcinoma: ESMO–ESDO Clinical Practice Guidelines for diagnosis, treatment and follow-up†. *Ann Oncol.* 2012;23(suppl. 7):vii33–vii40.

28. Siegel RL, Miller KD, Jemal A. Cancer Statistics, 2017. *CA Cancer J Clin.* 2017;67(1):7–30.

29. Strobel O, Berens V, Hinz U, et al. Resection after neoadjuvant therapy for locally advanced, "unresectable" pancreatic cancer. *Surgery.* 2012;152(3 Suppl 1):S33–S42.

30. Uesaka K, Boku N, Fukutomi A, et al. Adjuvant chemotherapy of S-1 versus gemcitabine for resected pancreatic cancer: a phase 3, open-label, randomised, non-inferiority trial (JASPAC 01). *Lancet.* 2016;388(10041):248–257.

31. Valle JW, Palmer D, Jackson R, et al. Optimal duration and timing of adjuvant chemotherapy after definitive surgery for ductal adenocarcinoma of the pancreas: ongoing lessons from the ESPAC-3 study. *J Clin Oncol.* 2014;32(6):504–512.

32. Von Hoff DD, Ervin T, Arena FP, et al. Increased survival in pancreatic cancer with nab-paclitaxel plus gemcitabine. *N Engl J Med.* 2013;369(18):1691–1703.

33. Wang-Gillam A, Li CP, Bodoky G, et al. Nanoliposomal irinotecan with fluorouracil and folinic acid in metastatic pancreatic cancer after previous gemcitabine-based therapy (NAPOLI-1): a global, randomised, open-label, phase 3 trial. *Lancet.* 2016;387(10018):545–557.

Anal Cancer 11

Chaoyuan Kuang and James J. Lee

INTRODUCTION

In the United States, anal cancer represents a rare malignancy and accounts for 2.5% of all gastro-intestinal malignancies; 8,200 new cases are diagnosed annually in the United States. The incidence has been increasing over the past four decades. The most significant risk factors are sexually transmitted viruses, tobacco smoking, and immunosuppression. Progress has been made over the years in the management of anal cancer. In the 1970s, treatment focused on abdomino-perineal resection (APR). Initially Nigro ND and colleagues at Wayne State employed preoperative chemotherapy with 5-FU and mitomycin (MMC) with radiation therapy (30 Gy) to improve on local control. Complete pathologic responses were discovered and ushered in the concept of definitive chemoradiation, which continues to be the mainstay of therapy for localized anal canal cancer. Since then, intensity-modulated radiation therapy (IMRT) and targeted biologic therapies have been recent advances which are not yet standard of care.

EPIDEMIOLOGY

The annual age-adjusted rates in the U.S. Surveillance, Epidemiology, and End Results (SEER) registry for 2009 to 2013 had dropped to 1.5 per 100,000 for males but increased to 2.1 for females. Cancers of the anus, anal canal, and anorectum are some of the few cancers that are more common in females than in males at nearly all ages. A potential reason for the rise in females may relate to the evolving sexual practices and association with anal HPV infections. Median age at diagnosis is 61. Advancing age is a risk factor for anal canal cancer. In certain populations such as HIV positive men who have sex with other men (MSM), the rate of anal cancer can be as high as 131 per 100,000.

ETIOLOGY AND RISK FACTORS

Several risk factors have been associated with the development of anal cancer:

- *Sexual activity*
  - 10 or more lifetime sexual partners
  - receptive anal intercourse before the age of 30
  - history of gonorrhea or syphilis or herpes simplex 2 or chlamydia
  - history of cervical cancer
- *Human papillomavirus infection.* Up to 93% of squamous cell carcinoma (SCC) of the anal canal has been associated with HPV infection, which is believed to cause tumor transformation by deregulating the cell cycle and evading immune surveillance. Women are more likely to have an HPV-associated anal cancer than men. Also HPV infection is more common in MSM. HPV 16 and 18 are the most frequently associated strains linked with anal cancer and account for 90% of anal cancers. HPV vaccination has been shown to reduce the risk of premalignant lesions (AIN 2/3).

- *HIV infection.* The incidence of anal cancer in HIV-infected MSM was found to be as high as 131 per 100,000 males in a recent study. The effect of HIV infection on incidence is less dramatic at 46 per 100,000 in other HIV-infected men and 30 per 100,000 in HIV-infected women. It is unknown whether HIV infection directly affects the pathogenesis or if the impact is through the interaction with HPV. Loss of T cell activity likely contributes to the failure of immune clearance of tumor cells.
- *Cigarette Smoking.* Case–control studies indicate increased risk in smokers and especially among current smokers.
- There are currently no guidelines for screening high risk individuals for anal cancer or AIN due to lack of proven benefit. A phase III trial is currently underway to examine whether chemical or surgical ablation versus observation of AIN in HIV positive patients increases the time to the development of anal carcinoma (NCT02135419).

PATHOLOGY

The anal canal measures approximately 3 to 4 cm in length. It extends from the anal verge to the puborectalis muscle of the anorectal ring. The dentate line is situated within the anal canal and the histology separates depending on the location above or below the dentate line. Proximal to the dentate, the histology is columnar epithelium, and distal to the dentate, the histology becomes squamous cell epithelium. The anal margin has been arbitrarily defined as an area within 5 cm of the anal verge.

Drainage proximal to the dentate line follows the distal rectum to the internal iliac lymph nodes (pudendal, hypogastric, and obturator). Drainage from the perianal skin, anal verge, and the region distal to the dentate line follows the superficial inguinal lymph nodes with some flow to the femoral nodes and external iliac lymphatics.

The anus comprises three different histologic types: (1) glandular, (2) transitional, and (3) squamous mucosa. Cancers arising from the transitional or squamous mucosa develop into squamous cell carcinomas. The basaloid or transitional carcinomas (formerly known as cloacogenic or junctional tumors) develop from the transitional mucosa. Those cancers developing above the dentate line are nonkeratinizing squamous cell carcinomas versus those distal to the dentate line are keratinizing squamous cell carcinomas. Tumors arising from the glandular mucosa of the anal canal develop into adenocarcinomas. Anal margin tumors develop within the hair-bearing skin distal to the transitional mucosa.

CLINICAL PRESENTATION

Rectal bleeding and anal discomfort are the two most common symptoms, occurring in over 45% and 30% of patients, respectively. Pruritus and discharge are other symptoms. Pain can be severe. Changes in bowel habits can be a presenting symptom, especially with proximal anal canal cancers. Patients may be asymptomatic as well.

MEDICAL WORKUP

Workup should include anoscope with biopsy (incisional), digital rectal examination (DRE), inguinal lymph node evaluation (biopsy or FNA of any suspicious lymph nodes), chest CT, abdominal/pelvic CT, or MRI. Pelvic examination should be performed on women including screening for cervical cancer. Consider HIV testing and CD4 levels for patients at risk. While PET/CT has not been validated as a tool for staging compared to CT in a prospective trial, PET/CT has resulted in up- and downstaging due to the presence or absence of positive lymph nodes and should be considered if advanced radiation techniques are planned. Full chemistries and CBC should be performed as well.

Staging is based on the seventh edition of the *American Joint Committee on Cancer* (AJCC), which employs a TNM system for the staging of anal canal cancers. T stage is based partly upon the size of the primary lesion or the invasion of nearby structures such as the bladder, prostate, vagina, or urethra.

The N stage is determined by the presence of perirectal, internal iliac, or inguinal lymph nodes. The M stage is based upon the presence or absence of distant metastases.

PROGNOSTIC FACTORS

- Tumor size. The size of the primary lesion has been shown to be one of the most significant factors in predicting local control and survival for lesions confined to the pelvis.
- Lymph nodes. The presence or absence of lymph nodes also has been shown to impact survival.
- Metastasis. The most significant prognostic risk factor for overall survival is the presence or absence of extrapelvic metastases.
- HIV status. High viral load and low CD4+ count in some series have predicted for survival and local control.
- Other: Hemoglobin levels ≤10 g/L, male gender, p16+ HPV status, and ulceration of the primary lesion have impacted prognosis in some studies.

TREATMENT

Surgery

Anal Canal Lesions

In the 1970s, surgical resection with an APR was considered standard of care. APR produced local control rates of 70%, and overall survival rates from 20% to 70% (average 50%). With inguinal lymph node involvement, some series showed 5-year survivals of 10% to 20%. After the 1974 publication by Nigro et al. showing complete pathologic response in three patients treated with chemoradiation, anal cancer patients are rarely treated with upfront surgery, and definitive chemoradiation remains the current standard of care. APR is reserved for salvage after failure with definitive chemoradiation or reserved for management of radiation complications.

Surgery alone with local excision may be considered with small, localized T1N0M0 squamous cell carcinomas of the anal canal. Several small retrospective series have demonstrated good local control and 5-year survival with such an approach. The key to offering local excision is patient selection. Patients with small tumors <2 cm, well differentiated, and no involvement of the sphincter may be considered candidates. Otherwise, chemoradiation should be offered.

Anal Margin Lesions

Early anal margin cancers have traditionally been treated with local excision. Such lesions behave more like a skin cancer, although this concept has never been validated prospectively. Wide local excision has been reserved mostly for well-differentiated T1N0M0 lesions with good local control. In a retrospective review of 48 patients with squamous cell carcinoma of the anal margin, 31 patients underwent local excision, and 11 were treated by APR. Local excision provided satisfactory results with a 5-year survival of 88%. However, larger lesions T2 or > or N+ should be treated with definitive chemoradiation.

Radiation Therapy

Since the Nigro et al.'s publication in 1974, radiation therapy has become the primary curative modality for the treatment of anal cancer. Radiation techniques have evolved over time and varying types of radiation therapy have been used including external beam radiation therapy (3D and IMRT), electrons, and brachytherapy.

Radiation alone has been used to treat early anal cancer (T1–T2N0M0) with relative success; most retrospective studies have demonstrated modest local control and 5-year survivals; however, not all studies show good local control with radiation alone. Tumors <2 cm appear to have better local control in particular. NCCN guidelines, however, recommend combined modality for even small T1N0M0 squamous cell carcinomas of anal canal. For the very elderly or those with significant comorbidities, radiation alone may be a reasonable approach.

Combined Radiation Therapy and Chemotherapy as Standard of Care

Nigro et al. at Wayne State developed the concept of treating anal cancer patients preoperatively in order to decrease APR failures. The treatment regimen was 5-FU 1,000 m^2 on days 1 to 4 and 29 to 32 and mitomycin-c 10 to 15 mg/m^2 on day 1, combined with moderate pelvic RT dose of 30 Gy. With the discovery of three pathologic complete responses after preoperative chemoradiation, the focus changed to preserving the sphincter using chemoradiation and reserving APR for salvage. Since Nigro et al.'s original publication, definitive chemoradiation therapy has become the standard. Several retrospective series have demonstrated the success achieved with chemoradiation therapy in terms of local control and overall survival (Table 11.1).

Radiation Therapy Alone versus Combined-Modality Therapy

Two prospective randomized trials have been conducted that have compared radiation alone versus chemoradiation (Table 11.1). The United Kingdom Coordinating Committee on Cancer Research (UKCCCR) trial enrolled patients with T1–T4, N0–N3, M0 anal cancer, and small number of anal margins and demonstrated improved local control and colostomy-free survival (CFS) with combined modality treatment (CMT) but no statistical difference in overall survival. Even for early anal cancer patients (T1–T2N0M0), there appeared to be a benefit favoring CMT on multivariate analysis.

The European Organization for Research and Treatment of Cancer (EORTC) conducted a similar trial comparing radiation alone to radiation with chemotherapy (5-FU and MMC), which also demonstrated an advantage toward CMT. This trial enrolled locally advanced anal canal cancer patients, T3–T4, N0–N3, and M0. Again, CMT showed a statistically significant advantage for CMT in terms of local control, colostomy rate, and disease-free survival (DFS) but not for overall survival. Thus, both the UKCCCR and EORTC trials established the principle that combined modality is superior to single modality radiation alone.

Value of MMC in the Combined-Modality Regimen

Due to the hematologic toxicity of MMC in CMT, two prospective phase III trials (RTOG/ECOG 8704 and RTOG 98-11) have evaluated the importance of MMC.

RTOG/ECOG 8704 was the first randomized trial to evaluate prospectively the importance of MMC in CMT and compared 5-FU and MMC with RT (standard arm) versus 5-FU and RT (experimental arm). The primary endpoint was DFS. At 4 years, DFS was 73% for 5-FU and MMC compared to 51% for 5-FU. Colostomy rate was 22% with 5-FU versus 9% with 5-FU, MMC ($P = 0.002$). Despite the higher toxicity of MMC, the authors concluded that MMC was still the preferred regimen, given the higher DFS and lower colostomy rate.

RTOG 98-11 was the second randomized trial to evaluate prospectively the role of MMC in CMT and compared 5-FU and MMC with concurrent radiotherapy (standard arm) versus induction 5-FU and CDDP followed by concurrent 5-FU and CDDP with radiotherapy (experimental arm). The primary endpoint was again DFS. With a median of 2.51 years, the initial report revealed no statistically significant difference in 5-year DFS (60% MMC vs. 54% CDDP), 5-year OS (75% MMC vs. 70% CDDP), 5-year local-regional control rates (25% MMC vs. 33% CDDP), or 5-year distant metastasis (DM) rates (15% MMC vs. 19% CDDP). The cumulative colostomy rate proved to be statistically significantly higher with CDDP, 19% versus MMC, 10%.

However, the updated RTOG 98-11 examined the long-term impact of treatment on survival (DFS, OS, CFS), as well as colostomy failure (CF), and locoregional failure (LRF), and DM. With longer follow-up, 5-FU/MMC regimen produced statistically significant improvement in DFS and OS for RT + 5-FU/MMC versus RT + 5-FU/CDDP (5-year DFS; 67.8% vs. 57.8%; $P = 0.006$; 5-year OS, 78.3% vs. 70.7%; $P = 0.026$). There was a trend toward statistical significance for CFS, LRF, and CF. Thus, the authors conclude that RT + 5-FU/MMC remains the preferred standard of care.

ACT II addressed two questions: (1) whether substituting CDDP for MMC improves the complete response rate and (2) whether two cycles of maintenance chemotherapy (5-FU/CDDP) reduce recurrences. The randomization employed a 2 × 2 factorial, and patients were randomized to 5-FU/MMC with concurrent radiotherapy (standard arm) or CDDP/5-FU with concurrent radiotherapy. Patients were

TABLE 11.1 Randomized Phase III Trials

Trial	No. of Pts	Eligible Pts	Study Design	Treatment	5-Y LFR	CR	5-Y OS	DFS/RFS	Colostomy Rate
UKCCCR	585	T1-T4, N0-N3 M0	RT vs. CRT	MMC 12 mg/m^2 d 1; 5-FU 1,000 mg/m^2 d 1-4, 29-32 RT 45 Gy/25#; 15 Gy boost	57%-RT; 32%-CRT ($P < 0.0001$)	CR at 6-wk post-Tx: 30%-RT 39%-CRT	5-y OS: 53%-RT 58%-CRT 10-y OS: 34%-RT 41.5%-CRT	3-y DFS: 38%-RT 56%-CRT 5-y RFS: 34%-RT 47%-CRT	5-y CFS: 37%-RT 47%-CRT
EORTC 22861 (1987–1994)	110	T3-T4 N0-N3 M0 or T1-T2 N1-N3 M0	RT vs. CRT	MMC 15 mg/m^2 day 1; 5-FU 750 mg/m^2 days 1-5, 29-33 RT 45 Gy/25#; 20 or 15 Gy boost	50%-RT 32%-CRT at 5 y $P = 0.02$	54%-RT 80%-CRT at 6 wk post-therapy	54%-RT 58%-CRT ($P = 0.17$)	Estimated improvement in DFS by 18% at 5 y	Estimated CFS improvement of 32% at 5 y
RTOG-8704/ECOG	291	T1-T4 N0-N1 M0	5-FU/RT vs. 5-FU/MMC/RT (if biopsy is +, 5-FU/CDDP + RT)	MMC 10 mg/m^2 d 1 and 29; 5-FU 1,000 mg/m^2 d 1-4, 29-32 RT 45-50.4 Gy/25-28#; if biopsy is positive, then 9 Gy boost	4-y LRF: 16%	CR at 4-6-wk post-Tx: 86%-5-FU 92.2%-MMC	71%-5-FU 78.1%-MMC	4-y DFS: 51%-5-FU 73%-MMC ($P = 0.0003$)	4-y CFS 22%-5-FU 9%-MMC ($P = 0.002$)
RTOG 98-11	644	T2-T4 N0-N3 M0	Neoadj CDDP/5-FU then CDDP/5-FU/RT vs. 5-FU/MMC/RT	Neoadj with CDDP 75 mg/m^2, 5-FU 1,000 mg/m^2 d 1-4, then CRT with 5-FU/CDDP vs. CRT with MMC 10 mg/m^2 d 1-4, 29-32; and 5-FU 1,000 mg/m^2 d 1-4, 29-32 Rt 45 Gy/25#; T3/T4, N+, or T2 with residual-received a boost to 54-59 Gy	71.9%-MMC 65%-CDDP ($P = 0.087$)	CR at 6-wk post-Tx: 30%-RT 39%-CRT	78.3%-MMMC 70.7%-CDDP ($P = 0.026$)	5-y DFS: 67.8%-MMC 57.8%-CDDP ($P = 0.006$)	5-y CFS: 71.9%-RT 65%-CRT ($P = 0.05$)

(continued)

TABLE 11.1 (Continued)

Trial	No. of Pts	Eligible Pts	Study Design	Treatment	5-Y LFR	CR	5-Y OS	DFS/RFS	Colostomy Rate
ACCORD-03	307	T ≥ 4 cm or T < 4 cm and N1–N3 M0	Arm A: Neoadj 5-FU/CDDP + Std RT Arm B: 5-FU/ CDDP + HD RT Arm C: 5-FU/ CDDP + Std RT Arm D: 5-FU/ CDDP + HD RT	Neoadj chemo: 5-FU 800 mg/m² d 1–4 and 29–32, CDDP 80 mg/m² d 1 and 29 CRT: 5-FU and CDDP – dose same Arms A and B: 45 Gy/25# to pelvis + std dose boost of 15 Gy or brachy boost (BT) Arms C and D: 45 Gy/25# to pelvis + high-dose boost of 20–25 Gy or BT;	A: 72% B: 87.6% C: 83.7% D: 78%	A: 92% B: 97% C: 86% D: 94%	A/B: 74.5% C/D: 71% (P = 0.81) A/C: 71% B/D: 74% (P = 0.43)	3-y DFS: A: 63.8% B: 78.1% C: 66.8% D: 62.3%	5-y CFS: A: 69.6% B: 82.4% C: 77.1% D: 72.7%
ACT II	940	T1–T4 N0–N3 M0	CDDP/5-FU-CRT vs. MMC/5-FU-CRT, then 4 wk later randomized to maintenance CDDP/5-FU vs. no maintenance	CDDP 60 mg/m² d 1 and 29, 5-FU 1,000 mg/m² d 1–4, d 29–32, and CRT; vs. MMC 12 mg/m² d 1, 5-FU 100 mg/m² d 1–4 and 29–32 CRT; maintenance chemo × 2 cycles = 5-FU 1,000 mg/ m² and CDDP 60 mg/m² RT 50.4 Gy/28#	11% MMC 13% CDDP	CR at 12-wk post-Tx: 94% 5-FU/ MMC/RT vs. 95% 5-FU/ CDDP/RT	3-y OS: 85% with maintenance; 84% without maintenance	3-y DFS: 75% MMC 75% CDDP	5% with maintenance; 4% without maintenance

UKCCCR, United Kingdom Coordinating Committee on Cancer Research; RTOG, Radiation Therapy Oncology Group; ECOG, Eastern Cooperative Oncology Group; ACT, Anal Cancer Trial; RT, radiation therapy; 5-FU, 5-fluorouracil; MMC, mitomycin C; CDDP, cisplatin; CRT, chemoradiation; Std RT, standard dose radiation therapy; HD RT, high-dose radiation therapy; LRF, local-regional failure; DFS, disease-free survival; CFS, colostomy-free survival; RFS, relapse-free survival; f/u, follow-up.

Adapted from Lim F, Glynne-Jones R. Chemotherapy/chemoradiation in anal cancer: a systematic review. *Cancer Treat Rev.* 2011;37:522.

then randomized to receive either two cycles of maintenance chemotherapy (CDDP/5-FU) or no main-tenance therapy. At 26 weeks, the complete response rate was 90.5% for MMC and 89.6% for CDDP (P =0.64). No statistically significant differences in terms of 3-year recurrence-free survival and overall survival were noted between CDDP and MMC regimens, nor between the maintenance and the no main-tenance arms. The authors again concluded that 5-FU/MMC with RT should remain the standard of care.

The data from ACT II and the updated RTOG 98-11 may seem to contradict one another: the CDDP arm in RTOG 98-11 appears to have a detrimental effect on DFS and OS, whereas the ACT II shows that CDDP may be at least equivalent to that of MMC. However, the trial designs were quite different. RTOG employed the use of neoadjuvant chemotherapy prior to the start of concurrent chemoradiotherapy. The prolongation of the overall treatment time may account for the inferior results of the CDDP arm. However, given the current data available, 5-FU/MMC should remain the standard of care.

In a single institution retrospective study comparing the efficacy of one cycle of MMC versus two cycles of MMC in combination with radiation, there was no significant difference in PFS (78% vs. 85%; $P = 0.39$) or OS (84% vs. 91%; $P = 0.16$). There were statistically significant fewer incidences of grade 2 or higher hematologic, dermatologic, and gastrointestinal toxicity in the single cycle versus the two cycles. While prospective multicenter data are lacking, this study suggests that a single cycle of MMC may be as efficacious as two cycles with less acute treatment-related toxicity.

Replacing 5-FU with Capecitabine

Capecitabine is a readily absorbed oral precursor of 5-FU with demonstrated efficacy and favorable side effect profile in the treatment of early stage or metastatic colorectal adenocarcinoma. Its theoretical benefit is that oral dosing will allow continuous therapeutic levels of drug during a treatment cycle, and preferential activation of capecitabine in tumor tissue over normal tissue enhances the therapeutic ratio. Clinical benefit of capecitabine has not yet been demonstrated with equal rigor in anal carcinoma as it has in colorectal cancer. Two phase II trials have demonstrated CR rates of 86% and 90% at 6 months, with almost no grade 4 toxicity in patient with stage I-IIIB anal carcinoma. NCCN guidelines currently recommend CMT with capecitabine/MMC as an alternative to 5-FU/MMC.

Acute Toxicity

Patients typically experience moderate to severe acute toxicities from the combination of both che-motherapy (5-FU and MMC) and radiation therapy. Side effects include nonhematologic toxicities (nausea/vomiting, abdominal pain, increased frequency of stool, diarrhea, skin irritation, fatigue, and weight loss) and hematologic toxicities (neutropenia, thrombocytopenia, anemia).

Toxic deaths from CMT have ranged from 0% to 5%. In the UKCCCR study, 6/116 (2%) experienced toxic death, mostly due to septicemia. The EORTC trial reported on 1 toxic death out 110 patients. In the RTOG 8704 study, four patients (3%) experienced death in the MMC arm. More recently, there were no reported toxic deaths in both RTOG 98-11 and ACT II trials. The ACCORD 03 trial, a four-arm ran-domized trial, showed similar toxic deaths across all four arms (A = 1 [1%], B = 2 [2.6%], C = 3 [3%], D = 1 [1%]). No patient required an APR for acute toxicity in any of the arms during the induction phase or the concurrent chemoradiation phase.

Late Toxicity

Late effects have not been well documented within the randomized trials. Part of the challenge in evaluating late effects is the differing toxicity scales used in the various trials. Early toxicity criteria used in the randomized trials did not allow for characterizing radiation-induced side effects.

Both the early EORTC and UKCCCR trials did not demonstrate a difference in long-term compli-cations between those receiving CMT versus RT alone. RTOG 8704 similarly revealed no significance difference in long-term toxicity between RT/5-FU and RT/5-FU/MMC, although two patients from each arm required stoma secondary to RT-related complications. In the RTOG 9811 update, the most com-mon types of late grade 3 or 4 toxicity included skin, small/large intestine, subcutaneous tissue, or other. There did not appear to be a difference between the MMC or CDDP arms for grade 3/4 toxic-ity (13.1% vs. 10.7%; $P = 0.35$). In the ACCORD 03 trial, late toxicities were primarily of grade 1 or 2. However, nine patients experienced grade 4 toxicities including necrosis, fistula, bleeding, or pain of whom five were treated with an APR and four underwent colostomy alone.

Chemoradiation in HIV-Positive Patients

The majority of retrospective studies suggest that HIV-positive patients do just as well with CMT as the general population. Those with CD4 counts of <200, however, may require a modification in their treatment regimen such as omission of MMC or a reduction in the RT field and/or dose.

Dose of Radiation

Local-regional failures occur in 20% to 30% after definitive chemoradiation. Because of such local-regional failures, RTOG 92-08, a phase II, dose escalation trial was designed to escalate dose to 59.4 Gy, with a mandatory treatment break of 2 weeks after the initial 36 Gy. The initial study included 47 patients with a mandatory break. The update of RTOG 92-08 analyzed not only the original 47 patients with the mandatory break but also analyzed 20 additional patients who did not have a planned break. Both groups of patients showed no difference in OS or LRF when compared historically to patients on RTOG 87-04 MMC arm. The higher dose likely did not result in improved outcomes because of the treatment break, which may have allowed for tumor repopulation and/or repair of sublethal damage.

The ACCORD-03 trial evaluated both the value of treatment intensification by induction chemotherapy (two cycles of 5-FU and CDDP) and radiation dose escalation by incorporating a 20 to 25 Gy boost in patients with locally advanced anal cancer patients (T2 > 4 cm or T3–T4Nx or any T, N1–N3, M0). The trial was conducted as a factorial 2 × 2 study (A = ICT; B = ICT +HDRT; C = reference arm = pelvic RT 45 Gy per 25 fractions with two cycles of 5-FU-CDDP + boost of 15 Gy; D = HDRT). High-dose RT (HDRT) incorporated a boost of 20 to 25 Gy. Thus, arms A and C received 60 Gy total and arms B and D received 65 to 75 Gy total. There appeared to be no difference in their primary endpoint of colostomy-free survival (CFS) at 3 years, or in any secondary endpoints such as response rate, toxicity, local control, or overall survival.

Although controversy exists regarding the optimal dose, a reasonable approach is to treat between 55 to 59 Gy (RTOG 98-11) if 3D conformal radiation is being contemplated and 54 Gy if dose painting IMRT (DP IMRT) is being employed per RTOG 0529.

Tumor Regression after Chemoradiation

After patients have completed definitive chemoradiation therapy, patients should be followed up clinically in 8 to 12 weeks after therapy. Cummings demonstrated that mean time for tumor regression was 3 months but regression of a tumor could occur for up to 12 months. Thus, if there is persistent disease at 8 to 12 weeks, patients should be followed up closely (every month) to document regression. As long as there is documented regression on serial examinations, patients may continue to be monitored. However, at any point if there is progression, then biopsy followed by salvage APR should be considered.

Targeted Therapy

Outcomes of several other types of solid tumors have benefited from targeted biologic therapy. However, use of targeted therapy has yet to reach phase III trials in anal carcinoma. Cetuximab is a monoclonal antibody, which blocks epidermal growth factor receptor (EGFR) from sending mitogenic signals via a KRAS dependent pathway. KRAS mutations are rare in anal carcinoma, making this pathway targetable in anal cancer. Reports of the phase II ECOG 3205 and AMC045 trial data evaluating safety and efficacy of cetuximab in addition to CMT with 5-FU/CDDP in both immunocompetent and HIV-positive patient with stage II–III anal carcinoma suggest improved rates of LRF compared to historical data, but also had high rates of grade 4 toxicity at 32% and 26% in EGOC 3205 and AMC045, respectively. A similar phase II trial, ACCORD 16, as well as a phase I trial both looking at safety and efficacy of a 5-FU/CDDP based regimen with cetuximab were terminated prematurely due to unacceptably high rates of grade 3/4 toxicity. Panitumumab is another EGFR antagonist. Preliminary results of a phase II trial (VITAL/GEMCAD 09-02) in which 36 patients with nonmetastatic anal carcinoma received panitumumab in addition to standard of care suggested an acceptable safety profile, with no treatment-related deaths, 8% grade 4 toxicity, and 56% CR rate at 8 weeks and 24 weeks.

Intratumoral HPV oncoproteins upregulate immune checkpoint proteins such as PD-L1 and promote immune resistance. Morris et al. reported the result of a phase II trial of nivolumab monotherapy in previously treated and immune therapy naïve patients (NCT02314169). Thirty-seven patients were enrolled and received at least one dose of nivolumab. Among the 37 patients, nine patients had responses (2 CR and 7 PR; ORR, 24%). Grade 3 adverse events were anemia ($N = 2$), fatigue ($N = 1$), rash ($N = 1$), and hypothyroidism ($N = 1$). No serious adverse events were reported.

TREATMENT OPTIONS ACCORDING TO STAGE

Stage 0

▪ Surgical resection is the treatment of choice for the lesions of the perianal area that does not involve the anal sphincter.

Stage I

▪ Small, well-differentiated tumors of the anal margin not involving the anal sphincter can be treated with wide local excision.
▪ All the other stage I tumors of the anal margin and anal canal are treated with chemoradiation with 5-FU/MMC or capecitabine/MMC.
▪ Patients who cannot tolerate chemotherapy, such as the very elderly or those with multiple comorbid conditions, may be treated with radiation alone.
▪ Surgical salvage with APR is reserved for residual cancer in the anal canal after chemoradiation.

Stages II to IIIB

▪ Chemoradiation with 5-FU/MMC or capecitabine/MMC is the recommended initial approach.
▪ Patients who cannot tolerate chemotherapy may be treated with radiation alone.
▪ Surgical salvage with APR is reserved for residual disease in the anal canal after chemoradiation.

Stage IV

There are limited data regarding the treatment of metastatic disease given the overall rarity of the disease. There are no available phase III data and only very limited phase II prospective data are available. The most widely used regimen is cisplatin plus 5-FU, which is the recommended as first-line therapy by NCCN. Response rates have been as high as 50% to 66% and median survivals of 12 to 34.5 months. Clinical trials should be encouraged. Palliative efforts remain an important component of care.

PERSISTENT OR RECURRENT ANAL CANCER

Surgery with APR is considered the treatment of choice for either persistent or recurrent disease and 20% to 40% of patients may achieve long-term control. For persistent disease, RTOG 8704 treated 22 patients with a 9 Gy boost with 5-FU and CDDP as salvage. Ultimately, 12 of 22 remained disease-free after surgical intervention. Given the limited data, surgery should remain the standard for chemoradiation failures.

Follow-Up

There are no prospective data regarding the optimal follow-up regimen. The ACT II trial did show that 29% of patient who did not achieve CR at 11 weeks achieved CR at 26 weeks. Based on these data, NCCN recommends an initial follow-up DRE in 8 to 12 weeks following completion of therapy. Patients with regression or no progression may be observed for up to 6 months to see if CR can be achieved and APR spared. If CR is achieved, then DRE, anoscopy, and inguinal lymph node palpation should be repeated every 3 to 6 months for 5 years. For T3–T4 or positive inguinal lymph nodes at diagnosis, one should consider chest/abd/pelvic imaging annually for 3 years. Patients with clear progression or relapse at any point require biopsy and restaging with CT or PET/CT and if progression or recurrence is proven, they should be considered for salvage APR.

Suggested Readings

1. Barnardi MP, Ngan SY, Michael M, et al. Molecular biology of anal squamous cell carcinoma: implications for future research and clinical intervention. *Lancet Oncol.* 2015;16(16):e611–e121.
2. Bartelink H, Roelofsen F, Eschwege F, et al. Concomitant radiotherapy and chemotherapy is superior to radiotherapy alone in the treatment of locally advanced anal cancer: results of a phase III randomized trial of the European Organization for Research and Treatment of Cancer Radiotherapy and Gastrointestinal Cooperative Groups. *J Clin Oncol.* 1997;15(5):2040–2049.
3. Bartelink H, Roelofsen F, Eschwege F, et al. Overexpression of p53 protein and outcome of patients treated with chemoradiation for carcinoma of the anal canal: a report of randomized trial RTOG 87-04. Radiation Therapy Oncology Group. *Cancer.* 1999;85(6):1226–1233.
4. Deutsch E, Lemanski C, Pignon JP, et al. Unexpected toxicity of cetuximab combined with conventional chemoradiotherapy in patients with locally advanced anal cancer: results of the UNICANCER ACCORD 16 phase II trial. *Ann Oncol.* 2013;24(11):2834–2838.
5. Feliu J, Garcia-Carbonero R, Capdevila J, et al. Phase II trial of panitumumab (P) plus mytomicin C (M), 5-fluorouracil (5-FU), and radiation (RT) in patients with squamous cell carcinoma of the anal canal (SCAC): safety and efficacy profile—VITAL study, GEMCAD 09-02 clinical trial. In: ASCO Annual Meeting. Chicago; 2014.
6. Garg MK, Zhao F, Sparano JA, et al. Cetuximab plus chemoradiotherapy in immunocompetent patients with anal carcinoma: a phase II eastern cooperative oncology group-American college of radiology imaging network cancer research group trial (E3205). *J Clin Oncol.* 2017;35(7):718–726.
7. Glynne-Jones R, Meadows H, Wan S, et al. EXTRA—a multicenter phase II study of chemoradiation using a 5 day per week oral regimen of capecitabine and intravenous mitomycin C in anal cancer. *Int J Radiat Oncol Biol Phys.* 2008;72(1):119–126.
8. Greenall MJ, Quan SH, Stearns MW, Urmacher C, DeCosse JJ. Epidermoid cancer of the anal margin. Pathologic features, treatment, and clinical results. *Am J Surg.* 1985;149(1):95–101.
9. Gunderson LL, Winter KA, Ajani JA, et al. Long-term update of US GI intergroup RTOG 98-11 phase III trial for anal carcinoma: survival, relapse, and colostomy failure with concurrent chemoradiation involving fluorouracil/mitomycin versus fluorouracil/cisplatin. *J Clin Oncol.* 2012;30(35):4344–4351.
10. James RD, Glynne-Jones R, Meadows HM, et al. Mitomycin or cisplatin chemoradiation with or without maintenance chemotherapy for treatment of squamous-cell carcinoma of the anus (ACT II): a randomised, phase 3, open-label, 2×2 factorial trial. *Lancet Oncol.* 2013;14(6):516–524.
11. Lim F, Glynne-Jones R. Chemotherapy/chemoradiation in anal cancer: a systematic review. *Cancer Treat Rev.* 2011;37(7): 520–532.
12. Morris VK, Salem ME, Nimeiri H, et al. Nivolumab for previously treated unresectable metastatic anal cancer (NCI9673): a multicentre, single-arm, phase 2 study. *Lancet Oncol.* 2017;18(4):446–453.
13. NCCN guidelines version 2.2017 Anal Carcinoma. NCCN Guidelines. http://www.nccn.org/. 2017.
14. Nigro ND, Vaitkevicius VK, Considine, Jr. B. Combined therapy for cancer of the anal canal: a preliminary report. *Dis Colon Rectum.* 1974;17(3):354–356.
15. Northover J, Glynne-Jones R, Sebag-Montefiore D, et al. Chemoradiation for the treatment of epidermoid anal cancer: 13-year follow-up of the first randomised UKCCCR Anal Cancer Trial (ACT I). *Br J Cancer.* 2010;102(7):1123–1128.
16. Olivatto LO, Vieira FM, Pereira BV, et al. Phase 1 study of cetuximab in combination with 5-fluorouracil, cisplatin, and radiotherapy in patients with locally advanced anal canal carcinoma. *Cancer.* 2013;119(16):2973–2980.
17. Oliveira SC, Moniz CM, Riechelmann R, et al. Phase II study of capecitabine in substitution of 5-FU in the chemoradiotherapy regimen for patients with localized squamous cell carcinoma of the anal canal. *J Gastrointest Cancer.* 2016;47(1):75–81.
18. Palefsky JM, Giuliano AR, Goldstone S, et al. HPV vaccine against anal HPV infection and anal intraepithelial neoplasia. *N Engl J Med.* 2011;365(17):1576–1585.
19. Peiffert D, Tournier-Rangeard L, Gerard JP, et al. Induction chemotherapy and dose intensification of the radiation boost in locally advanced anal canal carcinoma: final analysis of the randomized UNICANCER ACCORD 03 trial. *J Clin Oncol.* 2012;30(16):1941–1948.
20. Serup-Hansen E, Linnemann D, Hogdall E, Geertsen PF, Havsteen H. KRAS and BRAF mutations in anal carcinoma. *APMIS.* 2015;123(1):53–59.
21. Siegel RL, Miller KD, Jemal A. Cancer statistics, 2017. *CA Cancer J Clin.* 2017;67(1):7–30.
22. Silverberg MJ, Lau B, Justice AC, et al. Risk of anal cancer in HIV-infected and HIV-uninfected individuals in North America. *Clin Infect Dis.* 2012;54(7):1026–1034.
23. White EC, Goldman K, Aleshin A, Lien WW, Rao AR. Chemoradiotherapy for squamous cell carcinoma of the anal canal: comparison of one versus two cycles mitomycin-C. *Radiother Oncol.* 2015;117(2):240–245.
24. White EC, Khodayari B, Erickson KT, Lien WW, Hwang-Graziano J, Rao AR. Comparison of toxicity and treatment outcomes in HIV-positive versus HIV-negative patients with squamous cell carcinoma of the anal canal. *Am J Clin Oncol.* 2017;40(4):386–392.

Breast Cancer 12

Megan Kruse, Leticia Varella, Stephanie Valente, Paulette Lebda, Andrew Vassil, and Jame Abraham

INTRODUCTION

Breast cancer is the most common cancer among women worldwide and it accounts for 25% of all cancer diagnosed among women. It is second only to lung cancer as the leading cause of death from cancer in women in North America. When diagnosed early, breast cancer can be treated primarily using surgery, radiation, and systemic therapy. In Western countries at the time of diagnosis more than 90% of patients will have only localized disease. But many other parts of the world, about 60% of patients will have locally advanced or metastatic disease at the time of diagnosis.

EPIDEMIOLOGY

- In the United States, as per American Cancer Society, in 2017, an estimated 252,170 women and 2,470 men will be diagnosed with breast cancer.
- In addition, about 63,410 new cases of noninvasive (in situ) breast cancer will be diagnosed in 2017.
- In 2017, 40,610 women and 460 men are expected to die from breast cancer in the United States.
- As per International Agency for Cancer Research (IARC) about 1.7 million women will get a diagnosis of breast cancer worldwide in 2017 and about half a million will die globally from breast cancer.
- A U.S woman's lifetime risk of developing breast cancer is one in eight, or about 12% will develop breast cancer.
- There are currently more than 3.1 million breast cancer survivors in the United States in 2017.

RISK FACTORS

The risk factors for developing breast cancer in women are listed in Table 12.1. The etiologies of most breast cancers are unknown and sporadic. About 5% to 10% of breast cancers are familial or hereditary.

Genetics (For More Details Refer to Chapter 44 on Genetics)

- About 5% to 10% of all women with breast cancer may have a specific mutation in a single gene that is responsible for the breast cancer, with the most common mutations occurring in the BRCA1 or BRCA2 genes. Other genes implicated with breast cancer are PTEN (associated with Cowden syndrome), TP53 (associated with Li-Fraumeni syndrome), CDH1 (associated with hereditary diffuse gastric cancer syndrome), STK11, PALB2, CHEK2, and ATM.
- Individuals with these hereditary syndromes may develop cancers early in life or multiple cancers, including bilateral breast cancer.

TABLE 12.1 Risk Factors for Breast Cancer in Women

Increasing age
Family history of breast cancer at a young age
Genetic mutations such as BRCA1 or BRCA2 mutations
Increased mammographic breast density
Early menarche
Late menopause
Nulliparity
Older age at first child birth
Increased body mass index (BMI)
History of atypical lobular hyperplasia, atypical ductal hyperplasia, lobular carcinoma in situ (LCIS),
    or flat epithelial atypia
Prior breast biopsies
Long-term postmenopausal estrogen and progesterone replacement
Prior thoracic radiation therapy at age under 30

- Mutations of BRCA1 (chromosome 17q21) and BRCA2 (chromosome 13q12–13q13) are responsible for 85% of hereditary breast cancer. These genes are involved in DNA repair.
- Specific mutations of BRCA1 and BRCA2 are more common in women of Ashkenazi Jewish ancestry.
- Overall prevalence of disease-related mutation in BRCA1 has been estimated at 1 in 300, while BRCA2 is 1 in 800.
- The cumulative risk estimates for developing breast cancer by age 80 were 72% for BRCA1 carriers and 69% for BRCA2 carriers.
- The cumulative risk of a contralateral breast cancer 20 years after a first breast cancer was 40% for BRCA1 mutation carriers and 26% for BRCA2 mutation carriers.
- BRCA-related breast cancer is more likely to be triple negative particularly in the setting of BRCA1 mutations.
- The cumulative risk estimates for developing ovarian cancer by age 80 were 44% for BRCA1 mutation carriers and 17% for BRCA2 mutation carriers.

Indications for Genetic Testing

All patients should have a basic assessment for risk of a hereditary breast/ovarian cancer syndrome including documentation of personal and family history (both paternal and maternal sides) of malignancy. All patients with high risk for a hereditary syndrome based on personal/family history and age at diagnosis should undergo genetic counseling before undergoing the genetic test. The genetic counseling visit is an important step in addressing the patient's goals of testing and is an opportunity to address misconceptions/limitations of genetic testing. There are three possible outcomes of genetic testing for the BRCA mutations: positive, variant of uncertain significance, or negative. A negative result indicates no increased risk of breast cancer due to a germline mutation. A variant of uncertain significance (indeterminate) test result indicates that no conclusive evidence exists to indicate that the mutation does or does not carry an increased risk of the development of breast cancer due to an inherited genetic mutation. A positive result indicates that there exists a mutation in the patient's genes that has been associated with an inherited risk of developing breast cancer. In general, patients with a history suggestive of a single inherited cancer syndrome should have testing sent for that specific syndrome.

Multigene testing may be cost-effective and efficient if multiple different inherited cancer syndromes could be considered based on history or if single gene testing is negative in a patient with a compelling personal or family history suggestive of an inherited cancer syndrome. One concern with the multigene testing approach is the increased likelihood of detecting a variant of uncertain significance. This also increases the importance of appropriate genetic counseling in conjunction with genetic testing such that results are interpreted in the appropriate manner.

As per NCCN guidelines (accessed in July 2017), patients with breast cancer and one or more of the following features should undergo further genetic risk evaluation:

■ Early-age onset breast cancer (age ≤45)
■ Triple negative breast cancer (ER–, PR–, HER-2/neu-) diagnosed age ≤60
■ ≥2 breast primaries (with first diagnosed at age ≤50)
■ Diagnosed at age ≤50 with ≥1 close blood relative (first-, second-, or third-degree relative) with breast cancer at any age, pancreatic cancer, or prostate cancer (Gleason score ≥7)
■ Diagnosed at any age with ≥1 close blood relative with breast cancer diagnosed at age ≤50
■ Diagnosed at any age with ≥2 close blood relatives with breast cancer, pancreatic cancer, or prostate cancer (Gleason score ≥7) at any age
■ Personal history of ovarian cancer or ≥1 close blood relative with ovarian cancer, fallopian tube cancer, or primary peritoneal cancers diagnosed at any age
■ Ashkenazi Jewish descent
■ Personal history of male breast cancer or male breast cancer in close blood relative at any age

Management of Patients with Positive BRCA Test

Management recommendations for patients with a known genetic mutation are highly individualized and should be made by an expert. General recommendations include the following:

■ Clinical breast examination every 6 to 12 months, starting at age 25
■ Breast magnetic resonance imaging (MRI) with contrast starting at age 25 or earlier based on family history or mammogram if breast MRI is not available
■ Annual mammogram and annual breast MRI with contrast from age 30 to 75
■ Discuss option of bilateral prophylactic mastectomy on a case-by-case basis, since it could prevent breast cancer in >90% of patients with known BRCA1 or BRCA2 mutation
■ Recommend bilateral salpingo-oophorectomy (BSO) ideally between the ages of 35 and 40 or after completion of child bearing. BSO alone will reduce breast cancer risk by about 50%, but it may vary depending upon the specific genes and prevents ovarian cancer by about 95%.
■ Patients who defer BSO may consider concurrent trans-vaginal ultrasound and blood test such as CA-125, although it is not sufficiently sensitive or specific. This can be done at the discretion of the clinician, starting from the age of 30 and 35 years or 5 to 10 years prior to the earliest age of ovarian cancer in family history.

CHEMOPREVENTION

Risk Assessment

There are many risk models available to assess a women's risk for sporadic breast cancer, which accounts for 90% of the breast cancer. One of the most commonly used models is the Gail Risk model (https://www.cancer.gov/bcrisktool). It is a statistical model that calculates a woman's absolute risk of developing breast cancer by using the following criteria:

1. Age
2. Age at menarche
3. Age at first live birth
4. Number of previous biopsies
5. History of atypical ductal hyperplasia (ADH)
6. Number of first-degree relatives with breast cancer

This model is not intended to be used in patients with an existing history of invasive cancer, DCIS, or lobular carcinoma in situ (LCIS). It underestimates the risk of breast cancer in a person with hereditary breast cancer. It is used in calculating the risk in many breast cancer prevention studies including NSABP-P1 and NSABP-P2.

Prevention Studies

The National Surgical Adjuvant Breast and Bowel Project Breast Cancer Prevention Trial (P-1)

The National Surgical Adjuvant Breast and Bowel Project (NSABP) P-1 study showed a 49% reduction in the incidence of invasive breast cancer in high-risk subjects (based upon the Gail Risk Model) who took tamoxifen at a dose of 20 mg daily for 5 years. Women eligible for this trial were at least 35 years old and were assessed to have an absolute risk of at least 1.66% over the period of 5 years using the Gail model or a pathologic diagnosis of LCIS. Twenty-five percent of woman assigned to tamoxifen in this study discontinued the medication compared to 20% in the placebo group. Notable adverse events associated with tamoxifen therapy in this study include increased risk of endometrial cancer (particularly in women age 50 or older), cataracts, and venous thromboembolism (both deep venous thrombosis and pulmonary embolism). An update of results with 7 years of follow-up was published in 2005 showing a continued statistically significant improvement in rate of invasive breast cancer (risk ratio 0.57) and noninvasive breast cancer (risk ratio 0.63) with tamoxifen compared to placebo.

Use of tamoxifen for breast cancer risk reduction should be considered after weighing the risk benefit ratio for each patient. Women with a life expectancy of ≥10 years and no diagnosis/history of breast cancer who are considered at increased risk of breast cancer should receive individualized counseling to decrease breast cancer risk.

NSABP P-2: Study of Tamoxifen and Raloxifene

In the NSABP P-2 study, tamoxifen 20 mg daily was compared with raloxifene 60 mg daily in postmenopausal women with high risk of developing breast cancer (Gail risk model estimate of 5-year breast cancer risk of at least 1.66%). The results of the study revealed that raloxifene was equivalent to tamoxifen in preventing invasive breast cancer (about a 50% reduction). Raloxifene did not reduce the risk of DCIS or LCIS unlike tamoxifen.

Raloxifene has a better side effect profile, which resulted in a lower incidence of uterine hyperplasia, hysterectomy, cataracts, and a lower rate of thromboembolic events. In postmenopausal patients, due to equal efficacy and better side effect profile, raloxifene 60 mg daily could be used instead of tamoxifen for breast cancer prevention. A 2010 update of the NSABP P-2 study after a median follow-up of nearly 7 years confirmed no statistical difference between invasive breast cancer events in the tamoxifen- and raloxifene-treated patients. In addition, significant reductions in risk of endometrial cancer/hyperplasia as well as thromboembolic events were reported with raloxifene compared to tamoxifen.

Aromatase Inhibitors for Risk Reduction

Aromatase inhibitors were shown to decrease the incidence of contralateral breast cancer when used in the adjuvant setting (ATAC, BIG 1-98). These data led to the investigation of AI as chemoprevention for women at high-risk for developing breast cancer.

The MAP.3 trial evaluated the role of exemestane in a risk reduction setting, randomizing women at increased risk for breast cancer (based on age 60 or older, Gail 5-year risk score of at least 1.66%, prior atypical ductal/lobular hyperplasia or LCIS or DCIS status postmastectomy) to either exemestane or placebo. At a median follow-up of 3 years, it was found that exemestane reduced the relative incidence of breast cancers by 65% when compared to placebo. Exemestane was not associated with any significant serious side effects, although hot flashes and arthritis were very common in both the exemestane and placebo groups. Quality of life was minimally impacted by exemestane use with respect to menopausal symptoms.

In the randomized phase III IBIS II trial, postmenopausal women at increased risk of breast cancer (defined as significant family history, history of atypical hyperplasia, or LCIS, nulliparity or age at first birth of ≥ 30) were randomized to receive anastrozole or placebo for 5 years. Results showed a reduction in the risk of developing breast cancer (both invasive and noninvasive) of more than 50% (HR of 0.47) with use of anastrozole compared to placebo. Musculoskeletal events and vasomotor symptoms were significantly more common in patients receiving anastrozole rather than placebo.

Summary

In premenopausal women with increased risk of breast cancer as per the Gail risk model, it is reasonable to recommend tamoxifen 20 mg daily for 5 years. In postmenopausal women raloxifene and tamoxifen are equally effective, but raloxifene has been shown to have less side effects. Aromatase inhibitors can also be considered given the data from the MAP.3 and IBIS II trials; however, the FDA has not approved aromatase inhibitors in this setting. Any risk reduction approach should be carefully decided after a detailed risk versus benefit discussion with the patient.

BREAST CANCER SCREENING

Screening Mammograms

▪ Screening mammography has been shown to decrease breast cancer mortality in women between the ages of 40 and 70 years with an absolute mortality benefit of 1% for women screened annually for 10 years.

▪ Potential harms associated with screening mammography include overdiagnosis and treatment of cancers that would otherwise have been clinically insignificant in a woman's lifetime as well as the unnecessary anxiety and additional testing that is associated with false positive screening examination.

▪ The American Cancer Society recommends that women ages 40 to 44 should have the choice to start annual mammography screening and women ages 45 to 54 should receive annual mammograms. At age 55, the American Cancer Society suggests that women may switch to having mammograms every other year for breast cancer screening although annual screening may be continued if the patient desires.

▪ Women who are at higher than average risk of breast cancer (women with a family history of breast cancer, women with either the BRCA1 or the BRCA2 gene, women with a history of chest irradiation between the ages of 10 and 30, or women with a lifetime risk of breast cancer ≥20%) are recommended to initiate screening mammograms at age 25 to 30 or 10 years earlier than the age of the affected first-degree relative at diagnosis (whichever is later) or 8 years after radiation therapy, as per the American College of Radiology guidelines.

▪ Mammograms should be continued regardless of a woman's age, as long as she is in good health with an expected life expectancy of at least 10 years. Age alone should not be the reason to stop having regular mammograms. Women with serious health problems or short life expectancies should discuss with their doctors whether to continue having mammograms.

Digital Mammography

The diagnostic superiority of digital mammography was demonstrated in the Digital Mammographic Imaging Screening Trial (DMIST) published in 2005. This study concluded that the overall accuracy of digital and film mammography was similar however in pre- or peri-menopausal women under the age of 50 or women at any age with dense breasts, digital mammography more accurately detected of breast cancer.

Tomosynthesis

Digital breast tomosynthesis (DBT), commonly referred to as 3-D mammography, is an x-ray technique that uses a finite number of low-dose projections to reconstruct a series of thin-section images of the breast. The STORM (screening with tomosynthesis or standard mammography) trial was a large prospective Italian study that compared conventional screening digital mammography to combined digital mammography and DBT for breast cancer screening in an average risk population. The study demonstrated that detection of breast cancer significantly increased with the addition of DBT to conventional digital mammography. A 2014 study from Friedewald et al. also demonstrated that this technology can decrease the rate of recall for benign findings. As per discussion by Houssami and Skanne, it is important to note that integrated use of 2D mammography and DBT nearly doubles the overall radiation exposure, so careful consideration must be given of how to incorporate DBT to usual 2D screening. However, some DBT vendors have introduced synthetic 2D views which when used in place of conventional 2D images reduces the radiation dose of DBT combination examination.

Magnetic Resonance Imaging

While breast MRI has been shown to have a higher sensitivity than mammography, the specificity of breast MRI is lower, which can result in more false positives and therefore more biopsies. Patients need to be carefully selected for additional screening with breast MRI. In a high-risk population, the sensitivity of mammography when combined with MRI (92.7%) is higher than the sensitivity of mammography when combined with ultrasound (52%). Therefore, in women in whom supplemental screening is indicated, MRI is recommended when possible. According to the American Cancer Society recommendations, breast MRI can be used as an adjunct to screening mammography in high-risk women, specifically those with BRCA gene mutations (along with their untested first-degree relatives), those who received chest radiation between the ages of 10 and 30, and those whose lifetime risk of breast cancer exceeds 20%.

CLINICAL FEATURES OF BREAST CANCER

Clinical features may include a breast lump, skin thickening or alteration, peau d'orange, dimpling of the skin, nipple inversion or crusting (Paget disease), unilateral nipple discharge, and new onset pain. Patients may instead present with signs and symptoms of metastatic disease.

DIAGNOSIS

1. History and physical examination
2. Bilateral mammogram (80% to 90% accuracy)
3. Biopsy: Any distinct mass should be considered for a biopsy, even if the mammograms are negative
   The standard method of diagnosis for palpable lesions is
   * Core-needle biopsy
   The options in nonpalpable breast lesions are
   * Ultrasound-guided core-needle biopsy
   * Stereotactic core-needle biopsy under mammographic localization
   * Needle localization under mammography, followed by surgical excision
   * MRI-guided biopsy
4. Laboratory studies
   * Complete blood count, liver function tests, and alkaline phosphatase level can be considered depending upon the history and physical.
   * Routine use of breast cancer markers such as CA 27:29 and CA 15:3 is not recommended.
5. Pathology and special studies
   * Histology and diagnosis (invasive vs. in situ)
   * Pathologic grade of the tumor
   * Tumor involvement of the margin
   * Tumor size
   * Lymphovascular invasion
6. Estrogen receptor/progesterone receptor (ER/PR) status should be done in all tumors (both invasive and noninvasive) and biopsies of metastatic or recurrent (patients those who relapsed) lesions.
   * As per the ASCO/CAP guidelines (2010), ER/PR is considered as positive if ≥1% of tumor cell nuclei are immunoreactive.
7. HER-2/neu- testing (as per ASCO/CAP Guidelines 2013)
   * Positive for HER-2/neu- is either IHC 3 + (defined as uniform intense membrane staining of more than 30% of invasive tumor cells) or FISH amplified (ratio of HER-2/neu- to CEP17 of ≥2.0 or average HER-2/neu- gene copy number ≥6 signals/nucleus for those test systems without an internal control probe).

- Equivocal for HER-2/neu- is defined as either IHC 2 + or FISH ratio of <2 and average HER-2/neu- gene copy number of ≥ 4.0 and < 6.0 signals/nucleus for test systems without an internal control probe.
- Negative for HER-2/neu- is defined as either IHC 0–1 + or FISH ratio < 2 with an average HER-2/neu- gene copy number < 4 signals/nucleus for test systems without an internal control probe.

8. Indices of proliferation (e.g., mitotic index, Ki-67, or S phase) can be helpful. Ki-67 can be helpful in distinguishing luminal A versus B in ER/PR-positive lesions. Lack of standardization of Ki-67 testing limits its wide utilization in clinical practice.

9. Radiographic studies are performed on the basis of the findings of the history and physical examination, diagnostic breast imaging and blood tests. Appropriate imaging studies such as CT scan, ultrasound, MRI, or CT/PET scan can be considered as per the clinical indications. They are not routinely recommended for all patients.
    - As per the American Society of Clinical Oncology "Choosing Wisely" guidelines, it is not recommended that patients with DCIS or clinical stage I/ II disease receive staging PET, CT, or radionucleotide bone scan as there is no clear evidence indicating benefit, and unnecessary imaging can lead to unnecessary invasive procedures/radiation exposure, overtreatment or misdiagnosis.
    - The NCCN guidelines recommend that systemic imaging be considered in patients with locally advanced (Stage III) patients and in those with signs or symptoms suggestive of metastatic disease.

10. Breast MRI may be helpful in determining the extent of disease and to facilitate surgical planning in the following patients (as per NCCN guidelines):
    - Those with heterogenous and extremely dense mammographic tissue
    - Those with newly diagnosed invasive lobular carcinoma
    - Those with axillary nodal metastasis with unknown primary
    - Those who are candidates for neoadjuvant chemotherapy and as part of monitoring response to neoadjuvant therapy

- Evaluating the extent of disease in known cancer patients
    - Multifocal and multicentric disease
    - Pectoralis and chest wall involvement
- Postlumpectomy patients to evaluate residual disease (close or positive margins)
- Suspected recurrence of breast cancer
    - Inconclusive mammographic/clinical findings
    - Reconstruction with tissue flaps or implants
- Lesion characterization
- Inconclusive findings on mammogram, ultrasound, and physical examination

PATHOLOGY

Infiltrating or invasive ductal cancer is the most common breast cancer histologic type and comprises 70% to 80% of all cases (Table 12.2).

STAGING OF BREAST CANCER

For staging of breast cancer the American Joint Committee on Cancer (AJCC) manual, eighth edition, should be followed. This edition of the AJCC manual includes separate anatomic and prognostic staging group systems for breast cancer, reflecting the importance of biomarkers in breast cancer prognosis and treatment decisions. These biomarkers provide a sense of tumor biology. The traditional anatomic stage groups (including only the "TNM" or tumor size, nodal status, and metastasis categories) should now only be used in regions of the world where biomarker tests are not routinely available. The new eighth edition AJCC prognostic staging is the standard for cancer registries in the

TABLE 12.2 Pathologic Classification of Breast Cancer

Ductal
Intraductal (in situ)
Invasive with predominant intraductal component
Invasive, NOS
Comedo
Inflammatory
Medullary with lymphocytic infiltrate
Mucinous (colloid)
Papillary
Scirrhous
Tubular
Other
Other
Undifferentiated
Lobular
In situ
Invasive with predominant in situ component
Invasive
Nipple
Paget disease, NOS
Paget disease with intraductal carcinoma
Paget disease with invasive ductal carcinoma
Other types (not typical breast cancer)
Phyllodes tumor
Angiosarcoma
Primary lymphoma

NOS, not otherwise specified.

United States moving forward. This prognostic group staging system includes the TNM categories in addition to

1. Histologic grade
2. HER2 status
3. ER status
4. PR status
5. Oncotype Dx recurrence score (for certain TNM groups only)

Key stage changes that have occurred as a result of the eighth edition of the AJCC staging are summarized in Table 12.3.

Prognostic Factors

Anatomic features such as tumor size and lymph node status are important prognostic features. But biologic features of the tumor are equally important or possibly even more important than anatomic features.

TABLE 12.3 Key Stage Changes in AJCC Eighth Edition Breast Cancer Staging

Anatomic TNM Staging	Relevant Biomarkers in AJCC Eighth Edition	AJCC Seventh Edition Stage Group	AJCC Eighth Edition Prognostic Stage Group
T2N0M0	Grades 1–3 HER2 negative ER positive PR any Oncotype Dx Recurrence score <11	IIA	IA
T2N1M0	Grade 1 HER2 negative ER positive PR positive	IIB	IB
T2N1M0	Grade 2 HER2 positive ER positive PR positive	IIB	IB
T0-2N2M0	Grades 1–2 HER-2 positive ER positive PR positive	IIIA	IB
T3N1-2M0	Grades 1–2 HER2 positive ER positive PR positive	IIIA	IB
T1N0M0	Grades 1–3 HER2 negative ER negative PR negative	IA	IIA
T1N0M0	Grade 3 HER2 negative ER positive PR negative	IA	IIA
T1N0M0	Grade 3 HER2 negative ER negative PR positive	IA	IIA
T0-2N2	Grade 1 HER2 negative ER positive PR positive	IIIA	IIA
T0-1N1M0	Grade 2 HER2 negative ER negative PR negative	IIA	IIIA
T2N0M0	Grade 2 HER2 negative ER negative PR negative	IIA	IIIA

(*continued*)

TABLE 12.3 (Continued)

Anatomic TNM Staging	Relevant Biomarkers in AJCC Eighth Edition	AJCC Seventh Edition Stage Group	AJCC Eighth Edition Prognostic Stage Group
T2N0M0	Grade 3 HER2 negative ER positive PR negative	IIA	IIIA
T2N0M0	Grade 3 HER2 negative ER negative PR any	IIA	IIIA
T1-4N3M0	Grade 1 HER2 negative ER positive PR positive	IIIC	IIIA
T2N1M0	Grades 1–2 HER2 negative ER negative PR negative	IIB	IIIB
T2N1M0	Grade 3 HER2 negative ER positive PR negative	IIB	IIIB
T2N1M0	Grade 3 HER2 negative ER negative PR any	IIB	IIIC
T0-2N2M0	Grades 2–3 HER2 negative AND ER/PR negative OR ER positive/PR negative OR ER negative/PR any	IIIA	IIIC
T3N1-2M0	Grades 2–3 HER2 negative AND ER/PR negative OR ER positive/PR negative OR ER negative/PR any	IIIA	IIIC

1. Number of positive axillary lymph nodes
   * This is an important prognostic indicator. Prognosis is worse with increasing number of lymph nodes.
2. Tumor size
   * In general, tumors smaller than 1 cm have a good prognosis in patients without lymph node involvement.
3. Histologic or nuclear grade
   * Patients with poorly differentiated histology and high nuclear grade have a worse prognosis than others.
   * Scarff-Bloom-Richardson grading system and Fisher nuclear grade are commonly used systems. The modified Scarff-Bloom-Richardson grading system assigns a score (1 to 3 points) for features

such as size, mitosis, and tubule formation. These scores are added and tumors are labeled low grade (3 to 5 points), intermediate grade (6 to 7 points), or high grade (8 to 9 points).

4. ER/PR status
   - ER- and/or PR-positive tumors have better prognosis and these patients are eligible to receive endocrine therapy.

5. Histologic tumor type
   - Prognoses of infiltrating ductal and lobular carcinoma are similar.
   - Mucinous (colloid) and tubular histologies have better prognosis.
   - Inflammatory breast cancer is one of the most aggressive forms of breast cancer.

6. HER-2/neu expression
   - HER-2/neu overexpression is a poor prognostic marker and patients with HER-2/neu overexpression are candidates for HER-2/neu-targeted therapies. Availability of effective HER-2/neu-targeted therapies has revolutionized the treatment and outcome of HER-2/neu-positive breast cancer. Because of targeted therapies, for all practical purposes, HER-2/neu positivity can be considered as a good prognostic feature now.

7. Gene expression profiles
   - Oncotype DX is a diagnostic genomic assay based on reverse transcription polymerase chain reaction (RT-PCR) on paraffin-embedded tissue (Fig. 12.1). This assay was initially developed to quantify the likelihood of cancer recurrence in women with newly diagnosed, stage I or II, node-negative, ER-positive breast cancer. Patients are divided into low-risk, intermediate-risk, and high-risk groups on the basis of the expression of a panel of 21 genes. The recurrence score determined by this assay is found to be a better predictor of outcome than standard measures such as age, tumor size, and tumor grade.
   - The TAILORx study demonstrated excellent overall survival (OS), freedom from recurrence and invasive disease-free survival (DFS) at 5 years in "low risk" patients defined as those with a recurrence score of 0 to 10, all of whom received endocrine therapy only. Patients with recurrence score of 11 to 25 were randomly assigned to receive chemotherapy plus endocrine therapy or endocrine therapy alone, and outcome data on these patients is awaited. Studies have validated the role of Oncotype DX patients with ER-positive node-positive tumors and it can be used in selected settings. Oncotype DX testing has also been studied in DCIS where the resulting "DCIS score" quantifies the ipsilateral breast event risk for both invasive and noninvasive disease after surgical excision without radiation.
   - MammaPrint is a DNA microarray assay of 70 genes designed to predict the risk of recurrence of early-stage breast cancer. This testing classifies patients as low risk or high risk. There is no "intermediate" group as there is with the Oncotype. In February 2007, the FDA approved the use of MammaPrint in patients less than the age of 61, with a tumor size less than 5 cm and lymph node negative. The MINDACT study, which was published in 2016, was done to prospectively

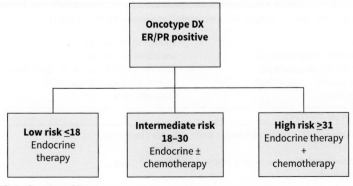

FIGURE 12.1 Oncotype DX assay.

assess the clinical utility of the MammaPrint in selecting early-stage patients with up to 3 axillary lymph nodes involved for adjuvant chemotherapy. The patients in this study had both genomic and clinical risk defined and those with discordant results (meaning low genomic risk /high clinical risk or high genomic risk/low clinical risk) were randomized to either receive chemotherapy or not. The primary endpoint of the study was survival without distant metastases in patients with high-risk clinical features and low-risk genomic features. It was found that 5-year metastasis-free survival in these patients was similar whether or not chemotherapy was given (absolute difference 1.5%).

An update to the ASCO clinical guidelines regarding use of MammaPrint was released in July 2017 stating that use of the MammaPrint can be considered to assist in decisions regarding adjuvant chemotherapy in ER-positive or PR-positive, HER2-negative, N0 or N1 breast cancer patients with high clinical risk of recurrence as described in the MINDACT study. For those who have low clinical risk of recurrence, use of MammaPrint is not recommended.

- Other genomic assays available for decision making in early breast cancer include the Breast Cancer Index, EndoPredict, PAM50 risk of recurrence score, Mammostrat and Urokinase plasminogen activator, and plasminogen activator inhibitor type 1. Each of these tests is intended to help clinicians identify patients with hormone receptor–positive, HER2-negative early-stage breast cancer who have a low risk of distant recurrence. This information can then be used to aide in making decisions regarding adjuvant systemic therapy.
- As per the 2016 ASCO clinical practice guideline on "use of biomarkers to guide decisions on adjuvant systemic therapy for women with early-stage invasive breast cancer," there is intermediate quality evidence for use of EndoPredict and Breast Cancer Index in ER/PR-positive, HER2-negative patients with node negative breast cancer to guide decisions on adjuvant systemic therapy. For the PAM50 risk of recurrence score, the evidence is considered high quality and recommendation for use in the above setting is strong.

Genomic Subtypes of Breast Cancer

Several distinct types of breast cancer are identified by gene expression studies. They differ markedly in prognosis and in the therapeutic targets they express (Table 12.4). The 5 main subtypes, known as the "intrinsic subtypes of breast cancer," are described here:

- **Luminal A and B subtypes:** Luminal A and luminal B subtypes express genes associated with luminal epithelial cells of normal breast tissue and overlap with ER-positive breast cancers defined by clinical assays. The luminal A subtype amounts to about 40% to 50% of cancers and has the best prognosis. These tumors are generally ER/PR-positive and HER-2 negative. Approximately 20% of breast cancers are of luminal B subtype, and they have worse prognosis compared to luminal A. The luminal B subtype tends to include tumors that are ER or PR positive and HER2-negative as well as those that are ER,

TABLE 12.4 Systemic Treatment Recommendations Based upon Subtypes

Luminal A	Endocrine therapy alone
Luminal B (HER-2/neu-negative)	Endocrine +/– Chemo
Luminal B (HER-2/neu-positive)	Chemo + anti-HER-2/neu-drugs endocrine therapy
HER-2/neu-positive (nonluminal)	Chemo + anti-HER-2/neu-drugs
Triple negative	Chemotherapy
Special Biologic Subtypes	
Endocrine responsive (cribriform, tubular, and mucinous)	Endocrine therapy
Endocrine nonresponsive (medullary, adenoid, and metaplastic)	Chemotherapy

PR, and HER2-positive. Luminal B cancers also tend to be higher grade tumors compared to luminal A cancers. Luminal A cancers are generally responsive to endocrine therapy while luminal B tumors may benefit from a combined approach including chemotherapy and endocrine therapy.

- **HER-2-enriched subtype:** The HER-2-enriched subtype comprises the majority of clinically HER-2/neu-positive breast cancers. It accounts for 10% to 15% of breast cancers. Not all HER-2/neu-positive tumors are HER-2/neu-enriched. About half of clinical HER-2/neu-positive breast cancers are HER-2/neu- enriched; the other half can include any molecular subtype including HER-2/neu-positive luminal subtypes. Those tumors that are ER/PR-negative and grade 3 tend to fall into the HER2-enriched subtype.

- **Basal-like subtype:** These tumors are usually ER-negative and characterized by low expression of hormone receptor–related genes. Up to 90% of triple negative breast cancers (those that are ER-negative, PR-negative, and HER2-negative) are classified in the basal-like subtype. They have a more aggressive clinical course with higher risk of relapse and derive benefit from chemotherapy.

- **Normal-like subtype:** This subtype is represented in a minority of breast cancers and is similar in biomarker profile to luminal A tumors but with a gene profile more consistent with normal breast tissue rather than a luminal A tumor.

MANAGEMENT

High-Risk Lesions

Patients with high-risk lesions may be eligible for breast cancer prevention studies. Tamoxifen and raloxifene are two FDA-approved drugs for breast cancer prevention in high-risk settings. As per the MAP.3 study exemestane was found to be effective in breast cancer prevention; however, the drug is not FDA approved for this indication. For breast cancer prevention, in premenopausal patients, tamoxifen is the drug of choice, but in postmenopausal patients, raloxifene or aromatase inhibitors can be used.

Atypical Ductal Hyperplasia (ADH)

- There is a 4- to 5-fold increase in the risk of developing breast cancer in patients with ADH.
- There is wide variation in the criteria used in the diagnosis of ADH.
- If diagnosis is made with core-needle biopsy, the presence of invasive cancer may be missed due to sampling error. As a result, surgical excision of the site of ADH is recommended.
- Fifteen percent to 30% of cases may be "upgraded" to diagnosis of invasive cancer.
- Clinical breast examination and mammogram are the preferred screening methods, role of MRI is under investigation.
- Tamoxifen 20 mg PO for 5 years: The NSABP P-1 study showed 86% reduction in the risk of developing invasive breast cancer in patients who received tamoxifen.
- The NSABP P-2 study showed similar efficacy for raloxifene 60 mg daily for 5 years, but with fewer adverse effects. Hence, in postmenopausal patients, raloxifene could be considered as the preferred treatment option.

Lobular Carcinoma In Situ

- LCIS is not considered a form of cancer, but rather a benign lesion that indicates an increased risk of developing invasive breast cancer. In the eighth edition of the AJCC staging system, Tis(LCIS) has been eliminated reflecting the nonmalignant nature of these lesions.

There is a 24% chance of developing breast cancer in patients within 10 years of developing LCIS.

- Classical LCIS is not managed with surgery; it is managed with close clinical follow-up. If the LCIS is pleomorphic or has necrosis, excision with negative margins can be considered.
- Patients with classical LCIS can be followed up by clinical breast examination every 4 to 12 months and annual mammogram. As per the American Cancer Society, there is insufficient data to recommend regular breast MRIs for all patients with LCIS although this can be considered on an individual basis.
- Tamoxifen or raloxifene (postmenopausal) may be used for prevention of breast cancer (56% reduction in risk as per the NSABP P-1 and P-2 studies).

Noninvasive Breast Cancer

Ductal Carcinoma In Situ

- The extensive use of mammograms has led to the increasing diagnosis of ductal carcinoma in situ (DCIS)
- Microcalcification or soft tissue abnormality is seen in the mammogram of DCIS.
- DCIS is considered a precursor lesion for invasive breast cancer
- Comedonecrosis and high nuclear grade have been associated with shorter time to recurrence but do not predict higher overall recurrence rates

Treatment of DCIS

In patients with ER positive DCIS, lumpectomy followed by radiation treatment followed by endocrine therapy for 5 years can be considered as the standard treatment approach.

- Based upon NSABP B-24, in premenopausal women with ER positive DCIS treated with lumpectomy, tamoxifen 20 mg daily for 5 years reduced the risk of breast cancer recurrence (ipsilateral and contralateral)
- Based upon NSABP B-35, in postmenopausal women with ER positive DCIS, anastrozole 1 mg daily resulted in improvement in breast cancer–free interval for women < 60 years. Based on this data, aromatase inhibitors can be used in postmenopausal patients with ER positive DCIS after lumpectomy.
- Mastectomy with or without lymph node evaluation can also be considered as a treatment option. In patients who undergo mastectomy, the role of endocrine therapy is limited. In selected patients, endocrine therapy can be considered for contralateral breast cancer prevention.
- Axillary lymph node evaluation is not recommended in pure DCIS without evidence of invasive cancer. In patients with DCIS on biopsy who are treated with mastectomy, a sentinel lymph node evaluation can be considered at the time of initial surgery as a future sentinel node evaluation would not be possible if invasive disease is found on final surgical pathology.
- NSABP B-43: study of trastuzumab in HER-2/neu-positive DCIS has completed and waiting for the results.

Invasive Breast Cancer

A multidisciplinary team should manage breast cancer, with the input from a radiologist, pathologist, breast surgeon, reconstructive surgeon, medical oncologist, and radiation oncologist. Other key members of the multidisciplinary team should include genetic counselors, psychologists, social workers, nurses, and navigators.

After the diagnosis of breast cancer with a core-needle biopsy or fine-needle aspiration cytology, it is important to confirm the histology, prognostic markers, and receptors. Various treatment options should then be discussed with the patient before the treatment plan is finalized.

Surgery

There are two components to surgical management of breast cancer: removal of the breast cancer and evaluation of lymph nodes.

Patients with DCIS or invasive cancer have two options for removing breast cancer, mastectomy, or lumpectomy. As per NSABP B-06 and EORTC 10801, 20 year local recurrence for mastectomy is 5%, for lumpectomy alone 40%, and lumpectomy with radiation is 14%. Despite these differences in local recurrence, there is no survival difference seen in patients who are treated with mastectomy versus lumpectomy and radiation therapy (breast conservation therapy [BCT]) and therefore both are offered as treatment options. Additionally, for those electing for BCT, adjuvant breast radiation is recommended.

In some cases, despite a desire for BCT, a mastectomy may be recommended. These include a contraindication to receiving radiation, multicentric disease, inflammatory breast cancer, or a large tumor in a small breast where resection would leave a cosmetically unpleasing result.

As per NCCN guidelines, contraindications for breast-conserving therapy requiring radiation therapy include

- Radiation therapy during pregnancy
- Widespread disease or calcifications that cannot be incorporated by breast conservation that achieves negative margins with a satisfactory cosmetic result
- Positive pathologic margin (no ink on tumor for invasive cancer, 2 mm margin for DCIS)
- Prior radiation therapy to the breast or chest wall
- Active connective tissue disease involving the skin (especially scleroderma and lupus)
- Tumors >5 cm

Women with a known genetic predisposition to breast cancer such as BRCA 1 or 2 have an increased risk of contralateral breast cancer or ipsilateral breast recurrence with breast-conserving therapy. Prophylactic bilateral mastectomy for risk reduction in these patients may be considered.

Sentinel Node Biopsy

The goal of sentinel lymph node biopsy (SLNB) is to provide prognostic information regarding the accurate pathologic staging of breast cancer. This information is used to guide additional management decisions. The SLN is defined as the main lymph node(s) that receives drainage directly from the primary tumor. SLN mapping and resection is the preferred method for staging the clinically negative axilla per NCCN guidelines. SLNB is performed by injection of technetium-labeled sulfur colloid, vital blue dye, or both around the tumor, or the subareolar area is taken up into the breast lymphatic system with a predominant pattern into the axilla. Nodes that contain dye or technetium are identified as the SLN. Identification rates of 92% to 98% of patients are the standard, especially when both techniques are used. If breast cancer were to spread, typically it would spread to the sentinel lymph node (SLN) first before moving to the other lymph nodes. This selective biopsy of potentially positive SLN, and sparing removal of negative lymph nodes decreases pain, sensation loss, and lymphedema compared to traditional axillary lymph node dissection (ALND).

The ACOSOG Z 0011 clinical trial showed that in patients with T1–T2 invasive breast cancer with clinically negative lymph nodes, found to have one to two positive lymph nodes on SLNB, there is no benefit in OS and DFS in performing a complete axillary node dissection. For patients who meet these criteria, a complete ALND can be potentially avoided.

Axillary Lymph Node Dissection

- Among patients with clinically negative axillary lymph nodes, 14% will have positive SLNB and will require additional axillary surgery.
- Axillary lymph node dissection (ALND) is complete surgical removal of level I and II axillary lymph nodes. The goal of ALND is to remove axillary burden of disease.
- A complete axillary node dissection is associated with approximately 10% to 25% risk of lymphedema, which can be mild to severe.

Reconstruction

Reconstructive surgery may be used for patients who opt for a mastectomy. It may be done at the time of the mastectomy (immediate reconstruction) or at a later time (delayed reconstruction). Patients diagnosed with early-stage breast cancer and electing to undergo a mastectomy should be offered immediate reconstruction as long as their comorbid conditions do not preclude this intervention. For patients with locally advanced or inflammatory breast cancer, undergoing mastectomy with delayed reconstruction may be the more appropriate management option.

Reconstruction can be done in one of two ways: implant-based (silicone or saline implants) or an autologous tissue graft. Examples of autologous tissue grafts include TRAM (transverse rectus abdominis myocutaneous) flaps, the latissimus dorsi flap, and the DIEP (deep inferior epigastric perforator) flap.

Radiotherapy

- Radiotherapy (RT) is an integral part of breast-conserving treatment (lumpectomy). It is associated with a large reduction in local recurrence and a positive impact on survival.
- Standard radiation is 45 to 50.4 Gy at 1.8 to 2 Gy per fraction to the whole breast. RT boost to the tumor bed cavity is recommended in patients at higher risk for local failure (based on age,

pathology, and margin status). The boost dose is 10 to 16 Gy at 2 Gy per fraction. An alternative hypofractionation schedule is 40 to 42.5 Gy at 2.66 Gy per fraction to the whole breast. This treatment method has been demonstrated to provide comparable cosmetic and oncologic results following breast-conserving surgery in patients with clear surgical margins and negative lymph nodes. Three-dimensional planning, inverse planning for intensity modulation, respiratory control, prone positioning, and proton therapy are techniques employed to minimize cardiac risks for whole breast and postmastectomy chest wall RT in patients with left-sided breast cancer.

■ RT is usually done after chemotherapy when systemic chemotherapy is indicated.
■ Postmastectomy radiation treatment to the chest wall, axillary, supraclavicular- and internal mammary lymph node regions decreases the risk of locoregional recurrence and improves survival in patients with multiple positive lymph nodes and patients with T3 or T4 tumors.
■ Two randomized trials showed improvement in OS for postmastectomy radiation in patients with one to three positive lymph nodes, and is being evaluated in more clinical trials. In selected patients, this should be discussed.
■ Other indications that may place patients at risk for local-regional failure and drive the decision for postmastectomy radiation include positive margins, extranodal extension and high-grade disease, young age and high-risk biology (e.g., triple-negative disease), and omission of axillary dissection after positive sentinel lymph node biopsy if sufficient information is present without needing to know if additional axillary lymph nodes are involved. ASCO (American Society of Clinical Oncology), ASTRO (American Society for Radiation Oncology), and SSO (Society of Surgical Oncology) updated guidelines for postmastectomy radiation therapy in 2016.
■ For patients receiving neoadjuvant chemotherapy, those who present with clinically node positive, cT3 or cT4 disease, will typically be recommended for postmastectomy radiation regardless of pathologic response outside of a clinical trial. Biopsy is recommended to confirm clinical suspicion of lymph node involvement prior to the initiation of chemotherapy.

Accelerated Partial Breast Irradiation

The primary goal of accelerated partial breast irradiation (APBI) is to shorten the duration of radiation therapy while maintaining adequate local control by targeting the lumpectomy cavity and adjacent at-risk tissue while sparing normal tissues. There are several APBI techniques currently in use and under study, including external beam radiation techniques, intraoperative radiation therapy, and brachytherapy; however, brachytherapy is the most widely used technique. Patients who are clinically felt to be at a lower risk recurrence outside of the lumpectomy site should be selected according to published criteria since the whole breast is not treated. ASTRO and SSO have published guidelines to aid in patient selection, e.g., older patients with Tis or T1 disease, screen-detected, low-intermediate grade, <2.5 cm with margins negative by at least 3 mm. The standard dose for balloon catheter brachytherapy is 34 Gy in 10 fractions delivered twice daily. Phase III data supports the use of intensity modulated external beam radiation therapy delivering 30 Gy in 5 fractions for select patients.

Intraoperative Radiation Therapy (IORT)

Intraoperative radiation therapy (IORT) delivers a concentrated dose of radiation to the tumor bed immediately after the tumor is removed. Two large studies evaluated the role of IORT in women with early-stage breast cancer. In the TARGIT-A study, women ages 45 or older were randomized to receive IORT or whole breast external beam radiation (WBRT) after lumpectomy. Survival rates were similar in both groups but local recurrence was more common in the IORT group. These findings are supported by the ELIOT trial results. In this study, women ages 48 to 75 with tumors ≤ 2.5 cm were randomized to IORT or WBRT, and survival rates were similar in both groups but local recurrence was more common in the IORT group.

Per the 2017 ASTRO/SSO APBI consensus statement update, IORT should be restricted to patients who are also suitable to partial breast radiation, and patients should be counseled that the risk of ipsilateral breast cancer might be higher with IORT.

Adjuvant Systemic Therapy

Adjuvant therapy decisions are made after carefully considering patient-related and tumor-related factors. Patient related factors include, age, comorbid conditions, performance status, patient preference,

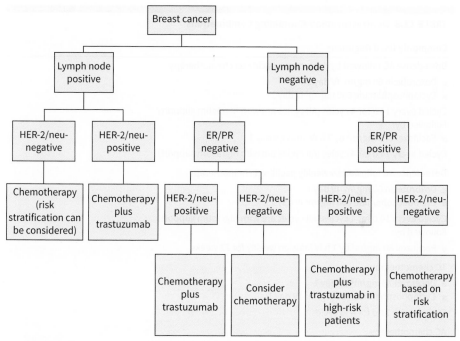

FIGURE 12.2 Algorithm for systemic adjuvant therapy.

risk–benefit discussion, and life expectancy. Tumor-related factors are tumor size, lymph node status (stage) ER/PR status, Her-2/neu, grade of the tumor and genomic expression profile (e.g.: Oncotype DX, MammaPrint, etc.) (Fig. 12.2).

General Principles of Adjuvant Therapy

1. All patients with breast cancer should be screened for potential clinical trials.
2. ER/PR-positive patients should be considered for antiestrogen therapy.
3. HER-2/neu-positive patients should be considered for HER-2/neu-targeted therapy.
4. Chemotherapy should be considered for the following patients (Table 12.3):
   a. ER/PR-negative patients
   b. Triple negative patients
   c. HER-2/neu-positive patients
   d. Node-positive patients
   e. High-risk patients based upon Oncotype DX, MammaPrint, or other prognostic classification

Adjuvant Therapy in HER-2/neu-Negative Patients

A variety of adjuvant regimens have been used across the world. Depending upon the biology of the tumor, stage of the disease, patient's health status, comorbid conditions, and chance of recurrence, an optimal regimen can be chosen (Table 12.5). There is no major difference in efficacy among the regimens.

Estrogen or progesterone receptor positive, HER-2 neu negative patients:

A nonanthracycline-containing regimen such as docetaxel and cyclophosphamide (TC) for four to six cycles can be used in ER positive patients who require systemic chemotherapy. The benefit of anthracycline-containing regimens in receptor positive patients is limited. This was illustrated in the ABC (anthracyclines in early breast cancer) trials (combined analysis of USOR 06-090, NSABP B-46

TABLE 12.5 Nontrastuzumab-Containing Combinations

Commonly Used Regimens

Dose-dense AC followed by dose-dense paclitaxel chemotherapy

- Doxorubicin 60 mg/m^2 IV day 1
- Cyclophosphamide 600 mg/m^2 IV day 1

Cycled every 14 d for 4 cycles (All cycles are with filgrastim support)
Followed by:

- Paclitaxel 175 mg/m^2 by 3 h IV infusion day 1

Cycled every 14 d for 4 cycles (All cycles are with filgrastim support)

Dose-dense AC followed by weekly paclitaxel chemotherapy

- Doxorubicin 60 mg/m^2 IV day 1
- Cyclophosphamide 600 mg/m^2 IV day 1

Cycled every 14 d for 4 cycles (All cycles are with filgrastim support)
Followed by:

- Paclitaxel 80 mg/m^2 by 1 h IV infusion weekly for 12 weeks

TC chemotherapy

- Docetaxel 75 mg/m^2 1V day 1
- Cyclophosphamide 600 mg/m^2 1V day 1

Cycled every 21 d for 4 -6 cycles

AC chemotherapy

- Doxorubicin 60 mg/m^2 IV day
- Cyclophosphamide 600 mg/m^2 IV day 1

Cycled every 21 d for 4 cycles

TAC chemotherapy

- Docetaxel 75 mg/m^2 IV day 1
- Doxorubicin 50 mg/m^2 IV day 1
- Cyclophosphamide 500 mg/m^2 IV day 1

Cycled every 21 d for 6 cycles (All cycles are with filgrastim support)

Other Regimens

FAC chemotherapy

- 5-Fluorouracil 500 mg/m^2 IV days 1 and 8 or days 1 and 4
- Doxorubicin 50 mg/m^2 IV day 1 (or by 72-h continuous infusion)
- Cyclophosphamide 500 mg/m^2 IV day 1

Cycled every 21 d for 6 cycles

CAF chemotherapy

- Cyclophosphamide 100 mg/m^2 PO days 1–14
- Doxorubicin 30 mg/m^2 IV days 1 and 8
- 5-Fluorouracil 500 mg/m^2 IV days 1 and 8

Cycled every 28 d for 6 cycles

CEF chemotherapy

- Cyclophosphamide 75 mg/m^2 PO days 1–14
- Epirubicin 60 mg/m^2 IV days 1 and 8
- 5-Fluorouracil 500 mg/m^2 IV days 1and 8

Cycled every 28 d for 6 cycles
With cotrimoxazole support

(continued)

TABLE 12.5 (Continued)

CMF chemotherapy
- Cyclophosphamide 100 mg/m² PO days 1–14
- Methotrexate 40 mg/m² IV days 1 and 8
- 5- Fluorouracil 600 mg/m² IV days 1 and 8

Cycled every 28 d for 6 cycles

AC followed by docetaxel chemotherapy
- Doxorubicin 60 mg/m² IV on day 1
- Cyclophosphamide 600 mg/m² IV day 1

Cycled every 21 d for 4 cycles
Followed by:
- Docetaxel 100 mg/m² IV on day 1

Cycled every 21 d for 4 cycles

EC chemotherapy
- Epirubicin 100 mg/m² IV day 1
- Cyclophosphamide 830 mg/m² IV day 1

Cycled every 21 d for 8 cycles

FEC followed by docetaxel
- 5-Fluorouracil 500 mg/m² IV day 1
- Epirubicin 100 mg/m² IV day 1
- Cyclophosphamide 500 mg/m² IV day 1

Cycled every 21 d for 3 cycles
Followed by:
- Docetaxel 100 mg/m² IV day 1

Cycled every 21 d for 3 cycles

FEC followed by weekly paclitaxel
- 5-Fluorouracil 600mg/m² IV day 1
- Epirubicin 90 mg/m² IV day 1
- Cyclophosphamide 600 mg/m² IV day 1

Cycled every 21 d for 4 cycles
Followed by:
- Paclitaxel100 mg/m² IV weekly for 8 weeks

FAC followed by weekly paclitaxel
- 5-Fluorouracil 500 mg/m2 IV days 1 and 8 or days 1 and 4
- Doxorubicin 50 mg/m2 IV day 1 (or by 72 h continuous infusion)
- Cyclophosphamide 500 mg/m² IV day 1

Cycled every 21 d for 4 cycles
Followed by:
- Paclitaxel 80 mg/m² by 1 h IV infusion weekly for 12 weeks

and NSABP B-49) where women with early-stage breast cancer were randomized to TC for six cycles versus standard anthracycline/taxane/cyclophosphamide based chemotherapy. This trial showed the anthracycline-based chemotherapy improved invasive DFS compared to TC for six cycles overall; however, in subgroup analysis, it was found that the benefit of anthracyclines for ER/PR-positive patients was most substantial for those with four or more lymph nodes involved. In high-risk (such as more than four nodes) ER/PR positive patients, an anthracycline-containing regimen such as dose dense AC followed by dose dense Paclitaxel or TAC regimen should be considered.

TABLE 12.6 Trastuzumab-Containing Regimens

AC followed by T chemotherapy with trastuzumab

- Doxorubicin 60 mg/m^2 IV day 1
- Cyclophosphamide 600 mg/m^2 IV day 1

Cycled every 21 d for 4 cycles

Followed by:

- Paclitaxel 80 mg/m^2 by 1 h IV weekly for 12 weeks

With:

- Trastuzumab 4 mg/kg IV with first dose of paclitaxel

Followed by:

- Trastuzumab 2 mg/kg IV weekly to complete 1 y of treatment (Alternative: trastuzumab 6 mg/kg IV every 21 days to complete 1 y of treatment)

TCH chemotherapy with trastuzumab

- Docetaxel 75 mg/m^2 IV day 1
- Carboplatin AUC 6 IV day 1

Cycled every 21 d for 6 cycles

With

- Trastuzumab 8 mg/kg IV day 1

Followed by:

- Trastuzumab 6 mg/kg IV every 3 weeks to complete 1 y of trastuzumab therapy

TCHP chemotherapy followed by trastuzumab (+/- pertuzumab)

- Docetaxel 75 mg/m^2 IV day 1
- Carboplatin AUC 6 IV day 1

Cycled every 21 d for 6 cycles

With

- Trastuzumab 8 mg/kg IV day 1
- Pertuzumab 840mg IV day 1

Followed by:

- Trastuzumab 6 mg/kg IV every 3 weeks to complete 1 y of trastuzumab therapy
- Pertuzumab 420mg IV every 3 weeks for 6 cycles (can also be continued to complete 1 y of dual HER2 blockade, if indicated)

Dose-dense AC followed by dose-dense paclitaxel chemotherapy with trastuzumab

- Doxorubicin 60 mg/m^2 IV day 1
- Cyclophosphamide 600 mg/m^2 IV day 1

Cycled every 14 d for 4 cycles

Followed by:

- Paclitaxel 175 mg/m^2 by 3 h IV infusion day 1

Cycled every 14 d for 4 cycles

(All cycles are with filgrastim support)

With

- Trastuzumab 4 mg/kg IV with first dose of paclitaxel

Followed by:

- Trastuzumab 2 mg/kg IV weekly to complete 1 y of treatment (Alternative: trastuzumab 6 mg/kg IV every 21 days to complete 1 y of treatment)

(Cardiac monitoring is recommended before and during treatment)

Paclitaxel chemotherapy and trastuzumab

- Paclitaxel 80 mg/ m^2 IV weekly for 12 weeks

With

- Trastuzumab 4 mg/kg IV with first dose of paclitaxel

Followed by:

- Trastuzumab 2 mg/kg IV weekly to complete 1 year of treatment. (Alternative: trastuzumab 6 mg/kg IV every 21 days to complete 1 y of treatment)

Adapted from NCCN 2017 Guidelines

Estrogen and progesterone receptor negative, HER-2/neu negative (Triple Negative) patients

These patients are often treated with anthracycline-based chemotherapy in the adjuvant setting; however, the ABC trials showed that the greatest benefit of anthracycline-containing chemotherapy for ER/PR-negative patients occurred when patients had one or more lymph nodes involved. For patients with lymph node negative or small tumors (less than 2 cm), TC chemotherapy for four to six cycles can be considered. In high-risk Triple Negative patients, anthracycline-containing regimens, such as Dose Dense AC followed by Dose Dense Paclitaxel or a TAC regimen should be considered. Role of carboplatin in adjuvant triple negative breast cancer is evaluated in NRG 003 clinical trial.

Adjuvant Therapy in HER-2/neu-Positive Patients

Incorporation of trastuzumab in the adjuvant therapy is the most important development in the treatment of breast cancer in the past 10 to 15 years. The clinical trials that initially showed benefit for the addition of trastuzumab to standard chemotherapy in treatment of HER2+ breast cancer (NSABP B-31 and NCCTG N9831) have published 10 year of follow-up showing 40% improvement in DFS and 37% improvement in OS. Many trastuzumab-containing regimens have been tested and all are equally effective (Table 12.6). The major difference between regimens is in the cardiac toxicity. Nonanthracycline-containing regimens (such as TCH from the BCIRG 006 trial) and the HERA trial regimens (the majority of which were anthracycline based but used sequential rather than concurrent trastuzumab) had less cardiac toxicity compared to other anthracycline-containing regimens. In the adjuvant setting, trastuzumab has only been tested in combination with chemotherapy.

Based upon the long-term follow-up of BCIRG 006 presented at the San Antonio Breast Cancer Symposium in 2015, a nonanthracycline regimen–containing TCH for six cycles could be considered for most patients with her-2 positive disease given the excellent outcomes. In very high-risk patients (multiple lymph nodes and very young patients), an anthracycline-containing regimen such as AC followed by TH or AC-THP can be considered after discussing about potential side effects such as cardiac toxicity and risk of secondary malignancies (MDS and AML).

The APHINITY study presented and published in June 2017, showed that the addition of adjuvant pertuzumab to standard adjuvant trastuzumab-containing regimen for HER2+ breast cancer resulted in a statistically significant, but a small 1.7% improvement in invasive DFS benefit predominantly in the lymph node positive and hormone receptor–negative patients. A 3.2% improvement in invasive DFS was seen in lymph node positive patients versus 0.5% improvement in lymph node negative patients and 1.6% improvement in invasive DFS improvement was seen in hormone receptor–negative patients compared to 0.5% improvement in hormone receptor–positive patients. Addition of pertuzumab was associated with a greater incidence of diarrhea. Given these results, use of adjuvant pertuzumab for one year in addition to trastuzumab can be considered in selected high-risk patients such as those with positive lymph nodes and those that are ER/PR-negative. The added cost should be considered before recommending pertuzumab in adjuvant setting.

In low-risk patients, especially patients with ER-positive, stage I or II tumors, weekly paclitaxel for 12 cycles with trastuzumab is a very reasonable option as per the APT (adjuvant paclitaxel and trastuzumab in node negative HER2 positive breast cancer) study.

Extended HER2-targeted therapy has also been investigated. The ExteNET study tested the irreversible pan-HER inhibitor neratinib 240 mg PO for 12 months in patients who completed standard trastuzumab-based adjuvant therapy and found a 2.3% benefit in 2-year invasive DFS for patients who received neratinib compared to placebo. Interestingly, pre-specified subgroup analysis showed greater benefit in hormone receptor–positive patients compared to hormone receptor–negative patients. Based on these results, the FDA approved neratinib 240 mg daily for 12 months for extended adjuvant treatment of early-stage HER2-positive breast cancer following adjuvant trastuzumab based therapy in July 2017.

Neoadjuvant or Preoperative Chemotherapy

Neoadjuvant or preoperative chemotherapy can be considered for patients with locally advanced breast cancer (IIB, IIIA, IIIB, IIIC), and inflammatory breast cancer. Response to neoadjuvant chemotherapy is much higher in triple negative and her-2 neu positive patients. In patients with stage III disease or inflammatory breast cancer, neoadjuvant therapy is the treatment of choice.

- Initial surgery is limited to biopsy to confirm the diagnosis and to identify the ER/PR, HER-2/neu-status, and other prognostic features.
- Preoperative evaluation of the breast mass by mammogram, ultrasound, or MRI is recommended.
- Systemic staging using CT scans or CT/PET scan can be considered for these patients before starting chemotherapy.
- Neoadjuvant chemotherapy can potentially reduce the size of the primary tumor so breast-conserving surgery can be performed.
- Complete pathologic response (pCR) is associated with better outcome compared with residual disease at the time of surgery as demonstrated in the NSABP B-18 and NSABP B-27 trials. These trials showed no difference in DFS or OS between the groups treated with neoadjuvant and adjuvant therapy.
- HER-2/neu-negative patients:
  - Usually, a preoperative regimen contains an anthracycline and a taxane. Any adjuvant regimen can be used in a neoadjuvant setting.
  - One of the largest neoadjuvant clinical trials is four cycles of AC followed by docetaxel for four cycles given every 3 weeks as per NSABP B-27 trial.
  - In the CALGB 40603 trial, the addition of carboplatin to an anthracycline-based neoadjuvant regimen in patients with triple-negative breast cancer was associated with improvement in pCR rates (41% vs. 54%). GeparSixto trials by the German Breast Cancer Group also showed similar high response with carboplatin in neoadjuvant setting.
  - In selected high-risk triple negative patients, it is very reasonable to consider adding carboplatin, especially if the tumor is not responding to standard anthracycline and taxane regimens.
- HER-2/neu-positive patients:
  - Any adjuvant trastuzumab-containing regimen can be used in a neoadjuvant setting.
  - Several clinical trials have shown an advantage for dual her-2 blockade in the neoadjuvant setting. Pertuzumab in combination with trastuzumab and docetaxel in the neoadjuvant setting was approved in 2013 based on the results of the phase II NeoSPHERE and TRYPHAENA trials. Lapatinib in combination with trastuzumab and paclitaxel in the neoadjuvant setting was studied in the NeoALTTO trial and was shown to be associated with higher rates of pCR than either anti-HER-2 drug alone.
  - In HER-2 positive patients with high-risk features (such as ER/PR negative, stage II and above) they may be treated with pertuzumab in addition to trastuzumab. Commonly used neoadjuvant regimens include TCHP for 6 cycles or AC followed by THP.

Adjuvant Endocrine Therapy

Unless there is a contraindication, endocrine therapy should be considered for all patients with ER-positive and/or PR-positive tumors. As per the Oxford overview analysis, tamoxifen can decrease mortality by about 30% and the risk of recurrence by 50% in hormone receptor–positive patients (Fig. 12.3 and Table 12.7).

Postmenopausal Women

Several large randomized studies have shown superiority of aromatase inhibitors (AIs) over tamoxifen in the adjuvant setting. If the patient has no contraindication, AIs are the preferred agents in postmenopausal patients. Anastrozole, letrozole, and exemestane are three third-generation AIs approved by the FDA for adjuvant use. The major side effects include arthralgia, osteopenia, osteoporosis, and fractures.

Anastrozole

One of the largest adjuvant breast cancer trials (ATAC) compared tamoxifen with anastrozole and combination of both anastrozole and tamoxifen. It was shown that anastrozole is superior to tamoxifen in improving DFS, reducing the incidence of contralateral breast cancer, and has a favorable side-effect profile. For postmenopausal patients, the recommended dose of anastrozole is 1 mg PO daily for 5 years; however, there has been much interest in extending adjuvant therapy to a duration of 10 years as described in the following "Extended Adjuvant Endocrine Therapy" section.

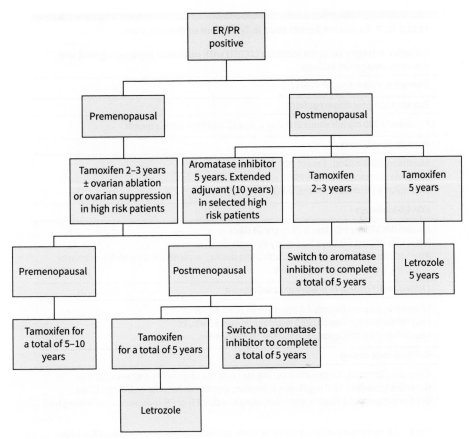

FIGURE 12.3 Adjuvant endocrine therapy.

Letrozole

BIG 1-98 showed a similar magnitude of improvement as anastrozole in the ATAC trial in DFS and a reduction of distant metastasis with letrozole. For postmenopausal patients, the recommended dose of letrozole is 2.5 mg PO daily for 5 years. Studies of extended adjuvant therapy with letrozole have been completed and are summarized below:

Switching from Tamoxifen to an Aromatase Inhibitor

In the IES study, exemestane therapy after 2 to 3 years of tamoxifen therapy significantly improved DFS and reduced the incidence of contralateral breast cancer as compared with the standard 5 years of tamoxifen therapy. The FDA has approved exemestane 25 mg daily after 2 to 3 years of tamoxifen in postmenopausal patients (total of 5 years of endocrine therapy).

The Italian tamoxifen anastrozole (ITA) trial, Austrian Breast Colorectal Study Group (ABCSG 8), and Arimidex, Noveldex (ARNO) study have shown an improvement in DFS and OS in patients who were initially treated with 2 to 3 years of tamoxifen and subsequently randomized to 2 to 3 years of anastrozole.

Extended Adjuvant Endocrine Therapy

The MA-17 study showed approximately 43% reduction in recurrence in postmenopausal patients receiving 2.5 mg of letrozole after completing 5 years of tamoxifen (extended adjuvant therapy). The

TABLE 12.7 Endocrine Agents Used in Treatment of Breast Cancer

Selective estrogen-receptor modifier (SERM) with combined estrogen agonist and estrogen antagonist activity

Tamoxifen (Nolvadex), 20 mg/d PO

Estrogen receptor downregulator

Fulvestrant 500 mg intramuscular day 1, day 15 and then once a month

Aromatase inhibitors

Anastrozole (Arimidex), 1 mg/d PO
Letrozole (Femara), 2.5 mg/d PO
Exemestane (Aromasin), 25 mg/d PO

CDK4/6 Inhibitors

Palbociclib 125 mg PO Days 1-21 every 28 days
Ribociclib 600 mg PO Days 1-21 every 28 days
Abemaciclib 150 mg twice a day (continuous dosing) in combination with fulvestrant or
      200 mg twice a day as single agent

LHRH agonist analog in premenopausal women

Leuprolide (Lupron Depot), 7.5 mg/dose IM monthly, or
Leuprolide (Lupron Depot), 22.5 mg/dose IM every 3 mo, or
Leuprolide (Lupron Depot), 30 mg/dose IM every 4 mo

GnRH agonist analog

Goserelin (Zoladex), 3.6 mg/dose s.c. implant into the abdominal wall every 28 d or
Goserelin (Zoladex), 10.8 mg/dose s.c. implant into the abdominal wall every 12 wk
Used in patients who have tumors that express either ER or PR receptors or both receptors

LHRH, luteinizing hormone–releasing hormone; GnRH, gonadotropin-releasing hormone; ER, estrogen receptor; PR, progesterone receptor.

MA.17R trial (an extension of the MA 17 trial) evaluated the role of 10 years of adjuvant letrozole in postmenopausal women. The five additional years of letrozole increased the 5 year DFS by 4% but only decreased the rate of distant recurrence by 1.1%.

The NSABP B-42 randomized phase III trial presented at the 2016 San Antonio Breast Cancer Symposium, however, did not show a DFS benefit with five additional years of adjuvant letrozole. Despite conflicting results of the MA-17R and NSABP B-42 studies, high-risk patients who are tolerating aromatase inhibitor well after 5 years, may consider continuing therapy for five additional years. Various biomarkers such as Breast Cancer Index (BCI) are being developed to aid in selecting patients who will benefit from extended adjuvant therapy.

Endocrine Therapy: Premenopausal Patients

Hormone receptor–positive, premenopausal patients are generally treated with tamoxifen (Fig. 12.3).

Tamoxifen

Tamoxifen is a selective estrogen-receptor modulator (SERM), with both estrogen agonist and antagonist potential. In premenopausal patients, tamoxifen 20 mg daily is the treatment of choice, unless the patient has any contraindications such as history of thromboembolic disease, stroke, or endometrial cancer. Major adverse effects include a higher incidence of cerebrovascular accidents, thrombosis, endometrial cancer, hot flashes, mood changes, and weight gain.

In general, tamoxifen is recommended for 5 years however many studies support a longer duration of treatment. In the ATLAS study, women who took tamoxifen for a total of 10 years rather than 5 had lower recurrence rate and increased OS. Extended adjuvant use of tamoxifen had little effect on recurrence or mortality rates from 5 to 9 years after diagnosis, but in the second decade following diagnosis, women who had continued tamoxifen treatment beyond 5 years had a 25% lower recurrence rate and a 29% lower breast cancer mortality rate. The results of the aTTom trial also demonstrated improved survival with 10 years of tamoxifen. Prolonged use of tamoxifen is associated with increased side effects (particularly endometrial carcinoma and PE); therefore, the decision to use tamoxifen for 10 years needs to be individualized, depending on the risk of recurrence and potential adverse effects.

Ovarian Ablation or Ovarian Suppression

The Oxford overview and several studies have found that premenopausal patients who stopped having periods after completion of chemotherapy have better survival than those who continued to have periods. Ovarian ablation can be achieved by surgery, radiation, or with LHRH agonists such as leuprolide, GNRH analogues such as goserelin.

The TEXT and SOFT trials, published in 2014, addressed the use of ovarian suppression as adjuvant therapy in premenopausal women with ER-positive breast cancer. In the TEXT trial, women were randomized to receive 5 years of tamoxifen with ovarian suppression or exemestane with ovarian suppression. In the SOFT trial, women were randomized to 5 years of tamoxifen, tamoxifen plus ovarian suppression, or exemestane plus ovarian suppression. DFS was higher in the exemestane plus ovarian suppression group comparing to the tamoxifen plus ovarian suppression group in both trials. In a subgroup analysis of the TEXT trial, younger women (under the age of 35 years) with high-risk disease warranting chemotherapy had higher DFS with exemestane and ovarian suppression compared to tamoxifen alone or tamoxifen with ovarian suppression. Based on these results, it is reasonable to consider exemestane with ovarian suppression for premenopausal women with high-risk disease, particularly those under the age of 35 years.

In general, we recommend use of monthly LHRH agonists such as leuprolide, GNRH analogues such as goserelin or surgical removal of ovaries for those patients who would benefit from ovarian suppression. In patients who are treated with GNRH analogues or LHRH agonists, it is important to make sure that they achieve a complete ovarian suppression by checking the serum estradiol, LH, and FSH although optimal frequency of this monitoring is unknown. Before a young woman decides to undergo bilateral oophorectomy, it is important to make sure that she understands the risks and benefits including its impact on quality of life. In this situation, it may be advisable to use medical ovarian suppression for a period of time, so potential side effects can be reversed with discontinuation of the medication.

Role of Adjuvant BisphosphCnate Therapy in Early Breast Cancer:

In an Oxford overview analysis including data from nearly 19,000 patients treated with adjuvant bisphosphonate therapy, significant reductions in distant breast cancer recurrence (particularly bone recurrence) and breast cancer mortality were found. These effects were limited to women who were postmenopausal when treatment was started. Based on this data, an update to the ASCO clinical practice guidelines occurred in July 2017. The guidelines now recommend that postmenopausal women with breast cancer who are candidates for adjuvant therapy be considered for treatment with either zoledronic acid (4mg IV every 6 months) or clodronate (1,600 mg PO daily). Optimal dosing during and intervals are not known although up to 5 years of treatment can be considered. Definition of menopause in this guideline includes both natural menopause and that induced by ovarian suppression or ablation.

BREAST CANCER IN PREGNANCY

- Breast cancer during pregnancy was initially thought to be more aggressive biologically; however, the overall poor outcome associated with breast cancer in pregnancy is likely related to more advanced stage at the time of diagnosis.
- Breast biopsy is safe in all stages of pregnancy and should be done for any mass concerning for cancer.

Treatment

- Lumpectomy and axillary node dissection can be performed in the third trimester, and radiation therapy can be safely delayed until after delivery.
- Modified radical mastectomy is the treatment of choice in the first and second trimesters because radiation treatment is contraindicated during pregnancy.

Chemotherapy

- Chemotherapy should not be administered during the first trimester.
- No chemotherapeutic agent has been found to be completely safe during pregnancy.
- An anthracycline combined with cyclophosphamide (e.g., AC given every 3 weeks for four cycles) has been used safely in the adjuvant or neoadjuvant setting during the second or third trimesters.
- Chemotherapy should be scheduled to avoid neutropenia and thrombocytopenia at the time of delivery.
- Paclitaxel is teratogenic and should not be used during pregnancy.
- Growth factors such as filgrastim and pegfilgrastim have been used in pregnancy when necessary; however, data regarding safety of use is limited to case reports and small retrospective series. The FDA considers these drugs as Category C.
- Her-2 targeted agents such as trastuzumab have been reported to cause oligo/anhydramnios and fetal renal failure, so it should be avoided during pregnancy.
- Tamoxifen is teratogenic and should not be used in pregnant women.
- Therapeutic abortion does not change the survival rate.

MALE BREAST CANCER

- Male breast cancer is uncommon.
- Risk factors include family history, germline mutation, especially BRCA2, Klinefelter syndrome, and radiation to the chest wall.
- Presence of gynecomastia is not a risk factor for breast cancer.
- It may present with a mass beneath the nipple or ulceration.
- The mean age of occurrence is 60 to 70 years.
- Eighty percent of male breast cancer is hormone-receptor positive.

Treatment

- Modified radical mastectomy.
- Lumpectomy is rarely done because it does not offer any cosmetic benefit.
- Systemic treatment with chemotherapy and endocrine therapy should follow the general guidelines for female patients.
- Tamoxifen 20 mg daily is the preferred endocrine therapy agent in male breast cancer.
- None of the adjuvant treatment modalities have been tested in a randomized clinical trial setting in men.

Phyllodes Tumor

A phyllodes tumor is clinically suspected when the tumor is growing rapidly and clinical and radiologic features suggestive of fibroadenoma. Phyllodes tumor is classified as benign, borderline, or malignant. It is treated with wide excision without an axillary node dissection. In patients who have recurrent phyllodes tumor, radiation therapy can be considered after wide excision. Role of chemotherapy in phyllodes tumor is limited. Patients with Li-Fraumeni syndrome have an increased risk for phyllodes tumors.

Paget's Disease of the Nipple

Paget's may present as bleeding, ulceration, or eczema-like changes of the nipple. Patients should be evaluated for any evidence of invasive or noninvasive breast cancer by appropriate imaging and biopsy as Paget's disease has been reported to occur with cancer elsewhere in the breast in up to 90% of cases. If the patient has only Paget disease of the nipple areolar complex (NAC), the patient can be treated with mastectomy with axillary lymph node dissection (ALND) or wide excision of the NAC and axillary node surgery with whole-breast radiation. Patients with invasive or noninvasive breast cancer should be managed accordingly.

METASTATIC BREAST CANCER

Principles of Treatment

1. Repeat biopsy to confirm the diagnosis of recurrent/metastatic breast cancer (Fig. 12.4).
2. Strongly recommend repeating all biomarkers including ER/PR and HER-2/neu.
3. All patients should be considered for clinical trials.
4. Genomic profiling using next generation sequencing can be considered if genomic-based clinical trials or targeted therapy options are available.
5. MSI (microsatellite instability) or MMR (mismatch repair deficient) testing can be considered in selected patients, especially patients with triple negative tumors or those who have limited standard treatment options available.
6. HER-2/neu-positive patients should be treated with HER-2/neu-targeted agents such as trastuzumab, pertuzumab, ado-trastuzumab emtansine (TDM-1), or lapatinib.
7. All ER/PR-positive, HER-2 neu negative patients should be considered for antiestrogen therapy with or without CDK 4/6 inhibitors such as palbociclib or ribociclib.
8. Premenopausal patients with ER-positive disease should be considered for ovarian suppression and endocrine therapy with or without CDK 4/6 inhibitors such as palbociclib or ribociclib.
9. In ER-positive patients, use of chemotherapy should be limited to those with visceral crisis or those who have progressed through various endocrine agents, CDK 4/6 inhibitors, or mTOR inhibitor treatments.
10. Since combination chemotherapy regimens have not shown DFS or OS benefit, patients should be treated with single agents in a sequential manner.
11. All patients with metastatic disease involving the bone should be considered for bone modifying agents such as bisphosphonates (zoledronic acid/pamidronate) or denosumab (RANK ligand inhibitor).

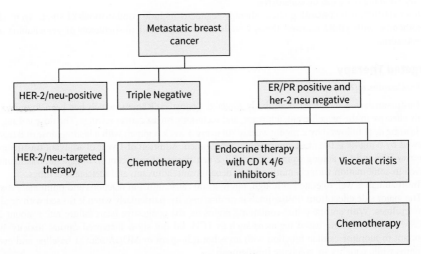

FIGURE 12.4 Algorithm for the management of metastatic breast cancer

12. Before starting treatment, a detailed assessment of comorbid conditions, performance status, patient preference, toxicities of the treatment, and risk versus benefit discussion should be done with each patient.
13. Goal of treatment should be discussed in detail with the patient, since it is palliative for majority of the patients.

Estrogen Receptor–Positive Metastatic Breast Cancer

- Endocrine therapy is the mainstay of treatment.
- Introduction of CDK 4/6 inhibitors such as palbociclib, ribociclib, and abemaciclib has revolutionized the treatment of estrogen receptor–positive metastatic breast cancer.
- Selection of endocrine therapy will depend upon the adjuvant or previous endocrine therapy, menopausal status, interval between completion of adjuvant therapy and development of metastatic disease.
- Premenopausal patients can be treated with tamoxifen or ovarian suppression and an aromatase inhibitor with palbociclib 125 mg daily (day 1 to 21 of a 28-day cycle) or ribociclib 600 mg daily (day 1 to 21 of a 28-day cycle).
- In postmenopausal patients, aromatase inhibitor with palbociclib or ribociclib should be considered as standard first-line treatment.
- Second-line options for those who progressed on an aromatase inhibitor or developed metastatic disease in less than 1 year on an AI, include fulvestrant as a single agent, fulvestrant with palbociclib, fulvestrant with abemaciclib, fulvestrant with anastrozole or exemestane with everolimus.
- Abemaciclib can be used as single-agent treatment for patients who have had disease progression on prior endocrine therapy and chemotherapy for metastatic disease.

HER-2-Positive Metastatic Breast Cancer

- Based upon the CLEOPATRA study, dual HER-2 blockade with trastuzumab and pertuzumab in combination with a taxane (THP) is considered standard treatment in first-line metastatic setting. The most commonly used regimen is docetaxel 75 mg/m2 with trastuzumab 8 mg/kg loading dose followed by 6 mg/kg and pertuzumab 480 mg loading dose followed by 420 mg given every 3 weeks with growth factor support. Weekly paclitaxel can be used rather than docetaxel in this setting.
- In the second-line setting, T-DM1 (Ado-trastuzumab emtansine 3.6 mg/kg every 3 weeks is recommended based upon the EMILIA trial.
- In the third-line setting, capecitabine 1000 mg/m^2 twice daily for 2 weeks on 1 week off plus lapatinib 1000 mg daily can be considered.
- Other trastuzumab-containing chemotherapy regimens include combinations of single agent chemotherapy with HER2-targeted therapy such as navelbine and trastuzumab or gemcitabine and trastuzumab.

Targeted Therapy

Trastuzumab (Herceptin)

Trastuzumab is a monoclonal antibody directed against HER2/neu, which has been found to be highly effective in the neoadjuvant, adjuvant, and metastatic breast cancer settings. The dose is 4 mg/kg as a loading dose followed by 2 mg/kg weekly. An every 3 week regimen with a loading dose of 8 mg/kg followed by 6 mg/kg is the most commonly used regimen. Addition of 1 year of adjuvant trastuzumab improves DFS and OS among women with HER-2/neu-positive breast cancer. In general, trastuzumab is given in combination with chemotherapy in neoadjuvant, adjuvant, and metastatic settings.

Trastuzumab is well tolerated although, rarely, it can cause infusion reactions and pulmonary toxicity. The major side effect from trastuzumab is cardiac toxicity, particularly when it is used with or after anthracyclines. With anthracycline-containing regimens, the congestive heart failure rate is about 2% to 4%. Nonanthracycline-based regimens such as TCH did not show increased cardiac toxicity. It is important to monitor cardiac function with an echocardiogram or MUGA scan at baseline and every 3 months while patients are receiving trastuzumab.

Pertuzumab (Perjeta)

Pertuzumab is a humanized monoclonal antibody that binds HER-2/neu at a different epitope of the HER-2/neu extracellular domain than that of trastuzumab. It prevents HER-2/neu from dimerizing with HER3. Similar to trastuzumab, pertuzumab causes antibody-dependent, cell-mediated cytotoxicity. Since pertuzumab and trastuzumab bind to different HER-2/neu epitopes and have complementary mechanisms of action, when pertuzumab is combined with trastuzumab, it provides a more comprehensive blockade of HER-2/neu signaling and results in greater antitumor activity in clinical trials. In the CLEOPATRA study, when pertuzumab was given with trastuzumab plus docetaxel, as compared with placebo plus trastuzumab plus docetaxel, in first-line treatment for HER-2/neu-positive metastatic breast cancer, it significantly prolonged progression-free survival (PFS). No additional cardiac toxicity was seen. The FDA-approved dose of pertuzumab is 840 mg, followed by 420 mg every 3 weeks.

Ado-trastuzumab Emtansine (Kadcyla)

Ado-trastuzumab emtansine is an antibody–drug conjugate composed of trastuzumab linked to a highly potent cytotoxic derivative of maytansine (DM1) by a stable linker. DM1 is a microtubule inhibitor. Trastuzumab targets the conjugate to HER-2/neu receptors and the stable linker releases the cytotoxic agent only when the compound is internalized through receptor endocytosis. Ado-trastuzumab emtansine (T-DM1) has been found to be active in trastuzumab- and lapatinib-resistant metastatic breast cancer, as well as in trastuzumab-naïve tumors.

Results of the phase III EMILIA trial that compared trastuzumab emtansine with capecitabine plus lapatinib in advanced HER-2/neu positive breast cancer showed a substantial improvement in PFS and OS with the conjugate, leading to FDA approval of T-DM1 in 2013. Final OS results of the EMILA trial published in 2017 continued to demonstrate an OS advantage of T-DM1 compared to capecitabine plus lapatinib, despite crossover that was allowed from the control group to T-DM1 following initial result reporting.

In the TH3RESA trial, patients with progressive disease after 2 or more anti-HER therapies were randomized to T-DM1 or treatment of physician's choice. The median PFS was significantly longer with T-DM1 (6.2 versus 3.3 months). In an update of OS results published in 2017, a 7 month OS benefit of T-DM1 was found (22.7 vs. 15.8 months) despite nearly 50% of patients crossing over from treatment of physician's choice to T-DM1.

The dose of ado-trastuzumab emtansine is 3.6 mg/kg IV every 3 weeks and it is extremely well tolerated in clinical trials. Side effects include thrombocytopenia and liver function abnormalities. No significant increase in cardiomyopathy or peripheral neuropathy was seen.

Lapatinib (Tykerb)

Lapatinib is a potent, small molecule inhibitor of the HER1 and HER2 tyrosine kinases. The inhibitory effects, though reversible, result in blockade of receptor-mediated activation and propagation of downstream signaling involved in regulation of cell proliferation and cell survival. The FDA-approved dose of lapatinib is 1,250 mg daily PO. The side effects include diarrhea and rash.

Neratinib (Nerlynx)

Neratinib is an irreversible small molecule inhibitor of HER1, 2, and 4, which was approved by the FDA in 2017 for the extended adjuvant treatment of patients with early-stage HER2-amplified breast cancer, following adjuvant trastuzumab-based therapy based on the results of the ExteNET. The FDA-approved dose of neratinib is 240 mg daily continuously for 1 year. The primary side effect of neratinib is diarrhea and antidiarrheal prophylaxis with loperamide is recommended during the first two cycles of treatment. Liver function tests should also be monitored during therapy with dose reduction occurring for severe hepatic impairment. The agent is also being studied for use in metastatic HER2-positive breast cancer in combination with T-DM1 (NSABP FB 10).

CDK 4/6 Inhibitors

Introduction of the novel class of drugs known as CDK 4/6 inhibitors is a major advancement in the treatment of hormone receptor–positive breast cancer. Palbociclib, ribociclib, and abemaciclib are the FDA-approved

CKD 4/6 inhibitors for the treatment of hormone receptor–positive metastatic breast cancer. Many ongoing clinical trials are studying the role of palbociclib, ribociclib, and abemaciclib in early breast cancer. Overall CD K4/6 inhibitors are well tolerated. Leukopenia is the most common class–related side effect but the incidence of febrile neutropenia is less than 2%. Abemaciclib causes more diarrhea.

Palbociclib (Ibrance)

Palbociclib is a cyclin-dependent kinase 4 and 6 inhibitor that has been used in the treatment of hormone-positive metastatic breast cancer in combination with endocrine therapy. In the phase II trial PALOMA-1, patients treated with letrozole and palbociclib had longer PFS as compared to letrozole alone (20.2 versus 10.2 months). These results led to FDA approval of palbociclib with letrozole in the first-line metastatic setting in February 2015. The recently published phase III study (PALOMA-2) confirmed this benefit, showing a median PFS of 24.8 months with letrozole plus palbociclib versus 14.5 months with letrozole alone.

In the PALOMA-3 study, patients with hormone-positive Her-2 negative breast cancer who had progressed during prior endocrine therapy were randomized to receive fulvestrant alone or fulvestrant with palbociclib. The median PFS was 9.5 months in the combination group and 4.6 months in the fulvestrant group. In February 2016, the FDA approved palbociclib in combination with fulvestrant for patients with advanced or metastatic hormone sensitive breast cancer with progression on prior endocrine therapy. The most notable side effect of palbociclib is neutropenia, which occurs in the vast majority of patients, although the neutropenic fever incidence in these studies were less than 2%. FDA-approved dose of palbociclib is 125 mg daily for 3 weeks and one week off, repeating every 4 weeks.

Ribociclib (Kisqali)

Ribociclib is also a cyclin-dependant kinase 4 and 6 inhibitor, which has been approved for use in combination with an aromatase inhibitor in the initial endocrine treatment of metastatic hormone receptor–positive breast cancer based on the results of the MONALEESA-2 trial. In this trial, postmenopausal woman with HR-positive, HER2-negative advanced, or metastatic breast cancer were treated with letrozole/ribociclib or letrozole/placebo as first-line therapy. It was found that the primary endpoint of PFS was significantly longer in the ribociclib-containing arm (not reached in the ribociclib arm vs. 14.7 months in the placebo arm) with 63% of patients free from progression at 18 months of follow-up versus 42% in the placebo group. The FDA-approved dose of ribociclib is 600 mg daily by mouth 3 weeks on followed by one week off treatment (with continuous aromatase inhibitor therapy). Notable side effects of this drug include neutropenia, Qt interval prolongation, diarrhea, and LFT elevation. Electrocardiogram monitoring is recommended during the first cycle of treatment to assess for Qt interval prolongation.

Abemaciclib (Verzenio)

Abemaciclib is the third cyclin-dependent kinase 4 and 6 inhibitor that is approved for use in advanced breast cancer. It can be used in combination with fulvestrant at a dose of 150 mg twice daily for disease progression following prior endocrine therapy or as a single agent at a dose of 200 mg twice daily for disease progression following prior endocrine therapy and chemotherapy in the metastatic setting. It is unique in its greater specificity for CDK 4 inhibition, which may translate into a different side effect profile than the other drugs in this class.

The phase II MONARCH 1 study, which used abemaciclib 200 mg PO twice a day as a single agent in previously treated hormone receptor–positive metastatic breast cancer, was initially presented at the 2016 American Society of Clinical Oncology meeting and recently published. In this study, a 20% objective response rate was found with over 40% of patients experiencing clinical benefit (including stable disease). In terms of side effects, abemaciclib is associated with less myelosuppression than the other medications in this class but is associated with more diarrhea, nausea, and vomiting.

Subsequently, the phase III MONARCH 2 study, which investigated abemaciclib 150 mg PO twice a day (continuous dosing) plus fulvestrant in HR-positive metastatic breast cancer patients previously treated with endocrine therapy, was published in June 2017 showing a significant improvement in PFS with the addition of abemaciclib to fulvestrant (16.4 vs 9.3 months, p<0.001). The response rate was also improved with the addition of abemaciclib. As seen in the MONARCH 1 study, common adverse events that occurred with abemaciclib included diarrhea, nausea, fatigue, and neutropenia. The MONARCH 3 study of abemaciclib plus a nonsteroidal aromatase inhibitor as initial treatment of HR-positive metastatic breast cancer is expected soon.

Other Agents

Fulvestrant (Faslodex)

Fulvestrant is an ER antagonist (ER down-regulator) and it is indicated in the treatment of hormone receptor–positive metastatic breast cancer in postmenopausal women with disease progression following antiestrogen therapy. Fulvestrant 500 mg should be administered intramuscularly into the buttocks slowly on days 1, 15, and 29 and once monthly thereafter. Side effects are mainly related to pain and injection site reaction.

Everolimus (Afinitor)

Everolimus is FDA approved for the treatment of postmenopausal women with advanced hormone receptor–positive, HER-2/neu-negative breast cancer in combination with exemestane after failure of treatment with letrozole or anastrozole. A randomized phase III study (BOLERO-2) showed everolimus 10 mg per day plus exemestane 25 mg per day improved PFS compared to placebo plus exemestane 25 mg per day. The most common adverse reactions in patients receiving everolimus and exemestane were stomatitis, infections, rash, fatigue, diarrhea, hyperglycemia, and pneumonitis.

Other Chemotherapy Agents Used for Breast Cancer

Capecitabine (Xeloda)

Capecitabine (Xeloda) is a fluoropyrimidine carbamate and it is an orally administered systemic prodrug of 5′-deoxy-5-fluorouridine (5′-DFUR), which is converted to 5-fluorouracil. It is indicated as monotherapy for metastatic breast cancer. The FDA-approved dose is 1,250 mg/m^2 twice a day given for 2 weeks on and 1 week off, repeating every 21 days. For practical purposes most clinicians use 1,000 mg/m^2 twice a day 2 weeks on 1 week off. The most common side effects are hand–foot syndrome and diarrhea. Patients should be educated about management of the hand–foot syndrome.

Eribulin (Halaven)

Eribulin mesylate is a nontaxane, tubulin-, and microtubule-targeting chemotherapeutic agent that binds directly with tubulin disrupting mitotic spindles and inhibits microtubule polymerization. A phase III study compared eribulin to treatment of physician's choice (TPC) in patients with locally recurrent or metastatic breast cancer previously treated with an anthracycline and a taxane. This study showed improvement in PFS and OS with eribulin. The most common side effects were neutropenia and peripheral neuropathy. Eribulin is the only chemotherapy agent that has shown a survival advantage in late lines of therapy for breast cancer. The FDA-approved dose of eribulin is 1.4 mg/m^2 administered on days 1 and 8 of a 21-day schedule.

Nab-Paclitaxel (Abraxane)

Nanoparticle albumin-bound paclitaxel (nab-paclitaxel) is a novel paclitaxel formulation that does not require cremophor or polysorbate 80 for solubilization, thus reducing solvent-related toxicity and micelle formation. The FDA-approved dose of nab-paclitaxel is 260 mg/m^2 every 3 weeks for the treatment of metastatic breast cancer. The side effects include neutropenia, peripheral neuropathy, nausea, etc. Due to lack of cremophor, nab-paclitaxel does not require premedication with steroids.

Ixabepilone (Ixempra)

This drug belongs to a novel class of drugs called epothilones. Epothilones are nontaxane microtubule-stabilizing agents. The tubulin-polymerizing activity of ixabepilone is stronger than paclitaxel. It has proven efficacy in taxane-resistant settings. Ixabepilone has low susceptibility to tumor resistance mechanisms such as P-glycoprotein (P-gp) and multidrug-resistance protein-1 (MRP1). The FDA-approved ixabepilone in combination with capecitabine in patients with meta-static or locally advanced breast cancer, who are resistant to or refractory to a taxane and anthra-cycline. Ixabepilone is also approved as monotherapy in patients who are resistant or refractory to taxane, anthracycline, and capecitabine. The dose is 40 mg/m^2 administered over 3 hours every 3 weeks. Patients should be premedicated with diphenhydramine and cimetidine an hour prior to the infusion with ixabepilone.

PARP Inhibitors

The poly(ADP-ribose) polymerase (PARP) enzymes function to help repair DNA. Inhibition of the PARP enzymes results in double stranded DNA breaks in dividing cells. In most cells, DNA double strand breaks are able to be repaired through homologous recombination however in BRCA1/2 defi-cient cells this mechanism is absent. Such cells rely on PARP enzymes for DNA repair and when these enzymes are inhibited, the cells will die. This concept is the foundation for use of PARP inhibitors in BRCA mutation positive–breast cancer patients. Other breast cancers may also be susceptible to PARP inhibition, particularly triple-negative breast cancer where homologous recombination defects may also be present.

Olaparib (Lynparza)

Olaparib is FDA approved for treatment of advanced ovarian cancer and primary peritoneal cancer with or without BRCA mutations. It has been studied in a variety of breast cancer settings and findings from the phase III OlympiAD metastatic breast cancer trial were recently published. In this study, meta-static breast cancer patients with germline BRCA mutations were randomized to receive either olaparib 300 mg twice daily or chemotherapy of physician's choice (capecitabine, eribulin, or vinorelbine). The study showed a statistically significant 3-month improvement in progression-free survival and 42% decrease in risk of disease progression or death with olaparib compared to standard chemotherapy. The response rate was higher in the olaparib-treated patients (60% vs. 29%) and grade 3 or higher adverse events occurred less frequently (37% vs. 50%).

Other PARP Inhibitors

Rucaparib and niraparib are other PARP inhibitors that have been approved for use in advanced ovarian cancer and are currently being studied in breast cancer. Veliparib is another PARP inhibitor that is not yet FDA approved but is actively being studied in breast cancer clinical trials. Talazoparib is a PARP inhibitor that is of particular interest due to its potent activity, thought to be mediated through an increase in "PARP trapping" in addition to PARP inhibition.

Immunotherapy in Breast Cancer

Interest in using immunotherapy, specifically checkpoint inhibitors, in breast cancer treatment has grown significantly in recent years. It is known that PD-1 is expressed in 20% to 30% of breast cancers with more frequent expression in HER2+ and triple-negative disease compared to hormone sensitive disease. Many studies of immunotherapy in breast cancer are ongoing, particularly in the triple-negative subset, and those that have been published to date show only modest activity of PD-1 and PD-L1 in the breast cancer population. In addition, there is no consistent correlation between PD-L1 expression and response to treatment in the available studies.

In the KEYNOTE-012 phase Ib study of pembrolizumab in advanced solid tumors, a response rate of 19% was seen among 27 metastatic triple-negative breast cancer patients enrolled. All patients in this study had PD-1 expression of ≥1%. The subsequent KEYNOTE-086 phase II trial of pembrolizumab, which was presented at the American Society of Clinical Oncology 2017 annual meeting, enrolled 170 previously treated metastatic triple negative breast cancer patients (PD-L1 positive and negative) and demonstrated an objective response rate of 5%.

May 2017 FDA approval of pembrolizumab for patients with unresectable or metastatic, microsatel-lite instability-high (MSI-H), or mismatch repair deficient (dMMR) solid tumors who have progressed on prior treatment and have no satisfactory treatment options has now raised the question of whether MSI/MMR testing should be done routinely in breast cancer patients. As the triple-negative patients are those breast cancer patients with the fewest satisfactory treatment options, one could make a case to test these patients for MSI/MMR in an attempt to obtain pembrolizumab, although the data for its efficacy in this population is not well defined.

The combination of chemotherapy with immunotherapy has been studied in a phase I trial of atezolizumab in combination with nab-paclitaxel in metastatic triple negative breast cancer with an encouraging response rate of 42% among 24 patients. This combination therapy is currently being evaluated in a global phase III randomized study (the Impassion130 trial). The combination of chemotherapy with immunotherapy has also demonstrated promising results in the neoadjuvant space where pembrolizumab was evaluated with standard neoadjuvant therapy as part of the ISPY-2 trial. In this study, both hormone-receptor positive breast cancers and triple negative breast cancers had an improvement in pathologic complete response with the addition of pembrolizumab to standard chemotherapy. These combinations will now be studied in the larger phase III setting.

Role of Next Generation Sequencing

Next generation sequencing (NGS) has become widely available with the advent of many commercial assays. These tests are often quite expensive and insurance coverage for them is inconsistent. In the metastatic breast cancer setting, NGS may help to identify targets for treatment that are accessible via clinical trial participation or by use of an FDA-approved medication in an off label manner. Despite the availability of these tests and enthusiasm surrounding their promise, evidence supporting the clinical utility of genomic testing in the metastatic breast cancer setting is lacking. When considering sending such testing, providers must counsel the patient on the likelihood of potentially actionable findings and the costs associated with testing.

The SAFIR-01 trial assessed clinical utility of genomic profiling in a metastatic breast cancer population. In this study, investigators profiled metastatic breast tumors prospectively and recorded responses based on treatment decisions guided by genomic analysis. Forty-six percent of patients were found to have actionable mutations and therapy was tailored based on these results for 13% of patients. Of the patients who received a "personalized" therapy, 9% had a partial response and 21% had stable disease for at least 16 weeks.

Multiple ongoing clinical trials, such as the NCI MATCH trial, are designed to pair patients with actionable genomic alterations with biologically rational treatments. As results of such studies become available, the clinical utility of NGS in various tumor types will be elucidated.

Supportive Care Agents

Bisphosphonates

- Bisphosphonates should be used in patients with bony metastatic disease because they prevent progression of lytic lesions, delay skeletal-related events, and decrease pain. However, the optimal frequencies of administration and duration of therapy are not known.
- Zoledronic acid (4 mg by 15-minute infusion) and pamidronate (90 mg by 2-hour infusion) are two available biphosphonates approved for bony metastatic disease.
- In the OPTIMIZE-2 trial, metastatic breast cancer patients with bone metastasis were randomized to receive zoledronic acid 4mg IV once every 4 weeks or once every 12 weeks for 1 year. The incidence of skeletal-related events and safety profile was similar for both groups. Based on these results, 12 week interval of dosing for zoledronic acid can be considered noninferior to 4 week interval of dosing.
- Osteonecrosis of the jaw (ONJ) is a very rare but a potential complication of long-term treatment with intravenous bisphosphonates.

Rank Ligand Inhibitor

The receptor activator of nuclear factor-κB (RANK), the RANK ligand (RANKL), and osteoprotegerin, a decoy receptor for RANK, regulate osteoclastogenesis and may play a key role in bone metastasis. Denosumab (XGEVA), a fully human monoclonal antibody that binds to and neutralizes RANKL, inhibits osteoclast function, prevents generalized bone resorption and local bone destruction, and has become a therapeutic option for preventing or delaying first on-study skeletal-related events in various malignancies.

It is approved for patients with bone metastasis from breast cancer, prostate cancer, and other solid tumors. The dose is 120 mg subcutaneous every 4 weeks. It can cause significant hypocalcemia. So patients should take appropriate calcium replacement. The incidence of osteonecrosis of the jaw is about 2.2% with denosumab. It does not have to be adjusted for renal impairment.

Central Nervous System Metastasis

Central nervous system (CNS) metastasis may consist of either parenchymal or leptomeningeal metastasis. The control of systemic disease is crucial to improving the survival of patients with resectable brain metastasis.

The standard treatment for multiple brain lesions remains whole-brain radiation (WBR) for symptom control, with no associated improvement in survival. The therapy for a single-brain metastasis remains either surgery or radiosurgery (Gamma Knife), with conflicting information as to the benefit of prior WBR. Leptomeningeal metastasis is conventionally treated with intrathecal chemotherapy, and may provide short-term symptom control. The superiority of intrathecal versus systemic chemotherapy in leptomeningeal metastasis is controversial. About 30% of HER-2/neu-positive patients will develop brain metatastic disease, and a lapatinib-containing regimen is an option in these patients as lapatinib is known to cross the blood brain barrier.

LOCALLY RECURRENT BREAST CANCER

After Mastectomy

- Eighty percent of local recurrences occur within 5 years.
- Treatment of choice is surgical excision and radiation therapy.
- Systemic therapy may be considered based upon ER/PR and HER-2 status. As per the CALOR study, a survival advantage was seen for patients who received systemic therapy after local recurrence. But maximum benefit was in triple negative or high risk patients.

After Lumpectomy

- Mastectomy is the treatment of choice for patients who have only isolated breast cancer recurrence.

Survivorship

Studies have suggested that up to 50% of cancer survivors experience late effects of cancer treatment. In breast cancer survivors, providers must consider the potential long-term impacts of chemotherapy, surgery, radiation, and endocrine therapy on the patient including risks of cardiac dysfunction, cognitive changes, depression, persistent fatigue, pain, neuropathy, lymphedema, premature menopause, sexual dysfunction, deterioration in bone health, and secondary malignancies.

As per the 2016 Commission on Cancer accreditation standards, a survivorship care plan should be provided to all patients at the completion of curative intent treatment with information including a personalized treatment summary with associated providers identified, guidance of signs of recurrence, information of long-term effects of treatment, guidelines for follow-up care and identification of support services available to the patient. Given the growing body of evidence supporting the importance of a healthy lifestyle, including maintaining an appropriate body weight and incorporating regular physical activity, in decreasing risk of cancer, oncologists should be mindful to ask questions regarding healthy lifestyle behaviors during routine follow-up.

Pregnancy after Breast Cancer

Many patients and oncologists harbor reservations about pregnancy following a breast cancer diagnosis for a variety of reasons. Two of the biggest concerns, particularly for hormone receptor–positive breast cancer survivors, are that pregnancy produces higher levels of estrogen, which could result in breast cancer cell growth and that pregnancy necessitates a gap in adjuvant endocrine treatment.

A large retrospective study presented at the American Society of Clinical Oncology 2017 meeting challenged these concerns by demonstrating that DFS 10 years following diagnosis was no different in survivors who became pregnant compared to those who did not become pregnant. Importantly, this held true when the estrogen receptor-positive cohort was analyzed individually. In secondary analyses, the timing of pregnancy (<2 years after diagnosis or >2 years after diagnosis) and breastfeeding did not affect DFS. The ongoing POSITIVE study will provide additional insight into the impact of interrupting adjuvant endocrine therapy during pregnancy for survivors of ER-positive breast cancer.

FOLLOW-UP FOR PATIENTS WITH OPERABLE BREAST CANCER (BASED ON ASCO GUIDELINES MARCH 2013)

1. History and physical examination every 3 to 6 months for the first 3 years, every 6 to 12 months for the next 2 years, and annually thereafter.
2. Physicians should counsel patients regarding symptoms of recurrence including new lumps, bone pain, chest pain, dyspnea, abdominal pain, and persistent headaches.
3. All women should be counseled to do monthly breast self-examination.
4. Annual mammogram of the contralateral and ipsilateral (remaining breast after lumpectomy) breast.
5. Regular gynecologic follow-up is recommended for all patients. Those who receive tamoxifen should be advised to report any unusual vaginal bleeding to their doctors.
6. Coordination of care: The risk of breast cancer recurrence continues through 15 years after primary treatment and beyond. Continuity of care for patients with breast cancer is recommended and should be performed by a physician experienced in the surveillance of patients with cancer and in breast examination, including the examination of irradiated breasts.
7. Follow-up by a PCP seems to lead to the same health outcomes as specialist follow-up with good patient satisfaction.
8. Routine blood tests including a complete blood count, liver function tests, and alkaline phosphatase levels are not recommended. Serum tumor markers (CA 27-29, and CA 15-3) are not recommended.
9. Chest X ray, ultrasound of the liver, breast MRI, bone scan, and CT scans of the chest, abdomen, pelvis, and brain or PET scans are not recommended routinely, but they are done if symptoms or laboratory abnormalities are present.

Suggested Readings

1. Adams S, Robinson Diamond J, Hamilton EP, et al. Phase Ib trial of atezolizumab in combination with nab-paclitaxel in patients with metastatic triple-negative breast cancer (mTNBC). Abstract presented at: ASCO Annual Meeting. 2016; Chicago, IL. Abstract 1009.
2. Adams S, Schmid P, Rugo H, et al. A phase 2 study of pembrolizumab (pembro) monotherapy for previously treated metastatic triple negative breast cancer (mTNBC): KEYNOTE-086 cohort A. Abstract presented at: ASCO Annual Meeting. 2017; Chicago, IL. Abstract 1008.
3. Aebi S, Gelber S, Anderson SJ, et al. Chemotherapy for isolated locoregional recurrence of breast cancer (CALOR): a randomized trial. *Lancet Oncol.* 2014;15:156–163.
4. Andre F, Bachelot T, Commo F et al. Comparative genomic hybridization array and DNA sequencing to direct treatment of metastatic breast cancer: a multicenter, prospective trial (SAFIR01/UNICANCER). *Lancet Oncol.* 2014;15(3):267–274.
5. Baselga J, Bradbury I, Eidtmann H, et al. Lapatinib with trastuzumab for HER2-positive early breast cancer (NeoALTTO): a randomised, open-label, multicentre, phase 3 trial. *Lancet.* 2012 Feb 18;379(9816):633–640.
6. Baselga J, Campone M, Piccart M, et al. Everolimus in postmenopausal hormone-receptor positive advanced breast cancer. *N Engl J Med.* 2012;366:520–529.
7. Baselga J, Cortes J, Kim SB, et al. Pertuzumab plus trastuzumab plus docetaxel for metastatic breast cancer. *N Engl J Med.* 2012;366:109–119.
8. Blum JL, Flynn PJ, Yothers G, et al. Anthracyclines in early breast cancer: the ABC trials- USOR 06-090, NSABP B-46-I/USOR 07132, and NSABP B-49. *J Clin Oncol.* 2017;35.

9. Chan A, Delaloge S, Holmes FA, et al. Neratinib after trastuzumab-based adjuvant therapy in patients with HER2-positive breast cancer (ExteNET): a multicentre, randomized, double-blind, placebo-controlled phase 3 trial. *Lancet Oncol*. 2016;17:367–377.

10. Chia S, Gradishar W, Mauriac L, et al. Double-blind, randomized placebo controlled trial of fulvestrant compared with exemestane after prior nonsteroidal AI therapy in postmenopausal women with hormone receptor-positive, advanced breast cancer: results from EFECT. *J Clin Oncol*. 2008;26:1664–1670.

11. Ciatto S, Houssami N, Bernardi D, et al. Integration of 3D digital mammography with tomosynthesis for population breast-cancer screening (STORM): a prospective comparison study. *Lancet Oncol*. 2013;14(7):583–589.

12. Coopey SB, Mazzola E, Buckley JM, et al. The role of chemoprevention in modifying the risk of breast cancer in women with atypical breast lesions. *Breast Cancer Res Treat*. 2012;136:627–633.

13. Cristofanilli M, Turner NC, Bondarenko I, et al. Fulvestrant plus palbociclib versus fulvestrant plus placebo for treatment of hormone-receptor-positive, HER2-negative metastatic breast cancer that progressed on previous endocrine therapy (PALOMA-3): final analysis of the multicentre, double-blind, phase 3 randomised controlled trial. *Lancet Oncol*. 2016 Apr;17(4):425–439.

14. Cuzick J, Sestak I, Forbes JF, et al. Anastrozole for prevention of breast cancer in high-risk postmenopausal women (IBIS-II): an international, double-blind, randomised placebo-controlled trial. *Lancet*. 2014 Mar 22;383(9922):1041–1048.

15. Dai X, Li T, Bai Z, et al. Breast cancer intrinsic subtype classification, clinical use and future trends. *Am J Cancer Res*. 2015;5(10):2929–2943.

16. Davies C, Pan H, Godwin J, et al. Long-term effects of continuing adjuvant tamoxifen to 10 years versus stopping at 5 years after diagnosis of oestrogen receptor-positive breast cancer: ATLAS, a randomised trial. *Lancet*. 2013 Mar 9;381(9869):805–816.

17. Dhesy-Thind S, Fletcher GG, Blanchette PS, et al. Use of adjuvant bisphosphonates and other bone-modifying agents in breast cancer: a cancer care Ontario and American Society of Clinical Oncology clinical practice guideline. *J Clin Oncol*. 2017;35:2062–2081.

18. Dickler MN, Tolaney SM, Rugo HS, et al. MONARCH 1: a phase II study of abemaciclib, a CDK4 and CDK6 inhibitor, as a single agent, in patients with refractory HR+/HER2- metastatic breast cancer. *Clin Cancer Res*. 2017;23(17):5218–5224.

19. Dieras V, Miles D, Verma S, et al. Trastuzumab emtansine versus capecitabine plus lapatinib in patients with previously treated HER2-positive advanced breast cancer (EMILA): a descriptive analysis of final overall survival results from a randomized, open-label, phase 3 trial. *Lancet Oncol*. 2017;18:732–742.

20. Early Breast Cancer Trialists' Collaborative Group (EBCTCG). Adjuvant bisphosphonate treatment in early breast cancer: meta-analyses of individual patient data from randomized trials. *Lancet*. 2015;386:1353–1361.

21. Emens LA, Adams S, Loi S, et al. Impassion130: a phase III randomized trial of atezolizumab with nab-paclitaxel for first-line treatment of patients with metastatic triple-negative breast cancer (mTNBC). Abstract presented at: ASCO Annual Meeting. 2016; Chicago, IL. Abstract TPS1104.

22. Fisher B, Costantino, Wickerham DL, et al. Tamoxigen for the prevention of breast cancer: report of the National Surgical Adjuvant Breast and Bowel Project p-1 study. *J Natl Cancer Inst*. 1998; 90:1371–1388.

23. Fisher B, Costantino J, Wickerham DL, et al. Tamoxifen for the prevention of breast cancer: current status of the National Surgical Adjuvant Breast and Bowel Project P-1 study. *J Natl Cancer Inst*. 2005;97(22):1652–1662.

24. Finn RS, Crown JP, Lang I, et al. The cyclin-dependent kinase 4/6 inhibitor palbociclib in combination with letrozole versus letrozole alone as first-line treatment of oestrogen receptor-positive, HER2-negative, advanced breast cancer (PALOMA-1/TRIO-18): a randomised phase 2 study. *Lancet Oncol*. 2015 Jan;16(1):25–35.

25. Finn RS, Martin M, Rugo HS, et al. Palbociclib and letrozole in advanced breast cancer. *N Engl J Med*. 2016 Nov 17;375(20):1925–1936.

26. Francis PA, Regan MM, Fleming GF, et al. Adjuvant ovarian suppression in premenopausal breast cancer. *N Engl J Med*. 2015 Jan 29;372(5):436–446.

27. Friedewald SM, Rafferty EA, Rose SL, et al. Breast cancer screening using tomosynthesis in combination with digital mammography. *JAMA*. 2014;311(24):2499–2507.

28. Geyer CE, Forster J, Lindquist D, et al. Lapatinib plus capecitabine for HER-2/neu-positive advanced breast cancer. *N Engl J Med*. 2006;355:2733–2743.

29. Gianni L, Pienkowski T, Im YH, et al. Efficacy and safety of neoadjuvant pertuzumab and trastuzumab in women with locally advanced, inflammatory, or early HER2-positive breast cancer (NeoSphere): a randomised multicentre, open-label, phase 2 trial. *Lancet Oncol*. 2012 Jan;13(1):25–32.

30. Gnant M, Mlineritsch B, Schippinger W, et al. Endocrine therapy plus zoledronic acid in premenopausal breast cancer. *N Engl J Med*. 2009;360:679–691.

31. Goss P, Ingle J, Ales-Martinez J, et al. Exemestane for breast-cancer prevention in postmenopausal women. *N Engl J Med*. 2011;364:2381–2391.

32. Goss PE, Ingle JN, Pritchard KI, et al. Extending aromatase-inhibitor adjuvant therapy to 10 years. *N Engl J Med*. 2016;375:209–219.

33. Gray RG, Rea D, Handley K, et al. aTTom: Long-term effects of continuing adjuvant tamoxifen to 10 years versus stopping at 5 years in 6,953 women with early breast cancer. *J Clin Onco.l* 2013;31:(suppl; abstr 5).

34. Harris LN, Ismaila N, McShane LM, et al. Use of biomarkers to guide decisions on adjuvant systemic therapy for women with early-stage invasive breast cancer: American Society of Clinical Oncology Clinical Practice Guideline. *J Clin Oncol.* 2016;34(10):1134–1150.

35. Hartmann LC, Degnim AC, Santen RJ, et al. Atypical hyperplasia of the breast-risk assessment and management options. *N Engl J Med.* 2015;372 :78–89.

36. Henry NL, Bedard PL, DeMichele A. Standard and Genomic Tools for Decision Support in Breast Cancer Treatment. 2017 ASCO Educational Book. asco.org/edbook

37. Himelstein AL, Foster JC, Khatcheressian JL, et al. Effect of longer-interval vs standard dosing of zoledronic acid on skeletal events in patients with bone metastases: A randomized clinical trial. *JAMA.* 2017 Jan 3;317(1):48–58.

38. Hortobagyi GN, Stemmer SM, Burris HA, et al. Ribociclib as first-line therapy for HR-positive, advanced breast cancer. *N Engl J Med.* 2016;375:1738–1748.

39. Hortobagyi GN, Van Poznak C, Harker WG, et al. Continued treatment effect of zoledronic acid dosing every 12 weeks vs 4 weeks in women with breast cancer metastatic to bone. The OPTIMIZE-2 randomized clinical trial. *JAMA Oncology.* 2017;3(7):906–912.

40. Houssami N, Skaane P. Overview of the evidence on digital breast tomosynthesis in breast cancer detection. *Breast J.* 2013;22:101–108.

41. Hu X, Huang W, Fan M. Emerging therapies for breast cancer. *J Hematol Oncol.* 2017;10:98

42. Jones SE, Savin MA, Holmes FA, et al. Phase III trial comparing doxorubicin plus cyclophosphamide with docetaxel plus cyclophosphamide as adjuvant therapy for operable breast cancer. *J Clin Oncol.* 2006;24:5381–5387.

43. Krop IE, Kim SB, González-Martín A, et al. Trastuzumab emtansine versus treatment of physician's choice for pre-treated HER2-positive advanced breast cancer (TH3RESA): a randomised, open-label, phase 3 trial. *Lancet Oncol.* 2014 Jun;15(7):689–699.

44. Krop IE, Kim SB, Gonzalez Martin A, et al. Trastuzumab emtansine versus treatment of physician's choice in patients with previously treated HER2-positive metastatic breast cancer (TH3RESA): final overall survival results from a randomised open-label phase 3 trial. *Lancet Oncol.* 2017:18:743–754.

45. Lambertini M, Kroman N, Ameye L, et al. Safety of pregnancy in patients with history of estrogen receptor positive (ER+) breast cancer: Long-term follow-up analysis from a multicenter study. *J Clin Oncol.* 2017. 35; suppl abstr LBA 10066.

46. Mainiero MB, Lourenco A, Mahoney MC, Newell MS, Bailey L, Barke LD et al. ACR Appropriateness criteria breast cancer screening. *J Am Coll Radiol.* 2013;10(1):11–14. doi: 10.1016/j.jacr.2012.09.036.

47. Martin M, Pienkowski T, Mackey J, et al. Adjuvant docetaxel for node-positive breast cancer. *N Engl J Med.* 2005;352:2302–2313.

48. Martin M, Segui M, Anton A, et al. Adjuvant docetaxel for high-risk, node-negative breast cancer. *N Engl J Med.* 2012;362:2200–2210.

49. Mehta R, Barlow W, Albain K, et al. Combination anastrozole and fulvestrant in metastatic breast cancer. *N Engl J Med.* 2012;367:435–444.

50. Miller K, Wang M, Gralow J, et al. Paclitaxel plus bevacizumab versus paclitaxel alone for metastatic breast cancer. *N Engl J Med.* 2007;357:2666–2676.

51. Morrow, M, Schnitt SJ, Norton L. Current management of lesions associated with an increased risk of breast cancer. *Nat Rev Clin Oncol.* 2015;12:227–238.

52. Moss S, Cuckle H, Evans A, et al. Effect of mammographic screening from age 40 years on breast cancer mortality at 10 years follow-up: a randomized controlled trial. *Lancet* 2006;368(9552):2053–2060.

53. Muss H, Berry D, Cirrincione C, et al. Adjuvant chemotherapy in older women with early stage breast cancer. *N Engl J Med.* 2009;360:2055–2065.

54. Nanda R, Chow L, Dees EC, et al. Pembrolizumab in patients with advanced triple-negative breast cancer: phase Ib KEYNOTE-012 study. *J Clin Oncol.* 2016;34(21):2460–2467.

55. Nanda R, Liu MC, Yau C, et al. Pembrolizumab plus standard neoadjuvant therapy for high-risk breast cancer (BC): Results from I-SPY 2. Abstract presented at: ASCO Annual Meeting. 2017; Chicago, IL. Abstract 506.

56. Pagani O, Regan MM, Walley BA, et al. Adjuvant exemestane with ovarian suppression in premenopausal breast cancer. *N Engl J Med.* 2014 Jul 10;371(2):107–118.

57. Patnaik A, Rosen LS, Tolaney SM, et al. Efficacy and safety of abemaciclib, an inhibitor of CDK4 and CDK6, for patients with breast cancer, non-small cell lung cancer, and other solid tumors. *Cancer Discov.* 2016;6(7):740–753.

58. Perez EA, Romond EH, Suman VJ, et al. Trastuzumab plus adjuvant chemotherapy for human epidermal growth factor receptor 2-positive breast cancer: planned joint analysis of overall survival from NSABP B-31 and NCCTG N9831. *J Clin Oncol.* 2014;32(33):3744–3753.

59. Piccart-Gebhart MJ, Holmes AP, Baselga J, et al. First results from the phase III ALTTO trial (BIG 2-06; NCCTG [Alliance] N063D) comparing one year of anti-HER2 therapy with lapatinib alone (L), trastuzumab alone (T), their sequence

(T→L), or their combination (T+L) in the adjuvant treatment of HER2-positive early breast cancer (EBC). *J Clin Oncol.* 32:5s, 2014 (suppl; abstr LBA4).

60. Piccart-Gebhart MJ, Procter M, Leyland-Jones B, et al. Trastuzumab after adjuvant chemotherapy in HER-2/neu-positive breast cancer. *N Engl J Med.* 2005;353:1659–1672.

61. Pisano ED, Gatsonis C, Hendrick E, et al. Diagnostic performance of digital versus film mammography for breast cancer screening. *N Engl J Med.* 2005;353: 1773–1793.

62. Rastogi P, Anderson SJ, Bear HD, et al. Preoperative chemotherapy: updates of National Surgical Adjuvant Breast and Bowel Project Protocols B-18 and B-27. *J Clin Oncol.* 2008 Feb 10;26(5):778–785.

63. Ravdin PM, Cronin KA, Howlader N, et al. The decrease in breast-cancer incidence in 2003 in the United States. *N Engl J Med.* 2007;356:1670–1674.

64. Robson M, Im S-A, Senkus E, et al. Olaparib for metastatic breast cancer in patients with a germline BRCA mutation. *N Engl J Med.* 2017;377(6):523–533.

65. Romond EH, Perez EA, Bryant J, et al. Trastuzumab plus adjuvant chemotherapy for operable HER-2/neu-positive breast cancer. *N Engl J Med.* 2005;353:1673–1684.

66. Saad A, Abraham J. Role of tumor markers and circulating tumors cells in the management of breast cancer. *Oncology* (Williston Park). 2008;22:726–731; discussion 734, 739, 743–744.

67. Schneeweiss A, Chia S, Hickish T, et al. Pertuzumab plus trastuzumab in combination with standard neoadjuvant anthracycline-containing and anthracycline-free chemotherapy regimens in patients with HER2-positive early breast cancer: a randomized phase II cardiac safety study (TRYPHAENA). *Ann Oncol.* 2013 Sep;24(9):2278–2284.

68. Seidman AD, Berry D, Cirrincione C, et al. Randomized phase III trial of weekly compared with every-3-weeks paclitaxel for metastatic breast cancer, with trastuzumab for all HER-2/neu- overexpressors and random assignment to trastuzumab or not in HER-2/neu- nonoverexpressors: final results of Cancer and Leukemia Group B protocol 9840. *J Clin Oncol.* 2008;26:1642–1649.

69. Sikov WM, Berry DA, Perou CM, et al. Impact of the addition of carboplatin and/or bevacizumab to neoadjuvant once-per-week paclitaxel followed by dose-dense doxorubicin and cyclophosphamide on pathologic complete response rates in stage II to III triple-negative breast cancer: CALGB 40603 (Alliance). *J Clin Oncol.* 2015 Jan 1;33(1):13–21.

70. Slamon D, Eiermann W, Robert N, et al. BCIRG 006: 2nd interim analysis phase III randomized trial comparing doxorubicin and cyclophosphamide followed by docetaxel (AC→T) with doxorubicin and cyclophosphamide followed by docetaxel and trastuzumab (AC→TH) with docetaxel, carboplatin and trastuzumab (TCH) in HER-2/neu-positive early breast cancer patients. *San Antonio Breast Cancer Symposium*; December 14–17, 2006. San Antonio, TX; 2006.

71. Slamon D, Eiermann W, Robert N, et al. Adjuvant trastuzumab in HER-2/neu-positive breast cancer. *N Engl J Med.* 2011;365:1273–1283.

72. Slamon DJ, Eiermann W, Robert NJ, et al. Ten year follow-up of BCIRG-006 comparing doxorubicin plus cyclophosphamide followed by docetaxel (AC→T) with doxorubicin plus cyclophosphamide followed by docetaxel and trastuzumab (AC→TH) with docetaxel, carboplatin and trastuzumab (TCH) in HER2+ early breast cancer. *San Antonio Breast Cancer Symposium*; Abstract S5-04, December 11, 2015.

73. Sledge GW, Toi M, Neven P et al. MONARCH 2: Abemaciclib in combination with fulvestrant in women with HR+/HER2-advanced breast cancer who had progressed while receiving endocrine therapy. *J Clin Oncol.* 2017;35:25, 2875–2884.

74. Solin L, Gray R, Baehner F, et al. A multigene expression assay to predict local recurrence risk for ducal carcinoma in situ of the breast. *J Natl Cancer Inst.* 2013; 105(10):701–710.

75. Sparano J, Wang M, Martino S, et al. Weekly paclitaxel in the adjuvant treatment of breast cancer. *N Engl J Med.* 2008;358:1663–1671.

76. Sparano JA, Gray RJ, Makower DF, et al. Prospective validation of a 21-gene expression assay in breast cancer. *N Engl J Med.* 2015;373:2005–2014.

77. Swayampakula AK, Dillis C, Abraham J. Role of MRI in screening, diagnosis and management of breast cancer. *Expert Rev Anticancer Ther.* 2008;8:811–817.

78. Tolaney SM, Barry WT, Dang CT, et al. Adjuvant paclitaxel and trastuzumab for node-negative, HER2-positive breast cancer. *N Engl J Med.* 2015;372:134–141.

79. Vaidya JS, Wenz F, Bulsara M, et al. Risk-adapted targeted intraoperative radiotherapy versus whole-breast radiotherapy for breast cancer: 5-year results for local control and overall survival from the TARGIT-A randomised trial. *Lancet.* 2014 Feb 15;383(9917):603–613.

80. Valdivieso M, Kujawa AM, Jones T, Baker LH. Cancer survivors in the United States: a review of the literature and a call to action. *Int J Med Sci.* 2012;9:163–173.

81. Valente SA, Levine GM, Silverstein MJ, et al. Accuracy of predicting axillary lymph node positivity by physical examination, mammography, ultrasonography, and magnestic resonace imaging. *Ann Surg Oncol.* 2012;19(6):1825–1830.

82. Verma S, Miles D, Gianni L, et al. Trastuzumab emtansine for HER-2/neu-positive advanced breast cancer. *N Engl J Med.* 2012;367:1783–1791.

83. Veronesi U, Orecchia R, Maisonneuve P, et al. Intraoperative radiotherapy versus external radiotherapy for early breast cancer (ELIOT): a randomised controlled equivalence trial. *Lancet Oncol.* 2013 Dec;14(13):1269–1277.

84. Veronesi U, Paganelli G, Viale G et al. A randomized comparison of sentinel-node biopsy with routine axillary dieesction in breast cancer. *N Engl J Med.* 2003; 349:546–553.

85. Vogel VG, Costantino JP, Wickerham DL, et al. Effects of tamoxifen vs raloxifene on the risk of developing invasive breast cancer and other disease outcomes: the NSABP study of tamoxifen and raloxifene (STAR) P-2 trial. *JAMA.* 2006; 295(23):2727–2741.

86. Vogel VG, Costantino JP, Wickerham DL, et al. Update of the national surgical adjuvant breast and bowel project study of tamoxifen and raloxifene (STAR) P-2 trial: preventing breast cancer. *Cancer Prev Res.* 2010; 3(6):696–706.

87. von Minckwitz G, Procter M, de Azambuja E, et al. Adjuvant pertuzuman and trastuzumab in early HER2-positive breast cancer. *N Engl J Med.* 2017;377(2):122–131.

88. Wang B, Chu D, Feng Y et al. Discovery and characterization of (8S,9R)-5-Fluoro-8-(4-fluorophenyl)-9-(1-methyl-1H-1,2,4-triazol-5-yl)-2,7,8,9-tetrahydro-3H-pyrido[4,3,2-de]phthalazin-3-one (BMN 673, Talazoparib), a Novel, Highly Potent, and Orally Efficacious Poly(ADP-ribose) Polymerase-1/2 Inhibitor, as an Anticancer Agent. *J Med Chem.* 2016;59(1):335–357.

89. Wimberly H, Brown JR, Schalper K, et al. PD-L1 expression correlates with tumor-infiltrating lymphocytes and response to neoadjuvant chemotherapy in breast cancer. *Cancer Immunol Res.* 2015;3: 326–332.

13 Renal Cell Cancer

Ramaprasad Srinivasan, Azam Ghafoor, and Inger L. Rosner

Renal cell cancer (RCC), a term that includes a variety of cancers arising in the kidney, comprises several histologically, biologically, and clinically distinct entities. Surgical resection for localized disease and immunotherapy for metastatic disease were the mainstays of therapy for RCC until the past decade or so. However, recent advances in our understanding of the molecular mechanisms underlying individual subtypes of the disease have led to newer, more effective, targeted approaches to managing metastatic RCC.

EPIDEMIOLOGY

- An estimated 64,000 new cases of cancer arising in the kidney and renal pelvis are expected in the United States in 2017, leading to more than 14,000 deaths.
- Incidence is higher in men, with a male:female ratio of 1.6:1.
- Incidence from 2004 to 2008 increased by 4.1% per year in men and 3.3% per year in women, largely due to an increase in diagnosis of early-stage disease. Mortality has decreased during the same period by 0.4% per year in men and 0.6% in women.
- Largely a disease of adulthood, with a peak incidence after the fifth decade of life, RCC may also occur in younger adults, children, and infants.

ETIOLOGY AND RISK FACTORS

Nonhereditary Risk Factors

- Tobacco use. Up to one-third of cases in men and one-fourth of cases in women may be linked to smoking.
- Hypertension.
- Occupational exposure to trichloroethylene, cadmium, asbestos, and petroleum products.
- Obesity.
- Chronic kidney disease and acquired cystic disease of the kidney associated with long-term dialysis.

Genetic Predisposition/Familial Syndromes

Several familial kidney cancer syndromes have been identified. Although they represent a minority of RCC patients, individuals affected by these heritable disorders have a predisposition for developing kidney cancer, which is often bilateral and multifocal. Systematic evaluation of at-risk families has helped elucidate the molecular mechanisms underlying the origins of several types of kidney cancer. Several forms of sporadic kidney cancer have histologically similar familial counterparts with which they share aberrant oncogenic pathways. The following familial kidney cancer syndromes have been described:

- *Von Hippel-Lindau (VHL) disease*
  - VHL is inherited in an autosomal-dominant pattern.
  - Affected individuals have a predilection for developing a variety of tumors, including bilateral, multifocal renal tumors (clear cell RCC), pancreatic neuroendocrine tumors, renal and pancreatic

cysts, CNS hemangioblastomas, retinal angiomas, pheochromocytomas, endolymphatic sac tumors, and epididymal/broad ligament cystadenomas.
- Genetic linkage analysis led to the identification of the *VHL* tumor suppressor gene located on chromosome 3p25. Affected individuals have a mutated/deleted allele of the *VHL* gene in their germ line. Acquisition of a somatic "second hit" that inactivates the normal copy of *VHL* leads to tumor formation in the affected organ(s).

■ *Hereditary papillary RCC (HPRC)*
- Affected individuals have bilateral, multifocal type 1 papillary RCC. There are no known extrarenal manifestations of this disease.
- The underlying genetic alteration is an activating germline mutation in the *MET* proto-oncogene, located on the long arm of chromosome 7, accompanied by a nonrandom duplication of the aberrant chromosome 7 (resulting in trisomy or polysomy 7).
- Patients usually present with renal tumors in or beyond the fifth decade of life, although an early-onset form that presents in the second or third decades has also been described.

■ *Birt-Hogg-Dube (BHD) syndrome*
- Affected individuals are at increased risk of developing cutaneous fibrofolliculomas, pulmonary cysts predisposing to the development of spontaneous pneumothoraces, and renal tumors.
- Several histologic types of renal tumors have been described in BHD, including chromophobe (34%), hybrid chromophobe-oncocytomas (50%), clear cell, papillary, and oncocytomas.
- The BHD gene, localized to chromosome 17p11, encodes a protein known as folliculin. Identification of somatic "second hit" mutations in *BHD/folliculin* indicates that this gene may function as a tumor suppressor.

■ *Hereditary leiomyomatosis and RCC (HLRCC)*
- Affected individuals have a predisposition to developing multiple cutaneous and uterine leiomyomas, as well as papillary RCC.
- Renal tumors are often solitary, but bilateral, multifocal disease has also been described.
- Histologically, these tumors are usually reminiscent of papillary type 2 RCC; may be mistaken for collecting duct RCC. The distinctive histopathologic hallmark of these tumors is the presence of a large nucleus with a prominent orangiophilic nucleolus surrounded by a halo.
- Tumors tend to metastasize early and have a characteristically aggressive clinical course.
- The underlying defect is a germline mutation in the gene encoding the Krebs cycle enzyme fumarate hydratase (FH), located on chromosome 1. Loss of fumarate hydratase and the accompanying alteration in Krebs cycle function result in a metabolic switch characterized by a reliance on aerobic glycolysis for cellular energy needs (Warburg effect). Other critical cellular events associated with loss of FH include dysregulated HIF1-α expression and downregulation of AMPK, a key cellular energy sensor.

■ *Succinate dehydrogenase associated RCC (SDH-RCC)*
- Succinate dehydrogenase is a multiunit mitochondrial enzymatic complex that catalyzes the conversion of succinate to fumarate in the Krebs cycle.
- Germline mutations in the genes encoding SDHA, SDHB, SDHC, and SDHD have been identified in patients with hereditary forms of kidney cancer. Patients with germline *SDHB* mutations are also at risk for developing pheochromocytomas and paragangliomas.
- Loss of SDH activity leads to impaired Krebs cycle function and leads to metabolic and biochemical alterations similar to those seen with FH inactivation.
- The precise histologic variants associated with SDH-RCC remain to be determined and may vary depending on the SDH subunit affected.

■ *Other genes associated with hereditary kidney cancer*
- Mutations in multiple genes involving the LKB1/TSC/mTOR are associated with familial forms of RCC.
- Mutations in the genes responsible for tuberous sclerosis complex (TSC1/2) have been associated with kidney cancer. While the majority of renal tumors resulting from TSC mutations are benign (angiomyolipomas), clear cell, papillary, and other subtypes of RCC have also been described.
- More recently, familial kidney cancer associated with mutations in the BAP1 gene has been recognized.

PATHOLOGIC CLASSIFICATION

Based on histopathologic features, RCC is divided into the following subtypes:

- Clear cell RCC. The most common variety, comprising 75% to 85% of all kidney cancers. Composed predominantly of cells with a clear cytoplasm.
- Papillary RCC. Further divided into type 1 and type 2 based on morphologic appearance. Represents approximately 10% to 15% of all kidney cancers.
- Chromophobe RCC. Represents approximately 5% of all malignant renal neoplasms. Characterized histologically by the presence of sheets of cells with pale or eosinophilic granular cytoplasm.
- RCC associated with HLRCC.
- Collecting duct RCC. Rare (<1%) variant believed to originate in the collecting system. Medullary RCC, which has some features suggestive of collecting duct RCC, is seen almost exclusively in patients with sickle-cell trait and is characterized by an aggressive clinical course.
- Unclassified. Represents approximately 3% to 5% of renal tumors. Lack distinct features of a particular subtype or variant.
- Renal tumors with sarcomatoid features do not comprise a separate entity. Instead, they represent sarcomatoid differentiation of one of the subtypes of RCC. Generally associated with poor prognosis.

MOLECULAR MECHANISMS

The identification of familial forms of kidney cancer was an important step in unraveling the complex aberrant pathways leading to the development of several types of both hereditary and sporadic RCCs. This has enabled the development of therapeutic agents that target pathways critical to the development and growth of these tumors.

Clear Cell RCC

- The vast majority of patients with sporadic clear cell RCC show evidence of *VHL* inactivation in tumor tissue (somatic alteration) resulting from either mutation or promoter hypermethylation. The absence of functionally active VHL protein has several consequences, the best understood of which is the accumulation of a group of transcription factors called hypoxia-inducible factors (HIF).
- Increased intracellular HIF leads to transcriptional upregulation of several proangiogenic growth and survival factors, such as vascular endothelial growth factor (VEGF), platelet-derived growth factor (PDGF), transforming growth factor-alpha (TGF-α), and the glucose transporter glut-1. This sequence of events appears to be important in the genesis and propagation of clear cell RCC.
- More recently, mutations in several genes associated with chromatin remodeling, including *PBRM1*, and *SETD2* and in the *BAP1* gene, which encodes a deubiquitinase, have been identified in some kidney tumors. The biologic significance of these alterations is being investigated.
- A recent effort at molecular characterization of ccRCC undertaken by The Cancer Genome Atlas (TCGA) reiterated the association of both *VHL* mutations and alterations in chromatin remodeling genes with clear cell RCC. In addition, high grade tumors and those attended by a poor prognosis demonstrated changes consistent with a glycolytic shift. Several components of these pathways are potential targets for novel therapeutic agents.

Type 1 Papillary RCC

- MET is a cell surface receptor normally activated on binding its ligand, hepatocyte growth factor (HGF). The HGF/ MET axis mediates a variety of biologic functions including cell growth, proliferation, and motility. Activating mutations in the *MET* proto-oncogene (which render the receptor constitutively active) are responsible for the bilateral, multifocal, type 1 papillary renal tumors seen in patients with HPRC.
- Activating somatic mutations in the tyrosine kinase domain of *MET* have also been identified in 10% to 15% of patients with sporadic papillary RCC. Duplication of chromosome 7, where genes for both MET and HGF are located, is seen more frequently than *MET* mutations in sporadic papillary tumors

(~70% in one series) and may represent an alternative mechanism for activation of the HGF/MET pathway. Gain of chromosome 17 has also been identified as a frequent event in type 1pRCC.
▪ Agents targeting the MET pathway are currently being evaluated in patients with papillary RCC.

Type 2 Papillary RCC

▪ Includes a heterogeneous group of tumors with papillary architecture but with features inconsistent with type 1 papillary tumors. Patients with HLRCC are at risk for developing renal tumors, which are sometimes described as type 2 papillary RCC.
▪ The underlying molecular defect in HLRCC-related tumors is the inactivation of the Krebs cycle enzyme fumarate hydratase, leading to accumulation of its substrate fumarate. Fumarate interferes with HIF degradation and leads to its accumulation and consequent transcriptional activation of its target genes (VEGF, PDGF, TGF-α, etc.). While no sporadic counterpart for this tumor has been described, it is speculated that some sporadic type 2 tumors may be associated with impaired Krebs cycle activity.
▪ A comprehensive molecular characterization of papillary renal tumors undertaken by TCGA has also identified changes involving CDKN2A, the NRF2 oxidative stress pathway and chromatin remodeling genes, particularly *SETD2*.

Chromophobe RCC

▪ The precise biochemical aberrations underlying chromophobe RCC are being investigated; however, patients with BHD often present with chromophobe renal tumors, and understanding the molecular alterations in BHD-associated tumors may provide some insight into those underlying sporadic chromophobe RCC.
▪ The gene for BHD (*folliculin*) appears to interact with the mTOR and AMPK pathways, which may be important in chromophobe tumors and, potentially, other histologic RCC subtypes seen in BHD.
▪ Molecular characterization of sporadic chromophobe RCC under the aegis of TCGA revealed loss of most or all of chromosomes 1, 2, 6, 10, 13, and 17. In addition, *TP53* was mutated in 32% of cases, and mTOR pathway changes occurred in 23% of cases. Mitochondrial DNA alterations as well as mutations in the TERT promoter were additional recurrent changes seen in these tumors.

Other Subtypes

▪ Other histologic subtypes of RCC include 1) medullary RCC, seen almost exclusively in association with sickle-cell trait, and 2) collecting duct RCC, which shares similarities with upper urinary tract tumors.
▪ Translocation RCCs are so named because of the presence in these tumors of characteristic translocations involving members of the microphthalmia transcription factor/transcription factor E (MITF/TFE). In its most common form, tumors exhibit translocations involving TFE3. These tumors are more common in children and young adults and can exhibit aggressive clinical behavior with a propensity for early metastasis.

CLINICAL PRESENTATION

▪ Many renal masses are found incidentally during evaluation for unrelated medical issues or metastatic foci.
▪ Only 10% of patients present with the classic triad of hematuria, pain, and flank mass.
▪ Initial presentation may be a paraneoplastic syndrome or laboratory abnormality, including elevated erythrocyte sedimentation rate, weight loss/cachexia, hypertension, anemia, hypercalcemia (ectopic release of PTH-like substance), elevated alkaline phosphatase, polycythemia (increased erythropoietin), and Stauffer's syndrome (reversible, hepatic dysfunction not related to hepatic metastasis that usually resolves once the primary tumor is removed).

- Approximately 50% of RCC patients present with localized disease, 25% with locally advanced disease, and 25% to 30% with metastatic disease. Of those without evidence of metastatic disease at presentation, approximately 30% will go on to develop metastases subsequently.
- Common sites of metastatic spread include lung (70% to 75%), lymph nodes (30% to 40%), bone (20% to 25%), liver (20% to 25%), and CNS.

DIAGNOSIS AND EVALUATION

- Initial workup for a patient with a renal mass includes a history and physical examination, complete blood count with differential, full chemistry panel, and PT/PTT.
- CT scan of the abdomen and pelvis, with and without contrast, is standard for evaluating the renal mass and regional lymph nodes. If the CT scan suggests renal vein and/or inferior vena cava involvement, an MRI of the abdomen and chest imaging is warranted.
- Chest x-ray is also recommended. Chest CT is indicated in the presence of an abnormal x-ray, a large primary tumor, or symptoms suggestive of pulmonary or mediastinal involvement such as cough, hemoptysis, or chest pain.
- Bone scan is indicated in patients with elevated alkaline phosphatase, hypercalcemia, pathologic fracture, or bone pain.
- MRI of the brain is usually reserved for patients with clinical features suggesting brain metastases, but is increasingly performed in some centers as part of initial staging in asymptomatic patients with known metastatic disease.

STAGING

The most commonly used system for staging RCC is the Tumor–Lymph Node–Metastasis (TNM) staging system outlined by the American Joint Committee for Cancer (AJCC). Stage I disease encompasses any tumor not greater than 7 cm in greatest dimension and is limited to the kidney. Stage II includes any tumor greater than 7 cm in greatest dimension but is limited to the kidney. Stage III disease is present if there are metastasis to regional lymph nodes, or the tumor extends into major veins or perinephric tissues but not the ipsilateral adrenal gland nor Gerota's fascia. Stage IV disease includes any distant metastasis or tumor invading beyond Gerota's fascia or contiguous extension into the ipsilateral adrenal gland.

PROGNOSTIC FACTORS

- Several tumor and patient characteristics appear to influence outcome for patients with localized kidney cancer. Nomograms based on factors such as tumor stage and nuclear grade, tumor histology, mode of presentation, and performance status are used to predict risk of disease recurrence following nephrectomy. Several such nomograms are currently available and are gaining acceptance in both clinical practice and clinical trial design as an effective means of risk stratification.
- In patients with metastatic disease, clinical characteristics (performance status, prior nephrectomy, number of metastatic sites, etc.) as well as laboratory parameters (serum lactate dehydrogenase, serum calcium, hemoglobin, etc.) are predictive of survival. A widely used prognostic model based on patients treated with either cytokines or chemotherapeutic agents (Memorial Sloan-Kettering Cancer Center prognostic criteria) implicates the following features with poor outcome:
  - Poor performance status (Karnofsky PS <80)
  - Elevated LDH (>1.5 × upper limit of normal)
  - Elevated corrected calcium (>10 mg/dL)
  - Low hemoglobin (<lower limit of normal)
  - Time for diagnosis to systemic therapy < 1 year

- The presence or absence of one or more of these prognostic features allows stratification of patients into the following prognostic categories:
  - Favorable: 0 risk factors, median survival 19.9 months
  - Intermediate: 1 or 2 risk factors, median survival 10.3 months
  - Poor: 3 to 5 risk factors, median survival 3.9 months
- With the advent of VEGF pathway antagonists, the role of the above prognostic criteria and risk stratification have been reexamined. Based on retrospective analyses, time from diagnosis to therapy, elevated calcium, decreased hemoglobin, and poor performance status remain important predictors of poor outcome; additionally, elevated neutrophil count and platelet count also portend poor prognosis in these models.

TREATMENT OF LOCALIZED RCC

Surgery

- For patients with early-stage localized RCC, surgical resection is often curative; for small renal masses (<4 cm) a partial nephrectomy/nephron sparing surgery is typically performed using an open, laparoscopic, or robotic-assisted approach.
- For tumors >4 cm, radical nephrectomy (open or laparoscopic procedure) is the treatment of choice. However, recent literature supports nephron-sparing procedures for tumors 4 to 7 cm in selected patients. Patients with primary tumors larger than 7 cm and disease localized to the kidney generally undergo a radical nephrectomy with curative intent.
- Active surveillance of small renal masses is also an alternative option in selected patients including the elderly and those with significant competing health risks and comorbidities.
- Less invasive techniques such as radiofrequency ablation and cryotherapy are being evaluated and may be effective in eradicating smaller renal tumors; however, studies demonstrate an increased risk of local recurrence when compared to surgery and long-term outcome data are lacking.

Adjuvant Therapy

Adjuvant Sorafenib or Sunitinib (ECOG-ACRIN E2805) (Table 13.2)

- VEGF TKI's sunitinib and sorafenib are FDA approved in advanced RCC.
- E2805: first phase 3 trial investigating the role of VEGFR inhibitors in the adjuvant setting in high-risk patients.
- 1,943 treatment naïve patients with high-risk, nonmetastatic RCC were randomized to 54 weeks of Sunitinib 50 mg/d (4 out of 6 week cycles), Sorafenib 400 mg twice/d continuously, or matched (sunitinib or sorafenib) placebo. A study amendment permitted reducing initial doses to Sunitinib 37.5 mg/d (or matched placebo) or sorafenib 400 mg/d (or matched placebo) due to toxicity and high rate of treatment discontinuations.
- The study included heterogeneous histologies (*clear cell and non-clear cell*) and staging groups: 9% of sunitinib and sorafenib patients were stage 1 (AJCC). There was an equal proportion of intermediate-high *versus* very-high risk (UCLA International Staging System risk stratification) in all treatment and placebo groups.
- Primary endpoint was DFS in the intention to treat patient population. Secondary endpoints were OS, DFS (clear cell), and adverse events classified by NCI CTCAE such as TKI-related hypertension, hand-foot syndrome, rash etc.
- After a median follow-up of 5.8 years, median DFS was not significantly different among sunitinib, sorafenib, or placebo groups (70.0 vs. 73.4 vs. 79.6 months, respectively). No benefit was demonstrated in a subgroup analysis in patients with clear cell histology in either treatment arm. Five-year OS also did not differ between the groups (sunitinib 77.9%; sorafenib 80.5%; placebo 80.3%).
- There were many dose reductions due to AEs. In patients starting on full doses, the overall treatment discontinuation rates were high (44% for sunitinib and 45% for sorafenib).
- Common AEs for sunitinib and sorafenib included hand–foot syndrome (15% and 33%, respectively), hypertension (17% and 16%), fatigue (18% and 7%), and rash (2% and 15%). Overall, there

was a high proportion of grade 3 or greater AEs in the two treatment arms (sunitinib 63%; sorafenib 72%). Despite starting-dose reductions, more than half of patients in each group experienced grade 3 or greater AEs.

- Subgroup analyses demonstrated no difference in DFS with patients who received full starting-dose versus reduced, starting-dose sunitinib or sorafenib (with trend favoring placebo at reduced doses), total dose received, or treatment duration.
- These data fail to provide data supporting the use of adjuvant sunitinib or sorafenib in high-risk RCC.

Adjuvant Sunitinib (S-TRAC trial)

- Sunitinib is approved as a first-line treatment option for metastatic RCC. The E2805 (see above) demonstrated no benefit with adjuvant sunitinib or sorafenib in locally advanced RCC.
- However, a recent phase 3 trial (S-TRAC: Sunitinib as adjuvant treatment for patients at high risk of recurrence of RCC following nephrectomy) highlighted the role of sunitinib in the adjuvant setting for nonmetastatic (locoregional) RCC with a high risk for relapse post nephrectomy.
- 615 treatment-naïve patients with nonmetastatic (locoregional), high-risk clear-cell RCC were prospectively randomized to Sunitinib 50 mg/d or placebo post nephrectomy. Treatment was administered for 4 weeks on followed by 2 weeks off for 1 year. Patients were randomized in a stratified fashion based on the University of California Los Angeles Integrated Staging System (UISS) high risk group.
- Primary endpoint was DFS. Secondary endpoints were OS (did not reach maturity), safety, HRQOL.
- After a median follow-up of 5.4 years in the sunitinib arm, the median DFS was significantly improved over placebo (6.8 vs. 5.6 years; HR 0.76). 36.6% of patient receiving sunitinib had a recurrence, second malignancy, or death compared to 47.1% in the placebo arm.
- Slightly more than half (54.2%) continued the initial dose of Sunitinib 50 mg/d, with 55.6% completing the actual treatment. The majority of discontinuations were due to AEs.
- A higher percentage of patients in the sunitinib arm encountered AEs than placebo (99.7% vs. 88.5%). Most common adverse events were diarrhea, PPE, hypertension, fatigue, nausea, dysgeusia, and mucosal inflammation. More grade 3 or greater AE's were reported in the sunitinib versus placebo arm (63.4% vs. 21.7%). There were 34.3% sunitinib dose reductions, 46.4% interrupted doses, and 28.1% treatment discontinuations. No treatment-related deaths were reported, and there were equivalent rates of *serious* AEs between the two arms.
- Adjuvant sunitinib improves median DFS with patients with locoregional, clear-cell RCC with a high risk for relapse post nephrectomy as compared to placebo. The long-term/overall survival benefit is not established and the toxicity profile may potentially limit its use in the nonmetastatic setting. Based on these data, the FDA recently approved the use of sunitinib in patients with RCC at high risk of recurrence

TREATMENT OF METASTATIC RCC

Surgery

- In selected patients with isolated metastases, surgical resection may provide extended disease-free periods. Five-year survival rates of 30% to 50% have been reported in retrospective analyses using this approach.
- Cytoreductive nephrectomy preceding systemic cytokine therapy has been the subject of several studies. At least two randomized phase 3 trials have demonstrated a survival advantage in patients receiving interferon-alpha (IFN-α) following nephrectomy versus patients receiving IFN-α alone. Careful patient selection is key to the success of this approach, and patients with limited metastatic burden, favorable tumor kinetics, and good performance status are most likely to benefit. Cytoreductive nephrectomy as a prelude to antiangiogenic targeted therapies is currently under

evaluation in randomized phase 3 trials, but appears to be associated with clinical benefit in retrospective analyses.
▪ Cytoreductive nephrectomy can be performed for palliation of intractable hematuria and pain associated with RCC.

Systemic Therapy

▪ Conventional cytotoxic chemotherapy is ineffective in the vast majority of patients with metastatic RCC (~5% to 6% overall response rate with single agent) and is not part of the standard approach to this disease. However, some patients with sarcomatoid variants of RCC are responsive to gemcitabine-based regimens.
▪ Targeted agents directed against the VEGF/PDGF and mammalian target of rapamycin (mTOR) pathways have been evaluated in patients with metastatic RCC and have largely supplanted cytokines as standard first-line agents in the management of clear cell RCC (Table 13.1). The standard initial approach for most patients with metastatic clear cell RCC is treatment with small molecule inhibitors of angiogenesis, although cytokine-based therapy with high-dose interleukin (IL)-2 should be considered in selected patients.
▪ Recent advances in our understanding of immune checkpoints have led to the development of novel immunotherapies in the management of clear-cell RCC. In addition, newer VEGFR inhibitors with a broader target profile, such as cabozantinib and lenvatinib have also been shown to have activity in patients who have progressed following first-line anti-angiogenic therapy.
▪ There are currently no standard treatments for non–clear cell variants, although several interesting mechanism-based approaches are under investigation.

VEGF Pathway Inhibitors

Up-regulation of proangiogenic factors such as VEGF and PDGF is an important consequence of VHL inactivation and provides the basis for the efficacy of anti-VEGF agents in clear cell RCC. Several agents targeting the VEGF pathway are approved by the US FDA for the treatment of metastatic RCC.

Sunitinib

▪ An oral tyrosine kinase inhibitor with potent activity against VEGF receptor 2 (VEGFR-2) and PDGF receptor (PDGFR).
▪ Initial single-arm phase 2 studies demonstrated a remarkably high overall response rate of 30% to 40% in patients with cytokine-refractory disease. A randomized phase 3 study comparing sunitinib with IFN-α in previously untreated clear cell RCC patients has demonstrated a significantly higher response rate (47% vs. 12%), improved progression-free survival (PFS) (median 11 vs. 5 months), and superior overall survival (OS) (26.4 vs. 21.8 months) with sunitinib.
▪ Dosage is 50 mg/d over 4 weeks, followed by a 2-week rest period.
▪ Fairly well tolerated by the majority of patients. Common side effects include hypertension, fatigue, cutaneous side effects (rash, hand–foot syndrome), gastrointestinal symptoms (nausea, vomiting, diarrhea, anorexia, constipation), and cytopenia.
▪ Sunitinib is one of the most widely used first-line agents in metastatic clear cell RCC.

Pazopanib

▪ Oral angiogenesis inhibitor that targets VEGFR-1, -2, and -3. Approved in 2009 by the FDA for the treatment of advanced RCC.
▪ In a phase III trial of patients with advanced RCC with 0 or 1 prior cytokine treatment comparing pazopanib versus placebo, PFS was higher in the pazopanib group (9.2 months) compared the placebo cohort (4.2 months). In subgroup analyses, the improvement on PFS was seen in both treatment-naïve patients and in those who had received prior cytokine therapy.
▪ Adverse reactions include diarrhea, hypertension, nausea, fatigue, and abdominal pain. Hepatotoxicity with elevated transaminases was seen, and a small number of deaths from hepatic failure were noted on study. Liver function should be carefully monitored while on therapy.

TABLE 13.1 Key Studies of Targeted Agents in Metastatic Renal Cell Carcinoma

Agent(s)	Phase	Study Population	# Of Patients	Overall Response Rate (RECIST)[a]	Median PFS (mo)[a]	Median OS (mo)[a]
First-line therapy						
Sunitinib vs. IFN-α	Randomized phase 3	Clear cell	750	**47% vs. 12%**	**11 vs. 5**	**26.4 vs. 21.08**
Tem vs. IFN-α vs. Tem+ IFN-α	Randomized phase 3	Poor prognosis, all subtypes	626	8.6% vs. 4.8% vs. 8.1%	5.5 vs. 3.1 vs. 4.7	**10.9 vs. 7.3** vs. 8.4
Bev + IFN-α vs. IFN-α	Randomized phase 3	Clear cell	649	**31% vs. 13%**	**10.2 vs. 5.4**	23.3 vs. 21.3
Bev + IFN-α vs. IFN-α	Randomized phase 3	Clear cell	732	**26% vs. 13%**	**8.5 vs. 5.2**	18.3 vs. 17.4
Pazopanib vs. Placebo	Randomized phase 3	Clear cell	233	**32% vs. 4%**	**11.1 vs. 2.8**	
Second-line and subsequent therapy						
Sunitinib	Single-arm phase 2	Clear cell, prior cytokines	63	40%	8.7	NA
Sunitinib	Single-arm phase 2	Clear cell, prior cytokines	106	44%	8.1	NA
Sorafenib vs. placebo	Randomized phase 3	Clear cell, prior cytokines	903	**10% vs. 2%**	**5.5 vs. 2.8**	17.8 vs. 15.2
Bev (10 mg/kg) vs. bev (3 mg/kg) vs. placebo	Randomized, phase 2	Clear cell, prior cytokines	116	**10% vs. 0% vs. 0%**	**4.8 vs. 3.0 vs. 2.5**	NA
Pazopanib vs. placebo	Randomized phase 3	Clear cell, prior cytokines	202	**29% vs. 3%**	**7.2 vs. 4.2**	
Everolimus vs. placebo	Randomized phase 3	Clear cell RCC, prior VEGF-targeted therapy	410	**1% vs. 0%**	**4.0 vs. 1.9**	NR vs. 8.8
Axitinib vs. sorafenib	Randomized phase 3	Clear cell, Prior VEGF,	723	**19% vs. 9%**	**6.7 vs. 4.7**	NA
Nivolumab vs. everolimus	Randomized Phase 3	mTOR or cytokine	821	**25% vs. 5%**	4.6 vs. 4.4	**25 vs. 19.6**
Lenvatinib + everolimus vs. everolimus	Randomized Phase 2	Clear Cell, prior VEGF-targeted therapy	153	**17% vs. 3%**	**14.6 vs. 5.5**	25.5 vs. 17.5
Cabozantinib vs. everolimus	Randomized phase 3	Clear cell Clear cell, prior VEGF-targeted therapy	658		**7.4 vs. 3.9**	**21.4 vs. 16.5**

[a]Statistically significant differences indicated in boldface type.

Bev, bevacizumab; IFN-α, interferon-alpha; NR, not reached; NA, not available; OS, overall survival; PFS, progression-free survival; tem, temsirolimus.

- Although the adverse events seen with sunitinib and pazopanib are similar, head-to-head comparison in randomized studies suggested that pazopanib was better tolerated, with both patients and physicians indicating a preference for this agent over sunitinib, based on better tolerability. Furthermore, in a phase 3 randomized study, the efficacy of pazopanib in clear cell RCC patients was shown to be non-inferior to that seen with sunitinib.

Axitinib

- A highly selective oral tyrosine kinase inhibitor that targets VEGFR 1, 2, and 3. Approved by the FDA in 2012 for the treatment of advanced RCC in patients who had previously failed cytokines or first line VEGFR targeted therapy.
- A phase III trial (AXIS) compared the efficacy of dose-escalated axitinib versus standard dose sorafenib following first line treatment with either sunitinib, bevacizumab plus IFN-α, temsirolimus, or cytokine therapy. The PFS was 6.7 months in the patients on axitinib versus 4.7 months in patients on sorafenib. In sub group analysis, the median PFS was consistently improved over the sorafenib group regardless of prior treatment, although the difference was more pronounced in patients who had received prior cytokine therapy.
- The agent appears to be fairly well tolerated. Adverse effects include hypertension, diarrhea, dysphonia, nausea, fatigue, and hand–foot syndrome.
- Treatment-related hypertension has been proposed as a clinically evaluable pharmacodynamic marker in patients receiving axitinib as well as other agents targeting the VEGF pathway. Retrospective studies demonstrate a correlation between the occurrence of hypertension (thought to indicate adequate plasma levels of the agent and consequently optimal inhibition of the VEGF pathway) and outcome.

Bevacizumab

- A monoclonal antibody against VEGF-A, approved by the FDA in 2009 for the treatment of advanced RCC in combination with IFN-α.
- A randomized, three-arm phase 2 study comparing two different doses of bevacizumab (10 mg/kg and 3 mg/kg i.v. every 2 weeks) and placebo in cytokine-refractory patients showed a PFS advantage favoring the 10 mg/kg arm (4.8 vs. 2.5 months).
- Two multicenter randomized phase 3 studies with similar trial designs comparing IFN-α alone (9 million IU s.c. 3 times per week) versus the same dose of IFN-α plus bevacizumab (10 mg/kg i.v. every 2 weeks) showed superior PFS in the combination arm (5.4 vs. 10.2 months). These improvements in PFS did not appear to translate into significant overall survival benefits in either of these trials.
- Side effects include hypertension, headache, epistaxis, headaches, proteinuria, and in some cases gastrointestinal perforation and difficulty with wound healing.

Sorafenib

- An oral tyrosine kinase inhibitor with activity against c-Raf, VEGFR-2, and PDGFR.
- A randomized phase 2 study showed significant improvement in PFS versus placebo (median 24 vs. 6 weeks) in patients with cytokine-refractory metastatic RCC. This finding was confirmed in a randomized phase 3 trial of sorafenib versus placebo (median PFS 5.5 vs. 2.8 months). OS was similar in the two groups (17.8 vs. 15.2 months) and may have been influenced by the trial's crossover design (patients progressing on placebo could cross over to the sorafenib arm).
- A randomized phase 2 study in metastatic, untreated clear cell RCC failed to demonstrate the drug's superiority over IFN-α.
- Typically administered at a dose of 400 mg twice a day. Adverse events are similar to those of sunitinib.
- Was considered a reasonable option for patients who have failed sunitinib and/or the other first-line agents; with the advent of several new agents with activity in the first- or second-line setting, the use of sorafenib is likely to be limited to those patients who have progressed on multiple prior therapies.

TABLE 13.2 Results from Key Studies of Adjuvant Targeted Agents in Renal Cell Carcinoma

Agent(s)	Phase	Study Population	# Of Patients	DFS (yr)*	5 Year OS (%)[a]
Sunitinib vs. Placebo (S-TRAC)[b]	Phase 3	Clear-cell RCC	615	**6.8 vs. 5.6**	Data not mature
Sunitinib vs. Sorafenib vs. Placebo (ECOG-ACRIN E2805)[c]	Phase 3	Clear and Non–clear Cell RCC	1943	5.8 vs. 6.1 vs. 6.6	77.9 vs. 80.5 vs. 80.3

[a]Statistically significant differences indicated in boldface type.

[b]Ravaud A, Motzer RJ, Pandha HS, et al. Adjuvant sunitinib in high- risk renal- cell carcinoma after nephrectomy. NEJM. December 2016;375(23):2246–2254.

[c]Haas NB, Manola J, Uzzo RG, et al. Adjuvant sunitinib or sorafenib for high- risk, non- metastatic renal- cell carcinoma (ECOG- ACRIN E2805): a double- blind, placebo- controlled, randomised, phase 3 trial. Lancet. 2016;387:2008– 2016.

Cabozantinib

- Oral multi-TKI (MET, VEGFR, AXL).
- A recent Phase 3 (METEOR trial) evaluated the efficacy of cabozantinib compared with everolimus (mTOR inhibitor) in 658 patients with advanced/metastatic clear-cell RCC, who progressed on prior VEGFR TKI; pts randomized to receive Cabozantinib 60 mg/d or Everolimus 10 mg/d.
- The trial demonstrated improved OS, PFS, and objective response with cabozantinib; OS was significantly increased with cabozantinib compared to everolimus (21.4 vs. 16.5 months). In general, more patients on the cabozantinib arm were alive at 6, 12, 18, and 24 months than the everolimus arm. Median PFS in all randomized patients was also considerably greater with cabozantinib versus everolimus (7.4 vs. 3.9 months). Finally, 17% of cabozantinib-treated patients and only 3% of everolimus-treated patients experienced an objective response.
- More grade 3 to 4 AE's were reported with cabozantinib than everolimus (71% vs. 60%). Common adverse events were hypertension, diarrhea, fatigue, palmar-plantar erythrodysethesia, anemia, hyperglycemia, and hypomagnesemia. Cabozantinib was also associated with serious adverse events such as abdominal pain (3%), pleural effusion (2%), pneumonia (2%), PE (2%), anemia (2%), and dyspnea (1%).
- Based on these data, the agent was approved for use in metastatic RCC following progression on front line VEGF-pathway directed therapy.
- Cabozantinib has also been evaluated in the front-line setting in a randomized phase 2 study compared to sunitinib (CaboSun). In this study, 157 patients with intermediate or poor risk (IMDC) metastatic clear cell RCC with no prior therapy were randomized to Cabozantinib 60 mg/d or Sunitinib 50 mg/d (4 weeks on, then 2 weeks break). Median PFS for cabozantinib versus sunitinib was 8.2 versus 5.6 months, respectively, and ORR was 33% versus 12%, respectively.

Lenvatinib

- Oral multi-TKI (VEGFR, FGFR, PDGFRα, RET, KIT).
- A recent phase 2 randomized study evaluated the efficacy of lenvatinib, together with everolimus, or each agent alone in 153 patients with advanced/metastatic, clear-cell RCC who progressed on prior anti-VEGF. Patients were randomized to Lenvatinib 18 mg/d plus Everolimus 5 mg/d, single agent Lenvatinib 24 mg/d, or standard dose Everolimus 10 mg/d alone. The primary endpoint was PFS.
- PFS in the combination (lenvatinib + everolimus) was better than with single-agent everolimus (14.6 vs. 5.5 months; HR 0.4; $P = 0.0005$). Objective response with combination therapy was 43% compared to 6% in the everolimus arm (rate ratio 7.2; $P < 0.0001$). The combination group had greater response duration. Furthermore, the combination group demonstrated greater OS benefit with respect to everolimus alone at post-hoc analysis (25.5 vs. 15.4 months; HR 0.51), but not significantly different at the primary data cutoff.

- There were more grade 3 or 4 AEs in the lenvatinib containing arm versus single-agent everolimus (71% combination vs. 50% everolimus). Most common grade 3 AEs in the lenvatinib-everolimus arm were diarrhea, fatigue, or hypertension; and anemia, dyspnea, hypertriglyceridemia, and hyperglycemia with everolimus alone.
- The combination of lenvatinib and everolimus has been approved by the US FDA for use in the second-line setting following progression on VEGF-pathway targeted therapy.

mTOR Pathway Inhibitors

The mTOR inhibitors temsirolimus and everolimus are rapamycin analogs believed to act at least in part by down-regulating mTOR-dependent translation of HIF.

Temsirolimus

- A prodrug of rapamycin-administered i.v.
- The most convincing evidence for the activity of this drug in RCC comes from a randomized phase 3 trial of 626 patients with previously untreated high-risk metastatic RCC (defined as the presence of three or more poor prognostic criteria). All histologic subtypes of RCC were included in this trial. Patients were randomized to receive temsirolimus 25 mg i.v. per week or temsirolimus 15 mg i.v. per week plus IFN-α (6 million IU 3 times/week) or IFN-α alone (18 million IU 3 times/week as tolerated). Single-agent temsirolimus was associated with significantly prolonged disease-free survival and OS compared to IFN-α alone (median OS 10.9 vs. 7.3 months). An exploratory subgroup analysis suggested that both patients with clear cell and those with non–clear cell RCC benefited from temsirolimus. The combined temsirolimus/IFN-α arm had superior disease-free survival compared to IFN-α alone, but there was no difference in OS between the two groups.
- Common adverse events include rash, fatigue, mucositis, hyperglycemia, hypercholesterolemia, and interstitial pneumonitis. Rapamycin analogs are also associated with a risk of immunosuppression.
- Single-agent temsirolimus is a reasonable option for patients with poor-prognosis RCC.

Everolimus

- An oral rapamycin analog.
- In a randomized phase 3 trial of metastatic RCC patients who had progressed on front-line VEGF-targeted therapy, everolimus improved disease-free survival compared to placebo (4 vs. 1.9 months).
- Side effects are similar to those of temsirolimus.
- Until recently, everolimus was a commonly used second-line option in patients with metastatic clear cell RCC. However, several recent studies demonstrating the superiority of immune checkpoint inhibitors as well as novel multikinase inhibitors in this setting have led to a reappraisal of the utility of everolimus in this setting. Everolimus may still be reasonable option in patients who have failed other available second- or third-line options.

Cytokines

Until the advent of VEGF-targeted therapy, cytokines were the mainstay of treatment for metastatic clear cell RCC. High-doses IL-2 and IFN-α are the most studied agents in this class.

IL-2

Since the early 1980s, numerous studies have demonstrated the efficacy of IL-2 in patients with metastatic RCC.

- High-dose IL-2 (600,000–720,000 IU/kg every 8 hours as tolerated up to a maximum 15 doses) has shown an overall response rate of 15% to 20%, with complete responses in 7% to 9% of patients. Since only a small subset of patients appears to benefit from this agent, no survival advantage has been demonstrated in randomized trials. However, most complete responses were durable, with very few recurrences noted during long-term follow-up. IL-2 is FDA-approved for treatment of RCC.
- Responses to IL-2 are best characterized in patients with clear cell histology; its role in other subtypes of RCC is unclear.

■ The major limitation of IL-2 is toxicity associated with the high-dose regimen. A high incidence of serious and life-threatening but often reversible complications (notably vascular-leak syndrome, hypotension, multiorgan failure, etc.) occurred in early trials, with resultant mortality rates of 1% to 5%. However, further experience with IL-2 has led to better management of side effects. A recent report of over 800 patients treated at the National Cancer Institute reported no treatment-related mortality.

■ IL-2 has been evaluated in combination with a variety of other modalities, including cellular therapy with lymphokine-activated killer cells and tumor-infiltrating lymphocytes, chemotherapy, interferon, etc. However, combining any of these therapies with high-dose IL-2 appears to provide no additional benefit.

■ Lower doses of either i.v. or s.c. IL-2 have been evaluated to determine if toxicity could be reduced without compromising efficacy. At least two randomized trials have demonstrated that lower-dose IL-2 leads to fewer responses and, more importantly, a decline in durable complete responses.

■ Despite the availability of newer, better tolerated, VEGF-targeted agents, high-dose IL-2 remains a reasonable first-line option for selected patients with metastatic clear cell RCC.

IFN-α

■ Overall response rate in treatment-naïve RCC patients treated with recombinant IFN-α is approximately 15%.

■ Administered s.c. in a variety of dosages (5 to 18 million IU) and regimens (3 to 5 times per week).

■ Limited long-term follow-up data; durable complete responses relatively rare.

■ Common side effects include constitutional symptoms, gastrointestinal toxicity, elevated hepatic transaminases, and bone marrow suppression.

■ Several studies evaluating combined IL-2 and IFN-α have demonstrated no survival benefit over single-agent cytokine therapy.

■ Single-agent IFN-α has fallen out of favor due to associated toxicity and the availability of more effective agents.

Allogeneic Stem Cell Transplantation

■ Investigated in metastatic RCC to test the hypothesis that this malignancy may be susceptible to alloimmune donor-mediated graft-versus-solid tumor effects.

■ Several groups have reported overall response rates of up to 30% to 40%, including some durable complete responses following nonmyeloablative or reduced-intensity conditioning peripheral blood stem cell transplants.

■ Transplant-related morbidity and mortality and the availability of HLA-matched donors are limitations to this current investigational approach.

PD-1/PD-1 L Inhibitors

■ Activation of inhibitory T cell receptors such as Programmed Death-1 (PD-1) is believed to play a major role in mediating resistance of some tumors to immune surveillance.

■ Inhibitors of PD-1 as well as one of its activating ligands, PDL-1, are currently undergoing clinical evaluation. Several recently completed studies have clearly established the activity of this class of agents in clear cell RCC, and nivolumab, a PD1 antibody has recently been approved by the US FDA for use in patients who have progressed on front-line antiangiogenic therapy.

Nivolumab

■ Humanized IgG4 (PD-1) immune checkpoint inhibitor.

■ Evaluated in a phase 3 study in 821 patients with advanced/metastatic clear-cell renal-cell carcinoma who had received prior antiangiogenic therapies. Pts randomized to nivolumab (3 mg/kg IV) every 2 weeks or Everolimus 10 mg/d.

■ The primary end point of overall survival clearly demonstrated the superiority of nivolumab over everolimus (medial OS 25 vs. 19.6 months; HR for mortality 0.73).

- Objective response rates (25% vs. 5%), were also higher with the nivolumab group, while median PFS was comparable in the two groups (4.6 vs. 4.4 months).
- Common adverse events with nivolumab were fatigue, nausea, and pruritus. A variety of autoimmune adverse events including pneumonitis, colitis, and hypophysitis were also associated with nivolumab but were generally amenable to medical management.
- Combinations of PD-1 or PD-L1 inhibitors with either other immune checkpoint inhibitors (such as anti-CTLA4 antibodies) or VEGF-pathway antagonists are currently under clinical evaluation.

Non–Clear Cell RCC

- There are currently no standard systemic options of proven benefit for the treatment of patients with advanced RCC of non–clear cell histology.
- Retrospective analyses and small phase 2 trials indicate that inhibitors of the VEGF and mTOR pathways are associated with modest activity in some subtypes. A subgroup analysis of patients from the phase 3 ARCC trial suggested that patients with poor-risk, non–clear cell RCC had better outcomes when treated with temsirolimus compared to interferon-α. The efficacy of the oral mTOR inhibitor, everolimus, is currently being evaluated in a phase 2 study in patients with papillary RCC.
- In a large phase 2 trial, foretinib, a novel inhibitor of MET and VEGFR2, was associated with activity in patients with papillary RCC, with an overall response rate of 13.5% and a median PFS of 9.3 months. Efficacy was most pronounced in patients with papillary type 1 RCC carrying a germline mutation in MET (overall response rate 50%), although patients without this alteration also appeared to benefit to some extent.
- Bevacizumab based combinations (bevacizumab plus erlotinib or bevacizumab plus everolimus) have shown efficacy in small nonrandomized phase 2 studies and warrant further investigation.
- A better understanding of the molecular changes driving individual subtypes of non-clear cell tumors is likely to lead to the development of mechanism-based treatment strategies for each histological/molecular variant.

Suggested Readings

1. Atkins MB, Dutcher J, Weiss G, et al. Kidney cancer: the Cytokine Working Group experience (1986–2001): part I. IL-2-based clinical trials. *Med Oncol*. 2001;18(3):197–207.
2. Childs R, Chernoff A, Contentin N, et al. Regression of metastatic renal-cell carcinoma after nonmyeloablative allogeneic peripheral-blood stem-cell transplantation. *N Engl J Med*. 2000;343(11):750–758.
3. Choueiri TK, Escudier B, Powles T, et al. Cabozantinib versus everolimus in advanced renal cell carcinoma (METEOR): final results from a randomised, open-label, phase 3 trial. *Lancet*. 2016; 17: 917–927.
4. Choueiri TK, Halabi S, Sanford BL, et al. Cabozantinib versus sunitinib as initial targeted therapy for patients with metastatic renal cell carcinoma of poor or intermediate risk: The Alliance A031203 CABOSUN trial. *J Clin Oncol*. 2017;(35):591–597.
5. Escudier B, Eisen T, Stadler WM, et al. Sorafenib in advanced clear-cell renal-cell carcinoma. *NEJM*. 2007;356(2):125–134.
6. Escudier B, Pluzanska A, Koralewski P, et al. Bevacizumab plus interferon alfa-2a for treatment of metastatic renal cell carcinoma: a randomised, double-blind phase III trial. *Lancet*. 2007;370(9605):2103–2111.
7. Flanigan RC, Salmon SE, Blumenstein BA, et al. Nephrectomy followed by interferon alfa-2b compared with interferon alfa-2b alone for metastatic renal-cell cancer. *NEJM*. 2001;345(23):1655–1659.
8. Fyfe GA, Fisher RI, Rosenberg SA, Sznol M, Parkinson DR, Louie AC. Long-term response data for 255 patients with metastatic renal cell carcinoma treated with high-dose recombinant interleukin-2 therapy. *J Clin Oncol*. 1996;14(8):2410–2411.
9. Grubb RL III, Franks ME, Toro J, et al. Hereditary leiomyomatosis and renal cell cancer: a syndrome associated with an aggressive form of inherited renal cancer. *J Urol*. 2007;177(6):2074–2079.
10. Haas NB, Manola J, Uzzo RG, et al. Adjuvant sunitinib or sorafenib for high-risk, non-metastatic renal-cell carcinoma (ECOG-ACRIN E2805): a double-blind, placebo-controlled, randomised, phase 3 trial. *Lancet*. 2016;387:2008–2016.
11. Hudes G, Carducci M, Tomczak P, et al. Temsirolimus, interferon alfa, or both for advanced renal-cell carcinoma. *NEJM*. 2007;356(22):2271–2281.
12. Latif F, Tory K, Gnarra J, et al. Identification of the von Hippel-Lindau disease tumor suppressor gene. *Science*. 1993;260(5112):1317–1320.
13. Linehan WM, Pinto PA, Srinivasan R, et al. Identification of the genes for kidney cancer: opportunity for disease-specific targeted therapeutics. *Clin Cancer Res*. 2007;13(2 Pt 2):671s–679s.
14. Linehan WM, Ricketts CJ. The metabolic basis of kidney cancer. *Semin Cancer Biol*. 2012 Jun 13. [Epub ahead of print].

15. Motzer RJ, Hutson TE, Glen H, et al. Lenvatinib, everolimus, and the combination in patients with metastatic renal cell carcinoma: a randomised, phase 2, open-label, multicentre trial. *Lancet.* 2015;16:1473–1482.
16. Motzer RJ, Escudier B, McDermott DF, et al. Nivolumab versus everolimus in advanced renal-cell carcinoma. *NEJM.* November 2015;373(19):1803–1813.
17. Motzer RJ, Escudier B, Oudard S, et al. Efficacy of everolimus in advanced renal cell carcinoma: a double-blind, randomised, placebo-controlled phase III trial. *Lancet.* 2008;372(9637):449–456.
18. Motzer RJ, Hutson TE, Tomczak P, et al. Sunitinib versus interferon alfa in metastatic renal-cell carcinoma. *NEJM.* 2007;356(2):115–124.
19. Motzer RJ, Mazumdar M, Bacik J, Berg W, Amsterdam A, Ferrara J. Survival and prognostic stratification of 670 patients with advanced renal cell carcinoma. *J Clin Oncol.* 1999;17(8):2530–2540.
20. Negrier S, Escudier B, Lasset C, et al. Recombinant human interleukin-2, recombinant human interferon alfa-2a, or both in metastatic renal-cell carcinoma. Groupe Francais d'Immunotherapie. *N Engl J Med.* 1998;338(18):1272–1278.
21. Ravaud A, Motzer RJ, Pandha HS, et al. Adjuvant sunitinib in high-risk renal-cell carcinoma after nephrectomy. *NEJM.* December 2016;375(23):2246–2254.
22. Ricketts CJ, Shuch B, Vocke CD, et al. Succinate dehydrogenase kidney cancer: an aggressive example of the Warburg effect in cancer. *J Urol.* 2012 Dec;188(6):2063–2071. doi: 10.1016/j.juro.2012.08.030. Epub 2012 Oct 18.
23. Rini BL, Escudier B, Tomczak P, et al. Comparative effectiveness of axitinib versus sorafenib in advanced renal cell carcinoma (AXIS): a randomized phase 3 trial. *Lancet.* 2011;378:1931–1939.
24. Rini BL, Halabi S, Rosenberg JE, et al. Phase III trial of bevacizumab plus interferon alfa versus interferon alpha monotherapy in patients with metastatic renal cell carcinoma: final results of CALGB 90206. *J Clin Oncol.* 2010;28:2137–2143.
25. Schmidt LS, Nickerson ML, Angeloni D, et al. Early onset hereditary papillary renal carcinoma: germline missense mutations in the tyrosine kinase domain of the met proto-oncogene. *J Urol.* 2004;172(4 Pt 1):1256–1261.
26. Schmidt LS, Nickerson ML, Warren MB, et al. Germline BHD-mutation spectrum and phenotype analysis of a large cohort of families with Birt-Hogg-Dube syndrome. *Am J Hum Genet.* 2005;76(6):1023–1033.
27. Sternberg CN, Davis IS, Mardiak J, et al. Pazopanib in locally advanced or metastatic renal cell carcinoma: results of a randomized phase III trial. *J Clin Oncol* 2010;28:1061–1068.
28. Yagoda A, Abi-Rached B, Petrylak D. Chemotherapy for advanced renal-cell carcinoma: 1983-1993. *Semin Oncol.* 1995;22(1):42–60.
29. Yang JC, Haworth L, Sherry RM, et al. A randomized trial of bevacizumab, an anti-vascular endothelial growth factor antibody, for metastatic renal cancer. *NEJM.* 2003;349(5):427–434.
30. Yang JC, Sherry RM, Steinberg SM, et al. Randomized study of high-dose and low-dose interleukin-2 in patients with metastatic renal cancer. *J Clin Oncol.* 2003;21(16):3127–3132.
31. Zbar B, Tory K, Merino M, et al. Hereditary papillary renal cell carcinoma. *J Urol.* 1994;151(3):561–566.

Prostate Cancer 14

Ravi A. Madan and William L. Dahut

EPIDEMIOLOGY

- Prostate cancer (CaP) is the most common noncutaneous malignancy and the second most frequent cause of cancer-related mortality in men in the United States; in 2017 there will be an estimated 161,360 men diagnosed with CaP and 26,730 deaths from the disease. A greater than 30% decline in incidence in recent years is likely due to decreased screening. The long-term implications of this remain unknown.
- The frequency of clinically aggressive disease varies geographically, but the frequency of occult tumors does not, suggesting the influence of environmental factors in the etiology of CaP.

RISK FACTORS

- Age: Risk increases progressively with age, with about 70% of cases in men over the age of 65.
- Family history: Risk increases 2-fold with a first-degree relative diagnosed with CaP, 5-fold with two first-degree relatives.
- Race: In the United States, incidence is highest among African Americans, followed by whites, then Asians. African-American men are more likely to be diagnosed with advanced disease and have a greater than 2-fold risk of death from the disease.
- Geography: Risk is lowest in Asia, high in Scandinavia and the United States.
- Diet: Consumption of red meat and animal fat has been associated with CaP, while eating cruciferous vegetables, soy products, and lycopene-containing tomato products may be protective.

Genetic Drivers: Emerging understanding about the underlying genetics of prostate cancer suggests that androgen receptor mutations drive the majority of advanced (metastatic, castration resistant) disease, but 20% to 30% of cases may have underlying DNA damage repair mutations. In addition, an analysis of 692 men with metastatic castration-resistant prostate cancer found that nearly 12% had inherited (germline) mutations in the DNA repair pathway. Retrospective data suggest that these defects in DNA repair may be prognostic for worse clinical outcomes in men with newly diagnosed disease.

CHEMOPREVENTION TRIALS

5-α Reductase Inhibitors

- Two clinical trials have evaluated the ability of 5-α reductase inhibitors to prevent CaP in asymptomatic men older than 50 years, although neither is approved for this purpose.
- In the Prostate Cancer Prevention trial, finasteride was compared to placebo in more than 9,000 men. There was a reduction in the incidence of CaP from 24.8% in the placebo arm to 18.4% in the finasteride arm within 7 years ($P < 0.001$).
- In the REDUCE trial, 8,321 men randomized to receive either dutasteride or placebo. Again, there was a reduction in the incidence of CaP in the treatment arm by 22.8% over the 4-year study period ($P < 0.001$).

- Both of these prevention studies found an increase in the percentage of aggressive tumors (Gleason score 7 to 10) in patients treated with the respective 5-α reductase inhibitors compared to the placebo. Subsequent pathology reviews of prostatectomy specimens did not confirm this increase, indicating potential sampling bias in the biopsies, perhaps due to a preferential reduction in normal versus tumor tissue caused by the effect of the 5-α reductase inhibitors.
- The US Food and Drug Administration (FDA) does not endorse either finasteride or dutasteride for the prevention of prostate cancer.

SCREENING

- Screening for CaP involves testing for levels of PSA and/or DRE. Screening of asymptomatic men is controversial. Debate centers on whether biologically and clinically significant cancers are being detected early enough to reduce mortality or, conversely, whether cancers detected by screening would cause clinically significant disease if left undetected and untreated. Autopsy series have shown that more men die with, rather than from, CaP, and the rate of occult CaP in men in their 80s is approximately 75%.
- The Prostate, Lung, Colon, and Ovary (PLCO) screening trial and the European Study on Screening for Prostate Cancer are evaluating clinical outcomes based on screening versus no screening. Data from the PLCO trial reveal that the rate of death from CaP was very low and did not differ significantly between subjects assigned to screening ($n = 38,340$) or no screening ($n = 38,343$), with nearly 15 years of follow-up. Despite these two large studies the evidence does not clearly support uniform population-based screening practices using PSA.
- Data from the European study suggest that PSA screening was associated with a reduction in the rate of death from CaP by 21% after a median follow-up of 13 years. These data indicate 781 men would need to be screened and 27 additional cases of CaP would need to be treated to prevent one death from CaP. Contamination from PSA screening outside the trial were less likely in Europe and could explain the differences with this study and the PLCO study.
- Controversy surrounds screening recommendations for prostate cancer in the United States. As of 2012, the US Prevention Services Task force recommends against PSA screening.
- The American Cancer Society suggests patients make an informed decision about PSA screening after a discussion with their health-care provider. Such decisions should be at age 50 for men who are healthy and expect to live 10 more years, at age 45 for men who are at high risk (African American or those with a first-degree relative having prostate cancer at an age under 65) or 40 for the highest-risk patients (multiple first-degree relatives having prostate cancer at an age under 65).
  - Most advocates of screening acknowledge the limited benefits in men who are over 75 years of age or men with less than 10 years of projected survival due to other comorbidities. It is likely that most men who fall in this category will not have their lifespan limited by CaP and thus screening may be unnecessary.

SIGNS AND SYMPTOMS

- Even with declines in PSA screening in the United States, most men are asymptomatic at diagnosis.
- Patients with local or regional disease may be asymptomatic or have lower urinary tract symptoms similar to those of benign prostatic hypertrophy or occasionally hematuria.
- Symptoms of metastatic disease include bone pain, changes in urination patterns, and weight loss; spinal cord compression is a rare but serious complication of metastatic disease.

WORKUP AND STAGING
Biopsy

- Abnormal PSA and/or DRE is followed by transrectal ultrasound with core biopsy. Historically, a PSA of >4 ng/mL was the threshold for biopsy, but current data suggest that cancers can be seen with lower PSA levels. In recent years a greater emphasis has also been placed on rate of PSA rise as a trigger for biopsy. A negative biopsy should prompt reassessment in 6 months with repeat biopsy as needed.

▪ There is an evolving role for combining magnetic resonance imaging (MRI) and ultrasound guided prostate biopsy in the diagnosis of prostate cancer. As opposed to random biopsies of the prostate, data from MRI imaging of the prostate is used to identify anatomic regions in the prostate that likely contain tumor. These regions can be deliberately oversampled during the biopsy procedure (informed biopsy) or using software that creates a fusion of the MRI image with real-time ultra sound, a targeted biopsy of the intraprostatic tumor can be done.

Pathology

▪ Ninety-five percent of CaPs are adenocarcinomas. Adenocarcinoma arises in the peripheral zone of the prostate in approximately 70% of patients.

▪ Small cell variants of prostate cancer are very rare and characterized by aggressive tumors with increased likelihood to have soft tissue metastasis, especially to the liver. These tumors may be more susceptible to DNA damaging agents (PARP-inhibitors or platinum agents) although randomized data in this population is lacking. It is important to note that adenocarcinoma with "neuroendocrine features" is more common than small cell variants and should be treated primarily as adenocarcinoma.

▪ Sarcoma, lymphoma, small cell carcinoma, and transitional carcinoma of the prostate are rare.

▪ Primary and secondary Gleason grades are determined by the histologic architecture of biopsy tissue. The primary grade denotes the dominant histologic pattern; the secondary grade represents the bulk of the nondominant pattern or a focal high-grade area. Primary and secondary grades range from 1 (well differentiated) to 5 (poorly differentiated). The combined grades comprise the GS (range 2 to 10). Gleason 6 or less are considered low risk, Gleason 7 is considered intermediate risk, and Gleason 8 to 10 is considered high risk.

▪ A new grading system has been proposed and is being increasingly incorporated into pathologic review of prostate tumors. This system is designed to subdivide Gleason 7 based on morphology and dominant pathology and perhaps separate Gleason 8 from Gleason 9 and 10.
  ● There is no role in re-evaluating GS once treatment has begun.

▪ At diagnosis, because of sampling bias, GS may change following radical prostatectomy (RP) (20% of scores are upgraded and up to 10% are downgraded).

▪ Prostatic intraepithelial neoplasia (PIN), and perhaps proliferative inflammatory atrophy (PIA), are considered precursor lesions.

Baseline Evaluation

▪ In candidates for local treatment, a bone scan is indicated for patients with bone pain, T3 or T4, GS >7, or PSA >10 ng/mL. There is no clinical evidence that a baseline bone scan improves survival in populations with better prognostic factors.

▪ In candidates for surgery, computed tomography (CT) or magnetic resonance imaging (MRI) of the abdomen and pelvis is obtained for T3 and T4 lesions, PSA >20 ng/mL, or GS >7 to detect enlarged lymph nodes. Endorectal MRI may help in determining the presence of extraprostatic extension. CT scans aid in treatment planning for radiation therapy (RT).

▪ Baseline laboratory tests include complete blood count, creatinine level, PSA (if not yet done), testosterone, and alkaline phosphatase level.

PROGNOSTIC FACTORS

▪ Stage at diagnosis
▪ Gleason Score
▪ PSA level
▪ Number of cores and percentage of each core involved

- Age at diagnosis
- Inherited genomic abnormalities

TREATMENT OF LOCALIZED DISEASE

Active Surveillance

For men aged 60 to 75 years with a >10-year life expectancy or low-grade (GS ≤ 6), T1c-T2a tumors, active surveillance is a reasonable alternative to immediate local therapy. In addition, men aged 50 to 60 years with those same features and low-volume (<3 cores, <50% of any one core involved) tumor may also be candidates for active surveillance. For patients with a <10-year life expectancy, CaP-specific mortality is very low and local definitive therapy may not be appropriate.

Surgery

Radical Prostatectomy

- Approaches include retropubic (RRP), perineal (RPP), or laparoscopic, with the latter often done with robotic assistance (RALP). Typical hospital stays are 1 to 2 days, with 7 to 14 days of urethral catheterization. Surgeries are somewhat longer with RALP, but hospital stays are usually shorter.
- Pelvic lymph node dissection may be performed at the time of RP in patients at high risk of developing positive lymph nodes, but may not be necessary in patients with T1c disease, PSA <10 ng/mL, and GS <7.
- Nerve-sparing RP may conserve potency in men with disease not adjacent to the neurovascular bundles that travel posterior-lateral to the prostate. The bilateral nerve-sparing technique is associated with 60% to 90% of patients recovering spontaneous erections versus only 10% to 50% with the unilateral technique. Both groups, however, may respond to oral therapy for erectile dysfunction.
- There is no role for neoadjuvant androgen-deprivation therapy (ADT) prior to RP, although ongoing studies in high-risk patients are evaluating ADT with modern antiandrogens (enzalutamide and abiraterone) to determine the potential to decrease or eliminate tumor prior to RP.
- Patients with microscopic lymph node metastasis diagnosed following RP may have a longer overall survival (OS) if given ADT rather than at time of clinical recurrence/metastatic disease.
- Salvage RP following RT may be done in select cases where local disease is organ confined. However, salvage RP is more technically demanding and is associated with higher morbidity.

Surgical Complications

- Immediate morbidity or mortality: less than 10%.
- Impotence: 20% to 60%, varying with age and extent of disease.
- Urinary incontinence: improves with time, generally less than 10% to 15% 2 years after surgery.
- Urinary structure: approximately 10%, most can be managed with simple dilatation.
- Inguinal Hernia: approximately 10%, but substantially less with minimally invasive surgery.
- The Prostate Cancer Outcomes Study found statistically significant differences in outcomes following RP or RT. For patients with normal baseline function, RP was associated with inferior urinary function, better bowel function, and similar sexual dysfunction compared with RT.

Radiation Therapy

Radiation Therapy as Definitive Therapy

- External beam RT (EBRT) targets the whole prostate, frequently including a margin of extraprostatic tissue, seminal vesicles, and pelvic lymph nodes.
- Higher doses given over approximately 8 weeks are associated with higher PSA control rates, but shorter courses of therapy are also under investigation.
- Three-dimensional (3D) conformal RT allows for maximal doses conforming to the treatment field, while sparing normal tissue.

▪ Intensity-modulated RT is a type of 3D conformal RT that is designed to conform even more precisely to the target.
▪ Proton beam irradiation focuses virtually greater energy within a very small area, thus theoretically minimizing damage to normal tissue.
▪ Stereotactic body radiotherapy (SBRT) may allow for higher doses of radiation to be given in less fractions.
▪ There is incomplete data comparing EBRT, proton and SBRT at this time and so patients should have discussions about the relative benefits of these options with their radiation oncologists.

RT with Adjuvant ADT

At least three randomized controlled trials have shown that combining ADT with RT in patients at high risk for recurrent disease (Table 14.1) improves OS. ADT is usually given during RT and for 2 to 3 years thereafter. It may also be used for 2 months prior to RT to help decrease tumor size and thus the target volume of RT. For patients with intermediate risk disease, 6 months of ADT has demonstrated improved outcomes as well.

RT with Adjuvant ADT and Chemotherapy

A randomized phase III trial suggested that in high risk patients, six infusions of docetaxel 75 mg/m^2 administered in 21-day cycles with prednisone starting 28 days after RT improved 4-year OS (93% vs. 86%; HR 0.49 using a one-sided 0.05 type I error and 90% power). One key limitation of this study was the use of a one-sided type I error, raising concerns about the robustness of the data. It remains unclear how widely adopted this approach is, but longer follow-up will certainly be of interest.

Brachytherapy

Interstitial brachytherapy with radioactive palladium or iodine seeds that delivers a much higher dose of radiation to the prostate is used in CaP patients with low-risk tumors and some intermediate-risk patients. Better definitions of tumor volume and radiation dosimetry have made this outpatient technique more accurate. CT and/or transrectal ultrasound are used to guide seed placement.

Combined EBRT and Brachytherapy

EBRT followed by brachytherapy boost is an increasingly used strategy. Preliminary clinical data support the safety and efficacy of this approach in a selected population of patients, but long-term follow-up and head to head comparisons is lacking. Nonetheless, many radiation oncologists are using this treatment combination in patients with high-risk disease.

TABLE 14.1 Risk Categories for Post-therapy Prostate-Specific Antigen Failure

	Low[a]	Intermediate[b]	High[b]
Stage	T1c, T2a	T2b	T2c
PSA	<10	10–20	>20
Gleason score	≤6	7	≥8

[a] All parameters required.

[b] Only one parameter required.

Adapted from D'Amico AV, Whittington R, Malkowicz SB, et al. Optimizing patient selection for dose escalation techniques using the prostate-specific antigen level, biopsy Gleason score, and clinical T-stage. *Int J Radiat Oncol Biol Phys.* 1999;45(5):1227–1233.

Adjuvant RT

- General indications for the use of adjuvant RT after RP include positive surgical margins, seminal vesicle involvement, and evidence of extracapsular extension. Nonetheless, the potential for cure with adjuvant RT will vary significantly from patient to patient and thus the risks and benefits of adjuvant RT should be evaluated in each case individually. Some studies have indicated that lower PSA and Gleason score have been associated with better disease-free survival.

Salvage RT

For select patients with rising PSA after RP and a high likelihood of organ-confined local recurrence (e.g., PSA <1.0 and slowly rising), salvage RT may be considered. However, there are limited data on which to make recommendations.

Complications of RT

Acute (Typically Resolve within 4 Weeks)

- Cystitis
- Proctitis/enteritis
- Fatigue

Long Term

- Impotence (30% to 45%)
- Incontinence (3%)
- Frequent bowel movements (10% more than with RP)
- Urethral stricture (RT delayed 4 weeks after transurethral resection of the prostate).

Focal Therapy for Disease Confined to a Region of the Prostate

Focal therapy for newly diagnosed CaP confined to a limited area of the prostate remains investigational. This strategy is different from other therapies for localized disease in that only a focal region of the prostate, as opposed to the entire glad, is targeted with hopes of limiting side effects. Cryosurgery destroys CaP cells through probes that subject prostate tissue to freezing followed by thawing. This procedure is associated with the high rates of erectile dysfunction due to freezing of the neurovascular bundle. Additional focal therapy strategies include thermal ablation via laser or high-intensity focused ultrasound among other techniques. There are limited data in highly selected populations on long-term outcomes for focal therapy. Thus, at most centers prostate focal therapies are largely reserved for consideration as salvage procedures.

COMPARISON OF PRIMARY TREATMENT MODALITIES

Comparing treatment modalities in terms of overall and disease-free survival is difficult because of the differences in study design, patient selection, and treatment techniques. Randomized trials are difficult to accrue to as patient choice for radiation or surgery can often not be overcome. Historical comparisons are flawed because patients with more comorbidities or advanced age often get radiation.

- While there are no satisfactory randomized trials comparing RT with RP, these approaches appear to have similar PSA-free survival (also called biochemical relapse-free survival) in appropriately matched patients at 5 years, but differ in type and frequency of side effects.
- In recent years, high risk patients who previously were treated predominantly with radiation and adjuvant ADT are increasingly having surgery. To some degree this is related to the emergence of MRI imaging where discrete lesions and possible extracapsular extension is better defined. Longer follow-up is required to determine the impact of surgery in this population.

FOLLOW-UP AFTER DEFINITIVE TREATMENT

- Patients treated with curative intent should have PSA levels checked at least every 6 months for 5 years, then annually. Annual DRE is appropriate for detecting recurrence.
- After RP, a detectable PSA suggests a relapse. PSA failure after RT is defined as 2 ng/mL over the nadir, whether or not the patient had ADT with RT.

TREATMENT FOR MEN WITH RISING PSA AFTER LOCAL THERAPY

- Treatment for patients who have rising PSA (biochemical failure) after local therapy has not been standardized and clinical trial data is incomplete (Fig. 14.1).
- Salvage RT, salvage RP, or salvage focal therapy (as previously described) may be offered to select patients with local recurrence.
- Men may live more than a decade after biochemical failure, thus a more conservative approach (e.g., surveillance, treating when symptomatic or based on PSA velocity) is a reasonable option for many men.
- Using PSA doubling time (i.e., less than 3 to 6 months) as a trigger to initiate ADT is frequently done in clinical practice; however, no randomized trials have prospectively evaluated this approach.

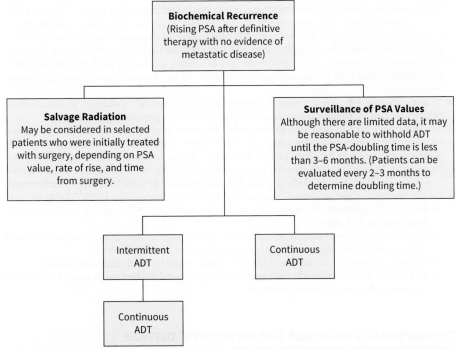

FIGURE 14.1 Treatment options for biochemical recurrence/nonmetastatic castration-sensitive prostate cancer. Continuous ADT employs repeated doses of GnRH agonists/antagonists to provide a constant testosterone suppression. Orchiectomy would also be an option. Intermittent ADT employs two or three-month doses of testosterone-lowering therapy, which are then discontinued if the PSA declines as expected. From there, PSA slowly recovers, lagging behind testosterone recovery. In selected patients, this approach can be used to alleviate some ADT toxicity. ADT is often reinstituted based on a PSA doubling time similar to the "surveillance of PSA" approach described in the figure.

Retrospective data suggests that a PSA doubling time of less than 3 to 6 months may be associated with development of metastatic disease visible on conventional imaging.

- ADT effectively lowers PSA; however, there are no definitive data indicating better survival with ADT than with no ADT in biochemical recurrent prostate cancer.
- Randomized data from over 1,300 subjects demonstrated that ADT given intermittently (in 8-month cycles) was non-inferior to continuous ADT in terms of OS. Intermittent ADT was predictably associated with better quality of life outcomes.
- Emerging imaging platforms that are more sensitive at detecting (micro) metastatic disease may alter how this stage of disease is managed in the future.

TREATMENT OF SYSTEMIC DISEASE EVOLUTION OF RESPONSE CRITERIA IN METASTATIC DISEASE

The Prostate Cancer Working Group 3 and the Implications for Clinical Practice

- As the understanding of CaP has evolved in the past decade, in the context of new available therapies and greater experience with older therapies, a consensus was generated by Prostate Cancer Working Group 3 (PSWG3) on determining response in clinical trials.
- Perhaps most importantly, PSA should not be used as the sole criteria to discontinue a therapy. Furthermore, the PSWG3 recommends that early changes in PSA and modest increases in pain, which could represent a tumor flare phenomenon, should not result in the discontinuation of therapy. This is especially important because PSA was not solely used to evaluate response of some of the latest therapies, thus discontinuing based on PSA alone could diminish the expected benefits of some therapies.
- For patients with metastatic CaP, objective changes on imaging studies (CT and bone scan) should be the primary criteria used to assess progression of disease in the absence of clear clinical progression of symptoms.
- To assess imaging, lymph nodes must be greater than 2 cm at baseline. In addition, physician discretion can be used for baseline lymph nodes less than 1.0 cm that grow to larger than 1.5 cm.
- Two new bone lesions on bone scan are required to document progressive disease, with one important exception. New lesions on the first bone scan should trigger another bone scan 6 or more weeks later, as these new lesions may have been present on the first scan, but missed on initial imaging or they may represent the "tumor flare phenomenon." If the second (and subsequent) bone scans show less than two new lesions and the patient is otherwise clinically stable, he should be considered to have stable disease.
- For the treatment of patients outside of clinical trials the implications of the PCWG3 are as follows:
  - Radiographic response criteria should be used to determine disease progression in metastatic CaP as opposed to PSA alone.
  - Initial changes on bone scan are not sufficient to remove patients from a treatment; patients could continue therapy if subsequent bone scans show less than two new lesions.
  - Changes in lymph nodes less than 2 cm in diameter should be interpreted with caution.
  - PSA should still be followed but interpreted with caution and not be used as a singular criteria to determine when to discontinue a therapy.

THERAPEUTIC STRATEGIES FOR METASTATIC DISEASE ANDROGEN-DEPRIVATION THERAPY

- ADT is the mainstay of treatment for metastatic CaP (Table 14.2), in addition to its potential role with localized disease and in neoadjuvant and adjuvant setting with RT.
- Bilateral surgical castration and depot injections of GnRH agonists (e.g., leuprolide, goserelin, and buserelin) and a GnRH antagonist (degarelix) provide equally effective testosterone suppression. Combined androgen blockade can be achieved by adding an oral androgen receptor antagonist (ARA; e.g., nilutamide, flutamide, and bicalutamide). However, this is controversial and provides little if any definitive survival benefit.

TABLE 14.2 Systemic Therapies for Prostate Cancer

Treatment	Dose	Most Common Side Effects
Bilateral orchiectomy	N/a	Impotence, loss of libido, gynecomastia, hot flashes, and osteoporosis
GnRH agonists (most common formulations)		
Goserelin acetate (Zoladex)	3.6 mg SC every month or 10.8 mg SC every 3 mo	Potential for tumor flare due to transient initial increase in testosterone, loss of libido, gynecomastia, hot flashes, and osteoporosis
Leuprolide acetate (Lupron)	7.5 mg SC every month or 22.5 mg i.m. every 3 mo, or 30 mg SC every 4 mo	Potential for tumor flare due to transient initial increase in testosterone, loss of libido, gynecomastia, hot flashes, and osteoporosis
GnRH agonist		
Degarelix (Firmagon)	240 mg SC initial dose followed by 80 mg SC every 28 d	Hot flashes, weight gain, erectile dysfunction, loss of libido, hypertension, hepatotoxicity, gyecomastia, and osteoporosis
Androgen receptor antagonists (ARAs)		
Bicalutamide (Casodex)	50 mg PO daily	Nausea, breast tenderness, hepatotoxicity, hot flashes, loss of libido, and impotence
Flutamide (Eulexin)	250 mg PO three times per day	Diarrhea, nausea, breast tenderness, hepatotoxicity, loss of libido, and impotence
Nilutamide (Nilandron)	150 mg PO daily	Visual field changes (night blindness or abnormal adaptation to darkness), hepatotoxicity, impotence, loss of libido, hot flashes, nausea, disulfiram-like reaction, and pulmonary fibrosis (rare)
Androgen biosynthesis inhibitors		
Ketoconazole (Nizoral)	200 or 400 mg PO 3 times a day with hydrocortisone 20 mg PO in the morning and 10 mg in the evening. (Ketoconazole is absorbed at an acidic pH; therefore, the concomitant use of H_2 blockers, antacids, or proton pump inhibitors should be avoided.)	Adrenal insufficiency is limited with physiologic dosing of hydrocortisone. Other side effects include impotence, pruritus, nail changes, adrenal insufficiency, nausea, emesis, and hepatotoxicity. (Ketoconazole is a potent inhibitor of CYP3A4, and thus multiple drug interactions are possible so review of medications is important.)
Abiraterone (Zytiga)	1,000 mg PO daily (on an empty stomach) Taken with prednisone 5 mg PO twice a day	Peripheral edema, hypertension, fatigue, hypokalemia, hypernatremia, increased triglycerides, hepatotoxicity, and hot flashes. (Abiraterone is a potent inhibitor of CYP3A4, and thus multiple drug interactions are possible, so review of medications is important.)

(continued)

TABLE 14.2 (Continued)

Treatment	Dose	Most Common Side Effects
Androgen receptor inhibitor		
Enzaluatmide	160 mg PO once daily	Fatigue, hot flashes, diarrhea, peripheral edema, fatigue, arthralgia, and musculoskeletal pain. Limited risk of seizures (less than 1%) but care should be taken in patients with seizure history or those who are on medications that may lower the seizure threshold
Immunotherapy		
Sipuleucel-T (Provenge)	Infusion of ≥50 million autologous CD54+ cells after ex vivo cellular processing given every 2 wk for three total doses	Fatigue, fever, chills, headache, nausea, emesis, myalgias, and infusion reaction symptoms
Chemotherapy regimens		
Docetaxel (Taxotere)	75 mg mg/m^2 IV every 21 d with prednisone 5 mg PO twice daily	Granulocytopenia, infection, anemia, fatigue, anemia, neutropenia, fluid retention, sensory neuropathy, nausea, fatigue, myalgia, and alopecia
Cabazitaxel (Jevtana)	25 mg mg/m^2 IV every 21 d with prednisone 5 mg PO twice daily	Myelosuppression, infection, fatigue/weakness, fever, diarrhea, nausea, emesis, peripheral neuropathy, arthralgias, peripheral edema, alopecia, and dyspepsia
Mitoxantrone (Novantrone)	12–14 mg mg/m^2 IV every 21 d with prednisone 5 mg PO twice daily	Edema, myelosuppresion, cardiac toxicity, fever, fatigue, alopecia, nausea, diarrhea, infection, and hepatotoxicity
Docetaxel (Taxotere) + carboplatin (Paraplatin)	Docetaxel at 60 mg/m^2 with carboplatin AUC 4 every 21 d with daily prednisone 5 mg PO twice daily	Myelosuppression, infection, hyperglycemia, hypoglycemia, pain, renal failure, and thrombosis. (These were seen in limited experience with 34 patients.)
Radiopharmaceuticals		
Radium 223	6 monthly infusions at 55 kBq (1.49 microcurie) per kg IV	Myelosuppression, nausea, diarrhea, emesis, peripheral edema

- GnRH agonists initially increase gonadotropin, causing a transient (~14 day) increase in testosterone that can lead to tumor flare. Tumor flare can be prevented by the use of an ARA, which binds to the androgen receptor (AR), effectively stopping the ability of the AR to activate cell growth. An ARA is often given for 1 to 2 weeks prior to GnRH agonist in patients at risk for complications (pain, obstruction, and cord compression) associated with tumor flare. For high-risk patients, bilateral orchiectomy can decrease testosterone more quickly.
- The use of the GnRH antagonist (degarelix) obviates the concern for tumor flare as it leads to more rapid reduction in testosterone without an initial increase in serum testosterone levels. For this reason, it may be preferred in the setting of initial treatment for men diagnosed with symptomatic metastatic disease.
  - CaP cells generally respond to ADT, producing durable remissions and significant palliation. Duration of response ranges from 12 to 18 months, with a limited number of patients having a complete biochemical response for several years. Ultimately, for most patients CRPC cells emerge and lead to disease progression.

- Continuing testosterone suppression after patients develop CRPC is also considered the standard of care for both nonmetastatic and metastatic disease. Androgens still play a very important role in driving the growth of CRPC, as evidenced by the benefits seen with new antiandrogen therapy (enzalutamide and abiraterone) in metastatic CRPC (mCRPC). Levels of AR and intracellular androgens within the tumor cells are significantly elevated in these patients and thus continuing ADT indefinitely in CRPC is recommended.

TREATMENT FOR METASTATIC CASTRATION-SENSITIVE PROSTATE CANCER

- This population of patients develop metastatic disease with normal levels of testosterone (i.e., while not on therapy with ADT). This population includes men who have metastatic disease at their primary diagnosis or those who develop it while in the follow-up after definitive therapy but are not receiving ADT.
- A randomized study ($n = 790$) established that six infusions of docetaxel (75 mg/m^2 every 3 weeks) substantially improved overall survival in this population 57.6 versus 44.0 months (HR 0.61). (Daily prednisone was not required.)
- Docetaxel was required to be initiated within 120 days of starting ADT in this population.
- A subgroup analysis with longer follow-up has suggested that patients with low volume disease (less than four bone lesions, no visceral disease or no disease beyond the spine or pelvis) did not benefit from the addition of docetaxel to ADT, perhaps calling into question the benefits in the "low volume" population.
- Emerging data from two additional studies in this population also indicates that abiraterone with ADT is superior to ADT alone. There is no clear evidence at this time as to which treatment, abiraterone or docetaxel is superior with ADT in this population.

TREATMENT OF NONMETASTATIC CASTRATION-RESISTANT PROSTATE CANCER AND THE USE OF SECOND-LINE ARAS

- Through the development of resistance mechanisms such as upregulation of the AR or intratumoral production of androgens, patients may develop progressive disease despite castration levels of testosterone (CRPC).
- For patients with a rising PSA but no evidence of metastatic disease ARAs can be added to ADT to provide a combined androgen blockade, which may delay disease progression or the development of metastasis.
- Upon progression of disease with ARA and ADT, it is important to note that up to 20% of patients treated with combined androgen blockade have a PSA decline of ≥50% upon discontinuation of oral ARA (range, 15% to 33%), although these declines generally last only 3 to 5 months. This proportion may be lower with shorter-term use ARA use. This ARA withdrawal response occurs within 4 to 6 weeks, depending on the ARA's half-life.
- Some patients with rising PSA (and still no evidence of metastasis) after ARA withdrawal may benefit from switching to other ARAs or initiating treatment with ketoconazole. A proportion of patients (35% to 50%) will have PSA declines with second-line and even third-line antiandrogen therapy.
- Emerging data suggests enzalutamide induces superior progression-free survival relative to bicalutamude in nonmetastatic castration resistant prostate cancer.

TREATMENT FOR METASTATIC CASTRATION-RESISTANT PROSTATE CANCER

Multiple treatment options are now available for the treatment of mCRPC as opposed to prior to 2010 when only docetaxel had demonstrated the ability to extend survival in this population. Given multiple forms of therapy including immunotherapy, chemotherapy, radiopharmaceuticals, and modern antiandrogen therapy, symptoms and pace of disease will likely dictate which treatments are most appropriate for each individual patient. At this time no standard sequence of therapy has been demonstrated as most effective (Fig. 14.2).

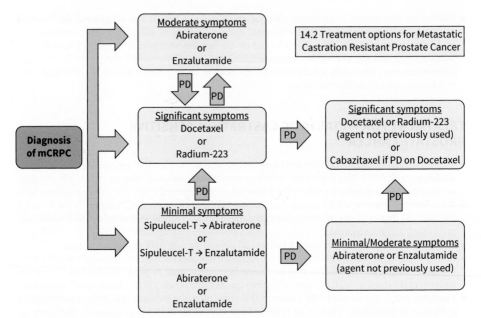

FIGURE 14.2 Suggested treatment approach for patients with metastatic castration-resistant prostate cancer. At this time there is no clear data on the optimal sequence in mCRPC. One strategy is to base treatment of mCRPC on presenting symptoms of the patient, selecting therapies that are less toxic for patients with minimal symptoms. Pace of disease should also be factored in, as rapidly progressing disease may require earlier chemotherapy, even before the onset of significant symptoms. Also, a brief previous response to ADT should temper the expectations for subsequent abiraterone or enzalutamide, as these particular disease manifestations may not be as dependent on the androgen receptor pathway for growth.

Immunotherapy

- Sipuleucel-T (Provenge)—is an activated cellular therapy that is derived from a patient's own immune cells, which are collected via leukapheresis. Once removed from circulation, the peripheral immune cells are sent to a central processing facility where they are exposed to a fusion peptide of PAP-GMCSF for 48 hours. The goal is to activate immune cells via ex vivo processing so that when they are reinfused into the patient, they generate an immune-mediated antitumor response.
- Although sipuleucel-T has been shown to improve survival versus placebo (25.8 vs. 21.7 months; HR 0.77; $P = 0.02$), it does not change short-term disease progression or cause decreases in PSA in most patients. For this reason, sipuleucel-T should ideally be followed by another therapy to provide short-term control and allow for the potential long-term effects, which can potentially improve survival. Patients whose disease on scans, PSA, and symptoms all remain stable after sipuleucel-T could be followed up closely until one of those parameters dictates the initiation of a subsequent therapy.
- Sipuleucel-T is indicated in patients with minimal symptoms related to their CaP. Although sipuleucel-T can be given 3 months after chemotherapy, given its delayed effects, it would seem most appropriate to give this treatment prior to chemotherapy.

Androgen Biosynthesis Inhibitor

- Abiraterone (Zytiga) is a selective and irreversible CYP17 inhibitor and significantly reduces secondary androgen production (including testosterone precursors dehydroepiandrosterone and androstenedione) from the adrenal glands and likely within CaP cells.

- Abiraterone has demonstrated improved OS in mCRPC patients relative to placebo regardless of previous chemotherapy.
- Abiraterone can be used in mCRPC patients who are chemotherapy-naïve and who have mild pain from their metastatic disease. It has been shown to delay the need for narcotics in this population.
- Abiraterone has also been shown to improve pain and quality of life in patients who have already received chemotherapy.
- Abiraterone requires co-administration of prednisone (10 mg daily) to limit treatment-related toxicity.

Androgen Receptor Inhibitor

- Enzaluatmide (Xtandi) is a modern version of the ARAs previously discussed although this agent has broader anti-AR properties beyond binding to the AR with greater binding affinity. It also significantly reduces AR translocation to the nucleus and limits DNA binding, and inhibits coactivator recruitment and receptor-mediated DNA transcription. In addition, enzalutamide has not demonstrated any agonist properties unlike previous ARAs.
- Like abiraterone, enzalutamide has demonstrated efficacy compared to placebo in men with mCRPC regardless of previous chemotherapy and can improve moderate levels of pain.
- Unlike abiraterone, enzalutamide does not require daily prednisone.
- Enzalutamide should not be used in patients with a seizure history or medications that may substantially lower the seizure threshold.

CHEMOTHERAPY FOR MCRPC

In spite of the advent of new antiandrogen therapies for mCRPC, chemotherapy is still important in treating symptomatic disease.

- Docetaxel (Taxotere)
  - Improved median OS from 16.5 months (mitoxantrone/prednisone) to 18.9 months ($P = 0.0005$) and improved quality of life (functional assessment of cancer therapy-prostate, 22% vs. 13%; $P = 0.009$). Although the absolute magnitude of the difference between the two arms was less than 3 months, it is important to note that the study did employ a cross-over meaning that patients not randomized to docetaxel initially may have received docetaxel when they had progressive disease.
  - Docetaxel is perhaps most appropriate for patients with mCRPC who have intermediate or significant levels of symptoms.
  - Docetaxel would also be a reasonable option for patients with rapidly progressing disease as determined by objective changes on imaging.
- Cabazitaxel (Jevtana)
  - This treatment became the second chemotherapy approved for CaP. A phase III study trial compared this taxane with mitoxantrone in patients who already received docetaxel. (Prednisone 5 mg twice daily was also given in both groups.) Cabazitaxel improved time to progression 2.8 versus 1.4 months ($P < 0.0001$) but also met the primary endpoint of the trial by extending survival 15.1 versus 12.7 months ($P < 0.0001$).
  - It is important to note that there was an 8% incidence of febrile neutropenia, and 2% of patients died from neutropenia-related infections. Thus serious consideration should be given for the use of growth factor support in appropriate patients.
  - A study comparing docetaxel and cabazitaxel as frontline chemotherapy for mCRPC did not find that cabazitaxel was superior.
- Mitoxantrone (Novantrone) + prednisone
  - Shown to improve quality of life, but not disease-free survival or OS, in two earlier randomized controlled trials versus steroids alone.
  - Mitoxantrone is stopped at a cumulative dose of 140 mg/m². Prochlorperazine is used as an antiemetic.
  - Mitoxantrone may be appropriate for symptomatic patients who have either progressed on or who are not candidates for taxane-based chemotherapy regimens.

- Docetaxel (Taxotere) + carboplatin
  - A single-arm phase II trial of patients ($n = 34$) who progressed on docetaxel-based chemotherapy evaluated this combination and showed a partial response rate of 14% with a median progression-free survival of 3 months and an OS of 12.4 months.
  - This combination may be most appropriate in patients who have a small cell variant of CaP (~2% of patients).

RADIOPHARMACEUTICALS FOR METASTATIC PROSTATE CANCER

- The radioisotopes strontium-89 (Metastron) and Samarium-153 lexidronam (Quadramet) have previously demonstrated palliative benefits in mCRPC patients with bone disease, but were frequently associated with substantial myelosuppression.
- The alpha-emitting radium-223 (Xofigo) has demonstrated the ability to have palliative benefits and, unlike its predecessors, the ability to extend OS in mCRPC. This benefit was seen in symptomatic patients regardless of previous chemotherapy.
- Radium-223 has less impact on the bone marrow, because alpha particles have a limited destruction radius, but anemia, thrombocytopenia, and leukopenia can still be encountered.
- Ultimately, radium-223 is commonly reserved for late stage, symptomatic patients because of the historic role of radioisotopes in mCRPC, but earlier use may be warranted. Safety data has suggested radium-223 can be safely given with abiraterone and enzalutamide, but it remains unclear if either combination is more beneficial than sequential use.

Emerging Option: Poly (adenosine diphosphate [ADP]-ribose) polymerase (PARP)-Inhibitors

- As described above, increasing data is suggesting that both germline defects and mutations in the DNA repair pathway are present in a subset of men with prostate cancer.
- Early phase II data has suggested that prostate cancer patients with germline or somatic mutations overwhelming response rates to PARP-inhibitors.
- Larger studies are ongoing and the FDA has granted breakthrough therapy status to olaparib.

SUPPORTIVE MEASURES

- Hot flashes from hormonal therapy are most commonly treated with low-dose venlafaxine or gabapentin with variable success. The potential side effects of these medicines also have to be taken into account when using them to treat hot flashes.
- Painful gynecomastia, often seen when ARAs are used alone, can be prevented with EBRT to the breasts (2 to 5 fractions) or may be treated with tamoxifen.
- Testosterone-lowering therapy causes a decrease in estradiol, needed to maintain bone density, which may lead to osteoporosis. Many specialists recommend that patients receiving ADT should be given daily vitamin D and calcium supplements unless contraindicated. Obtain baseline bone mineral density before starting long-term ADT. Treatment with bisphosphonates should be considered in patients with low bone mineral density.

MANAGEMENT OF BONE METASTASES

- While narcotics can be used to alleviate bone pain, the anti-inflammatory effects of NSAIDs should not be overlooked in patients with bone metastasis as a first-line measure.
- RT directed to painful spinal cord metastases provides palliation in approximately 80% of patients. Side effects generally are limited to fatigue and anemia that are usually reversible. Generally, the painful vertebral lesion and the two vertebrae superior to and inferior to the lesion are treated with 30 Gy.

The spinal cord can tolerate radiation up to approximately 50 Gy, so retreatment of some lesions may be considered.

▪ Bisphosphonates inhibit osteoclastic bone resorption and can decrease skeletal-related events in patients with advanced metastatic CRPC. Zoledronic acid 4 mg IV every 3 to 4 weeks has been approved for this indication. Side effects include infusion-related myalgias, renal dysfunction, and osteonecrosis of the jaw. Dose should be adjusted for renal insufficiency.

▪ Denosumab (Xgeva) is a fully humanized antibody that binds to RANK-ligand that is crucial in the function of osteoclasts, which play a vital role in bone resorption. Even though it is mechanistically different from bisphosphonates, there is a similar incidence of osteonecrosis of the jaw.

▪ In light of the potential toxicity and the benefits, treatment with bisphosphonates or RANK-ligand inhibitor could be considered for patients with disease in the spine and other weight-bearing bones of the pelvis and lower extremities.

SPINAL CORD COMPRESSION

▪ Vertebral column metastases impinging on the spinal cord can cause spinal cord compression, an oncologic emergency common in patients with CaP who have widespread bone metastases.

▪ Pain is an early sign of spinal cord compression in more than 90% of patients. Muscle weakness or neurologic abnormalities are other indicators of spinal cord compression, along with weakness and/or sensory loss corresponding to the level of spinal cord compression, which often indicate irreversible damage. Genitourinary, gastrointestinal, and autonomic dysfunction are late signs; spinal cord compression usually progresses rapidly at this point.

▪ Diagnosis requires a thorough history and physical, with special attention to musculoskeletal and neurologic examinations. The standard for diagnosing and localizing spinal cord compression is MRI, usually with gadolinium. A myelogram may be used in patients with contraindications to MRI such as a pacemaker.

▪ High-dose steroids should be started (e.g., dexamethasone ≥24 mg IV followed by 4 mg IV or PO every 6 hours) as soon as history or neurologic examination suggests spinal cord compression.

▪ Neurologic/orthopedic surgeons and/or radiation oncologists should be consulted soon after diagnosis.

Suggested Readings

1. Antonarakis ES, Feng Z, Trock BJ, et al. The natural history of metastatic progression in men with prostate-specific antigen recurrence after radical prostatectomy: long-term follow-up. *BJU Int.* 2012;109(1):32–39.
2. Antonarakis ES, Lu C, Wang H, et al. AR-V7 and resistance to enzalutamide and abiraterone in prostate cancer. *N Engl J Med.* 2014;371(11):1028–1038.
3. Beer TM, Armstrong AJ, Rathkopf DE, et al. Enzalutamide in metastatic prostate cancer before chemotherapy. *N Engl J Med.* 2014;371(5):424–433.
4. Bolla M, Collette L, Blank L, et al. Long-term results with immediate androgen suppression and external irradiation in patients with locally advanced prostate cancer (an EORTC study): a phase III randomised trial. *Lancet.* 2002;360(9327):103–106.
5. Bolla M, Gonzalez D, Warde P, et al. Improved survival in patients with locally advanced prostate cancer treated with radiotherapy and goserelin. *N Engl J Med.* 1997;337(5):295–300.
6. Bolla M, van Poppel H, Tombal B, et al. Postoperative radiotherapy after radical prostatectomy for high-risk prostate cancer: long-term results of a randomised controlled trial (EORTC trial 22911). *Lancet.* 2012;380(9858):2018–2027.
7. Crawford ED, Eisenberger MA, McLeod DG, et al. A controlled trial of leuprolide with and without flutamide in prostatic carcinoma. *N Engl J Med.* 1989;321(7):419–424.
8. de Bono JS, Logothetis CJ, Molina A, et al. Abiraterone and increased survival in metastatic prostate cancer. *N Engl J Med.* 2011;364(21):1995–2005.
9. de Bono JS, Oudard S, Ozguroglu M, et al. Prednisone plus cabazitaxel or mitoxantrone for metastatic castration-resistant prostate cancer progressing after docetaxel treatment: a randomised open-label trial. *Lancet.* 2010;376(9747):1147–1154.
10. Eisenberger MA, Blumenstein BA, Crawford ED, et al. Bilateral orchiectomy with or without flutamide for metastatic prostate cancer. *N Engl J Med.* 1998;339(15):1036–1042.
11. Epstein JI, Zelefsky MJ, Sjoberg DD, et al. A contemporary prostate cancer grading system: A validated alternative to the Gleason score. *Eur Urol.* 2016 Mar;69(3):428–435.

12. Gleave M, Goldenberg L, Chin JL, et al. Natural history of progression after PSA elevation following radical prostatectomy: update. *J Urol.* 2003;169(4):A690.
13. Granfors T, Modig H, Damber JE, Tomic R. Combined orchiectomy and external radiotherapy versus radiotherapy alone for nonmetastatic prostate cancer with or without pelvic lymph node involvement: a prospective randomized study. *J Urol.* 1998;159(6):2030–2034.
14. Hanks GE, Pajak TF, Porter A, et al. Radiation Therapy Oncology Group. Phase III trial of long-term adjuvant androgen deprivation after neoadjuvant hormonal cytoreduction and radiotherapy in locally advanced carcinoma of the prostate: the Radiation Therapy Oncology Group Protocol 92-02. *J Clin Oncol.* 2003;21(21):3972–3978.
15. Hoskin PJ, Motohashi K, Bownes P, et al. High dose rate brachytherapy in combination with external beam radiotherapy in the radical treatment of prostate cancer: initial results of a randomized phase three trial. *Radiother Oncol.* 2007;84(2):114–120.
16. Hurwitz MD, Halabi S, Archer L, et al. Combination external beam radiation and brachytherapy boost with androgen deprivation for treatment of intermediate-risk prostate cancer: long-term results of CALGB 99809. *Cancer.* 2011;117(24):5579–5588.
17. Kantoff PW, Higano CS, Shore ND et al. Sipuleucel-T immunotherapy for castration-resistant prostate cancer. *N Engl J Med.* 2010;363(5):411–422.
18. Klotz L, Boccon-Gibod L, Shore ND, et al. The efficacy and safety of degarelix: a 12-month, comparative, randomized, open-label, parallel-group phase III study in patients with prostate cancer. *BJU Int.* 2008;11:1531–1538.
19. Lawton CA, Winter K, Murray K, et al. Updated results of the phase III Radiation Therapy Oncology Group (RTOG) trial 85-31 evaluating the potential benefit of androgen suppression following standard radiation therapy for unfavorable prognosis carcinoma of the prostate. *Int J Radiat Oncol Biol Phys.* 2001;49(4):937–946.
20. Lippman SM, Klein EA, Goodman PJ, et al. Effect of selenium and vitamin E on risk of prostate cancer and other cancers: the Selenium and Vitamin E Cancer Prevention Trial (SELECT). *JAMA.* 2009;301(1):39–51.
21. Mateo J, Carreira S, Sandhu S, et al. DNA-repair defects and olaparib in metastatic prostate cancer. *N Engl J Med.* 2015;373(18):1697–1708.
22. Messing E, Manola J, Sarosdy M, et al. Immediate hormonal therapy compared with observation after radical prostatectomy and pelvic lymphadenectomy in men with node positive prostate cancer: results at 10 years of EST 3886. *J Urol.* 2003;169(suppl 4):A1480.
23. Moyer VA, Force USPST. Screening for prostate cancer: U.S. Preventive Services Task Force recommendation statement. *Ann Intern Med.* 2012;157(2):120–134.
24. Na R, Zheng SL, Han M, et al. Germline Mutations in ATM and BRCA1/2 Distinguish Risk for Lethal and Indolent Prostate Cancer and are Associated with Early Age at Death. Eur Urol. 2016.
25. Nilsson S, Franzén L, Parker C, et al. Bone-targeted radium-223 in symptomatic, hormone-refractory prostate cancer: a randomised, multicentre, placebo-controlled phase II study. *Lancet Oncol.* 2007;8(7):587–594.
26. Parker C, Nilsson S, Heinrich D, et al. Alpha emitter radium-223 and survival in metastatic prostate cancer. *N Engl J Med.* 2013;369(3):213–223.
27. Pinsky PF, Prorok PC, Yu K, et al. Extended mortality results for prostate cancer screening in the PLCO trial with median follow-up of 15 years. *Cancer.* 2017;123(4):592–599.
28. Pritchard CC, Mateo J, Walsh MF, et al. Inherited DNA-repair gene mutations in men with metastatic prostate cancer. *N Engl J Med.* 2016;375(5):443–453.
29. Pilepich MV, Caplan R, Byhardt RW, et al. Phase III trial of androgen suppression using goserelin in unfavorable-prognosis carcinoma of the prostate treated with definitive radiotherapy: report of Radiation Therapy Oncology Group Protocol 85-31. *J Clin Oncol.* 1997;15(3):1013–1021.
30. Pilepich MV, Winter K, Lawton C, et al. Androgen suppression adjuvant to definitive radiotherapy in prostate carcinoma—long-term results of phase III RTOG 85-31. *Int J Radiat Oncol Biol Phys.* 2005;61(5):1285–1290.
31. Robinson D, Van Allen EM, Wu YM, et al. Integrative clinical genomics of advanced prostate cancer. *Cell.* 2015;161(5):1215–1228.
32. Ross RW, Beer TM, Jacobus S, et al. A phase 2 study of carboplatin plus docetaxel in men with metastatic hormone-refractory prostate cancer who are refractory to docetaxel. *Cancer.* 2008: 112(3):521–526.
33. Ryan CJ, Smith MR, Fizazi K, et al. Abiraterone acetate plus prednisone versus placebo plus prednisone in chemotherapy-naive men with metastatic castration-resistant prostate cancer (COU-AA-302): final overall survival analysis of a randomised, double-blind, placebo-controlled phase 3 study. *Lancet Oncol.* 2015;16(2):152–160.
34. Saad F, Gleason DM, Murray R, et al. A randomized, placebo-controlled trial of zoledronic acid in patients with hormone-refractory metastatic prostate carcinoma. *J Natl Cancer Inst.* 2002;94(19):1458–1468.
35. Sandler H, Hu C, Rosenthal S, Sartor O, Gomella L, Amin M. A phase III protocol of androgen suppression (AS) and 3DCRT/IMRT versus AS and 3DCRT/IMRT followed by chemotherapy (CT) with docetaxel and prednisone for localized, high-risk prostate cancer (RTOG 0521). *J Clin Oncol.* 2015;33(suppl):abstr LBA5002.

36. Scher HI, Fizazi K, Saad F, et al. Increased survival with enzalutamide in prostate cancer after chemotherapy. *N Engl J Med.* 2012;367(13):1187–1197.
37. Scher HI, Morris MJ, Stadler WM, et al. Trial design and objectives for castration-resistant prostate cancer: updated recommendations from the prostate cancer clinical trials working group 3. *J Clin Oncol.* 2016;34(12):1402–1418.
38. Schroder FH, Hugosson H, Roobol MJ, et al. Screening and prostate-cancer mortality in a randomized European study. *N Engl J Med.* 2009;360(13):1320–1328.
39. Smith MR, Saad F, Coleman R, et al. Denosumab and bone-metastasis-free survival in men with castration-resistant prostate cancer: results of a phase 3, randomised, placebo-controlled trial. *Lancet.* 2012;379(9810):39–46.
40. Siddiqui MM, Rais-Bahrami S, Turkbey B, et al. Comparison of MR/ultrasound fusion-guided biopsy with ultrasound-guided biopsy for the diagnosis of prostate cancer. *JAMA.* 2015;313(4):390–397.
41. Tannock IF, De Wit R, Berry WR, et al. Docetaxel plus prednisone or mitoxantrone plus prednisone for advanced prostate cancer. *N Engl J Med.* 2004;351(15):1502–1512.

15 Bladder Cancer

Andrea B. Apolo, Piyush K. Agarwal, and William L. Dahut

EPIDEMIOLOGY

Estimates are that in the United States, 79,030 individuals were diagnosed with bladder cancer in 2017, and that 16,870 died from the disease. Worldwide, more than 430,000 individuals are diagnosed with bladder cancer each year. The male:female ratio is 3:1, with a peak occurrence in the seventh decade of life, making bladder cancer the fourth and eighth most commonly diagnosed cancer in men and women, respectively.

ETIOLOGY

- Cigarette smoking is the most common cause of bladder cancer. In fact for smokers, the risk of developing bladder cancer is twice what it is for nonsmokers. Smoking explains a similar proportion of bladder cancer in both sexes (50% in men and 52% in women). The histology of both urothelial and squamous cell cancer (SCC) of the bladder reveals an association with the duration and amount of cigarette smoking.
- Occupational exposures to chemical carcinogens are associated with an increased risk of bladder cancer. Workers exposed to arylamines in the dye, paint, rubber, textile, and leather industries are at increased risk.
- Analgesics: The abuse of the analgesic phenacetin (banned by the U.S. Food and Drug Administration [FDA] in 1983) is associated with an increased risk of urothelial cancers, especially in the renal pelvis.
- Treatment-related risks: Prior treatment with pelvic radiation and cyclophosphamide increases the risk of urothelial cancers.
- Chronic infections or inflammation: In endemic areas, chronic infection with *Schistosoma haematobium* predisposes patients to develop SCC of the bladder due to squamous metaplasia, as well as urothelial carcinoma. Individuals with an ongoing source of inflammation (i.e., a chronic indwelling catheter) have a higher incidence of bladder cancer, especially SCC, than the general population. Progressive inflammation of the renal parenchyma also occurs in patients with Balkan nephropathy, predisposing patients to low-grade cancers of the upper urinary tract.
- Hereditary nonpolyposis colorectal cancer (HNPCC), or Lynch syndrome: An autosomal-dominant germline mutation in mismatch repair genes, predominantly in MSH2 rather than MSH1. HNPCC increases the lifetime risk of urothelial carcinoma of the ureter and renal pelvis. Individuals with HNPCC can develop upper urinary tract tumors at a younger age and an almost equal gender ratio compared to the general population.
- Thiazolidinediones such as pioglitazone and rosiglitazone used as second-line treatment of type II diabetes mellitus are associated with an increased risk of bladder cancer. In June 2011, the FDA warned that use of pioglitazone (Actos) for more than one year may be associated with an increased risk of bladder cancer.
- Arsenic-contaminated drinking water: Epidemiological studies provide solid evidence of the association of arsenic-contaminated drinking water and bladder cancer.

■ Aristolochic acid may be found in Chinese herbal remedies such as fangchi. It is associated with urothelial carcinoma, particularly upper-tract tumors. Aristolochic acid-associated tumors tend to develop in younger female patients.

PATHOLOGY

■ Most urothelial carcinomas originate in the bladder, but may also occur in the urethra or upper urinary tract, including the renal pelvis and ureter. These tumors are less common, accounting for 5% to 10% of all urothelial carcinomas.
■ Urothelial carcinoma, previously called transitional cell carcinoma, accounts for 90% to 95% of all bladder tumors in the United States. Other bladder cancer histologies include 5% SCC, 1% to 2% adenocarcinomas (including urachal), and approximately 1% small-cell tumors. Urothelial tumors often have divergent histologies, including urothelial carcinoma and squamous, sarcomatoid, adenocarcinoma, and/or nested micropapillary subtypes.
■ Carcinomas in situ (CIS) are flat tumors that usually present as diffuse urothelial involvement in patients with non–muscle-invasive bladder cancer (NMIBC). CIS increases the risk of subsequent invasive disease and recurrence, alone or in association with NMIBC.
■ Papillary tumors have a fibrovascular core and are typically raised on a stalk that can invaginate into the surface layer, lamina propria, or muscularis propria. They can be either low- or high-grade and have a risk of recurrence and progression over time.
■ Patients with upper-tract urothelial tumors have a 20% to 40% incidence of synchronous or metachronous bladder cancer. Patients with bladder cancer have about a 1% to 4% incidence of synchronous or metachronous upper-tract tumor.

CLINICAL FEATURES

■ Approximately 85% of patients have painless gross or microscopic hematuria; 20% of patients have symptoms of bladder irritability.
■ Patients with invasive disease may present with flank pain due to ureteral obstruction leading to hydronephrosis.
■ Patients with advanced disease may present with constitutional symptoms such as weight loss, abdominal pain, or bone pain.

SCREENING

Microscopic or gross hematuria is the most common presenting symptom in patients with bladder cancer. Studies evaluating the role of screening for bladder cancer have examined the utility of conventional Hemastix testing. However, because hematuria per se is nonspecific, patients who test positive for hematuria need to undergo further tests to determine its etiology. Other noninvasive screening methods include urine cytology or urine-based markers. Markers such as nuclear matrix protein 22, bladder-tumor antigen, cytokeratins, and many others have widely variable sensitivity and specificity. In contrast, fluorescence in situ hybridization (FISH) testing for four molecular alterations in urine (Urovysion) is extremely sensitive, with specificity rivaling urine cytology. However, FISH is expensive and can produce anticipatory positive results that predate the actual development of visible tumor. Therefore, definitive diagnosis is best established by cystoscopy and biopsy.

DIAGNOSIS AND STAGING WORKUP

■ Diagnostic workup of a patient with suspected bladder cancer should begin with an office cystoscopy and urine cytology.

- If a bladder mass is detected, the patient should undergo transurethral resection of the bladder tumor (TURBT) for full primary tumor staging. The TURBT specimen should include muscle to accurately assess the depth of tumor invasion. A repeat TURBT is recommended in the case of T1 high-grade disease, even if muscle is present in the specimen, as T1 tumors can be understaged by TURBT, and a repeat TURBT has prognostic value in predicting response to intravesical therapy.
- TURBT is performed with an examination under anesthesia (EUA). The EUA is important in clinical staging as it can detect locally advanced bladder cancer by assessing for invasion into adjacent organs, extravesical extension, and abdominal or pelvic sidewall extension. A bladder fixed on EUA suggests that it may be surgically unresectable.
- The upper tracts should also be evaluated by computerized tomography (CT) urography, ureteroscopy, retrograde pyelogram, intravenous pyelography, or magnetic resonance (MR) urogram. It is especially important to fully investigate the upper tracts of patients with positive cytology and normal cystoscopy. When CIS is detected, multiple random biopsies should be obtained to assess the extent of involvement.
- In patients with high-grade and/or invasive tumors, radiologic assessment should be performed with a high-resolution CT of the chest, abdomen, and pelvis with i.v. contrast, or MR of the abdomen and pelvis with gadolinium, and CT of the chest without i.v. contrast (if the patient has renal insufficiency) to assess for local lymph node involvement, upper tract disease, and distant metastases.
- The value of FDG-PET/CT for initial staging is still under investigation, but it appears to be a good adjunct (not a substitute) to anatomical imaging with high-resolution CT or MR.
- A ^{99m}Tc bone scan is recommended for patients with elevated blood alkaline phosphatase or bone pain. NaF-PET/CT to assess bone disease is also under investigation in bladder cancer.

TUMOR STAGING AND GRADING

- The staging of bladder cancer (Table 15.1) is the most important independent prognostic variable for progression and overall survival (OS). Bladder cancers are classified as non–muscle-invasive, muscle-invasive, and metastatic (Fig. 15.1).
- NMIBCs account for ~70% of all bladder cancers. They involve only the mucosa (Ta; ~60%) or submucosa (T1; ~30%) and flat CIS (Tis; ~ 0%). Most NMIBCs recur within 6 to 12 months at the same stage, but 10% to 15% of patients may develop invasive or metastatic disease.
- The grading of bladder cancer has prognostic significance for recurrence and progression of NMIBC. In 1973, the World Health Organization (WHO) graded tumors as papillomas and grade 1 to 3 urothelial tumors. In a 2004 revision of this system, the WHO classified papillomas as papillary urothelial neoplasms of low malignant potential. Grading of actual urothelial tumors was simplified to low-grade (WHO 1973 grade 1 or 2) or high-grade (WHO 1973 grade 2 or 3).
- Risk factors for recurrence and progression in NMIBC include high-grade disease, multifocal disease, tumors > 3 cm, CIS tumors, and T1 tumors.
- Muscle-invasive bladder cancers (MIBCs) invade the muscularis propria (T2), perivesical tissues (T3), or adjacent structures (T4a). Patients with muscle-invasive disease have a 50% likelihood of occult distant metastases at diagnosis.

TABLE 15.1 Stage Grouping of Carcinoma of the Bladder by TNM Involvement

	T1	T2	T3	T4a	T4b
N0	Stage I	Stage II	Stage III		
N1-3					
M1		Stage IV			

Bladder Cancer Management by Stage

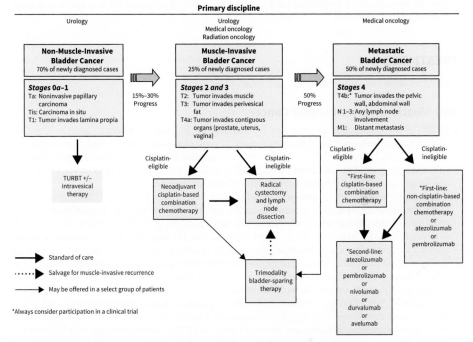

FIGURE 15.1 Management of bladder cancer differs significantly depending on stage. This algorithm depicts the treatment of non–muscle-invasive, muscle-invasive, and metastatic bladder cancer. *T4b, if tumor responds to systemic chemotherapy, consolidation with radical cystectomy may be considered.

- Tumors that invade the abdominal wall or pelvic sidewall and are fixed or immobile during EUA are staged as T4b tumors and are categorized as unresectable metastatic disease. Node-positive disease is categorized as stage IV bladder cancer (Fig. 15.1).
- The usual sites of metastases are pelvic lymph nodes, liver, lung, bone, soft tissue, adrenal glands, and peritoneum/omentum.

PROGNOSIS

- Major prognostic factors are tumor stage at diagnosis and degree of tumor differentiation.
- Five-year survival rates for patients with NMIBC, MIBC, and metastatic bladder cancer are 95%, 50%, and 6%, respectively. Median OS for NMIBC is 10 years, with a natural history characterized by recurrence of non–muscle-invasive tumor or progression to muscle-invasive disease. Non–muscle-invasive tumors recur in 60% to 70% of cases, about one third of which progress to a higher stage or grade. OS varies significantly in patients with metastatic urothelial cancer undergoing first-line treatment with chemotherapy. To better predict OS in these patients, Memorial Sloan Kettering Cancer Center (MSKCC) developed a prognostic model based on two pretreatment risk factors: a Karnofsky Performance Status of <80%, or the presence of visceral metastases (liver, lung, or bone). By the MSKCC prognostic model, no risk factors = median OS of 33 months; one risk factor = median OS of 13.4 months; and two risk factors = median OS of 9.3 months (P = 0.0001). An update of the MSKCC model included four pretreatment variables: visceral metastases, performance status, albumin, and hemoglobin. This four-variable prognostic model for patients with metastatic urothelial

carcinoma has a statistical significance for predicting OS that is superior to the two-variable model, and can predict survival probabilities at 1, 2, and 5 years as well as median OS in patients with metastatic urothelial carcinoma.

TREATMENT

Figure 15.1 shows an algorithm for the treatment of bladder cancer.

Non–Muscle-Invasive Bladder Cancer

- TURBT is the cornerstone of treatment for NMIBC (Ta, T1, and Tis bladder cancers). A second TURBT may be performed for high-grade tumors. Beyond observation after TURBT, intravesical chemotherapy may be indicated. Close follow-up is recommended for high-risk tumors (high-grade Ta, CIS, and high-grade T1), with urine cytology and cystoscopy every 3 to 6 months for the first 2 years and longer subsequent follow-up intervals after 2 years, as appropriate.
- Intravesical chemotherapy is primarily an adjunct or prophylaxis following TURBT, employed to lower the incidence of disease recurrence and/or progression. Intravesical chemotherapy is indicated for low-risk disease (low-grade Ta and T1), while intravesical bacillus Calmette-Guerin (BCG) is recommended for high-risk disease (high-grade Ta and T1, and CIS). Chemotherapeutic agents instilled intravesically include thiotepa, doxorubicin, epirubicin, and, most commonly, mitomycin C. Data suggest that currently available intravesical chemotherapeutic agents are equally effective but differ in toxicity. Although no standardized dosing or scheduling has been established for intravesical chemotherapy, a meta-analysis showed that one dose of cytotoxic chemotherapy reduced the risk of recurrence by 39%. Patients with low-grade solitary papillary tumors particularly benefited. Thus, in addition to observation after TURBT, an option for a low-grade, clinical stage Ta lesion would be single-dose intravesical chemotherapy within 24 hours of TURBT. Immunotherapy with BCG has statistically significant clinical benefits, including complete response in CIS (70% to 75%) and reduced recurrence in high-grade Ta or T1 (20% to 57%), but has shown no consistent reduction in tumor progression unless combined with maintenance BCG administered as per the Southwest Oncology Group (SWOG) protocol described by Lamm et al. Recurrent or persistent high-grade tumors may require a second induction of BCG. Tumors that do not respond to two induction courses of BCG or one induction course of BCG and one maintenance course of BCG are considered BCG-refractory, and radical cystectomy is advised. Intravesical valrubicin is FDA-approved for patients with BCG-refractory tumors who refuse or are intolerant of cystectomy. Other agents used in this population include gemcitabine and BCG⁺ interferon-α-2b. Clinical trials are ongoing for patients with BCG-refractory or BCG-unresponsive tumors who refuse radical cystectomy.
- Early radical cystectomy is indicated for BCG-refractory CIS or high-grade lesions that recur after BCG immunotherapy. High-grade T1 and CIS lesions have a propensity to progress and even metastasize.

Muscle-Invasive Bladder Cancer

- Radical cystectomy with bilateral lymph node dissection is the standard therapy for MIBC. In men, the surgery involves radical cystoprostatectomy. A total urethrectomy is indicated if the prostatic urethra is involved. In women, radical cystectomy involves wide excision of the bladder, urethra, uterus, adnexa, and anterior vaginal wall.
- Preserving the bladder with definitive chemoradiotherapy is an alternative to radical cystectomy. The two most common approaches include protocols developed at Massachusetts General Hospital, the University of Paris, and the University of Erlangen. In the Mass General and University of Paris protocols, patients undergo complete TURBT followed by an induction dose of chemoradiotherapy, and are then assessed for response. Patients who achieve a complete response then undergo consolidative chemoradiotherapy for bladder preservation; patients who do not achieve a complete response are referred for radical cystectomy with curative intent. In the University of Erlangen protocol, patients receive a full dose of chemoradiotherapy up-front, and then are evaluated for therapeutic response. Patients who do not achieve a complete response then undergo radical cyctectomy. Cisplatin is the

most common radiosensitizer used in this trimodal therapy; however, many patients are cisplatin-ineligible due to impaired renal function or poor performance status. For these patients, a combination of fluorouracil and mitomycin is an alternative treatment. Patients with multifocal disease, CIS, or hydronephrosis are not ideal candidates for definitive trimodal therapy. For these patients, chemotherapy combined with radiotherapy significantly improves locoregional control of MIBC without a significant increase in toxicity.

- Neoadjuvant cisplatin-based chemotherapy prior to definitive therapy improves survival in patients with T2 to T4a MIBC. A trial by the Medical Research Council and the European Organization for Research and Treatment of Cancer tested neoadjuvant cisplatin, methotrexate, and vinblastine (CMV) prior to definitive cystectomy or radiotherapy. Mature results from this trial showed an absolute survival benefit of 6% and a relative reduction in the risk of death from bladder cancer of 16% at 10 years in 976 randomized patients with MIBC. A similar survival benefit was seen in a U.S. Intergroup randomized trial (SWOG-8710) of neoadjuvant methotrexate, vinblastine, doxorubicin, and cisplatin (MVAC). A meta-analysis of >3,000 MIBC patients who received cisplatin-based neoadjuvant chemotherapy also showed a survival benefit of 6% and a 14% reduction in risk of mortality at 5 years, indicating that cisplatin-eligible patients should receive neoadjuvant chemotherapy prior to definitive therapy. In the United States, gemcitabine and cisplatin (GC) are frequently used in the neoadjuvant setting instead of MVAC or CMV. GC is equivalent to MVAC in the metastatic setting, but has not been studied in a randomized phase III trial in the neoadjuvant setting. Perioperative therapies for cisplatin-ineligible patients are still under investigation. There are no data supporting the administration of non-cisplatin-based neoadjuvant chemotherapies, such as carboplatin combinations.
- Data for adjuvant cisplatin-based chemotherapy are less compelling; thus, this regimen should not replace neoadjuvant chemotherapy. However, some patients benefit from cisplatin-based adjuvant chemotherapy, including those who did not receive neoadjuvant chemotherapy and have extensive disease discovered on radical cystectomy. Unfortunately, bladder cancer patients are usually elderly and tend to have multiple comorbidities, making adjuvant chemotherapy after radical cystectomy a challenge. Furthermore, patients may not be able to tolerate chemotherapy after surgery due to delayed healing and/or postsurgical complications.

Metastatic Bladder Cancer

First-Line Therapy (Tables 15.2 and 15.3)

- Dose-dense MVAC and GC are standard first-line chemotherapy regimens for metastatic urothelial carcinoma. MVAC is the most active regimen, with response rates of 40% to 72%.
- A randomized study of standard MVAC (4-week regimen) versus dose-dense MVAC (ddMVAC) (2-week regimen with growth factor support) showed that treatment could be completed faster, with less toxicity and better outcome, by eliminating day 15 and 22 of methotrexate and vinblastine. ddMVAC is used almost exclusively in clinical practice.
- GC has been shown to be equivalent to standard MVAC in OS, time to treatment failure, and response rates, with less toxicity. ddMVAC has not been compared to GC in a randomized study. GC is more commonly used, given its favorable toxicity profile.
- A randomized controlled study of ddMVAC versus ddGC showed that the regimens were comparable in OS and progression-free survival, but that ddGC had a better toxicity profile. However, this study halted randomization early due to poor accrual.
- Triplet chemotherapy combination regimens such as paclitaxel, gemcitabine, and cisplatin (PCG) have shown increased response in some patients, but their impact on survival is unclear (Table 15.2). In one study, the PCG arm had more febrile neutropenia than the GC arm (13.2% vs. 4.3%; $P < 0.001$). There are no data showing that carboplatin can be effectively substituted for cisplatin. Before it closed prematurely due to poor accrual, an Eastern Cooperative Oncology Group phase III study of MVAC versus carboplatin and paclitaxel demonstrated a nonstatistically significant difference in median OS of 15.4 months for the MVAC arm versus 13.8 months for the carboplatin-paclitaxel arm ($P = 0.65$), with toxicity favoring the carboplatin-paclitaxel arm. Therefore, carboplatin should be substituted for cisplatin only in patients deemed cisplatin-ineligible.

TABLE 15.2 Randomized Phase III Studies of Cisplatin-Based Chemotherapy in Metastatic Bladder Cancer

First Author, Year	Regimen	No. of Patients	Overall Response Rate (%)	Median Survival (mo)	P Value
Bamias, 2012	ddMVAC vs.	66	60	19	0.98
	ddGC	64	65	18	
Bellmunt, 2012	GC vs. gemcitabine/	314	44	12.7	0.075
	cisplatin/ paclitaxel	312	56	15.8	
Dreicer, 2004	MVAC vs.	44	40	14.2	0.41
	paclitaxel/ carboplatin	41	28	13.8	
Bamias, 2004	MVAC vs.	109	54	14.2	0.025
	docetaxel/cisplatin	111	37	9.3	
Sternberg, 2001	MVAC VS.	129	50	14.1	0.122
	ddMVAC	134	62	15.5	
von der Maase, 2000	MVAC vs.	202	46	14.8	0.750
	GC	203	49	13.8	
Loehrer, 1992	MVAC vs.	120	39	12.5	<0.0002
	cisplatin	126	12	8.2	
Logothetis, 1990	MVAC vs.	55	65	12.6	<0.05
	CISCA	55	46	10	

CISCA, cyclophosphamide, cisplatin, doxorubicin; dd, dose-dense.

Cisplatin-Ineligible Patients

- Patients are considered cisplatin-ineligible if they have poor performance status, renal insufficiency, hearing loss, neuropathy, or class III heart failure.
- A randomized phase II/III study in cisplatin-ineligible patients examined gemcitabine and carboplatin versus methotrexate, carboplatin, and vinblastine (M-CAVI). Median OS was 9.3 months in the gemcitabine and carboplatin arm versus 8.1 months in the M-CAVI arm ($P = 0.64$). Severe toxicity was seen in 9.3% of patients in the gemcitabine and carboplatin arm versus 21.2% of patients in the M-CAVI arm. These results demonstrated no difference between the two carboplatin-based regimens relative to survival outcome; however, more severe toxicity was associated with the M-CAVI regimen.
- Immunotherapy with checkpoint inhibition of the PD-1/PD-L1 pathway has demonstrated rapid, durable responses in metastatic urothelial carcinoma. Two checkpoint inhibitors, atezolizumab and pembrolizumab, are FDA-approved for first-line treatment of metastatic urothelial carcinoma in cisplatin-ineligible patients (Table 15.4).
- Atezolizumab is a humanized IgG1 monoclonal antibody (mAb) targeting PD-L1. Cohort 2 of the IMvigor 210 trial enrolled 123 treatment-naïve patients. Of these, 119 were cisplatin-ineligible and received atezolizumab as first-line treatment. The objective response rate (ORR) was 23% and median OS was 15.9 months, with no enrichment of clinical activity by PD-L1 immunohistochemistry (IHC) expression. Incidence of adverse events of any grade was 66%. Fatigue, diarrhea, and pruritus occurred in ≥10% of patients, and grade 3/4 adverse events occurred in 16% of patients, most commonly fatigue and elevated ALT and AST (3% each).
- Pembrolizumab is a humanized IgG4 mAb targeting PD-1. The phase II KEYNOTE-052 study assessed pembrolizumab as first-line therapy in 370 cisplatin-ineligible patients with metastatic urothelial carcinoma. The ORR was 27%, with high-level PD-L1 IHC expression predicting patients most likely to respond to treatment. Adverse events of any grade were seen in 62% of patients; 16% had grade ≥3 adverse events.

TABLE 15.3 Common Chemotherapy Regimens for Urothelial Carcinoma

Regimen	Dosing	Duration (days)	Setting
Gemcitabine + cisplatin	Gemcitabine, 1,000 mg/m² IV days 1 and 8 Cisplatin, 70 mg/m² IV day 1	21	Neoadjuvant and first line
MVAC	Methotrexate, 30 mg/m² IV days 1, 15, and 22 Vinblastine, 3 mg/m² IV days 2, 15, and 22 Doxorubicin, 30 mg/m² IV day 2 Cisplatin, 70 mg/m² IV day 2	28	Neoadjuvant and first line
ddMVAC	Methotrexate, 30 mg/m² IV day 1 Vinblastine, 3 mg/m² IV day 1 Doxorubicin, 30 mg/m² IV day 1 Cisplatin, 70 mg/m² IV day 1 Pegfilgrastim day 2	14	Neoadjuvant and first line
CMV	Methotrexate, 30 mg/m² IV days 1 and 8 Vinblastine, 4 mg/m² IV days 1 and 8 Cisplatin, 100 mg/m² IV infusion over 4 hours on day 2, ≥ 12 hours after methotrexate and vinblastine	21	Neoadjuvant and first line
Docetaxel + cisplatin	Docetaxel, 75 mg/m² slow IV infusion over 1 hour day 1 Cisplatin, 75 mg/m² IV day 1	21	First line
Paclitaxel + carboplatin	Paclitaxel, 200 mg/m² IV infusion over 3 hours on day 1 Carboplatin AUC of 5 mg/mL/minute IV after paclitaxel	21	Cisplatin-ineligible First line
ITP	Ifosfamide, 1,500 mg/m²/d IV days 1–3 Mesna, 300 mg/m² IV 30 minutes before ifosfamide, then 300 mg/m² IV 4 and 8 hours after ifosfamide; 600 mg/m² p.o. 4 and 8 hours after ifosfamide Paclitaxel, 200 mg/m² IV infusion over 3 hours day 1 Cisplatin, 70 mg/m² IV day 1 Pegfilgrastim day 2	21	Non-urothelial carcinoma histology First line

AUC, area under the curve; CMV, cisplatin, methotrexate, vinblastine; dd, dose-dense; ITP, ifosfamide, paclitaxel, cisplatin; IV, intravenous; MVAC, methotrexate, vinblastine, doxorubicin, cisplatin; p.o., by mouth.

TABLE 15.4 Reported Trials of PD-1/PD-L1 Inhibitors Leading to FDA Approval in Urothelial Carcinoma

	Pembrolizumab	Atezolizumab	Nivolumab	Durvalumab	Avelumab	Atezolizumab	Pembrolizumab
NCT number	NCT02256436	NCT02108652	NCT02387996	NCT01693562	NCT01772004	NCT02108652	NCT02335424
Authors	Bellmunt, et al.	Rosenberg, et al.	Galsky, et al.	Hahn, et al.	Apolo, et al.	Balar, et al.	Balar, et al.
FDA approval	May 2017	May 2016	February 2017	May 2017	May 2017	April 2017	May 2017
Phase	III	II	II	I/II	I	II	II
Dose and schedule	200 mg q3w	1,200 mg q3w	3 mg/kg q2w	10 mg/kg q2w	10 mg/kg q2w	1,200 mg q3w	200 mg q3w
N	542	310	265	182	161	119	370
ORR (%)	Pembro: 21.1 / Chemo: 11.4	15	19.6	17.6	17.4	23	24
ORR	Pembro: 21.6 / Chemo: 6.7	26	28.4	27.4	25.4	28	39
PD-L1+ (%)							
PR (%)	Pembro: 14.1 / Chemo: 8.1	10	17.4	14.3	11.2	13	19
CR (%)	Pembro: 7 / Chemo: 3.3	5	2.3	3.3	6.2	9	5
PD-L1+ assay and cutoff for positivity	Dako 22C3: TC and IC ≥ 10%	Ventana SP142: IC0 (<1%) IC1 (≥1%/<5%) IC2/3 (≥5%)	Dako 28-8: TC ≥ 5%	Ventana SP263 TC and IC ≥ 25%	Dako 73-10: TC ≥ 5%	Ventana SP142: IC0 (<1%) IC1 (≥1%/<5%) IC2/3 (≥5%)	Dako 22C3: TC and IC ≥ 10%
PD-L1+ prevalence (%)	Pembro: 27.4 / Chemo: 33.1	32.2 (IC2/3)	30.5	52	32.9	27	22
PFS (mo)	Pembro: 2.1 / Chemo: 3.3	2.1	2.0	1.5[a]	1.7	2.7	2
OS (mo)	Pembro: 10.3 / Chemo: 7.4	11.4	8.7	18.2[a]	7.4	15.9	NR
Grade 3/4 AEs (%)	Pembro: 15 / Chemo: 49.4	16	17.8	13.6[a]	8.4[b]	16	16

[a] Based on cohort of 191 patients (including nine chemotherapy-naive patients) treated with durvalumab.

[b] Based on cohort of 249 patients (88 with <6 months follow-up) treated with avelumab.

AEs, adverse events; CR, complete response; FDA, U.S. Food & Drug Administration; NR, not reported; ORR, objective response rate; OS, overall survival; PD-L1+, programmed death-ligand 1-positive; PFS, progression-free survival; PR, partial response.

Second-Line Therapy

▪ Five checkpoint inhibitors (atezolizumab, nivolumab, durvalumab, avelumab, and pembrolizumab) have demonstrated clinical efficacy in the second-line setting in patients with metastatic urothelial carcinoma, with comparable ORRs of 15% to 20% (Table 15.4). Atezolizumab, nivolumab, durvalumab, and avelumab received accelerated FDA approval, while pembrolizumab gained regular approval for the treatment of metastatic MIBC or metastatic progression within 12 months of neoadjuvant/adjuvant platinum-based chemotherapy.

  • **Atezolizumab.** The phase II IMvigor 210 trial of atezolizumab reported a 15% overall ORR, and 26% ORR in patients with higher PD-L1 IHC expression (IC2/3 defined as ≥5% of cells). Median OS was 7.9 months overall, 11.4 months in the IC2/3 group, and 8.8 months in the IC1/2/3 group. Grade 3 to 4 treatment-related adverse events, of which fatigue was the most common, occurred in 16% of patients. Grade 3 to 4 immune-mediated adverse events occurred in 5% of patients, with pneumonitis, increased AST and ALT, rash, and dyspnea being the most common.

  • **Nivolumab.** The phase II CheckMate 275 study investigated the safety and efficacy of nivolumab, mAb to PD-1, in 265 patients with metastatic urothelial carcinoma who had received prior treatment. The ORR was 20% in all patients (7 complete responses and 46 partial responses) and 16% and 24% in patients with negative (≤1%) and positive (>1%) PD-L1 IHC expression on tumor cells, respectively. Median OS was 8.7 months overall and 6.0 and 11.30 months in PD-L1$^-$ and PD-L1$^+$ patients, respectively. Grade ≥ 3 adverse events occurred in 18% of patients, with fatigue and diarrhea each in 2% of patients.

  • **Pembrolizumab.** The phase III KEYNOTE-045 trial compared single-agent pembrolizumab versus the physician's choice of chemotherapy (paclitaxel, docetaxel, or vinflunine) in 542 patients with metastatic urothelial carcinoma post-platinum-based chemotherapy. The ORR was 21% versus 11% ($P = 0.0011$) and median OS was 10.3 versus 7.4 months (HR 0.73; $P = 0.0022$), respectively. There was a lower incidence of adverse events of any grade (61% with pembrolizumab vs. 90% with chemotherapy), including grade ≥3 adverse events (15% and 49% for pembrolizumab and chemotherapy, respectively).

  • **Durvalumab.** A phase I/II study of durvalumab in 182 patients with metastatic urothelial carcinoma who had progressed after platinum-based chemotherapy reported an ORR of 17%; 3.7% of patients had a complete response. Among the 191 patients included in the safety analysis, grade 3 to 4 adverse events occurred in 7% and two deaths were treatment-related.

  • **Avelumab.** An anti-PD-L1 mAb has been shown to induce antibody-dependent cell-mediated cytotoxicity of tumor cells in preclinical studies. The JAVELIN Solid Tumor phase I trial investigated the safety and clinical activity of avelumab in patients with metastatic urothelial carcinoma post-platinum-based chemotherapy. An initial cohort ($n = 44$) showed encouraging antitumor responses and a manageable safety profile, leading to the addition of an efficacy cohort of 205 patients. A pooled analysis of the initial and efficacy cohorts showed an ORR of 17% in patients with ≥6 months of follow-up. The ORR in patients with or without baseline visceral metastases was 14% and 38%, respectively. Median OS in all post-platinum avelumab-treated patients was 7 months. Adverse events of any grade occurred in 67% of patients and included infusion-related reactions, fatigue, and rash (≥10%); 7% of patients had grade ≥ 3 treatment-related adverse events, including fatigue (≥1%). In Europe, vinflunine is approved as second-line treatment for metastatic bladder cancer, based on a randomized phase III study of vinflunine plus best supportive care (BSC) versus BSC alone. In the intent-to-treat population, OS was not statistically significant ($P = 0.287$). However, multivariate Cox analysis adjusted for prognostic factors did reveal a statistically significant difference for vinflunine plus BSC versus BSC alone. Median OS for vinflunine plus BSC was 6.9 versus 4.3 months for BSC alone ($P = 0.040$).

▪ Response rates to second-line chemotherapy are low (5% to 20%). Common treatment involves single-agent taxanes or pemetrexed.

Suggested Readings

1. Adjuvant chemotherapy in invasive bladder cancer: a systematic review and meta-analysis of individual patient data Advanced Bladder Cancer (ABC) Meta-analysis Collaboration. *Eur Urol.* 2005;48(2):189–199; discussion 99–201.

2. Antoni S, Ferlay J, Soerjomataram I, Znaor A, Jemal A, Bray F. Bladder cancer incidence and mortality: a global overview and recent trends. *Eur Urol.* 2017;71(1):96–108.

3. Apolo A, Ellerton J, Infante J, et al. Updated efficacy and safety of avelumab in metastatic urothelial carcinoma (mUC): Pooled analysis from 2 cohorts of the phase 1b Javelin solid tumor study. *J Clin Oncol.* 2017;35S:abstr 4528.

4. Apolo AB, Grossman HB, Bajorin D, Steinberg G, Kamat AM. Practical use of perioperative chemotherapy for muscle-invasive bladder cancer: summary of session at the Society of Urologic Oncology annual meeting. *Urol Oncol.* 2012;30(6):772–780.

5. Apolo AB, Infante JR, Balmanoukian A, et al. Avelumab, an anti-programmed death-ligand 1 antibody, in patients with refractory metastatic urothelial carcinoma: results from a multicenter, phase Ib study. *J Clin Oncol.* 2017;35(19):2117–2124.

6. Apolo AB, Ostrovnaya I, Halabi S, et al. Prognostic model for predicting survival of patients with metastatic urothelial cancer treated with cisplatin-based chemotherapy. *J Natl Cancer Inst.* 2013;105(7):499–503.

7. Bajorin DF, McCaffrey JA, Dodd PM, et al. Ifosfamide, paclitaxel, and cisplatin for patients with advanced transitional cell carcinoma of the urothelial tract: final report of a phase II trial evaluating two dosing schedules. *Cancer.* 2000;88(7):1671–1678.

8. Balar A, Castellano D, O'Donnell P, et al. Pembrolizumab as first-line therapy in cisplatin-ineligible advanced urothelial cancer: Results from the total KEYNOTE-052 study population. *J Clin Oncol.* 2017;35(suppl 6):abstr 284.

9. Balar AV, Bellmunt J, O'Donnell PH, et al. Pembrolizumab (pembro) as first-line therapy for advanced/unresectable or metastatic urothelial cancer: Preliminary results from the phase 2 KEYNOTE-052 study. *Ann Oncol.* 2016;27(suppl 6):abstr LBA32_PR.

10. Balar AV, Galsky MD, Rosenberg JE, et al. Atezolizumab as first-line treatment in cisplatin-ineligible patients with locally advanced and metastatic urothelial carcinoma: a single-arm, multicentre, phase 2 trial. *Lancet.* 2017;389(10064):67–76.

11. Bamias A, Aravantinos G, Deliveliotis C, et al. Docetaxel and cisplatin with granulocyte colony-stimulating factor (G-CSF) versus MVAC with G-CSF in advanced urothelial carcinoma: a multicenter, randomized, phase III study from the Hellenic Cooperative Oncology Group. *J Clin Oncol.* 2004;22(2):220–228.

12. Bamias A, Dafni U, Karadimou A, et al. Prospective, open-label, randomized, phase III study of two dose-dense regimens MVAC versus gemcitabine/cisplatin in patients with inoperable, metastatic or relapsed urothelial cancer: a Hellenic Cooperative Oncology Group study (HE 16/03). *Ann Oncol.* 2013;24(4):1011–1017.

13. Bellmunt J, de Wit R, Vaughn D, et al. Keynote-045: open-label, phase III study of pembrolizumab versus investigator's choice of paclitaxel, docetaxel, or vinflunine for previously treated advanced urothelial cancer. SITC Annual Meeting Abstracts. 2016:abstr 470.

14. Bellmunt J, von der Maase H, Mead GM, et al. Randomized phase III study comparing paclitaxel/cisplatin/gemcitabine and gemcitabine/cisplatin in patients with locally advanced or metastatic urothelial cancer without prior systemic therapy: EORTC Intergroup Study 30987. *J Clin Oncol.* 2012;30(10):1107–1113.

15. Bladder Cancer Practice Guidelines: National comprehensive cancer network. 2017. Available at: http://www.nccn.org. Accessed June 2017.

16. De Santis M, Bellmunt J, Mead G, et al. Randomized phase II/III trial assessing gemcitabine/carboplatin and methotrexate/carboplatin/vinblastine in patients with advanced urothelial cancer who are unfit for cisplatin-based chemotherapy: EORTC study 30986. *J Clin Oncol.* 2012;30(2):191–199.

17. Dreicer R, Manola J, Roth BJ, et al. Phase III trial of methotrexate, vinblastine, doxorubicin, and cisplatin versus carboplatin and paclitaxel in patients with advanced carcinoma of the urothelium. *Cancer.* 2004;100(8):1639–1645.

18. Edge S, Compton C. The American Joint Committee on Cancer: the 7th edition of the AJCC cancer staging manual and the future of TNM. *Ann Surg Oncol.* 2010;17:1471–1474.

19. Freedman ND, Silverman DT, Hollenbeck AR, Schatzkin A, Abnet CC. Association between smoking and risk of bladder cancer among men and women. *JAMA.* 2011;306(7):737–745.

20. Galsky MD, Hahn NM, Rosenberg J, et al. Treatment of patients with metastatic urothelial cancer "unfit" for Cisplatin-based chemotherapy. *J Clin Oncol.* 2011;29(17):2432–2438.

21. Galsky MD, Iasonos A, Mironov S, et al. Prospective trial of ifosfamide, paclitaxel, and cisplatin in patients with advanced non-transitional cell carcinoma of the urothelial tract. *Urology.* 2007;69(2):255–259.

22. Galsky MD, Retz MM, Siefker-Radtke A, et al. Efficacy and safety of nivolumab monotherapy in patients with metastatic urothelial cancer (mUC) who have received prior treatment: results from the phase II CheckMate 275 study. *Ann Oncol.* 2016;27(suppl 6):abstr LBA31-PR.

23. Garcia del Muro X, Marcuello E, Gumá J, et al. Phase II multicentre study of docetaxel plus cisplatin in patients with advanced urothelial cancer. *Br J Cancer.* 2002;86(3):326–330.

24. Griffiths G, Hall R, Sylvester R, Raghavan D, Parmar MK. International phase III trial assessing neoadjuvant cisplatin, methotrexate, and vinblastine chemotherapy for muscle-invasive bladder cancer: long-term results of the BA06 30894 trial. *J Clin Oncol.* 2011;29(16):2171–2177.

25. Grossman HB, Natale RB, Tangen CM, et al. Neoadjuvant chemotherapy plus cystectomy compared with cystectomy alone for locally advanced bladder cancer. *N Engl J Med.* 2003;349(9):859–866.

26. Hahn N, Powles T, Massard C, et al. Updated efficacy and tolerability of durvalumab in locally advanced or metastatic urothelial carcinoma (UC). *J Clin Oncol.* 2017;35S:abstr 4525.

27. Han RF, Pan JG. Can intravesical bacillus Calmette-Guerin reduce recurrence in patients with superficial bladder cancer? A meta-analysis of randomized trials. *Urology.* 2006;67(6):1216–1223.

28. Herr HW, Bochner BH, Dalbagni G, Donat SM, Reuter VE, Bajorin DF. Impact of the number of lymph nodes retrieved on outcome in patients with muscle invasive bladder cancer. *J Urol.* 2002;167(3):1295–1298.

29. Herr HW, Donat SM, Bajorin DF. Post-chemotherapy surgery in patients with unresectable or regionally metastatic bladder cancer. *J Urol.* 2001;165(3):811–814.

30. James ND, Hussain SA, Hall E, et al. Radiotherapy with or without chemotherapy in muscle-invasive bladder cancer. *N Engl J Med.* 2012;366(16):1477–1488.

31. Key Statistics for Bladder Cancer: American Cancer Society. Last revised January 5, 2017. Available at: https://www.cancer.org/cancer/bladder-cancer/about/key-statistics.html. Accessed June 2017.

32. Koga F, Kihara K. Selective bladder preservation with curative intent for muscle-invasive bladder cancer: a contemporary review. *Int J Urol.* 2012;19(5):388–401.

33. Lamm DL, Blumenstein BA, Crissman JD, et al. Maintenance bacillus Calmette-Guerin immunotherapy for recurrent TA, T1 and carcinoma in situ transitional cell carcinoma of the bladder: a randomized Southwest Oncology Group Study. *J Urol.* 2000;163(4):1124–1129.

34. Loehrer PJ, Sr., Einhorn LH, Elson PJ, et al. A randomized comparison of cisplatin alone or in combination with methotrexate, vinblastine, and doxorubicin in patients with metastatic urothelial carcinoma: a cooperative group study. *J Clin Oncol.* 1992;10(7):1066–1073.

35. Logothetis CJ, Dexeus FH, Finn L, et al. A prospective randomized trial comparing MVAC and CISCA chemotherapy for patients with metastatic urothelial tumors. *J Clin Oncol.* 1990;8(6):1050–1055.

36. Massard C, Gordon M, Sharma S, et al. Safety and efficacy of durvalumab (MEDI4736), an anti–programmed cell death ligand-1 immune checkpoint inhibitor, in patients with advanced urothelial bladder cancer. *J Clin Oncol.* 2016;34:3119–3125.

37. Montironi R, Lopez-Beltran A. The 2004 WHO classification of bladder tumors: a summary and commentary. *Int J Surg Pathol.* 2005;13(2):143–153.

38. Neoadjuvant chemotherapy in invasive bladder cancer: update of a systematic review and meta-analysis of individual patient data advanced bladder cancer (ABC) meta-analysis collaboration. *Eur Urol.* 2005;48(2):202–205; discussion 5–6.

39. Plimack ER, Bellmunt J, Gupta S, et al. Safety and activity of pembrolizumab in patients with locally advanced or metastatic urothelial cancer (KEYNOTE-012): a non-randomised, open-label, phase 1b study. *Lancet Oncol.* 2017;18(2):212–220.

40. Plimack ER, Hoffman-Censits JH, Viterbo R, et al. Accelerated methotrexate, vinblastine, doxorubicin, and cisplatin is safe, effective, and efficient neoadjuvant treatment for muscle-invasive bladder cancer: results of a multicenter phase II study with molecular correlates of response and toxicity. *J Clin Oncol.* 2014;32(18):1895–1901.

41. Powles T, Eder JP, Fine GD, et al. MPDL3280A (anti-PD-L1) treatment leads to clinical activity in metastatic bladder cancer. *Nature.* 2014;515(7528):558–562.

42. Rosenberg JE, Hoffman-Censits J, Powles T, et al. Atezolizumab in patients with locally advanced and metastatic urothelial carcinoma who have progressed following treatment with platinum-based chemotherapy: a single-arm, multicentre, phase 2 trial. *Lancet.* 2016;387(10031):1909–1920.

43. Sharma P, Callahan MK, Bono P, et al. Nivolumab monotherapy in recurrent metastatic urothelial carcinoma (CheckMate 032): a multicentre, open-label, two-stage, multi-arm, phase 1/2 trial. *Lancet Oncol.* 2016;17(11):1590–158.

44. Small EJ, Lew D, Redman BG, et al. Southwest Oncology Group Study of paclitaxel and carboplatin for advanced transitional-cell carcinoma: the importance of survival as a clinical trial end point. *J Clin Oncol.* 2000;18(13):2537–2544.

45. Sternberg CN, de Mulder P, Schornagel JH, et al. Seven year update of an EORTC phase III trial of high-dose intensity M-VAC chemotherapy and G-CSF versus classic M-VAC in advanced urothelial tract tumours. *Eur J Cancer.* 2006;42(1):50–54.

46. Sylvester RJ, van der Meijden AP, Witjes JA, Kurth K. Bacillus calmette-guerin versus chemotherapy for the intravesical treatment of patients with carcinoma in situ of the bladder: a meta-analysis of the published results of randomized clinical trials. *J Urol.* 2005;174(1):86–91; discussion-2.

47. von der Maase H, Hansen SW, Roberts JT, et al. Gemcitabine and cisplatin versus methotrexate, vinblastine, doxorubicin, and cisplatin in advanced or metastatic bladder cancer: results of a large, randomized, multinational, multicenter, phase III study. *J Clin Oncol.* 2000;18(17):3068–3077.

16 Testicular Carcinoma

Kevin R. Rice, Michelle A. Ojemuyiwa, and Ravi A. Madan

INTRODUCTION

Germ cell tumors (GCT) comprise 95% of testicular neoplasms. Testicular GCT is the most common malignancy in men between the ages of 20 and 35, but represents only 1% of all malignancies in males. The disease is believed to originate from the malignant transformation of primordial germ cells that may occur early in embryonic development. Testicular GCT is divided in seminoma and nonseminomatous germ cell tumors (NSGCT) due to distinct clinical behavior and treatment paradigms. As late as the 1970s, metastatic testicular carcinoma was associated with a 20% survival. However, subsequent demonstration of testicular cancer's marked sensitivity to cisplatin-based chemotherapeutic regimens has led to cancer-specific survival rates of >99% for early-stage disease and >90% for disseminated testicular cancer. Given these high cure rates, a considerable amount research effort has been directed at minimizing treatment-related toxicity, improving functional outcomes, and appropriately tailoring post diagnosis/treatment surveillance based on likelihood of recurrence. Despite these favorable outcomes, one cannot overemphasize the importance of rigorous adherence to the latest guidelines for post-treatment surveillance in maximizing oncologic and functional outcomes.

CLINICAL FEATURES

Epidemiology

- It was estimated that in 2016 there would be 8720 new cases of testicular carcinoma and 380 deaths due to the disease in the United States.
- Testicular cancer accounts for 1% of all malignancies in men but the majority of cases occur between the ages of 20 to 35 years. NSGCT peaks in the third decade while seminoma peaks in the fourth decade. Testicular GCT is rare after age 40.
- There is significant variability in the incidence by ethnicity with American Caucasians being 5 times more likely than African Americans, 4 times more likely than Asian Americans, and 1.3 times more likely than Hispanics to develop testicular GCT.
- For unclear reasons, the incidence of testicular cancer has been increasing over the past four to five decades in most western countries.

Risk Factors

- Cryptorchidism: Cryptorchid testis, defined as a maldescended testis located above the external inguinal ring, is associated with a 4- to 6-fold increase in the risk of testicular cancer with intra-abdominal testes having a higher risk than inguinal testes. Performance of orchiopexy before puberty is now thought to decrease risk of GCT development. There is also an increased risk of developing GCT in the normally-descended contralateral testis.
- Second primary tumors: Synchronous or metachronous testicular carcinoma may occur in the contralateral testis in a few group of patients; 1% to 5% of patients have bilateral disease at presentation.

After treatment of testicular cancer, patients should be counseled that they have an approximately 2% chance of metachronous contralateral GCT.

▪ Intratubular germ cell neoplasia (ITGCN): A premalignant condition seen in 90% of testicular carcinomas (not typically seen with spermatocytic seminoma). The finding of ITGCN on testis biopsy is associated with an at least 50% chance of development of ipsilateral GCT at 5 years and 70% at 7 years. ITGCN is believed to be present in at least 5% of contralateral testicles at the time of orchiectomy for GCT.

▪ Hereditary: Despite the overwhelming evidence of a strong familial component to the risk of testicular carcinoma, to date, no definite oncogene has been identified. About 1.4% of patients with testicular carcinoma have a positive family history of the disease. A son of an affected father has a 4- to 6-fold increased risk while for a brother of an affected sibling the risk increases to 8- to 10-fold. The risk is reportedly greater than 70-fold in monozygotic twins.

▪ Chromosomal abnormalities: Klinefelter syndrome has been shown to be associated with increased risk of primary mediastinal germ cell tumors in a few case series and surveys. Similar studies have also suggested the possibility of an increased risk of testicular cancer with Down syndrome. Additionally, disorders of sexual differentiation (DSD) are associated with a variable increased risk of developing GCT when a Y-chromosome is present. The typical pre-GCT neoplasm in these patients is gonadoblastoma. For this reason, prophylactic gonadectomy is often recommended before puberty for abnormal or streak gonads.

▪ Viral infections: Possible associations between Epstein-Barr (EBV), Cytomegalovirus (CMV), and human immunodeficiency virus (HIV) and testicular cancer have been reports, although most associations are modest or inconclusive. The risk of seminomatous testicular tumors is considerably higher in HIV-infected men compared to age-matched HIV-negative men. There are also recent reports of non-Hodgkin lymphoma of the testicles in patients with HIV infection.

▪ Hypospadias: Analyses of data from Danish health registry have suggested a potential association between hypospadias and testicular tumor.

The opinions expressed in this chapter represent those of the authors and do not necessarily represent official positions or opinions of the US government or of the U.S. Department of Health and Human Services.

Presentation

▪ Asymptomatic testicular nodule or swelling (painful in 10% to 20% of patients)
▪ Feeling of testicular heaviness, dull ache, and/or hardness (up to 40% of patients)
▪ Disease at extragonadal site (5% to 10% of patients; symptoms vary with site):
  ● Dyspnea, cough, or hemoptysis (pulmonary metastases)
  ● Weight loss, anorexia, nausea, abdominal, or back pain (retroperitoneal adenopathy)
  ● Mass or swelling in neck (left-sided supraclavicular lymphadenopathy)
  ● Superior vena cava syndrome due to mediastinal disease
▪ Rare presentations:
  ● Urinary obstruction
  ● Headaches, seizures, or other neurologic complaints due to brain metastases
  ● Bone pain due to bone metastases
  ● Gynecomastia due to elevated β-human chorionic gonadotropin (β-HCG).
  ● Anti-Ma2-associated paraneoplastic encephalitis

DIFFERENTIAL DIAGNOSIS

▪ Epididymitis (initial diagnosis and treatment in 18% to 33% of testicular cancer patients)
▪ Testicular trauma (GCT often comes to attention after trauma to the testis)
▪ Orchitis, hydrocele, varicocele, or spermatocele
▪ Paratesticular neoplasm (can be benign or malignant)
▪ Testicular torsion

- Lymphoma or leukemia
- Metastasis from other tumors including melanoma or lung cancer
- Infectious diseases including tuberculosis and tertiary syphilis causing gumma

DIAGNOSIS

The initial evaluation of a suspicious testicular mass should include measurement of serum tumor markers—alphafetoprotein (AFP), beta-human chorionic gonadotropin (β-HCG), and serum lactate dehydrogenase (LDH) and —testicular ultrasound, and a chest x-ray. Subsequently, if findings support a testicular tumor, a radical inguinal orchiectomy should be performed. Postoperatively, if germ cell tumor is confirmed, an abdominopelvic CT scan should be performed and serum tumor markers should be repeated. Chest CT should be performed for abnormalities on preoperative chest film, pulmonary symptoms, or if retroperitoneal/abdominal disease is noted on staging CT of the abdomen/pelvis. Brain imaging is generally only indicated for neurologic symptoms or for high-stage disease with markedly elevated serum tumor markers. This is particularly important in the setting of significant HCG elevation, as this usually indicates the presence of choriocarcinoma, which has a propensity for widespread hematogenous dissemination.

Goals

- Expediency—Every testicular mass requires a timely workup to exclude testicular carcinoma. Delay in diagnosis can lead to disease progression, increasing treatment toxicity and leading to poorer oncologic and functional outcomes. Thus, urgent referral to urology should be standard.
- Appropriate diagnostic evaluation—Avoid unnecessary diagnostic tests in patients where the diagnosis of testicular cancer is unclear. Similarly, avoid unnecessary imaging in low-stage, low-risk patients (i scans or CNS imaging).
- Fertility—If future paternity is desired by the patient, provide him the opportunity and resources to bank sperm prior to orchiectomy in all but the most advanced and ominous cases.
- Appropriate surgical approach—radical inguinal orchiectomy is the standard of care. There is no role for transscrotal orchiectomy, biopsy, or fine-needle aspiration due to potential scrotal contamination, inadequate local control of the spermatic cord, and inadequate tissue sampling.

Laboratory

Serum α-Fetoprotein (AFP)

- A glycoprotein with a half-life of approximately 4 to 6 days.
- Commonly produced by the fetal yolk sac, liver, and gastrointestinal tract.
- Should not be elevated in serum of healthy men. Can be elevated in setting of liver disease/malignancy. Alcohol intake should be determined and a liver function panel should be sent in cases of mild elevation.
- Can be produced by yolk sac tumor and embryonal cell carcinoma.
- Not present in patients with pure seminoma. Elevated serum α-fetoprotein (AFP) levels indicate a nonseminomatous component to the patient's testicular cancer. Thus, patients with AFP elevation should be managed as NSGCT even when testicular specimen demonstrates pure seminoma.

Serum β-Human Chorionic Gonadotropin

- Secreted by syncytiotrophoblasts; half-life of 0.5 to 1.5 days.
- Most commonly elevated tumor marker in patients with testicular cancer.
- Present in choriocarcinomas; may be modestly elevated in approxiatel 15% of pure seminomas due to presence of syncytiotrophoblastic blood islands.
- High levels may lead to gynecomastia.
- False positives may be seen in patients with low testosterone due to cross reactivity of luteinizing hormone (LH) with the β-HCG assay. Thus, if β-HCG is elevated after orchiectomy for solitary testicle

or if remaining testicle is atrophic/soft, serum testosterone should be analyzed and if low, IM testosterone 200 mcg should be administered. β-HCG can then be rechecked in 1 week.

Serum Lactate Dehydrogenase
- Nonspecific tumor marker in testicular cancer
- Elevated in 80% of metastatic seminomas and 60% of advanced nonseminomatous tumors
- Reflects overall tumor burden, tumor growth rate, and cellular proliferation

Imaging
- Testicular Ultrasound: evaluates for the presence of testicular parenchymal abnormality.
- Chest x-ray: Posterior–anterior and lateral film evaluation for pulmonary metastases and evidence of mediastinal adenopathy if widened mediastinum is seen.
- Computerized tomography (CT): CT scans of chest, abdomen, and pelvis determine extragonadal metastasis and are the most effective modality for staging the disease. However, a plain posterior anterior film of the chest can be substituted for the Chest CT in clinical stage I disease to minimize radiation load.
- Magnetic resonance imaging (MRI): Testicular MRI may provide additional information if ultrasound is indeterminate, although this scenario is extremely rare. MRI of the brain is necessary only when there are symptoms involving the central nervous system (e.g., headache, neurologic deficit, seizure).
- Positron emission tomography (PET) scan: PET scans are not indicated in primary staging, but may have limited utility for characterizing postchemotherapy/postradiotherapy residual masses in pure seminoma patients (see below). The routine use of PET scans has not been shown to improve outcome in NSGCT.

Pathology
Patients with testicular masses should have surgical exploration, with complete removal of the testis and spermatic cord up to the internal inguinal ring. Transscrotal orchiectomy or testicular biopsy are not recommended due to incomplete control of the spermatic cord in the inguinal canal as well as the theoretical risk of scrotal seeding of tumor cells.

- GCTs can be composed of pure histologies or combinations of 5 histologic subtypes Table 16.1:
  - Seminoma
  - Embryonal cell carcinoma
  - Yolk sac tumor
  - Choriocarcinoma
  - Teratoma
- Immunohistochemical staining can be used to distinguish the different histologic subtypes of testicular carcinoma. While an experienced genitourinary pathologist is able to distinguish subtypes of GCT based on morphologic features alone in the great majority of cases, immunohistochemical staining can be used to confirm diagnoses in difficult cases.
- Several genes (either deleted or amplified) located on isochromosome 12p have been implicated in the malignant transformation of primordial germ cells. Among patients with familial testicular germ cell tumors compatible with X-linked inheritance, evidence suggests the presence of a susceptibility gene on chromosome Xq27.

STAGING
Staging is in accordance with the American Joint Committee on Cancer tumor/node/metastasis (TNM) criteria.

- T classification is based on pathological finding after radical orchiectomy, hence pT nomenclature. pT0 means there is no evidence of disease. pTis refers to intratubular germ cell neoplasia or carcinoma in situ. pT1 refers to disease limited to the testis and epididymis without lymphovascular

TABLE 16.1 Histopathologic Characteristics of Testicular tumors

Tumor Type	Percentage	Pathologic Feature(s)	Percentage
Germ cell tumors	95	Seminomas	40–50
Single cell–type tumors	60	Primordial germ cell	
Mixed cell–type tumors	40	Nonseminomas	50–60
		Embryonal cell tumors	
		Yolk sac tumors	
		Teratomas	
		Choriocarinomas	
Tumors of gonadal stroma	1–2	Leydig cell	
		Sertoli cell	
		Granulosa cell	
		Primitive gonadal structures	
Gonadoblastoma	1	Germ cell + stromal cell	

invasion, although it may invade the tunica albuginea but the tunica vaginalis. pT2 tumor is similar to pT1 but with lymphovascular invasion or the involvement of the tunica vaginalis. In pT3 tumor, there is invasion of the spermatic cord with or without lymphovascular invasion. Involvement of the scrotum with or without lymphovascular invasion is designated as pT4. pTx is used when the primary tumor cannot be assessed.

- N classification is based on lymph node involvement and may be pathologic (pN) or clinical. When there is no regional lymph node involvement, the N0 designation is used. N1 refers to metastasis with a lymph node mass of 2 cm or less in greatest dimension. N2 is a lymph node metastasis or multiple lymph nodes metastasis with any one mass greater than 2 cm but not more than 5 cm in greatest dimension. Lymph node metastasis greater than 5 cm is termed N3. If a lymph node metastasis is ascertained pathologically after surgery, it is termed as pN nomenclature is used. pN0 means no evidence of lymph node involvement, while pN1 refers to involvement of less than 5 lymph nodes with none greater than 2 cm. Likewise, pN2 is similar to N2 but also include the involvement of more than 5 lymph nodes, none more than 5 cm or evidence of extra nodal extension. pN3 has similar definition as N3. When regional lymph nodes cannot be assessed the Nx or pNx designation is used.

- M classification is based on the extent of distant metastasis. M0 means there is no distant metastasis, while M1, which is further divided to M1a and M1b, signifies distant metastasis. M1a refers to nonregional nodal or pulmonary metastasis, while M1b indicates distant metastasis other than nonregional lymph nodes and lung.

- Unique to testicular germ cell tumors is the use of serum tumor markers in the staging process. S0 refers to normal serum levels of tumor markers. S1 indicates that the lactate dehydrogenase (LDH) is <1.5 times the upper limit of normal, BHCG is <5,000 milli-international units/ml, and AFP is <1000 ng/ml. S2 is used when the LDH is between 1.5 and 10 times the upper limit of normal, or B-HCG is between 5,000 and 50,000 milli-international units/mL, or AFP 1,000 to 10,000 ng/mL. S3 refers to LDH >10 times the upper limit of normal, or BHCG >50,000 milli-international units/mL or AFP >10, 000 ng/mL. Sx refers to tumor markers not available or not completed.

- The TNM classification is then used in the anatomic stage grouping as follows:
  - Stage I: pT1-4, N0, M0, Sx/S0
    - Stage Ia: pT1, N0, M0, Sx/0
    - Stage Ib: pT2-4, N0, M0, Sx/0
    - Stage IS: Any p T/Tx, N0, M0, S1-3
  - Stage II: Any pT/Tx, N1-3, M0, Sx/S0-1
    - Stage IIa: Any pT/Tx, N1, M0, S0-1
    - Stage IIb, Any pT/Tx, N2, M0, S0-1
    - Stage IIc, Any pT/Tx, N3, S0-1

- Stage III: Any pT/Tx, any N, M1, Sx/S0-3
  - Stage IIIa: Any pT/Tx, Any N, M1a, S0-1
  - Stage IIIb: Any pT/Tx, AND N0-3, M1a, S2 OR N1-3, M0, S2
  - Stage IIIc: Any pT/Tx, N0-3, M1b, Any S OR M1a, S3 OR N1-3, Any M and S3

PROGNOSIS

- Patients with clinical stage Ia and Ib GCT have a 99% to 100% survival. The prognosis for patients with metastatic disease GCT can be estimated by utilizing the international germ cell consensus classification system developed by the International Germ Cell Cancer Collaborative Group (IGCCCG) and published in 1997. This system utilizes postorchiectomy levels of tumor markers, site of primary tumor (for NSGCT) and the site of metastasis (pulmonary vs. nonpulmonary visceral metastases) to predict the progression-free survival (PFS) and overall survival (OS) (Table 16.2).
- The 5-year PFS and 5-year OS for disseminated seminomatous and nonseminomatous germ cell tumors are given in Table 16.3. However, it should be noted that many patients included in development and validation of the IGCCCG model were treated in the early cisplatin-era. Thus, survival is likely underestimated in this model. For example, a more contemporary review of 273 poor risk patients treated at a referral center revealed IGCCCG poor risk patients to demonstrate a 73% 5-year OS and 58% 5-year PFS.

TREATMENT MODALITIES

Radical inguinal orchiectomy is the preferred surgical approach for all patients with a testicular mass for reasons described previously. This is both a diagnostic and therapeutic procedure. Adjuvant therapy,

TABLE 16.2 International Consensus Risk Classification for Germ Cell Tumors

Prognosis	Nonseminoma	Seminoma
Good	Testis/retroperitoneal primary. No nonpulmonary visceral metastases. AFP <1,000 mg/mL; HCG <5,000 international units/L (1,000 mg/mL); LDH <1.5 × ULN (56% of all nonseminomas)	Any primary site. No nonpulmonary visceral metastases. Normal AFP; any concentration of HCG; any concentration of LDH (90% of all seminomas)
Intermediate	Testis/retroperitoneal primary. No nonpulmonary visceral metastases. AFP ≥1,000 and ≤10,000 ng/mL or HCG ≥5,000 milli-International units/milliliter (mIU/mL) and ≤50,000 international units/L or LDH = 1.5 × NL and ≥10 × NL (28% of all nonseminomas)	Any primary site. No nonpulmonary visceral metastases. Normal AFP; any concentration of HCG; any concentration of LDH (10% of all seminomas)
Poor	Mediastinal primary or nonpulmonary visceral metastases or AFP >10,000 ng/mL or HCG >50,000 international units/L (10,000 ng/mL) or LDH >10 × ULN (16% of all nonseminomas)	No patients classified as poor prognosis

LDH, lactate dehydrogenase; HCG, human chorionic gonadotropin; AFP, α-fetoprotein; ULN, upper limit of normal; NL, normal limit.

TABLE 16.3 Expected Survival for Disseminated Disease

Prognosis	5-y Progression-Free Survival (%)		5-y Overall Survival (%)	
	Seminoma	Nonseminoma	Seminoma	Nonseminoma
Good	82	89	86	92
Intermediate	67	75	72	80
Poor[a]	—	41	—	48

[a]There is no poor prognosis category for seminoma.

which may include chemotherapy, radiotherapy, or further surgery, is tailored to the disease stage and histology. Radiation therapy is only offered to pure seminoma patient due to known radiosensitivity and very low likelihood of radioresistant (and chemoresistant) teratomatous elements. The need for adjuvant therapy after orchiectomy in clinical stage I disease is generally not recommended in pure seminoma and Stage Ia NSGCT patients. The use of adjuvant therapy in Stage Ib NSGCT is controversial.

Pure Seminoma

Adjuvant treatment options for seminoma are outlined in Figure 16.1.

Stage I

- Orchiectomy is curative in 80% to 85% of patients with clinical stage (CS) I seminoma.
- Postorchiectomy management options include 1) surveillance, 2) radiotherapy, and 3) single agent carboplatin.

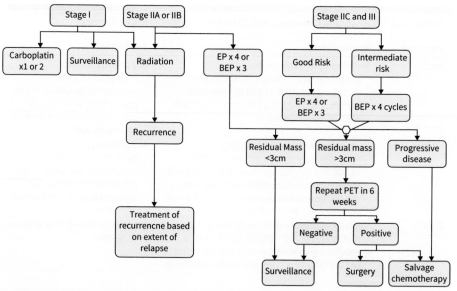

FIGURE 16.1 Adjuvant treatment options for seminoma. Radiation*, radiation therapy to para-aortic lymph nodes; BEP, bleomycin, etoposide, and cisplatin; EP, etoposide, and cispaltin; PET positron emission tomography.

- Risk factors for recurrence of CS I seminoma include primary tumor size of >4cm and rete testis invasion. When one or both factors are present, recurrence rate increases to approximately 30%.
- Adjuvant treatment with radiotherapy to the para-aortic lymph nodes or single agent carboplatin both increase recurrence-free survival (RFS) to approximately 94%.
- With a recurrence rate of <20% and OS of 99% to 100% regardless of postorhiectomy management strategy, active surveillance is the preferred postorchiectomy management option. Risk-adapted utilization of postorhiectomy adjuvant therapy is generally not recommended. Rather, physicians and patients must discuss the short-term and long-term advantages and disadvantages of surveillance versus chemotherapy or radiation in CS I seminoma. All patients must understand the need to comply with surveillance protocols.
- Disease relapse typically occurs in the retroperitoneal lymph nodes and nearly all patients are successfully salvaged with radiation or chemotherapy.

Stage IIA–B

- For stage IIA–B seminoma, postorchiectomy-managed options include external beam radiation or induction cisplatin-based chemotherapy (IGCCCG good risk). Both radiation therapy (30 Gy for stage IIA; 36 Gy for stage IIB) to ipsilateral iliac and retroperitoneal lymph nodes ("modified dog-leg") and induction chemotherapy are associated with a 90% RFS.
- In general, radiation therapy is preferred for stage IIA patients. However, in select stage IIA cases where radiation is contraindicated (i.e., horseshoe kidney, inflammatory bowel disease, or history of abdominal/retroperitoneal radiation) or when the patient's preference is to avoid radiation, IGCCCG good risk cisplatin-based chemotherapy is appropriate. For stage IIB serminoma, IGCCCG good risk cisplatin-based chemotherapy can be utilized as an equivalent (and perhaps superior) alternative to radiation therapy.
- Patients with stage II seminoma may be treated with IGCCCG good risk chemotherapy regimens, which include three cycles of bleomycin, etoposide, and cisplatin (BEP) or four cycles of etoposide and cisplatin (EP).
- There is no evidence that the combination of both radiation and chemotherapy increases RFS or OS.

Stage IIC–III

Stages IIC and III seminoma are curable in most cases. Even intermediate risk pure seminoma is associated with a >70% 5-year cancer-specific survival. These patients should be managed with full induction courses of cisplatin-based chemotherapy following radical orchiectomy. Patients with IGCCCG good risk disease may be treated with three cycles of BEP or four cycles of EP; intermediate risk patients (non-pulmonary visceral metastases) should be treated with four cycles of BEP or four cycles of etoposide, ifosfamide, and cisplatin (VIP) if bleomycin is contraindicated.

Management of residual retroperitoneal masses after radiation and/or chemotherapy:

- In most cases, a residual mass after treatment of seminoma with radiation or systemic chemotherapy does not indicate persistent disease. Rather, it tends to be a manifestation of the dense desmoplastic reaction that this tumor has to treatment. In series where resections have been performed, the rate of persistent viable tumor was <10%. The likelihood of persistent seminoma seems to correlate with the size of the residual mass. A cut point of 3 cm has been proposed.
- For residual masses <3 cm in greatest dimension, observation is recommended.
- For residual masses >3cm, a PET scan should be performed at least 6 weeks from completion of induction chemotherapy or radiation. If negative, observation is recommended. If positive, treatment options include salvage chemotherapy (standard or high dose) or postchemotherapy (PC)-RPLND (Retroperitoneal lymph node dissection) in select cases where disease appears easily resectable as judged by an experienced urologic oncologist.

Nonseminoma

Adjuvant treatment options for stages I, II, and III nonseminoma are outlined in Figures 16.2 and 16.3.

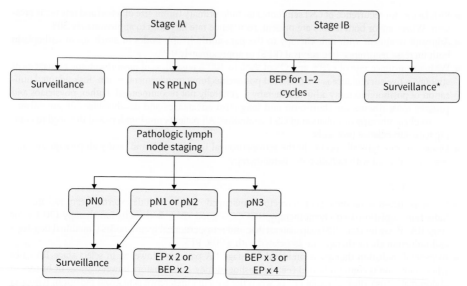

FIGURE 16.2 Adjuvant treatment options for stage I nonseminoma. RPLN, never sparing retroperitoneal lymph node dissection; BEP, bleomycin, etoposide, and cisplatin; EP, etoposide and cisplatin.
* For T2 lesions only

Stage IA–B

- Stage I NSGCT (including pure testicular seminomas with elevated levels of serum AFP) has a 99% to 100% survival regardless of postorchiectomy management option. Overall chance of recurrence/occult disease is approximately 25% to 30%. Risk factors for recurrence/occult disease increases with lymphovascular invasion (LVI) and/or embryonal predominance (>40% of primary tumor). Patients that have LVI and/or embryonal predominance have a >50% chance of recurrence. Those with neither risk factor have an approximately 15% chance of recurrence.
- Management options include 1) surveillance, 2) primary RPLND, and 3) systemic chemotherapy.
- Surveillance has become the preferred option for patients without the risk factors listed above. Surveillance is a reasonable option for patients with risk factors for recurrence given the fact that while primary RPLND and adjuvant chemotherapy can improve RFS, they have no effect on cancer-specific survival in this population.
- RPLND was traditionally the preferred approach given that most small volume regional lymph node metastases remain curable with RPLND alone. Some experts continue to advocate for primary RPLND in CS IB patients. This surgery is utilized based on the predictable lymphatic spread from the testicles to the retroperitoneum and the fact that regionally metastatic testicular cancer remains largely curable with surgery alone. Generally, the main advantage/goal of primary RPLND is avoidance of chemotherapy. In the absence of adjuvant post-RPLND chemotherapy, patients with pN0 disease have a 10% chance of recurrence (usually pulmonary), those with pN1-2 disease have a 30% to 50% chance of recurrence. Two cycles of cisplatin-based chemotherapy (BEP or EP) virtually eliminate chance of recurrence in patients with pN1-2 disease at primary RPLND. However, adjuvant chemotherapy after primary RPLND has no effect on cancer-specific survival, which should approach 100%. Adjuvant chemotherapy is an option, but is generally not recommended for pN1 disease. Utilization of adjuvant chemotherapy for pN2 disease varies from center to center. Patients found to have pN3 disease at primary RPLND should have full induction chemotherapy (BEPx3 or EPx4), although this situation is vanishingly rare with sensitivity of preoperative CT for retroperitoneal metastases.

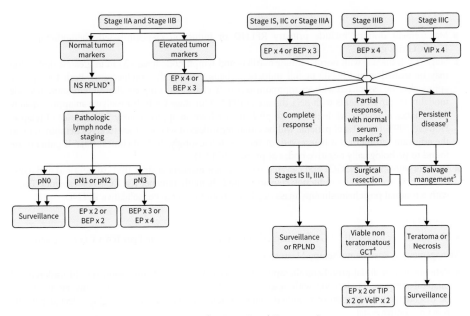

FIGURE 16.3 Adjuvant treatment options for stage II and III nonseminoma.
1. Complete response, negative markers
2. Partial response residual masses, normal tumor markers
3. Incomplete response (persistent tumor markers)
4. Viable nonteratomatous germ cell tumor includes yolk sac, embryonal, choricarcinoma, or seminoma
5. Depends on prognosis, treatment options include clinical trial, salvage chemotherapy, or salvage resection
* Nerve sparing retroperitoneal lymph node dissection (NS-RPLND)
Adapted from National Comprehensive Cancer Network (NCCN).

- Adjuvant chemotherapy: BEPx1 or BEPx2 has been recommended by some experts for CS I patients with LVI or embryonal predominance given the 50% chance of disease recurrence. Proponents of this approach cite the fact that surgeons who can properly perform an RPLND are not available at all centers and that treatment in the adjuvant setting avoids three to four cycle induction with cisplatin-based chemotherapy in patient's destined to recur on surveillance. Opponents to such risk-adapted utilization of adjuvant chemotherapy cite the 99% to 100% CSS regardless of approach and propose that avoiding chemotherapy entirely in 50% of patients who are not destined to recur may be more beneficial than avoiding one to two additional cycles of chemotherapy in the 50% of patients destined to recur on surveillance.
- Several factors must be considered before choosing active surveillance. These include the patient's level of anxiety, compliance, and access to a facility with experienced physicians, radiologists, and CT scanners to detect recurrence. Interestingly, sequelae of treatment, rather than fear of recurrence have been demonstrated to have a negative impact on quality of life in GCT tumor patients. Additionally, there are no reliable predictors of patient compliance.

Stage IS

- Patients with Stage IS disease have elevated postorchiectomy serum tumor markers but no radiographically measurable metastatic disease outside of the testicle.
- Management is full induction chemotherapy per IGCCCG risk group.
- RPLND should not be performed due to unacceptably high relapse rate outside of the retroperitoneum.

Stage II

- Management options include primary RPLND or induction cisplatin-based chemotherapy per IGCCCG risk group.
- Stage IIA–B disease with normal tumor markers and lymph node mass ≤3 cm in greatest dimension may be treated with RPLND or full induction chemotherapy after orchiectomy. Both therapeutic approaches are associated with an approximately 65% chance of complete clinical remission to single modality therapy. Patients with pN1 disease at RPLND for stage CS II disease have an approximately 30% chance of relapse while those with pN2 disease have an approximately 50% chance of relapse. However, 99% to 100% of patients will be cured regardless of whether they receive chemotherapy in the adjuvant setting or if it is reserved for relapse. Interestingly, 20% of clinical stage II patients are found to pathologically negative nodes at primary RPLND.
- Patients with stage II NSGCT and elevated serum tumor markers or stage IIB/C tumors and nodal disease >3 cm should receive induction cisplatin-based chemotherapy per IGCCCG risk category. Those with a residual postchemotherapy mass of ≥1 cm should undergo consolidative RPLND.

Stage III

- The majority of stage III NSGCT remain curable and should be treated per IGCCCG risk group.

Management of Postchemotherapy Masses in NSGCT:

- Patients with residual postchemotherapy masses >1 cm in greatest dimension should undergo full bilateral template PC-RPLND with resection of all residual masses. Tumorectomy alone should be discouraged. Utilization of modified unilateral template PC-RPLND in highly selected patients remains controversial.
- Management of patients with complete clinical response (no residual masses >1 cm in greatest dimension) to induction chemotherapy is somewhat controversial. Although most experts agree that observation of these patients is safe citing a 97% 15-year CSS in one large study, some experts advocate for consolidative PC-RPLND in all patients who had a retroperitoneal mass prior to chemotherapy.
- Patients with brain metastases at diagnosis should receive an IGCCCG Poor Risk chemotherapy regimen (BEPx4 in most patients). While multimodality treatment is often necessary, treatment should be individualized based primarily on response to chemotherapy, but also on the location and surgical resectability of residual lesions as determined by neurosurgery. Utilization of stereotactic radiation therapy has been described, but the specific role remains to be defined. While whole brain radiotherapy has been used extensively in the past, the survival benefit of this modality has not been clear and it can be associated with significant long-term neurologic sequelae.

Histology at PC-RPLND

- In general histology of residual masses are fibrosis 40% to 45%, teratoma in 40% to 45%, and viable nonteratomatous GCT 10% to 15% of the time.
- Patients found to have fibrosis or teratoma without viable GCT at PC-RPLND demonstrate a >95% 5-year CSS. Those with viable GCT have a 60% to 70% 5-year CSS.
- Adjuvant EPx2 can be delivered to minimize chance of relapse in patients with viable nonteratomatous GCT. However, it may not provide any benefit in patients with complete resection of all gross disease, viable malignancy involving <10% of the specimen, and history IGCCCG good risk disease at presentation as patients with these favorable risk factors demonstrate a 90% 5-year RFS.

Chemotherapy Regimens

Commonly used chemotherapy regimens (Table 16.4) include BEP and EP. VIP and VeIP are used less often.

Follow-Up

Appropriate surveillance of patients with testicular cancer is essential and should be determined by the tumor's histology, stage, and treatment (Tables 16.5 and 16.6).

TABLE 16.4 Commonly Used Chemotherapeutic Agents and Regimens

Agent	Dose	Schedule
BEP	Bleomycin, 30 units IV weekly on days 1, 8, and 15 (can also be administered on days 2, 9, and 16) Etoposide, 100 mg/m² IV daily × 5 d Platinol (cisplatin), 20 mg/m² IV daily × 5 d	2 to 4 cycles administered at 21-d intervals
EP	Etoposide, 100 mg/m² IV daily × 5 d Platinol (cisplatin), 20 mg/m² IV daily × 5 d	4 cycles administered at 21-d intervals
VIP[a]	VePesid (etoposide), 75 mg/m² IV daily × 5 d Ifosfamide, 1.2 g/m² IV daily × 5 d Platinol (cisplatin), 20 mg/m² IV daily × 5 d Mesna, 400 mg IV bolus prior to first ifosfamide dose, then 1.2 g/m² IV infused continuously daily for 5 d	4 cycles administered at 21-d intervals
VeIP[b]	Velban (vinblastine), 0.11 mg/kg on days 1 and 2 Ifosfamide, 1.2 g/m² IV daily × 5 d Platinol (cisplatin), 20 mg/m² IV daily × 5 d Mesna, 400 mg IV bolus prior to first ifosfamide dose, then 1.2 g/m² IV infused continuously daily for 5 d	3 to 4 cycles administered at 21-d intervals
TIP[b]	Taxol (paclitaxel), 175 mg/m² IV on day 1 Ifosfamide, 1 g/m² daily × 5 d Platinol (cisplatin), 20 mg/m² daily × 5 d Mesna, 400 mg IV bolus prior to first ifosfamide dose, then 1.2 g/m² IV infused continuously daily for 5 d	4 cycles administered at 21-d intervals

[a] May be used in patients with contraindications to bleomycin.
[b] Generally reserved for tumors that recur after prior chemotherapy.
d, days; IV, intravenous.

Salvage Therapy

▪ Salvage therapy is usually reserved for disease that has not had a durable response to primary chemotherapy with platinum-based regimen. Such patients may also be considered for a clinical trial especially if they have poor prognostic features.
▪ Conventional dose regimens incorporate ifosfamide and cisplatin with either vinblastine (VeIP) or paclitaxel (TIP).
▪ High-dose chemotherapy with autologous bone marrow or peripheral stem cell has demonstrated superior oncologic outcomes to standard-dose salvage therapy particularly when used as second-line treatment. Thus, it has replaced standard dose treatment in a significant number of patients—particularly with cisplatin-refractory or cisplatin-resistant disease.
▪ Agents currently under investigation include gemcitabine, paclitaxel, epirubicin, and oxaliplatin.

High-Dose Chemotherapy with Autologous Hematopoietic Stem Cell Rescue

▪ The benefit of high-dose chemotherapy with hematopoietic stem cell rescue (HDT) as first-line salvage therapy has been shown in nonrandomized trials but not in randomized phase III studies (Table 16.7).
▪ In a large retrospective study, 5-year survival was 53% with HDT as the first salvage therapy.

TABLE 16.5 Surveillance Schedule for Seminoma

Year	H&P, Markers (interval in months)	ABD/Pelvic CT (interval in months)	CXR
Stages I (active surveillance)			
1	3–6	3, 6, 12	As clinically indicated
2–3	6–12	6–12	
4–5+	12	12–24	
Stages IA, IB, IS (post radiation)ᵃ			
1–2	6–12	12	As clinically indicated
3–10	12	12 (up to year 3)	
Stages IIA, nonbulky IIB (post radiation or chemotherapy)			
1	3	3, 6–12	6
2–5	6	12 (at 4 yrs as clinically indicated)	6 upto year two
6–10	12		
Stages IIB, IIC, III (post radiation or chemotherapy)			
1	2	At 3 to 6 months, then	2
2	3	as clinical indicated	3
3–4	6	*PET as clinical indicated	Annual

H&P, history and physical; CXR, chest x-ray; ABD, abdomen; CT, computed tomography.

Adapted from National Comprehensive Cancer Network (NCCN) guidelines. There is considerable interinstitutional variation in the standard of follow-up care, with little evidence that different schedules lead to different outcomes.

ᵃ Surveillance schedule for stages IA and IB (postchemotherapy) is similar.

- Cisplatin refractory germ cell tumors are less likely to have durable response to HDT as compared with tumors that are not refractory to cisplatin.
- HDT should be considered in patients with germ cell tumors that are refractory to primary chemotherapy or those that failed first-line conventional salvage chemotherapy.

Late Relapse

- Defined as recurrent GCT >24 months after complete remission to primary therapy.
- Relatively poor prognosis with reported 5-year CSS of 60% to 70% in most series.
- Tends to be chemorefractory in patients with prior receipt of cisplatin-based chemotherapy. Thus, initially management should be surgical resection in patients with disease is deemed resectable. Chemotherapy can be utilized to cytoreduce unresectable masses prior to consolidative resection where possible.
- Most common histologies are yolk sac tumor and teratoma
- AFP is often elevated (reflecting high prevalence of yolk sac tumor).
- Disproportionally high rate of GCT with somatic-type malignancy (i.e., sarcoma, primitive neuroectodermal tumor, adenocarcinoma).

Extragonadal Germ Cell Tumors:

- Germ cell tumors can arise anywhere along the path of migration of the primordial germ cells from the pineal gland, down through the midline to the gonads. The most common locations of

TABLE 16.6 Surveillance Schedule for Nonseminoma

Year	H&P, Markers (interval in months)	ABD/Pelvic CT (interval in months)	CXR
Stages I (active surveillance)			
1	2	4–6	At 4 and 12
2	3	6–12	12
3	4–6	12	12
4	6		12
5	12		12
Stages IB (active surveillance)			
1	2	4	2
2	2	4–6	3
3	4–6	6	4–6
4	4	12	6
5	12		12
Stages IB treated with 1–2 cycles of adjuvant BEP chemotheraphy			
1	3	12	6–12
2	3	12	12
3–4	6		
5	12		
Stages II–III nonseminoma that has shown a complete response to chemotherapy, with or without post-chemotherapy RPLND			
1	2	6	6
2	3	6	6
3–4	6		12
5	6		12
Stage IIA–B nonseminoma, after primary RPLND and treatment with adjuvant chemotherapy			
1	6	After RPLND	6
2	6	As clinically indicated	12
3–5	4-6 (annually after year 5)		12
Stage IIA–B nonseminoma, after primary RPLND and not treated with adjuvant chemotherapy			
1	2	3–4	2–4
2	3	As clinically indicated	3–6
3	4		12
4	6		12
5	12		12

H&P, history and physical; CXR, chest x-ray; ABD, abdomen; CT, computed tomography.

Adapted from National Comprehensive Cancer Network (NCCN) guidelines. There is considerable interinstitutional variation in the standard of follow-up care, with little evidence that different schedules lead to different outcomes.

extragonadal GCTs are the anterior mediastinum and retroperitoneum. It should be noted that up to 70% of primary retroperitoneal GCTs are thought to represent the metastatic spread of a burned out testicular germ cell tumor.

▪ Primary mediastinal GCTs should be distinguished from benign or malignant tumors. About 80% of mediastinal germ cell tumors are benign.

TABLE 16.7 Commonly Used High-Dose Regimens

Agent/Dose	Schedule
IU regimen	
Carboplatin 700 mg/m² IV on days 1, 2, and 3	2 cycles given at 14-d interval. Autologous peripheral stem cell infusion on day 6 of each cycle
Etoposide 750 mg/m² IV on days 1, 2, and 3	
MSKCC regimen	
Paclitaxel 200 mg/m² over 24 h on day 1	2 cycles given at 14-d interval. Leukapheresis on days 11–13
Ifosfamide 2,000 mg/m² over 4 h daily on days 2–4 with mesna	
Followed by	
Carboplatin AUC 7--8 IV daily on days 1–3	3 cycles given at 14-d to 21-d interval. Autologous peripheral stem cell infusion on day 5 of each cycle
Etoposide 400 mg/m² IV daily on days 1–3	

IU, Indiana University; MSKCC, Memorial Sloan-Kettering Cancer Center.

- While the prognosis of seminoma is not thought to be affected by site of disease, primary mediastinal NSGCT carries a distinctly poorer prognosis than testicular primaries. These tumors are often refractory to cisplatin-based chemotherapy, particularly in the salvage setting. In fact, the futility of high dose chemotherapy in most of these patients has led some experts to recommend against its utilization in this setting given its toxicity.

Therapy-Related Toxicity

Complications of RPLND

- Overall complication rates have been reported to range from 10% to 20% with major complication rates of <10%.
- Complications are more common with PC-RPLND than primary RPLND.
- Mortality rate for primary RPLND is 0% and <1% for PC-RPLND.
- Most common complications include wound infections and pulmonary complications, which occur in <5% of patients.
- Chylous ascites, symptomatic lymphocele, or postoperative small bowel obstruction occurs in <3% of patients.
- Utilization of modified unilateral templates as well as sparing of the L1-4 postganglionic sympathetic fibers preserves postoperative antegrade ejaculation in nearly all patients where these techniques can be employed. However, nerve-sparing and/or modified template dissections are not always possible or appropriate in the postchemotherapy setting.

Fertility

Although 70% to 80% of patients treated with chemotherapy may recover sperm production within 5 years, sperm banking should be discussed with all patients desiring to father children after therapy.

■ At diagnosis, approximately 45% of patients have oligospermia, sperm abnormalities, or altered follicular-stimulating hormone levels due in part to the association of testicular cancer with conditions such as cryptorchidism or testicular atrophy.

■ Orchiectomy may further impair spermatogenesis.

■ Almost all patients become azospermic or oligospermic during chemotherapy.

■ Children of treated patients do not appear to have an increased risk of congenital abnormalities.

Pulmonary Toxicity

■ Bleomycin may cause pneumonitis and pulmonary fibrosis, which is now rare, but may be fatal in up to 50% of patients.

■ More frequently, asymptomatic decreases in pulmonary function resolve after completion of bleomycin therapy.

■ Bleomycin should be discontinued if early signs of pulmonary toxicity develop or if there is a decline of ≥40% in diffusing capacity of lung for carbon monoxide (DLCO).

■ Routine pulmonary function tests are rarely indicated and should be reserved for patients with signs and symptoms of pulmonary toxicity (e.g., dry rales or pulmonary lag on physical examination or dyspnea on exertion).

■ Corticosteroids may be used to reduce lung inflammation if pulmonary toxicity occurs.

■ Smokers treated with bleomycin should be particularly discouraged from tobacco use and alternatives to bleomycin-containing regimens should be considered (i.e., EPx4 in good risk patients and VIPx4 in intermediate and poor risk patients).

■ Retrospective studies have suggested that low fraction of inspired oxygen and conservative intravascular volume management during PC-RPLND may reduce the incidence of postoperative bleomycin-induced pulmonary toxicity.

Nephrotoxicity

■ Cisplatin-based chemotherapy may result in decreased glomerular filtration rate, which can be permanent in 20% to 30% of patients.

■ Hypokalemia and hypomagnesemia are also frequent manifestations of altered kidney function in these patients.

Neurologic Toxicity

■ Cisplatin-based chemotherapy may result in persistent peripheral neuropathy in 20% to 30% of patients.

■ Cisplatin-induced neuropathy is sensory and distal. Peripheral digital dysesthesias and paresthesias are the most common manifestations.

■ Polymorphism in the glutathione S-transferase gene may increase the susceptibility to cisplatin-induced neurotoxicity.

■ Ototoxicity in the form of tinnitus or high-frequency hearing loss, usually outside the frequency of spoken language, may be seen in up to 20% of the patients treated with cisplatin-based regimen. The risk increases with increasing number of treatment cycles.

Cardiovascular Toxicity

■ Bleomycin, cisplatin, and radiation alone or in combination can increase the risk of cardiovascular disease.

■ Angina, myocardial infarction, and sudden cardiac death are increased by up to twofold.

■ The risk of hypertension, hypercholesterolemia, and insulin resistance is increased in patients with testicular cancer treated with chemotherapy.

■ Patients are also at increased risk of thromboembolism and Raynaud phenomenon.

Secondary Malignancies

- Secondary malignancies are associated with the use of cisplatin, etoposide, and radiation. Patients treated for testicular cancer with these agents reportedly have a 1.7-fold increase in their risk of developing a secondary malignancy.
- The increased risk of second malignancy may persist for up to 35 years after the completion of chemotherapy or radiotherapy for testicular carcinoma.
- Alkylating agents such as cisplatin may lead to a myelodysplastic syndrome within 5 to 7 years that can eventually progress to leukemia. Topoisomerase inhibitors such as etoposide may cause secondary leukemias within 3 years.
- There is an increased incidence of solid tumors in previous radiation fields, including the bladder, stomach, pancreas, and kidney.

Suggested Readings

1. Albers P, Albrecht W, Algaba F, et al. Guidelines on Testicular Cancer: 2015 Update. *Eur Urol.* 2015;68:1054.
2. Beard CJ, Gupta S, Motzer RJ, et al. Follow-up management of patients with testicular cancer: a multidisciplinary consensus-based approach. *J Natl Compr Canc Netw.* 2015;13:811–822.
3. CR Nichols, B Roth, P Albers, et al. Active surveillance is the preferred approach to clinical stage I testicular cancer. *J Clin Oncol.* 2013;31:3490–3493.
4. De Santis M, Becherer A, Bokemeyer C, et al. 2-18fluoro-deoxy-D-glucose positron emission tomography is a reliable predictor for viable tumor in postchemotherapy seminoma: an update of the prospective multicentric SEMPET trial. *J Clin Oncol.* 2004 Mar;22(6):1034–1039.
5. de Wit R, Fizazi K. Controversies in the management of clinical stage I testis cancer. *J Clin Oncol.* 2006;24:5482–5492.
6. Ehrlich, Yaron et al. Advances in the treatment of testicular cancer. *Transl Androl Urol.* 2015;4(3):381–390.
7. Einhorn LH, Williams SD, Chamness A, et al. High-dose chemotherapy and stem-cell rescue for metastatic germ-cell tumors. *N Engl J Med.* 2007;357:340–348.
8. Farmakis D, Pectasides M, Pectasides D. Recent advances in conventional-dose salvage chemotherapy in patients with cisplatin-resistant or refractory testicular germ cell tumors. *Eur Urol.* 2005;48:400–407.
9. Fizazi K, Pagliaro L, Laplanche A, et al. Personalised chemotherapy based on serum tumor marker decline in poor-prognosis germ-cell tumours (GETUG13): a phase 3, multicentre, randomised trial. *Lancet Oncol.* 2014;15:1442–1450.
10. Greene MH, Kratz CP, Mai PL, et al. Familial testicular germ cell tumors in adults: 2010 summary of genetic risk factors and clinical phenotype. *Endocr Relat Cancer.* 2010;17:R109–R121.
11. Huddart RA, Norman A, Shahidi M, et al. Cardiovascular disease as a long-term complication of treatment for testicular cancer. *J Clin Oncol.* 2003;21:1513–1523.
12. International Germ Cell Cancer Collaborative Group. International Germ Cell Consensus Classification: a prognostic factor-based staging system for metastatic germ cell cancers. *J Clin Oncol.* 1997;15:594–603.
13. J Beyer, P Albers, R Altena, et al. Maintaining success, reducing treatment burden, focusing on survivorship: highlights from the third European consensus conference on diagnosis and treatment of germ-cell cancer *Ann Oncol.* 2013;24:878–888.
14. Kollmannsberger C, Tyldesley S, Moore C, et al. Evolution in management of testicular seminoma: population-based outcomes with selective utilization of active therapies. *Ann Oncol.* 2011;22:808.
15. Kondagunta GV, Bacik J, Sheinfeld J, et al. Paclitaxel plus ifosfamide followed by high-dose carboplatin plus etoposide in previously treated germ cell tumors. *J Clin Oncol.* 2007;25:85–90.
16. Kopp HG, Kuczyk M, Classen J, et al. Advances in the treatment of testicular cancer. *Drugs.* 2006;66:641–659.
17. Middleton WD, Teefey SA, Santillan CS. Testicular microlithiasis: prospective analysis of prevalence and associated tumor. *Radiology.* 2002;224:425–428.
18. Nasser H, Hanna MD, and Lawrence H. Einhorn MD. Testicular cancer - Discoveries and updates. *N Engl J Med.* 2014;371:2005–2016.
19. National Comprehensive Cancer Network guidelines available online at: http://www.nccn.org/professionals/physician_gls/f_guidelines.asp
20. Oliver RT, Mead GM, Rustin GJ, et al. Randomized trial of carboplatin versus radiotherapy for stage I seminoma: mature results on relapse and contralateral testis cancer rates in MRC TE19/EORTC 30982 study (ISRC TN27163214). *J Clin Oncol.* 2011;29:957–962.
21. Oliver T. Conservative management of testicular germ-cell tumors. *Nat Clin Pract Urol.* 2007;4:550–560.
22. Pagliano LC, Logothetis CJ, et al. Cancer of the testis. In: DeVita VT, Lawrence TS, Rosenberg SA, eds. *Cancer, Principles and Practice of Oncology.* 10th ed. Philadelphia, PA: Lippincott Williams & Wilkins; 2015.
23. Rajpert-De-Meyts E, McGlynn KA, Okamoto K, et al. Testicular germ cell tumors. *Lancet.* 2016;387:1762–1774.

24. Schnack TH, Poulsen G, Myrup C, et al. Familial congregation of cryptorchidism, hypospadias, and testicular germ cell cancer: a nationwide cohort study. *J Natl Cancer Inst.* 2012;102:187–192.
25. Siegel R, Naishadham D, Jemal A. Cancer statistics, 2013. *CA Cancer J Clin.* 2013;63:11–30.
26. Testicular Cancer Treatment (PDQ)—National Cancer Institute. Available at: https://www.cancer.gov/types/testicular/hp/testicular-treatment-pdq
27. van den Belt-Dusebout AW, de Wit R, Gietema JA, et al. Treatment-specific risks of second malignancies and cardiovascular disease in 5-year survivors of testicular cancer. *J Clin Oncol.* 2007;25:4370–4378.
28. Weir HK, Marrett LD, Moravan V. Trends in the incidence of testicular germ cell cancer in Ontario by histologic subgroup, 1964-1996. *CMAJ.* 1999;160:201–205.

17 Ovarian Cancer

Jung-min Lee and Elise C. Kohn

BACKGROUND AND EPIDEMIOLOGY

- Ovarian cancer is the most common cause of gynecologic cancer death, and fifth leading cause of cancer death in women in the United States.
- In 2016, approximately 22,280 cases were diagnosed in the United States, resulting in 14,240 deaths, a pattern that has been relatively stable for at least two decades.
- The median age at diagnosis is 63, with approximately 70% of new diagnoses at or beyond 55 years of age.
- Lifetime risk of developing an epithelial ovarian cancer (EOC) is approximately 1 in 70 (1.4%). It can be as high as 60% and 30% for patients with germline deleterious *BRCA1* and *BRCA2* mutation (*gBRCAm*), respectively.
- The majority of EOCs (~75%) are diagnosed at advanced stage (III/IV; Fig. 17.1).
- The EOC overall 5-year survival is 45%, with >75% of early-stage (stage I) patients alive at 5 years.

MOLECULAR AND CELLULAR PATHOLOGY

- Epithelial histology accounts for 90% of all ovarian cancers.
- EOCs are graded using a two-type grade classification system of low grade and high grade (and ungraded clear cell).
- EOCs consist of several molecular-pathological entities:
  - Low malignant potential (borderline; LMP) neoplasms account for approximately 15% of EOCs. They are defined by limited layers of stratified epithelial proliferation, without ovarian stromal invasion. They can progress to invasive low-grade serous malignancies.
  - Low-grade serous ovarian cancer (LGSOC) may be found concomitant and/or in continuity with serous LMP cancers. BRAF V600E and KRAS mutations can be found in up to 70% of serous LMP tumors with the frequency dropping to approximately 40% in invasive low-grade cancers. LGSOC is more slowly growing and has been inferred to be less susceptible to cytotoxic chemotherapy.
  - Clear cell and low-grade endometrioid cancers may be contiguous and progress from ovarian endometriosis. They share up to 40% somatic mutation in ARID1a, and may be found as a mixed subtype. Clear cell cancers are more aggressive and have a worse outcome in early stage than other non–high-grade serous EOC.
  - Primary mucinous and transitional cell carcinomas. These are extremely rare. True mucinous carcinoma of the ovary must be separated anatomically and histopathologically from mucinous cancers of other origins, especially appendiceal malignancies. Nearly 80% of mucinous ovarian cancers have KRAS mutation. If there is extension beyond the ovary, the appendix must be cleared of malignancy for a pathologic conclusion of mucinous carcinoma of the ovary.
  - High-grade serous or endometrioid ovarian cancer (HGSOC) are now shown to originate in the serous epithelium of the fallopian tube.
    - Dysregulating mutations in *TP53* is a ubiquitous and in some cases, defining, event.

234

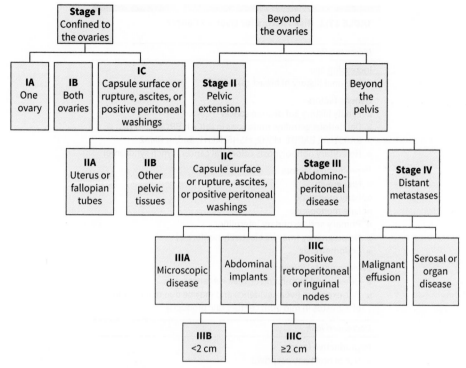

FIGURE 17.1 A flow chart for ovarian cancer the International Federation of Gynecology and Obstetrics (FIGO) staging. Patients are staged at diagnosis based on the extent of the spread of the ovarian cancer. Correct staging is critical as it impacts treatment decisions.

- HGSOC are more aggressive and disseminate early within the abdominal cavity upon presentation, although parenchymal invasion is often a late event.
- HGSOC, fallopian tube, and primary peritoneal carcinomas are now considered a single clinical entity ("EOC").
- Mixed Muellerian malignant tumor or carcinosarcoma is a variant of EOC with sarcomatous appearing histology and carcinomatous molecular changes. It appears to be an aggressive variant of HGSOC.
■ The remaining 10% of ovarian cancers consist of sex-cord stromal or germ cell histology.
- Sex-cord stromal tumors are mesenchymal and include granulosa cell and Sertoli–Leydig cell tumors. They are most often benign and can begin at post puberty. Granulosa cell tumors account for 70% of sex-cord stromal tumors and may produce estrogen. Sertoli–Leydig cell tumors may produce testosterone.
- Germ cell neoplasms include dysgerminoma, teratoma, and yolk sac (endodermal sinus) tumors. Malignant germ cell tumors are treated similarly to testicular cancer.

RISK FACTORS

■ Table 17.1 lists risk factors for ovarian cancer.
■ gBRCAm women have high lifetime risk for the development of EOC, up to 60% for *BRCA1* and 40% for *BRCA2*, respectively.
■ Women with a strong family history without an identified deleterious germline mutation also have a high lifetime risk for the development of EOC.

TABLE 17.1 Risk Factors for Ovarian Cancer

Increased Risk

Increasing age
■ Personal history of breast cancer

Genetic factors
■ Family history 3of ovarian cancer
■ Deleterious germline mutations in BRCA1, BRCA2, PALB2, RAD51c/d, BARD1, MSH2, MSH6, MLH1, and/or PMS2
■ Hereditary nonpolyposis colorectal cancer (Lynch syndrome)

Reproductive factors
■ Nulligravity
■ Early menarche
■ Late menopause
■ Primary and secondary infertility
■ No pregnancy (may be electively nonfertile)
■ Endometriosis

Environmental factors
■ Obesity and high-fat diet (weak evidence)
■ Talc exposure (weak evidence and may be due to inclusion of asbestos in mid-20th century talc products)

Decreased Risk

Reproductive factors
■ Use of oral contraceptives
■ Pregnancy/multiparity
■ Breastfeeding

Gynecologic surgery
■ Salpingo-oophorectomy
■ Tubal ligation

PREVENTION

■ The use of oral contraceptives is protective against EOC for the general population. Increasing duration of use is associated with larger reductions in EOC risk.
■ Risk reduction salpingo-oophorectomy (RRSO) has been shown to reduce the lifetime risk of ovarian/tubal/peritoneal cancer to less than 5% in high-risk women. RRSO is recommended for high-risk women defined as those with familial ovarian cancer syndromes, and/or gBRCAm. Surgery is recommended after completion of childbearing and, where feasible, approximately 10 years earlier than the age of diagnosis of the youngest affected family member.
■ The use of salpingectomy without oophorectomy remains controversial and untested. If used, it should be considered in women of childbearing potential who wish to have children after which oophorectomy should be done.
■ RRSO has been shown to decrease the risk of breast cancer up to 50% in gBRCAm carriers.
■ RRSO is not recommended for women at average risk.

SCREENING

■ The FDA released a formal recommendation *against* using any screening tests for ovarian cancer on September 7, 2016.

- The 2012 Reaffirmation Recommendation Statement of the U.S. Preventive Services Task Force reiterated its recommendation against screening for EOC in women who are asymptomatic and without known genetic mutations that increase its risk.
  - Mounting evidence suggests that annual screening with transvaginal ultrasonography (TVU) and serum cancer antigen 125 (CA-125) does not reduce mortality. High false-positive rates leading to intervention are associated with subsequent harm, such as unnecessary surgical intervention.
- Women with a family history of breast/ovarian cancer should be offered genetic counseling and genetic testing if interested.
- Familial ovarian cancer syndrome patients and known *gBRCA*m carriers who have not undergone RRSO may be offered screening consisting of a pelvic examination, TVU, and a CA-125 blood test every 6 months beginning between the ages of 30 and 35 years, or 5 and 10 years earlier than the earliest age of first EOC diagnosis in the family. There are no data demonstrating survival benefit of screening high-risk patients.
- Women with high-risk families in whom deleterious mutations are not found (*BRCA1*, *BRCA2* or Lynch syndrome–associated genes) can be referred for panel testing for lower abundance deleterious germline mutations. Absent such testing and confirmation of a genetic risk, such women are treated similarly to those in whom genetic risk is identified. RRSO is recommended; absent RRSO, screening as for high-risk women is reasonable.

SERUM BIOMARKERS

- CA-125 is a high-molecular-weight glycoprotein and marker of epithelial tissue turnover produced by ovarian, endocervical, endometrial, peritoneal, pleural, colonic, and breast epithelia.
  - CA-125 is increased in approximately 50% of early-stage and >90% of advanced-stage serous and endometrioid EOC.
  - Specificity of CA-125 for ovarian cancer is poor. It can be increased in many benign conditions, such as endometriosis, first trimester pregnancy, pelvic inflammatory disease, uterine fibroids, benign breast disease, cirrhosis, and in response to pleural or peritoneal effusions of any cause, and other epithelial malignancies.
  - CA-125 is FDA approved for use as a biomarker for monitoring EOC response to treatment and recurrence. It is neither approved nor recommended for screening.
  - The reliability of following CA-125 concentrations during molecularly targeted therapy is unknown.
- Human epididymis protein 4 (HE4) is a glycoprotein also expressed in some EOC. It is increased in >50% of tumors that do not also express CA-125. HE4 testing is FDA approved as a biomarker for monitoring EOC recurrence and response to treatment. It is neither approved nor recommended for screening.

DIAGNOSIS AND EVALUATION

- EOC is not a silent disease. Symptoms are present, though nonspecific.
- Several studies suggest usefulness of a Symptom Index Tool to identify women who may have EOC: new (within 1 year) and persistent (more than 12 times/month) pelvic/abdominal pain, increased abdominal size/bloating, difficulty eating/feeling full, and urinary urgency/frequency should trigger evaluation by a gynecologic oncologist.
- Stromal tumors can produce virilization, precocious puberty, amenorrhea, and/or postmenopausal bleeding, depending on patient age, and type and amount of ectopic hormone produced.
- The preoperative workup of a patient with a suspected ovarian malignancy is summarized in Table 17.2.
- Early referral to a gynecologic oncologist is strongly recommended.
- Diagnosis can be made by laparoscopy, or biopsy, especially in situations where surgical extirpation may not be considered optimally done and neoadjuvant therapy is being considered. The extent and quality of surgical debulking has a prognostic role.

TABLE 17.2 Workup for Patient with a Pelvic Mass and/or Suspected EOC

History of present illness, attention to issues related to Symptom Index Tool (see text)
Family history
Gynecologic history
Physical examination, including cervical scraping for PAP smear

Labwork: full panels with added:
- Consider CA-125 (not diagnostic)
- β-HCG (should be used to rule out pregnancy in women of childbearing potential; if the germ cell tumor is considered depending upon age and presentation)
- AFP (germ cell consideration; depending upon age and presentation)

Imaging[a]
- Transvaginal/abdominal ultrasound (may skip to CT if high index of suspicion, ascites, etc.)
- CT abdomen/pelvis with oral and IV contrast
- Chest x-ray (chest CT is not done)

[a] Value of PET and MRI uncertain; PET/CT interpretability may be compromised by lack of IV and oral contrast.

TREATMENT

Surgery

- Proper EOC diagnosis and staging require tissue.
- Standards of care are now either primary debulking or tissue sampling for diagnosis with interim debulking after initiating neoadjuvant chemotherapy.
  - Primary debulking surgery includes laparotomy with en bloc TAH/BSO tumor removal, abdominal fluid sampling, tumor debulking, and pathologic assessment of the abdomen, including diaphragms, paracolic gutters, and serosal surfaces. Unilateral salpingo-oophorectomy can be considered in women with stage I grade 1/2 tumors who wish to preserve fertility. Completion of salpingo-oophorectomy is recommended upon completion of child-bearing.
  - Interval debulking uses the same complete extent of surgery, but occurs after 3–4 cycles of neoadjuvant therapy.
  - The goal of surgery, whether primary or interval, is "R0" or no visible disease. Optimal debulking remains no lesion greater than 1cm residual in largest diameter. Data indicate better outcome for women undergoing surgical debulking by a gynecologic oncologist.
- Stage I disease with favorable prognostic features (grade 1/2, stage IA/B, non–clear cell histology) can be treated by surgery alone.

Initial Chemotherapy

- The current international consensus standard of care for all stage IC and stages II–IV is adjuvant chemotherapy. That chemotherapy should include a platinum and a taxane and should be administered for 6 cycles, with fewer cycles considered acceptable for IC (GOG-157).
- Neoadjuvant chemotherapy (NACT) can be administered with interval debulking for advanced-stage patients. In such cases the total neoadjuvant and adjuvant exposure should be 6 to 8 cycles of combination chemotherapy. NACT with interval debulking has been shown to be noninferior to primary debulking surgery and adjuvant chemotherapy.
- Adjuvant chemotherapy remains the recommendation for all histologic types, types I and II, ovarian cancers.
- Combination intraperitoneal/intravenous chemotherapy with platinum and taxane has been shown in numerous trials to be superior to intravenous chemotherapy in optimally debulked advanced stage ovarian cancer patients.

- Dose-dense paclitaxel/carboplatin therapy is not superior to every 3-week paclitaxel therapy, although it appears that every 3 weekly paclitaxel/carboplatin with bevacizumab is superior to 3 weekly paclitaxel/carboplatin in a post hoc unplanned subset analysis (GOG0262).
- NACT and adjuvant chemotherapy regimens are summarized in Table 17.3.
- Paclitaxel and docetaxel have been shown to yield similar outcomes in adjuvant therapy (SCOTROC1).
- Carboplatin dosing should be based on the Calvert formula for calculating AUC (http://ctep.cancer.gov/content/docs/Carboplatin_Information_Letter.pdf) dosing of carboplatin [AUC × (GFR + 25)], where GFR is the calculated glomerular filtration rate. If a patient's GFR is estimated based on serum creatinine measurements by an isotope dilution mass spectrometry (IDMS) method, FDA recommends that physicians consider capping the dose of carboplatin for desired exposure (AUC) to avoid potential toxicity due to overdosing.
- Patients can demonstrate hypersensitivity to paclitaxel with the initial treatment doses due to an anaphylactoid reaction to either the paclitaxel and/or its vehicle. Treatment can be changed to docetaxel, which has a different vehicle if premedication with steroids, H1 and H2 blockers, and/or slower infusion is not sufficiently protective.
- Platinum hypersensitivity is an anaphylactic, true atopic reaction and presents in later cycles (usually >6 to 10 exposures).
  - Cisplatin and carboplatin can be cross-substituted, depending on the severity of the reaction. The two agents can have cross-sensitivity because the bioactive moiety is the same.
  - Women having a history of platinum allergy may be retreated using slow infusion and premedication with steroids and H1/H2 blockers.
- Phase III studies suggest that bevacizumab given during adjuvant carboplatin/paclitaxel and in maintenance prolongs PFS and does not improve OS (GOG218 and ICON7).
- A meta-analysis of six randomized maintenance trials confirmed no improvement in OS (HR 1.07; 95% CI, 0.91 to 1.27; N = 902). This analysis did not include bevacizumab maintenance therapy.

Recurrent or Persistent Disease

- Recurrence occurs in >80% of stage III/IV patients; recurrent EOC is not curable, although subsequent complete remissions may occur.
- No OS benefit was observed in a RCT comparing early treatment of relapse (based upon increased CA-125 alone) versus observation until symptoms or physical examination trigger disease assessment (MRC OV05/EORTC 55955).
- Secondary cytoreduction surgery can be considered for women with recurrence-free intervals of ≥12 months. Its value is being examined in an ongoing phase III trial (GOG-0213).
- Patients with a progression-free interval of ≥6 months have platinum-sensitive disease, although this is a continuum. Second-line platinum-based therapy, single agent or combination, improves survival in women with platinum-sensitive EOC (Table 17.3).
- Recurrence within 6 months of, or progression on, initial platinum-based chemotherapy is defined as platinum-resistant disease.
- Sequential single-agent chemotherapy is preferred for platinum-resistant/refractory patients, due to increased toxicity without sufficient evidence of increased benefit of combinations (Table 17.3).
- Cisplatin/gemcitabine is the one combination chemotherapy regimen with RCT-documented benefit.
- Topotecan, pegylated liposomal doxorubicin, or weekly paclitaxel with bevacizumab has been shown to be superior on PFS to chemotherapy alone and is licensed in the United States (AURELIA).

Use of Molecularly Targeted Agents

- Bevacizumab has modest single agent activity in relapsed ovarian cancer, both platinum sensitive and platinum resistant. It is licensed in the United States and Europe in combination with chemotherapy for platinum-resistant recurrent EOC (Table 17.3).
- PARP inhibitors have demonstrated clinical activity in recurrent EOC with gBRCAm. Olaparib is licensed in the United States for gBRCAm carriers with EOC who had more than three chemotherapy treatment (Table 17.3).
- Clinical trials investigating other targeted agents and immunotherapy either in combination or single agents are ongoing.

TABLE 17.3 Adjuvant Chemotherapy and Therapy for Recurrent Disease

Neoadjuvant or Adjuvant Chemotherapy

Indication	Treatment	Supporting Data
Neoadjuvant chemotherapy (NACT), stage III/IV	IV carboplatin (AUC5 or 6) and paclitaxel at 175 mg/m^2 every 21 d	NACT followed by interval debulking surgery was not inferior to PDS → adjuvant chemotherapy Patients who cannot tolerate IP therapy or bulky stage IIIC/IV EOC: OS HR = 0.98 (90% confidence interval [CI] 0.84–1.13; P = 0.01), PFS HR = 1.01 (90% CI 0.89–1.15) CHORUS (Lancet, 2015): stage III/IV, non-inferiority study: OS HR=0.87 (90% CI 0.72–1.05): median OS 24.1 (NACT) vs. 22.6mo (PDS)
Optimally debulked advanced stage III	IV paclitaxel at 135 mg/m^2 over 24 hours on day 1; IP cisplatin at 100 mg/m^2 on day 2 and IP paclitaxel at 60 mg/m^2 on day 8	GOG172: median PFS 18.3 (IV) vs. 23.8 mo (IV/IP; P = 0.05); median OS 49.7 (IV) vs. 65.6 mo (IV/IP; P = 0.03) 10 yr follow-up (GOG114 and 172) median OS 51.4 mo (IV) vs. 61.8 (IV/IP; adjusted HR = 0.77; 95% CI, 0.65 to 0.90; P =0.002)
Dose-dense weekly paclitaxel	Weekly paclitaxel at 80 mg/m^2 with carboplatin (AUC6)	Japanese GOG3016 study: median PFS 28.20 (dose- dense) vs. 17.52 mo (q3wk; HR = 0.76, 95%CI 0.62-0.91, P=0.0037)P = 0.0015); Median OS at 3 y 72.1%100.5 (dose- dense) vs. 65.1%62.0 mo (q3wk; HR = 0.79, 95% CI 0.63-0.99, P=0.039) P = 0.03)
	Weekly paclitaxel at 80 mg/m^2 with carboplatin (AUC6) +/- bevacizumab	GOG0252: Overall, no PFS benefit: 14.7 (dose-dense) vs. 14.0 mo (q3wk; HR=0.89, p=0.18). Subgroup analysis: with bevacizumab; no PFS benefit; 14.9 (dose-dense) vs. 14.7 mo (q3wk; HR=0.99) without bevacizumab: PFS benefit; 14.2 (dose-dense) vs. 10.3 mo (q3wk; HR=0.62, 95% CI (0.40-0.95, P=0.03)
Maintenance therapy	Bevacizumab during adjuvant carboplatin/paclitaxel and for maintenance therapy; doses: GOG 218 (15 mg/kg) ICON 7 (7.5 mg/kg)	GOG218 and ICON7: bevacizumab prolongs PFS but does not improve OS. It is not approved for maintenance in the US. Approved by the EMA for high-risk EOC

Recurrent or Persistent Disease

Indication	Treatment	Supporting Data
Platinum-sensitive disease	Platinum-based combination therapy (with pegylated liposomal doxorubicin, gemcitabine, or taxane)	ICON-4, AGO-OVAR-2.2, OCEANS GCIG, CALYPSO: 70% of patients >2 y from initial treatment will respond to retreatment. Carboplatin/paclitaxel or carboplatin/gemcitabine are better than carboplatin alone; carboplatin/doxil is better tolerated and equivalent otherwise to carboplatin/paclitaxel

(continued)

TABLE 17.3 (Continued)

Recurrent or Persistent Disease

Indication	Treatment	Supporting Data
	Platinum-based chemotherapy+targeted therapy combination/targeted therapies	ICON6: platinum-based chemotherapy+cediranib vs. chemotherapy alone: median PFS; 11.1 vs. 8.7 mo (HR=0.57, p<0.00001; not licensed) Additional studies ongoing; SOLO2: olaparib vs. single agent chemotherapy in gBRCAm carriers, ARIEL (rucaparib) and NRG-GY004 olaparib+cediranib vs. platinum-based chemotherapy)
Platinum-resistant/ refractory disease	Single-agent chemotherapy: pegylated liposomal doxorubicin (PLD), topotecan, gemcitabine, taxotere, oral etoposide, weekly paclitaxel, hexamethylmelamine, and/or consideration of hormone ablation with letrozole/anastrazole or tamoxifen; experimental therapy	
	Bevacizumab+chemotherapy (PLD, topotecan or weekly paclitaxel) for platinum-resistant recurrent EOC patients who had no more than two prior chemotherapies	AURELIA: PFS benefit; 6.7 (bevacizumab+ chemotherapy) vs. 3.4 mo (chemotherapy alone; HR=0.48; 95% CI: 0.38-0.60; P=0.001)
Maintenance in platinum-sensitive recurrent disease	Olaparib 400mg capsules BID as the first therapy for the maintenance treatment in *gBRCAm* carriers with HGSOC, fallopian tube or primary peritoneal cancer. *Olaparib is licensed in the US only for gBRCAm carriers with EOC who had more than three chemotherapy treatments and not for maintenance use*	Study 19: PFS benefit after platinum-based chemotherapy; 11.2 (olaparib maintenance) vs. 4.3 mo (placebo; HR=0.18; 95% CI 0.10-0.31; P<0.0001)
	Bevacizumab (15 mg/kg on day 1 every 3 wk), concurrent with carboplatin/ gemcitabine for 10 cycles maximum, followed by bevacizumab alone until disease progression	OCEANS: PFS only benefit for carbo/ gemcitabine with maintenance bevacizumab (HR = 0.48; median PFS = 12.4 mo vs. 8.4 mo; P < 0.0001). No OS benefit 33.6 vs. 32.9 HR=0.95, p=0.65 GOG 213: PFS benefit for carbo/ paclitaxel with maintenance bevacizumab (HR=0.61; median PFS 13.8 vs 10.4 mo; p<0.0001) surgical randomization still ongoing

Nonepithelial Ovarian Cancer

- Most patients with ovarian germ cell tumors are diagnosed with early-stage disease. Lymph node metastases are rare. Unilateral salpingo-oophorectomy, if contralateral ovary is uninvolved, is possible in women who wish to preserve fertility.
- BEP chemotherapy (bleomycin/etoposide/cisplatin) should be considered after surgery for germ cell tumors: nondysgerminoma, all but stage I grade 1 disease, and ≥stage II dysgerminoma.
- Most ovarian sex-cord stromal tumors are low grade, early stage at presentation, and have excellent survival. Radiation to gross residual tumors and hormonal therapy with progestin for granulosa cell tumors are considered after surgical resection.
- Many malignant stromal tumors including granulosa cell tumors produce estrogen; hence, evaluation of the endometrium for malignant change is needed.

Radiation

Radiation therapy (RT) plays a limited role in the treatment of EOC in the United States. Tumors of ovarian and tubal origin are sensitive to RT. RT should be considered for solitary metastases with functional consequences (brain metastases, distal bowel obstruction, bleeding).

Experimental Therapy/Immunotherapy

Patients with ovarian cancer of all stages, at diagnosis and at recurrence, should be encouraged to participate in clinical trials (www.clinicaltrials.gov).

SUPPORTIVE CARE

Common Treatment Toxicities

- Myelosuppression: Carboplatin-related bone marrow suppression is a cumulative toxicity (**see Chapter 34**).
- Nausea/vomiting: Carboplatin is less emetogenic than cisplatin. Both acute and delayed nausea/vomiting should be monitored and addressed therapeutically (**see Chapter 38**).
- Renal dysfunction
  - Great care should be taken in patients with borderline or abnormal renal function.
  - Serum creatinine-based calculations of GFR underestimate renal dysfunction in patients who have received platinums.
- Neurotoxicity
  - Both platinums and taxanes cause neuropathy. Platinums cause demyelinating injury and can leave long-lasting neuro-residuals. Taxanes and other chemotherapies cause axonal degeneration, which is recoverable.
  - Grade 3 to 4 neuropathy can have long-term effects and may require substitution or discontinuation of the offending agent(s). Dose modification of drugs with grade 2 neuropathy may be needed to avoid grade 3 to 4 neuropathy.
- Perforation
  - Bevacizumab causes a 5% to 11% risk of gastrointestinal perforation in EOC patients.
  - Possible risk factors for perforation include previous irradiation, tumor involving bowel, and early tumor response.
- Obstruction
- Patients can present with both bowel and urinary tract obstruction. Presenting symptoms include nausea, vomiting, abdominal pain, abdominal distention, abdominal and/or back pain, and infrequent bowel movements or urination.
- Initial treatment for bowel obstruction may be conservative, with bowel rest and nasogastric suction, but many patients will require bypass surgery.
- The aggressiveness of intervention should be balanced with the patient's prognosis, health status, and goals of care. Management with analgesics, antiemetics, anticholinergics, etc. and/or endoscopic placement of drainage tubes are options for poor surgical candidates.

▪ Urinary obstruction may be relieved with ureteral stents or nephrostomy, depending on the location, length, and severity of the obstruction.
▪ Occasionally, RT to a particular mass causing obstruction may be appropriate.

SUMMARY

▪ EOC is the most common cause of death among women with gynecologic malignancies and the fifth leading cause of cancer death in women in the United States.
▪ Limited disease with high-risk features and advanced disease need adjuvant paclitaxel/carboplatin.
▪ For women who experience a recurrence, the selection of therapy is commonly based upon response to initial platinum-based treatment.

ACKNOWLEDGMENT

This work was supported by the Intramural Program of the Center for Cancer Research, National Cancer Institute and the Cancer Therapy Evaluation Program, Division of Cancer Treatment and Diagnosis, National Cancer Institute.

Suggested Readings

1. Aghajanian C, Blank SV, Goff BA, et al. OCEANS: a randomized, double-blind, placebo-controlled phase III trial of chemotherapy with or without bevacizumab in patients with platinum-sensitive recurrent epithelial ovarian, primary peritoneal, or fallopian tube cancer. *J Clin Oncol.* 2012;30:2039.
2. Armstrong DK, Bundy B, Wenzel L, et al. Intraperitoneal cisplatin and paclitaxel in ovarian cancer. *N Engl J Med.* 2006;354:34–43.
3. Bristow RE, Zahurak ML, Diaz-Montes TP, et al. Impact of surgeon and hospital ovarian cancer surgical case volume on in-hospital mortality and related short-term outcomes. *Gynecol Oncol.* 2009;115:334–338.
4. Burger RA, Brady MF, Bookman MA, et al. Incorporation of bevacizumab in the primary treatment of ovarian cancer. *N Engl J Med.* 2011;365:2473.
5. Frederick PJ, Ramirez PT, McQuinn L, et al. Preoperative factors predicting survival after secondary cytoreduction for recurrent ovarian cancer. *Int J Gynecol Cancer.* 2011;21(5):831–836.
6. Goff BA, Mandel LS, Drescher CW, et al. Development of an ovarian cancer symptom index. *Cancer.* 2007;109:221–227.
7. Hunn J, Rodriguez GC. Ovarian cancer: etiology, risk factors, and epidemiology. *Clin Obstet Gynecol.* 2012;55(1):3–23.
8. Kim G, Ison G, McKee AE, et al. FDA approval summary: olaparib monotherapy in patients with deleterious germline BRCA-mutated advanced ovarian cancer treated with three or more lines of chemotherapy. *Clin Cancer Res.* 2015;21(19):4257–4261.
9. Kurman RJ, Shih IM. Pathogenesis of ovarian cancer: lessons from morphology and molecular biology and their clinical implications. *Int J Gynecol Pathol.* 2008;27:151–160.
10. Ledermann J, Harter P, Gourley C, et al. Olaparib maintenance therapy in platinum-sensitive relapsed ovarian cancer. *N Engl J Med.* 2012;366:1382–1392.
11. Moyer VA. U.S. Preventive Services Task Force. Screening for Ovarian Cancer: U.S. Preventive Services Task Force Reaffirmation Recommendation Statement. *Ann Intern Med.* 2012;157(12):900–904.
12. National Comprehensive Cancer Network. NCCN Clinical Practice Guidelines in Oncology (NCCN Guidelines®) *Ovarian Cancer. Version 4.* 2017. Available at: https://www.nccn.org/professionals/physician_gls/pdf/ovarian.pdf. Last accessed on November 14, 2017.
13. Pujade-Lauraine E, Hilpert F, Weber B, et al. Bevacizumab combined with chemotherapy for platinum-resistant recurrent ovarian cancer: The AURELIA open-label randomized phase III trial. *J Clin Oncol.* 2014.
14. Pujade-Lauraine E, Wagner U, Aavall-Lundqvist E, et al. Pegylated liposomal doxorubicin and carboplatin compared with paclitaxel and carboplatin for patients with platinum-sensitive ovarian cancer in late relapse. *J Clin Oncol.* 2010;28(20):3323–3329.
15. Rustin GS, Van der Burg ME, Griffin CL, et al. Early versus delayed treatment of relapsed ovarian cancer (MRC OV05/EORTC 55955): a randomized trial. *Lancet.* 2010;376:1155–1163.
16. Vergote I, Trope C, Amant F, et al. Neoadjuvant chemotherapy or primary surgery in stage IIIC or IV ovarian cancer. *N Engl J Med.* 2010;363:943–953.

18 Endometrial Cancer

Kristen P. Zeligs and Christina M. Annunziata

EPIDEMIOLOGY

- Endometrial cancer is the most commonly diagnosed gynecologic malignancy in developed countries, and is the fourth most common cancer in women in the United States, comprising 7% of all new cancer cases in women.
- Approximately 60,050 new cases of uterine cancer will be diagnosed in 2016 in the United States. One in 36 women will be diagnosed with endometrial cancer during her lifetime.
- This cancer is slightly more common in Caucasian women who have a 2.8% lifetime risk of developing uterine cancer compared with a 2.5% lifetime risk for African-American women.
- The incidence is 26.0 per 100,000 white women per year, compared to 24.6 per 100,000 African-American women per year.
- Although incidence is 1.4 times higher in white women than in African-American women, the 5-year survival rate is lower in African-American women than in white women (66% vs. 86%).
- An estimated 10,470 deaths are expected in 2016 due to this malignancy, accounting for 1.8% of all cancer deaths in women.
- The mortality rate continues to decline, likely because of increased awareness of symptoms such as abnormal uterine bleeding.
- Peak incidence is in the sixth and seventh decades of life, with a median age at diagnosis of 62 years.

RISK FACTORS

- Most risk factors for the development of endometrial cancer are related to prolonged exposure to unopposed estrogen, whether endogenous or exogenous which acts to stimulate the endometrium.
- Causes of unopposed endogenous estrogen excess:
  - Chronic anovulation (e.g., polycystic ovary syndrome).
  - Anovulatory menstrual cycles. Estrogen-producing tumors (e.g., granulosa cell tumor of the ovary).
  - Excessive peripheral conversion of androgens to estrone in adipose tissue: Being overweight by 20 to 50 pounds increases risk 3-fold and being overweight by >50 pounds increases risk 10-fold. Each 5 kg/m^2 increase in BMI is associated with 30% to 60% increased risk of endometrial cancer.
  - Advanced liver disease.
  - Early menarche and late menopause: Menopause in women older than 52 years increases risk by 2.4-fold.
  - Irregular menses, infertility, and nulliparity: Nulliparous women have twice the risk of developing uterine cancer compared to women with one child and thrice the risk compared to women who give birth to five or more children.
- Unopposed exogenous estrogen sources:
  - Systemic unopposed estrogen therapy increases the risk of endometrial cancer by up to 20-fold, with the increasing risk correlating with the duration of use. Concomitant administration of progestin mitigates this risk.

- Tamoxifen (TAM), although an estrogen antagonist in the breast, has an estrogen-agonist effect on the endometrium. Most studies have found that the increased relative risk (RR) of developing endometrial cancer for women taking TAM is two to three times higher than that of age-matched population depending on the drug dose and length of exposure. Additionally, the ability of TAM to induce endometrial cancer appears to differ between premenopausal and postmenopausal women, with no difference in rates between women 49 years and younger but by a 4.01 RR in women 50 years or older. Women taking TAM should be informed about the risks of endometrial proliferation, endometrial hyperplasia, endometrial cancer, and uterine sarcomas, and any abnormal uterine bleeding should be evaluated.
- Type II diabetes mellitus (DM), possibly related to the effects of hyperinsulinemia.
- Hypertension.
- Hereditary factors (accounts for 3% to 5% of cases of uterine cancer):
  - Personal history of breast, ovarian, or colorectal cancer.
  - Personal or family history consistent with hereditary nonpolyposis colorectal cancer (HNPCC) (Lynch II syndrome) is associated with a RR of 1.5 for development of endometrial cancer in the premenopausal years and a 15% to 66% lifetime risk (dependent on the mismatch repair (MMR) mutation).
  - History of endometrial cancer in a first-degree relative increases risk 3-fold.
  - History of colorectal cancer in a first-degree relative increases risk of endometrial cancer 2-fold.

PROTECTIVE FACTORS

- Oral contraceptives:
  - There is a 50% decrease in RR when oral contraceptives that include a progestin are used for at least 12 months.
  - Protection lasts for at least 10 years after discontinuation of oral contraceptive.
  - Similar protection has been observed with long-term use (≥10 years) of hormone replacement therapy that includes daily progestin.
- Physical activity: Lack of sufficient activity (20 minutes or more of vigorous physical activity at least three times per week) has been associated with a 30% to 40% increased risk of endometrial cancer.
  - It is estimated that if women exercised vigorously five or more times per week and sat for 4 or fewer hours per day, then 34% of endometrial cancers could be avoided.
- Cigarette smoking appears to have a modest protective role. However, this is strongly outweighed by the significantly increased risk of lung cancer and other diseases.

DIAGNOSIS AND SCREENING

- There are no cost-effective screening techniques for early detection of endometrial cancer in asymptomatic women. The diagnosis is based on evaluation of signs and symptoms.
- Women with HNPCC can have greater than a 60% lifetime risk of developing endometrial cancer, and the disease often occurs 10 to 20 years earlier than nonhereditary cancers. The American Cancer Society (ACS), therefore, recommends that women with HNPCC be offered annual screening with endometrial biopsy and/or transvaginal ultrasound starting at age 35. Prophylactic hysterectomy and bilateral salpingo-oophorectomy (BSO) should also be considered as a risk-reducing treatment option for women with Lynch Syndrome who have completed childbearing.
- Women taking TAM should have a gynecologic evaluation according to the same guidelines for women not taking TAM. Routine endometrial surveillance has not proved to be effective in increasing the early detection of endometrial cancer in women using TAM and is not recommended.

Signs and Symptoms

- Abnormal uterine bleeding to include postmenopausal bleeding is the most common symptom of endometrial cancer, seen in approximately 90% of cases.
- Premenopausal women with prolonged and/or heavy menses or intermenstrual spotting should undergo endometrial biopsy.
- Ten percent of cases present with profuse serous or serosanguinous discharge.
- All postmenopausal women with uterine bleeding should be evaluated for endometrial cancer (10% of these patients will ultimately be diagnosed with the malignancy).
- Biopsy is also recommended for women taking estrogen therapy for menopausal symptoms who have withdrawal bleeding.
- Asymptomatic patients with abnormal glandular tissue on Pap smear should be evaluated for endometrial cancer.
- All postmenopausal women with endometrial cells on Pap smear should be evaluated for malignancy.
- Approximately 10% of uterine cancer cases are detected by Pap smear. Pap smear alone, however, is not an adequate tool for detecting endometrial malignancy.
- Palpable, locally advanced tumor detected on pelvic examination is suggestive of endometrial cancer. Common distant sites of metastases include lung, inguinal, and supraclavicular lymph nodes (LNs), liver, bones, brain, and vagina. Signs and symptoms of advanced disease, manifested in <10% of cases, include
  - Bowel obstruction
  - Jaundice
  - Ascites
  - Pain

Procedures

- Endometrial sampling via an in-office endometrial biopsy is the preferred diagnostic test for symptomatic patients with abnormal uterine bleeding. Endometrial biopsy is generally a well-tolerated outpatient procedure and has a diagnostic accuracy of 93% to 98% when compared with subsequent findings of hysterectomy or dilation and curettage (D&C).
- Women with postmenopausal bleeding may be initially assessed with either an endometrial biopsy or transvaginal ultrasound. When ultrasound measurement of endometrial thickness is less than or equal to 4 mm, endometrial sampling is not required because the incidence of malignancy is rare in these cases. However, if postmenopasual bleeding persists, endometrial sampling should be performed.
- Patients taking TAM tend to have thicker endometrium than women who do not take TAM. In this setting, there is no consensus on the cutoff thickness of endometrial stripe that would indicate a need for endometrial biopsy.

HISTOLOGY

Subtypes

Subtypes of endometrial cancer include endometrioid (75% to 80%), uterine papillary serous (5% to 7%), clear cell (1% to 5%), mucinous (5%), squamous (<1%), undifferentiated, and mixed. Endometrial carcinoma is also divided into pathogenetic Types I and II:

- Type I tumors, the more common type of endometrial carcinoma, occur more often in younger of perimenopausal women and tend to be better differentiated than type II tumors. Most are estrogen dependent, and many have positive estrogen and progesterone receptors. Type I tumors are more often associated with DM and obesity and tend to have better prognosis.
- Type II endometrial carcinomas are poorly differentiated or of papillary serous or clear cell histology. These tumors tend to occur in older, thin, postmenopausal women with no source of excess estrogen,

arising in the background of atrophic endometrium. Type II tumors are associated with a poorer prognosis than Type I tumors.

- African-American women with endometrial carcinoma have a poorer prognosis because of disproportionately higher percentage of type II carcinomas.

Characteristics of both types of tumors is delineated below:

- Type I Endometrial Carcinomas:
  - Endometrioid histology
  - More differentiated (lower grade, higher progesterone receptor [PR] levels)
  - Less myometrial invasion (lower stage at presentation)
  - Younger patients
  - Genetic aberrations: Mutations in K-ras, β-catenin, PI3K, PTEN, ARID1A, and microsatellite instability and DNA mismatch repair defects
- Type II Endometrial Carcinomas:
  - Nonendometrioid histology (serous, clear cell)
  - Commonly associated with p53 mutations (serous), chromatin-remodeling and ubiquitin ligase complex genes (CHD4, FBXW7, and SPOP)
  - Aneuploid (grade 3)
  - Her2/neu overexpressed

Special Considerations

- Adenomatous hyperplasia is an estrogen-dependent lesion that could be seen along with type I but not with type II endometrial carcinoma.
- Women with the serous subtype are at increased risk of developing a concurrent or subsequent breast cancer—breast cancer is diagnosed in 20% to 25% of patients with serous subtype compared to 3% with endometrioid subtype.

PRETREATMENT EVALUATION

- Physical examination with particular attention to the size and mobility of the uterus and the presence of extrauterine masses or ascites.
- Cervical cancer screening with Pap test.
- Routine blood and urine studies.
- Chest x-ray should be performed to rule out pulmonary metastasis and to evaluate the cardiorespiratory status of the patient. Additional imaging studies to include pelvic or abdominal imaging to assess myometrial invasion or cervical involvement are unnecessary if surgical staging is planned.
- Routine age-appropriate health maintenance: If HNPCC is suspected, colonoscopy should be performed before planning treatment.
- Evaluation of specific symptoms or physical examination findings as indicated.

STAGING

- Endometrial carcinoma is surgically staged according to the joint 2010 International Federation of Gynecology and Obstetrics (FIGO)/TNM classification system.
- Staging for endometrial carcinoma is surgical and is based on information from hysterectomy, BSO, peritoneal cytology, and pelvic and periaortic LN dissection.
- Endometrial cancer distribution by stage:
  - Stage I: 70% to 75%
    - IA: Tumor confined to the uterus, no or <1/2 myometrial invasion
    - IB: Tumor confined to the uterus, >1/2 myometrial invasion
  - Stage II: 10% to 15%
    - II: Cervical stromal invasion, but not beyond uterus

- Stage III: 5% to 10%
  - IIIA: Tumor invades serosa or adnexa
  - IIIB: Vaginal and/or parametrial involvement
  - IIIC1: Pelvic LN involvement
  - IIIC2: Para-aortic LN involvement, with or without pelvic node involvement
- Stage IV: <5%
  - IVA: Tumor invasion bladder mucosa and/or bowel mucosa
  - IVB: Distant metastases including abdominal metastases and/or inguinal LNs

PROGNOSTIC FACTORS

Uterine

- The prognosis of endometrial carcinoma is determined primarily by disease stage and histology (including both grade and histologic subtype).
- Five-year survival (%) distribution by stage:
  - Stage I: 81% to 91%
  - Stage II: 71% to 79%
  - Stage III: 30% to 60%
  - Stage IV: 14% to 25%
- Histology—serous and clear cell have a worse prognosis; squamous and undifferentiated behave aggressively.
- Tumor hormone-receptor status: The presence and levels of estrogen receptor (ER)/PR are inversely proportional to histologic grade and are associated with longer survival.
- Tumor size: Tumors >2 cm have worse prognosis.
- Vascular-space invasion: Rate of disease recurrence is approximately 25%.

Extrauterine

- Positive peritoneal cytology: Rate of disease recurrence is approximately 15%.
- LN metastasis:
  - Involvement of pelvic LN or peritoneal metastases: Approximately 25% risk of recurrence
  - Metastasis to para-aortic LN: Risk increases to 40%
  - Adnexal metastasis: Approximately 15% risk of recurrence
  - Myometrial invasion
  - Older age is associated with worse prognosis

CATEGORIZING A PATIENT'S RISK BASED ON HISTOLOGY AND STAGE

Patients with endometrial cancer are stratified into the following categories based on their risk of disease recurrence:

- Low-risk: grade 1 endometrial cancer of endometrioid histology with disease confined to the endometrium (subset of stage IA).
- Intermediate-risk: endometrial cancer that is confined to the uterus but invades the myometrium (stage IA or stage IB) or demonstrates occult cervical stromal invasion (stage II). Within this subgroup, there are additional adverse prognostic factors used to further stratify women into high- and low-intermediate risk. These include deep myometrial invasion, grade 2 or 3 histology, or the presence of lymphovascular space invasion within the cancer.
- High-risk: stage III or higher endometrial cancer regardless of histology or grade. Women with serous or clear cell histology are categorized as high-risk regardless of stage.

Additional prognostic considerations that influence decision of adjuvant therapy include lower uterine segment involvement, positive peritoneal cytology, older age, African-American race, and molecular prognostic factors.

MANAGEMENT

- Endometrial cancer is usually treated with surgery, radiation, hormones, and/or chemotherapy, depending on the stage of disease.
- Surgery is the cornerstone of staging and therapy for most patients with endometrial cancer. Treatment is stratified based on the risk of disease recurrence, which is determined using the stage of disease, histology of the tumor, and other pathologic factors.
- Total extrafascial hysterectomy with BSO with pelvic and para-aortic lymph node dissection (LND) is the standard staging procedure for endometrial carcinoma.
- One of the most important prognostic factors for endometrial carcinoma is the presence of extra-uterine disease, particularly pelvic and para-aortic LN metastases. The approach to LN assessment is controversial, particularly in women presume to have early-stage disease.
- The rate of nodal spread varies with tumor stage and grade. The risk is 3% to 5% in patients with well-differentiated superficially invasive tumors, but as high as 20% in poorly differentiated deeply invasive disease. The presence of any of the following variable indicates a high-risk of nodal disease, even in apparent stage I disease; therefore, the presence of any of these features suggests a benefit for surgical resection of the LNs:
  - Serous, clear cell, or high-grade histology
  - Myometrial invasion >50%
  - Large tumors (>2 cm in diameter or filling the endometrial cavity)
- There is ongoing controversy over whether pelvic and para-aortic LN sampling or complete LND should be performed.
- Decisions about adjuvant therapy are based upon clinicopathologic factors (e.g., grade, tumor size, and patient's age). Other factors may also impact adjuvant therapy decisions (e.g., lower uterine segment involvement, positive peritoneal cytology).

TREATMENT GUIDELINES

- Endometrial hyperplasia with atypia: Total abdominal hysterectomy (TAH) with or without BSO (dependent on post menopausal status) is the treatment of choice for patients who are not planning future pregnancy.
- Endometrial carcinoma: Therapy should be individualized for endometrial carcinoma using risk based on histology and stage. The following guidelines may be generally employed:
  - Low risk: TAH/BSO with no adjuvant treatment (unless patients are interested in and are candidates for fertility-sparing options). Pelvic nodes are often removed for staging purposes, and sentinel LN mapping may be considered. This treatment can be considered adequate for low-risk patients with the following:
    - Grade 1, well-differentiated endometrioid histology tumors confined to the endometrium (a subset of stage IA).
    - Negative peritoneal cytology. If no peritoneal fluid is found during surgery, peritoneal washing with normal saline should be done.
    - No lymphovascular-space invasion.
- Intermediate risk: surgical staging including a radical TAH/BSO combined with para-aortic and selective pelvic LN sampling or dissection, and pelvic washings followed by postoperative adjuvant RT. Some clinicians may offer adjuvant chemotherapy (with or without RT) to women with higher risk intermediate-risk endometrial cancer, although the benefit of this approach is not yet clear.

■ High risk: surgical staging (see above) followed by adjuvant chemotherapy, which has shown a survival advantage. While adjuvant RT reduces the risk of local recurrence it is not entirely clear whether there is an additional benefit to adjuvant RT. Clinical trials are strongly encouraged for these patients (including enrollment in GOG 258).

Adjuvant Therapies

Chemotherapy

Adjuvant chemotherapy is recommended for women with advanced extrauterine disease (stage III), and improves both progression-free survival (PFS) and overall survival (OS), regardless of whether RT is used (GOG 122, GOG 184). Regimens of choice include the following:

■ TC (paclitaxel 175 mg/m^2 and carboplatin AUC 5) for six cycles showed response rates ranging from 47% to 87%. Gynecologic Oncology Group (GOG) 209 demonstrated non-inferiority of TC to TAP (equivalent overall response rate, similar PFS, but with less toxicity when compared to TAP).
■ TAP (doxorubicin 45 mg/m^2, cisplatin 50 mg/m^2 on day 1; paclitaxel 160 mg/m^2 on day 2) for six cycles with G-CSF support.
■ Chemotherapy has shown a survival advantage over whole abdominal irradiation (WAI) in advanced endometrial carcinoma (GOG 122).
■ AP (doxorubicin 60 mg/m^2, cisplatin 50 mg/m^2 for seven cycles, plus one additional cycle of cisplatin alone) was compared to WAI (30 Gy in 20 fractions with a 15 Gy boost to pelvic and para-aortic nodes). Better progression-free and overall survival was seen in the chemotherapy arm.
■ One randomized study of platinum-based chemotherapy in stage I uterine papillary serous carcinoma showed improvement in disease-free and overall survival.

Radiation Therapy

Radiation therapy (RT) may be used alone in women with high-risk cancer confined to the endometrium. It may be considered in patients with extrauterine disease confined to the pelvic LNs. RT reduces risk of local recurrence. Current American Society for Radiation Oncology (ASTRO) guidelines recommend the use of radiotherapy in addition to chemotherapy in patients with Stage III disease, particularly in women with a good performance status. RT reduces the risk of local recurrence. RT is associated with early and late toxicity. Strategies include the following:

■ Whole pelvic RT: 45 to 50 Gy external beam radiation (EBRT) along with vaginal irradiation with vaginal cylinder or colpostats to bring the vaginal surface dose to 80 to 90 Gy (5-year disease-free survival of 80% and locoregional control of 90%).
■ Vaginal brachytherapy: May be administered alone if patient has undergone complete surgical staging to confirm that disease is confined to the uterus.
■ WAI (reserved for more aggressive, nonendometrioid histologies).
■ Preoperative intracavitary radiation plus EBRT: This method is a combination of preoperative intracavitary radiation (consisting of uterine tandem and vaginal colpostat insertions with a standard Fletcher applicator delivering 20 to 25 Gy to a point A) and EBRT (40 to 45 Gy with standard fractionation delivered to multiple fields). In patients with extensive cervical involvement precluding initial hysterectomy, EBRT should be followed in 4 to 6 weeks by hysterectomy and BSO with periaortic LN sampling. This approach can provide 5-year disease-free survival of 70% to 80%.

Combined Chemotherapy and RT

■ May decrease local recurrence rate, which can be as high as 50% with chemotherapy alone.
■ To date studies of radiotherapy combined with chemotherapy have shown a benefit to PFS but no definite increase in overall survival. GOG 249, GOG 258, and PORTEC III studies are currently under way to address the role of combined chemotherapy and radiotherapy in the management of endometrial cancer.
■ Radiation may be administered after completion of 6 cycles of chemotherapy, "sandwiched" in between 3 cycles of chemotherapy before and after radiation treatment, or concurrently.

Special Considerations

■ Low-risk, low-grade patients who still desire fertility can be managed with progestational agents such as levonorgestrel-releasing intrauterine system (e.g., Mirena IUD), with appropriate follow-up to ensure a response to therapy.

■ Low-risk patients who are not surgical candidates can be treated with RT alone; however, this may achieve a lower cure rate than surgery.

■ Combined surgery and EBRT has a higher complication rate than either treatment alone (e.g., bowel complications, 4%). Therefore, special attention should be given to appropriate patient selection and choice of surgical techniques. Fewer complications are seen with retroperitoneal approach and with LN sampling versus LN dissection.

■ Pelvic surgery has an increased risk of thrombophlebitis in the pelvis and lower extremities; hence, low-dose heparin or compression stockings should be used.

■ The subgroup of women with isolated ovarian metastasis has a relatively better prognosis. However, some believe that this represents double primary tumors rather than true metastasis from primary endometrial cancer. Five-year disease-free survival ranges between 60% and 82%, depending on histologic grade and depth of myometrial invasion. Pelvic radiation doses of 45 to 50 Gy are given in standard fractionation, with vaginal boost with cylinder or colpostats adding 30 to 35 Gy to the vaginal surface.

■ If tumor extends to the pelvic wall, patients should be considered inoperable and treated with RT.

■ When parametrial extension is present, preoperative RT (external and intracavitary) is applied.

■ Patients who are not candidates for either surgery or RT are treated with progestational agents (see the subsequent text).

Stage IVB and Recurrent Disease

Therapy recommendations depend on sites of metastasis or recurrent disease and disease-related symptoms. All patients should be considered for clinical trials.

Local Recurrence

■ Pelvic exenteration: This method can be considered for patients with disease extending only to the bladder or rectum or for isolated central recurrence after irradiation. Occasional long-term survival has been reported.

■ RT: Palliative radiation is applied for localized recurrences, for example, pelvic LN (EBRT together with brachytherapy boost), para-aortic LN, or distant metastases. For isolated vaginal recurrence, irradiation may be curative if not previously administered.

Distant Metastasis: Systemic Therapy

Hormonal therapy produces responses in 15% to 30% of patients and is associated with survival twice as long as in nonresponders. On average, responses last for 1 year. Hormonal therapy is used for endometrioid histologies only (not for clear cell, serous, or carcinosarcoma). Tumor tissue should be checked for ER and PR levels, since hormone-receptor levels and degree of tumor differentiation correlate well with response. Hormonal therapy is preferred as first-line intervention for recurrent or metastatic endometrial cancer due to its lower toxicity profile and response rate similar to chemotherapy. Options include the following:

■ Megestrol acetate (Megace), 160 to 320 mg daily, is the preferred initial regimen.

■ Medroxyprogesterone acetate (Depo-Provera), 400 to 1,000 mg IM weekly for 6 weeks and then monthly.

■ Oral medroxyprogesterone (Provera), 200 mg PO daily works equally well as 1,000 mg per day.

■ TAM, 20 mg PO BID, may be given as second-line with or without a progestin (medroxyprogesterone acetate 200 mg per day). Addition of progestin may improve response rate when used with TAM 40 mg per day PO).

■ Aromatase inhibitors (e.g., anastrozole, letrozole) are currently being evaluated and to date have response rates of 10%.

■ There is no role for hormonal therapy in the adjuvant setting to treat early-stage disease.

Chemotherapy

There are no FDA-approved chemotherapy agents for the treatment of recurrent and metastatic endometrial cancer. However, the following regimens are typically used.

- Single-agent therapy
  - Options include cisplatin, carboplatin, doxorubicin, paclitaxel, topotecan, bevacizumab, and temsirolimus.
  - Response rates 17% to 28%; partial responses of short duration (<6 months); overall survival 9 to 12 months.
- Combination chemotherapy
  - Multi-agent chemotherapy regiments are preferred, if tolerated.
  - Response rates 36% to 67%; partial responses are short duration (4 to 8 months).
  - Overall survival not improved over single-agent therapy.
  - Combinations may include carboplatin/paclitaxel, cisplatin/doxorubicin, cisplatin/doxorubicin/paclitaxel, carboplatin/paclitaxel, ifosfamide/paclitaxel.
  - Paclitaxel-containing regimens may improve response and progression-free intervals; overall survival advantages may be seen in time. Such regimens may include TAP (doxorubicin 45 mg/m², cisplatin 50 mg/m² on day 1; paclitaxel 160 mg/m² on day 2) or TC (paclitaxel at 175 mg/m² followed by carboplatin AUC of 5 to 7, every 4 weeks).

Less well-studied treatment regimens have been proposed:

- Chemotherapy in conjunction with hormonal therapy.
  - Response rates may be slightly higher than with either therapy alone.
  - Overall survival may also be improved.
- The addition of medroxyprogesterone (200 mg daily) to cyclophosphamide, doxorubicin, and 5-FU, followed by TAM 20 mg daily for 3 weeks was tested in a small clinical trial of 46 women. Overall survival was 14 months compared to 11 months with chemotherapy alone.
- Targeted agents:
  - Bevacizumab may be given in the recurrent setting following progression after cytotoxic chemotherapy. Trials are in progress looking at bevacizumab in combination with carboplatin and paclitaxel.
  - mTOR inhibitors such as temsirolimus are being investigated in phase II trials.

Estrogen-Replacement Therapy

Estrogen-replacement therapy for patients with endometrial cancer remains controversial.

Post-therapy Surveillance

- Most recurrences are seen in the first 3 years after primary therapy (>50% of recurrences occur within 2 years and approximately 75% within 3 years of initial treatment).
- NCCN guidelines for post-therapy surveillance of endometrial cancer include
  - History and physical examination, every 3 to 6 months for 2 years, then annually. Up to 70% of patients with recurrent disease will report symptoms of vaginal bleeding, pain, cough, or weight loss.
  - Imaging as clinically indicated.
  - Genetic counseling or testing is advised in patients <50 years of age with a significant family history and/or pathologic features suggestive of Lynch syndrome, e.g., MSI-high.

Suggested Readings

1. American Cancer Society. *Cancer Facts and Figures 2016*. Atlanta, GA: American Cancer Society; 2016. Available at: http://www.cancer.org/research/cancerfactsstatistics/cancerfactsfigures2016. Last accessed October 1, 2016.
2. FIGO Committee on Gynecologic Oncology. Revised FIGO staging for carcinoma of the vulva, cervix and endometrium. *Int J Gynecol Obstet.* 2014;125:97–98.
3. NCCN Clinical Practice Guidelines in Oncology: Uterine Cancers. Version 2.2016. Available at: http://www.nccn.org/professionals/physician_gls/PDF/uterine.pdf. Last accessed October 1, 2016.

4. Park CA, Apte S, Acs G, et al. Cancer of the endometrium. In: Abeloff MD, Armitage JO, Niederhuber JE, et al., eds. *Abeloff's Clinical Oncology.* 4th ed. New York: Churchill Livingstone; 2008.
5. Prat J, Gallardo A, Cuatrecasas M, et al. Endometrial carcinoma: pathology and genetics. *Pathology.* 2007;39(1):72–87.
6. Trope CG, Alektiar KM, Sabbatini P, et al. Corpus: epithelial tumors. In: Hoskins WJ, Perez CA, Young RC, Barakat RR, Markman M, Randall ME, eds. *Principles and Practice of Gynecologic Oncology.* 5th ed. Philadelphia, PA: Lippincott Williams and Wilkins; 2009;683–732.
7. SGO Clinical Practice Endometrial Cancer Working Group. Endometrial cancer: a review and current management strategies: part I. *Gynecol Oncol.* 2014 Aug;134(2):385–92.
8. SGO Clinical Practice Endometrial Cancer Working Group. Endometrial cancer: a review and current management strategies: part II. *Gynecol Oncol.* 2014 Aug;134(2):393–402.

19 Cervical Cancer

Sarah M. Temkin and Charles A. Kunos

EPIDEMIOLOGY

- Uterine cervix cancer represents the fourth most common cancer in women, and the seventh overall, representing an estimated 527,624 new cancer cases from around the world in 2012.
- There were an estimated 265,672 deaths from uterine cervix cancer worldwide in 2012, making it the fourth most common lethal cancer in women and 10th overall. Uterine cervix cancer accounts for 8% of all female cancer-related deaths.
- Among American women, uterine cervix cancer is the third most common cancer of the genital system, with an estimated 12,990 new cases and 4,120 deaths estimated in 2016.
- Papanicolaou (Pap) smear screening has lowered the incidence and mortality of invasive uterine cervix cancer by almost 75% over the past 50 years; however, nearly 85% of cases occur in less developed regions where Pap screening may not be available.
- Uterine cervix cancer incidence among American women continues to decline but remains disproportionately high among subpopulation (American blacks, Hispanics of any race, Asian/Pacific Islander Americans, American Indian/Alaskan Natives).
- In developed socioeconomic regions, the cumulative risk of uterine cervix cancer by age 75 years is 0.9% and the mortality risk is 0.3%; in less developed regions, those same risks are 1.9% and 1.1%, respectively.

RISK FACTORS

Human Papillomavirus

- Human papillomavirus (HPV) infection is the most important factor in disease progression to uterine cervix cancer. Up to 90% of uterine cervix cancers retain HPV DNA in the malignant cell phenotype.
- Over 170 HPV subtypes are known, and about 40 subtypes infect the genital system.
- HPV virus subtypes associated with high risk for uterine cervix cancer include types 16, 18, 31, 33, 35, 39, 45, 51, 52, 56, 58, and 59. A 9-valent HPV vaccine includes HPV 6, 11, 16, 18, 31, 33, 45, 52, and 58 virus-like particles.
- HPV types 16 and 18 account for 70% of uterine cervix cancer incidence.
- In the United States, up to 50% of sexually active young women will be HPV (+) within 36 months of sexual activity; however, most women clear the infection within 8 to 24 months.
- HPV prevalence in regions with a high incidence of uterine cervix cancer is 10% to 20%, while in regions with a lower incidence of uterine cervix cancer, HPV prevalence is 5% to 10%.
- The HPV oncogenic phenotype involves HPV E6 protein, which inactivates p53, and HPV E7 protein, which inactivates pRb. Resulting loss of a G1/S cell cycle checkpoint leads to unregulated DNA replication, favorable for viral DNA duplication and implicated in malignant transformation of uterine cervix cells.

▪ It is not known whether HPV subtyping of invasive uterine cervix cancer impacts clinical outcome or cancer care provider management. For women with high-grade squamous intraepithelial lesions (HSIL), the presence of high-risk HPV subtypes elevates the hazard for invasive uterine cervix cancer.

Demographic, Personal, or Sexual Risk Factors

▪ Risk of invasive uterine cervix cancer is largely influenced by HPV exposure, vaccination, and screening as well as immune response to HPV infection.

▪ Demographic risk factors include race (elevated among Hispanics of any race, American blacks, and American Indian/Alaskan Natives), low socioeconomic status (reflective of poverty and poor education status), and immigration from high-HPV prevalence or low-screening worldwide regions.

▪ Personal risk factors include early onset of coitus (relative risk [RR] is 2-fold for younger than 18 years compared to 21 years or older), multiple sex partners (RR is 3-fold with six or more partners compared to one partner), and a history of sexually transmitted infections.

▪ Among males with multiple sex partners (a known risk factor for HPV infection), penile circumcision appears to reduce the risk of uterine cervix cancer in their female partners.

▪ A "current smoker" status raises the RR of squamous cell uterine cervix cancer 4-fold and has been shown to accelerate progression of dysplasia to invasive carcinoma 2-fold.

▪ Additional risk factors include multiparity (RR = 3.8), use of oral contraceptives for more than 5 years (RR of 1.90), and immunosuppression.

▪ Renal transplantation (RR = 5.7) and HIV infection (RR = 2.5) increase the risk of uterine cervix cancer—a uterine cervix cancer diagnosis identifies an indicator condition for acquired immunodeficiency syndrome [AIDS] in human immunodeficiency virus [HIV]-positive women according to 1993 Centers for Disease Control and Prevention criteria.

SCREENING

▪ Joint national guidelines provide the following consensus screening recommendations:
  ● Uterine cervix cancer screening of women in the general population should begin no sooner than age 21.
  ● Women aged 21 to 29 should be screened with cervical cytology alone every 3 years.
  ● In women aged 30 to 65, cotesting with cervical cytology and HPV testing every 5 years is preferred. Continued screening with cervical cytology every 3 years is acceptable.
  ● Screening should end at age 65 in women with negative prior screening and no history of HSIL. Likewise, it should end in women who have had a (total) hysterectomy with removal of the cervix and no prior history of HSIL.

▪ Cervical cytology should be described using the 2001 Bethesda System detailing specimen adequacy and interpretation.

▪ Interpretation is divided into nonmalignant findings and epithelial cell abnormalities including squamous and glandular abnormalities.

▪ Adenocarcinoma incidence has been increasing over past three decades because Pap screening is often inadequate for detecting endocervical lesions; however, HPV screening and vaccine may decrease both squamous and adenocarcinoma rates.

PRECURSOR LESIONS

▪ Mild, moderate, and severe cervical dysplasias are categorized as low-grade squamous intraepithelial lesions (LSIL, formerly CIN 1) or HSIL (formerly CIN 2 or 3).

▪ Mild-to-moderate dysplasias are more likely to regress than progress. Nevertheless, the rate of progression of mild dysplasia to severe dysplasia is 1% per year; the rate of progression of moderate dysplasia to severe dysplasia is 16% within 2 years and 25% within 5 years.

▪ Untreated carcinoma in situ has a 30% probability of progression to invasive cancer over a 30-year observation period.

SIGNS AND SYMPTOMS

- HSIL and early uterine cervix cancer are often asymptomatic.
- In symptomatic patients, abnormal vaginal bleeding (i.e., postcoital, intermenstrual, or menorrhagia) is the most common symptom and may lead to anemia-related fatigue.
- Vaginal discharge (serosanguinous or yellowish, sometimes foul smelling) may represent a more advanced lesion.
- Pain in the lumbosacral or gluteal area may suggest hydronephrosis caused by tumor, or tumor extension to lumbar nerve roots.
- Bladder or rectum symptoms (hematuria, rectal bleeding, etc.) may indicate organ invasion.
- Persistent, unilateral, or bilateral leg edema may indicate lymphatic and venous blockage caused by extensive pelvic sidewall nodal or tissue disease.
- Leg pain, edema, and hydronephrosis are characteristic of advanced-stage disease (IIIB).

DIAGNOSTIC WORKUP

- History and physical examination should include bimanual pelvic and rectovaginal septum examinations. These are usually normal with stage IA disease (microscopic invasion only).
- The most frequent examination abnormalities include visible cervical lesions or abnormalities on bimanual pelvic examination.
- About 15% of adenocarcinomas have no visible lesion because the carcinoma is within the endocervical canal.

Standard Diagnostic Procedures

- Cervical cytology for routine screening and in the absence of a gross lesion
- Cervical biopsy of any gross lesion (perhaps by colposcopy)
- Conization for subclinical tumor, or after negative biopsy when malignancy is suspected
- Conization for microinvasive cancer to assist in primary treatment triage
- Endocervical curettage for suspected endocervical lesions
- Cystoscopy and proctoscopy for symptoms worrisome for bladder or rectal tumor extension

Radiologic Studies

- Because of the limits of low-resource regions, International Federation of Gynecology and Obstetrics (FIGO) clinical staging limits radiographic imaging for staging purposes to chest x-ray, intravenous pyelography (IVP), and barium enema.
- If available for treatment planning purposes, computed tomography (CT), positron emission tomography (PET), PET/CT, or magnetic resonance imaging (MRI) are informative.
- MRI is the best for delineating soft-tissue or parametrial tissue invasion.
- CT or PET/CT is useful to evaluate initial pelvic or para-aortic lymph node involvement.

Laboratory Studies

- Complete blood count to evaluate for anemia
- Blood chemistries to evaluate for renal function
- Liver function tests to evaluate synthetic and metabolic factors

HISTOLOGY

- Cervical carcinoma often originates at a squamous-columnar cell junction of the uterine cervix, by name, the transformation zone.
- Seventy-five percent to 80% of uterine cervix cancers are of squamous cell histology; the remaining 20% to 25% are mostly adenocarcinomas or adenosquamous carcinomas.

STAGING

▪ Because the global burden of uterine cervix cancer occurs in low-resource regions where abilities to surgically stage women with disease may be limited, uterine cervix cancer is clinically staged. The 2010 FIGO definitions and staging system are accepted uniformly. This system has been endorsed by the American Joint Committee on Cancer (AJCC).

▪ Laparoscopy, lymphangiography, CT, CT/PET, and/or MRI have all been used for primary treatment planning.

PROGNOSTIC FACTORS

▪ Major prognostic factors include clinical stage, lymph node involvement, tumor volume (or >4 cm in unidimensional measurement), depth of cervical stroma invasion, lymphovascular space invasion (LVSI), and to a lesser extent histologic type and grade.

▪ Stage is the most important prognostic factor, followed by lymph node involvement.

▪ Five-year survival based on the extent of tumor at diagnosis:
  ● Uterine cervix confined: 92%
  ● Pelvis-contained: 56%
  ● Extrapelvic metastatic disease: 16.5%
  ● Unstaged at diagnosis: 60%

MODE OF SPREAD

▪ Disease spread is orderly, occurring first along lymphovascular planes to involve parametrial tissues. Disease may extend to the vaginal mucosa or the uterine corpus. Disease spread to adjacent organs is typically by direct extension.

▪ Ovarian involvement by direct extension of uterine cervix cancer is rare (0.5% of squamous cell carcinomas (SCCs), 1.7% adenocarcinomas).

▪ Lymphatic dissemination most commonly involves pelvic lymph nodes first and then para-aortic lymph nodes. Skip para-aortic nodal lesions occur.

▪ Vascular spread is late in the disease process, and metastases occur in lung, liver, and bone.

▪ Risk of pelvic lymph node metastases increases with increasing depth of tumor invasion, tumor bulk, and presence of LVSI.

TREATMENT

High-Grade Intraepithelial Lesions/Carcinoma in Situ

▪ AJCC includes stage 0 for in situ disease (Tis), while FIGO no longer includes stage 0 (Tis).

▪ Noninvasive lesions can be treated with electrosurgical excision, cryotherapy, laser excision or ablation, surgical conization, or other surgical procedures.

▪ A one-step diagnostic and therapeutic option is the loop electrosurgical excision procedure (LEEP), which allows excision of the entire transformation zone of the cervix with a low-voltage diathermy loop.

▪ A cold-knife conization (CKC) excises the transformation zone with a scalpel, avoiding cautery artifact on the surgical margins. In the majority of situations, LEEP may be an acceptable alternative to CKC because it is a quick, outpatient procedure requiring only local anesthesia.

▪ When margin status will dictate the need for, and type of, additional therapy, as in cases of adenocarcinoma in situ or microinvasive SCC, a CKC is preferred.

▪ Extrafascial (i.e., simple or total) hysterectomy is preferred for management of adenocarcinoma in situ in women who have completed childbearing. If preservation of fertility is desired, conization with negative margins followed by surveillance is reasonable.

Invasive Uterine Cervix Cancer

- Treatment for each clinical stage varies depending on the size of the tumor (Figure 19.1). Smaller tumors may be treated surgically or with radiation. Larger tumors are usually only treated with radio-chemotherapy (or, radiation alone in special circumstances).
- Results from five randomized phase III trials demonstrated an overall survival (OS) advantage for cisplatin-based chemotherapy co-administered with radiotherapy when compared to radiation-only therapy. These trials demonstrated a 30% to 50% risk reduction overall for death in women with FIGO stages IB2 to IVA tumors, or in women with FIGO stages I to IIA tumors with poor prognostic factors (i.e., pelvic lymph node involvement, parametrial disease, and positive surgical margins).
- Based on these data, the National Cancer Institute issued a clinical alert informing cancer care providers that a strong consideration should be given to adding cisplatin-based chemotherapy to radiotherapy in the treatment of invasive uterine cervix cancer.
- The most common regimen for concurrent radiochemotherapy is once-weekly cisplatin, 40 mg/m^2 IV (maximum 70 mg) for six weekly cycles during daily radiation therapy.
- Alternatively, cisplatin with 5-FU given every 3 to 4 weeks during radiation is acceptable.

Stage IA1

- Prior to initial therapy, the most important factors confounding cancer care include (1) a woman's fertility desires, (2) medical operability, and (3) presence of LVSI at biopsy.
- For women with no LVSI and negative histopathological margins on their LEEP or CKC specimen, and who have completed childbearing, a simple hysterectomy is indicated.

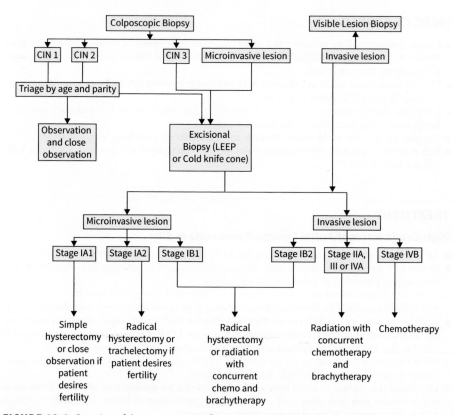

FIGURE 19.1 Overview of the management of preinvasive and invasive lesions of the cervix.

- For those with LVSI or positive margins, a modified radical hysterectomy with pelvic lymph node dissection is indicated.
- For those who wish to preserve fertility, a conization with negative margins, followed by observation is adequate therapy. However, if margins are positive, options include radical trachelectomy or repeat cone biopsy.
- Para-aortic lymph node dissection is reserved for patients with known or suspected nodal disease.

Stages IA2, IB1, IIA1 (Early-Stage Disease)

- General options for early-stage disease include the following:
  - Fertility sparing—radical trachelectomy and pelvic lymph node dissection with (or without) para-aortic lymph node dissection
  - Modified radical hysterectomy and pelvic lymph node dissection with para-aortic lymph node dissection for known or suspected nodal disease
  - Definitive radiochemotherapy
- All options are equally effective but differ in associated morbidity and complications.
- For early-stage uterine cervix cancers, primary surgery is often recommended.
- Optimal therapy selection depends on patient's age and childbearing plans, disease stage, current comorbidities, and the presence of histologic characteristics associated with the increased risk of recurrence.

Stage IB2 or IIA2 (Bulky Disease)

- General options for bulky disease include the following:
  - Definitive radiochemotherapy (whole pelvic radiation and brachytherapy), or
  - Radical hysterectomy plus pelvic lymph node dissection with para-aortic lymph node dissection for known or suspected nodal disease.
- Radiologic imaging (including PET/CT) is recommended for assessing bulky disease.
- Radiochemotherapy has been shown to improve patient survival.

Surgery

- Adjuvant hysterectomy after primary radiochemotherapy appears to improve pelvic control, but not OS and has increased morbidity. Adjuvant surgery (i.e., after pelvic radiotherapy) is not routinely performed but may be considered in patients with residual tumor confined to the cervix or in patients with suboptimal brachytherapy because of vaginal anatomy.
- Laparoscopic and robotic approaches are associated with shortened recovery time, decreased hospital stay, and less blood loss. They are used routinely in many institutions with promising early outcome data.
- Radical trachelectomy is a fertility-preserving surgery, which may be an option for small-volume, early-stage disease (IA1–IB1).
- Para-aortic lymph node sampling may be indicated in patients with positive pelvic nodes, clinically enlarged nodes, or patients with large-volume disease.

Indications for Adjuvant Therapy

- High risk for recurrent disease:
  - Positive or close margins
  - Positive lymph nodes
  - Positive parametrial involvement
- Intermediate risk for recurrent disease:
  - LVSI
  - Deep stromal invasion (greater than one-third)
  - Large tumor size (greater than 4 cm)

Adjuvant Therapy

- Women who undergo a modified radical hysterectomy should receive adjuvant radiochemotherapy treatment in the presence of risk factors (listed above).

- For women with intermediate risk factors, a randomized trial demonstrated that adjuvant RT improved progression-free survival (PFS), with a trend toward improved OS.
- For women with high risk factors, a randomized trial demonstrated that adjuvant radiochemotherapy was associated with an improved PFS and OS.

■ If definitive radiotherapy is chosen over radical hysterectomy, concurrent cisplatin-based chemotherapy should be administered.

Stages IIB, III, IV

■ Patients with stage IIB to IVA disease (commonly referred to as locally advanced-stage disease) should be treated with tumor volume–directed radiotherapy and concurrent cisplatin-based chemotherapy.
■ Radiologic imaging (PET/CT) and potentially surgical staging (i.e., extraperitoneal or laparoscopic lymph node dissection) are recommended to assess lymph node involvement and serves as a guide to radiation therapy portal design.
■ Patients with stage IVA disease (bowel or bladder mucosa invasion), who are poor candidates for radiochemotherapy (i.e., acute or chronic pelvic inflammatory disease, coexistent pelvic mass), may be candidates for pelvic exenteration surgery.
■ Patients who have distant metastasis (IVB disease) should receive systemic and/or biologic agent chemotherapy with (most often) or without (less often) pelvis-directed radiation therapy.

Radiation Therapy

■ For definitive treatment, pelvic external beam radiation therapy (EBRT) with intracavitary brachytherapy is used routinely.
■ High (>8000 cGy) radiation dose may be delivered to central primary tumors through use of EBRT and intracavitary brachytherapy. EBRT alone often cannot achieve these doses due to intervening normal tissues (e.g., small bowel, large bowel, and bladder).
■ In select cases of very early disease (stage IA2) brachytherapy alone may be an option.
■ Pelvic inflammatory disease, inflammatory bowel disease, and pelvic kidney are relative contraindications to conventional pelvic radiation, but may not impede intensity modulated radiation therapy (IMRT).
■ CT-based treatment planning is considered standard-of-care for EBRT.
■ EBRT should encompass gross disease (vaginal margin 3 cm from tumor), parametrial tissues, uterosacral ligaments, and presacral, external/internal iliac, and obturator lymph nodes. For patients at high risk for lymph nodes involvement, the radiation field should also cover common iliac lymph nodes. If common iliac or para-aortic lymph node involvement is clinically suspected, extended-field radiation that raises the superior radiation portal boundary up at least to the level of renal vessels is recommended.
■ Both high-dose brachytherapy (isotope ^{192}Iridium; rate 200 to 300 cGy per hour) and low-dose brachytherapy (isotope ^{137}Cesium; rate 40 to 70 cGy per hour) are used. Either brachytherapy source or technique are acceptable.
■ Determining maximum effective dose to the primary tumor, as well as to the bladder and rectum, is of primary importance. A typical regimen of EBRT is 4000 to 5000 cGy plus 3000 to 4000 cGy point A brachytherapy, for a total dose of 8000 to 9000 cGy to point A.
■ Point A is located 2 cm cephalad and 2 cm lateral to the cervical OS. Anatomically, it correlates with the boundary between the lateral uterine cervix and the medial edge of parametrial tissue, an anatomic point where the ureter and uterine artery cross.
■ A parametrial boost (900 to 1440 Gy) by EBRT may be applied to point B (defined as 5 cm lateral to patient midline and corresponding to the pelvic sidewall lymph nodes).
■ Radiation treatment is equivalent to surgery for stages IB and IIA, with identical 5-year OS and disease-free survival. Expected cure rate is 75% to 80% (85% to 90% in small-volume disease).
■ A study by the Radiation Therapy Oncology Group (RTOG 79-20) showed a 11% 10-year survival advantage for patients with IB2, IIA, and IIB disease treated with prophylactic para-aortic nodal (extended field RT) and total pelvic irradiation compared to those treated with pelvic irradiation alone.

- Multivariate analyses have shown that a total dose of >8500 cGy intracavitary radiation to point A (locally advanced stage only), radiosensitizers like cisplatin, and overall treatment time of <8 weeks are associated with improved pelvic tumor control and survival in women with uterine cervix cancer. Treatment times beyond 8 weeks (56 days) result in an up to 1% decline, per extended treatment day, in recurrence-free survival.

Palliative Chemotherapy

- No standard chemotherapy regimen has been shown to produce prolonged complete remissions.
- Combination platinum-based chemotherapy has demonstrated improved response rates in randomized trials compared to single-agent therapy.
- Cisplatin/paclitaxel demonstrated higher response rate and improved PFS compared to single-agent cisplatin in Gynecologic Oncology Group (GOG) 169. Preliminary data from a Japanese randomized trial demonstrate equivalency of carboplatin/paclitaxel with cisplatin/paclitaxel.
- Cisplatin/topotecan demonstrated superior response rate, PFS, and median survival compared to single-agent cisplatin in GOG 179.
- A comparison trial of cisplatin/topotecan, cisplatin/gemcitabine, and cisplatin/vinorelbine compared to a control arm of cisplatin/paclitaxel was halted when the experimental arms were not superior to the control. Cisplatin/paclitaxel had the best response rate, 29.1%.
- Based on the above, cisplatin/paclitaxel and carboplatin/paclitaxel are the most commonly used regimens for metastatic and recurrent uterine cervix cancer. Cisplatin/topotecan, cisplatin/gemcitabine, or single-agent therapies are reasonable alternatives.
- The most active single agents include
  - cisplatin (response rate 20% to 30%)
  - carboplatin (response rate 15% to 28%)
  - ifosfamide (response rate 15% to 33%)
  - paclitaxel (response rate 17% to 25%)
- Other agents with activity include irinotecan, vinorelbine, gemcitabine, bevacizumab, docetaxel, 5-FU, mitomycin, topotecan, and pemetrexed.
- The benefit of chemotherapy with or without radiation versus best supportive care in this patient population has not yet been established.

Special Considerations

- Recent studies have clearly demonstrated the deleterious effect of anemia on patients receiving radiation therapy. Hemoglobin levels <10 g/dL at the time of radiation therapy impede local disease control and survival. Blood transfusions to raise hemoglobin levels above 10 g/dL are recommended.
- Some patients with small-volume disease in para-aortic lymph nodes and controllable pelvic disease can potentially be cured. Removal of grossly involved para-aortic lymph nodes prior to radiotherapy may be therapeutic.
- Toxicity from extended-field radiation exceeds that of pelvic radiation alone, but most commonly is seen in women with prior abdominopelvic surgery.
- Different surgical techniques affect the incidence of complications secondary to para-aortic lymph node extended-field radiation. For example, extraperitoneal lymph node sampling leads to fewer radiation-related posttherapy complications than transperitoneal lymph node sampling.
- IMRT has been shown to reduce sequelae of pelvic and extended-field radiation therapy. Clinical trials evaluating IMRT are underway in this patient population.

Recurrent Disease

- A 10% to 20% recurrence rate has been reported in stage IB to IIA women with negative nodal sampling treated by primary surgery or radiation therapy.
- Up to 70% of women with stage IIB, III, or IVA disease with or without positive nodal sampling exhibit recurrences.
- Intrapelvic recurrences are symptomatic, with 80% to 90% detected by 2 years posttherapy.

- In the recurrence setting, favorable prognostic factors include central pelvis disease site, disease not fixed to the pelvic sidewall, the posttherapy disease-free interval is 6 months or longer, and the recurrent tumor measures less than 3 cm.
- More than 90% of women with distant extrapelvic recurrence die of disease within 5 years.
- For stage I-IIA disease, the predominant anatomic site of recurrence is local (vaginal apex) or intrapelvic (pelvic sidewall).
- Multiple studies have shown that the distribution of recurrence site as
  - Central pelvis (vaginal apex)—22% to 56%
  - Regional pelvis (pelvic sidewall)—28% to 37%
  - Distant extrapelvic metastasis—15% to 61%
- Women with positive lymph nodes at initial diagnosis, particularly para-aortic lymph node involvement, have a higher risk of distant metastases as compared to women with negative lymph nodes.
- No curative therapy is available for metastatic disease. In direct contrast, intrapelvic recurrence can potentially be treated with curative intent.
- Surgical resection of limited metastatic disease, such as in the lung, may result in prolonged clinical remission.
- For patients with intrapelvic recurrence after radical surgery, cisplatin-based radiochemotherapy has a 40% to 50% durable control rate and long-term survival rate.
- Pelvic exenteration (resection of the bladder, rectum, vagina, uterus/cervix) is a preferred treatment for centrally located recurrent disease after primary radiation therapy, with a 32% to 62% 5-year survival in select women. Reconstructive procedures include continent urinary conduit, end-to-end rectosigmoid reanastomosis, and myocutaneous graft for a neovagina.
- High-dose intraoperative radiation therapy combined with surgical resection is offered by some centers for patients whose tumors extend close to the pelvic sidewalls.
- Chemotherapy for distant recurrent disease is palliative, not curative, demonstrating low response rates, short response duration, and low OS rates (see the Palliative Chemotherapy section). Cisplatin is the most active single agent, with a median survival of seven months.
- Factors associated with higher likelihood of recurrence to cisplatin-based combination chemotherapy include
  - American black race
  - Performance status 1 or 2
  - Disease in the pelvis
  - Prior treatment by cisplatin-containing regimen
  - Relapse within one year of initial diagnosis
- Chemotherapy-naive patients have a higher response rate than those exposed to chemotherapy as part of their initial treatment.

TREATMENT DURING PREGNANCY

- Uterine cervix cancer is the most common gynecologic malignancy associated with pregnancy, ranging from 1 in 1,200 to 1 in 2,200 pregnancies.
- No therapy is warranted for preinvasive lesions; colposcopy, but not endocervical curettage, is recommended to rule out invasive cancer.
- Conization is reserved for suspicion of invasion or for persistent cytologic evidence of invasive cancer in the absence of colposcopic confirmation. Management of dysplasia is usually postponed until postpartum.
- Treatment of invasive cancer depends on the tumor stage and the fetus's gestational age. If cancer is diagnosed before fetal maturity, immediate appropriate cancer therapy for the relevant stage is recommended. However, with close surveillance, delay of therapy to achieve fetal maturity is a reasonable option for patients with stage IA and early IB disease. For more advanced disease, delaying therapy is not recommended unless diagnosis is made in the final trimester. When the fetus reaches acceptable maturity, a cesarean section precedes definitive treatment.

TREATMENT OF HIV (+) WOMEN

▪ HIV-infected women (or immunocompromised) should undergo uterine cervix cancer screening twice in the first year after diagnosis and then annually.

▪ Each examination should include a thorough visual inspection of the anus, vulva, vagina, as well as the uterine cervix.

▪ The American College of Obstetricians and Gynecologists and the Centers for Disease Control do not endorse HPV testing in the triage of HIV-infected patients. This conflicts with 2006 American Society for Colposcopy and Cervical Pathology Consensus Guidelines, which endorse similar management of patients irrespective of HIV status.

▪ Treatment of preinvasive lesions and uterine cervix cancers in HIV (+) patients is the same as in HIV-negative patients, though response to therapy is usually poorer.

▪ Incidence of HSIL is four- to five-times higher in HIV (+) women compared to HIV-negative women with high-risk behaviors.

▪ Among HIV-infected women, rates of oncogenic HPV and HSIL increase with diminished CD4 counts and higher circulating HIV RNA levels.

▪ Women with HIV are more likely to have persistent HPV and HSIL than uninfected women.

▪ Although anti-retroviral therapy has altered the natural history of HIV, its effect on HPV and HPV-associated neoplasia is less clear.

FOLLOW-UP AFTER PRIMARY THERAPY

▪ Eighty percent to 90% of recurrences occur within 2 years of completing therapy suggesting a role for increased surveillance during this period.

▪ Follow-up visits, including thorough physical examination, should occur every 3 to 6 months in the first 2 years posttherapy, every 6 to 12 months for the following 3 years then annually to detect any potentially curable recurrences.

▪ Additionally, patients should have annual cervical or vaginal cytology, though an exception can be made for those that have undergone pelvic radiation.

▪ There are insufficient data to support the routine use of radiographic imaging; chest x-ray, CT, and PET or PET/CT should only be used if recurrence is suspected.

▪ Patients should be counseled about signs and symptoms of recurrence to include persistent abdominal and pelvic pain, leg symptoms such as pain or lymphedema, vaginal bleeding or discharge, urinary symptoms, cough, weight loss, and anorexia.

PREVENTION

▪ The efficacy of HPV vaccination against HSIL and cancer has been demonstrated in multiple studies since 2002. Advisory Committee on Immunization Practices of the Centers for Disease Control and Prevention recommend that females aged 9 to 12 years of age be vaccinated by the three (3) dose regimen. Vaccine administrations to "catch up" occur through age 26 in females. The 9-valent HPV vaccine is most commonly administered.

Suggested Readings

1. ACOG Practice Bulletin No. 117. Gynecologic care for women with human immunodeficiency virus. *Obstet Gynecol.* 2010;116(6):1492–1509.
2. ACOG Practice Bulletin Number 131. Screening for cervical. *Obstet Gynecol.* 2012;120(5):1222–1238.
3. Berrington de Gonzalez A, Green J. Comparison of risk factors for invasive squamous cell carcinoma and adenocarcinoma of the cervix: collaborative reanalysis of individual data on 8,097 women with squamous cell carcinoma and 1,374 women with adenocarcinoma from 12 epidemiological studies. *Int J Cancer.* 2007;120(4):885–891.
4. de Sanjose S, Quint WG, Alemany L, et al. Human papillomavirus genotype attribution in invasive cervical cancer: a retrospective cross-sectional worldwide study. *Lancet Oncol.* 2010;11(11):1048–1056.

5. Holowaty P, Miller AB, Rohan T, et al. Natural history of dysplasia of the uterine cervix. *J Natl Cancer Inst.* 1999;91(3):252–258.
6. Kaplan JE, Benson C, Holmes KH, et al. Guidelines for prevention and treatment of opportunistic infections in HIV-infected adults and adolescents: recommendations from CDC, the National Institutes of Health, and the HIV Medicine Association of the Infectious Diseases Society of America. *MMWR Recomm Rep.* 2009;58(RR-4):1–207; quiz CE1–4.
7. Keys HM, Bundy BN, Stehman FB, et al. Cisplatin, radiation, and adjuvant hysterectomy compared with radiation and adjuvant hysterectomy for bulky stage IB cervical carcinoma. *N Engl J Med.* 1999;340(15):1154–1161.
8. Keys HM, Bundy BN, Stehman FB, et al. Radiation therapy with and without extrafascial hysterectomy for bulky stage IB cervical carcinoma: a randomized trial of the Gynecologic Oncology Group. *Gynecol Oncol.* 2003;89(3):343–353.
9. Kitagawa R, Katsumata N, Ando M, et al. A multi-institutional phase II trial of paclitaxel and carboplatin in the treatment of advanced or recurrent cervical cancer. *Gynecol Oncol.* 2012;125(2):307–311.
10. Kunos CA, Radivoyevitch T, Waggoner S, et al. Radiochemotherapy plus 3-aminopyridine-2-carboxaldehyde thiosemi-carbazone (3-AP, NSC #663249) in advanced-stage cervical and vaginal cancers. *Gynecol Oncol* 2013;130(1):75–80.
11. Long HJ III, Bundy BN, Grendys EC Jr, et al. Randomized phase III trial of cisplatin with or without topotecan in carcinoma of the uterine cervix: a Gynecologic Oncology Group Study. *J Clin Oncol.* 2005;23(21):4626–4633.
12. Markowitz LE, Dunne EF, Saraiya M, et al. Quadrivalent human papillomavirus vaccine: recommendations of the Advisory Committee on Immunization Practices (ACIP). *MMWR Recomm Rep.* 2007;56(RR-2):1–24.
13. McCredie MR, Sharples KJ, Paul C, et al. Natural history of cervical neoplasia and risk of invasive cancer in women with cervical intraepithelial neoplasia 3: a retrospective cohort study. *Lancet Oncol.* 2008;9(5):425–434.
14. Moore DH, Blessing JA, McQuellon RP, et al. Phase III study of cisplatin with or without paclitaxel in stage IVB, recurrent, or persistent squamous cell carcinoma of the cervix: a gynecologic oncology group study. *J Clin Oncol.* 2004;22(15): 3113–3119.
15. Morris M, Eifel PJ, Lu J, et al. Pelvic radiation with concurrent chemotherapy compared with pelvic and para-aortic radiation for high-risk cervical cancer. *N Engl J Med.* 1999;340(15):1137–1143.
16. NCCN Clinical Practice Guidelines in Oncology: Cervical Cancer. 2012; Version 1.2018. Available at: https://www.nccn.org/professionals/physician_gls/default.aspx. Last accessed November 14, 2017.
17. Peters WA III, Liu PY, Barrett RJ II, et al. Concurrent chemotherapy and pelvic radiation therapy compared with pelvic radiation therapy alone as adjuvant therapy after radical surgery in high-risk early-stage cancer of the cervix. *J Clin Oncol.* 2000;18(8):1606–1613.
18. Rogers L, Siu SS, Luesley D, et al. Radiotherapy and chemoradiation after surgery for early cervical cancer. *Cochrane Database Syst Rev.* 2012;5:CD007583.
19. Rose PG, Bundy BN, Watkins EB, et al. Concurrent cisplatin-based radiotherapy and chemotherapy for locally advanced cervical cancer. *N Engl J Med.* 1999;340(15):1144–1153.
20. Rotman M, Sedlis A, Piedmonte MR, et al. A phase III randomized trial of postoperative pelvic irradiation in Stage IB cervical carcinoma with poor prognostic features: follow-up of a gynecologic oncology group study. *Int J Radiat Oncol Biol Phys.* 2006;65(1):169–176.
21. Salani R, Backes FJ, Fung MF, et al. Posttreatment surveillance and diagnosis of recurrence in women with gynecologic malignancies: Society of Gynecologic Oncologists recommendations. *Am J Obstet Gynecol.* 2011;204(6):466–478.
22. Saslow D, Solomon D, Lawson HW, et al. American Cancer Society, American Society for Colposcopy and Cervical Pathology, and American Society for Clinical Pathology screening guidelines for the prevention and early detection of cervical cancer. *Am J Clin Pathol.* 2012;137(4):516–542.
23. Tewari KS, Sill MW, Long HJ, et al. Improved survival with bevacizumab in advanced cervical cancer. *N Engl J Med.* 2014;370(8):734–743.
24. Walboomers JM, Jacobs MV, Manos MM, et al. Human papillomavirus is a necessary cause of invasive cervical cancer worldwide. *J Pathol.* 1999;189(1):12–19.
25. Wright TC Jr, Massad LS, Dunton CJ, et al. 2006 consensus guidelines for the management of women with abnormal cervical cancer screening tests. *Am J Obstet Gynecol.* 2007;197(4):346–355.

Vulvar Cancer **20**

Kristen P. Zeligs and Christina M. Annunziata

EPIDEMIOLOGY

- Vulvar cancer is the fourth most common gynecologic cancer, accounting for 5% of all female genital tract malignancies.
- A total of 5,950 new cases and 1,110 deaths from vulvar cancer were projected for 2016.
- It is most frequently diagnosed in postmenopausal women, with a median age of diagnosis of 68 years.
- One in 333 (0.3%) women will be diagnosed with vulvar cancer during her lifetime (2.4 per 100,000 women per year in the United States).
- The rate of vulvar cancer has remained stable over the past 20 years, however the incidence of its precursor (vulvar intraepithelial neoplasia 3) has doubled.

ETIOLOGY AND RISK FACTORS

Two independent pathways of vulvar carcinogenesis are felt to exist currently: the first related to human papillomavirus (HPV) infection and the second related to disorders of chronic inflammation (e.g. vulvar dystrophy) or autoimmune processes. Premalignant lesions of the vulva, collectively known as vulvar high-grade squamous intraepithelial lesions (HSIL) or VIN 2/3, are linked to HPV DNA in 70% to 80% of cases. However, the association between HPV and vulvar cancer is observed less frequently, with only 40% to 60% of vulvar cancers testing positive on molecular analysis for HPV DNA (most commonly HPV subtypes 16 and 33). Vulvar cancers not associated with HPV infection often are associated with vulvar dystrophies, most commonly lichen sclerosus and squamous cell hyperplasia.

Risk Factors

- Vulvar high-grade squamous intraepithelial lesions (VIN 2/3) increase the risk of development of invasive vulvar cancer.
- Other risk factors include cigarette smoking, vulvar dystrophies (e.g., lichen sclerosus), VIN or CIN, HPV infection, prior history of cervical cancer, immunodeficiency disorders (e.g., HIV), and Northern European ancestry.

HISTOLOGY

- Squamous cell carcinomas (SCCs) constitute >90% of cases.
- Melanomas constitute 5% to 10% of cases.
- The remainder of tumor types include basal cell carcinoma, sarcoma, extramammary Paget's disease, and Bartholin gland adenocarcinoma.

VULVAR SQUAMOUS CELL CARCINOMA

Vulvar SCC is commonly indolent, with slow extension and late metastases. Signs and symptoms in order of decreasing frequency are pruritus, mass, pain, bleeding, ulceration, dysuria, and discharge. Many patients are asymptomatic. A synchronous second malignancy is found in up to 22% of patients with vulvar SCC (most commonly, cervical cancer).

Diagnostic Workup

- Biopsy must include adequate tissue to determine histology and grade, depth of invasion, and stromal reaction present.
- Use of colposcopy following application of 5% acetic acid solution is helpful in delineating multifocal lesions, which occur in 5% of cases.
- Cystoscopy, proctoscopy, chest x-ray, and intravenous urography should be performed as needed based on the extent of disease.
- Suspected bladder or rectal involvement must be biopsied.
- If invasive disease is present, detailed pelvic exam in addition to pelvic and abdominal imaging with PET/CT or MRI should be performed to assess deep and pelvic lymph nodes (LNs).

Indications for Excisional Biopsy of Vulvar Lesions

- Any gross lesion
- Red, white, dark brown, or black skin patches
- Areas firm to palpation
- Pruritic, tingling, or bleeding lesions
- Any nevi in the genital tract
- Enlarged or thickened areas of Bartholin glands, especially in postmenopausal women

Location and Metastatic Spread Pattern of Vulvar SCC

- Vulvar SCC is found on
  - The labia majora in 50% of cases
  - The labia minora in 15% to 20% of cases
  - The clitoris and perineum in rare cases
- Vulvar SCC tends to grow locally via direct extension to nearby structures (e.g., vagina, urethra, clitoris, anus), with early spread to inguinal, femoral, and pelvic LNs.
- Hematogenous spread occurs late in the course of disease and is rare in patients without inguinofemoral LN involvement.
- Inguinal and femoral LV involvement is the most important prognostic factor for survival.

Staging

- Vulvar cancer is a surgically staged disease. The revised 2014 FIGO staging system is as follows:
  - Stage I: Tumor confined to the vulva
    - IA: Lesions ≤2 cm in size, confined to the vulva or perineum, and with stromal invasion ≤1.0 mm, no nodal metastasis
    - IB: Lesions >2 cm in size or with stromal invasion >1.0 mm, confined to the vulva or perineum, and with negative nodes
  - Stage II: Tumor of any size with extension to adjacent perineal structures (lower 1/3 urethra, lower 1/3 vagina, anus) with negative nodes
  - Stage III: Tumor of any size with or without extension to adjacent perineal structures (lower 1/3 urethra, lower 1/3 vagina, anus) with positive inguinofemoral LNs
    - IIIA: (i) With one LN metastasis (≥5 mm), or (ii) 1 to 2 LN metastasis (es) (<5 mm)
    - IIIB: (i) With two or more LN metastases (≥5 mm), or (ii) three or more LN metastases (<5 mm)
    - IIIC: With positive nodes with extracapsular spread

- Stage IV: Tumor invades other regional or distant structures
  - IVA: Tumor invades any of the following: (i) upper urethral and/or vaginal mucosa, bladder mucosa, rectal mucosa, or fixed to pelvic bone, or (ii) fixed or ulcerated inguinofemoral LNs
  - IVB: Any distant metastasis including pelvic LNs

Prognosis and Survival

- Survival depends on stage, LN involvement, depth of invasion, structures involved, and tumor location.
- LN metastases are related to tumor size (>4 cm is associated with 30% to 50% rate of inguinofemoral metastases), clinical stage, and depth of invasion.
- 5-year overall survival ranges from 70% to 93% in patients without LN involvement to 25% to 41% for those with LN involvement.
- Studies suggest a high overall incidence of local recurrence following primary surgical treatment. Disease presence at the excised tumor margin has been postulated as a significant prognostic factor for recurrence.

Management

Vulvar Intraepithelial Neoplasia 2/3

Therapeutic options are based on individual patient need and can include any of the following:

- Surgical excision (e.g., wide local excision, skinning vulvectomy)
- Laser ablation
- Pharmacologic treatment (topical imiquimod, cidofovir, or 5-FU cream)

Recurrences are seen in up to 35% of women regardless of initial treatment modality. The most common sites of recurrence are perineal skin and clitoral hood.

Invasive cancer is present in 10% to 22% of women with VIN on initial biopsy, thus surgical excision (where additional pathologic specimen can be evaluated) should be treatment of choice if patient has any risk factors for invasive disease.

Stage I (lesions confined to vulva)

- ≤1 mm depth of invasion (stage IA): wide local excision
  - Excise down to inferior fascia of urogenital diaphragm.
  - Strive for 1–2 cm clear margins to minimize risk of local recurrence.
  - No inguinofemoral lymphadenectomy (LND) or sentinel lymph node biopsy (SNLB) necessary.
- > 1 mm depth of invasion (stage IB): wide local excision + inguinofemoral LND versus SLNB
  - Ipsilateral inguinofemoral LND for lateral lesions (located ≥2 cm from vulvar midline).
  - Bilateral inguinofemoral LND for centrally located lesions.
  - SNLB is an emerging technique in early-stage vulvar cancer and may obviate the need for full nodal dissections in many women. SNLB can be offered to patients with vulvar cancer if tumor diameter is <4 cm, >1 mm depth of invasion, no palpable LNs, unifocal disease, and surgeon has sufficient expertise.
  - Patients with close or positive surgical tumor margins (<8 mm from tumor) can undergo re-resection or, if unresectable, adjuvant radiation therapy (RT).

Special Considerations

- Poor surgical candidates can be treated with chemoradiation, achieving long-term survival.
- Surgical complications include mortality (2% to 5%), wound breakdown or infection, sepsis, thromboembolism, chronic leg lymphedema (use of separate incision for the groin LN dissection reduces wound breakdown and leg edema), urinary tract infection, stress urinary incontinence, and poor sexual function.

Stage II

- Modified radical vulvectomy (hemivulvectomy if possible) and bilateral inguinofemoral LND if ≥1 cm of negative margins can be achieved with preservation of midline structures.
- Adjuvant RT is recommended for women with no LN involvement on LND in the presence of additional risk factors to include: tumor size >4 cm, close tumor margins (≤8 mm), lymphovascular invasion, depth of invasion, or spray/diffuse pattern of invasion.

Stage III (Inguinofemoral LN Involvement)

- Modified radical vulvectomy and bilateral inguinofemoral LND are standard.
- Adjuvant chemoradiation is recommended for women with involved LNs, and most commonly involves Cisplatin 40 mg/m^2 concurrently with RT to the inguinal, external iliac, internal iliac, and obturator regional bilaterally.

Stage IVA

- Radical vulvectomy and bilateral inguinofemoral lymphadenectomy can be used if ≥1 cm of negative margins can be achieved with preservation of midline structures.
- As in stage II and III vulvar cancers, adjuvant chemoradiation is recommended for women with LN involvement or surgical margins <8 mm.
- Neoadjuvant chemoradiation, with cisplatin concurrently with RT to the vulva, groin, and LNs, may improve operability and should be considered in patients with
  - Anorectal, urethral, or bladder involvement
  - Disease fixed to the bone
  - Gross inguinal or femoral LN involvement

Special Considerations

- Management of positive groin nodes: Positive LNs require RT to primary tumor/groin/pelvis + concurrent chemotherapy.
- Suggested doses of localized adjuvant radiation are 45 to 50 Gy.
- Neoadjuvant chemoradiation can be used in stages III and IV disease to improve the operability of the tumor. Recent GOG trials have successfully used cisplatin and 5-FU concurrently with RT.
- Patients with inoperable disease can achieve long-term survival with radical chemoradiation therapy.
- Radiation fraction size of ≤180 cGy has been proven to minimize the radiation complication rate (i.e., late fibrosis, atrophy, telangiectasia, and necrosis). Total doses of 54 to 65 Gy should be used.
- Radical vulvectomy and pelvic exenteration are not commonly used due to extensive morbidity and uncertain survival benefit.

Stage IVB (Metastatic) and Recurrent Disease

Therapy recommendations depend on sites of metastasis or recurrent disease and disease-related symptoms. All patients should be considered for clinical trials.

- Distant metastasis or recurrence: RT for locoregional control/symptom palliation and/or chemotherapy or best supportive care. Chemotherapy choices for advanced, recurrent/metastatic disease commonly include cisplatin, cisplatin/vinorelbine, or cisplatin/paclitaxel. These patients are also appropriate candidates for clinical trials.
- If recurrence is confined locally to the vulva (and LNs are clinically negative), radical excision and unilateral or bilateral inguinofemoral LND (if not done prior) may be employed. This should be followed by RT +/- concurrent chemotherapy if LNs are found to be surgically positive or surgical margins are positive.
- Patients with recurrence in groin LNs who have not undergone prior RT can undergo resection of positive LNs +/- inguinofemoral LND followed by RT +/– concurrent chemotherapy

VERRUCOUS CARCINOMA

■ Variant of SCC with distinctive cauliflower-like features of vulvar lesions.
■ Verrucous carcinoma is very rare and can be confused with condyloma acuminatum because of an exophytic growth pattern.
■ It is locally destructive and rarely metastasizes.
■ It is associated with HPV type 6.
■ The main treatment is surgery. LN dissection is of questionable value unless LNs are obviously involved. Radiation therapy is contraindicated because it is ineffective and can potentially lead to more aggressive disease.

PAGET DISEASE

■ Characterized by preinvasive lesions.
■ Most frequent symptoms include pruritus, tenderness, or vulvar lesions (i.e., "red velvet," hyperemic, well-demarcated, thickened lesions with areas of induration and excoriation).
■ Can be associated with underlying adenocarcinoma of the vulva (1% to 2%). Although Paget disease is histologically a preinvasive disease locally, it should be treated with radical wide local excision, as with other vulvar malignancies. Patients require radical excision, often with intraoperative frozen section confirmation of clear margins, because microscopic disease often extends beyond the gross visual margin observed by the operating surgeon.

MALIGNANT MELANOMA

■ Malignant melanoma of the vulva is a rare tumor (representing 5% of all melanoma cases and 5% to 10% of primary vulvar neoplasms).
■ Most melanomas are located on the labia minora and clitoris.
■ Prognosis depends on size of lesion and depth of invasion.
■ Staging of malignant melanoma is the same as for skin melanoma.
■ Suggested therapy is radical vulvectomy with inguinal and pelvic lymphadenectomy, although there is a current trend toward a more conservative approach. For most well-demarcated lesions, 2 cm margins are suggested for thin (up to 7 mm) lesions and 3 to 4 cm margins for thicker lesions.

BARTHOLIN GLAND ADENOCARCINOMA

■ Adenocarcinoma of the Bartholin gland is a very rare tumor (1% of all vulvar malignancies).
■ Peak incidence is in women in their mid-60s.
■ Enlargement of the Bartholin gland area in postmenopausal women requires evaluation for malignancy with biopsy.
■ Therapy includes radical vulvectomy with wide excision to achieve adequate margins and inguinal lymphadenectomy.

Basal Cell Carcinoma

■ The natural history and therapeutic approach for basal cell carcinoma are similar to those for primary tumors seen in other sites (i.e., wide local excision).

Suggested Readings

1. American Cancer Society. Cancer Facts and Figures 2016. Atlanta, GA: American Cancer Society; 2016. Available at: http://www.cancer.org/research/cancerfactsstatistics/cancerfactsfigures2016. Last accessed October 1, 2016.

2. DiSaia PJ, Creasman WT. *Clinical Gynecologic Oncology*. 5th ed. St. Louis: Mosby; 1997.
3. FIGO Committee on Gynecologic Oncology. Revised FIGO staging for carcinoma of the vulva, cervix and endometrium. *Int J Gynecol Obstet* 2014;125:97–98.
4. Jhingran A, Russell AH, Seiden MV, et al. Cancer of the cervix, vulva, and vagina. In: Abeloff MD, Armitage JO, Niederhuber JE, et al., eds. *Abeloff's Clinical Oncology*. 4th ed. Philadelphia, PA: Churchill Livingstone; 2008.
5. Moore DH, Koh WJ, McGuire WP, et al. In: Hoskins WJ, Perez CA, Young RC, Barakat RR, Markman M, Randall ME, eds. *Principles and Practice of Gynecologic Oncology*. 5th ed. Philadelphia, PA: Lippincott Williams and Wilkins; 2009: 553–590.
6. Nash JD, Curry S. Vulvar cancer. Surg Oncol Clin N Am. 1998;7(2):335–346.
7. National Cancer Institute Physician Data Query website. http://cancer.gov/cancertopics/types/vulvar
8. NCCN Clinical Practice Guidelines in Oncology: Vulvar Cancer (Squamous Cell Carcinoma). Version 1.2016. Available at: http://www.nccn.org/professionals/physician_gls/PDF/vulvar.pdf. Last accessed October 1, 2016.

Sarcomas and Malignancies 21 of the Bone

Dale R. Shepard

EPIDEMIOLOGY

Sarcomas are tumors of mesenchymal tissues and represent about 1% of adult cancers and about 10% of pediatric cancers. Of these sarcomas, about 80% are in soft tissues and about 20% are in bone.

SOFT TISSUE SARCOMA

Clinical Presentation

Patients with soft tissue sarcomas rarely have constitutional symptoms, such as weight loss or increased fatigue. They may experience pain, paresthesia, or edema from compression by an enlarging tumor. While soft tissue sarcomas can occur throughout the body, the majority of them are in the extremities. In one series of 4500 sarcomas, 46% were in the groin, thigh, or buttock; 13% in the upper extremity; 18% in the torso, and 13% in the retroperitoneum. Red flags that suggest presence of a soft tissue sarcoma include

- Mass greater than 5 cm in size
- Rapid growth of the mass
- Mass that is deep to the fascia
- New pain in a previously painless mass
- Recurrence of a mass

Pathology

The World Health Organization classifies soft tissue sarcomas into over 100 subtypes based on histology with designation based on the presumed tissue of origin, such as liposarcoma, synovial sarcoma, fibrosarcoma, peripheral nerve sheath tumors, or angiosarcoma. Pathology should be reviewed by a center that specializes in sarcoma to ensure the proper diagnosis based on morphology, immunohistochemistry, and molecular genetic studies. Soft tissue sarcomas are characterized by the FNCLCC grading system developed by the French Federation of Cancer Centers Sarcoma Group.

Diagnosis

Patients with a suspected sarcoma of the extremity should have an MRI of the primary site. Masses in the abdomen or retroperitoneum can be assessed with CT scans. A CT of the chest should be obtained for staging since this is a frequent site of metastases for soft tissue sarcoma. PET scans may help in some situations, such as distinguishing a neurofibroma from a malignant peripheral nerve sheath tumor, but PET scans should not be obtained as a part of routine staging. Imaging of the CNS is not a part of routine staging and should only be obtained if there is a clinical suspicion for metastasis.

271

Tumors should be sampled with image-guided core needle biopsies or an incisional biopsy with a preference for a needle biopsy. The biopsy should be along the axis of a planned resection, if possible. A sentinel lymph node biopsy should be obtained in patients with enlarged nodes by palpation or imaging and sarcomas likely to have lymphatic spread (rhabdomyosarcoma, angiosarcoma, clear cell sarcoma, epithelioid sarcoma, or synovial sarcoma). There are no serum or plasma biomarkers that should be used for diagnosis, assessing treatment response, or monitoring for recurrence of disease.

Treatment

Surgery is the treatment of choice for patients with a primary sarcoma of the extremity or the trunk. Negative surgical margins are associated with improved overall survival and surgery is usually done with at least a 1 cm margin with consideration for presence of bone or fascia as a margin. Involvement of the bone or vasculature or the inability to achieve proper margins requires discussion of amputation. Radiation therapy with image-guided external beam radiation should be considered either preoperatively or postoperatively for patients with intermediate or high-grade soft tissue sarcomas. Brachytherapy is an alternative for radiotherapy delivery at the time of surgery either alone or in combination with external beam radiation. Neoadjuvant radiation therapy should also be considered for patients with low-grade tumors if this may improve the likelihood for appropriate surgical margins.

There are conflicting data for the use of neoadjuvant or adjuvant chemotherapy for patients with soft tissue sarcoma of an extremity. A meta-analysis of 1953 patients enrolled in 18 trials failed to show a survival benefit for treatment with adjuvant doxorubicin, but there was a significant hazard ratio for the combination of doxorubicin and ifosfamide. However, a separate pooled analysis of 2 large trials of patients treated with adjuvant doxorubicin and ifosfamide was negative. Trials have not identified the patients most likely to benefit from adjuvant chemotherapy with inconsistent data on the importance of completeness of resection, tumor size, and tumor grade. Ideally, adjuvant chemotherapy would be given in the setting of a clinical trial. Similarly, there is no consensus in the literature on the role of neoadjuvant chemotherapy. Even trials enriched for large- or high-grade tumors or utilizing chemotherapy thought to be more specific, for the tumor histology failed to show a benefit. As with adjuvant chemotherapy, neoadjuvant chemotherapy should only be used on a case-by-case basis or as part of a clinical trial.

Surgical resection is the only potentially curative treatment for retroperitoneal sarcomas. Surgery for these tumors often requires a multidisciplinary team with planned mobilization, resection, or repair of adjacent organs in order to get appropriate margins with an en bloc resection. Preoperative radiation therapy should be given to patients with intermediate- or high-grade soft tissue sarcoma with consideration of intraoperative radiation. Postoperative radiation requires higher doses and increased risk for toxicity to normal tissue. Patients with an unresectable retroperitoneal sarcoma may benefit from systemic chemotherapy to allow for resection in those who respond. In a phase III trial comparing doxorubicin to doxorubicin and ifosfamide in patients with soft-tissue sarcoma, the response rate was 14% and 25%, respectively. Patients should receive the combination of doxorubicin and ifosfamide to optimize the likelihood of subsequent resection. There are no data to support the use of adjuvant chemotherapy for patients with an R0 or R1 resection of a retroperitoneal sarcoma.

There is a lack of histology-specific treatment for most patients with metastatic soft-tissue sarcoma. The initial treatment for most patients is doxorubicin-based therapy. In a trial enrolling patients with numerous subtypes of soft tissue sarcoma, addition of the platelet-derived growth factor receptor (PDGFR) inhibitor olaratumab to doxorubicin resulted in an 18% response rate and improved overall survival (OS) from 14.7 to 26.5 months. Clinical trials should always be considered for patients with metastatic soft tissue sarcoma, but some additional chemotherapy regimens are listed in Table 21.1.

RHABDOMYOSARCOMA

Clinical Presentation

Rhabdomyosarcoma is the most common soft tissue tumor in children accounting for about half of soft tissue sarcomas in this population; however, these are still rare with an incidence of about 350 new

TABLE 21.1 Chemotherapy Regimens for Patients with Metastatic Soft Tissue Sarcoma

Chemotherapy	Indication
Gemcitabine/docetaxel	May have more activity in leiomyosarcoma
Paclitaxel	May be the best initial therapy for angiosarcoma
Pazopanib	Patients with nonlipogenic sarcomas
Trabectedin	Patients with liposarcoma or leiomyosarcoma
Eribulin	Patients with liposarcoma
Sunitinib	Initial therapy for alveolar soft part sarcoma or malignant solitary fibrous tumor
Sirolimus	Initial therapy for perivascular epithelioid cell differentiation (PEComa)

TABLE 21.2 Most Common Sites of Rhabdomyosarcoma, Frequency and Clinical Presentation

Site	Frequency (%)	Presentation/Symptoms
Head and Neck	35–40	Proptosis (orbit), discharge, painless mass
Genitourinary	25	Hematuria, urinary obstruction, vaginal discharge
Extremities	20	Painless mass with erythema of overlying skin

cases in the United States per year. Only 2% to 5% of rhabdomyosarcoma occurs in adults, most often as a head and neck tumor.

As with other soft tissue sarcomas, patients with rhabdomyosarcoma may be asymptomatic or they may have signs and symptoms related to the site of the disease (Table 21.2).

A prognostic stratification has been developed based on stage, clinical group, site of disease, size of tumor, age, histology, presence of metastatic disease, and involvement of lymph nodes. Patients with an excellent prognosis based on this stratification have a >85% event-free survival. Patients with a very good prognosis and good prognosis have a 70% to 85% and 50% to 50% event-free survival, respectively. A poor prognosis is associated with a <30% event-free survival.

Factors associated with poorer prognosis in patients with a relapse of rhabdomyosarcoma include

- Metastatic disease
- Prior alkylating agents and radiation therapy
- Alveolar histology
- Shorter time to relapse
- Higher stage/clinical group at diagnosis

Pathology

Rhabdomyosarcoma is a tumor of mesenchymal origin that is characterized by myogenic differentiation. Morphologically, rhabdomyosarcoma resembles other tumors, such as lymphoma, mesenchymal chondrosarcoma, and Ewing family sarcomas making it important that the pathology be reviewed at a center with expertise in sarcoma. Rhabdomyosarcoma will usually stain for actin, myosin, desmin, myoglobin, and MyoD. There are pleomorphic and nonpleomorphic rhabdomyosarcomas.

Among nonpleomorphic rhabdomyosarcoma, 80% of patients have an embryonal subtype and about 15% of patients have an alveolar subtype. The embryonal subtype is characterized by 11p15.5 loss of heterogeneity and hyperdiploid DNA. The alveolar subtype is characterized by PAX3/FKHR t(2, 13)(Q35;q14) and PAX3/FKHR t(1:13)(p36;q14) translocations and tetraploid DNA.

Diagnosis

Open biopsy is the preferred approach for tissue diagnosis and should be undertaken at an oncology center, where diagnostic material can be optimally used and the initial surgical approach can be

TABLE 21.3 Chemotherapy Regimens for Patients with Newly Diagnosed Rhabdomyosarcoma

Prognosis Group	Regimen
Low risk (excellent prognosis)	VA for 15 cycles OR VAC/VA for 8 cycles
Low risk (very good prognosis)	VAC for 15 cycles
Intermediate risk (good prognosis)	VAC for 14 cycles OR VAC/VI for 14 cycles
High risk (poor prognosis)	VAC for 14 cycles

VA (vincristine and dactinomycin); VAC (vincristine, dactinomycin, cyclophosphamide); VI (vincristine and irinotecan).

determined by a multidisciplinary team responsible for the patient's subsequent treatment. Patients should have an MRI or CT of the primary site of disease and a PET/CT scan or bone scan to assess for metastatic disease.

Treatment

Pleomorphic rhabdomyosarcoma should be treated as a soft-tissue sarcoma. The diversity of primary sites, distinctive surgical approaches and radiotherapy regimens for each primary site, subsequent site-specific rehabilitation, and potential treatment-related sequelae underscore the importance of patients with nonpleomorphic rhabdomyosarcoma consulting with or being treated at a medical center that has appropriate experience in surgery, radiation therapy, and medical oncology. Tumors should only be resected if there is no evidence of adenopathy or metastatic disease and the surgery would not lead to excessive morbidity. Due to poor survival with surgery alone, rhabdomyosarcoma is usually treated with a combination of surgery, radiation therapy, and chemotherapy. This combination therapy is determined by the estimated risk of recurrence.

Patients with rhabdomyosarcoma usually have a very long course of treatment. Those with low-risk, intermediate-risk, or high-risk disease receive chemotherapy for 24 to 45 weeks with radiation therapy starting at week 13 (Table 21.3). Most patients also receive radiation therapy starting at week 13 of their therapy, so consultation with radiation oncology as part of a multidisciplinary team is important.

OSTEOSARCOMA

Osteosarcoma, a primary malignancy of the bone, represents 1% of all cases of cancer diagnosed in the United States annually. This cancer primarily affects adolescents with a peak incidence between ages 13 and 16 and adults over 65 years of age. It is the most common primary cancer of the bone in children and young adults. While a primary cancer in children and young adults, osteosarcoma in adults is often secondary to prior radiation or the presence of Paget's disease.

Clinical Presentation

In children, osteosarcoma is most common in the metaphysis of long bones. In adults, osteosarcoma is more common in the axial skeleton or at sites of either prior radiation or abnormalities of the bone. Most patients present with localized pain, often with a long period of pain with intermittent severity. Fever, weight loss, and fatigue are rare. Patients generally develop a soft tissue mass that is painful to palpation. Fifteen to twenty percent of patients have metastatic disease at the time of diagnosis.

Diagnosis

The primary differential diagnosis for patients with osteosarcoma is Ewing sarcoma, lymphoma, and metastatic disease. Plain radiographs may show either a lytic or sclerotic appearance or periosteal elevation from tumor penetration of the cortical bone. Workup should include an MRI of the involved bone, a CT of the lungs, and a bone scan or PET/CT to assess for metastatic disease. A biopsy is required to confirm the diagnosis. The biopsy should be done carefully with consideration of how it may impact subsequent definitive surgery and either be a surgical or core biopsy. Patients of reproductive age should have a discussion about fertility.

Pathology

Osteosarcomas are of mesenchymal origin and can differentiate to fibrous tissue, cartilage, or bone. Histologically, osteosarcomas have a sarcomatous stroma with tumor osteoid and bone. There are no translocations or molecular abnormalities that define osteosarcoma. Osteosarcoma can be defined as low grade with intramedullary and surface involvement, periosteal, high-grade intramedullary, and surface or extraskeletal osteosarcoma. Extraskeletal osteosarcomas are soft-tissue sarcomas that don't involve the bone or periosteum, but produce bone, osteoid, or chondroid material.

Treatment

Amputation and limb-sparing resection incorporate wide en bloc excision of the tumor with the biopsy site through normal tissue planes, leaving a cuff of normal tissue around the periphery of the tumor. Wide excision with negative margins improves local tumor control. Limb-sparing surgery is now the preferred approach for 70% to 90% of patients with osteosarcoma due to improved functional outcome. Reconstruction may involve allografts or customized prosthetic devices.

Patients with low-grade osteosarcoma of the intramedullary or surface of the bone or with periosteal osteosarcoma should undergo wide excision of the tumor with consideration of adjuvant chemotherapy for those with periosteal osteosarcoma (Table 21.4). If these patients have a high-grade tumor on excision, they should receive chemotherapy.

Patients with a high-grade osteosarcoma involving the intramedullary or surface of the bone should receive neoadjuvant chemotherapy. Those with an unresectable tumor after neoadjuvant chemotherapy should receive radiation therapy or additional chemotherapy. Patients with a resectable tumor after the neoadjuvant chemotherapy should have a wide excision. Further therapy is based on the surgical margins and response to therapy with poor response defined as >10% viable tumor in the resected tumor. Treatment options for patients with positive margins include additional surgery, radiation therapy, and adjuvant chemotherapy. Patients with negative surgical margins should receive adjuvant chemotherapy with either the initial neoadjuvant regimen or a different regimen based on the treatment response.

TABLE 21.4 Chemotherapy Options for Patients with Osteosarcoma

First-line chemotherapy (neoadjuvant or adjuvant therapy or metastatic disease)
Doxorubicin and cisplatin
Doxorubicin, cisplatin, high-dose methotrexate
Doxorubicin, cisplatin, high-dose methotrexate, ifosfamide

Second-line/Subsequent therapy
Docetaxel and gemcitabine
Etoposide and cyclophosphamide
Etoposide and high-dose ifosfamide
Gemcitabine
Radium-223
Sorafenib

Patients with metastatic disease at the time of diagnosis should have consideration of resection or stereotactic radiation for pulmonary, visceral, or skeletal metastases followed by chemotherapy. Patients with unresectable disease should receive chemotherapy or radiation therapy with reassessment for resectability of the metastatic disease.

Patients with an extraosseous osteosarcoma should have their tumor treated as a soft-tissue sarcoma.

EWING FAMILY OF TUMORS (EFT)

The EFT comprises Ewing sarcoma of the bone, peripheral primitive neuroectodermal tumors (PNET), and extraosseous Ewing sarcoma. These tumors have similar immunohistochemical and histologic features and chromosomal translocations suggesting they are derived from a common cell of origin. The EFT is the second most common primary bone tumor in children and adolescents.

Clinical Presentation

EFT are most common in the long bones of the extremities and the bones of the pelvis. In a review of nearly 1000 patients with EFT, 54% of patients had disease in the axial skeleton with 42% in the appendicular skeleton. Typical symptoms of EFT is localized pain or swelling that may be present for weeks to months with an increase in intensity over time. Pain may be worse with exercise or at night. Patients may have a mass that is tender to palpation with some localized erythema. Fatigue, weight loss, and fever can occur, but are rare. Approximately 20% of patients with EFT have overt metastases at diagnosis with metastatic disease more common in patients with tumors in the pelvis. Of the patients with metastatic disease, about 50% have lung metastases and about 40% have multiple bone lesions and diffuse bone marrow involvement. The peak incidence is in those between 10 and 15 years of age with 30% of cases in those greater than 20 years of age.

Diagnosis

Patients with EFT should have a history and physical, an MRI with contrast of the primary site, a CT of the chest, and a PET/CT or a bone scan to determine the presence of metastatic disease. Patients preferably have an open biopsy for the tissue diagnosis, ideally at an oncology center where the diagnostic material can be optimally assessed and the initial surgical approach can be determined by a multidisciplinary team responsible for the patient's subsequent treatment. Needle biopsy may restrict access to fresh and frozen tissue for cytogenetic and molecular genetic investigations that are necessary to diagnose an EFT. Patients should have a consultation about fertility, unless past the age of reproductive potential.

Pathology

Morphologically, EFT are similar to other small, round, blue cell tumors including lymphoma, small cell osteosarcoma, undifferentiated neuroblastoma, desmoplastic small round cell tumors, and rhabdomyosarcoma. EFT can be diagnosed by the presence of *EWSR1* translocations, the most common being t(11;22)(q24;q12) leading to the *EWSR1-FLI1* gene fusion.

Treatment

Many patients with EFT with apparently localized disease at the time of diagnosis have subclinical micrometastases. Patients with EFT should be treated with a multidisciplinary approach including systemic chemotherapy, surgery, and radiation therapy.

Patients with localized or metastatic EFT should be treated initially with combination chemotherapy for at least 12 weeks (Table 21.5). Patients should be restaged with MRI and/or CT of the primary site, a CT of the chest and possibly PET/CT or bone scan to determine treatment response.

Patients with stable disease or a treatment response following the initial chemotherapy should undergo wide excision, continue with definitive radiation and chemotherapy or, in some cases, amputation. Patients with positive margins after wide resection should have adjuvant chemotherapy and radiation therapy with adjuvant chemotherapy alone in patients with negative margins. Patients requiring

TABLE 21.5 Chemotherapy Options for Patients with EFT

First-line therapy for neoadjuvant or adjuvant therapy

VAC/IE (vincristine, doxorubicin, and cyclophosphamide alternating
  with ifosfamide and etoposide)
VAI (vincristine, doxorubicin, and ifosfamide)
VIDE (vincristine, ifosfamide, doxorubicin, and etoposide)

First-line therapy for metastatic disease at diagnosis

VAC
VAC/IE
VAI
VIDE

Second-line therapy for relapsed/refractory or metastatic disease

Cyclophosphamide and topotecan
Irinotecan and temozolomide
Etoposide and high-dose ifosfamide
Gemcitabine and docetaxel

amputation as local therapy should receive adjuvant chemotherapy with radiation therapy for positive margins.

Patients with progressive disease after their initial chemotherapy should consider radiation therapy or surgery to the primary site of disease for palliation followed by additional chemotherapy.

Suggested Readings

1. Arndt CA, Crist WM. Common musculoskeletal tumors of childhood and adolescence. *N Engl J Med.* 1999;341:342–352.
2. Biermann JS, Adkins DR, Agulnik M. Bone Cancer. *J Natl Compr Can Netw.* 2013;11:688–723.
3. Biermann JS, Chow W, Reed DR. Bone Cancer. *J Natl Compr Can Netw.* 2017;15:155–167.
4. Carvajal R, Meyers P. Ewing's sarcoma and primitive neuroectodermal family of tumors. *Hematol Oncol Clin North Am.* 2005;19(3):501–525, vi–vii.
5. Cutts S, Andrea F, Piana R, Haywood R. The management of soft tissue sarcomas. *Surgeon.* 2012;10(1):25–32. doi:10.1016/j.surge.2011.09.006.
6. Dangoor A, Seddon B, Garrand C, et al. UK Guidelines for the management of soft tissue sarcomas. *Clin Sarcoma Res.* 2016;6:20.
7. Ferrari S, Palmerini E. Adjuvant and neoadjuvant combination chemotherapy for osteogenic sarcoma. *Curr Opin Oncol.* 2007;19(4):341–346.
8. Fletcher CDM, Bridge JA, Hogendoorn PCW, Mertens F eds. World Health Organization classification of tumours of soft tissue and bone, 4th edn. Lyon: IARC Press, 2013.
9. Gerrand C, Athanasou N, Brennan B, et al. UK Guidelines for the management of bone sarcomas. *Clin Sarcoma Res.* 2016;6:7.
10. Grohar PJ, Helman LJ. Prospects and challenges for the development of new therapies for Ewing sarcoma. *Pharmacol Ther.* 2013;137(2):216–224.
11. Gustafson P, Dreinhofer KE, Rydholm A. Soft tissue sarcoma should be treated at a tumor center. A comparison of quality of surgery in 375 patients. *Acta Orthop Scand.* 1994;65:47–50.
12. Huh WW, Skapek SX. Childhood rhabdomyosarcoma: new insight on biology and treatment. *Curr Oncol Rep.* 2010;12(6):402–410.
13. Kim SY, Helman LJ. Strategies to explore new approaches in the investigation and treatment of osteosarcoma. *Cancer Treat Res.* 2009;152:517–528.
14. Lawrence, W., Jr., et al. (1987). Adult soft tissue sarcomas. A pattern of care survey of the American College of Surgeons. *Ann Surg.* 205(4):349–359.
15. Le Cesne A, Ouali M, Leahy MG. Doxorubicin-based adjuvant chemotherapy in soft tissue sarcoma: pooled analysis of two STBSG-EORTC phase III clinical trials. *Ann Oncol.* 2014;25:2425–2432.

16. Mirabello L, Troisi RJ, Savage SA. Osteosarcoma incidence and survival rates from 1973 to 2004: Data from the surveillance, epidemiology, and end results program. *Cancer*. 2009;115:1531–1543.
17. NCCN Clinical Practice Guidelines in Oncology. Soft Tissue Sarcoma. V.1.2018. https://www.nccn.org/professionals/physician_gls/PDF/sarcoma.pdf
18. Rosen G, Marcove RC, Huvos AG et al. Primary osteogenic sarcoma: eight-year experience with adjuvant chemotherapy. *J Cancer Res Clin Oncol.* 1983;106 Suppl;55–67.
19. Rothermundt C, Whelan JS, Dileo P, et al. What is the role of routine follow-up for localized limb soft tissue sarcomas? A retrospective analysis of 174 patients. *Br J Cancer*. 2014;110:2420–2426.
20. Rubin BP. Recent progress in the classification of soft tissue tumors: the role of genetics and clinical implications. *Curr Opin Oncol*. 2001;13:256–260.
21. Tap WD, Jone RL, Van Tine BA, et al. Olaratumab and doxorubicin versus doxorubicin alone for treatment of soft-tissue sarcoma: an open-label phase 1b and randomized phase 2 trial. *Lancet* 2016;388:488–497.
22. von Mehren M, Randall RL, Benjamin RS. Soft tissue sarcoma, Version 2.2016, NCCN Clinical Practice Guidelines in Oncology. *J Natl Compr Canc Netw*. 2016;14:758–786.
23. Woll PJ, Reichardt P, Le Cesne A, et al. Adjuvant chemotherapy with doxorubicin, ifosfamide, and lenograstim for resected soft-tissue sarcoma (EORTC 62931): a multicentre randomized controlled trial. *Lancet Oncol* . 2012;13;10;1045–1054.

Skin Cancers and Melanoma **22**

Upendra P. Hegde and Sanjiv S. Agarwala

INTRODUCTION

The skin is the largest organ of the human body, embryologically derived from the neuroectoderm and the mesoderm, eventually organized into epidermis, dermis, and subcutis.

Cancer of the skin arises from the cell types of structures in all the three layers (Table 22.1).

Direct exposure of the skin to sun's ultraviolet radiation and a wide variety of environmental carcinogens predisposes to genetic damage and increased risk of cancer. Skin cancers are best divided into melanoma and nonmelanoma.

MELANOMA

Melanoma arises from the melanocyte, a neural crest–derived cell that migrates during embryogenesis predominantly to the basal layer of the epidermal skin and less commonly to the other tissues in the body such as mucosa of the upper aerodigestive and the lower genitourinary tract, the meninges, and the ocular choroid, where melanoma is rarely encountered.

Epidemiology

- Melanoma ranks as the 5th and 7th leading type of cancer in US men and women, respectively.
- Incidence is high in young, middle age, and elderly subjects.
- Estimated lifetime risk of developing invasive melanoma in US whites is about 1 in 33 in males and 1 in 52 in women.
- In 2017, 87,110 new cases of invasive melanoma are expected to be diagnosed in the US with 9,73010,130 subjects projected to die from it.
- The incidence of melanoma is higher in men than women, Northern than Eastern and Central Europeans and more than 10 times greater in whites than in blacks.
- Australia has the highest incidence of melanoma in the world, approximately 40 cases compared to 23.6 cases among US whites per 100,000 population per year.
- The rate of rise in melanoma incidence has decreased from 6% a year in the 1970s to 3% a year between 1980 and 2000 and stabilized after that period in younger subjects.
- In white males over 50 years of age, the incidence continues to climb at the fastest rate.
- The median age at diagnosis and death from melanoma is 63 and 69 years, respectively.
- The percent of cutaneous melanoma deaths is highest among people aged 75 to 84 years.

Etiology

- Ultraviolet rays' exposure is a major risk factor for melanoma development and is related to (Fig. 22.1)
  - Intermittent intense exposure
  - Exposure at a young age
  - Fair skin, blue eyes, blonde or red hair, propensity for sunburns, and inability to tan

TABLE 22.1 Cell of Epidermis, Dermis, and Respective Tumor Types

Cells of Epidermis	Tumor-Type/ Incidence	Cells of Dermis	Tumor-Type[a]
Melanocytes	Melanoma 5%–7%	Fibroblasts	Benign and malignant fibrous tumor
Epidermal basal cells	Basal cell carcinoma 60%	Histiocytes	Histiocytic tumor
Keratinocytes	Squamous cell carcinoma 30%	Mast cells	Mast cell tumor
Merkel cells	Merkel cell tumor 1%–2%	Vasculature	Angioma, Angiosarcoma, Lymphangioma
Langerhans cells	Histiocytosis X <1%	Lymphocytes	Non-Hodgkin lymphoma
Appendage cells	Appendageal tumors <1%	—	—

[a] Incidence of tumors in dermis <1% each type.

Familial Melanoma

- About 5% to 10% of melanomas are familial among which up to 40% have hereditary basis.
- A tumor suppressor gene cyclin-dependent kinase inhibitor 2A (CDKN2A).
- is the most commonly implicated gene located on the short arm of chromosome 9, which could be either mutated or suppressed by epigenetic silencing.
- The protective effect of CDKN2A is mediated by encoded protein p16^{INK4A}.
- Other candidate genes in this category include cyclin-dependent kinase 4 (CDK4) and CDKN2A/p14 alternate reading frame CDKN2A/ARF.
- Mutations in the telomere-related genes such as POT1, shelterin complex genes, and TERT have been identified in families with clusters of cutaneous melanoma.
- A high-risk variant of the α-melanocyte-stimulating hormone receptor gene (MC1R) located on chromosome 16q24 and associated with red hair and freckles confer high risk of familial melanoma in families segregating the CDKN2A gene.
- Hereditary basis of melanoma should be suspected in the following circumstances:
  - Individuals with three or more primary cutaneous melanomas
  - Melanoma at a young age and a family history of melanoma (mean age between 30 and 40)
  - Individuals with cutaneous melanoma and a family history of at least one invasive melanoma and two or more other diagnoses of melanoma and/or pancreatic cancer among first- or second-degree relatives on the same side of the family
  - Melanoma associated in patients with dysplastic nevi and atypical nevi
- Precursor lesions of melanoma include the following:
  - Dysplastic nevi genetic locus of which resides on short arm of chromosome 1
  - Congenital nevi and acquired melanocytic nevi

Risk Factors for Cutaneous Melanoma

- Xeroderma pigmentosum (caused by mutations in UV damage repair genes)
- Familial atypical mole melanoma syndrome (FAMMS)
- Advanced age and immune-suppressed states
- Melanoma in a first-degree relative and previous history of melanoma

Common Chromosomal Abnormalities in Melanoma

- Early chromosomal abnormalities:
  - Loss of 10q and 9p

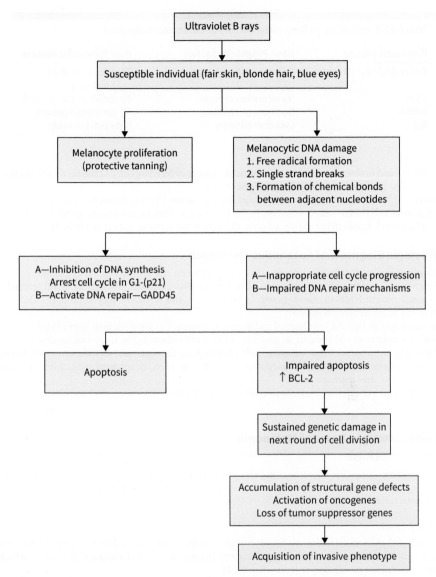

FIGURE 22.1 Model of ultraviolet B light–mediated pathogenesis of cutaneous melanoma.

- Late chromosomal abnormalities:
  - Deletion of 6q, 11q23
  - Loss of terminal part of 1p
  - Duplication of chromosome 7

Clinical Features of Cutaneous Melanoma (ABCDE)

- Most cutaneous melanoma lesions are pigmented and display asymmetry (A), irregular borders (B), variegate colors (C) with shades of brown, black, pink, white, red, or blue have diameter of at least

TABLE 22.2 Independent Prognostic Factors of Cutaneous Melanoma

Prognostic Factors	Good Prognostic Factors	Poor Prognostic Factors
Tumor thickness (Breslow)	Thin tumor (tumor ≤1 mm deep)	Thick tumor (tumor >1 mm deep)
Ulceration	No ulceration of tumor	Tumor ulceration present
Mitosis	No tumor cell mitosis	Tumor mitosis present
Age	Less than 60 years	Sixty years or over

6 mm (D) and evolve in size, color, nodularity, ulceration, or bleeding (E). Cutaneous melanoma may be painless or, at times, cause itching and discomfort.
- Rarely (<1%) cutaneous melanomas lack pigment (amelanotic) posing diagnostic challenges.
- Cutaneous melanoma is more common in the lower extremities in women, the trunk in men, and head and neck region in the elderly subjects although it can occur anywhere in the body.

Pathologic Diagnosis of Cutaneous Melanoma

- Morphologically identified melanoma cells express vimentin and are negative for cytokeratin.
- Diagnosis is confirmed by the detection of melanoma-associated antigens such as S-100, premelanosomal protein HMB-45, nerve growth factor receptor, and tyrosinase-related protein 1 (MEL-5) detected by immunohistochemistry.
- In melanoma in situ, the transformed melanocyte is restricted to the epidermal layer of skin.
- Invasive melanoma is defined by its invasion of the dermis quantified by Clark and Breslow.
- Histologic characteristics (microstaging) help prognosticate the tumor and include, tumor thickness, mitosis, ulceration, Clark levels, vascular or perineural invasion, lymphocyte infiltration, morphologic variants, and regression.
- Independent variables of melanoma prognosis are Breslow thickness, mitosis, ulceration, and older age (Table 22.2).

Clinico-histologic Types of Melanoma

Breslow Thickness

Breslow used an ocular micrometer to measure the vertical depth of penetration of tumor from the granular layer of the epidermis or from the base of the ulcerated melanoma to the deepest identifiable contiguous melanoma cell.

Clark Levels

Clark et al. subdivided melanoma invasion of the papillary dermis into a deep group in which tumor cells accumulate at the junction of the papillary and reticular dermis and a superficial group in which tumor cells did not invade deeper layers (Fig. 22.2).

Principles of American Joint Committee on Cancer (AJCC) Melanoma Staging

Melanoma stage is based on the information derived from three key categories (**TNM**):

- (**T**) Tumor characteristics on microscopic examination
- (**N**) Nodes—status of the regional lymph node metastasis
- (**M**) Distant metastasis—either present or absent

In AJCC staging, melanoma is divided into four stages:

- Stage I—Thin melanoma (subdivided into IA and IB)

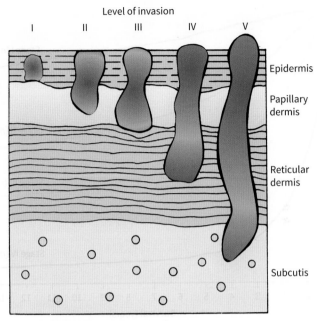

FIGURE 22.2 Schematic diagram of Clark levels of invasion.

- Stage II—Deeper melanoma without lymph node metastasis (subdivided into IIA, IIB, and IIC)
- Stage III—Melanoma spread to regional lymph nodes (subdivided into IIIA, IIIB, and IIIC)
- Stage IV—Distant metastasis (subdivided into M1a, M1b, and M1c)

  The following factors are taken into consideration for subdividing each stage into A, B, or C:

- Stages IA and IB: Depth of invasion, ulceration, and mitosis
- Stages IIA, IIB, and IIC: Depth of invasion, presence, or absence of ulceration.
- Stages IIIA, IIIB, and IIIC: Depth, ulceration of the primary melanoma, number of lymph node metastases, microscopic versus macroscopic (clinically palpable) lymph nodes, intralymphatic metastases (in transit metastasis), or satellite lesions.

  Sentinel lymph node biopsy (SLNB) is recommended for detection of occult melanoma metastasis in a lymph node when clinical examination is negative.

- Sentinel lymph node is not usually recommended in a thin melanoma ≤1mm deep, without mitosis or ulceration since in such a case lymph node metastasis is rare.
- The sensitivity of finding melanoma cells or clusters in a sentinel lymph node is enhanced by subjecting it for immunohistochemical staining of melanoma-associated antigens.
- Dividing stage IV melanoma into M1a, M1b, and M1c helps characterize prognosis:
  - M1a—Metastasis to the distant lymph node and subcutaneous tissues (favorable stage IV)
  - M1b—Lung metastasis (intermediate prognosis)
  - M1c—Non–lung visceral metastasis such as liver, bone, brain, and other organs (poor prognosis)
  - Serum enzyme lactate dehydrogenase enzyme (LDH) if elevated upgrades M1a and M1b to M1c

Prediction of Patient Outcome Based on AJCC Melanoma Staging 2009 (Figure 22.3)

- Low risk: Stages I and IIA (melanoma-specific mortality less than 25% at 20 years)
- Medium to high risk: Stages IIB, IIC, and III (melanoma-specific mortality between 55% and 75% at 20 years)
- Poor risk: Stage IV (melanoma-specific mortality more than 90% at 5 years)

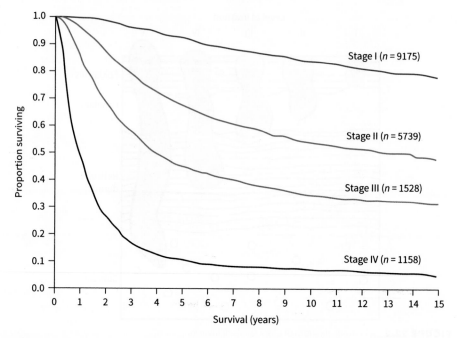

FIGURE 22.3 Relationship between the stage of melanoma and survival (20-year follow-up). (Kaplan-Meier survival curves adapted from Balch CM, Gershenwald JE, Soong S-J, et al. Final version of 2009 AJCC melanoma staging and classification. *J Clin Oncol.* 2009; 27:6199–6206.)

Cutaneous Melanoma: Prevention and Early Diagnosis

Public health education measures specific for melanoma include emphasis on spreading awareness of melanoma as a serious cancer, focus on its risk factors such as ultraviolet light exposure and tanning booth use, preventive strategies such as sun avoidance techniques, light clothing, sun screen use, and early diagnosis by periodic self-skin and total body skin examinations (TBSE).

TBSE performed by a dermatologist provides the opportunity to identify suspicious skin lesions for biopsy and early diagnosis.

- Digital photography helps to track suspicious skin lesions over time in patients with multiple nevi or dysplastic nevus syndrome.
- Dermoscopy (epiluminescence microscopy) improves diagnostic sensitivity, and utilizes either a dermatoscope or 10× ocular scope (microscope ocular eyepiece held upside down) to visualize structures and patterns in pigmented skin lesions not discernible to the eye.

Cutaneous Melanoma Management

An algorithm for melanoma management is presented in Figure 22.4.
Primary surgical treatment: Principles

- Complete excision of primary melanoma confirmed by comprehensive histologic examination of the entire excised specimen and assessment of melanoma metastasis to the regional lymph node (except in stage IA where the risk is low) forms the basis of surgical treatment.
- Recommendations for extent of surgical margins vary by depth of cutaneous melanoma (Table 22.3), but risk of local recurrence relates to completeness rather than extent of surgical margins.

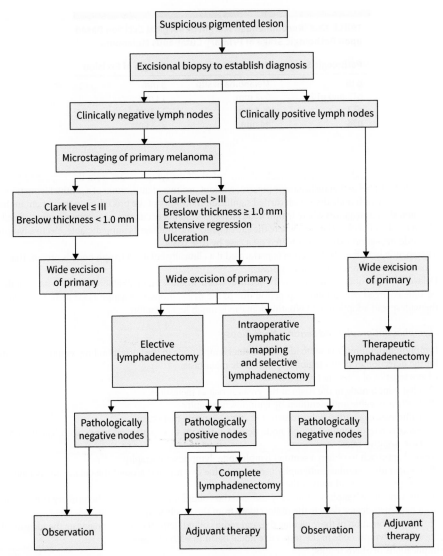

FIGURE 22.4 Algorithm for cutaneous melanoma management.

Assessment of the Regional Lymph Node Metastasis and Lymph Node Dissection: Principle

▪ The risk of regional lymph node metastasis is directly proportional to the depth of invasion, tumor ulceration, and mitosis, all reflecting tumor biology.

Historically, complete excision of primary cutaneous melanoma is followed with elective, therapeutic, or delayed lymph node dissection from the respective basin.

TABLE 22.3 Recommended Margin of Surgical Excision Based upon Pathologic Stage of Primary Cutaneous Melanoma

Pathologic Stage	Tumor Thickness	Margin of Excision
p tis	Melanoma in situ	5 mm
pT1 and pT2	0–2 mm	1 cm
pT3	2–4 mm	1–2 cm
pT4	>4 mm	2–3 cm

- Elective lymph node dissection consists of removal of all the lymph nodes from the respective basin grounded on a belief that metastasis is present, without positive identification of a sentinel lymp node.
  - Elective lymph node dissection carried significant morbidity of the procedure to the patient in the clinical circumstances where lymph node metastasis did not occur and is no longer recommended.
  - In head and neck melanoma where the site of lymphatic drainage is unpredictable, elective lymph node dissection may be considered on a case by case basis.
- Therapeutic lymph node dissection is performed if a clinically enlarged lymph node is present that is considered or proven to harbor metastasis.
- Delayed lymph node dissection is performed when initially nonpalpable regional lymph nodes become enlarged over a follow-up period due to the delayed onset of lymph node metastasis. With the widespread adoption of SLNB, this scenario is much less common.

Lymphoscintigraphy and Sentinel Node Biopsy

- Lymphoscintigraphy is a tool to identify sentinel lymph node in the corresponding lymph node basin for the detection of occult regional lymph node metastasis.
- Characteristics of a sentinel lymph node:
  - First lymph node in the basin at the greatest risk of metastasis.
  - Easily accessible and identified by lymphoscintigraphy.
  - Pathologic evaluation helps to detect occult melanoma metastasis.
  - Success rate of sentinel lymph node detection is 95% in experienced hands with less than 5% false negative rates.
- Surgical approach to obtain a sentinel lymph node: lymphoscintigraphy
  - Preoperative lymphoscintigraphy uses a vital blue dye injected around the cutaneous melanoma that provides a road map of the lymph node basin.
  - Intraoperative lymphoscintigraphy uses a radio colloid injection around the primary tumor, and a handheld device detects the radioactivity from the involved lymph node.
  - The combination of the vital blue dye and radio colloid helps the surgeon navigate the identity of sentinel lymph node in the respective nodal basin in 95% of cases.
- Implications of SLNB results:
  - Only those patients with melanoma metastasis to the sentinel lymph node (positive sentinel lymph node) will undergo complete lymph node dissection.
  - A negative sentinel lymph node saves the patient the morbidity of lymph node dissection.
  - SLNB–guided information about the extent of lymph node metastasis helps in prognostication of primary melanoma and reduces the risk of recurrence in the lymph node basin. Its impact on overall survival is not clear.

The Multicenter Selective Lymphadenectomy Trial I (MSLT-1) was designed to find if SLNB followed by early complete lymph node dissection would have an overall survival benefit in patients with intermediate thickness melanoma (1.2 to 3.5 mm depth).

- The results showed improved 5-year disease-free survival (83.2% vs. 53.4%) in subjects assigned to lymphoscintigraphy whose SLNB was negative for metastasis compared to those whose sentinel lymph nodes were positive.

- A subgroup analysis was suggestive of the improved melanoma specific five-year survival for patients with node-positive microscopic disease who underwent immediate lymph node dissection compared to the observation arm who underwent lymph node dissection upon macroscopic lymph node metastasis (72.3% vs. 52.4%), but this did not translate into an overall melanoma-specific survival benefit in the intention-to-treat population.

We should include MSLT-2 results as they will be available soon.

Ongoing debate about SLNB and completion lymphadenectomy:

- Is completion lymphadenectomy necessary in all sentinel lymph node positive tumors?
- Can tumor bulk in sentinel lymph node determine need for completion lymphadenectomy?
- Melanoma Sentinel Lymphadenectomy Trial (MSLT-2) is evaluating the therapeutic benefit of completion lymphadenectomy after positive SLNB. Patients with positive SLNB are randomized to either completion lymphadenectomy or nodal observation by periodic ultrasound. The results are awaited.
- The German DECOG study group randomized cutaneous melanoma patients with a positive sentinel lymph node to either completion lymphadenectomy or nodal observation. In a short median follow-up of 34 months, there were no differences in recurrence-free survival, distant metastases-free survival or melanoma-specific survival.
- The Sunbelt Melanoma Trial reported no difference in overall survival after complete lymph node dissection compared to observation after positive SLNB (although the study was underpowered and this was not be the main objective of the study).
- EORTC 1208 Minitub is a prospective registry that aims to examine which cutaneous melanoma patients with sentinel lymph node metastasis will benefit from completion lymph node dissection based on sentinel lymph node tumor burden.

Adjuvant Treatment of Melanoma in Patients at Risk of Recurrence after Surgery

Adjuvant treatment of melanoma is recommended in stage IIB, IIC, and III patients since follow-up studies following surgical treatment of cutaneous melanoma showed a high rate of relapse and melanoma specific mortality (35% to 75%).

Interferon alpha (IFNα-2b) as adjuvant treatment of cutaneous melanoma: Principles based on antiproliferative and immunomodulatory effects, prolonged use of IFNα-2b (high dose, low dose, intermediate dose for variable periods of time) has been extensively studied in an adjuvant setting after surgery and approved by the FDA in the adjuvant setting (Table 22.4).

- High dose IFNα-2b treatment conferred consistent relapse and disease-free survival benefits in multiple trials.
- Its impact upon overall survival has been variable and less consistent.

TABLE 22.4 FDA-approved Adjuvant Therapy in Cutaneous Melanoma

Study Group	Treatment Regimen
EORTC 18071 Ipilimumab vs. placebo	Ipilimumab Induction phase: Ipilimumab 10mg/Kg IV every 3 weeks for four doses Maintenance phase: Ipilimumab 10mg/Kg every 12 weeks for up to 3 years
ECOG E 1684 Interferon alpha vs. observation	High-dose interferon treatment Induction phase: IFN-α 2b, 20 million units/m2/dose IV, 5 d/wk × 4 wk (total dose/wk, 100 million units/m2), followed by Maintenance phase: IFN-α 2b, 10 million units/m² SC, three times/wk for 48 wk (total dose/wk, 30 million units/m²) vs. observation

ECOG, Eastern Cooperative Oncology Group; EORTC, European Organization for the Research and Treatment of Cancer; IV intravenous; SC subcutaneous.

- Reducing the dose (low dose) or duration (induction only) of IFNα-2b for one month does not provide clinical benefit compared to high dose treatment.
- Pegylated form of IFN-α (slow release) given subcutaneously once weekly for up to 5 years conferred relapse-free survival advantage without overall survival benefit.
- The predominant toxicities of high-dose IFNα-2b include severe flu-like symptoms, chronic fatigue, nausea, bone marrow suppression, liver toxicity, and depression that adversely affect quality of life and may compromise the intended benefit.

The decision to use interferon in the adjuvant setting of cutaneous melanoma treatment should be based on the perceived relative merits of disease control, quality of life, and financial cost.

Ipilimumab (anti CTLA-4 antibody) as an adjuvant therapy of melanoma: Principles based on the survival benefit conferred by Ipilimumab in about 25% of patients in metastatic melanoma, it was investigated as a candidate in the adjuvant setting.

- Ipilimumab administered intravenously at a dose of 10 mg/kg body weight every 3 weeks for four doses (induction phase) followed by same dose given every 12 weeks for up to 3 years (maintenance phase) improved relapse-free survival and overall survival compared to placebo.
- At a median follow-up of 27.4 months, relapse-free survival was 26.1 months following Ipilimumab versus 17.1 months in patients receiving placebo (HR 0.75, P=.0013).
- At 5 years of follow-up, Ipilimumab treatment-led recurrence-free survival was translated into distant metastasis-free survival and overall survival compared to placebo. The overall survival rate at 5 years was 65.4% in the Ipilimumab group, as compared with 54.4% in the placebo group (hazard ratio for death from any cause, 0.72, $P = 0.001$).
- Ipilimumab-induced survival advantage occurred in all subgroups of stage III patients including those with microscopic as well as macroscopic recurrences and irrespective of ulceration of the primary melanoma. Ipilimumab was FDA approved for stage III melanoma in 2016 (Table 22.4).
- Serious autoimmune side effects referred to as immune-related adverse events (irAE) of Ipilimumab led to discontinuation of treatment in 52% of patients (39% patients in induction phase and 13% during maintenance phase).
- Common irAE involved gastrointestinal system (16%), liver (11%), and endocrine organs (8%).
- Five patients (1%) died of severe irAE including 3 from colitis two of whom had perforation, 1 patient of myocarditis and 1developed Guillain-Barré syndrome and multi-organ failure.

Biochemotherapy as adjuvant treatment of cutaneous melanoma: Principles

Biochemotherapy produced favorable response rates and occasional durable responses in newly diagnosed metastatic melanoma patients leading to its study in the adjuvant setting.

- Biochemotherapy administered every 3 weeks with G-CSF support for three cycles was compared to high dose interferon α 2b treatment.
- The results showed a significant relapse-free survival advantage for biochemotherapy without overall survival benefit but it also caused severe grade 3/4 toxicities.

Some of the ongoing clinical trials in adjuvant treatment of melanoma:

- A phase III ECOG 1609 trial is comparing two doses of ipilimumab (3 mg/kg and 10 mg/kg) to high-dose interferon. This study may help find the optimal dose of ipilimumab as compared to high-dose interferon alpha.
  - A randomized, double-blind phase III trial of the EORTC Melanoma Group is studying the anti PD-1 agent pembrolizumab versus placebo after complete resection of high-risk stage III melanoma. The primary end point is recurrence-free survival, secondary end points are distant metastases-free survival and overall survival. Patients will be stratified by PD-L1 expression. At relapse, patients will be unblended and allowed to cross over to the active treatment arm if on placebo.
  - COMBI-AD is an ongoing phase III trial that plans to randomize 852 patients with stage III BRAF V600E/K mutation-positive melanoma to combined dabrafenib and trametinib versus placebo. The primary end point is RFS.
  - BRIM-8 plans to randomize 725 patients with stage IIC and III BRAF V600 mutation-positive melanoma to adjuvant vemurafenib versus placebo. The primary end point is DFS.

Role of Radiation Therapy in Melanoma

Radiation therapy of melanoma may be used in the following clinical scenarios:

- Bulky and/or four or more lymph node metastasis or extracapsular spread in a lymph node
- Local recurrence of melanoma in a previously dissected lymph node basin
- After surgical resection of desmoplastic melanoma with neurotropism
- Pain relief of melanoma metastasis to the musculoskeletal region
- Brain metastasis of melanoma

Radiation therapy in brain metastasis of melanoma includes the following:

- Whole-brain radiation if multiple and/or large size brain metastases are present.
- Stereotactic brain radiation is preferred in small-sized or fewer (two to three) brain metastases.

Results of studies by Skibber et al. and others suggest that external radiation to the whole brain after resection of solitary brain metastasis of malignant melanoma has survival benefits.

Isolated Limb Perfusion or Infusion as a Treatment of Melanoma: Principles

To deliver maximally tolerated chemotherapy in patients with locally advanced and metastatic melanoma to a regionally confined tumor area such as a limb while limiting systemic toxicity.

- Isolated limb perfusion (ILP): Involves hyperthermia and oxygenation of the circulation that potentiates the tumoricidal effects of the chemotherapeutic agents such as melphalan (L-PAM), thiotepa, mechlorethamine with or without tumor necrosis factor (TNF-α), and IFN-γ.
- Isolated limb infusion (ILI): Is a simplified and minimally invasive procedure developed at the Sydney Melanoma Unit (SMU) intended to obtain the benefits of ILP without major disadvantages. It is a low-flow ILP procedure performed via percutaneous catheters without oxygenation.

Both procedures may help improve the patient's quality of life by controlling the local pain following effective shrinkage of local tumor metastasis that is not possible with surgery or at high risk of recurrence after surgery. It does not provide a survival advantage.

Potential complications of the procedure include ischemia of the limb, peripheral neuropathy, and bone marrow suppression.

Management of Patients with Metastatic Melanoma

The management options for a patient with metastatic melanoma have expanded following the recent FDA approvals of immune based and targeted therapy (Figure 22.5). Surgery has a role in resection of isolated metastasis while chemotherapy may have a role in palliative treatment of selected patients who have failed upfront therapy.

Immune-based Therapy of Metastatic Melanoma: Principles

- Melanoma is considered to be one of the best models of an immunogenic tumor attracting lymphocytes at both the primary and metastatic sites.
- A number of well-defined melanoma antigens have been identified both at a protein and gene level that evoke a cellular immune-based antimelanoma response (Table 22.5).
- Antigen-specific CD8+ Cytotoxic T lymphocytes (CTLs) lead the antimelanoma response with critical help from CD4+ helper T cells and antigen-presenting cells (APCs).

Activation of CTLs against melanoma requires two signals: Priming and activation

- Signal 1: Priming of CD8+ or CD4+ CTL requires presentation of melanoma antigen (peptide epitope) either by the tumor cell or by the APCs at the MHC class I or MHC class II molecules, respectively, to the T-cell receptor of CD8+ CTL or CD4+ T cells.
- Signal 2: Activation of antigen primed CD8+ or CD4+ CTL requires co-stimulatory signaling through binding of its CD28 molecules with costimulatory molecules B7.1 (CD80) and B7.2 (CD86) on the APCs forming a tight synapse between the two cells critical for signal transduction to the T cell nucleus.
- The transcribed genes include cytokines and effector molecules necessary for T cell growth, proliferation and survival as well as tumor killer activity.

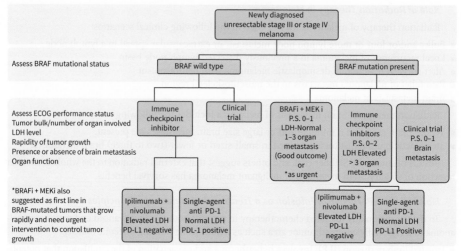

FIGURE 22.5 Algorithm for treatment of newly diagnosed unresectable stage III/IV melanoma.

TABLE 22.5 Melanoma-associated Antigens, Peptides, and Presenting MHC Molecules

Melanoma Antigens	Peptides	Presenting MHC Molecules
MAGE-A1[a]	EADPTGHSY	HLA-A1 & B37
MAGE-A1[a]	TSCILESLFRAVITK	HLA-DP4
MAGE-A3[a]	EVDPIGHLY	HLA-A1
NY-ESO-1[a]	SLLMWITQC	HLA-A2
NY-ESO-1[a]	MPFATPMEA	HLA-B51
Melan-A/MART-1[b]	EAAGIGILTV	HLAB35
Melan-A/MART-1[b]	ILTVILGVL	HLA-A2
Tyrosinase[b]	MLLAVLYCL	HLA-A2
Gp100/pmel17[b]	KTWGQYWQV	HLA-A2
β-Catenin[c]	SYLDSGIHF	HLA-A24

[a] Shared antigens; [b] differentiation antigens; [c] mutated antigens.

- Activated CD8+ CTLs kill tumor cells directly through production of perforins and granzyme and indirectly by the elaboration of secreted cytokines such as TNF-α, IFN γ, granulocyte-macrophage colony stimulating factor (GMCSF), and IL-2 all which help shape the composition of tumor immune microenvironment.

Immune-based Treatment Strategies of Metastatic Melanoma: Two Approaches

Specific immunity evoked by melanoma vaccines:

- Administration of one or more (monovalent or polyvalent) melanoma antigens as a tumor vaccine either directly or after being pulsed on to monocyte-derived APCs (dendritic cell vaccine) in the subcutis or in the dermis evoke melanoma antigen specific CTLs.
- Adjuvants are intended to enhance the immune response and are either premixed with vaccine or preapplied to the skin at the site of the vaccine.

TABLE 22.6 FDA-approved Systemic Immune Therapy of Metastatic Melanoma

High dose IL-2	Pembrolizumab	Nivolumab	Ipilimumab +Nivolumab
High-dose IL-2 administered at 600,000 to 720,000 units per kilogram by 15 min bolus intravenous infusion every 8 h on days 1 to 5 and 15 to 19. Treatment courses were repeated at 8- to 12-wk intervals in responding patients until complete response is achieved or toxicity sets in that the physician decides to stop treatment for safety reasons	2mg/Kg dose IV over 30 min every 3 wks for up to 2 y unless disease progression or unacceptable toxicity occurred	3mg/kg IV over 30 min every 2 wks for up to 2 y unless disease progression or unacceptable toxicity occurred	**Induction phase:** Ipilimumab 3 mg/Kg IV over 90 min plus nivolumab 1mg/Kg IV over 30 min every 3 wks x 4 doses, followed by **Maintenance phase:** Nivolumab at 3mg/ Kg IV every 2 wks for up to 2 y unless disease progression or unacceptable toxicity occurred

Although successful in a mouse model, induction of antimelanoma specific immunity by vaccine treatment has been unpredictable and not uniformly successful in humans. Also, generation of melanoma-specific T-cell activity did not always correlate with patient responses.

Nonspecific immunity (Table 22.6) involves

- Re-activation by T cell growth factors of melanoma antigen sensitized effector T cells or
- Releasing inhibition of immune checkpoint inhibitors on activated T cells

Biologic Agents in the Treatment of Metastatic Melanoma

IFN-α was the first recombinant cytokine investigated in phase I and II clinical trials of patients with metastatic melanoma based on its antiproliferative and immunomodulatory effects.

- Initial studies showed response rates of about 15% in patients with metastatic melanoma.
- One-third of these responses were complete and durable.
- Responses could be observed up to 6 months after the therapy was initiated.
- Small volume disease and uninterrupted use resulted in pronounced responses.
- These results could not be reproduced in subsequent randomized phase III studies.
- Essentially, IFN-α is rarely used as primary therapy for metastatic melanoma.

Interleukin 2 (IL-2) is a T cell growth factor produced by T lymphocytes that help growth and expansion of T cells including antigen-specific CD8+ CTL precursors and LAK cells.

Multiple large single institution studies confirmed the ability of high dose IL-2 to cure metastatic melanoma in a small subset of patients leading to its FDA approval in 1998 to treat this disease.

- The overall response rate is about 16% that include complete response of about 6%.
- Responses are more common in patients with subcutaneous, lymph node, and lung metastasis.
- Complete responses are durable in the majority of patients leading to potential cure.
- Good baseline performance and treatment naive status are predictive of response.

Toxicity of high dose IL-2 is dose limiting and is mediated by endothelial damage that result in vascular leak in multiple organs. Common manifestations of toxicity include the following:

- High fevers and nausea, vomiting, diarrhea (gastrointestinal), hypotension, cardiac arrhythmias (cardiac), hypoxemia, pleural effusions (pulmonary), azotemia and renal failure (renal), confusion and delirium (central nervous system).
- IL-2 induced defects of neutrophil chemotaxis function require prompt management of infections with antibiotics.

- Common autoimmune side effects include hypothyroidism, vitiligo anduveitis although a number of other unusual manifestations are described and require prompt management.
- Patients with active comorbidities involving heart, lung, kidney, and liver or those with untreated hemorrhagic brain metastasis with vasogenic edema are excluded from high dose IL-2 treatment due to elevated risk of life-threatening complications.

Lower doses of IL-2 administered either subcutaneously or as a continuous intravenous infusion at 9 to 18 million international units/m2/day for 4 to 5 days have been studied in patients not eligible for high-dose IL-2 treatment. Although total response rates as high as 20% have been reported, complete responses appear to be lower than those with high-dose.

Barriers to Achieving a Successful Immune Response in Melanoma: Immune Regulation and Tolerance

Antigen activated CTLs are "highly regulated" or held in check by a number of biological processes so as to prevent body injury associated with uncontrolled inflammation. These regulatory processes arise from mechanisms either intrinsic to CTL or by a negative influence imposed by regulatory T cells (immune system) or tumor or its microenvironment.

Intrinsic T cell regulation by immune checkpoints:

- Cytotoxic T-lymphocyte-associated antigen-4 (CTLA- 4) is a high affinity molecule rapidly expressed by activated T lymphocytes to mediate CTL inhibition by outcompeting CD28 molecule for binding to costimulatory molecules CD80 and CD86 on antigen-presenting cells.
- Programmed cell death protein-1 (PD-1) receptor is expressed on activated CTL that traffic into tumor tissue intending to destroy it. The PD-1 receptor is expressed by CTL in response to immune stimulatory cytokines (such as interferons) or constitutively in response to inhibitory ligands PD-L1 and PD-L2 expressed on tumor or antigen presenting cells. Ligation of PD-L1/L2 with PD-1 results in CTL exhaustion, premature death, and abrogation of anti-melanoma tumor activity.

Extrinsic mechanisms that regulate the immune response: regulatory T cells

- CD8+ CTL responses are regulated by thymus-derived, naturally occurring CD4+CD25+ T cells referred to as nTreg as well as by CD4 + T cells that acquire inhibitory properties upon encountering antigen, referred to as induced T regulatory cells (iTreg).
- Regulatory T cells cause CTL inhibition through inhibitory cytokines or directly by contact inhibition mediated by transcription factor FOXP3.

Tumor and its immune microenvironment mediated immune tolerance:

- Antigen presentation to CTL is seriously compromised by downregulation of MHC class I molecules by tumor and antigen-presenting cells.
  - Immune tolerance is facilitated by inhibitory cytokines such as IL-10, TGF beta, IL-6, and VEG-F produced by tumor cells, hypoxemia, and myeloid-derived suppressive cells.
  - Indoleamine 2,3-dioxygenase (IDO) is an immune suppressive molecule secreted by the tumor cells, stromal cells, macrophages, and APC in the tumor microenvironment that starve T cells from an important amino acid tryptophan critical for a rate-limiting step in the de-novo biosynthesis of nicotinamide adenine dinucleotide (NAD). Additionally, accumulation of N-formyl-kynurenine, an IDO induced by product of tryptophan catabolism, inhibit T cell activity.

Reactivating antimelanoma immunity by inhibiting immune checkpoint on T cells: Successful reactivation of antimelanoma immunity is become possible by effective blockade of inhibitory immune checkpoints (CTLA-4 and PD-1) expressed on activated T cell through monoclonal antibodies. Two classes of monoclonal antibodies are approved by the FDA (Table 22.7).

- Ipilimumab is an IGG1 monoclonal antibody designed to block inhibitory checkpoint CTLA-4 antigen on activated CD8+ CTLs leading to their reactivation.
- Pembrolizumab and Nivolumab are two highly selective humanized IgG4-kappa isotype antibodies against PD-1 receptor expressed on the membrane of activated CTLs designed to block its engagement with its two known inhibitory ligands, PD-L1 and PD-L2. The interruption of the PD-1-PD-L1/2 axis reverses adoptive T cell resistance and restores antimelanoma activity.

TABLE 22.7 FDA-approved Immune Therapy and Their Efficacy in Metastatic Melanoma

Treatment	Complete Remission	Partial Remission	Stable Disease	Clinical Benefit	MPFS Months	MOS Months	1-year Survival	2- and 3-year Survival Rates
High-dose Interleukin-2 (IL-2)	6%	10%	NA	20%	13.1	11.4	50%	6%
Ipilimumab	1.5%	9.5%	17.5%	28.5%	2.9	10.1	45.6%	23.5%
Pembrolizumab	6.1%	26.8%	16.7%	56.7%	4.1	NR	68.4%	
Nivolumab	7.6%	32.4%	16.7%	56.7%	5.1	NR	72.9%	NA
Ipilimumab + Nivolumab	11.5%	46.2%	13.1%	70.8%	11.5	NR	NR	
T-VEK* (intra-tumoral injection)	10.8%*	15.6%	NR	26.4%				

Ipilimumab treatment of melanoma: In two large randomized phase III clinical trials, ipilimumab improved both progression-free and overall survival in patients with unresectable stage III and stage IV melanoma compared to a glycoprotein 100 (gp100) peptide vaccine or chemotherapy.

In March 2011, ipilimumab was approved by the FDA for the treatment of unresectable stage III or IV melanoma administered intravenously at 3 mg/kg dose every 3 weeks for four doses.

Important facts about ipilimumab treatment of patients with metastatic melanoma:

- Objective responses occur in between 10% and 16% patients while about 15% of patients develop stabilization of the disease resulting in long-term survival benefit in 20% to 25% of patients.
- Immune responses sometimes continued beyond 24 weeks converting nonresponsive disease to stable, stable disease to partial, and partial responses to complete responses.
- Responses are seen in treatment naïve or previously treated patients including those with high-risk visceral metastasis and elevated serum LDH levels.
- The onset of response is slow and mediated by antigen-specific tumor infiltrating CD8+ CTLs consistent as the proposed mechanism.
- Reinduction therapy with ipilimumab at the time of disease progression can result in further benefit in a proportion of patients (reinduction is not FDA approved).
- The effect on overall survival is independent of age, sex, baseline serum LDH levels, metastatic stage, and previous treatment with IL-2 therapy.
- The non-specific activation of pre-sensitized CTL against both tumor as well as host (shared antigens) resulted in loss of self-tolerance manifesting as serious irAEs in organs.
- Ipilimumab caused irAE in about 60% but grade 3/4 toxicity occurred in 20% to 30% patients.
- Common irAEs involve skin, gastrointestinal tract, liver, and endocrine organs although careful symptom evaluation is important to detect other organ involvement.
- Skin irAEs manifest as rashes and are first to appear after 3 to 4 weeks of treatment followed by colitis, liver (hepatitis), and endocrine organ involvement in that order.
- Colitis symptoms should be distinguished from diarrhea by the presence of fever, abdominal cramps, distension and blood in stools as they can progress to intestinal obstruction or perforation.
- Patient education about toxicity is critical, and prompt reporting of side effects improves outcomes from early initiation of immune suppressive treatment.
- Oral steroids at 1–2 mg/kg dose or its parenteral equivalent followed by gradual taper remain first line of treatment of irAE and best managed with a multidisciplinary team approach.
- Patients not responsive to steroids within 2 to 3 days may need to be administered higher level of immune suppression with agents such as anti–TNF-alpha antibody infliximab, antimetabolite mycophenylate mofetil, calcineurin inhibitor tacrolimus, and cyclosporine. Rarely, T-cell depleting antibody such as anti-thymocyte globulin has been used to achieve effective T cell suppression
- The median time to resolution of severe irAEs of grade 2, 3, or 4 after initiation of immune-suppressive therapy is about 6.3 weeks and sometimes longer.

Anti PD-1 treatment of metastatic melanoma: Phase I/II and randomized phase III studies of anti PD-1 agents Pembrolizumab and Nivolumab in treatment naïve and previously treated patients reported response rates between 52% to 38%, respectively.

- Responses were seen in those with high risk features such as visceral metastasis (stage M1c), elevated LDH, and those with history of brain metastasis.
- The effect on overall survival is independent of age, sex, baseline LDH levels, stage, and previous treatment with ipilimumab therapy.
- Responses were durable even after stopping treatment leading to progression-free and overall survival.
- Common irAE included skin rashes, fatigue, diarrhea, and pruritus while serious grade 3/4 toxicity in 5% to 15% patients was lower than seen with ipilimumab treatment (20% to 30%).
- Unusual irAE included autoimmune pneumonitis (presenting as cough, shortness of breath, and even fatal respiratory failure) and endocrine toxicity that appeared higher than with anti CTLA-4 antibody. Unusual irAEs included diabetes mellitus, nephritis besides others.
- Management principle of irAEs of anti PD-1 are same as that of ipilimumab (see above).

Combined Immune Checkpoint Inhibition and Metastatic Melanoma: Principles

Hypothesis: Since CTLA-4 and PD-1 are two nonredundant inhibitory pathways affecting activated CTL, their combined inhibition might result in superior antimelanoma response.

- Proof of this hypothesis obtained in preclinical models was confirmed in humans.
- Phase I/II as well as randomized phase III studies showed superior clinical benefit of iIpilimumab + nivolumab compared to single agent nivolumab or ipilimumab. The response rates were higher including complete responses of 11% to 22% and progression-free survival reached highest ever compared to single agents (11.5 vs. 6.9 vs. 2.9 months, respectively).
- Onset of responses was earlier and the majority of responses were deep (more than 80% tumor reduction) and durable although follow-up studies await its impact on overall survival.
- The adverse prognostic effects of elevated LDH and negative PD-L1 expression affecting single agent ipilimumab or nivolumab treatment were not seen with the combination.
- Serious irAE were much higher with ipilimumab + nivolumab versus ipilimumab (54% vs.24%).
- irAE led to discontinuation of treatment in 36.4% patients receiving ipilimumab + nivolumab.
- The combined use of ipilimumab and nivolumab was approved by the FDA for the treatment of immune checkpoint inhibitor naïve unresectable stage III or IV melanoma.
- The choice between using monotherapy with a PD-1 inhibitor or combination anti-CTLA4 and PD-1 remains controversial. Data on PDL-1 staining of tumors suggest that patients with low staining (less than 1%) may benefit from combined blockade while those with high staining (>5%) may do well with monotherapy.

Oncolytic Therapy and Antimelanoma Immune Responses: Principles

Oncolytic therapy is intralesional injection of agents that may produce both, a local and a systemic response. They could be viral or nonviral based.

Oncolytic viruses are modified live viruses designed to selectively replicate in tumor cells after intratumoral administration leading to release of tumor antigens in the proximity of tumor and evoking regional and systemic anti melanoma immunity. The immune response is facilitated by insertion and expression of gene encoding human granulocyte macrophage colony stimulating factor (GM-CSF), local production of which help recruit and activate antigen-presenting cells.

T–VEC is a first in class FDA-approved agent for intratumoral injection and contains a modified herpes simplex virus (HSV) type I through the deletion of two nonessential viral genes.

- Functional deletion of herpes virus neurovirulence factor gene (ICP34.5) attenuates viral pathogenicity and enhances tumor-selective replication.
- Deletion of the ICP47 gene helps to reduce virally mediated suppression of antigen presentation and increases the expression of the HSV US11 gene.

A multicenter, open-label study assigned eligible surgically unresectable stage IIIB, IIIC, or IV melanoma patients suitable for direct or ultrasound-guided injection of T-VEC (at least one cutaneous, subcutaneous, or nodal lesion or aggregation of lesions more than or equal to 10 mm in diameter) versus subcutaneous injection of recombinant GM-CSF at a dose of 125 microgram/M^2 randomly at a two-to-one ratio every 3 weeks after the first dose and then every 2 weeks until tumor progression or occurrence of toxicity.

- Overall response rate was 26.4% with T-VEC versus 5.7% with GM-CSF, with durable responses of at least six months duration seen in 16.3% and 2.1% in each arms, respectively.
- Unresectable and treatment naive IIIB, IIIC, and IV M1a patients experienced more benefit compared to previously treated patients or stage IV M1b or M1c patients.
- Systemic immune effects were seen in 15% uninjected measurable lesions in systemic visceral sites that shrunk by > or = 50% size.
- Side effects of T-VEC were minor and included chills, fever, injection-site pain, nausea, influenza-like illness and fatigue. Vitiligo was reported in 5% of patients.
- Grade 3/4 irAE were seen respectively in 11% and 5% patients after TVEC and GM-CSF.
- A pattern of pseudo progression seen in some responding patients suggested continued treatment in clinically stable patients even if lesions appeared to grow or new lesions appeared.

- Vitiligo and increased numbers of MART-1 specific T cells as well as decreased CD4+ and CD8+ FoxP3+ regulatory T cells in injected lesions suggested systemic antitumor immunity.
- Several other oncolytic agents are in clinical trials at this time both as monotherapy and in combination with checkpoint inhibitors.

Adaptive Cell Therapy of Metastatic Melanoma: Principles

Adaptive cell therapy refers to boosting antitumor immunity by transfer of autologous melanoma specific T cells obtained from the tumor (tumor infiltrating lymphocytes) or peripheral blood, back to the patient after their expansion ex vivo to large numbers. Conditioning regimens help provide space and growth factors for survival of the infused T cells. This treatment is based on the following fundamental facts:

- In animal systems tumors can be controlled with adoptively transferred syngeneic T cells.
- T cells capable of recognizing autologous tumors in humans exist and they can be activated and expanded ex vivo, as well as engineered to express a set of highly avid T cell receptors for targeting tumor expressed epitopes displayed canonically on their MHC molecules.

Pioneered at the National Cancer Institute, response rates of as high as 50% were seen with this treatment modality with durable responses in subset of patients refractory to other treatments.

Targeted Therapy of Melanoma: Principles

Targeted therapy of melanoma is based upon a better understanding of functional cellular genetic machinery critical for transducing signals of cellular growth from outside of the cells to the nucleus leading to the transcription of key genes important for maintaining cellular homeostasis through control of proliferation, differentiation, and cell death.

- The mitogen-activated protein kinase (MAPK) pathway is an important signaling cascade containing Ras/Raf/MEK/ERK proteins.
- B-Raf is a serine/threonine kinase occupying a central place in the MAPK pathway that harbors activating mutations in 50% to 60% of cutaneous melanomas conferring RAS independent proliferation and survival of melanoma cells.
- Molecular identity of BRAF mutations led to its targeted inhibition through the design of small inhibitory molecules.
- About 90% of mutations in BRAF result in the substitution of glutamic acid for valine at codon 600 (BRAF V600E). Other BRAF mutations include V600K and V600D/V600R variants.
- Vemurafenib (first-in-class) and Dabrafenib are two FDA-approved reversible oral small molecule BRAF kinase inhibitors that selectively target cells harboring BRAF mutation. The resulting tumor cell death and inhibition of growth translated into survival in patients.
- Results from randomized clinical trials showed high response rates of up to 55%, and tumor stabilization of 30% for a clinical benefit to 80% to 90% of metastatic melanoma patients resulting in improved progression-free and overall survival compared to dacarbazine treatment (Table 22.8).

The FDA-approved vemurafenib at a dose of 960 mg administered orally twice a day while dabrafenib is approved at a dose of 150 mg administered orally twice a day for metastatic melanoma.

Important facts about BRAF kinase inhibitor treatment of metastatic melanoma:

- The survival benefit of vemurafenib and dabrafenib was observed in each pre-specified subgroup according to age, sex, performance status, tumor stage, serum levels of lactate dehydrogenase, and geographic region.
- Patient compliance with medication is important to maintain continued inhibition of MAPK pathway in tumor cells to ensure continued clinical benefit to the patient.
- Acquired drug resistance to BRAF inhibitor agent frequently leads to treatment failures due to resumption of increased signaling through the MAPK pathway.
- Mechanisms underlying acquired drug resistance include mutations of NRAS (17%), KRAS (2%), BRAF splice variants (16%), BRAF amplifications (13%), MEK 1/2 mutations (7%), and non-MAPK pathway alterations (11%) that include upregulation of platelet-derived growth factor receptor beta (PDGFRβ) and alterations in the PI3K-AKT pathway.

TABLE 22.8 FDA-approved Targeted Therapy of BRAF Mutant Melanoma and Their Clinical efficacy

Treatment	Complete remission	Partial remission	Stable disease	MPFS months	MOS months	12 month Survival (%)	24 month Survival (%)	2 and 3 year survival rates
Vemurafenib 960mg PO BID	8%	44%	30%	7.3	13.6	65%	38%	NA
Dabrafenib 150mg PO BID	3%	47%	42%	5.1	18.7	68%	NA	42%
Trametinib 2mg PO daily	2%	20%	56%	4.8	16.1	NA	NA	NA
Dabrafenib 150mg PO BID+ Trametinib 2mg PO daily	13%	51%	26%	11.4	25.1	74%	50%	51%
Vemurafenib 960mg PO BID+ Cobimetinib	16%%	54%	18%	12.3	22.3	75%	49%	NA

- Toxicities of BRAF inhibitor agents include hyperproliferative skin lesions such as hyperkeratosis, keratoacanthoma, squamous cell carcinoma, and palmar-plantar erythrodysesthesia believed to be due to paradoxical activation of the MAPK pathway in normal cells bearing wild-type BRAF. Secondary cancers occur in RAS mutated organs.
- Photosensitivity, muscle pain, arthralgia, pruritus, fatigue, alopecia, diarrhea, and nausea and electrolyte abnormalities were other side effects.
- Fever is a side effect seen with dabrafenib in 16% to 26% patients (grade 2/3 in 11% patients).
- Caution must be used with concomitant use of medications affecting CYP3A4, CYP2C8, and CYP2C9 metabolic pathways for concerns of change in dabrafenib concentrations leading to its inefficacy or toxicity.
- Toxicity led to modification or interruption of vemurafenib dose in about 38% of patients and dose reductions and discontinuation of dabrafenib in 28% and 3%, respectively.

MEK is the downstream of BRAF and a therapeutic gene target in the MAPK pathway. Trametinib and cobimetinib are two orally selective reversible kinase inhibitors targeting MEK1 and MEK2 activation leading to decreased phosphorylated ERK and thus decreased tumor growth.

- In a large phase III open-label trial of patients diagnosed with BRAF-mutated metastatic melanoma, trametinib treatment resulted in 22% responses and 56% stabilization of disease translating into both progression and overall survival survival benefit compared to dacarbazine chemotherapy. Trametinib is approved for the treatment of metastatic melanoma for patients not able to tolerate BRAF inhibitor agents.
- Side effects were skin rash, diarrhea, peripheral edema, fatigue, and dermatitis acneiform.
- No squamous cell carcinoma or hyperproliferative skin lesions occurred.
- Ocular events such as blurred vision and reversible chorioretinopathy in 9% of patients.
- Cardiac toxicity in 7% patients included decreased ejection fraction, ventricular dysfunction.
- Toxicity led to dose interruptions and dose reductions in 35% and 27% of patients, respectively.

Combined inhibition of mutated BRAF and downstream MEK protein consolidates inhibition of MAP kinase pathway leading to delayed emergence of resistance to BRAF inhibitor. In two large randomized phase III studies, combined BRAF and MEK inhibition resulted in higher overall response rate of about 69% compared to dabrafenib alone (53%) and translated into superior progression-free and overall survival with combination compared to single agent dabrafenib.

- The incidence of cutaneous hyperproliferative lesions and squamous cell carcinoma decreased dramatically consistent with blockade by MEK inhibition of paradoxical activation of MAPK pathway BRAF wild-type cells.
- Incidence of fever increased in dabrafenib plus trametinib (71%) compared to 24% for single agent dabrafenib.
- Fever is believed to be likely from a metabolite of dabrafenib (hydroxyl dabrafenib) clearance of which might be impaired in the presence of a MEK inhibitor.
- 58% of patients on combined dabrafenib/trametinib required dose reduction and 7% discontinued treatment permanently out of which pyrexia contributed in 4%.
- Pyrexia management following dabrafenib or dabrafenib/trametinib consists of holding dabrafenib if fever is over 38.5°C while trametinib is continued till fever resolved. Nonsteroidal anti-inflammatory agents (NSAID) or acetaminophen are used for short-term fever management but lower dose steroids, sometimes even prophylactically, may be used for persistent fevers.
- Brain metastasis of melanoma: The high incidence of brain metastasis of melanoma is reflected by the 50% to 55% melanoma patients documented to have brain metastasis in autopsy studies. Unlike systemic chemotherapy, both immune checkpoint inhibitor agents and BRAF targeting agents have documented intracranial effects in patients with brain metastasis. Dabrafenib has a 39% response rate in patients with brain metastasis that was durable and concordant with systemic effects while both pembrolizumab and ipilimumab have reported activity of 22% to 24%, respectively, in the brain that is concordant with systemic activity. Although smaller metastasis respond better, occasional responses are seen in larger tumors as well, resulting in survival benefit to patients. A number of clinical trials are actively investigating ways to improve outcomes in patients diagnosed with brain metastasis of melanoma using newer agents.

TABLE 22.9 Combination Chemotherapy Regimens of Metastatic Melanoma

Chemotherapy Regimens	Treatment Description	Response Rates (%)
CVD (M.D. Anderson Cancer Center)	Cisplatin, 20 mg/m^2/d IV for 4 d (2, 3, 4, 5) (total dose/cycle, 80 mg/m^2) Vinblastine, 1.6 mg/m^2/d IV for 5 d (1, 2, 3, 4, 5) (total dose/cycle, 8 mg/m^2) Dacarbazine, 800 mg/m^2 IV on day 1 (total cycle dose 800 mg/m^2) cycle repeats every 21 d	21–48
CBDT (the Dartmouth regimen)	Cisplatin, 25 mg/m^2/d IV for 3 d (1, 2, 3) (total dose/cycle, 75 mg/m^2) Carmustine,150 mg/m^2 IV day 1 (every odd-numbered cycle, i.e., every 43 d total dose every two cycles, 150 mg/m^2 Dacarbazine, 220 mg/m^2/d IV for 3 d (1, 2, 3) (total dose/cycle, 660 mg/m^2) Tamoxifen, 10 mg twice daily PO during the therapy Cycle repeated every 21 d	19–55

IV, intravenous; PO, per oral.

Chemotherapy of Metastatic Melanoma: Single-Agent Chemotherapy

Chemotherapy of melanoma does not lead to durable responses and therefore does not confer survival advantage to patients. A chemotherapy option might be used as a bridge to potentially effective experimental treatments in patients who fail presently available treatment of melanoma.

Dacarbazine is the only FDA-approved chemotherapeutic agent for melanoma treatment that has a response rate of about 10% to 20% without overall survival benefit.

Temozolomide is a synthetic analog of Dacarbazine that is orally bioavailable, crosses the blood–brain barrier, has comparable efficacy, and has a reduced toxicity profile.

Combination therapy results in higher response rates and toxicity without survival advantage.

Combination Chemotherapy Regimens of Metastatic Melanoma (Table 22.9)

- M.D. Anderson regimen: cisplatin, vinblastine, dacarbazine (CVD)
- Dartmouth regimen: cisplatin, carmustine, dacarbazine, and tamoxifen (CBDT)
- A phase III multicenter randomized clinical trial of dacarbazine alone versus the Dartmouth regimen in patients with metastatic melanoma showed higher response rates of 25% to 30% and increased toxicity with Dartmouth regimen without significant survival benefit.
- A phase III trial of melanoma patients treated with nab-paclitaxel (abraxane) versus dacarbazine showed improved progression free-survival for nab-paclitaxel compared to dacarbazine. Although a trend toward improved overall survival was seen, this did not achieve statistical significance

Combining Chemotherapy and Biologic Agents in Metastatic Melanoma (Table 22.10)

Bio-chemotherapy: Rationale

- Preclinical studies suggested that combining chemotherapeutic and biologic agents (bio-chemotherapy) may confer additive or synergistic effects against melanoma.
- Chemotherapeutic and biologic agents have different mechanisms of anti-melanoma effects.
- There are no overlapping toxicity or cross-resistance.
- Falkson et al. reported the outcome of patients with metastatic melanoma treated with either dacarbazine alone or a combination of dacarbazine and IFN-α-2b. The results indicated a response rate

TABLE 22.10 Biochemotherapy of Metastatic Melanoma

Biologic and Chemotherapeutic Agents	Response Rates
Cisplatin 20 mg/m² days 1, 2, 3, 4	Overall response rate of 64%
Vinblastine 1.6 mg/m² days 1, 2, 3, 4	Complete response rate of 21%
Dacarbazine, 800 mg/m² day 1	Partial response of 43%
Recombinant IL-2, administered IV as continuous 24 h infusion at 9 MIU/m² days 1, 2, 3, 4	
IFN-α 2b, 5 MIU/m², SC days 1, 2, 3, 4, 5	
Cycle repeated every 21 d	

MIU, million international units; IV, intravenous; SC, subcutaneous.

TABLE 22.11 Relationship of Depth and Diameter of Uveal Melanoma and Survival

Uveal Choroidal Melanoma (size)	Diameter (mm)	Depth (mm)	10-y Survival (%)
Small	<10	<3	80
Medium	10–15	3–5	60
Large	>15	>5	34.8

NR, not reached, NA, data not available, MPFS, median progression-free survival, MOS, median overall survival.

and median survival of 20% and 9.6 months, respectively, with dacarbazine alone compared to a 53% and 17.6 months, respectively, in patients receiving both these agents.
- The CVD regimen of chemotherapy plus continuous intravenous infusion of moderate dose IL- 2 and –IFN-α administered subcutaneously showed high response rates and durable survival of between 10% and 20% in selected patients (Table 22.10).

- The toxicity associated with bio-chemotherapy regimens and the lack of reproducibility of survival benefit among investigators has dampened interest in its universal use.
- A meta-analysis of 18 clinical trials and a phase III randomized clinical trial comparing bio-chemotherapy to CVD chemotherapy in stage IV melanoma confirmed high response rates of 40% to 50% and increased toxicity with bio-chemotherapy without overall survival advantage.

Uveal Choroidal Melanoma

Uveal choroidal melanoma is the most common primary malignancy of the eye.
- Estimated incidence in the United States is six to seven cases per 1 million people.
- Depth and diameter determine the treatment indication and prognosis (Table 22.11).
- Benign choroidal nevi are up to 5 mm and 1 mm in diameter and depth, respectively.
- Monosomy of chromosome 3 is a common cytogenetic abnormality and confers poor disease-free survival and high risk of death from melanoma.
- Other cytogenetic abnormalities involve chromosomes 1, 6, and 8.
- The most common site of metastasis is the liver, although in later stages the tumor can spread to other sites such as the lungs, bones, and skin.

Management of Uveal Choroidal Melanoma

- Local ablative treatment such as brachytherapy (iodine-125 plaque therapy), photo-radiation, cryotherapy, and ultrasonic hyperthermia.
- Surgical treatments that include local resection, or enucleation of the eye.

- Systemic chemotherapy or biologic therapy is ineffective in metastatic uveal melanoma.
- Experimental therapies for liver metastasis include in situ ablative therapies such as radiofrequency ablation and isolated perfusion using melphalan.

A randomized trial evaluated the use of liver chemosaturation with melphalan using a specialized approach of isolating the liver using a system of catheters (PHP, percutaneous hepatic perfusion) in patients with melanoma (mostly uveal) metastasis to the liver. The trial showed high response rates and improved liver-specific progression-free survival.

Follow-up of patients with uveal choroidal melanoma after local treatment includes close surveillance for liver metastasis with liver function tests and imaging studies of the liver that include sonography every 6 months in the first 5 years for early diagnosis of liver metastasis. However, late relapses may occur.

Indications for Enucleation of the Eye

- Tumor growing in a blind eye
- Melanoma involving more than half of the iris
- Tumor involving the anterior chamber of the eye or extraocular extension
- Failure of previous local therapy

NONMELANOMA SKIN CANCER

There are two major types of nonmelanoma skin cancers: basal cell carcinoma (BCC) and squamous cell carcinoma (SCC). Together they account for nearly 1 million cases in the United States per year. A weakened immune system is believed to play an important role in their causation due to their prevalence in immune suppressive states such as aging populations and transplant recipients. Histologically, regressing nonmelanoma skin cancers show infiltration of the tumor by activated T cells and cytokines such as IFN-α, TNF-β, and IL-2.

Basal Cell Carcinoma (BCC)

- BCC is the commonest cancer in the US white population of over 50 years of age, accounting for 75% of the 1 million new cases of nonmelanoma skin cancers.
- BCCs are keratinocyte tumors most commonly diagnosed in people of European ancestry.
- Ultraviolet rays are the most important risk factor followed by ionizing radiation and arsenic.
- Usual location of BCC is the skin of the head and neck region (sun-exposed area).
- BCC is highly cured by surgery and death rate is very low despite its high incidence.
- When locally advanced or metastatic (rare occasions), local invasion can lead to tissue destruction that makes surgical treatment difficult and outcomes poor.

Clinical Presentations of BCC

- Typical presentation of BCC is a shiny pink translucent papule with telangiectasia while other types include nodular variants (at times pigmented), sclerosing or morphea type (might go undiagnosed for longer time) and less commonly, hyperkeratotic type affecting head and neck region.

Surgery is the primary treatment modality and may include Mohs surgery.

BCC as a Heritable Disorder

- A rare familial presentation of BCC is called basal cell nevus syndrome (BCNS) also known as Gorlin syndrome characterized by a high incidence of BCCs and medulloblastomas.
- Autosomal dominant inheritance results from uncontrolled activation of the Hedgehog (Hh) signaling pathway.
- The genetic defect underlying this condition is linked to mutation of a tumor suppressor gene called patched 1 (PTCH1) mapped to human chromosome 9q22.
- The mutations of PTCH1 and TP53 genes critical to BCC carcinogenesis are believed to be produced by exposure to UV radiation, elucidating the role of UV exposure in its causation.

Squamous Cell Carcinoma (SCC)

- Usually found as single or multiple lesions in elderly white men with sun-damaged skin.
- Common sites include back of the hand, forearm, face, and neck.
- Presents as a firm, indurated, expanding nodule, often at the site of actinic keratosis.
- Nodules may be ulcerated, and regional lymph nodes may be enlarged.

Squamous Cell Carcinoma of a Muco-cutaneous Site

- Common in elderly men with history of smoking, alcohol use, chewing of tobacco or betel nut.
- Mouth and lower lip are common sites where it typically start as an ulcerated nodule or erosion.
- Other sites of origin include the sole of the foot (verrucous form) and male genitalia related to human papillomavirus in underlying condylomata of Buschke-Lowenstein tumor.

Diagnosis of Nonmelanoma Skin Cancer

- A detailed history should include ethnic background, and skin type as well as duration of the skin lesion, pain, itching, and recent changes.
- Excessive exposure to sun, radiation and arsenic, and occupational and recreational activities.
- Examination of scalp, ears, palms, soles interdigital areas and mucous membranes, assess extent of sun damage (i.e., solar elastosis, scaling, erythema, telangiectasia, and solar lentigines)
- Assessment of the locoregional lymph nodes and distant metastases

Diagnosis: An excisional or incisional biopsy in a small or large tumor, respectively, is obtained for histologic diagnosis. A shave biopsy may be used in noduloulcerative, cystic, or superficial lesions.

Complete surgical resection with negative margins of at least 4–6 mm is recommended with regional lymphadenectomy if melanoma metastasis to the regional lymph node/nodes is present.

Mohs Surgery

- Mohs Surgery allows excision of the tumor until negative margins are achieved. It includes micrographic surgery guided by frozen section to ascertain complete resection.
- Superficial BCC: Imiquimod is an FDA-approved agent for the treatment of superficial BCC when used in cream form. The drug works via toll-like receptor agonist activity and causes stimulation of the innate and adaptive immune system. Common side effects include local skin rashes, burning sensation, erythema, edema, induration, erosion, and pruritus.

Radiation Therapy

X-rays delivered at a total dose of 2,000 to 3,000 cGy penetrate up to 2 to 5 mm, the level to which most of the basal cell and squamous cell carcinomas infiltrate. The total dose is divided into multiple smaller doses, usually over 3 to 4 weeks, to reduce side effects.

Hedgehog Signaling and Targeted Therapy of Locally Advanced and Metastatic BCC

- Hh signaling is a pivotal abnormality in BCC resulting in carcinogenesis due to uncontrolled proliferation of the basal cells of the epidermis.
- The Hh pathway is activated after binding of Hh ligand to the PATCHED 1 protein encoded by PTCH1 tumor suppressor gene present on target cells.
- In the absence of excessive Hh ligand, PTCH1 inhibits a downstream protein called smoothened (SMO) and prevents its translocation into the cilium.
- Binding of the Hh ligand to PTCH1 inhibits its protective activity of inhibiting SMO allowing uninhibited SMO to translocate to the primary cilium.
- Downstream effects of SMO activity lead to increased transcription factors GLI1 and GLI2, both of which cause transcription of gene important in proliferation and cell survival.

Approximately 90% of sporadic BCCs have at least one allele of PTCH1 mutated, while about 10% of BCCs have mutations in the downstream SMO protein that makes SMO resistant to inhibition by PTCH1. Targeted therapy of BCC is directed toward inhibition of Hh signaling.

- Cyclopamin (plant alkaloid) is a competitive inhibitor of SMO signaling that binds directly to the protein PTCH1 or SMO and cause regression of the tumor upon local application.
- Vismodegib (first-in-class) and sonidegib are two FDA-approved small molecule inhibitors of SMO for metastatic or locally advanced BCC.
- In locally advanced BCC, vismodegib at a daily 150 mg oral dose produced a response rate of 58% with median duration of response of about 12.8 months.
- Vismodegib has lower activity in metastatic BCC (response 30%, median duration 7.6 months)
- Oral daily administration of sonidegib at 200 mg in locally advanced or metastatic BCC showed response rate of 58% that coincided with decrease in GLI1 expression in the tumor.
- Hh inhibitor treatment is continued daily till disease progression or intolerable toxicity occurs.
- Common toxicity of Hh inhibitors includes alopecia, dysgeusia (taste disturbance), muscle spasms, fatigue, weight loss, and hair loss. Vesmodegib led to serious adverse events in 25% of patients that included deaths.
- Sonidegib also cause nausea, anorexia, vomiting, myalgia and raised serum creatinine kinase. Grade 3/4 toxicities include weight loss, myalgia, hyperbilirubinemia, dizziness, and fatigue.
- Adverse events result in discontinuation of treatment in a significant number of patients (63%)
- Acquired mutations of SMO result in resistance to the treatment and recurrence of disease.
- Anti-fungal agents itraconazole and pociconazole have anti SMO effects and show promising activity in BCC refractory to vesmodegib or sonidegib treatment.

Isolated reports published in the literature indicate efficacy of anti PD-1 agents in patients with metastatic BCC and SCC leading to design of clinical trials to explore their benefit in such patients.

MERKEL CELL CARCINOMA

Merkel cell carcinoma occurs due to the neoplastic proliferation of the Merkel cells located in the basal layer of the epidermis and hair follicles. These cells, which originate from the neural crest, are a member of the amine precursor uptake and decarboxylation cell system (APUD). Merkel cells serve as tactile sensory cells in lower animals and they function as a mechanoreceptor in humans.

Characteristics of Merkel Cell Tumors

- Common in older patients in chronically sun-damaged skin of the head and neck region.
- Less common sites are extremities and genitalia.
- Typical presentation is a 0.5 to 1 cm intracutaneous, firm, bluish-purple, nontender nodule.
- Histologically, a small round cell tumor containing neurosecretory cytoplasmic granules that may look similar to small cell carcinoma, melanoma, Ewing sarcoma, and lymphoma.
- Tumor cells stain positive for neuron-specific enolase and anticytokeratin antibody CAM 5.2.
- Polyomaviral DNA integration in >90% of tumor cells supports its role in etiology.
- Incidence in elderly suggests clinical relevance of the weakened aging immune system.
- Early spread occurs to locoregional lymph nodes and hematogenously to the distant sites.

Management of Merkel Cell Carcinoma (MCC): Surgery

- Complete surgical excision of the tumor with lymph node assessment for metastasis by the sentinel lymph node procedure forms the primary treatment.
- In the absence of systemic metastasis, if sentinel lymph node is positive, lymph node dissection from the respective lymph node basin is recommended as in cutaneous melanoma.
- Adjuvant radiation to the excised site of primary tumor is recommended to prevent local recurrence arising from incomplete resection of tumor or larger size tumor (2 cm or more).

Metastatic MCC: Cisplatin and etoposide is the preferred first line chemotherapy combination as tumor also responds to other chemotherapy agents such as adriamycin, cyclophosphamide, vincristine, and irinotecan.

- In metastatic MCC high response rates of 50% to 60% are obtained with cisplatin and etoposide combination but frequent recurrences limit median survival to between 8 and 10 months.

Immune therapy of metastatic Merkel cell carcinoma: Immune checkpoint inhibitor treatment studies show PD-L1 is expressed in the tumor microenvironment that accompanies the findings of inflammation. The infiltrating T lymphocytes demonstrate Polyoma virus large T antigen specific T cells that exhibit exhaustion markers such as PD-1 and TIM-3. Targeting PD-1-PDL-1/2 pathway by anti PD-1 and anti PD-L1 agents is now possible and show promising results.

- In a phase II study of pembrolizumab in metastatic MCC, objective responses of 56% included complete responses of 16%, with progression-free survival at 6 months of 67%.
- Avelumab is a fully human anti PD-L1 IgG1 monoclonal antibody that activate CTL by blocking PD-1-PD-L1 interaction as well as by antibody-mediated cellular toxicity (ADCC).
- In a phase II open label study of avelumab at 10 mg/kg dose every 2 weeks in refractory MCC, objective response rate was 31.8% (28.5% complete remissions). The responses were ongoing in 82% patients and 92% of responses were durable for at least 6 months.
- Serious irAE occurred in 5 patients (6%) that included enterocolitis, infusion-related reaction, elevated aminotransferases, chondrocalcinosis, synovitis, and interstitial nephritis in one each.

RARE TUMORS ARISING FROM THE SKIN

Rarely, tumors arise from skin appendages such as in hair follicles, arrector pili muscles, apocrine sweat glands and sebaceous glands. Most of these tumors are benign. The treatment principle is complete surgical excision and lymph node assessment as in melanoma.

Dermatofibrosarcoma Protuberans:

A rare fibro histiocytic tumor of the skin and subcutaneous tissue affecting trunk and extremities, demonstrating slow growth and intermediate malignant potential. The t (17:22) cytogenetic abnormality is present in more than 90% patients.

- The translocation t(17;22) between chromosomes 17 and 22 places platelet-derived growth factor-β (PDGF-β) under the control of COL1A1, resulting in upregulation, expression, and activation of tyrosine kinase PDGF-β.
- Imatinib Mesylate is a potent and specific inhibitor of PDGFR-β that is effectively used in neoadjuvant settings and in patients with recurrent disease after surgery.

Suggested Readings

1. Balch CM, Gershenwald JE, Soong S-J, et al. Final version of 2009 AJCC melanoma staging and classification. *J Clin Oncol.* 2009; 27:6199–6206.
2. Breslow A. Thickness, cross-sectional areas and depth of invasion in the prognosis of cutaneous melanoma. *Ann Surg.* 1970 ;172(5):902–908.
3. Chapman PB, Hauschild A, Robert C, et al. Improved survival with Vemurafenib in melanoma with BRAF V600E mutation. *N Engl J Med.* 2011; 364:2507–2516.
4. Davies H, Bignell GR, Cox C, et al. Mutations of the BRAF gene in human cancer. *Nature.* 2002; 417:949–954
5. Eggermont AM, Chiarion-Sileni V, Grobb JJ, et al. Prolonged survival in stage III melanoma with Ipilimumab adjuvant therapy. *N Engl J Med.* 2016; 375:1845–1855.
6. Flaherty KT, Infante JR, Daud A, et al. Combined BRAF and MEK inhibition in melanoma with BRAF V600 mutations. *N Engl J Med.* 367; 18:1694–1703.
7. Ghussen F, Krüger I, Smalley RV, et al. Hyperthermic perfusion with chemotherapy for melanoma of the extremities. *World J Surg.*1989;13(5):598–602.
8. Hamid O, Robert C, Daud A, et al. Safety and tumor responses with Lambrolizumab (Anti-PD-1) in melanoma. *N. Engl J Med.* 2013; 369:134–144.
9. Hodi FS, O'Day SJ, McDermott DF, et al. Improved survival with ipilimumab in patients with metastatic melanoma. *N Engl J Med.* 2010; 363:711–723.
10. Larkin J, Chiarion-Sileni V, Gonzalez JJ, et al. Combined Nivolumab and Ipilimumab or monotherapy in untreated melanoma. *N Engl J Med.* 2015; 373:23–34.
11. Leachman SA, Carucci J, Kohlmann W, et al. Selection criteria for genetic assessment of patients with familial melanoma. *J Am Acad Dermatol.* 2009; 61:677. el-1–14.

12. Legha SS, Ring S, Bedikian A, et al. Treatment of metastatic melanoma with combined chemotherapy containing cisplatin, vinblastine, dacarbazine (CVD) and biotherapy using interleukin 2 and interferon alpha. *Ann Oncol.* 1996; 7:827–835.

13. Low JA, de Sauvage FJ. Clinical experience with Hedgehog pathway inhibitors. *J Clin Oncol.* 2010; 28:5321–5326.

14. Marquette A, Bagot M, Bensussan A, et al. Recent discoveries in the genetics of melanoma and their therapeutic implications. *Arch Immunol Ther Exp.* 2007; 55:363–372.

15. McDermott D, Lebbe C, Hodi SF, et al. Durable benefit and the potential for long-term survival with immunotherapy in advanced melanoma. *Cancer Treatment Rev.* 2014; 40:1056–1064.

16. Morton DL, Thompson JF, Cochran AJ, et al. Sentinel-node biopsy or nodal observation in melanoma. *N Engl J Med.* 2006; 355:1307–1317.

17. Mukherji B, Chakraborty NG, Sporn JR, et al. Induction of peptide antigen reactive cytolytic T cells following immunization with MAGE-1 peptide pulsed autologous antigen presenting cells. *Proc Natl Acad Sci U S A.* 1995; 92:8078–8082.

18. O'Day SJ, Hamid O, Urba WJ. Targeting cytotoxic T-lymphocyte antigen-4 (CTLA-4): a novel strategy for the treatment of melanoma and other malignancies. *Cancer.* 2007; 110:2614–2627.

19. Robert C, Schachter J, Long GV, et al. Pembrolizumab versus Ipilimumab in advanced melanoma. *N Engl J Med .* 2015; 372:2521–2532.

20. Rosenberg SA, Yang JC, Topalian SL, et al. Treatment of 283 consecutive patients with metastatic melanoma or renal cell cancer using high-dose bolus interleukin 2. *JAMA.* 1994; 271:907–913.

21. Santa Cruz DJ, Hurt MA. Neoplasms of skin [chapter 2] In: Sternberg SS. *Diagnostic surgical pathology* 2nd ed. Vol.1. New York: Raven Press; 1994:57–102.

22. Schadendorf D, Hodi SF, Robert C, et al. Pooled analysis of long-term survival data from phase II and phase III trials of Ipilimumab in unresectable or metastatic melanoma. *J Clin Oncol.*2015;33:1889–1894.

23. Spain L, Diem S, Larkin J. Management of toxicities of immune checkpoint inhibitors. *Cancer Treatment Rev.* 2016; 44:51–60.

24. Takahira T, Oda Y, Tamiya S, et al. Detection of COL1A1-PDGFB fusion transcripts and PDGFB/PDGFRB mRNA expression in dermatofibrosarcoma protuberans. *Mod Pathol.* 2007; 20:668–675.

23 Acute Leukemia

Aaron T. Gerds and Mikkael A. Sekeres

INTRODUCTION

Acute leukemia represents a very aggressive, malignant transformation of an early hematologic precursor. The malignant clone is arrested in an immature blast form, proliferates abnormally, and no longer has the ability to undergo maturation. In contrast, the chronic leukemias are characterized by resistance to apoptosis and by accumulation of nonfunctional cells, with the emphasis on proliferation, in contrast to the block in differentiation seen with acute leukemias. Accumulation of the blasts within the bone marrow results in progressive hematopoietic failure, with associated infection, anemia, and thrombocytopenia. These are the complications that often prompt evaluation in newly diagnosed patients.

Acute leukemia continues to be a grave diagnosis because of its rapid clinical course. Patients, particularly those who are younger, require aggressive and urgent evaluation and treatment initiation. As a general rule, treatment is expected to improve quality of life and prolong survival. Unfortunately, many patients present at an advanced age and with comorbid conditions, making cytotoxic approaches difficult. Older or unwell patients who are given the best supportive care survive for a median of only a few months.

The immature, clonally proliferating cells that form blasts are derived from myeloid or lymphoid cell lines. Transformation of granulocyte, RBC, or platelet (myeloid) precursors results in acute myeloid (myelogenous) leukemia (AML). Acute lymphoblastic (lymphocytic) leukemia (ALL) originates from B or T lymphocytes. This general division has implications for different treatment and diagnostic approaches. It is the first step in classifying the leukemic process occurring in the patient.

EPIDEMIOLOGY

- Estimated new cases in the United States in 2016 are 19,950 for AML (1.2% of all new cancer cases) and 6,590 for ALL (0.4% of all new cancer cases).
- AML accounts for 10,430 deaths and ALL accounts for 1,430 deaths annually in the United States.
- The risk of developing AML increases with advanced age, the median age being 67 years.
- Seventy-five percent of newly diagnosed patients with AML are older than 60 years.
- ALL is more common in children; 60% to 70% are diagnosed in patients younger than 20 years.

RISK FACTORS

Most patients will have no identifiable risk for developing acute leukemia. Table 23.1 lists the conditions that are associated with an increased risk for developing acute leukemia. Most epidemiologic studies have evaluated the relationship between the risk factors and AML. The conditions that are most commonly associated with AML are chemotherapy or radiation therapy for other cancers (which account for >90% of therapy-related AML), followed by environmental exposures, such as chronic benzene exposure or exposure to ionizing radiation.

TABLE 23.1 Risk Factors for Acute Leukemia

Exposure

Ionizing radiation, benzene, cytotoxic drugs, alkylating agents, cigarette smoking, ethanol use by the mother

Acquired disorders

Myelodysplastic syndrome, paroxysmal nocturnal hemoglobinuria, polycythemia vera, chronic myelogenous leukemia, myeloproliferative disorders, idiopathic myelofibrosis, aplastic anemia, eosinophilic fasciitis, myeloma, primary mediastinal germ cell tumor (residual teratoma elements evolve into myeloid progenitors that evolve into AML years later)

Genetic predisposition

Down syndrome, Fanconi anemia, Diamond-Blackfan anemia, Kostmann syndrome, Klinefelter syndrome, chromosome 21q disorder, Wiskott-Aldrich syndrome, ataxia-telangiectasia, dyskeratosis congenita, combined immunodeficiency syndrome, von Recklinghausen disease, neurofibromatosis 1, Shwachman syndrome

Familial

Nonidentical sibling (1:800), monozygotic twin (1:5), first-degree relative (three times increased risk)

Infection

Human T-cell leukemia virus and T-cell ALL

AML, acute myeloid leukemia; ALL, acute lymphoblastic leukemia.

Ionizing Radiation Exposure Explored in Atomic Bomb Survivors

- Ionizing radiations have a latency period of 5 to 20 years and a peak period of 5 to 9 years in atomic bomb survivors.
- They exhibit a 20- to 30-fold increased risk of AML and chronic myelogenous leukemia (CML).

Chemotherapy

- Therapy-related AML may account for 10% to 20% of new cases.
- Leukemia associated with alkylating agents may be associated with cytogenetic changes of chromosomes 5, 7, and 13. Often there is a multiyear, latent-phase myelodysplastic syndrome preceding the development of AML.
- Topoisomerase II agents, often with an abnormal chromosome 11q23 in the blasts, can rapidly evolve after initial therapy, at a median of 2 years following exposure.
- Previous, high-dose therapy with autologous transplant leads to a cumulative risk of 2.6% by 5 years, especially with total body irradiation (TBI)-containing regimens.

CLINICAL SIGNS AND SYMPTOMS

- Ineffective hematopoiesis: Results from marrow infiltration by the malignant cells and a block in differentiation
  - Anemia: Pallor, fatigue, and shortness of breath, rarely myocardial infarction or stroke
  - Thrombocytopenia: Epistaxis, petechiae, and easy bruising
  - Neutropenia: Fever and pyogenic infection

- Infiltration of other organs
  - Skin: Leukemia cutis in 10%
  - Gum hypertrophy: Especially in monocytic leukemias
  - Myeloid (granulocytic) sarcoma: Localized tumor composed of blast cells; <1% will present with prominent extramedullary disease; imparts poorer prognosis; occasionally associated with chromosome 8; 21 translocation; approach to treatment is the same as with overt bone marrow involvement with AML
  - Enlarged liver, spleen, and lymph nodes: Common in ALL, occasionally in monocytic leukemia
  - Thymic mass: Present in 15% of ALL in adults
  - Testicular infiltration: Also a site of relapse for ALL (sanctuary site)
  - Retinal involvement
- Central nervous system (CNS) and meningeal involvement
  - 5% to 10% of ALL cases at diagnosis; <5% AML, associated with inv (16), high blast count, or myeloid sarcoma abutting spine
  - Cerebrospinal fluid (CSF) analysis and prophylaxis are given in every patient with ALL to decrease CNS relapse
  - Symptoms: Headache and cranial nerve palsy, but mostly asymptomatic
- Disseminated intravascular coagulation (DIC) and bleeding
  - Common with acute promyelocytic leukemia (APL) or other AML with blasts whose cytoplasms contain granules; the mechanism is related to tissue factor release by granules and fibrinolysis; generally improves with all-trans retinoic acid (ATRA, for APL only), the early initiation of which is imperative
  - Can be present in AML inv (16) or monocytic leukemias or can be related to sepsis
- Patients may present with the medical emergencies of tumor lysis syndrome or leukostasis (reviewed later in this chapter)

DIAGNOSTIC EVALUATION

- A complete history and physical examination are an essential part of diagnosis of acute leukemia, including a detailed family history and history of previous chemotherapy or radiation therapy, or of environmental exposures.
- Complete blood count (CBC), differential and manual examination of peripheral smear, and peripheral blood flow cytometry are considered when circulating blasts are sufficiently abundant to rapidly establish a diagnosis.
- Coagulation tests include prothrombin time (PT), partial thromboplastin time (PTT), D-dimer, and fibrinogen.
- Complete metabolic panel with calcium, magnesium, phosphorus, and uric acid. Pseudohyperkalemia, as well as a spuriously low glucose and P_{O2} (partial pressure of oxygen) can occur with a high blast count.
- Bone marrow biopsy and aspirate (with analysis for morphology), cytogenetics, flow cytometry, and cytochemical stains (Sudan black, myeloperoxidase, acid phosphatase, and specific and nonspecific esterase) are used for diagnosis.
- Human leukocyte antigen (HLA) testing of patients who are transplant candidates—the test is performed before the patient becomes cytopenic. Specimen requirements are minimal when DNA-based HLA typing is performed.
- Hepatitis B and C, and human immunodeficiency virus antibody titers are obtained.
- Pregnancy test (β-human chorionic gonadotropin), if applicable.
- Electrocardiogram (ECG) and analysis of cardiac ejection fraction should be done prior to the treatment with anthracyclines only if a patient has symptoms or a history of heart disease.
- Lumbar puncture: Performed when signs and symptoms of neurologic involvement are present. Thrombocytopenia and fibrinogen should be corrected prior to the procedure, which should be performed after reduction of peripheral blast count to avoid theoretical inoculation of blasts into uninvolved CSF. Obtain cell count, opening pressure, protein level, and submit cytocentrifuge specimen for cytology or flow cytometry.

- Central venous access should be obtained. An implanted port-type catheter is not recommended. Coagulation abnormalities should be corrected if present. It is often possible to initiate induction therapy with normal peripheral veins and await subsidence of coagulopathy to reduce risk of procedural complications.
- Supplemental fluorescent in situ hybridization (FISH) or other assay for *PML-RARa*, or t(15;17), is performed when APL is suspected; and testing for *BCR-ABL1*, or t(9;22), is performed when CML in blast phase or ALL is suspected.
- Cytogenetic (metaphase karyotype) and gene mutation analysis of blasts are essential for risk-stratification and are needed to determine subsequent management.

INITIAL MANAGEMENT

The initial management of acute leukemia involves the following:

- Hydration with IV fluids (2 to 3 L/m^2 per day).
- Tumor lysis prophylaxis and relevant laboratory monitoring should be started.
- Blood product support: Suggestions for prophylactic transfusions are a hemoglobin level of <8 g/dl and a platelet level of <10,000/uL. Platelet transfusion threshold can be higher in the context of fever or bleeding, cryoprecipitate can be used if fibrinogen level is <normal, and fresh frozen plasma (FFP) can be used to immediately correct significantly elevated levels of PT and PTT. Platelet transfusion threshold should be increased in APL patients to <50,000/uL. The minimum "safe" platelet level required to prevent spontaneous hemorrhage is not known. Additional platelet optimization strategies include avoidance of nonsteroidal anti-inflammatory drugs (NSAIDs), aspirin, and clopidogrel-like agents. Deep venous thrombosis prophylaxis with anticoagulants or leg compression devices should be avoided.
- Blood products should be irradiated and given with a WBC filter (leukopoor).
- Episodes of fever require blood and urine cultures, followed by treatment with appropriate antibiotics, particularly in the setting of neutropenia, (see Chapter 37), and imaging.
- Therapeutic anticoagulation should be given with extreme caution in patients during periods of extreme thrombocytopenia. Adjustment of prophylactic platelet transfusion thresholds or anticoagulants may be required.
- Suppression of menses: High doses of an oral contraceptive pill (containing 35 mcg ethinyl estradiol taken two to four times per day) can be used for heavy or irregular uterine bleeding during chemotherapy. Leuprolide acetate 7.5 mg intramuscularly every 28 days can also be used to suppress menses.

Tumor Lysis Syndrome

- Tumor lysis syndrome can be spontaneous or can be induced by chemotherapy.
- Risk factors include elevated uric acid, high WBC count, elevated lactate dehydrogenase (LDH), and high tumor burden.
- Laboratory tests indicate elevated potassium (or low potassium with monocytic leukemias), LDH, phosphorus, and uric acid, with a resulting decrease in calcium.
- Patients should be initiated on allopurinol 300 mg daily until WBC falls to below normal levels.
- For hydration, alkalinizing fluids (0.5 NS with 50 mEq sodium bicarbonate, D5W with up to 150 mEq sodium bicarbonate) could be considered to increase solubility of uric acid, minimizing intratubular precipitation. Caution should be taken as alkalizing the urine also promotes calcium–phosphate complex deposition, and normal saline is a viable alternative.
- Uricolytic agents (rasburicase) can be considered if the patient has hyperuricemia (>12) and an elevated creatinine on presentation or has hyperuricemia uncontrolled with allopurinol. Prophylactic rasburicase is not necessary with proper uric acid monitoring, due to quick onset of action of rasburicase.
- Hemodialysis may be required in refractory cases or urgently in the setting of life-threatening hyperkalemia, or volume overload if oliguric (see Chapter 39).

Leukostasis

- Occurs with elevated blast counts.
- Symptoms result from capillary plugging by leukemic cells.
- Common signs: dyspnea, headache, confusion, chest pain, and/or hypoxia.
- Initial treatment includes aggressive hydration, chemotherapy to rapidly lower the circulating blast percentage (e.g., oral hydroxyurea), or leukapheresis if readily available.
- Transfusions should be avoided, as these may increase viscosity.
- Leukapheresis has not been shown to be superior to chemotherapy for the treatment of leukostasis. If used, it may be repeated daily in conjunction with chemotherapy until the blast count is <50,000. Leukapheresis should not be used for patients with APL, because it may worsen the intrinsic coagulopathy associated with this subtype of leukemia.

CLASSIFICATION

Acute Myeloid Leukemia

Over time, the pathologic classification system from the World Health Organization (WHO) has replaced the French-American-British (FAB) one. The WHO classification system emphasizes recurrent karyotypic and genetic abnormalities over morphology, due to their prognostic relevance (Table 23.2), while still retaining elements of the FAB system to further stratify cases without recurrent genetic

---

TABLE 23.2 The World Health Organization (WHO) Classification of Acute Myeloid Leukemia

AML with recurrent genetic abnormalities

AML with t(8;21)(q22;q22.1);*RUNX1-RUNX1T1*
AML with inv(16)(p13.1q22) or t(16;16)(p13.1;q22);*CBFB-MYH11*
APL with *PML-RARA*
AML with t(9;11)(p21.3;q23.3);*MLLT3-KMT2A*
AML with t(6;9)(p23;q34.1);*DEK-NUP214*
AML with inv(3)(q21.3q26.2) or t(3;3)(q21.3;q26.2); *GATA2, MECOM*
AML (megakaryoblastic) with t(1;22)(p13.3;q13.3);*RBM15-MKL1*
Provisional entity: AML with BCR-ABL1
AML with mutated *NPM1*
AML with biallelic mutations of *CEBPA*
Provisional entity: AML with mutated RUNX1
AML with myelodysplasia-related changes
Therapy-related myeloid neoplasms
AML, not otherwise specified (NOS)
AML with minimal differentiation (FAB M0)
AML without maturation (FAB M1)
AML with maturation (FAB M2)
Acute myelomonocytic leukemia (FAB M3)
Acute monoblastic/monocytic leukemia (FAB M5)
Pure erythroid leukemia (FAB M6)
Acute megakaryoblastic leukemia (FAB M7)
Acute basophilic leukemia
Acute panmyelosis with myelofibrosis
Myeloid sarcoma

AML, acute myeloid leukemia; FAB, French-American-British.

abnormalities. Marrow blasts should comprise 20% of the nucleated cells within the aspirate unless t(8;21) or inv(16) is present. The blasts may be characterized as myeloid lineage by the presence of Auer rods; a positive myeloperoxidase, Sudan black, or nonspecific esterase stain; and the immunophenotype shown by flow cytometry. Cell surface markers associated with myeloid cell lines include CD13, CD33, CD34, c-kit (CD117), and HLA-DR. Monocytic markers include CD64, CD11b, and CD14. CD41 (platelet glycophorin) is associated with megakaryocytic leukemia, and glycophorin A is present on erythroblasts. HLA-DR–negative blast phenotype is commonly seen in APL and serves as a rapidly available test corroborating suspicion of this subtype requiring a specific induction therapy.

Acute Lymphoblastic Leukemia

The WHO classification of ALL broadly divides the disease into B-cell, T-cell, and NK-cell leukemias, with subsets being defined by recurrent genetic abnormalities, in particular the presence of BCR-ABL (the *Philadelphia chromosome*). Immunophenotyping of B-lineage ALL reveals the typical lymphoid markers CD19, CD20, CD10, TdT, and immunoglobulin. T-cell markers include TdT, CD2, CD3, CD4, CD5, and CD7. Burkitt-cell leukemia is characterized by a translocation between chromosome 8 (the *c-myc* gene) and chromosome 14 (immunoglobulin heavy chain), or between chromosome 8 and chromosomes 2 or 22 (light chain) regions.

PROGNOSTIC GROUPS

Acute Myeloid Leukemia

Patients who are older (>60 years) and those with an elevated blast count at diagnosis (>20,000) have a worse prognosis. Therapy-related AML and those with a prior history of myelodysplastic syndromes (MDS) have a worse chance of obtaining a complete remission (CR) and shorter long-term survival. Table 23.3 illustrates the prognostic groups according to cytogenetics and molecular markers.

Acute Lymphoblastic Leukemia

As in AML, patients with ALL have a worse prognosis when presenting with advanced age or an elevated WBC count. Burkitt-cell (mature B-cell) leukemia or lymphoma has an improved prognosis with intensive chemotherapy and CNS treatments; it usually has a translocation involving chromosome 8q24. Table 23.4 lists the prognostic groups according to cytogenetic analysis.

The presence of t(9;22) (Philadelphia chromosome, Ph, BCR-ABL1 fusion) is the most common abnormality in adults, occurring in 20% to 30% of patients with ALL and in up to 50% of patients in the B-cell lineage. Long-term survival is dismal in this group, if treated by chemotherapy alone. The introduction of tyrosine kinase inhibitors into treatment regimens have improved outcomes, and patients are recommended to undergo allogeneic transplantation if they have a suitable candidate in first CR. Ph-like (also called BCR/ABL1-like) ALL lacks the hallmark BCR-ABL1 oncoprotein; however, it shares a similar gene expression profile and poor prognosis as Ph-positive ALL. This subtype of ALL frequently harbors *IKZF1* and *CRLF2* alterations; and comprises 10% to 15% of pediatric patients, and 20% to 30% of adolescents and adults with B-cell ALL.

TREATMENT

Acute Myeloid Leukemia (Excluding Acute Promyelocytic Leukemia)

The goal of "induction" chemotherapy is to obtain a remission, which is correlated with improved survival. Complete response (CR) is defined as the elimination of the malignant clone (marrow blasts <5%) and recovery of normal hematopoiesis (absolute neutrophil count [ANC] >1,000/uL and platelet count >100,000/uL). Patients typically have a leukemia cell burden of approximately 10×10^{12} that is reduced to approximately 10×10^9 by induction. This residual disease may be undetectable

TABLE 23.3 Risk Groups in Newly Diagnosed Adult Acute Myeloid Leukemia

Risk Category	Genetic abnormality
Favorable	t(8;21)(q22;q22.1); *RUNX1-RUNX1T1*
	inv(16)(p13.1q22) or t(16;16)(p13.1;q22); *CBFB-MYH11*
	Mutated *NPM1* without *FLT3*-ITD or with *FLT3*-ITD[lowa]
	Biallelic mutated *CEBPA*
Intermediate	Mutated *NPM1* and *FLT3*-ITD[higha]
	Wild-type *NPM1* without *FLT3*-ITD or with *FLT3*-ITD[lowa] (without adverse-risk genetic lesions)
	t(9;11)(p21.3;q23.3); *MLLT3-KMT2A*[b]
	Cytogenetic abnormalities not classified as favorable or adverse
Adverse	t(6;9)(p23;q34.1); *DEK-NUP214*
	t(v;11q23.3); *KMT2A* rearranged
	t(9;22)(q34.1;q11.2); *BCR-ABL1*
	inv(3)(q21.3q26.2) or t(3;3)(q21.3;q26.2); *GATA2,MECOM(EVI1)*
	−5 or del(5q); −7; −17/abn(17p)
	Complex karyotype,[c] monosomal karyotype[d]
	Wild-type *NPM1* and *FLT3*-ITD[higha]
	Mutated *RUNX1*[¶]
	Mutated *ASXL1*[¶]
	Mutated *TP53*

[a] Low, low allelic ratio (<0.5); high, high allelic ratio (≥0.5)

[b] t(9;11)(p21.3;q23.3) takes precedence over rare, concurrent adverse-risk gene mutations

[c] Three or more unrelated chromosome abnormalities in the absence of one of the WHO-designated recurring translocations or inversions, that is, t(8;21), inv(16) or t(16;16), t(9;11), t(v;11)(v;q23.3), t(6;9), inv(3) or t(3;3); AML with *BCR-ABL1*

[d] Defined by the presence of 1 single monosomy (excluding loss of X or Y) in association with at least 1 additional monosomy or structural chromosome abnormality (excluding, t(8;21), inv(16) or t(16;16))

[¶] These markers should not be used as an adverse prognostic marker if they co-occur with favorable-risk AML subtypes

TABLE 23.4 Prognostic Groups by Cytogenetics in Adult Acute Lymphoblastic Leukemia

Poor Risk	Good Risk
t(9;22) (Philadelphia (Ph) chromosome)	8q24 translocations
t(4;11)	t(12;21)
Hypodiploid	t(10;14)
t(1;19)	t(7;10)
9p abnormalities (del(9p), add(9p), der(9)t(V;9)(V;p), i(9q))	
Intrachromosomal amplification of chromosome 21 (iAMP21)	

morphologically, but will certainly lead to relapse in a few months if more therapy is not administered. Additional intensive "post-remission" or "consolidation" cycles of chemotherapy are given to further reduce the residual burden in the hope that host immune mechanisms can suppress the residual leukemia population, thereby leading to sustained, maintenance-free remission. The general approach to induction chemotherapy for adults is shown in Table 23.5. All patients should be considered for clinical trials if available.

TABLE 23.5 Standard Induction for Acute Myeloid Leukemia

"7 + 3," 7 d of infusional cytarabine and 3 d of anthracycline
Cytarabine 100–200 mg/m² daily as continuous infusion × 7 d with
    Idarubicin 12 mg/m² daily bolus for 3 d
      OR
    Daunorubicin 60–90 mg/m² daily bolus for 3 d

TABLE 23.6 Consolidation for Acute Myeloid Leukemia

Age <60
Cytarabine 3 g/m² infused over 3 h, q12h on days 1, 3, and 5 (six doses)
Creatinine 1.5–1.9 mg/dL: Decrease cytarabine 1.5 g/m² per dose
Age >60
"5 + 2": Cytarabine 100 mg/m² daily as continuous infusion for 5 d and anthracycline (idarubicin 12 mg/m² or daunorubicin 45–90 mg/m²) bolus daily for 2 d
OR
Intermediate-dose cytarabine: 1–1.5 g/m² q12h on days 1, 3, 5 OR 1–1.5 g/m² daily × 4–5 days

In general

- Addition of high-dose cytarabine (HiDAC) or etoposide has been evaluated in published regimens for induction, but have not been conclusively been shown to be superior to the backbone of 3 days of an anthracycline and 7 days of cytarabine.
- The FLT3-inhibitor midostaurin may be added to chemotherapy and is associated with improved survival in patients whose blasts express this marker.
- Bone marrow aspiration should be repeated at approximately day 14 of induction chemotherapy. If significant residual blasts are present (generally defined as >5%), induction chemotherapy should be repeated ("7 + 3," or can consider "5 + 2" in Table 23.6 for older or frail patients). If significant disease is present (<50% reduction in disease volume), a change in the regimen to age-appropriate HiDAC may be considered.
- Older patients (>60 years) may benefit from intensive induction and consolidation treatment. Post-remission cytarabine requires dose reduction due to CNS toxicity.
- Older patients or patients who decline intensive induction chemotherapy (i.e., 7 + 3) may be candidates for therapy with low-dose cytarabine or hypomethylating agents (azacitidine or decitabine). These agents have lower CR rates (approximately 10% to 20%) but lower therapy-related mortality, and may be administered in the outpatient setting.

Supportive Care

- Infection is a major cause of morbidity and mortality. Prophylactic antibacterials (quinolones), anti-fungals (itraconazole, fluconazole, or posaconazole), and antivirals (acyclovir) may be given during these periods of prolonged neutropenia. Broad-spectrum antimicrobials are used for neutropenic fever (see Chapter 36).
- Growth factors such as granulocyte colony-stimulating factor (G-CSF) can be considered in the setting of neutropenia and severe infection. They may be used rarely to aid in count recovery. Patients should be off growth factors for a minimum of 7 days prior to a bone marrow biopsy that is being used to document remission as it can confound the interpretation of bone marrow morphology.
- Steroid eye drops are required during HiDAC infusions to reduce the risk of exfoliative keratitis.

Acute Myeloid Leukemia Postremission Therapy (Excluding Acute Promyelocytic Leukemia)

The consolidation options for those patients who enter CR are shown in Table 23.6. HiDAC especially may benefit those patients with good-risk disease [t(8;21), inv(16), *NMP1* mutated/*FLT3* wild type]. These good-risk patients should not receive allogeneic transplantation in CR1. Consolidation usually consists of four cycles (the minimum effective dose and the number of cycles are not clear). Older patients do not seem to benefit from more than one to two consolidation cycles of a lower-dosed cytarabine-based regimen. Patients with preceding MDS or poor-risk cytogenetics should receive an allogeneic transplantation in CR1, if possible. Patients with intermediate-risk cytogenetics should be considered for an allogeneic transplant, especially if they have a matched sibling donor, though it remains unclear if this provides an advantage for this sub-population over standard chemotherapy consolidation. Gene mutations may assist in the proper identification of standard-risk patients who would or would not benefit from allogeneic transplant in CR1 (see the Allogeneic Transplantation section).

Acute Promyelocytic Leukemia, t(15;17)

The t(15;17) brings together the retinoic acid receptor-α and the promyelocytic leukemia genes, allowing for transduction of a novel protein (PML-RARα). The protein plays a role in blocking differentiation of the promyelocyte, thereby promoting abnormal accumulation within the marrow space. Because the characteristic translocation occurs in this subgroup of AML, therapy incorporates all-*trans* retinoic acid (ATRA) and/or arsenic trioxide (ATO), which act as differentiating agents. Table 23.7 shows a treatment summary in APL.

- Therapy with ATRA should be started immediately upon suspicion of APL; therapy can be tailored pending genetic confirmation.
- ATRA + ATO is used for low to intermediate risk patients (WBC ≤10 x10^9/L at presentation) as well as an alternative option for higher-risk patients unable to tolerate anthracyclines.
- ATRA + chemotherapy (anthracycline and cytarabine) is used for higher-risk patients (WBC >10 x10^9/L)
- Time to attain remission may be more than 30 days and a bone marrow biopsy is not performed on day 14.
- PCR should be followed for PML-RARα: Reinduction therapy or allogenic transplantation should be considered if PCR is still positive postconsolidation (but not postinduction); levels should be followed during the maintenance phase. A return of the transcript to positive heralds relapse.

TABLE 23.7 Treatment of Acute Promyelocytic Leukemia

	Low to Intermediate Risk	High Risk
Induction	ATRA + ATO	ATRA + anthracycline (idarubicin or daunorubicin) +/- cytarabine Or ATRA + idarubicin + ATO
Consolidation	ATRA + ATO (28 weeks)	ATRA + anthracycline × 3 cycles +/– cytarabine Or Arsenic × 2 cycles followed by anthracycline × 2 cycles
Maintenance (2 y)	None	ATRA 45 mg/m² daily for 15 d q3mo + Mercaptopurine 50 mg/m² daily + MTX 15 mg/m² weekly

ATRA, all-trans retinoic acid; ATO, arsenic trioxide; 6-MP, 6-mercaptopurine; MTX, methotrexate.

- ATRA (or ATO) syndrome (differentiation syndrome) consists of capillary leak and cytokine release resulting in fever, leukocytosis, respiratory compromise (dyspnea and infiltrates), weight gain, effusions (pleural and pericardial), renal failure, and hypotension. This syndrome occurs in upwards of 25% of patients during induction, with peak occurrences between 1 and 3 weeks into therapy, and is associated with a rapidly rising neutrophil count. Treat with dexamethasone 10 mg IV BID × 3 days, and then taper over 2 weeks. Discontinuation of ATRA can be considered in severe cases. ATRA may still be safely employed in consolidation or maintenance-phase therapy because the ATRA syndrome is limited to the induction-period neutrophilia.
- A similar differentiation syndrome, not involving ATRA, is seen with the use of arsenic trioxide.
- Prognosis with APL is very good, with >90% of patients attaining a CR and >70% long-term disease-free survival.
- Patients are typically classified as high-risk (WBC ≥10,000), intermediate-risk (WBC< 10,000 and platelets ≤40), or low-risk (WBC <10,000 and platelets >40) disease at diagnosis.

Relapsed Disease

- ATO 0.15 mg/kg/day until second CR.
- Median of 57 days to remission.
- Baseline electrolytes (Ca, K, Mg), creatinine, and ECG (for prolonged QT interval).
- Monitoring: At least weekly electrolytes and ECG. Keep K >4.0 mEq/L and Mg >2.0 mg/dL and reassess if QTc interval >500.
- Patients commonly develop APL differentiation syndrome similar to ATRA.
- Eighty-five percent of patients achieve CR.
- Arsenic trioxide may be given as consolidation at a dose of 0.15 mg/kg/day, 5 days per week (Monday through Friday) for 25 doses.
- Patients achieving CR (PCR negative) should receive consolidation with an autologous transplant, if eligible. Patients with persistent positive PCR results should be considered for an allogeneic transplant.

Relapsed or Refractory Acute Myeloid Leukemia

Relapse of AML after initial CR is common (60% to 80% of all cases). Relapse occurring within 6 months of induction or a patient never attaining remission with induction (refractory disease) complicates many re-induction attempts. The prognosis for long-term survival in this subset of patients is poor with chemotherapy alone, and all patients who are able to tolerate the treatment should be evaluated for allogeneic transplantation. Some treatment approaches are described below.

- Reinduction with "7 + 3" or HiDAC.
- Reinduction may be an option for those patients who relapse more than 6 to 12 months after initial induction.
- Subsequent remissions are usually of shorter duration (<50% of the duration of the preceding remission).
- Etoposide, mitoxantrone, ± cytarabine (EM or MEC).
- FLAG: fludarabine, cytarabine, and G-CSF (can be combined with idarubicin or mitoxantrone).
- Clofarabine +/– cytarabine or cyclophosphamide.
- FLT3 inhibitors may have activity (sorafenib, midostaurin, and quizartinib), but are currently investigational in this setting.
- In cases of isolated CNS relapse, it should be considered that systemic relapse almost always follows soon and that a systemic therapy is also required.

Acute Lymphoblastic Leukemia

General scheme: induction, consolidation, maintenance, and CNS treatment.

Several strategies exist for the treatment of adult ALL. Table 23.8 illustrates the hyper-CVAD (cyclophosphamide, vincristine, doxorubicin, and dexamethasone) regimen used at many North American centers. Modification of the Larson regimen reported by Cancer and Leukemia Group B (CALGB, now Alliance for Clinical Trials in Oncology) Study 19802, shown in Table 23.9, is

TABLE 23.8 The Hyper-CVAD and MTX/HIDAC Regimen

Cycles 1, 3, 5, and 7
Cyclophosphamide 300 mg/m² IV over 3 h q12h days 1–3 (six doses)
Mesna 600 mg/m²/d IV as continuous infusion days 1–3
Vincristine 2 mg IV days 4 and 11
Doxorubicin 50 mg/m² IV day 4
Dexamethasone 40 mg PO daily days 1–4 and 11–14
G-CSF 10 µg/kg/d SQ starting after chemotherapy
Cycles 2, 4, 6, and 8
Methotrexate 200 mg/m² IV over 2 h on day 1, followed by
Methotrexate 800 mg/m² IV over 22 h on day 1
Leucovorin 50 mg starting 12 h after methotrexate completed, followed by leucovorin 15 mg every 6 h × eight doses, dose adjusted on the basis of methotrexate levels
Cytarabine 3 g/m² IV over 2 h every 12 h on days 2 and 3 (four doses)
Methylprednisolone 50 mg IV twice daily days 1–3
G-CSF 10 µg/kg/d SQ starting after chemotherapy
CNS prophylaxis[a]
Methotrexate 12 mg intrathecal (IT) on day 2
Cytarabine 100 mg IT on day 8
Maintenance therapy[b] *(POMP) × 2 y*
Mercaptopurine 50 mg PO three times daily
Methotrexate 20 mg/m² PO weekly
Vincristine 2 mg IV monthly
Prednisone 200 mg/d for 5 d each month
Dosage adjustments
Vincristine reduced to 1 mg if bilirubin 2–3 mg/dL (omitted if bilirubin >3 mg/dL)
Doxorubicin decreased to 50% for bilirubin 2–3 mg/dL, decreased to 25% if bilirubin 3–5 mg/dL, and omitted if bilirubin >5 mg/dL
Methotrexate reduced to 50% if creatinine clearance 10–50 mL/min, and a decrease to 50%–75% for delayed excretion, nephrotoxicity, or grade ≥3 mucositis with prior courses
High-dose cytarabine decreased to 1 g/m² if patient ≥60 y, creatinine ≥1.5 mg/dL, or MTX level >20 µmol/L at the completion of the MTX infusion

[a]Dosing interval based on risk stratification (see text).

[b]Maintenance therapy is not given in Burkitt-cell leukemia/lymphoma.

G-CSF, granulocyte colony-stimulating factor; CNS, central nervous system; MTX, methotrexate.

also commonly used. Other options based on the Hoelzer and Linker regimens are also available. Burkitt-cell leukemia (mature-B ALL, FAB L3) can be treated with hyper-CVAD without maintenance therapy but requires aggressive CNS treatment to prevent relapse. Adolescent and young adult patients (age ≤40) with ALL should be treated with a pediatric-like regimen such as CALGB 10403.

Supportive Care

The regimens described previously incorporate growth factors to reduce neutropenia and allow more scheduled chemotherapy to proceed. All patients will require blood product support at some point

TABLE 23.9 The Modified Larson Regimen

Modules A1 and A2

Cyclophosphamide 1,000 mg/m² IV day 1[a]
Daunorubicin 60 mg/m² IV days 1–3[a]
Vincristine 1.5 mg/m² (capped at 2 mg) IV days 1, 8, 15, 22
Prednisone 60 mg/m²/d PO days 1–21[a]
L-Asparaginase (*Escherichia coli*) 6,000 IU/m² SQ/IM days 5, 8, 11, 15, 18, 22
G-CSF 5 µg/kg/d SQ starting day 4

Module B1 and B2

Methotrexate 15 mg intrathecal (IT) day 1
Cyclophosphamide 1,000 mg/m² IV day 1
Cytarabine 2,000 mg/m²/d IV days 1–3
G-CSF 5 µg/kg/d SQ starting day 4

Module C1 and C2

IT Methotrexate 15 mg days 1, 8, 15
Vincristine 1.5 mg/m² (capped at 2 mg) IV days 1, 8, 15
Methotrexate 1,000 mg/m² IV over 4 hours days 1, 8, 15
Methotrexate 25 mg/m² PO q 6 hours x 4 doses beginning 6 hours after initiation of IV methotrexate
  on days 1, 8, 15
Leukovorin 25 mg /m² IV on days 2, 9, 16; given 30 hours after initiation of IV methotrexate, followed
  by leukovorin 5 mg/m² PO q 6 hours until methotrexate level is <0.05 uM

Prolonged maintenance (continue until 24 mo after diagnosis)

Vincristine 2 mg IV day 1 of every 4 wk
Prednisone 60 mg/m²/d PO days 1–5 of every 4 wk
6-Mercaptopurine 60 mg/m²/d PO days 1–28
Methotrexate 20 mg/m² PO days 1, 8, 15, 22

[a]Dosage reductions for age >/=60 y: no cyclophosphamide, daunorubicin 60 mg/m² days 1–3, and prednisone 60 mg/m² days 1–7.

CNS, central nervous system.

during the treatment. Those patients treated with hyper-CVAD receive prophylactic antimicrobials (i.e., levofloxacin 500 mg daily, fluconazole 200 mg daily, and valacyclovir 500 mg daily).

Central Nervous System Disease

▪ The CNS is a sanctuary site.
▪ CNS disease is diagnosed by the presence of neurologic deficits at diagnosis *or* by five or more blasts per microliter of CSF.
▪ Therapy for CNS disease is intrathecal (IT), methotrexate (MTX), or cytarabine (Ara-C), often alternating. These will be given twice weekly until disease clears, then weekly for 4 weeks, and then resume the prophylaxis schedule. Radiation (fractionated to 2,400 to 3,000 cGy) can also be considered, being aware of potential late-term cognitive toxicities.
▪ Prophylaxis decreases CNS relapse from 30% to <5%. The prophylactic chemotherapy schedule is dependent on the relapse risk.
▪ In the hyper-CVAD regimen, patients with high-risk disease (i.e., LDH level >2.3 times upper limit of normal or elevated proliferative index) should receive eight prophylactic IT treatments, and those

with low-risk disease (no factors) receive six prophylactic IT treatments. Patients with mature B-cell disease or a history of documented CNS involvement will require 16 IT therapies. No prophylactic cranial irradiation is given.

Relapsed Acute Lymphoblastic Leukemia

The bone marrow is the most common site of relapse, but relapse can occur in the testes, eye, and CNS. Patients with late relapse (more than 6 months to 1 year from induction) may respond to rein-duction with the original regimen. Early relapse or refractory disease will require changing the treat-ment plan and evaluation for allogeneic transplantation. Several chemotherapy options are available, including

- Blinatumomab
- HiDAC with or without idarubicin, mitoxantrone, or fludarabine
- Methotrexate, vincristine, asparaginase (not PEG), steroids (MOAD)
- Dasatinib, imatinib, or nilotinib (if Ph-positive)
- Hyper-CVAD, if not given initially
- Vinorelbine with mitoxantrone, fludarabine, steroids, or rituximab
- Nelarabine
- Clofarabine +/– cytarabine or cyclophosphamide
- Liposomal vincristine
- Investigational monoclonal antibody agents (e.g., inotuzumab ozogamicin)
- Chimeric Antigen Receptor (CAR) T-Cells

Use of Targeted and Immunotherapy in Acute Lymphoblastic Leukemia

1. Blinatumomab (Blincyto)
   - Bispecific T-cell engager (BiTE) monoclonal antibody directed at both CD19 on B-cell ALL cells, and CD3 on the patient's T-cells, which enables the T-cells to recognize the malignant B-cells that express CD19. After the T-cell links with the malignant cell, it is activated and exerts cytotoxic activity on the ALL cell.
   - Compared to cytarabine-based therapy, blinatumomab was shown to have an improved CR with full hematologic recovery (34% versus 16%), as well as CR with incomplete hematologic recovery (44% versus 25%), leading to an improved overall survival in a randomized study.
   - It is given as a continuous intravenous infusion over 4 weeks, followed by a two-week treatment-free interval; maintenance treatment may continue as 4-week continuous infusions every 12 weeks.
   - Unique and serious side effects include cytokine release syndrome and neurological toxicities. Patients are hospitalized for the first 9 days of the continuous infusion to monitor for cytokine release syndrome and neurologic toxicity.
2. Rituximab (Rituxan)
   - Anti-CD20 chimeric murine–human monoclonal antibody
   - Given in addition to the previously noted regimens in front-line treatment, if CD20+
3. Imatinib, dasatinib, nilotinib, bosutinib, and ponatinib
   - Tyrosine kinase inhibitors targeting the Philadelphia chromosome [t(9;22)].
   - Dasatinib or imatinib should be considered in addition to previously noted regimens in front-line treatment, if Ph positive.
   - Role in maintenance therapy is unknown, but could be considered.
   - May be used as treatment or palliation in combination with steroids for patients unable to tolerate aggressive chemotherapy.
   - Choice of tyrosine kinase inhibitor agent should be selected based on BCR/ABL mutation analysis.
4. Chimeric Antigen Receptor (CAR) T-cells
   - This technology involves collecting a patient's T-cells, "reprograming" them with a genetically engineered immunoreceptor using a viral vector, expanding them, then reinfusing them into the patient.

- Studies with CD19-directed CAR T-cells are ongoing, and are available only at certain centers with infrastructure for cellular therapy.
- A pilot study evaluated the use of CD19-directed CAR-T cells in 30 children and adults with relapsed or refractory ALL (10% primary refractory, and 60% with relapse after allogeneic transplantation). A CR was seen in 90% of patients with an estimated 6-month event-free survival of 67%, and overall survival of 78%.
- As with blinatumomab, cytokine-release syndrome and neurological toxicities do occur early in the treatment course. Severe cytokine-release syndrome can be treated with the anti-interleukin-6 receptor antibody tocilizumab.
- Relapses were a result of tumor cell evasion of the CAR T-cells (loss of expression of CD19).
- Larger trials with long-term follow-up are needed to verify the efficacy of this treatment.
- Three second-generation CAR T-cell products are in advanced phases of development.

TRANSPLANTATION

Autologous Transplantation

- Autologous transplant appears to have minimal benefit in acute leukemia in CR1.
- Autologous transplant could be considered for patients achieving CR2, without availability of an allogeneic donor.
- It may be performed in older patients (age >60).

Allogeneic Transplantation

- Allogeneic transplant has the added benefit of "graft versus leukemia" effect.
- In the setting of unrelated donor searches, the prolonged time needed to identify a donor needs to be considered at the time of diagnosis. Referral to a transplant center is preferred as early as possible in the treatment plan.
- It is considered for all patients with relapsed or refractory disease, as it is the option that may yield long-term survival.
- It is performed in the first CR or early in the course for those patients with poorer-risk cytogenetics or transformation from MDS.
- Patients with good-risk AML [t(8;21), inv(16)), *NPM1* mutated] or APL [t(15;17)] should not be transplanted in CR1.
- Patients with intermediate-risk cytogenetics may be offered allogeneic transplant, especially if they have a sibling donor, though superiority to standard postremission chemotherapy has not been demonstrated prospectively in this group.
- Gene mutations may be able to help stratify intermediate-risk patients with normal cytogentics as having a poorer or more favorable outcome, assisting in the decision of the usefulness of transplantation in CR1. Patients with *NPM1* and *CEBPA* mutations (without *FLT3*-ITD mutations) may have a good prognosis and may not benefit from transplant in CR1. *FLT3*-ITD mutations are a negative predictor of outcome.
- When transplanted in CR1, overall survival is 50% to 60%; it decreases to 25% to 40% when performed for patients in CR2, and is <10% for patients with refractory disease.
- Reduced-intensity conditioning transplantation is reasonable for those patients unable to proceed with ablative treatment secondary to comorbidities or advanced age.
- In a randomized fashion, BMT-CTN 0901 evaluated the role of reduced-intensity conditioning compared to myeloablative preparative regimens for allogeneic transplant in patients with AML. This study was stopped early because of high relapse incidence with reduced intensity versus myeloablative conditioning (48.3% versus 13.5%). Overall survival was higher with myeloablative regimens, but not significantly. Reduced intensity conditioning resulted in lower complication rates, but due to the higher relapse rates, there was a statistically significant advantage in relapse-free survival with myeloablative conditioning.

PROGNOSIS AND SURVIVAL

Adults with acute leukemia remain at high risk for disease-related and treatment-related complications. In AML, the prognostic characteristics of the disease are associated with survival. Good-risk AML is associated with an 80% to 90% CR rate, and long-term disease-free survival is 60% to 70% in younger patients treated with HiDAC. Poor-risk features are associated with only a 50% to 60% chance of obtaining a CR, and a high risk of relapse is observed in those patients who enter CR. Additionally, gene mutations have been identified as correlating with prognosis in AML, especially in the intermediate-risk group in which cytogenetics cannot guide postremission therapy. In these patients, *FLT3*-ITD and *TP53* mutations confer a poor prognosis. In patients who are *FLT3*-ITD negative, *NPM1* and *CEBPA* identify a good prognostic subgroup.

CR and long-term outcome have improved for adult patients with ALL who were receiving intensive courses of chemotherapy. With the hyper-CVAD and modified Larson regimens, 85% to 90% of patients will obtain a CR with a median duration of CR of 30 months. Five-year survival is approximately 40%.

Suggested Readings

1. Arber DA, Orazi A, Hasserjian R, et al. The 2016 revision to the World Health Organization classification of myeloid neoplasms and acute leukemia. *Blood.* 2016 May 19;127(20):2391–2405.
2. Burnett AK, Milligan D, Prentice AG, et al. A comparison of low-dose cytarabine and hydroxyurea with or withoutall-trans retinoic acid for acute myeloid leukemia and high-risk myelodysplastic syndrome in patients not considered fit for intensive treatment. *Cancer.* 2007 Mar;109(6):1114–1124.
3. Byrd J, Mrozek K, Dodge R, et al. Pretreatment cytogenetic abnormalities are predictive of induction success, cumulative incidence of relapse, and overall survival in adult patients with de novo acute myeloid leukemia: results from Cancer and Leukemia Group B (CALGB 8461). *Blood.* 2002;100:4325–4336.
4. Curran E, Stock W. How I treat acute lymphoblastic leukemia in older adolescents and young adults. *Blood* 2015 125:3702-3710.
5. Döhner H, Estey E, Grimwade D, et al. Diagnosis and management of AML in adults: 2017 ELN recommendations from an international expert panel. *Blood.* 2017 Jan 26;129(4):424–447.
6. Dombret H, Seymour JF, Butrym A, et al. International phase 3 study of azacitidine vs conventional care regimens in older patients with newly diagnosed AML with >30% blasts. *Blood.* 2015 Jul 16;126(3):291–299.
7. Fernandez HF, Sun Z, Yao X, et al. Anthracycline dose intensification in acute myeloid leukemia. *N Engl J Med.* 2009;361:1249–1259.
8. Gerds, AT, Appelbaum F. To transplant or not to transplant for adult acute myeloid leukemia: an ever-evolving decision. *Clin Adv Hematol Oncol.* 2012 Oct;10(10):655–662.
9. Grimwade D, Walker H, Harrison G, et al. The predictive value of hierarchical cytogenetic classification in older adults with acute myeloid leukemia (AML): analysis of 1065 patients entered into the United Kingdom Medical Research Council AML11 trial. *Blood.* 2001;98:1312–1320.
10. Kantarjian H, Stein A, Gökbuget N, et al. Blinatumomab versus chemotherapy for advanced acute lymphoblastic leukemia. *N Engl J Med.* 2017;376(9):836.
11. Kantarjian H, Thomas D, O'Brien S, et al. Long-term follow-up results of hyperfractionated cyclophosphamide, vincristine, doxorubicin, and dexamethasone (Hyper-CVAD), a dose intensive regimen, in adult acute lymphoblastic leukemia. *Cancer.* 2004;101:2788–2801.
12. Litzow MR, Ferrando AA. How I treat T-cell acute lymphoblastic leukemia in adults. *Blood* 2015 126:833–841.
13. Lo-Coco F, Avvisati G, Vignetti M, et al. Retinoic acid and arsenic trioxide for acute promyelocytic leukemia. *N Engl J Med.* 2013 Jul 11;369(2):111–121.
14. Majhail NS, Farnia SH, Carpenter PA, et al. Indications for autologous and allogeneic hematopoietic cell transplantation: Guidelines from the American Society for blood and marrow transplantation. *Biol Blood Marrow Transplant.* 2015 Nov;21(11):1863–1869.
15. Maude SL, Frey N, Shaw PA, et al. Chimeric antigen receptor T cells for sustained remissions in leukemia. *N Engl J Med.* 2014;371(16):1507.
16. Powell BL, Moser B, Stock W, et al. Arsenic trioxide improves event-free and overall survival for adults with acute promyelocytic leukemia: North American Leukemia Intergroup Study C9710. *Blood.* 2010;116:3751–3757.
17. Rousselot P, Coudé MM, Gokbuget N, et al. Dasatinib and low-intensity chemotherapy in elderly patients with Philadelphia chromosome-positive ALL. *Blood.* 2016 Aug;128(6):774–782.
18. Rowe JM, Buck G, Burnett AK, et al. Induction therapy for adults with acute lymphoblastic leukemia; results of more than 1500 patients from the international ALL trial: MRC UKALL XII/ECOG E2993. *Blood.* 2005;106:3760–3767.

19. Schlenk R, Dohner K, Drauter J, et al. Mutations and treatment outcome in cytogenetically normal acute myeloid leukemia. *N Engl J Med.* 2008;358:1909–1918.

20. Sekeres MA, Gerds AT. Mitigating fear and loathing in managing acute myeloid leukemia. *Semin Hematol.* 2015 Jul;52(3):249–255.

21. Stock W, Johnson JL, Stone RM, et al. Dose intensification of daunorubicin and cytarabine during treatment of adult acute lymphoblastic leukemia: results of Cancer and Leukemia Group B Study 19802. *Cancer.* 2013 Jan 1;119(1):90–98.

22. Stock W, La M, Sanford B, et al. What determines the outcomes for adolescents and young adults with acute lymphoblastic leukemia treated on cooperative group protocols? A comparison of Children's Cancer Group and Cancer and Leukemia Group B studies. *Blood.* 2008;112:1646–1654.

23. Thomas D, Faderl S, Cortes J, et al. Treatment of Philadelphia chromosome-positive acute lymphoblastic leukemia with hyper-CVAD and imatinib mesylate. *Blood.* 2004;103:4396–4407.

24. Thomas D, Faderl S, O'Brien S, et al. Chemoimmunotherapy with hyper-CVAD plus rituximab for the treatment of adult Burkitt and Burkitt-type lymphoma or acute lymphoblastic leukemia. *Cancer.* 2006;106:1569–1580.

25. Welch JS, Petti AA, Miller CA, et al. TP53 and Decitabine in Acute Myeloid Leukemia and Myelodysplastic Syndromes. *N Engl J Med.* 2016;375(21):2023.

24 Chronic Lymphoid Leukemias

Neel Trivedi and Chaitra Ujjani

INTRODUCTION

Chronic lymphocytic leukemia (CLL) is the most common form of leukemia in the western world. Major advances in the management of CLL over the past decade resulting in an improved patient outcome include more accurate diagnostic techniques, validated prognostic studies, better supportive care, and improved treatment regimens with targeted therapies. This chapter will focus on CLL and include information on two other chronic lymphoid malignancies, prolymphocytic leukemia (PLL) and hairy cell leukemia (HCL).

PRESENTATION AND DIAGNOSIS

The estimated incidence of CLL in the United States for 2016 was 18,960 cases. It tends to be a disease of the elderly, with a median age at diagnosis of 70 years. The disease affects men twice as often as women. Although about half of the patients present with an asymptomatic lymphocytosis, symptoms typically associated with disease include recurrent infections and constitutional symptoms such as fatigue, weight loss, fevers, chills, and night sweats. Other clinical features include nontender lymphadenopathy, splenomegaly, autoimmune hemolytic anemia (AIHA), pure red cell aplasia, or immune-mediated thrombocytopenia.

According to the guidelines published by the National Cancer Institute-Sponsored Working Group (NCI-WG), diagnostic criteria for CLL include the following:

- Absolute lymphocytosis ($\geq 5 \times 10^3/\mu L$), with a morphologically mature appearance, often with smudge cells.
- Monoclonal B-cell phenotype by flow cytometry: CD19, CD23, and CD5 with low levels of CD20 and surface immunoglobulin. Expression of CD38 and Zeta-associated protein-70 (ZAP-70) is not diagnostic for CLL, but has prognostic implications.
- Molecular cytogenetics, although not necessary for diagnosis, can identify prognostic chromosomal abnormalities and help distinguish CLL from other lymphoid disorders.
- As flow cytometry can be performed on peripheral blood, a bone marrow biopsy is not necessary to make the diagnosis. If a bone marrow biopsy is performed, the degree of lymphocytic involvement should be greater than 30% in order to confirm the diagnosis. Less than 30% involvement would indicate a diagnosis of small lymphocytic lymphoma (SLL). A bone marrow biopsy can be helpful in ascertaining the cause of cytopenias and should be considered in patients with anemia or thrombocytopenia. In addition, a bone marrow biopsy should be performed prior to and after treatment in order to evaluate for response.

STAGING AND PROGNOSIS

The most commonly used staging methods include the Rai, modified Rai, and the Binet staging systems. Prognosis based on the modified Rai staging system is outlined in Table 24.1. There are a number of

TABLE 24.1 Staging and Prognosis of Chronic Lymphocytic Leukemia

Rai	Modified Rai	Criteria	Median Survival[a]
0	Low risk	Lymphocytosis only ($\geq 15 \times 10^3/\mu L$ in peripheral blood)	>10 y
1	Intermediate risk	Lymphocytosis with enlarged nodes	7 y
2	Intermediate risk	Lymphocytosis with increased splenic or hepatic size	
3	High risk	Lymphocytosis with anemia (Hgb ≤ 11 g/dL)	5 y
4	High risk	Lymphocytosis with thrombocytopenia ($\leq 100 \times 10^3/\mu L$)	

[a]Survival as reported in the original publication.

Hgb, hemoglobin.

prognostic factors for CLL. Those associated with an inferior outcome include the cytogenetic abnormalities detected by fluorescent in situ hybridization of deletion (del) 11q and del 17p, an elevated serum β-2-microglobulin level ≥ 4 mg/L, unmutated immunoglobulin variable region heavy chain genes (IgVH), overexpression of the ZAP-70 >20%, expression of CD38 >30%, and advanced-stage disease. NOTCH1 and SFB3B1 mutations have also been identified as poor prognostic markers. Trisomy 12 and normal cytogenetics are associated with an intermediate outcome, while del 13q is associated with a favorable outcome. The utility of these factors lies in prognosis and choice of regimen. They are not used to determine when to initiate treatment.

Computerized tomography (CT) is not required at diagnosis or for staging purposes, but may be useful to evaluate the presence of internal enlarged lymph nodes unable to be palpated by physical examination. Patients with clinical stage 0 disease, but stage I by CT, often behave more like the latter. Contrast-enhanced CT has a higher sensitivity of detecting CLL than PET/CT. At this time there is no role for positron emission tomography (PET) scanning in CLL, except to assess for a potential transformation to a high-grade lymphoma.

COMPLICATIONS

Patients with CLL can develop infections, high-grade transformation, and are at an increased risk for other malignancies. Hematologic complications include anemia or thrombocytopenia due to marrow involvement, treatment effect, splenic sequestration, AIHA, pure red cell aplasia, and immune-mediated thrombocytopenia. AIHA can be due to the CLL itself or to fludarabine, which is commonly used in the treatment of this disease. Pure red cell aplasia, although rare, is possibly caused by suppressor T cells. Cyclosporine may be effective with a reticulocyte response within a few weeks. Frequent infections, often sinopulmonary, are often related to immunosuppressive treatments, hypogammaglobulinemia, inadequate humoral response, and impaired complement activation. Transformation to Richter syndrome (large B-cell lymphoma), PLL, ALL, and multiple myeloma occurs in 10% to 15% of cases. Patients are also at increased risk of developing other malignancies of sites such as the gastrointestinal tract, lung, and skin. Other chemotherapeutics, such as cyclophosphamide or chlorambucil, are associated with secondary malignancies such as AML and MDS.

TREATMENT

CLL often exhibits an indolent course, not requiring treatment at diagnosis. The indications for treatment of CLL per the NCI-Sponsored WG guidelines include the following:

- Significant and persistent fatigue
- Unintentional weight loss of ≥10% in previous 6 months
- Persistent fevers >100.5°F or 38.0°C for 2 or more weeks without evidence of infection
- Night sweats for more than 1 month without evidence of infection
- Autoimmune anemia or thrombocytopenia poorly responsive to steroids
- Progressive marrow failure with worsening or new anemia or thrombocytopenia
- Progressive splenomegaly (>6 cm below costal margin) or lymphadenopathy (>10 cm)
- Progressive lymphocytosis: Increase >50% in 2 months or doubling time <6 months

The appropriate choice of front-line therapy for CLL is dependent on a number of patient-specific factors including age, comorbidities, performance status, and cytogenetic abnormalities. Recent advances in the field have provided oncologists with a variety of options including small molecule inhibitors and newer anti-CD20 antibodies in addition to the previously established chemoimmunotherapy regimens (Table 24.2).

Chemoimmunotherapy

Chlorambucil (Chl) had been the mainstay of treatment for CLL until the arrival of fludarabine (F) and bendamustine (B). Each agent has individually shown superiority to chlorambucil in terms of overall response rate (ORR) and progression-free survival (PFS). Combination with rituximab (R) has also shown significant activity in patients with previously untreated disease. The ORR of FR was 90% (complete remission (CR) 47%); whereas the combination of BR produced an ORR of 88% (CR 23%). The addition of cyclophosphamide (C) to FR has demonstrated ORRs of 90% to 95% (CR 44% to 72%). Based on these data, the German CLL Study Group conducted the CLL-10 study, which compared FCR to BR in physically fit, previously untreated patients with few comorbidities and lacking del 17p. While the ORRs were similar between the arms (FCR 95% vs. BR 96%), the CR + CRi (complete remission with incomplete count recovery) rate and median PFS favored FCR (CR 40% vs. 31% p = .03, PFS 55 vs. 42 months, p<0.001). FCR, however, was associated with significantly greater ≥ grade 3 neutropenia and infection, particularly in patients >65-years-old. BR is preferred for the elderly and those with comorbidities based on the toxicity profile, but can be offered to younger patients as there was no difference in OS between the arms. FCR can be considered for younger, fit patients, particularly those who possess the mutated IGVH gene based on a lengthy median PFS, greater than 15 years. Patients with white blood cell counts >50,000/μL and/or bulky disease should receive tumor lysis prophylaxis with allopurinol and aggressive hydration. Patients receiving bendamustine should not receive allopurinol, however, given the risk of Stevens-Johnson syndrome.

Chlorambucil alone or in combination with an anti-CD20 monoclonal antibody is an option for patients who are unable to tolerate more aggressive chemotherapy regimens. Ofatumumab, a second-generation anti-CD20 antibody with stronger complement dependent cytotoxicity compared to rituximab, was initially approved for fludarabine and alemtuzumab-refractory CLL based on an ORR of 58% (0% CR) and median PFS of 5.7 months. (Alemtuzumab is an anti-CD52 antibody no longer commercially available for CLL.) In the COMPLEMENT-1 trial, compared to single-agent chlorambucil, the combination of chlorambucil and ofatumumab produced a superior ORR (82% vs. 69%, p = 0.001), CR rate (14% vs. 1%), and median PFS (23 vs. 15 months, p<0.001). Obinutuzumab is a type II, glycoengineered, third-generation anti-CD20 monoclonal antibody with stronger antibody-dependent cellular cytotoxicity and apoptosis than rituximab, which has also been evaluated with chlorambucil. The agents were combined (Chl-Ob) and compared to Chl-R and single-agent chlorambucil in the front-line phase III CLL-11 study. The Chl-Ob arm demonstrated superiority to Chl-R in terms of ORR (78% vs. 65%), CR (21% vs. 7%), and median PFS (27 vs. 15 months, p<0.001). Obinutuzumab and ofatumumab each gained approval in combination with chlorambucil for patients who were not fit to be candidates for aggressive chemotherapy based on these data. Antimicrobial prophylaxis against varicella zoster, Pneumocystis jirovecii, and other fungi should be considered for each patient based on their functional immune status.

Small Molecule Inhibitors

Aside from chemoimmunotherapy, there have been several advances in the treatment of CLL, mainly due to the arrival of small molecule inhibitors. These agents target intracellular mediators of tumor cell proliferation and survival. They provide an advantage over chemoimmunotherapy in that they have considerable activity in patients with traditionally poor prognostic markers, including del 17p, del 11q, and unmutated IgVH. In addition, they are orally bioavailable. These agents require indefinite therapy, however, until progression or unacceptable toxicity.

Ibrutinib is an irreversible, selective inhibitor of the Bruton's tyrosine kinase (BTK). It was initially approved for the treatment of relapsed and refractory CLL based on a phase II study of 85 patients, demonstrating an ORR of 71%. The approval was contingent on the RESONATE study, a phase III comparison of ibrutinib and ofatumumab, which demonstrated ibrutinib's superiority in terms of ORR (63% vs. 4%, p<0.001), PFS (not reached vs. 8.1 months, P<0.001), and OS (1-yr OS 90% vs. 81%, p = .005). Given the activity noted in the RESONATE-17 trial of 144 patients with relapsed/refractory CLL/SLL characterized by del 17p (ORR 83%, 24-month PFS 63%), ibrutinib acquired a front-line indication for this population as well. Its front-line indication was expanded based on the RESONATE II study, which compared ibrutinib to chlorambucil in patients above age 65 with previously untreated CLL/SLL. The trial found that patients in the ibrutinib arm experienced a higher ORR (86% vs. 35%, P<0.001), longer median PFS (not reached vs. 19 months), and greater estimated 2-year OS (at 24 months 98% vs. 85%, P = 0.001). Ibrutinib was well tolerated by the elderly study population with fewer patients discontinuing treatment due to adverse events in the ibrutinib arm than in the chlorambucil arm (9% versus 23%). The most common adverse events with ibrutinib are diarrhea, fatigue, and cough; whereas common serious adverse events include neutropenia, anemia, and hypertension. An increased risk of bleeding has also been reported with ibrutinib due to inhibition of platelet signaling and platelet adhesion on von Willebrand factor. The majority of patients experience mild bruising or petechiae but rare, major hemorrhage has been reported as well. Caution should be taken with concomitant anticoagulation. Additionally, atrial fibrillation was noted in up to 7% of patients.

Idelalisib is an inhibitor of the delta isoform of phosphoinositide 3'-kinase (PI3K). It was approved in combination with rituximab for the treatment of relapsed CLL based on a phase III trial of rituximab with or without idelalisib in patients who were deemed unfit for cytotoxic chemotherapy. The idelalisib plus rituximab arm had a significantly higher ORR (81% vs. 13%, P<0.001), increased PFS (93% vs. 46% at 24 weeks, P<0.001), and greater 1-year OS at 12 months (92% vs. 80%, P = 0.02). The most common adverse events were pyrexia, fatigue, and nausea. Serious adverse events with idelalisib include pneumonitis, hepatitis, and colitis. These adverse events typically can be managed with drug interruption, dose reduction, and supportive care including steroids; however, some patients will require discontinuation of therapy. Both idelalisib and ibrutinib can trigger a demargination of lymphocytes into the peripheral bloodstream with initiation of therapy. In the absence of other concerning findings, the resulting lymphocytosis should not be considered a sign of disease progression. It is a benign finding that resolves in the majority of patients despite continuing the medication. Distinct from the BCR pathway is the BCL-2 family of proteins, which tightly regulate apoptosis. Venetoclax is a selective, second-generation inhibitor of BCL2, an anti-apoptotic protein that is overexpressed in CLL and thought to contribute to chemotherapy resistance. Venetoclax was approved for patients with previously treated CLL characterized by del 17p based on a single-arm phase II study of 106 patients demonstrating an ORR of 80% and CR+CRi of 7.5%. The median duration of response had not been reached at one year of follow-up. The most common severe adverse events were related to myelosuppresssion, which occurred primarily within the first month of therapy and resolved over time. Due to the profound, rapid activity of the drug, venetoclax requires a dose ramp-up over 5 weeks in conjunction with aggressive tumor lysis prophylaxis and rigorous monitoring to prevent serious clinical consequences of tumor lysis syndrome including cardiac arrhythmia and acute renal failure.

Despite the multiple effective treatment options for CLL, patients inevitably relapse and require additional therapy. All patients should be evaluated for new cytogenetic abnormalities with initiation of each line of therapy, as up to 50% of patients can develop the del 17p mutation over time. Patients with relapsed CLL can be retreated with a prior chemoimmunotherapy regimen if a durable response was achieved or a small molecule inhibitor (Table 24.2). Patients who progress on a small molecule inhibitor can be effectively treated with an alternative oral inhibitor. At this time the only therapy that has been proven to be potentially curative in CLL is allogeneic stem cell transplantation. However, this is often not an option for the elderly population that CLL typically affects or patients with multiple comorbidities.

TABLE 24.2 Treatment Options for Chronic Lymphocytic Leukemia

Front-line

Regimen	Mechanism of Action	Dosing
Fludarabine and rituximab (FR)	F: purine analog R: anti-CD20 antibody	F 25 mg/m² IV days 1–5 R 375 mg/m² IV day 1 q4wk × 6 cycles
Fludarabine, cyclophosphamide, and rituximab (FCR)	F: purine analog C: alkylating agent R: anti-CD20 antibody	Cycle 1: F 25 mg/m² IV days 2–4 C 250 mg/m² IV days 2–4 R 375 mg/m² IV day 1 Cycles 2–6: F 25 mg/m² IV days 1–3 C 250 mg/m² IV days 1–3 R 500 mg/m² IV day 1 q4wk × 6 cycles
Bendamustine and rituximab (BR)	B: alkylating agent R: anti-CD20 antibody	Cycle 1: B 90 mg/m² IV days 1–2 R 375 mg/m² IV day 1 Cycles 2–6: B 90 mg/m² IV days 1–2 R 500 mg/m² IV day 1 q4wk × 6 cycles
Chlorambucil and ofatumumab (Chl-Of)	Chl: alkylating agent Of: anti-CD20 antibody	Cycle 1: Chl 10 mg/m² PO days 1–7 Of 300 mg IV day 1 and 1000 mg IV day 8 Cycles 3–12: Chl 10 mg/m² PO days 1–7 Of 1000 mg IV day 1 q4wk x 12 cycles
Chlorambucil and obinutuzumab (Chl-Ob)	Chl: alkylating agent Ob: anti-CD20 antibody	Cycle 1: Chl 0.5 mg/kg PO days 1 and 15 Ob 100 mg IV day 1, 900 mg IV day 2, and 1000 mg IV days 8 and 15 Cycles 2–6: Chl 0.5 mg/kg PO days 1 and 15 Ob 1000 mg IV day 1 q4wk × 6 cycles
Ibrutinib	Bruton's tyrosine kinase inhibitor	420 mg PO daily until disease progression

Treatment Options for Relapsed/Refractory Disease		
Regimen	*Mechanism of Action*	*Dosing*
FR, FCR, Chl-+anti-CD20 monoclonal antibody	See above	See above
BR	See above	Cycle 1: B 70 mg/m² IV days 1–2 R 375 mg/m² IV day 1 Cycles 2–6: B 70 mg/m² IV days 1–2 R 500 mg/m² IV day 1 q4wk × 6 cycles

TABLE 24.2 (Continued)

Front-line		
Ibrutinib	Bruton's tyrosine kinase inhibitor	420 mg PO daily until disease progression
Idelalisib and rituximab (Id-R)	Id: PI3-kinase inhibitor R: anti-CD20 antibody	Id 150 mg PO twice daily until disease progression R 375 mg/m² IV day 1 and 500 mg/m² q2wk for 4 doses then q4wk for 3 doses (total of 8 infusions)
Venetoclax	BCL-2 antagonist	<u>Week 1:</u> 20 mg PO daily <u>Week 2:</u> 50 mg PO daily <u>Week 3:</u> 100 mg PO daily <u>Week 4:</u> 200 mg PO daily <u>Week 5 and beyond:</u> 400 mg PO daily until disease progression Allopurinol, hydration, and electrolyte monitoring based on risk for TLS (see package insert)
Stem cell transplantation		Patients with multiple relapses; relapsed younger del 17p patients. Allogeneic transplantation with nonmyeloablative approaches allow older patients and patients with comorbidities to undergo transplant; toxicities: opportunistic infections and GVHD

IV, intravenously; SC, subcutaneously; PO, by mouth; F, fludarabine; C, cyclophosphamide; B, bendamustine; Chl, chlorambucil; Of, ofatumumab; Ob, obinutuzumab; Id, idelalisib; TLS, tumor lysis syndrome; del: deletion; GVHD, graft vs. host disease.

OTHER CHRONIC LYMPHOID LEUKEMIAS

Other rare lymphoid malignancies include PLL (Table 24.3) and HCL (Table 24.4). PLL presents similarly to CLL, and can be of either T-cell or B-cell origin. PLL typically presents with >90% circulating prolymphocytes, whereas CLL has <55% prolymphocytes. PLL can occur de novo or rarely, from CLL, and has a poorer prognosis. HCL is a de novo process. It is highly treatable with cladribine, pentostatin, α-interferon, and rituximab.

TABLE 24.3 Prolymphocytic Leukemia

Clinical findings	Hepatosplenomegaly; very high lymphocyte count; patients with T-PLL may have pleural effusion and skin lesions
Clinical course	B-PLL: variable course; indolent in some, while others with anemia, thrombocytopenia, and a high lymphocyte count have a shorter survival T-PLL: more aggressive than B-PLL or CLL

(continued)

TABLE 24.3 (Continued)

Morphology	Large cells with abundant cytoplasm and prominent nucleolus within a convoluted nucleus with immature chromatin
Phenotypic features	B-PLL: surface expression of CD19, CD20, CD22, CD79a, FMC 7, bright IgM, and/or IgD; occasional ZAP-70, CD38, CD5, CD23, negative for CD11c, CD103, cyclin D1 T-PLL: surface expression of CD52, CD2, CD3, CD5, CD7, occasionally CD4 and/or CD8; rearrangement of the T-cell–receptor gene
Treatment	B-PLL: anecdotal reports of treatment with nucleoside analogs and monoclonal antibodies T-PLL: alemtuzumab, pentostatin, allogeneic stem cell transplantation for patients who achieve a CR and are eligible

CLL, chronic lymphocytic leukemia; B-PLL, B-cell prolymphocytic leukemia; T-PLL, T-cell prolymphocytic leukemia; sIg, surface immunoglobulin; CR, complete response.

TABLE 24.4 Hairy Cell Leukemia

Clinical findings	Male predominance, pancytopenia, splenomegaly, B symptoms, infections Less often: lymphadenopathy, necrotizing vasculitis, lytic bone abnormalities, effusions
Morphology	Lymphocytes with cytoplasmic projections, TRAP-stain positive
Bone marrow	Aspiration frequently unsuccessful, "dry tap" secondary to fibrosis; marrow biopsy reveals "hairy" cells and classic "fried-egg" appearance
Immunology	CD11c, CD20, CD25, CD103, and CD123
Treatment indications	Symptomatic splenomegaly or lymphadenopathy, neutropenia ($<1.0 \times 10^9$/mL) with repeated infections, symptomatic anemia (Hgb <11 g/dL), bleeding due to thrombocytopenia ($<100 \times 10^9$/mL), constitutional symptoms
Treatment	First-line Cladribine: ORR: 80%–95%, dose: 0.1 mg/kg/d by CIV days 1–7 Pentostatin: ORR: 75%–80%, dose: 4 mg/m^2 IV q2wk for 3–6 mo Relapsed/recurrent disease Retreatment with nucleoside analogs Interferon-α: ORR: 75%–90%, dose: 2 million units/m^2 SC three times/wk Splenectomy is reserved for those with symptomatic splenomegaly, pancytopenia despite other chemotherapeutics, and as a temporizing measure in symptomatic pregnant women Rituximab RR: 24%–80%, dose: 375 mg/m^2 IV qwk for four doses Investigational BL22, an anti-CD22 monoclonal antibody linked to pseudomonas exotoxin A ORR 72% (CR 47%) in cladribine-refractory patients Vemurafenib, a BRAF inhibitor ORR 96% (CR 35%), dose: 960 mg orally twice daily

TRAP, tartrate-resistant acid phosphatase; sIg, surface immunoglobulin; Hgb, hemoglobin; CIV, continuous intravenous infusion; ORR, overall response rate; CR, complete response.

Suggested Readings

1. Burger JA, Tedeschi A, Barr PM, et al. Ibrutinib as initial therapy for patients with chronic lymphocytic leukemia. *N Engl J Med.* 2015;373(25):2425–2437.
2. Byrd JC, Brown JR, O'Brien S, et al. Ibrutinib versus ofatumumab in previously treated chronic lymphoid leukemia. *N Engl J Med.* 2014:371(3):213–223.
3. Byrd JC, Furman RR, Coutre SE, et al. Targeting BTK with ibrutinib in relapsed chronic lymphocytic leukemia. *N Engl J Med.* 2013;369(1):32–42.
4. Byrd JC, Furman RR, Coutre SE, et al. Three-year follow-up of treatment-naive and previously treated patients with CLL and SLL receiving single-agent ibrutinib. *Blood.* 2015
5. Byrd JC, Peterson BL, Morrison VA, et al. Randomized phase 2 study of fludarabine with concurrent versus sequential treatment with rituximab in symptomatic, untreated patients with B-cell chronic lymphocytic leukemia: results from Cancer and Leukemia Group B 9712 (CALGB 9712). *Blood.* 2003;101(1):6–14.
6. Cheson BD, Byrd JC, Rai KR, et al. Novel targeted agents and the need to refine clinical end points in chronic lymphocytic leukemia. *J Clin Oncol.* 2012;30(23):2820–2822.
7. Cheson BD, Fisher RI, Barrington SF, et al. Recommendations for initial evaluation, staging, and response assessment of Hodgkin and non-Hodgkin lymphoma: the Lugano classification. *J Clin Oncol.* 2014;32(27):3059–3068.
8. Chiaretti S, Marinelli M, Del Giudice I, et al. NOTCH1, SF3B1, BIRC3 and TP53 mutations in patients with chronic lymphocytic leukemia undergoing first-line treatment: correlation with biological parameters and response to treatment. *Leuk Lymphoma.* 2014;55(12):2785–2792.
9. Dearden CE, Matutes E, Cazin B, et al. High remission rate in T-cell PLL with Campath-1H. *Blood.* 2001;98:1721–1726.
10. Döhner H, Stilgenbauer S, Benner A, et al. Genomic aberrations and survival in CLL. *N Engl J Med.* 2000;343:1910–1916.
11. Dreger P, Döhner H, Ritgen M, et al. Allogeneic stem cell transplantation provides durable disease control in poor-risk CLL. *Blood.* 2010;116(14):2438–2447.
12. Eichhorst B, Fink AM, Bahlo J, et al. First-line chemoimmunotherapy with bendamustine and rituximab versus fludarabine, cyclophosphamide, and rituximab in patients with advanced chronic lymphocytic leukaemia (CLL10): an international, open-label, randomised, phase 3, non-inferiority trial. *Lancet Oncol.* 2016;17:928–942.
13. Else M, Dearden CE, Matutes E, et al. Long-term follow-up of 233 patients with HCL, treated initially with pentostatin or cladribine, at a median of 16 years from diagnosis. *Br J Haematol.* 2009;145(6):733–740.
14. Fischer K, Cramer P, Busch R, et al. Bendamustine in combination with rituximab for previously untreated patients with CLL (GCLLSG). *J Clin Oncol.* 2012;30(26):3209–3216.
15. Furman RR, Sharman JP, Coutre SE, et al. Idelalisib and rituximab in relapsed chronic lymphocytic leukemia. *N Engl J Med.* 2014;370(11):997–1007.
16. Gidron A, Tallman MS. 2-CdA in the treatment of HCL. *Leuk Lymphoma.* 2006;47(11):2301–2307.
17. Goede V, Fischer K, Busch R, et al. Obinutuzumab plus chlorambucil in patients with CLL and coexisting conditions. *N Engl J Med.* 2014;370(12):1101–1110.
18. Grever M, Kopecky K, Foucar M, et al. Randomized comparison of pentostatin versus interferon alfa-2a in previously untreated patients with HCL. *J Clin Oncol.* 1995;13:974–982.
19. Grever MR, Lozanski G. Modern strategies for HCL. *J Clin Oncol.* 2011;29(5):583–590.
20. Hallek M, Cheson BD, Catovsky D, et al. Guidelines for the diagnosis and treatment of CLL: a report from the IW-CLL updating the NCI-WG 1996 guidelines for CLL. *Blood.* 2008;111(12):5446–5456.
21. Hillmen P, Robak T, Janssens A, et al. Chlorambucil plus ofatumumab versus chlorambucil alone in previously untreated patients with chronic lymphocytic leukaemia (COMPLEMENT 1): a randomised, multicentre, open-label phase 3 trial. *The Lancet.* 2015;385(9980):1873-1883.
22. Knauf WU, Lissichkov T, Aldaoud A, et al. Phase III randomized study of bendamustine compared with chlorambucil in previously untreated patients with chronic lymphocytic leukemia. *J Clin Oncol.* 2009;27(26):4378–4384.
23. Levade M, David E, Garcia C, et al. Ibrutinib treatment affects collagen and von Willebrand factor-dependent platelet functions. *Blood.* 2014;124(26):3991–3995.
24. O'Brien S, Jones JA, Coutre SE, et al. Ibrutinib for patients with relapsed or refractory chronic lymphocytic leukaemia with 17p deletion (RESONATE-17): a phase 2, open-label, multicentre study. *Lancet Oncol.* 2016:1–13.
25. Rai K, Peterson B, Appelbaum F, et al. Long-term survival analysis of the North American Intergroup Study C9011 comparing fludarabine and chlorambucil in previously untreated patients with CLL. *Blood.* 2009;114(22):Abstract 536.
26. Rai KR, Peterson BL, Appelbaum FR, et al. Fludarabine compared with chlorambucil as primary therapy for chronic lymphocytic leukemia. *N Engl J Med.* 2000;343(24):1750–1757.
27. Rassenti LZ, Jain S, Keating MJ, et al. Relative value of ZAP-70, CD38, and immunoglobulin mutation status in predicting aggressive disease in CLL. *Blood.* 2008;112(5):1923.

28. Sawada K, Fujishima N, and Hirokawa M. Acquired pure red cell aplasia: updated review of treatment. *Br J Haematol.* 2008;142(4): 505–514.
29. Siegel RL, Miller KD, Jemal A. Cancer statistics, 2016. *CA Cancer J Clin.* 2016;66(1):7–30.
30. Stilgenbauer S, Eichhorst B, Schetelig J, et al. Venetoclax in relapsed or refractory chronic lymphocytic leukaemia with 17p deletion: a multicentre, open-label, phase 2 study. *Lancet Oncol.* 2016;17(6):768–778.
31. Thompson PA, Tam CS, O'Brien SM, et al. Fludarabine, cyclophosphamide, and rituximab treatment achieves long-term disease-free survival in IGHV-mutated chronic lymphocytic leukemia. *Blood.* 2016;127(3):303–309.
32. Tiacci E, Park JH, De Carolis L, et al. Targeting Mutant BRAF in Relapsed or Refractory Hairy-Cell Leukemia. *N Engl J Med.* 2015;373(18):1733.
33. Tsimberidou AM, Keating MJ. Richter syndrome: biology, incidence and therapeutic strategies. *Cancer.* 2005;103:216–228.

Chronic Myeloid Leukemias **25**

Samer A. Srour and Muzaffar H. Qazilbash

EPIDEMIOLOGY

Chronic myeloid leukemia (CML) is a clonal myeloproliferative neoplasm characterized by dysregulated proliferation of mature granulocytes secondary to deregulated tyrosine kinase. It was first described in Europe during the 1840s as reviewed by Geary and Deininger, and currently accounts for 15% to 20% of newly diagnosed leukemia in adults with a median age of 54 years. The age-adjusted incidence of CML is 3.3 per one million person-years, with male predominance. The average person's lifetime risk of being diagnosed with CML is about 1 in 625, and there has been a notable increase in the incidence and prevalence of CML over last decade, likely related to increased use of Philadelphia (Ph) chromosome testing and improved survival with the use of tyrosine kinase inhibitors (TKIs), respectively.

PATHOPHYSIOLOGY

CML is a clonal disorder of hematopoietic stem cells. The reciprocal translocation between the long arms of chromosomes 9 and 22 [t(9;22)], the Ph chromosome, is the initiating event and the diagnostic hallmark of CML. This translocation results in the transfer of the Ableson (ABL) gene on chromosome 9 to an area of chromosome 22 termed the breakpoint cluster region (BCR), resulting in the BCR-ABL fusion gene. This fusion gene results in the expression of the constitutively active protein tyrosine kinase, BCR-ABL1 oncogene, which plays the central role in the pathogenesis of CML leading to an uncontrolled proliferation of granulocytes, predominantly neutrophils but also eosinophils and basophils at various maturation stages. The BCR-ABL1 gene fusion is present in all CML patients, and the majority express the 210 kDa oncoprotein, while less than 10% express either the 190 kDa or 230 kDa oncoprotein. The different-molecular-weight isoforms are generated due to different breakpoints and mRNA splicing. Patients who lack BCR-ABL1 are considered atypical CMLs, and an alternative diagnosis to BCR-ABL-positive CML should be sought. If left untreated, majority of patients with chronic phase (CP) CML will progress to accelerated phase (AP) and/or blast phase (BP), which is likely a multistep process that remains poorly understood. However, it is notable that the bulk of genetic changes occur in transition from CP-CML to AP, and that clonal evolution plays a major role in progression to BP.

DIAGNOSIS AND CLINICAL FEATURES

Symptoms and Signs

Patients with CML present in the CP in over 85% of cases, and the diagnosis is mostly incidental. Up to 50% of patients are asymptomatic at presentation. Symptoms are usually related to underlying cytopenias or splenomegaly. The following are the common symptoms at presentation:

- Fatigue and malaise
- Anorexia and weight loss

- Sweats and low-grade fever
- Left upper quadrant discomfort/early satiety associated with splenomegaly
- Dyspnea on exertion
- Bleeding

Laboratory Features

The diagnosis of CML may be accomplished with peripheral blood testing. An elevated white blood cell count with a left shift, including higher than normal percentages of basophils, eosinophils, myelocytes, and metamyelocytes, in addition to thrombocytosis are suggestive of CML. Although identification of Ph chromosome on cytogenetic analysis or the detection of BCR-ABL fusion transcript by fluorescence in situ hybridization (FISH) analysis or polymerase chain reaction (PCR) in peripheral blood may be sufficient for initial presumptive diagnosis, a bone marrow aspiration/biopsy and cytogenetic analysis are mandatory before initiation of treatment for staging purposes and to detect chromosomal abnormalities other than Ph chromosome. This would guide the choice of initial therapy and subsequent disease monitoring, including clonal evolution. The absolute value of the transcript level by PCR testing is not important for initial diagnosis or staging, but it is essential for subsequent evaluation of response.

Differential Diagnosis

- Leukoerythroblastic reaction in response to infection, inflammation, or malignancy
- Chronic myelomonocytic leukemia
- Juvenile myelomonocytic leukemia
- Chronic eosinophilic leukemia
- Chronic neutrophilic leukemia
- Atypical CML
- Idiopathic myelofibrosis
- Essential thrombocytosis
- Polycythemia vera

STAGING AND PROGNOSTIC FACTORS

CML is characterized by three distinct clinical phases. Minor differences in defining disease stages exist among study groups, but the World Health Organization (WHO) classification is widely adopted (Table 25.1). In the recently published 2016 revised WHO classification, no major changes were noted in defining the 3 CML phases but "provisional" criteria were added to AP definition to include failure of tyrosine kinase treatment and/or acquisition of BCR-ABL1 mutations while on treatment. While over 85% of patients are diagnosed in the more indolent stage termed CP, if left untreated most patients will eventually progess within 3 to 5 years to an AP, followed by an aggressive blastic phase. Twenty to 25% of patients can progress directly from CP to BP, which is characterized by ≥20% blasts in the bone marrow or peripheral blood, or the development of extramedullary disease outside of the spleen.

Prognosis of patients with CML has improved markedly over past 2 decades with the introduction of TKIs, leading to 10-year survival rates exceeding 80% for CML patients in CP, but remains relatively poor for those in AP or BP. Risk stratification scores are commonly used for patients in CP. The Sokal and Hasford risk scores are derived from patients treated with conventional chemotherapy or recombinant interferon alpha (rIFNα), and use clinical and laboratory features at diagnosis such as age, spleen size, platelet count, and peripheral blood blasts, eosinophils and basophils (Table 25.2). The Sokal score has been shown to correlate with both, the response rates to imatinib mesylate (IM) and survival outcomes. The 6-year follow-up data from the IRIS trial (International Randomized Study of Interferon vs. STI571) confirmed the prognostic value of the Sokal scoring system; the 6-year overall survival (OS) and event-free survival (EFS) estimates were 94% and 91%, respectively, for low-risk patients; 87% and 81% for intermediate-risk patients, respectively; and 76% and 67% for high-risk patients, respectively. More recently, the European Treatment and Outcome Study (EUTOS) and the EUTOS long term survival (ELTS) scores were introduced, but are not commonly used in the United States.

TABLE 25.1 World Health Organization (WHO) Criteria for Chronic Myeloid Leukemia Stages

Stage	Features
Chronic phase	Blast cells in blood or marrow <10%
	Basophils in blood <20%
	Platelets >100 × 10^9/L
Accelerated phase[*]	Blast cells in blood or marrow 10%–19%
	Basophils in blood 20% or more
	Persistent thrombocytopenia (<100 x 10^9/L) unrelated to therapy
	Thrombocytosis (>1000 x 10^9/L) unresponsive to therapy
	Persistent or increasing splenomegaly and/or WBC (>10 x 10^9/L) count unresponsive to therapy
	Additional clonal chromosomal abnormalities at diagnosis or any evidence of new clonal chromosomal abnormality while on treatment
Blastic phase	Blast cells in blood or bone marrow ≥20%
	Extramedullary blast proliferation
	Large foci or clusters of blasts in the bone marrow biopsy

[*]"Provisional" response-to-tyrosine kinase inhibitor (TKI) criteria were added in the 2016 revised WHO classification to define accelerated phase CML. These included: Hematologic resistance to the first TKI (or failure to achieve a complete hematologic response to the first TKI); or any hematological, cytogenetic, or molecular indications of resistance to 2 sequential TKIs; or occurrence of 2 or more mutations in BCR-ABL1 during TKI therapy.

TABLE 25.2 Sokal and Hasford Risk Indexes

Risk Category	Risk Index	Median Survival
Sokal		
Low	<0.8	5 y
Intermediate	0.8–1.2	3.5 y
High	>1.2	2.5 y
Hasford		
Low	≤780	98 mo
Intermediate	781–1,480	65 mo
High	>1,480	42 mo

Sokal risk index was defined based on patients treated with conventional chemotherapy. Hasford risk index was defined based on patients treated with rIFNα-based regimens.

Sokal score: EXP [0.0116 × (age – 43.4) + 0.0345 × (spleen size [cm below costal marigin] – 7.51) + 0.188 × [(platelet count/700)^2 – 0.563] + 0.0887 × (myeloblasts – 2.1)].

Hasford score: [0.666 when age ≥50 y + 0.042 × (spleen size [cm below costal marigin]) + 1.0956 (when platelet count ≥ 1,500 × 10^9/L) + 0.0584 × myeloblasts + 0.2039 (when basophils ≥3%) + 0.0413 × eosinophils (%)]× 1,000.

Additional cytogenetic abnormalities may develop in over 80% of patients in the accelerated and blast crisis phases. Clonal cytogenetic evolution, while on treatment, confers a worse prognosis especially when it includes one of the "major route" abnormalities such as trisomy 8, trisomy 19, duplication of the Ph chromosome, and isochromosome 17q. The depth and timing of hematologic, cytogenetic, and molecular responses to treatment is correlated with prognosis as well.

TREATMENT

Historically, treatment options for CML included conventional cytotoxic chemotherapy (such as hydroxy-urea and busulfan), interferon α, and allogeneic hematopoietic stem cell transplantation which remains the only potentially curative option. The introduction of TKIs have revolutionized the treatment of CML in the past two decades leading to practice changes in treatment algorithms, treatment goals, monitoring tools, and the expectations of patients and physicians. The mainstay of frontline CML therapy is currently IM or one of the second-generation TKIs such as nilotinib and dasatinib. The more recently approved agents, bosutinib and ponatinib, are mostly used for subsequent lines of treatment, or in some individual cases as frontline. The newer agents can overcome some of the genetic mutations that underly TKI resistance, and can lead to quicker and deeper cytogenetic and molecular remissions when compared to IM. Omacetaxine, a subcutaneously bioavailable semisynthetic form of homoharringtonine, was recently approved for CML treatment in patients who had progressed after treatment with at least two TKIs.

Hydroxyurea

Hydroxyurea is a cytotoxic antiproliferative agent that is administered orally and is used when a patient has an elevated white blood cell count ($>80 \times 10^9$/L) to allow rapid control of blood counts. It induces hematologic responses in 50% to 80% of patients and is continued until confirmation of diagnosis; however, it does not alter disease course. Allopurinol may be added to prevent tumor lysis syndrome when starting hydroxyurea.

Interferon

Recombinant IFNα-based regimens were the standard therapy for chronic-phase CML before the discovery of IM. Majority of patients achieved complete hematologic remission (CHR), but complete cytogenetic responses (CCyR) were noted in minority of patients. While effective and even curative in some patients, with earlier studies showing that 10-year OS exceeding 70% for those who achieve CCyR, these agents had significant adverse effects that greatly impair the quality of life and adherence to treatment. IFN is no longer recommended for fronline treatment in CML. However, it can be considered in specific circumstances such as during pregnancy given its relative safety compared to TKIs.

Tyrosine Kinase Inhibitors

Imatinib Mesylate

With the advent of IM, CML had set the bar for how a malignancy could be effectively treated with targeted therapy, and ushered a new era of research in this field. IM is a phenylaminopyrimidine derivative that inhibits the BCR-ABL tyrosine kinase by competitive binding at the ATP-binding site. Although active in all phases of CML, the most durable responses are seen in newly diagnosed patients in CP. Results of the pivotal IRIS trial established the superiority of IM, and at 8-year follow-up, the estimated EFS was 81%, freedom from progression to CML-AP or CML-BP 92%, and OS 85%. When only CML-related deaths were considered, OS reached 93%. An estimated 7% of patients progressed to accelerated-phase CML or blast crisis. As a result, IM 400 mg daily was established as the standard of care for patients with newly diagnosed chronic-phase CML. The most common adverse events seen with IM are skin rash, muscle cramps, edema, myelosuppression, diarrhea, and liver function test abnormalities.

The high rate of complete cytogenetic response with IM has shifted the goal of therapy to achieving molecular responses measured by PCR. Response criteria are summarized in Table 25.3. Duration of remission and survival are related to the depth of molecular response achieved. As more information has become available, the responses to TKI therapy have become the most important marker of overall prognosis. This makes molecular monitoring an essential component of CML management. More recently monitoring schema have become available that help to determine when a second-generation TKI would be appropriate as well as timing to refer for allogeneic stem cell transplant. If there is suboptimal response to IM, BCR-ABL1 kinase domain mutational analysis is indicated and treatment options include an increase in IM dose, switching to a second-generation TKI, and an early referral for allogeneic transplant. At this time there are no definite data favoring one option over another although the failure of IM predicts for poorer prognosis. Most experts refer patients for stem cell transplant evaluation after suboptimal response to 2 TKIs. The revised and updated LeukemiaNet treatment recommendations based on initial and subsequent response are summarized in Table 25.4 and 25.5.

TABLE 25.3 Response Criteria

Complete hematologic response (CHR)	WBC < 10 × 10⁹/L
	No immature granulocytes
	Less than 5% basophils,
	Platelets <450×10⁹/L
	Spleen nonpalpable
Complete cytogenetic response (CCyR)	No Ph+ metaphases
Partial cytogenetic response (PCyR)	1%–35% Ph+ metaphases
Minor cytogenetic response (mCyR)	36%–65% Ph+ metaphases
Minimal cytogenetic response (minCyR)	66%–94% Ph+ metaphases
No cytogenetic response (NoCyR)	≥95% Ph+ metaphases
Major molecular response (MMR)	BCR-ABL: ABL ≤0.1% on the International scale
Complete molecular response (CMR)	BCR-ABL transcript undetectable by RT-Q-PCR

TABLE 25.4 Definition of the Response to Frontline Treatment with Any Tyrosine Kinase Inhibitor

	Warnings	Failure	Optimal Response
Baseline	High-risk chronic myeloid leukemia or—clonal abnormalities in Ph+ cells	Not applicable	Not applicable
3 Mo	BCR-ABL1 >10%and/or Ph+ 36%–95%	No hematologic response and/or Ph+ >95%	BCR-ABL1 ≤10% and/or Ph+ ≤35%
6 Mo	BCR-ABL1 1%–10% and/or Ph+ 1%–35%	BCR-ABL1 >10% and/or Ph+ >35%	BCR-ABL1 <1% and/or Ph+ 0%
12 Mo	BCR-ABL1 >0.1%–1%	BCR-ABL1 >1% and/or Ph+ >0%	BCR-ABL1 ≤0.1%
Then, and at any time	Clonal abnormalities in Ph- cells (–7, or 7q–)	Loss of any aforementioned responses and/or acquisition of either BCR-ABL1 mutations and/or clonal chromosomal abnormalities in Ph+ cells	BCR-ABL1 ≤0.1%

The definitions are the same for patients in chronic phase, accelerated phase, and blastic phase and apply also to second-line treatment, when first-line treatment was changed for intolerance. The response can be assessed with either a molecular or a cytogenetic test, but both are recommended whenever possible.

Adapted from Baccarani M, Deininger MW, Rosti G, et al. European LeukemiaNet recommendations for the management of chronic myeloid leukemia: 2013. *Blood*. 2013;122: 872–884.

TABLE 25.5 Treatment Recommendations for Second Line and Subsequent Treatment for Chronic Phase Chronic Myeloid Leukemia*

Second line, secondary to intolerance to the first TKI
Any alternative TKI approved in the first line setting (imatinib, dasatinib, nilotinib)
Second line, secondary to failure of imatinib first line
One of the second generation TKIs (dasatinib, niltotinib, bosutinib)
HLA typing for patient and siblings
Second line, secondary to failure of dasatinib first line
One of the alternative second generation TKIs (niltotinib, bosutinib)
HLA typing for patient and siblings; search for an unrelated stem cell donor and consider allogeneic
    stem cell transplantation
Second line, secondary to failure of nilotinib first line
One of the alternative second generation TKIs (dasatinib, bosutinib)
HLA typing for patient and siblings; search for an unrelated stem cell donor and consider allogeneic
    stem cell transplantation
Third line, secondary to failure of and/or intolerance to 2 previous TKIs
Any alternative second or third generation TKI or omacetaxine
Allogeneic stem cell transplantation is recommended to all eligible patients
Any line, detection of T315I mutation
Ponatinib or omacetaxine
HLA typing for patient and siblings; search for an unrelated stem cell donor and consider allogeneic
    stem cell transplantation

Abbreviations: TKI, tyrosine kinase inhibitor.

*Taken into consideration the National Comprehensive Cancer Network (NCCN V1.2016) Guidelines and the European LeukemiaNet recommendations.

Second and Third Generation Tyrosine Kinase Inhibitors

Second-generation TKIs include dasatinib, nilotinib, and bosutinib that are more potent than IM. Dasatinib and nilotinib are approved for frontline therapy by the U.S. Food and Drug Administration. There remains no consensus on the preferred first line TKI, although there are experts who would advocate starting therapy with a second-generation TKI in light of better complete cytogenetic response and major molecular response (>75%) and lower rates of transformation to advanced phases with the newer agents. However, IM has the advantage of having the longest safety data, with expectations to be available in a generic form in the near future, and to-date there is no overall survival benefit shown with the use of the second generation TKIs. Awaiting longer term safety and efficacy data, baseline patient- and disease-factors as well as the availability, cost, and distinct safety profile for first and second generation TKIs may influence initial choice of treatment. Dasatinib can be associated with significant pleural effusions, increased bleeding risk secondary to platelet aggregation inhibition, and pulmonary artery hypertension, and hence it should be avoided in patients with underlying lung disease and/or at increased risk for bleeding. Nilotinib has been associated with prolonged QT interval, increased risk of vascular events (including peripheral artery occlusive disease), hyperglycemia, and pancreatitis; therfore, in presence of an alternative its use should be avoided in patients with cardiac arrhythmias, peripheral vascular disease, uncontrolled diabetes, and/or pancreatitis.

Bosutinib, a dual kinase inhibitor, has proven activity in imatinib-resistant CML patients with CCyR of approximately 40%. Bosutinib is not active against the T315I mutation, however it has shown activity in patients with BCR-ABL1 mutations resistant to dsastinib (F317L) and nilotinib (Y253H and F359C/I/V). There are several third-generation TKIs in the pipeline. These agents have activity against the BCR-ABL/T315I mutation that is mainly responsible for resistance to IM and second-generation TKIs. Ponatinib was approved recently by the FDA for use in patients failing second-generation TKIs or with the BCR-ABL/T315I mutation. Ponatinib has shown potent activity against several other BCR-ABL1 mutations. Because of its serious cardiovascular events, ponatinib use is limited to patients who have failed other TKIs and/or have T315I mutation. Recent data suggested a decreased risk of cardiovascular events at lower doses, and hence ongoing studies are assessing efficacy and safety of reduced-dose ponatinib. As more information is gathered regarding mutational status, better decisions can be made on the optimal TKI selection for CP patients. Currently, mutational status is checked at the time of failure of initial TKI therapy; however, the argument can be made that ascertaining mutational status at diagnosis leads to a decreased rate of failure and hence a better durable response by choosing the right TKI while the disease is at its earliest stage. This is a topic of ongoing clinical trials. For patients who are diagnosed in AP or BP, a second-generation TKI alone or combined with cytotoxic chemotherapy is recommended, followed by allogeneic stem cell transplant for eligible patients.

Omacetaxine

Homoharringtonine is a natural alkaloid that is obtained from various Cephalotaxus species and its mechanism of action is through inhibition of protein synthesis and promotion of apoptosis. The semisynthetic derivative, omacetaxine, has been shown to have benefit in IM-resistant CML and for those patients with T315I mutation. Evidence is based on two phase 2 studies. The first study examined the use of omacetaxine in patients with IM-resistant CML harboring T315I mutation and showed favorable complete hematologic response, major CyR and CCyR in 77, 23, and 16 percent, respectively. The second phase 2 study included patients who had failed or were intolerant to at least 2 TKIs. The CHR, MCyR, and CCyR were 70, 18, and 9 percent, respectively, with a median duration of response of 11 months. In a pooled analysis from the two aforementioned studies, omacetaxine was found to be effective in patients with advanced phase CML, particularly the AP with median PFS and OS of 4.8 and 17.6 months, respectively. The most frequent grade 3/4 toxicities are thrombocytopenia, neutropenia, anemia, and diarrhea. Omacetaxine is FDA approved for CML patients in CP or AP who had failed or were intolerant to at least two TKIs.

Allogeneic Stem Cell Transplantation

Allogeneic stem cell transplantation has been long shown to be the only potentially curative treatment for CML, and remains the most viable treatment option for patients diagnosed in AP, BP, or with known resistant mutations against TKIs. Despite the advances made with TKIs and long-term remissions exceeding 10 years in some patients, there is a consensus that current treatment is not curative, and should be continued indefinitely given the high risk of relapse after stopping TKIs. CML is a disease in which graft versus leukemia plays an important role and there are extensive reports of the use of donor lymphocyte infusions leading to durable complete remissions. An analysis from the Center for International Blood and Marrow Transplant Research (CIBMTR) reported outcomes on 2,444 patients who received myeloablative allogeneic stem cell transplant in first CP and survived in continuous complete remission for ≥5 years. OS for the entire patient population was 94% at 10 years and 87% at 15 years. Compared to matched general population, these patients had a 2.5 times higher risk of death at 10 years due to complications such as multiorgan failure, infection, graft versus host disease, relapsed disease, and secondary malignancies. However, mortality rates approached that of the general population at 15 years post–allogeneic transplant for those who survived. Improvements in HLA typing, management of infections, supportive care, conditioning regimens, and immunosuppressive agents have contributed to a significant improvement in transplant outcomes. Reduced-intensity regimens have been safely used in older patients and patients with comorbidities. In recent years, advances in alternative donor transplantation including the use of mismatched related donors and unrelated umbilical cord blood as stem cell sources have made allogeneic transplants available to patients that previously were unable to find a matched related or unrelated donor. Interestingly, patients who were resistant to TKIs prior to transplant become responsive posttransplant, which has prompted a number of studies that are evaluating the role of TKIs in the posttransplant setting.

Summary

Imatinib, dasatinib, and nilotinib are all approved and acceptable options for newly diagnosed chronic-phase CML. Treatment choice should be individualized based on cost, patient characteristics, and drug safety profile. After the failure of imatinib as frontline therapy, a second generation TKI such as dasatinib or nilotinib is recommended. When a second generation TKI is used as frontline therapy and fails, an alternate second generation TKI may be used. These patients may also be considered for allogeneic stem cell transplantation and/or enrollment in clinical trials. Ponatinib is considered after failure of other TKIs and is the treatment of choice for patients with T315I mutation. Omacetaxine is indicated for patients who have failed or are intolerant to at least two previous TKIs and is effective for patients with T315I mutation. Allogeneic stem cell transplantation remains the preferred choice for eligible high-risk patients such as those who have failed two TKIs, harbor T315I mutations, and those with advanced-stage CML.

Suggested Readings

1. Arber DA, Orazi A, Hasserjian R, et al. The 2016 revision to the World Health Organization classification of myeloid neoplasms and acute leukemia. *Blood.* 2016;127: 2391–2405.
2. Baccarani M, Deininger MW, Rosti G, et al. European LeukemiaNet recommendations for the management of chronic myeloid leukemia: 2013. *Blood.* 2013;122: 872–884.
3. Branford S. Chronic myeloid leukemia: molecular monitoring in clinical practice. *Hematology Am Soc Hematol Educ Program.* 2007;2007:376–383.
4. Breccia M, Alimena G. How to treat CML patients in the tyrosine kinase inhibitors era? From imatinib standard dose to second generation drugs front-line: unmet needs, pitfalls and advantages. *Cancer Lett.* 2012;322(2):127–132.
5. Champlin R, de Lima M, Kebriaei P, et al. Nonmyeloablative allogeneic stem cell transplantation for chronic myelogenous leukemia in the imatinib era. *Clin Lymphoma Myeloma.* 2009;9(suppl 3):S261–S265.
6. Cortes J, Kantarjian H. How I treat newly diagnosed chronic phase CML. *Blood.* 2012;120(7):1390–1397.
7. Druker BJ, Guilhot F, O'Brien SG, et al. Five-year follow-up of patients receiving imatinib mesylate for chronic myeloid leukemia. *N Engl J Med.* 2006;355:2408–2417.
8. Druker BJ, Talpaz M, Resta DJ, et al. Efficacy and safety of a specific inhibitor of the BCR-ABL tyrosine kinase in chronic myeloid leukemia. *N Engl J Med* 2001;344:1031–1037.
9. Goldman JM, Majhail NS, Klein JP, et al., Relapse and late mortality in 5-year survivors of myeloablative allogeneic hematopoietic cell transplantation for chronic myeloid leukemia in first chronic phase. *J Clin Oncol.* 2010;2811:1888-1895.
10. Gratwohl A, Brand R, Apperley J, et al. Allogeneic hematopoietic stem cell transplantation for chronic myeloid leukemia in Europe 2006: transplant activity, long-term data and current results. An analysis by the Chronic Leukemia Working Party of the European Group for Blood and Marrow Transplantation (EBMT). *Haematologica.* 2006;91:513–521.
11. Hasford J, Pfirrmann M, Hehlmann R, et al. A new prognostic score for survival of patients with chronic myeloid leukemia treated with interferon alfa. Writing Committee for the Collaborative CML Prognostic Factors Project Group. *J Natl Cancer Inst.* 1998;90:850–858.
12. Hehlmann R, Hochhaus A, Baccarani M, European LeukemiaNet. Chronic myeloid leukaemia. *Lancet.* 2007;370:342–350.
13. Jabbour E, Kantarjian H. Chronic myeloid leukemia: 2016 update on diagnosis, therapy and monitoring. *Am J Hematol.* 2016;91:252–265.
14. Kebriaei P, Detry MA, Giralt S, et al. Long-term follow-up of allogeneic hematopoietic stem-cell transplantation with reduced-intensity conditioning for patients with chronic myeloid leukemia. *Blood.* 2007;110:3456–3462.
15. O'Brien S, Radich JP, Abboud CN, et al. Chronic myelogenous leukemia, version 1.2015. *J Natl Compr Canc Netw.* 2014;12:1590–1610.
16. Rowley JD. A new consistent chromosomal abnormality in chronic myelogenous leukaemia identified by quinacrine fluorescence and Giemsa staining. *Nature.* 1973;243:290–293.
17. Sawyers CL. Chronic myeloid leukemia. *N Engl J Med.* 1999;340:1330–1340.
18. Shah NP. Medical management of CML. *Hematology Am Soc Hematol Educ Program.* 2007;2007:371–375.
19. Silver RT, Woolf SH, Hehlmann R, et al. An evidence-based analysis of the effect of busulfan, hydroxyurea, interferon, and allogeneic bone marrow transplantation in treating the chronic phase of chronic myeloid leukemia: developed for the American Society of Hematology. *Blood.* 1999;94:1517–1536.
20. Smith CC, Shah NP. Tyrosine kinase inhibitor therapy for chronic myeloid leukemia: approach to patients with treatment-naive or refractory chronic-phase disease. *Hematology Am Soc Hematol Educ Program.* 2011;2011:121–127.
21. Sokal JE. Prognosis in chronic myeloid leukaemia: biology of the disease vs. treatment. *Baillieres Clin Haematol.* 1987;1:907–929.
22. Srour SA, Devesa SS, Morton ML, et al. Incidence and patient survival of myeloproliferative neoplasms and myelodysplastic/myeloproliferative neoplasms in the United States, 2001-12. *Br J Haematol.* 2016;174:382–396.

Chronic Myeloproliferative Neoplasms **26**

Yogen Saunthararajah

INTRODUCTION

Chronic myeloproliferative neoplasms (MPNs) are clonal diseases of myeloid precursors that stand out clinically because of an increase in at least one peripheral blood count or a substantial increase in bone marrow fibrosis. The World Health Organization (WHO) recognizes the following entities (Table 26.1):

1. Chronic myelogenous leukemia (CML), *BCR-ABL* positive
2. Chronic neutrophilic leukemia (CNL)
3. Polycythemia vera (PV)
4. Primary myelofibrosis (PMF)—PMF, prefibrotic early stage; PMF, overt fibrotic stage
5. Essential thrombocythemia (ET)
6. Chronic eosinophilic leukemia, not otherwise specified (NOS)
7. MPN, unclassifiable

CML is discussed in Chapter 25 because of its unique treatment paradigm. This chapter is limited to a discussion of the three "classical" and more common MPNs: PV, ET, and PMF. These three neoplasms share clinical characteristics, including propensities to thrombosis and hemorrhage, splenomegaly, debilitating systemic symptoms, cytopenias of some lineages, and a risk of leukemic transformation. The overlap in clinical features, which sometimes confounds attempts at disease classification, reflects overlap at the level of causative mutations, illustrated by a common high frequency of the *JAK2* V617F mutation. Common biologic strands are revealed also by evolution of both PV and ET into PMF in some patients, and a common risk for transformation into acute myeloid leukemia (AML). Overlap can also occur with myelodysplastic syndromes (MDS), and MDS/MPN overlap neoplasm is a classification recognized by the WHO.

PATHOPHYSIOLOGY AND DIAGNOSIS

Molecular Mechanism

The MPNs are clonal diseases driven by combinations of molecular abnormalities, most of which can be found in all the MPN subtypes, although individual mutations do have specific clinicopathologic associations. For example, the *JAK2* mutation that substitutes phenylalanine for valine at position 617 (V617F) causes cytokine-independent (constitutive) activation of downstream messengers through the JAK-STAT, PI3K, and AKT pathways and is found in 95% of patients with PV and 50% to 60% with ET or idiopathic myelofibrosis. Mutated *JAK2* is found in >50% of patients with Budd-Chiari syndrome suggestive of a masked myeloproliferative disorder. The *CSF3R* mutation is strongly linked with CNL. Inactivating mutations in *EZH2* (a polycomb repressor complex component which is also deleted by chromosome 7q loss) are more evenly distributed, but do have an association with increased platelet

TABLE 26.1 The 2016 World Health Organization Classification Scheme for Myeloid Neoplasms (Sub-types of AML and MDS Not Shown)

1. Myeloproliferative neoplasms (MPN)
   3.1   Chronic myeloid leukemia (CML), *BCR-ABL*⁺
   3.2   Polycythemia vera (PV)
   3.3   Essential thrombocythemia (ET)
   3.4   Primary myelofibrosis (PMF)PMF, prefibrotic/early stage; PMF, overt fibrotic stage
   3.5   Chronic neutrophilic leukemia (CNL)
   3.6   Chronic eosinophilic leukemia, not otherwise specified (NOS)
   3.7   MPN, unclassifiable
2. MDS/MPN
   4.1   Chronic myelomonocytic leukemia (CMML)
   4.2   Juvenile myelomonocytic leukemia
   4.3   Atypical chronic myeloid leukemia (aCML), *BCR-ABL*⁻
   4.4   MDS/MPN with ring sideroblasts and thrombocytosis (MDS/MPN-RS-T)
   4.5   MDS/MPN unclassifiable
3. Myeloid neoplasms associated with eosinophilia and abnormalities of *PDGFRA, PDGFRB,* or *FGFR1*
   5.1   Myeloid neoplasms associated with *PDGFRA* rearrangement
   5.2   Myeloid neoplasms associated with *PDGFRB* rearrangement
   5.3   Myeloid neoplasms associated with *FGFR1* rearrangement (8p11 myeloproliferative syndrome)
4. Myelodysplastic syndromes (MDS)
5. Acute myeloid leukemia (AML)

counts. Inactivating mutations in another polycomb repressor component *ASXL1* are highly associated with PMF, and interestingly, with transformation of PV or ET into PMF. Thus, the improving knowledge regarding the molecular basis of MPNs is useful for diagnosis and prognosis (Table 26.2), and hopefully increasingly useful in guiding therapy. Testing for the *JAK2* V617F mutation by different techniques (polymerase chain reaction, restriction enzyme digestive pyrosequencing) is sensitive and specific, and readily available as a diagnostic tool.

Diagnosis and Distinguishing between the MPNs

The clinical presentation of MPNs can be with incidentally noted abnormal blood counts with patterns that vary depending on the particular MPN (Table 26.3). Distinctive clinical features relate to these lineage changes and splenomegaly.

■ **Symptoms and Signs:** Increased red blood cell (RBC) mass and thus viscosity in PV can produce symptoms such as headaches, vertigo, tinnitus, and blurred vision, as well as arterial or venous thrombotic events. Another characteristic of PV in some patients is pruritus (histamine release) aggravated by hot water. Increased number of abnormal platelets in ET can cause arterial thrombotic events such as cerebrovascular ischemia, digital ischemia/erythromelalgia, and spontaneous abortions. Anemia in patients with MF may cause fatigue and shortness of breath, and splenomegaly can cause abdominal discomfort or early satiety. Hypermetabolic symptoms such as weight loss and sweating can be seen in MF but also in the other MPNs. Symptom burden can be semi-quantified using the MPN Symptom Assessment form for 20 items (MPN-SAF). Obviously prior transfusion and treatment history is highly pertinent information.

■ **Bone marrow aspirate and biopsy:** Morphologic examination should incorporate trichome and reticulin stains. Standard metaphase karyotyping can be supplemented with fluorescence in situ hybridization (FISH) especially if *BCR-ABL*⁺ CML is in the differential diagnosis.

TABLE 26.2 WHO Diagnostic Criteria for Polycythemia Vera (PV), Essential Thrombocythemia (ET), and Primary Myelofibrosis (PMF)

	PV (Requires all 3 Major, or First 2 Major and the Minor Criterion	ET (Requires All 4 Major Criteria, or First 3 Major and the Minor Criterion)	PMF (Requires All 3 Major and at Least 1 Minor Criteria)
Major criteria	**1.** Hgb >16.5 g/dL (men), >16.0 g/dL (women) OR Hematocrit >49% (men), >48% (women) OR increased red cell mass >25% above mean normal predicted value **2.** BM biopsy showing hypercellularity for age with trilineage growth (panmyelosis) including prominent erythroid, granulocytic, and megakaryocytic proliferation with pleiomorphic, mature megakaryocytes **3.** Presence of *JAK2V617F* or *JAK2* exon 12 mutation	**1.** Platelet count ≥450 × 10⁹/L **2.** BM biopsy showing proliferation mainly of megakaryocytes with large and mature morphology; no significant increase or left shift in neutrophil or erythroid proliferation, and very rarely minor (grade 1) increase in reticulin fibers. **3.** Not meeting WHO criteria for *BCR-ABL*⁺CML, PV, PMF, MDS, or other myeloid neoplasms **4.** Presence of *JAK2, CALR, or MPL* mutation	**1.** Megakaryocyte proliferation and atypia (pre PMF=without reticulin fibrosis>grade1; overt PMF=reticulin and/or collagen fibrosis ≥grade2), accompanied by increased age-adjusted BM cellularity, granulocytic proliferation, and often, decreased erythropoiesis **2.** Not meeting WHO criteria for *BCR-ABL*⁺CML, PV, ET, MDS, or other myeloid neoplasms. **3.** Presence of *JAK2, CALR or MPL* mutation OR in the absence of these mutations, presence of another clonal marker OR absence of minor reactive BM reticulin fibrosis
Minor criteria	**1.** Subnormal serum erythropoietin level	**1.** Presence of a clonal marker or absence of evidence for reactive thrombocytosis	**1.** Anemia, not attributed to comorbidity **2.** Leukocytosis ≥11 x 10⁹/L **3.** Palpable splenomegaly **4.** LDH above upper limit of normal **5.** Leukoerythroblastosis (criterion for overt PMF)

▪ **Molecular testing:** For *JAK2* V617F mutation, and if negative, for *CALR* and *MPL* mutations if clinical impression is of ET or MF, and for *JAK2* Exon 12 mutations if clinical impression is of PV.
▪ **Other relevant labs:** Besides complete blood counts with differentials and peripheral smear, reticulocyte counts, LDH and D-dimer levels can be useful parameters to assist with evaluation and tracking of tumor burden and risks over-time. Serum erythropoietin levels and iron studies are pertinent also to diagnosis and management. Finally, human leukocyte antigen (HLA) testing and evaluation by a stem cell transplant team is appropriate for patients with PMF who might be stem cell transplant candidates.
▪ **Risk stratification** is discussed below in the context of management.

Diagnosis summary

As outlined earlier, there is overlap in the molecular underpinnings of MPNs, and thus, not surprisingly, in clinical behaviors. Nonetheless, the various MPN individual diagnoses do have differing types of complication, risks of complication, and prognoses. For example, prefibrotic (early) PMF, distinguishable from ET on the basis of BM morphology, has a higher risk of progressing to overt PMF or AML and has poorer survival than ET. Thus, there is clinical and treatment value in establishing a best-fit

TABLE 26.3 Distinguishing Clinical Features of the Myeloproliferative Neoplasms

	CML	PV	ET	PMF
Hematocrit	N or ↓	↑↑	N	↓
WBC count	↑↑↑	↑	N	↑ or ↓
Platelet count	↑ or ↓	↑	↑↑↑	↑ or
Splenomegaly	++++	+	+	++++
Cytogenetic abnormality	Ph chromosome	±	–	±
LAP score[a]	↓	↑↑	N or ↑	N or ↑
Marrow fibrosis	±	± or ↓	±	++++ (Dry tap)
Marrow cellularity	↑↑↑ Myeloid	↑↑	↑↑ Megakaryocytes	N or ↓
Basophils ≥2%	+	±	±	Usually +

[a] See Chapter 24.

CML, chronic myeloid leukemia; PV, polycythemia vera; ET, essential thrombocytopenia; MF, myelofibrosis; N, normal; WBC, white blood cell; LAP, leukocyte alkaline phosphatase; MPN, myeloproliferative neoplasm.

specific diagnosis. CML should be ruled out by performing a FISH analysis for *BCR-ABL* in JAK2 mutation-negative thrombocytosis or bone marrow fibrosis. Even with a positive JAK2 mutation or other clinical and peripheral blood observations to favor a particular MPN classification, bone marrow biopsy with cytogenetic analysis is recommended, to not miss a diagnosis of CML or MDS with accompanying prognostic and treatment implications. Platelet function tests or bleeding times are of little use in diagnosing or in guiding the management of MPNs.

PROGNOSIS

Median Survivals

- Patients with PV have a median survival of 1.5 to 13 years. In a recent multicountry prospective study of 1,638 patients with PV, the 5-year event-free survival was 82%, with a relatively low risk of death from cardiovascular disease and a high risk of death from noncardiovascular causes (mainly hematologic transformations).
- Patients with ET have a median survival of more than 10 years.
- Patients with MF have a median survival between 3 and 5 years.

Rate of Transformation to Acute Leukemia

- The estimated incidence of acute leukemia in 1,638 patients with PV prospectively followed in the European collaboration study on low-dose aspirin in polycythemia (ECLAP) study was 1.3%, with an estimated annual incidence of 0.5 per 100,000 per year. Older age and exposure to P32, busulfan, or pipobroman were independent risk factors.
- The cumulative rate of transformation for patients with ET is 2% to 4%, respectively, at 10 and 20 years from diagnosis.
- The cumulative rate of transformation for patients with MF is 10% at 10 years (please also see discussions on treatment regarding transformation risk).

Transformation of PV or ET into PMF

Both PV and ET may progress to post-PV PMF or post-ET PMF, previously referred to as the spent phase, which clinically resembles PMF and is characterized by progressive cytopenias, splenomegaly, and marrow fibrosis. The cumulative rate of transformation is 5% and 10% at 10 to 20 years, respectively, for ET, and 10% to 20% for the same time line for PV.

Risk Factors for Thrombosis

In two prospective studies, the ECLAP study and the MRC-PT1, the cumulative rate of cardiovascular events in patients with PV ranged from 2.5% to 5% per patient-year and from 1.9% to 3% per patient-year for patients with ET. Arterial thrombosis accounts for 60% to 70% of the events, and is the major cause of death.

- In PV, older age (>60), a hematocrit ≥45%, and a previous history of thrombosis are risk factors. Surgery should be avoided in patients until a hematocrit <45% has been maintained for more than 2 months.
- In ET, age over 60 years and the presence of other cardiovascular risk factors (e.g., smoking and previous thrombosis) increase the risk for thrombosis.

    In ET, an association between platelet count and thrombosis has not been established, but platelet cytoreduction on treatment with hydroxyurea (HU) has been associated with a *reduced* risk.

Risk Factors for Hemorrhage

- In ET, a platelet count >2 × 10^6/μL is a risk factor for hemorrhage (please also see the recommendations regarding treatment).

TREATMENT

As a general principle, treatment for PV, ET, PMF, or overlaps thereof is aimed at (i) alleviating the particular symptoms present in the individual patient (e.g., symptoms from splenomegaly, pruritus, cytopenias) and (ii) anticipating and preventing potential life-threatening complications or risks such as thrombosis or hemorrhage. Accordingly, management is guided by formal assessments of risk as described below. Bone marrow transplantation is a potentially curative option that should be considered for some patients with PMF. Following is a definition of risk categories and recommended treatments, with an overview provided in Table 26.4.

Polycythemia Vera

- **Low risk:** Age <60 years and no personal history of vascular events, and who do not have additional risk factors for cardiovascular disease. Recommended treatment: phlebotomy alone (target hematocrit <45%) with or without low-dose aspirin (81–100 mg/day).
- **High risk:** Age ≥60 years and/or a prior history of thrombosis. Recommended treatment: HU (with or without concomitant phlebotomy) and low-dose aspirin.

Maintaining a hematocrit <45% dramatically decreases the incidence of thrombotic complications. This is important, since in PV, 35% of initial thrombotic events are fatal. A randomized study of 518 patients with PV has shown that treatment with low-dose aspirin (100 mg per day) lowers the risk of cardiovascular death, nonfatal myocardial infarction, and nonfatal stroke. For females, a lower threshold of <42% can be considered, especially if there are persistent or progressive symptoms.

- **Post-PV/ET PMF:** Please see PMF management.
- **Pruritus:** Intractable pruritus responds to IFN-α in up to 81% of patients. In low-risk patients in whom IFN-α is not indicated, paroxetine, a selective serotonin reuptake inhibitor, can alleviate symptoms in most cases.
- **Hyperuricemia:** Allopurinol should be started before chemotherapy to decrease the risk of urate nephropathy (300 mg per day given orally; dose reduction needed in renal insufficiency).

Essential Thrombocythemia

Treatment is primarily directed at preventing thrombosis and/or hemorrhage, and risk stratification is mostly a means to guide the use of cytoreductive treatments, to avoid potential risks of triggering more aggressive transformation of disease by unnecessary early application of cytotoxic/cytostatic treatment with hydroxyurea. Other cardiovascular risk factors should be concurrently managed.

- **Very Low risk:** Age ≤60 years, no *JAK2* mutation, no history of thrombosis.

TABLE 26.4 Current Management Depending on Risk Stratification in PV, ET, and MF

Risk Category	PV	ET	PMF
Low	Low-dose aspirin (81–100 mg/day) + phlebotomy to maintain hematocrit <45% (consider <42% for females or if symptoms persist or progress)	Observation or low-dose aspirin (also for very low risk)	Individualize per predominant symptoms (e.g., anemia, splenomegaly, constitutional). Managing patients with both splenomegaly and cytopenias is where difficulties arise—consider pegylated IFN-α or DNMT1-depleting drugs (decitabine or 5-azacytidine) in such subjects. Please see text
Intermediate		Low-dose aspirin ± hydroxyurea	Consider stem cell transplant in transplant eligible intermediate-2 or high-risk subjects.
High	Low-dose aspirin + phlebotomy + hydroxyurea. Alternative to hydroxyurea for cytoreduction are IFN-α or ruxolitinib	Low-dose aspirin + hydroxyurea. Alternative to hydroxyurea for cytoreduction is IFN-α especially for patients <60 years old	

PV, polycythemia vera; ET, essential thrombocytopenia; PMF, myelofibrosis.

Recommended treatment: observation or low-dose aspirin, especially if there are symptoms or cardiovascular risk factors (e.g., smoking). Cytoreductive therapy is not an upfront consideration, but could be needed for progressive increase in platelet counts to $\geq 1,500 \times 10^9$/L. In this instance, also consider possibility of acquired von Willebrand's disease (ristocetin cofactor activity <30%). Other reasons to consider cytoreductive therapy are symptomatic splenomegaly or thrombocytosis, B-symptoms, new thrombosis or hemorrhage, or progressive thrombocytosis or leukocytosis. If cytoreductive treatment needed, consider IFN-α rather than hydroxyurea in these younger patients.

■ **Low risk:** As above but with *JAK2* mutation.

Recommended treatment: As above.

■ **Intermediate risk:** Age >60 years, no JAK2 mutation, no history of thrombosis.

Recommended treatment: Aspirin 81–100 mg. In addition, cytoreductive therapy with hydroxyurea or IFN-α could be an upfront consideration.

■ **High risk:** Age >60 years and/or a previous history of thrombosis.

Recommended treatment: Aspirin 81–100 mg/day and in addition, cytoreduction with hydroxyurea or IFN-α.

A randomized trial of hydroxyurea versus placebo in 114 high-risk patients showed a significant reduction of thrombotic events in the treatment arm (3.6% vs. 24%). The hydroxyurea dose was adjusted to achieve a platelet count of $<600 \times 10^9$/L. Anagrelide is a nonmutagenic orally active agent that produces selective platelet cytoreduction by interfering with megakaryocyte maturation. In a randomized study of 809 patients with high-risk ET, hydroxyurea plus low-dose aspirin was superior to anagrelide plus low-dose aspirin. IFN-α can also effectively cause platelet cytoreduction and is preferred in younger patients. The therapeutic target platelet count in this trial was <400 × 10⁹/L. Plateletpheresis is used as an emergency therapy when ongoing thrombosis cannot be adequately managed with chemotherapy and antithrombotic agents.

Myelofibrosis

Risk stratification by the Dynamic International Prognostic Scoring System Plus (DIPSS Plus) determines whether a patient should be considered upfront for stem cell transplant if they are a transplant candidate (for DIPSS intermediate-2 or high-risk patients). Otherwise, for low risk or intermediate-1 risk patients, or non-transplant candidate higher risk patients, management is directed toward relieving symptoms caused by splenomegaly or cytopenias, and decreasing risk of further progression.

▪ Risk stratification by DIPSS Plus: one point each for age >65 years, white blood cell count >25 × 10⁹/L, circulating blast cells ≥1%, presence of constitutional symptoms, unfavorable karyotype, platelet count <100 × 10⁹/L, and transfusion dependence, and two points for hemoglobin <10 g/dL.

Low risk: 0 points, median survival 20 years. *Intermediate risk-1*: 1 point, median survival 6.5 years. *Intermediate risk-2*: 2 to 3 points, median survival 2.9 years. *High risk*: 4 to 6 points, median survival 1.7 years.

Anemia: Androgens (e.g., danazol) combined with prednisone (prednisone is tapered after a few weeks) is an option, with the caution that danazol can potentially exacerbate thrombotic risk. There is some data to support use of lenalidomide (especially if there is a 5q– chromosome abnormality) or thalidomide combined with prednisone, although again, possible increase in thrombotic risk should be considered with thalidomide, and results have been mixed. Erythropoietin replacement is a consideration in patients with inappropriately low erythropoietin levels (<500 mU/mL in the setting of anemia can be considered as inappropriately low). DNMT1-depleting drugs (decitabine or 5-azacytidine) that are approved for treatment of MDS can also alleviate anemia and thrombocytopenia in PMF, and can be considered, although the optimal doses and regimens to use, especially for decitabine, are still being evaluated, with lower dose, more frequent administration likely to be more rational based on mechanism of action (5-azacytidine and decitabine are both pro-drugs that are metabolized differently and it is possible that decitabine could have more activity than 5-azacytidine in the context of PMF cellular metabolism). Transfusion needs may diminish after splenectomy (see below). Iron chelation may be indicated for transfusion-dependent patients.

Splenomegaly: Options include JAK2 inhibitor (ruxolitinib) if there is no significant anemia and platelets are >50 x10⁹/L, although the currently approved dosages may be unnecessarily high, and it may be appropriate to start with lower than standard dosages with an escalation if necessary. The main cautions are that ruxolitinib has a high chance of lowering platelet and hemoglobin levels, which is why it may be appropriate to sometimes start at lower than approved doses in the package insert, and for rebound disease growth and inflammatory symptoms if the drugs are discontinued abruptly (dosage should be tapered off rather than abruptly discontinued). Lenalidomide can be considered if there is a 5q– abnormality. HU can be considered, with dose modifications depending on cytopenias. Difficulties arise when confronted with symptomatic splenomegaly and clinically significant anemia or thrombocytopenia. Other treatment options to consider in this circumstance, with an eye to ongoing clinical trials, are pegylated IFN-α or DNMT1-depleting drugs (decitabine or 5-azacytidine). Splenectomy is an option to alleviate pain and early satiety, depending on local surgical experience and thus surgical risk. Secondary progressive hepatomegaly is a potential long-term complication of splenectomy. Increasing white blood cell counts and platelet counts after splenectomy may necessitate HU therapy. Also a possible consideration depending on local expertize is splenic artery embolization via interventional radiology. Analgesia may be required for splenic infarct pain, whether or not a patient has splenic artery embolization.

Curative therapy: Allogeneic transplantation should be considered for intermediate-2 or high risk patients who are transplant candidates. Five-year survivals with a related or an unrelated matched transplant have been reported at 54% and 48%, respectively, by the European Group for Blood and

Marrow Transplantation (EBMT). A recommendation for transplantation is not clear-cut in lower risk patients because the median survival in this group is >14 years with non-transplant therapy. In other words, risk classification should be considered, and although the outcome with transplantation is adversely affected by risky characteristics, risk factors such as hemoglobin level <10 g/dL; white blood cell count <4 × 10³/µL or >30 × 10³/µL; more than 10% of circulating blasts, promyelocytes, or myelocytes; or abnormal cytogenetics should prompt consideration for transplantation. Pretransplantation splenectomy, although not necessary in every patient, is associated with faster engraftment and can be considered in those with massive splenomegaly. Marrow fibrosis is reversible with transplantation.

Suggested Readings

1. Arber DA, Orazi A, Hasserjian R, Thiele J, Borowitz MJ, Le Beau MM, Bloomfield CD, Cazzola M, Vardiman JW. The 2016 revision to the World Health Organization classification of myeloid neoplasms and acute leukemia. *Blood.* 2016 May 19;127(20):2391–2405.
2. Gangat N, Caramazza D, Vaidya R, et al. DIPSS plus: a refined dynamic international prognostic scoring system for primary myelofibrosis that incorporates prognostic information from karyotype, platelet count, and transfusion status. *J Clin Oncol.* 2011;29(4):392–397.
3. Harrison CN, Campbell PJ, Buck G, et al. Hydroxyurea compared with anagrelide in high-risk essential thrombocythemia. *N Engl J Med.* 2005;353:33–45.
4. Landolfi R, Marchioli R, Kutti J, et al. Efficacy and safety of low-dose aspirin in polycythemia vera (ECLAP study). *N Engl J Med.* 2004;350:114–124.
5. Saunthararajah Y, Maciejewski J. Polycomb segment myeloid malignancies. *Blood.* 2012;119(5):1097–1098.
6. Spivak J. Polycythemia vera: myths, mechanisms, and management. *Blood.* 2002;100:4272–4290.
7. Vannucchi AM, Harrison CN. Emerging treatments for classical myeloproliferative neoplasms. *Blood.* 2017 Feb 9;129(6):693–703.

Multiple Myeloma 27

Arjun Lakshman and Shaji K. Kumar

INTRODUCTION

Multiple myeloma (MM) is characterized by clonal proliferation of plasma cells in the bone marrow, often producing a monoclonal immunoglobulin. This can result in hypercalcemia, renal dysfunction, anemia, or extensive skeletal destruction with osteolytic lesions that are the major presenting signs of the disease. Unlike most other malignancies, diagnosis requires the presence of these clinical features and its attribution to clonal plasma cell proliferation. Recently, the diagnostic criteria have been updated to include biomarkers predictive of high risk of developing the above clinical features. Newer active agents and autologous stem cell transplantation (ASCT) have led to improvement in outcomes, from a median survival of 3 years in the late 1990s to nearly 8 years currently, a metric that continues to get better.

EPIDEMIOLOGY

MM accounts for 1.8% of all cancers and about 10% of all hematologic malignancies. In 2017, it is estimated that 30,280 new cases and 12,590 deaths from MM will occur in the United States. The annual age-adjusted incidence in the United States is approximately 6.6 per 100,000 and has remained stable over time. The median age at diagnosis is about 69 years and MM is slightly more common in men than in women (1.6:1). Incidence in the African American population is two- to threefold higher than that in Caucasians, whereas it is lower in Asians. The risk of developing MM is approximately 3.7-fold higher in individuals with a first-degree relative of MM.

PATHOPHYSIOLOGY

MM is characterized by the proliferation and accumulation of clonal plasma cells in the bone marrow. Almost all patients with MM evolve from an underlying, asymptomatic monoclonal gammopathy of undetermined significance (MGUS). Prevalence of MGUS is over 3% above the age of 50 years, and the rate of progression to MM is roughly 1% per year, a risk that does not change with time from diagnosis. Studies suggest that patients with myeloma typically have MGUS for an average of 15 years before development of symptomatic myeloma. Some patients may also develop an intermediate, more advanced stage referred to as smoldering multiple myeloma (SMM) that is defined clinically (Table 27.1). The risk of progression of SMM to symptomatic myeloma is about 10% per year over the first 5 years after diagnosis, about 3% per year for the next 5 years, and 1% per year from then on.

The clonal plasma cells in myeloma are characterized by recurrent genetic abnormalities, with the majority having one or more well-characterized abnormalities. Five recurrent translocations involving the heavy chain locus on chromosome 14 have been identified and are present in approximately 40% of all patients. Trisomies of odd-numbered chromosomes are detected in nearly half of the patients, with monosomies or deletions of other chromosomes overlapping with these two sets of abnormalities. The clinical features of MM are a result of bone marrow infiltration by the malignant clone, damage from high levels of immunoglobulins or free light chains (FLCs) in the circulation or glomeruli, the secretion of osteoclast-activating factors such as RANKL (receptor activator of nuclear factor-κB ligand) and MIP-1 (macrophage inflammatory protein-1) with resultant bone damage, decreased production of the natural RANKL inhibitor OPG (osteoprotegerin), overexpression of dickkopf 1 inhibiting osteoblast differentiation and new bone formation, and impaired immunity, both cell-mediated and humoral.

CLINICAL FEATURES

Bone pain, particularly in the back or chest, and less often in the extremities, is present in nearly 60% of patients with MM. Patients may present with pathologic fractures and can also have loss of height

TABLE 27.1 International Myeloma Working Group Criteria for Diagnosis of Multiple Myeloma and Related Plasma Cell Disorders

Terminology	Definition
Non-IgM monoclonal gammopathy of undetermined significance (MGUS)[a]	■ Serum monoclonal protein (non-IgM type) <3 g/dL AND ■ Clonal bone marrow plasma cells <10% AND ■ Absence of end-organ damage [hypercalcemia, renal insufficiency, anemia, and bone lesions (CRAB)] attributable to the plasma cell proliferative disorder
Smoldering multiple myeloma	■ Serum monoclonal protein (IgG or IgA) ≥3 g/dL, or urinary monoclonal protein ≥500 mg/24 hours and/or clonal bone marrow plasma cells 10%–60% AND ■ Absence of myeloma defining events or amyloidosis
Multiple myeloma	■ Clonal bone marrow plasma cells ≥10% or biopsy-proven bony or extramedullary plasmacytoma[b] AND ■ One or more of the myeloma defining events (MDEs): 1. Evidence of end organ damage attributable to the underlying plasma cell proliferative disorder, specifically: 　a. Hypercalcemia: serum calcium >1 mg/dL higher than the upper limit of normal or >11 mg/dL 　b. Renal insufficiency: creatinine clearance <40 mL per minute or serum creatinine >2 mg/dL 　c. Anemia: hemoglobin >2 g/dL below the lower limit of normal, or a hemoglobin <10 g/dL 　d. Bone lesions: one or more osteolytic lesions on skeletal radiography, computed tomography (CT), or positron emission tomography-CT (PET-CT) 2. One or more of the biomarkers of malignancy 　a. Clonal bone marrow plasma cell percentage ≥60% 　b. Involved: uninvolved serum free light chain (FLC) ratio ≥100 (involved free light chain level must be >10 mg/dL) 　c. >1 focal lesions on magnetic resonance imaging (MRI) studies
Light chain MGUS	■ Abnormal free light chain (FLC) ratio (<0.26 or >1.65) AND ■ Increased level of the appropriate involved light chain (increased kappa FLC in patients with ratio >1.65 and increased lambda FLC in patients with ratio <0.26) AND ■ No immunoglobulin heavy chain expression on immunofixation AND ■ Absence of end-organ damage attributable to the plasma cell proliferative disorder AND ■ Clonal bone marrow plasma cells <10% AND ■ Urinary monoclonal protein <500 mg/24 hours

(continued)

TABLE 27.1 (Continued)

Terminology	Definition
Solitary plasmacytoma[c]	▪ Biopsy proven solitary lesion of clonal plasma cells involving bone or soft tissue AND ▪ No evidence of clonal plasma cells in bone marrow AND ▪ Normal skeletal survey and MRI (or CT) of spine and pelvis (except for the primary solitary lesion) AND ▪ Absence of end-organ damage (hypercalcemia, renal insufficiency, anemia, or bone lesions) attributable to a lymphoplasma cell proliferative disorder

[a] IgM MGUS is defined by IgM monoclonal protein <3g/dL in serum, <10% bone marrow infiltration by lymphoplasmacytic cells and absence of any end organ damage that can be attributed to underlying lymphoproliferative disorder.

[b] Approximately 4% of patients may have fewer than 10% bone marrow plasma cells since marrow involvement may be focal, or they may have multifocal plasmacytomas. Such patients should undergo repeat bone marrow biopsy or CT/MRI guided biopsy of a bony or extramedullary lesion.

[c] Solitary plasmacytoma with minimal marrow involvement is defined as a biopsy proven bony or soft tissue plasmacytoma with <10% clonal bone marrow plasma cells, and no other myeloma defining event other than the primary solitary lesion. Solitary lesion with ≥10% clonal plasma cells is considered as multiple myeloma.

Adapted from Rajkumar SV, Dimopoulos MA, Palumbo A, et al. International Myeloma Working Group updated criteria for the diagnosis of multiple myeloma. *Lancet Oncol.* 2014;15:e538–548.

because of vertebral collapse. Other common clinical features include fatigue (32%), weight loss (24%), normocytic normochromic anemia (73%), and hypercalcemia (28%). MM can also result in a low anion gap due to severe hypercalcemia and/or the cationic immunoglobin molecule. Renal insufficiency is seen in almost half the patients with MM at diagnosis and is commonly caused by hypercalcemia and related dehydration, or light chain cast nephropathy. Other etiologies may include renal amyloidosis, light chain deposition disease, cryoglobulinemia, or drug-induced kidney injury. In some patients, concurrent light chain amyloidosis can cause nephrotic syndrome (<5%). Acquired Fanconi syndrome with glycosuria, phosphaturia, and aminoaciduria can also occur with MM. MM patients are at an increased risk for infection due to impaired lymphocyte function, suppression of normal plasma cell function, and hypogammaglobulinemia. Patients can also present with radiculopathy or spinal cord compression that can result from compression of nerve roots by paravertebral plasmacytoma or by a fractured vertebral body. Peripheral neuropathy can be present at diagnosis, and can be related to the monoclonal protein or to concomitant amyloidosis.

DIAGNOSIS AND WORKUP

Diagnosis of MM requires evidence of clonal plasma cell proliferation with the presence of end-organ damage (hypercalcemia, renal insufficiency, anemia, or bone lesions) attributable to the plasma cell disorder or presence of biomarkers predicting for a high risk of progression to symptomatic myeloma. The criteria for diagnosis of monoclonal gammopathies were recently updated by the International Myeloma Working Group (IMWG) and are shown in Table 27.1. When MM is suspected, the diagnostic workup should include a thorough history and physical examination with specific attention to complaints of bone pain, constitutional symptoms, neurologic symptoms, and infections. In addition, for diagnosis and staging, these labs should be performed: complete blood count with differential; serum electrolytes, blood urea nitrogen, serum creatinine, calcium, phosphate, magnesium, uric acid, albumin, β_2-microglobulin, lactate dehydrogenase, serum protein electrophoresis (SPEP) and immunofixation

(IFE), serum FLC assay, 24-hour urine protein electrophoresis (UPEP) and IFE, quantitative immuno-globulins, radiographic skeletal survey, and bone marrow aspirate and biopsy with interphase fluores-cent in situ hybridization (FISH) testing of the plasma cells.

SPEP is useful in detecting and quantifying the presence of an intact monoclonal protein (M-protein) that is visualized as an M-spike in the gamma region. Serum IFE confirms the presence of the monoclo-nal immunoglobulin and, more importantly, determines its type (Fig. 27.1). SPEP and/or serum IFE is sometimes inadequate as approximately 15% of patients have only light chains (light chain myeloma), which may rapidly be cleared from the plasma to the urine. Hence, serum FLCs, UPEP, and/or urine IFE should be performed in all patients.

SPEP detects an M-spike in 82% of patients with MM. Addition of serum IFE increases the sensitiv-ity to 93%. The sensitivity increases to 97% or more if either the serum FLC assay or 24 hour UPEP/urine IFE is performed in addition. Patients who lack detectable M-protein by any of these tests, but have end-organ damage and clonal plasma cells in the bone marrow, are considered to have nonsecre-tory myeloma. The circulating M-protein on IFE is IgG in 52% of cases, IgA in 21%, light chain only (kappa or lambda) in 16%, IgD in 2%, and biclonal in 2%. IgM myeloma is exceedingly rare and is seen in <1% of cases. Kappa is the predominant light chain isotype compared with lambda (ratio 2:1), except in IgD myeloma, where lambda isotype is more common.

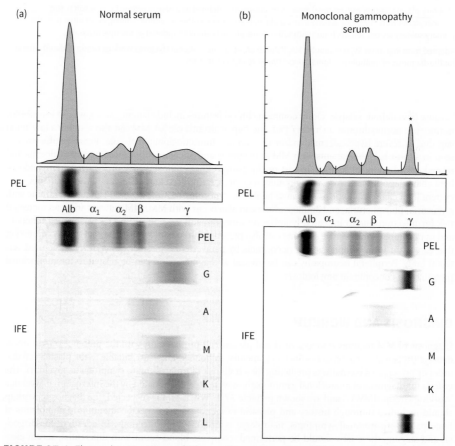

FIGURE 27.1 Electrophoretic pattern of (A) normal human serum and (B) immunoglobulin G (IgG lambda) multiple myeloma. Asterisk indicates M spike in the gamma region.

Bone marrow studies should include FISH testing designed to detect t(11;14), t(4;14), t(14;16), t(6;14), t(14;20), hyperdiploidy, 1q amplification, 1p deletion, and deletion 17p for risk stratification. Conventional metaphase cytogenetics is productive in only a third of the patients given the low proliferative rate of plasma cells, and can provide limited prognostic value and is increasingly being discarded in favor of FISH and newer approaches. Gene expression profiling, when available, may also be considered for additional prognostic information. More recently, mutation panels that examine the plasma cells for common recurrent mutations have become available, but the clinical utiity remains to be demonstrated.

Radiologic changes seen on a skeletal survey include punched-out lytic lesions, severe osteopenia or osteoporosis, and pathologic fractures. There is increasing use of whole-body low dose CT scan given the higher sensitivity of this technique in detecting myeloma bone lesions. A nuclear medicine bone scan is not useful in MM because lytic lesions are not visualized on bone scans. Routine fluoro-deoxyglucose positron emission tomography/computed tomography (PET-CT) and magnetic resonance imaging (MRI) scans are not needed for every patient, but are indicated when symptomatic areas show no abnormality on a radiographic skeletal survey or when there is uncertainty about the true extent of bone disease on radiographs alone. Another indication where these scans should be utilized is when solitary plasmacytoma is suspected, to reliably rule out bony or extramedullary disease. Imaging studies also play a key role in identifiying patients with SMM who are at high risk of progression to myeloma, as well as discriminating between SMM and active MM based on the revised diagnostic criteria. Any patient with significant back pain should also undergo MRI of the spine to evaluate for cord compression.

STAGING

Two main staging systems exist for MM that primarily reflect tumor burden: the International staging system (ISS) that is based on laboratory values and the Durie-Salmon staging system, predominantly a clinical system. Both of these provide prognostic information but are not helpful in making therapeutic choices. Of these, the ISS had become the preferred staging system because of its simplicity and lack of subjectivity (Table 27.2). Recently, the ISS staging system has been revised with the inclusion of cytogenetic abnormalities and LDH, resulting in an improved prognostic and staging system that incorporates some aspects of diease biology.

PROGNOSIS

Prognosis in myeloma depends on host factors (age, performance status, and comorbidities), stage, disease aggressiveness, and response to therapy. Other laboratory parameters such as creatinine, calcium, lactate dehydrogenase, immunoglobulin subtype, plasmablastic morphology, circulating plasma cells, and C-reactive protein have also been shown to be independent risk factors for survival in myeloma. A high plasma-cell proliferative rate also strongly predicts poor prognosis, but this test is not commonly available. A risk stratification model based on independent molecular cytogenetic markers to assess disease aggressiveness has been found useful for both prognosis and therapeutic decision-making. Newly diagnosed patients can be stratified using these markers as having standard-, intermediate-, and high-risk disease based on the Mayo stratification of myeloma and risk-adapted therapy (mSMART) classification (Table 27.3). The IMWG criteria groups patients into standard risk and high risk myeloma based on age, disease stage, and cytogenetic abnormalities (Table 27.2). Median survival varies from 8 to 10 years for standard-risk patients versus 2 to 3 years for high-risk myeloma. Major progresses has been made in understanding the impact of genomic abnormalities on the outcome of patients in MM. Gene expression profiling has identified several signatures that allow for prognostication in patients with myeloma and at least two of these are available for use in the clinic.

TABLE 27.2 Staging and Risk stratification of Multiple Myeloma

Stage	Criteria	Percentage of Patients	Median Survival (mo)
	Durie and Salmon Staging[a]		
I	Low measured myeloma cell mass—all of the following: Hemoglobin >10g/dL Serum calcium <12 mg/dL On x-ray, normal bone structure, or solitary plasmacytoma only Low M-component production (IgG<5g/dL, IgA<3g/dL, and Urine M-component <4g/24 hours)		
II	Intermediate myeloma cell mass—Fitting neither stage I or stage III		
III	High myeloma cell mass—one or more of the following: Hemoglobin <8.5g/dL Serum calcium >12mg/dL Advanced lytic bone lesions High M-component production (IgG>7g/dL, IgA>5g/dL, and Urine M-component >12g/24 hours)		
	International Stating System (ISS)		
I	Serum β_2-microglobulin <3.5 mg/L Serum albumin ≥3.5 g/dL	28	62
II	Not fitting stage I or III	33	44
III	Serum β_2-microglobulin ≥5.5 mg/L	39	29
	Revised International Staging System (R-ISS)[b]		
I	ISS stage I and no high-risk cytogenetics by FISH and normal LDH	28%	Not reached
II	Not R-ISS stage I or II	62%	83
III	ISS stage III and either high-risk cytogenetics by FISH or high LDH	10%	43
	International Myeloma Working group risk stratification		
Low risk	ISS I/II and absence of t(4;14), del(17p), and +1q21 and age<55 years	20%	>120
Standard risk	Neither high risk nor low risk	60%	72
High risk	ISS II/III and t(4;14) and/or del(17p)	20%	24

FISH- interphase fluorescent in situ hybridization; LDH- lactate dehydrogenase.

[a] Durie and Salmon stages are subdivided into A (serum creatinine<2 mg/dL) and B (serum creatinine ≥2mg/dL).

[b] High-risk cytogenetics on FISH of plasma cells is defined as presence of del(17p) and/or t(4;14) and/or t(14;16).

Adapted from 1. Durie BG, Salmon SE. A clinical staging system for multiple myeloma. Correlation of measured myeloma cell mass with presenting clinical features, response to treatment, and survival. *Cancer* 1975; 36:842; 2. Greipp PR, San Miguel J, Durie BG, et al. International staging system for multiple myeloma. *J Clin Oncol*. 2005;23(15):3412–3420.; 3. Palumbo A, Avet-Loiseau H, Oliva S, et al. Revised International Staging System for Multiple Myeloma: A Report from International Myeloma Working Group. *J Clin Oncol*. 2015;33:2863; and 4. Chng WJ, Dispenzieri A, Chim C-S, et al. IMWG consensus on risk stratification of multiple myeloma. *Leukemia*. 2014; 28(2):269–277.

TABLE 27.3 Mayo Stratification of Myeloma and Risk-Adapted Therapy (mSMART) classification of Multiple Myeloma

	High Risk	Intermediate Risk[a]	Standard Risk[a,b]
Incidence	20%	20%	60%
Median overall survival (years)	3	4–5	8–10
Characteristic	Del 17p[c]	t(4;14)	All others
	t(14;16)[c]	Del 13 or hypodiploidy by	including:
	t(14; 20)[c]	conventional karyotyping	Hyperdiploidy
	High-risk signature	Plasma cell labelling index ≥3%	t(11;14)[d]
	on gene expression		t(6;14)
	profiling		

Chromosomal abnormalities are based on FISH analysis unless specified.

[a] A subset of patients will be classified as high risk by gene expression profiling.

[b] Lactate dehydrogenase >upper limit of normal and beta-2-microglobulin >5.5 mg/dL may indicate worse prognosis.

[c] Trisomies may ameliorate the high risk.

[d] t(11;14) may be associated with plasma cell leukemia.

Adapted from Mikhael JR, Dingli D, Roy V, et al. Management of newly diagnosed symptomatic multiple myeloma: updated Mayo Stratification of Myeloma and Risk-Adapted Therapy (mSMART) consensus guidelines 2013. *Mayo Clin Proc.* 2013;88(4):360–376 and www.msmart.org.

TREATMENT

General

Monoclonal Gammopathy of Undetermined Significance

Risk-stratification models have been proposed for predicting the progression of monoclonal gammopathy of undetermined significance (MGUS) and assist in detecting patients with higher risk of progression to myeloma. Patients with all three risk factors consisting of a serum M-protein ≥1.5 g/dL, IgA or IgM MGUS, and an abnormal serum FLC ratio have a risk of progression at 20 years of 58%, compared with 37% when two risk factors are present, 21% when one risk factor is present and only 5% when none of the risk factors are present. Patients with MGUS should be monitored indefinitely without treatment because 20% to 25% of them will eventually progress to myeloma at a rate of approximately 1% per year. Patients should have SPEP and/or UPEP repeated 3 to 6 months atfer initial diagnosis, and if stable can be followed every year for high- or intermediate-risk patients and every 2 to 3 years for low-risk patients (no risk factors present) or when evolution to myeloma is suspected. Treatment is not indicated unless it is part of a clinical trial.

Smoldering (Asymptomatic) Multiple Myeloma

These patients should also be observed closely without therapy, but they have a higher risk of progression to myeloma than MGUS (10% per year vs. 1% per year). These patients should have SPEP, UPEP, complete blood count, and calcium and creatinine measurement 2 to 3 months after the initial diagnosis. If the results are stable, the studies should be repeated every 4 to 6 months during the first year and, if stable, evaluation can be lengthened to every 6 to 12 months. Currently, treatment is indicated only when there is evidence of progression to symptomatic disease, or as a part of clinical trial, although there is increasing thought that treating high risk patients early (before they develop symptomatic disease) may lead to better outcomes.

Solitary Plasmacytoma

Patients suspected to have a solitary plasmacytoma should have a PET scan performed to conclusively rule out other lesions, once the initial lesion is biopsied and confirmed to be a plasmacytoma. The initial evaluation is similar to that for myeloma, including a bone marrow aspirate and biopsy. These patients are primarily treated with radiation therapy to the affected area and surgery is reserved for specific situations such as bone lesions with extensive destruction that require stabilization or soft tissue masses with pressure symptoms. After completion of treatment, patients should be followed by regular monitoring of M-protein and imaging studies as indicated, given the risk of progression to MM. Older patients, plasmacytoma of bone, especially of the axial skeleton, persistent monoclonal protein after radiation therapy, presence of marrow involvement, increased angiogenesis in the plasmacytoma and presence of circulating plasma cells, all suggest a higher risk of progression.

Multiple Myeloma

The treatment approaches for myeloma has undergone significant shifts in the last decade, primarily driven by the increased availability of new drugs, development of effective multidrug combinations, and the concept of prolonged therapy. The introduction of novel, highly active drugs such as thalidomide, bortezomib, and lenalidomide along with the increasing application of stem cell transplantation has significantly improved the outcome of patients with MM. More recently newer drugs like carfilzomib, pomalidomide, ixazomib, panobinostat, and the monoclonal antibodies daratumumab and elotuzumab have become available for management of relapsed disease, allowing for better disease control than had been possible in the past. There is increasing use of aggressive multidrug treatment upfront to achieve deep responses or sequential disease control approach emphasizing quality of life and prolonged survival. In particular, patients with high-risk disease have better long-term OS if they achieve a deep response, justifying an aggressive strategy upfront. The treatment choice for symptomatic myeloma patients largely depends on eligibility for stem cell transplantation and risk stratification (Fig. 27.2). In the transplant-eligible patients, the current approach includes initial therapy with a triplet combination, followed by ASCT which is followed by maintenance therapy of variable duration. In transplant-ineligible patients, initial therapy typically uses a doublet or dose-adjusted triplet combinations, given for a defined duration followed by the maintenance for variable duration. Eligible patients should always be considered for enrollment in clinical trials that evaluate novel treatment strategies.

As a result of the improved therapies, we have been able to achieve deep responses, not previously seen with the older therapies. This exposed the limitations of the previous response assessment approaches that relied primarily on the serologic and/or urine monoclonal protein assessment along with marrow assessment using methods with low sensitivity. This coupled with improvements in flow cytometry as well as the development of next generation sequencing to identify VDJ recombination regions have allowed us to detect extremely low levels of tumor cell involvement in the marrow with detection of 1 clonal plasma cell in 10^5 to 10^6 nucleated cells. This sensitive marrow assessment has been combined with imaging in the revised IMWG response criteria to assess the extramedullary compartment to provide a more thorough evaluation of disease status. The recently revised criteria by the IMWG for evaluating response to treatment and progression in myeloma patients are outlined in Table 27.4.

Initial Therapies

Induction Treatment for Patients Eligible for Transplantation

Initial therapy of myeloma has moved from doublets of thalidomide, lenalidomide or bortezomib and dexamethasone to triplets that incorporate one or more of different drug classes in addition to dexamethasone. A summary of these regimens is shown in Table 27.5.

Commonly Used Combinations for Upfront Treatment

The most commonly used induction therapy in the US is the combination of bortezomib, lenalidomide and dexamethasone. This combination is very effective with over 90% of the patients obtaining a partial response to therapy and over a third reaching complete response in some of the trials. In a phase 3 trial, VRd was associated with improved PFS and OS, supporting its use as the current standard of care. European trials have predominantly used the combination of bortezomib, thalidomide and dexamethasone (VTd) in their phase 3 trials as induction therapy, and this regimen is very effective in inducing responses in newly diagnosed MM. Another regimen that has been

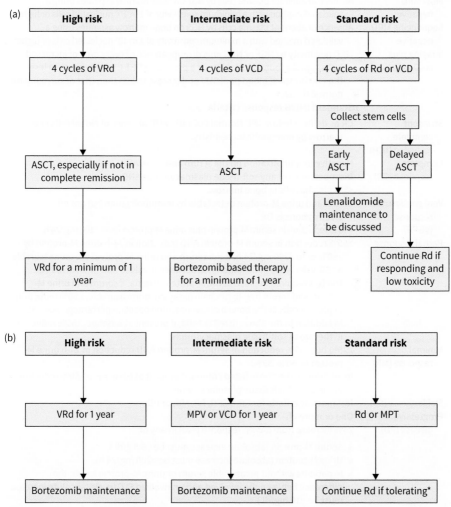

FIGURE 27.2 A suggested treatment algorithm for newly diagnosed multiple myeloma patients. Transplant-eligible (A) and transplant-ineligible (B). All patients should receive supportive care and must be considered for bisphosphonate treatment and clinical trials. High risk includes patients with del(17p), t(14;16) or t(14;20); intermediate risk includes patients with t(4;14); and standard risk includes patients with t(911;14), t(6;14) or trisomies. ASCT, autologous stem cell transplantation; VRd, bortezomib, lenalidomide, and dexamethasone; KRd, carfilzomib, lenalidomide, and dexamethasone; Rd, lenalidomide, and dexamethasone. (Adapted from Kumar SK, Rajkumar SV, Kyle RA, et al. *Nat rev Dis Primers*. 2017;3:10746.)

TABLE 27.4 International Myeloma Working Group Consensus Criteria for Response Assessment

Response Subcategory	Response Criteria
	IMWG MRD criteria (requires a complete response as defined below)
Sustained MRD negative	MRD negative in the marrow (NGF, NGS, or both) AND by imaging, confirmed at least 1 year apart.
Flow MRD negative	Absence of aberrant plasma cells by NGF on bone marrow aspirates using a validated method with a minimum sensitivity of 1 in 10^5 nucleated cells or higher.
Sequencing MRD negative	Absence of aberrant plasma cells by NGS on bone marrow aspirates using a validated method with a minimum sensitivity of 1 in 10^5 nucleated cells or higher.
Imaging plus MRD negative	MRD negativity by NGF or NGS plus disappearance of every area of increased tracer uptake found at baseline or a preceding PET-CT or decrease to less than mediastinal blood pool SUV or decrease to less than that of surrounding normal tissue.
	Standard IMWG response criteria
Stringent complete response (sCR)	CR as defined below AND Normal FLC ratio AND absence of clonal cells in bone marrow by immunohistochemistry.
Complete response (CR)	Negative immunofixation on the serum and urine AND Disappearance of any soft-tissue plasmacytomas AND <5% plasma cells in bone marrow.
Very good partial response (VGPR)	Serum and urine M-protein detectable by immunofixation but not on electrophoresis OR ≥90% reduction in serum M-protein plus urine M-protein level <100 mg/24 h.
Partial response (PR)	≥50% reduction in serum M-protein AND reduction in 24-h urine M-protein by ≥90% or to <200 mg/24 h. If the serum and urine M-protein are unmeasurable, a ≥50% decrease in the difference between involved and uninvolved FLC levels is required in place of the M-protein criteria. If serum and urine M-protein and serum free-light-chain assay are unmeasurable, ≥50% reduction in plasma cells in the bone marrow provided baseline percentage was ≥30%. In addition to the above listed criteria, if present at baseline, ≥50% reduction in the size of soft-tissue plasmacytomas.
Minimal response (MR)	≥25% but ≤49% reduction of serum M-protein AND reduction in 24-h urine M-protein by 50%–89%. In addition to the above listed criteria, if present at baseline, a ≥50% reduction in the size of soft tissue plasmacytomas.
Stable disease (SD)	Not meeting criteria for CR, VGPR, PR, MR, or PD.
Progressive disease (PD)	One or more of: 25% increase from lowest response level in any of:

- Serum M-protein (absolute increase must be ≥0.5 g/dL).
- Urine M-protein (absolute increase must be ≥200 mg/24 h).
- In patients without measurable serum or urine M-protein levels, the difference between the involved and uninvolved FLC levels (absolute increase must be >10 mg/dL).
- In patients without measurable serum or urine M-protein levels, and without measurable involved FLC levels, bone marrow plasma cell percentage (absolute increase must be ≥10%).

Development of new lesion(s), ≥50% increase from nadir in SPD of >1 lesion, or ≥50% increase in the longest diameter of a previous lesion >1 cm in short axis; ≥50% increase in circulating plasma cells (minimum of 200 cells per μL) if this is the only measure of disease.

(continued)

TABLE 27.4 (Continued)

Response Subcategory	Response Criteria
Clinical relapse	One or more of:
	CRAB features related to underlying plasma cell proliferative disorder.
	New soft tissue plasmacytomas or bone lesions.
	Definite increase (>50% and ≥1 cm) in size of existing plasmacytomas or bone lesions.
	Hypercalcemia (>11 mg/dL).
	Decrease in hemoglobin >2g/dL (not related to therapy or a cause other than myeloma).
	Rise in serum creatinine ≥2 mg/dL attributable to myeloma.
	Hyperviscosity related to serum paraprotein.
Relapse from CR[a]	One or more of:
	Reappearance of serum or urine M-protein by immunofixation or electrophoresis. Development of ≥5% plasma cells in the bone marrow. Any other sign of progression.
Relapse from MRD[a]	One or more of:
	Loss of MRD negativity.
	Reappearance of serum or urine M-protein by immunofixation or electrophoresis. Development of ≥5% plasma cells in the bone marrow. Any other sign of progression.

[a] To be used for calculation of disease-free survival only; progression should be defined using criteria for progressive disease.

IMWG, International Myeloma Working Group; MRD, minimal residual disease; NGF, next generation flow; NGS, next generation sequencing; PET-CT, positron emission tomography-computed tomography; SUV, standardized uptake value; FLC, free light chain; SPD, sum of the products of the maximal perpendicular diameters; CRAB, calcium elevation, renal failure, anemia, lytic bone lesions. All response categories require two consecutive assessments made at any time before the institution of any new therapy. All categories also require no known evidence of new or progressive bone lesions or extramedullary plasmacytomas if radiographic studies were performed. Radiographic studies are not required to satisfy the response requirements. Bone marrow assessments need not be confirmed. Each category other than SD will be considered unconfirmed until the confirmatory test is performed.

Adapted from Kumar S, Paiva B, Anderson KC, et al. International Myeloma Working Group consensus criteria for response and minimal residual disease assessment in multiple myeloma. *Lancet Oncol.* 2016;17(8):e328–46.

commonly used around the globe is the combination of bortezomib, cyclophosphamide and dexamethasone (VCd). All the recent regimens have used dexamethasone weekly compared to the earlier use of 4 days on-4 days off regimen, with phase 3 trials demonstrating an improved OS associated with lower dose of dexamethasone. It is also important to note that use of bortezomib has shifted to mostly subcutaneous use due to reduced risk of neuropathy with preserved efficacy. Other regimens that have been studied in phase 2 and 3 trials include cyclophosphamide and dexamethasone with lenalidomide (CRd) or thalidomide (CTd), and lenalidomide, adriamycin, and dexamethasone (RAD). Four drug regimens adding cyclophosphamide to VRd or VTd have also been studied in phase 2 trials.

Novel Combinations in Clinical Trials

The past few years have witnessed an ongoing effort to further improve the efficacy of the induction regimens by adding new drug classes to the upfront combinations. Carfilzomib with lenalidomide (KRd) or cyclophosphamide (KCd) have led to high response rates in phase 2 trials, and large phase 3

TABLE 27.5 Currently Recommended Regimens for Induction Therapy in Transplant-Eligible Myeloma Patients

Regimen	OR (CR + VGPR+PR)[a]	CR + VGPR[a]	Reference(s)
VRD	94%–100%	58%–74%	(Richardson, Weller et al. 2010, Roussel, Lauwers-Cances et al. 2014)
VCRD vs. VRD vs. VCD-mod[b] (EVOLUTION)	88% vs. 85% vs. 100%	58% vs. 51% vs. 53%	(Kumar, Flinn et al. 2012)
VRD vs. Rd[c] (SWOG S0777)	81% vs. 71%	43% vs. 32%	(Durie, Hoering et al. 2017)
VRD-ASCT vs. VRD (IFM 2009)	NA	47% vs. 45%	(Attal, Lauwers-Cances et al. 2017)
VTD vs. TD	93% vs. 79%	62% vs. 28%	(Cavo, Tacchetti et al. 2010)
VTD vs. TD (PETHEMA/GEM)	85% vs. 62%	60% vs. 29%	(Rosiñol, Oriol et al. 2012)
vtD vs. VD (IFM 2007-02)	88% vs. 81%	49% vs. 36%	(Moreau, Avet-Loiseau et al. 2011)
VTD vs. VCD (IFM2013-04)	92% vs. 83%	66% vs. 56%	(Moreau, Hulin et al. 2016)
VCD	84%–88%	61%	(Einsele, Liebisch et al. 2009, Reeder, Reece et al. 2009)
PAD vs. VAD (HOVON-65/ GMMG-HD4)	78% vs. 54%	42% vs. 14%	(Sonneveld, Schmidt-Wolf et al. 2012)
PAD vs. VCD (GMMG MM5)	72% vs. 78%	34% vs. 37%	(Mai, Bertsch et al. 2015)
RD vs. high-dose dexamethasone (S0232)	78% vs. 48%	63% vs. 16%	(Zonder, Crowley et al. 2010)
Rd vs. RD (E4A03)	70% vs. 81%	40% vs. 50%	(Rajkumar, Jacobus et al. 2010)
VD vs. VAD (IFM2005-01)	78% vs. 63%	38% vs. 15%	(Harousseau, Attal et al. 2010)
KRd	97%–100%	85%–88%	(Jakubowiak, Dytfeld et al. 2012, Zingone, Kwok et al. 2013)
IRd	90%	35%	(Kumar, Berdeja et al. 2014)

[a] The results given are for best response after induction unless specified otherwise.

[b] VCD-mod included an extra dose of cyclophosphamide 500mg/m^2 on day 15 in addition to the doses on days 1 and 8 in VCD.

[c] The response rates indicate the best responses for patients after VRD or Rd induction for 6 cycles followed by Rd maintenance and followed up for a median of 55 months.

OR, overall response; CR, complete response; PR, partial response; VGPR, very good partial response; VRD, bortezomib, lenalidomide, and dexamethasone; VCRD, bortezomib, cyclophosphamide, lenalidomide, and dexamethasone; VCD, bortezomib, cyclophosphamide, and dexamethasone; VTD, bortezomib, thalidomide, and dexamethasone; vtD, contains reduced doses of bortezomib and thalidomide, and dexamethasone; TD, thalidomide and dexamethasone; VD, bortezomib and dexamethasone; PAD, bortezomib, doxorubicin, and dexamethasone; VAD, vincristine, doxorubicin, and dexamethasone; RD, lenalidomide and high-dose dexamethasone; Rd, lenalidomide and low-dose dexamethasone; KRd, carfilzomib, lenalidomide, and dexamethasone; and IRd, ixazomib, lenalidomide, and dexamethasone.

trials are ongoing. Ixazomib has been combined with lenalidomide and dexamethasone (IRd) providing a well-tolerated and efficacious all-oral regimen. The monoclonal antibodies daratumumab and elotuzumab have both been combined with lenalidomide in newly diagnosed MM and studied in large phase 3 trials, the results of which are awaited. Typically, patients receive 4 to 6 cycles of induction therapy and proceed to SCT. The ideal duration of induction therapy remains a subject of debate with retrospective trials demonstrating no impact of the initial response on the outcomes of transplantation and early data from a phase 3 trial suggesting that it may have a beneficial impact, albeit in the context of relatively less effective initial therapy.

Autologous Stem Cell Transplantation

The initial results showing benefit of ASCT in patients with MM when compared to those receiving conventional chemotherapy were published in 1996 and 2003. The Inter Groupe Francophone du Myelome 90 (IFM 90) trial and the Medical Research Council Myeloma VII Trial demonstrated that high-dose therapy (HDT) followed by ASCT improves response rate and overall survival (by approximately 12 months) compared to conventional chemotherapy in myeloma patients younger than 65 years with good performance status (Table 27.6). However, two clinical trials published later failed to show an OS benefit in patients receiving HDT with ASCT. One of them showed a trend to better EFS and a longer period without symptoms or treatment related toxicity. The IFM 95 trial showed that 200 mg/m^2 of melphalan is less toxic and at least as effective a conditioning regimen as total body irradiation of 8 Gy with 140 mg/m^2 melphalan before ASCT. Although ASCT is commonly performed following three to four cycles of induction chemotherapy, a randomized trial comparing early versus late transplantation demonstrated that ASCT could be delayed until relapse without compromising survival provided that the stem cells are harvested and cryopreserved early in the disease course. Therefore, the timing of ASCT is based on patient preference and other conditions, including response to initial induction therapy.

The above mentioned trials were conducted when novel agents including thalidomide, lenalidomide and bortezomib were not available. Novel agent-based chemotherapy improves EFS and are associated with deeper responses compared to conventional chemotherapy prior to ASCT. In the IFM 2005-01 trial where patients were randomized to bortezomib with dexamethasone (VD) or conventional chemotherapy (vincritine, doxorubicin and dexamethasone; VAD) before ASCT, the overall response in the VD arm was better, and there was a trend toward improved PFS in the VD arm-36 months compared to 29.7 months in the VAD arm (P=0.064). In the PETHEMA/GEM study, patients receiving bortezomib, thalidomide and dexamethasone (VTD) had a PFS of 56 months compared to 28.2 months in the thalidomide with dexamethasone (TD) arm and 35.3 months in the conventional therapy with bortezomib arm. Multiple trials have compared ASCT with novel agent-based chemotherapy as a consolidation strategy. In the RV-MM-EMN-441trial, patients received Rd as induction and (single or double) ASCT was compared with CRd as consolidation strategy, followed by R-maintenance. The patients in the ASCT arm had improved PFS (43.3 vs. 28.6 months) and an improved OS at 4 years (86% vs. 73%). In the GIMEMA RV-209 trial enrolling patients with age ≤65 years, and comparing melphalan, with prednisolone and lenalidomide (MPR) against ASCT as consolidation followed by lenalidomide maintenance, both PFS (22.4 vs. 43 months) and OS (65% vs. 82% at 4 years) were prolonged in patients in the ASCT arm. Another study which compared bortezomib, with melphalan and prednisolone (VMP) against single or double ASCT, found deeper responses and improved PFS (44 months vs. not reached) in patients in the ASCT arm. Finally, in the IFM DFCI 2009 study, VRD followed by ASCT and lenalidomide maintenance resulted in higher rates of CR (59% vs. 48%) and improved PFS (50 vs. 36 months), with similar rates of OS at 3 years (88%) when compared to RD consolidation and lenalidomide maintenance. These studies show that consolidation with SCT provides a clear PFS benefit even when compared to novel agent based chemotherapy. The recent trials may show an OS benefit as the long term follow-up data are available. Hence HDT with ASCT, either early or at first relapse is the current standard of care in treatment of MM.

The question of using single versus tandem (planned second HDT and SCT done within 6 months of the first ASCT) SCT in MM is controversial. The IFM 94 trial and the Bologna 96 clinical study showed that double (tandem) transplantation is superior to single autologous transplantation after conventional chemotherapy, providing benefit in PFS as well as OS. However, the GMMG-HD2 trial which randomized patients after conventional chemotherapy to single HDT with ASCT or tandem SCT did not show any difference in EFS or OS. The BMT CTN 0702 (STaMINA) trial which addressed the role of tandem SCT in the era of novel agents, randomized patients after an ASCT to lenalidomide (R)

TABLE 27.6 Results for Chemotherapy versus High-Dose Therapy (HDT) Followed by Stem Cell Transplantation (SCT)

Treatment	OR (CR + PR)	CR	Median EFS/ PFS (months)	Median OS (months)	Reference
CC vs. SCT (IFM 90)	57% vs. 81%	5% vs. 22%	18 vs. 28	44 vs. 57	(Attal, Harousseau et al. 1996)
CC vs. SCT (MRC7)	48% vs. 86%	8% vs. 44%	20 vs. 32	42 vs. 54	(Child, Morgan et al. 2003)
CC vs. SCT (MAG)	58% vs. 62%	4% vs. 6%	18.7 vs. 25.3	47.6 vs. 47.8	(Fermand, Katsahian et al. 2005)
CC vs. SCT (SWOG9321)	76% in both arms	11% in both arms	14% vs. 17% at 7 y	38% at 7 years in both arms	(Barlogie, Kyle et al. 2006)
CC vs. VD, followed by SCT (IFM 2005-01)	77% vs. 80%	9% vs. 16%	29.7 vs. 36.0	77% and 81% at 3 years	(Harousseau, Attal et al. 2010)
CC+V vs. TD vs. VTD, followed by SCT (PETHEMA/GEM)	NA	38% vs. 24% vs. 46%	35.3 vs. 28.2 vs. 56.2	70% vs. 65% vs. 74% at 4 years	(Rosiñol, Oriol et al. 2012)
MPR vs. SCT (GIMEMA RV-MM-PI-209)	91% vs. 93%	18% vs. 23%	22.4 vs. 43.0	65% vs. 82% at 4 years	(Palumbo, Cavallo et al. 2014)
CRd vs. single or double SCT (RV-MM-EMN-441)	89% vs. 91%	50% vs. 54%	28.6 vs. 43.3	73% vs. 86% at 4 years	(Gay, Oliva et al. 2015)
VMP vs. single or double SCT (EMN02/HO95 MM)	89% vs. 97%	33% vs. 42%	44 vs. not reached	NA	(Cavo, Palumbo et al. 2016)
VRD-SCT vs. VRD alone, followed by lenalidomide maintenance (IFM 2009)	99% vs. 97%	59% vs. 48%	50 vs. 36	81% vs. 82% at 4 years	(Attal, Lauwers-Cances et al. 2017)

OR, overall response; CR, complete response; PR, partial response; CC, conventional chemotherapy; SCT, stem cell therapy; EFS, event-free survival; PFS, progression-free survival; OS, overall survival; VD, bortezomib and dexamethasone; V, bortezomib; TD, thalidomide and dexamethasone; VTD, bortezomib, thalidomide, and dexamethasone; MPR, melphalan, prednisolone, and lenalidomide; CRd, cyclophosphamide, lenalidomide, and dexamethasone; and VMP, bortezomib, melphalan, and prednisolone.

maintenance, VRD consolidation and R maintenance, or a tandem ASCT followed by R maintenance and showed similar PFS (52% vs. 57% vs. 56% at 38 months) and OS at interim analysis, further suggesting that a tandem ASCT may not have distinct advantage over single ASCT. The EMN02 trial, on the other hand showed a PFS advantage for tandem transplant, especially in patients with high-risk myeloma. This is consistent with a meta-analysis of European randomized trials, which showed better OS with the tandem approach, among patients with t(4;14) or del17p. Tandem ASCT should be considered as an option, especially for patients younger than 60 years who fail to achieve very good partial response after first ASCT (Table 27.7).

TABLE 27.7 Results for Single versus Double Autologous Stem Cell Transplantation (ASCT)

Treatment	OR (CR + PR)	CR + VGPR/ nCR	Median EFS (mo)	Median OS (mo)	TRM	Reference
Single vs. double ASCT (IFM 94)	84% vs. 88%	42% vs. 50%	25 vs. 30	48 vs. 58	4% vs. 6%	(Attal, Harousseau et al. 2003)
Single vs. double ASCT (Bologna 96)	NA	33% vs. 47%	23 vs. 35	65 vs. 71	3% vs. 4%	(Cavo, Tosi et al. 2007)
Single ASCT vs. double ASCT (GMMG HD2)	93% vs. 91%	CR- 16% vs. 19%	25.0 vs. 28.7	73 vs. 75.3	2% vs. 5%	(Mai, Benner et al. 2016)
Single ASCT with VRD consolidation vs. double ASCT vs. single ASCT only, and R maintenance (BMT CTN 0702/ STaMINA)	NA	NA	57% vs. 56% vs. 52% at 38 mo	86% vs. 82% vs. 83% at 38 mo	3 vs. 4 vs. 1	(Stadtmauer, Pasquini et al. 2016)

OR, overall response; CR, complete response; PR, partial response; VGPR, very good partial response; nCR, near complete response; EFS, event-free survival; OS, overall survival; TRM, treatment-related mortality; ASCT, autologous stem cell transplantation; IFM, InterGroupe Francophone du Myelome; GMMG, German-speaking Myeloma Multicentre Group; VRD, bortezomib, lenalidomide, and dexamethasone; R, lenalidomide; and STaMINA, stem cell transplantation for multiple myeloma incorporating novel agents.

Initial Treatment for Patients Not Eligible for Transplantation

For a long time, melphalan-based regimens formed the workhorse for therapy in patients with MM who were ineligible for an SCT. Addition of novel agents to melphalan resulted in deeper responses and improvement in PFS and OS. Currently, novel agent-based triplets are the preferred initial therapy in this group of patients. The recommendations are based on trials conducted in transplant-ineligible patients as well as trials which included a significant proportion of patients with advanced age. (Table 27.8) These regimens include VRd, VTd, VCd, IRd, and KRd. In general, the newer agents improve PFS and OS in transplant-ineligible patients, but with a significant increased risk of toxicity. In the SWOG S0777 trial, VRd improved PFS and OS in patients with age 65 years or more. IRd, an all-oral, triplet combination has shown 73% PFS and 83% OS at 1 year in elderly patients in a phase I/II study and may be an attractive option in transplant-ineligible patients. The doses of individual drugs in triplets can be modified to limit toxicity. Reduced intensity regimens using a single novel agent such as Rd or Vd should be reserved for patients with significant comorbidities who cannot tolerate triplets. In the FIRST trial, continuous Rd was better than fixed duration Rd (72 weeks) and MPT with respect to PFS (25.5 months vs. 20.7 months vs. 21.2 months), and the Rd arm showed better OS at 4 years compared to MPT. In the UPFRONT trial, VD was comparable to VTD and VMP in terms of PFS (14.7 months vs. 51 months vs. 17.3 months) and OS (49.8 months vs. 51 months vs. 53.1 months). MP alone may still be considered in elderly patients without access to or are not candidates for novel agents due to advanced age or comorbidities.

TABLE 27.8 Regimens Evaluated in Newly Diagnosed Transplant-Ineligible Patients with Multiple Myeloma

Regimen	OR (CR + PR)	CR + VGPR	Median EFS/ PFS/TTP (months)	Median OS (months)	Reference(s)
Rd-continuous vs. Rd for 18 mo vs. MPT (FIRST)	75% vs. 73% vs. 62%	44% vs. 43% vs. 28%	25.5 vs. 20.7 vs. 21.2	59% vs. 56% vs. 51% at 48 months	(Benboubker, Dimopoulos et al. 2014)
VD vs. VTD vs. VMP (UPFRONT)	73% vs. 80% vs. 70%	37% vs. 51% vs. 41%	14.7 vs. 15.4 vs. 17.3	49.8 vs. 51 vs. 53.1	(Niesvizky, Flinn et al. 2015)
VCD	95%	70%	12	NA	(Jimenez Zepeda, Duggan et al. 2014)
IRd[a]	88%	71%	73% at 12 months	83% at 12 months	(Kumar, Berdeja et al. 2014)
KRd[b]	97%–100%	85%–91%	80% at 36 months	100% at 36 months	(Zingone, Kwok et al. 2013, Dytfeld, Jasielec et al. 2014)
KMP vs. VMP (CLARION)	84% vs. 79%	NA	22.3 vs. 22.1	NA	(Facon, Lee et al. 2017)
MPT vs. MP (GISMM2001-A)	70% vs. 48%	29% vs. 11%	22 vs. 14.5	45 vs. 48	(Palumbo, Bringhen et al. 2008)
MPT vs. MP (IFM 99-06)	76% vs. 35%	47% vs. 7%	27 vs. 18	52 vs. 33	(Facon, Mary et al. 2007)
VMP vs. MP (VISTA)	74% vs. 39%	41% vs. 8%	24 vs. 17	83% vs. 70% at 24 months	(San Miguel, Schlag et al. 2008)
MPR	81%	48%	92% at 12 months	100% at 12 months	(Palumbo, Falco et al. 2007)

[a] Data for evaluable patients with age ≥65 years enrolled in the trial.

[b] Data for PFS and OS are from Dytfeld et al

OR, overall response; CR, complete response; PR, partial response; VGPR, very good partial response; EFS, event-free survival; PFS, progression-free survival; TTP, time to progression; OS, overall survival; Rd, lenalidomide and low dose dexamethasone; MPT, melphalan, prednisone, and thalidomide; VD, bortezomib and dexamethasone; VTD, bortezomib, thalidomide, and dexamethasone; VMP, bortezomib, melphalan, and prednisolone; VCD, bortezomib, cyclophosphamide, and dexamethasone; IRd, ixazomib, lenalidomide, and dexamethasone; KRd, carfilzomib, lenalidomide, and dexamethasone; MP, melphalan and prednisone; and MPR, melphalan, prednisolone, and lenalidomide.

For patients at risk of DVT and in patients with renal insufficiency, VCd or Vd is preferred; for patients with history of peripheral neuropathy, Rd can be considered; if costs are a concern, MPT is least expensive; if oral therapy is desired, MPT or MPR would be good choice.

Maintenance Therapy

Multiple trials have evaluated the role of lenalidomide and bortezomib in post-ASCT maintenance therapy as well as in patients receiving non-transplant primary therapy (Table 27.9). In patients undergoing ASCT, lenalidomide maintenance has shown a consistent PFS benefit. The IFM2005-02 trial showed a PFS of 41 months vs. 23 months in lenalidomide maintenance versus placebo arms, with a comparable 3 year OS of 80% and 84%, respectively. The CALGB 100104 trial showed

TABLE 27.9 Randomized Trials Evaluating Maintenance in Transplant and Non-transplant Setting

	Median PFS (months)	OS	Second primary malignancy	Reference
Maintenance after ASCT				
R maintenance vs. placebo (IFM2005-02)	41 vs. 23	80% and 84% at 3 years	3.1 vs. 1.2 per 100 patient years	(Attal, Lauwers-Cances et al. 2012)
R maintenance vs. placebo (CALGB 100104)	46 vs. 27	88% vs. 80% at 3 years	8% vs. 3%	(McCarthy, Owzar et al. 2012)
ASCT vs. MPR followed by R maintenance vs. no maintenance (GIMEMA RV-MM-PI-209)	41.9 vs. 21.6	88% vs. 79% at 3 years	5 patients in either arm	(Palumbo, Cavallo et al. 2014)
VAD+ASCT and thalidomide maintenance vs. PAD+ASCT and Bortezomib maintenance (HOVON-65/ GMMG-HD4)	28 vs. 35	55% vs. 61% at 5 years	NA	(Sonneveld, Schmidt-Wolf et al. 2012)
Maintenance after non-transplant primary treatment				
MP followed by placebo vs. MPR vs. MPR followed by R maintenance (MM-015)	13 vs. 14 vs. 31	66% vs. 62% vs. 70% at 3 years	3% vs. 7% vs. 7% at 3 years	(Palumbo, Hajek et al. 2012)
Rd for 72 weeks vs. Rd indefinitely (FIRST)	20.7 vs. 25.5	56% vs. 59% at 4 years	6% vs. 3%	(Benboubker, Dimopoulos et al. 2014)

PFS, progression-free survival; OS, overall survival; ASCT, autologous stem cell transplant; R, lenalidomide; MPR, melphalan, prednisolone and lenalidomide; VAD, vincristine, doxorubicin and dexamethasone; PAD, bortezomib, doxorubicin and dexamethasone; MP, melphalan and prednisolone; and Rd, lenalidomide and dexamethasone.

improvement in PFS (46 months vs. 27 months) as well as OS (88% vs. 80% at 3 years) in patients receiving lenalidomide maintenance compared to placebo after ASCT. A better PFS (41.9 months vs. 21.6 months) was also observed in patients receiving lenalidomide maintenance who were randomized after ASCT or MPR for consolidation. A recently published meta-analysis which included the above three studies showed a median PFS of 52.8 months for the maintenance group and 23.5 months for the placebo/observation group. The OS was not reached in the lenalidomide group compared to 86 months in the placebo/observation group. Second primary malignancies were common in lenalidomide group (6.1% vs. 2.8%). However the risk of developing progressive MM was lower and the time to death from MM was longer in patients receiving lenalidomide maintenance. Only one randomized study has been published which evaluates the role of long term bortezomib therapy after ASCT. The HOVON-65/ GMMG-HD4 trial randomized patients to bortezomib-based and conventional therapy followed by ASCT. This was followed by bortezomib and thalidomide respectively as maintenance in the two arms. The PFS was better in the bortezomib arm (35 months vs. 28 months) and the incidence of peripheral neuropathy was lower with bortezomib. Bortezomib significantly improved PFS and OS in high risk sub-groups including patients with renal failure at diagnosis and those with a del(17p) on FISH.

Lenalidomide has shown improvement in PFS in at least two clinical trials in patients who do not receive ASCT as part of the primary therapy. The MM-015 trial assigned patients randomly to MP followed by placebo vs. MPR vs. MPR followed by lenalidomide maintenance. The patients in the maintenance arm had prolonged PFS (13 months vs. 14 months vs. 31 months) while there was no improvement in OS at 3 years. In the FIRST trial, patients who had lenalidomide indefinitely had better PFS (25.5 months vs. 20.7 months) when compared to those who received lenalidomide for a fixed duration. In both these studies, the incidence of second primary cancers was higher in the lenalidomide maintenance arm. The UPFRONT trial is the only study which has used bortezomib maintenance in the transplant-ineligible population. Patients received VD, VTD, or VMP for induction, followed by bortezomib maintenance. Bortezomib sustained the responses or deepened the responses during maintenance with little additional toxicity.

In summary, potential risks and benefits, patient characteristics that influence outcomes and patient preference should be taken into consideration while making a decision to institute maintenance therapy. Maintenance with lenalidomide is preferred after upfront therapy irrespective of the use of ASCT. Bortezomib is a viable alternative, especially in patients who have renal dysfunction, those with del(17p) or for patients who are intolerant to lenalidomide.

Supportive Measures

Intravenous pamidronate given monthly reduces bone pain and the incidence of pathologic fractures and the need for surgery or irradiation to the bone in patients with advanced myeloma. A randomized trial demonstrated that zoledronic acid is as effective as pamidronate in reducing skeletal complications, in addition to having the advantage of a shorter administration time. However, zoledronic acid is associated with an increased risk of osteonecrosis of the jaw (ONJ) when compared to pamidronate. The long term outcomes of MRC Myeloma IX trial, which randomized patients with MM regardless of bone lesions, showed improved PFS and OS, and higher rates of ONJ in patients receiving zoledronic acid. Based on the above trials and a meta-analysis that demonstrated benefit of bisphosphonates, they are recommended in all patients with MM regardless of the presence of bone disease. Patients should have a dental examination prior to therapy and should be monitored for ONJ and renal dysfunction during therapy. Bisphosphonate should be given monthly for 2 years. After 2 years, patients can get less frequent infusions or it can be stopped. Bisphosphonates should be restarted at relapse. In a recently reported randomized trial, the RANK-ligand inhibitor denosumab was non-inferior to zoledronic acid with respect to the time to first skeletal-related event. Denosumab was associated with lower rates of renal adverse events, especially in those with a creatinine clearance ≤60 mL/min.

Infection prophylaxis is crucial during induction therapy. All patients should receive antibacterial prophylaxis with single strength sulfamethoxazole/trimethoprim daily for 4 months. A quinolone or penicillin can be substituted for patients with sulfa allergy or when lenalidomide is used in the induction regimen. Intravenous immunoglobulin therapy may be useful in patients with recurrent life threatening infections and immunoparesis. Herpes zoster prophylaxis with acyclovir 400 mg twice a day or valacyclovir 500 mg daily should be used in patients receiving bortezomib- or daratumumab-containing regimens. For patients on long-term, high-intensity steroid treatment, *Pneumocystis jiroveci* prophylaxis with sulfamethoxazole/trimethoprim is recommended. Inhaled pentamidine monthly can be substituted for patients with sulfa drug allergy.

Other supportive measures in myeloma include adequate analgesia with or without local irradiation for bone pain, limited field radiation or surgery for spinal cord compression, vertebroplasty or kyphoplasty for vertebral compression fractures, surgical stabilization for impending pathologic fractures, erythropoietin for anemia blood product transfusions, treatment and prevention of hypercalcemia, avoidance of dehydration by a high fluid intake of approximately 3 L per day to maintain renal function, and dialysis if necessary.

Prophylactic anticoagulation to decrease the risk of thrombotic complications is recommended for myeloma patients receiving therapy. The National Cancer Center Network (NCCN) guidelines for cancer-associated venous thromboembolic disease can be used to choose thromboprophylaxis. Patients receiving immunomodulatory drug-based therapy or with one individual risk factor should receive prophylaxis with aspirin (81 to 325 mg once daily). Low-molecular-weight heparin (equivalent of enoxaparin 40 mg per day) or warfarin (INR: 2–3) is recommended for patients with ≥2 patient-related risk factors, or those receiving highly thrombotic therapy [an immunomodulatory drug in combination with high-dose dexamethasone (≥480 mg/month), or doxorubicin, or multi-agent chemotherapy].

REFRACTORY OR RELAPSED DISEASE

Relapsed MM is defined as previously treated MM that progresses (biochemical progression or clinical relapse) and requires salvage therapy. MM is said to be refractory to a drug if the patient fails to attain at least a minimal response to therapy, or attains a response, but progresses while on therapy or within 60 days of therapy. Almost all patients with MM relapse after primary therapy. Even with the availability of multiple active agents, the outcome of patients who have relapsed multiple times and are refractory to multiple drugs is poor. In a recent study, patients refractory to a proteasome inhibitor and an immunomodulatory drug, had received at least 3 prior therapies, and were exposed to an alkylating agent had a median OS of only 13 months and a PFS of 5 months.

All patients with relapsed MM should undergo a comprehensive evaluation for factors that aid in deciding the choice of therapy and defining the prognosis. This would include bone marrow biopsy with FISH testing for high-risk secondary cytogenetic abnormalities like del(17p), 1q gain, 1p deletion and MYC rearrangement, serum LDH, flow cytometry for circulating plasma cells, and an appropriate imaging such as whole body PET-CT for evaluation of extramedullary disease. High-risk cytogenetic abnormalities, circulating plasma cells, extramedullary plasmacytoma(s), elevated LDH, refractoriness to primary therapy, and relapse within 18 months of an ASCT indicate high-risk disease and require aggressive therapy. All patients should be encouraged to explore the option of enrolling in a clinical trial investigating newer drugs and drug combinations. Drug regimens tested in phase 3 trials in patient with relapsed and/or refractory multiple myeloma (RRMM) are shown in Table 27.10. In general, patients who are relapsing while off therapy can be treated with the primary therapy if it had provided a good response earlier. Patients who relapse while on therapy or within 6 months of last therapy should receive a triplet regimen containing ≥1 agents belonging to separate classes of drugs or at least drugs belonging to the next generation within the same class. Doublets have shown efficacy in clinical trials, but should be reserved for patients who cannot tolerate a triplet. IRd/ICd and ERd are triplet combinations that may be tolerated in frail patients. Patients who did not receive an upfront ASCT should be considered for ASCT after re-induction. Patients who had received an ASCT as part of primary therapy would benefit from ASCT if they had derived a meaningful PFS from their first ASCT. In patients who are refractory to multiple agents, efforts should be made to choose drug combinations that contain as many drugs as possible to which the patient is not refractory. Aggressive therapies like VTD PACE or its modifications may be used in patients with quadruple refractory disease, secondary plasma cell leukemia, or extensive extramedullary disease, for cytoreduction and as a bridge to transplant.

The ASPIRE trial compared KRd with Rd in patients with RRMM, and patients receiving KRd showed an improved PFS (26.3 months vs. 17.6 months). On subgroup analysis, the benefit was sustained in patients who had ≥2 prior lines of therapy and in those exposed to thalidomide, lenalidomide, or bortezomib. In the TOURMALINE-MM1 study, IRd when compared to Rd improved PFS (20.6 months vs. 14.7 months) in patients with RRMM, including patients with high-risk cytogenetics, with only minor additional toxicity.

TABLE 27.10 Phase III Clinical Trials in Relapsed and/or Refractory Multiple Myeloma

Regimen	OR (CR + VGPR+PR)	CR + VGPR	Median EFS/ PFS (months)	Median OS (months)	Reference(s)
Vd vs. D (APEX)	38% vs. 18%	7% vs. 1%	7 vs. 5.6	80% vs. 66% at 12 months	(Richardson, Sonneveld et al. 2005)
RD vs. D (MM-009)	61% vs. 19%	24% vs. 2%	11.1 vs. 4.7	29.6 vs. 20.2	(Weber, Chen et al. 2007)
RD vs. D (MM-010)	60% vs. 24%	24% vs. 5%	11.3 vs. 4.7	Not reached vs. 21	(Dimopoulos, Spencer et al. 2007)
V-PLD vs. V	44% vs. 41%	275 vs. 19%	9.3 vs. 6.5	76% vs. 65% at 15 months	(Orlowski, Nagler et al. 2007)
VTD vs. TD (MMVAR/IFM 2005-04)	87% vs. 72%	56% vs. 35%	19.5 vs. 13.8	71% vs. 65% at 24 months	(Garderet, Iacobelli et al. 2012)
V+Vorinostat vs. V (VANTAGE 088)	56% vs. 41%	NA	7.6 vs. 6.8	Not reached vs. 28	(Dimopoulos, Siegel et al. 2013)
Pd vs. D (MM-003)	31% vs. 10%	6% vs. <1%	4.0 vs. 1.9	12.7 vs. 8.1	(San Miguel, Weisel et al. 2013)
Pano-VD vs. Vd (PANORAMA1)	61% vs. 55%	285 vs. 16%	12.0 vs. 8.1	40.3 vs. 35.8	(San-Miguel, Hungria et al., San-Miguel, Hungria et al. 2014)
KRd vs. Rd (ASPIRE)	87% vs. 67%	70% vs. 40%	26.3 vs. 17.6	73% and 65% at 24 months	(Stewart, Rajkumar et al. 2015, Dimopoulos, Stewart et al. 2017)
ERd vs. Rd (ELOQUENT-2)	79% vs. 66%	33% vs. 28%	19.4 vs. 14.9	60% vs. 53% at 36 months	(Lonial, Dimopoulos et al. 2015, Dimopoulos, Lonial et al. 2017)
Kd vs. Vd (ENDEAVOR)	77% vs. 63%	545 vs. 29%	18.7 vs. 9.4	47.6 vs. 40	(Dimopoulos, Moreau et al. 2016, Dimopoulos, Goldschmidt et al. 2017)
IRd vs. Rd (TOURMALINE MM1)	78% vs. 72%	48% vs. 39%	20.6 vs. 14.7	Not reached	(Moreau, Masszi et al. 2016)
Pd (Phase 3b) (STRATUS)	33%	8%	4.6	11.9	(Dimopoulos, Palumbo et al. 2016)
DVd vs. Vd (CASTOR)	83% vs. 63%	59% vs. 29%	Not reached vs. 7.2	Not reached	(Palumbo, Chanan-Khan et al. 2016)
DRd vs. Rd (POLLUX)	93% vs. 76%	76% vs. 44%	Not reached vs. 18.4	92% and 87% at 12 months	(Dimopoulos, Oriol et al. 2016)

Vd, bortezomib and dexamethasone; D, dexamethasone; RD, lenalidomide and dexamethasone; V-PLD, bortezomib, pegylated liposomal doxorubicin, and dexamethasone; V, bortezomib; VTD, bortezomib, thalidomide, and dexamethasone; TD, thalidomide and dexamethasone; Pd, pomalidomide and dexamethasone; Pano-VD, Panobinostat, bortezomib, and dexamethasone; KRd, carfilzomib, lenalidomide, and dexamethasone; ERd, Elotuzumab with lenalidomide and dexamethasone; Kd, carfilzomib and dexamethasone; IRd, ixazomib, lenalidomide, and dexamethasone; DVd, daratumumab, bortezomib, and dexamethasone; and DRd, daratumumab, lenalidomide, and dexamethasone.

Adapted from Dingli D, Ailawadhi S, Bergsagel L, et al. Therapy for relapsed multiple myeloma: Guidelines from the Mayo stratification for myeloma and risk-adapted therapy. *Mayo Clin Proc.* 2017;92(4):578–598.

Of particular interest in therapy of MM is the arrival of targeted molecular and cellular therapies. Daratumumab, an anti-CD38, humanized IgG-kappa monoclonal antibody is active as single agent as well as in combination in MM. The CASTOR trial compared DVd with Vd in patients with RRMM not refractory to bortezomib, while POLLUX compared DRd against Rd in patients not refractory to lenalidomide. Both these studies have shown a PFS benefit in interim analysis (61% vs. 27% 1 year PFS in CASTOR, and 83% vs. 60% in POLLUX) as well as deep responses of which many were MRD-negative responses. The hazard ratios for progression or death seen in CASTOR (0.39) and POLLUX (0.37) were unprecedented in trials of relapsed MM. These results form the basis of our recommendation for using daratumumab-based combinations at first relapse. Elotuzumab, an anti-SLAMF7 monoclonal antibody is approved for use in combination with Rd, and isatuximab, another anti-CD38 monoclonal antibody, is under clinical trial. The early results from clinical trials of anti-BCMA (B-cell maturation antigen) chimeric antigen receptor-T (CAR-T) cells in RRMM are promising. In a single center, single arm study of 19 patients, 6 of 7 patients who had a follow-up beyond six months achieved MRD-negative status and 12 patients with follow-up less than 6 months achieved a near-CR. In a multicenter trial, in which 11 patients have been treated so far, 2 out of 6 evaluable patients achieved an MRD-negative status and overall response rate was 100%. Venetoclax, a small molecule inhibitor of BCL-2, showed a higher overall response (40%) in patients with t(11;14) compared to patients without t(11;14) (8%) in a phase I study. In combination with bortezomib, venetoclax has been studied in a phase 1 trial with high response rates. As more data becomes available, targeted therapies may change the treatment paradigm for MM and allow individualization of therapeutic choices.

Myeloablative as well as non-myeloablative allogeneic stem cell transplantation may benefit a small percentage of patients with relapsed MM because of a powerful graft-versus-myeloma effect, with attendant risks of transplant-related mortality and graft-versus-host disease. Allogeneic transplantation especially under the purview of a clinical trial may be considered as a salvage option in younger, fit patients, with high-risk markers who are refractory to commonly used regimens.

CONCLUSION

Recent advances in understanding of tumor biology, availability of newer drugs and widespread use of ASCT are improving the survival in patients with MM. Novel agent-based triplets form the backbone of initial therapy as well as the treatment of relapsed disease. Monoclonal antibodies are a recent addition to the therapeutic armamentarium, with the potential to induce deep and lasting remissions. However, a proportion of patients have high-risk features and their outcomes are poor. Development of biomarkers and targeted drug development are necessary to improve the survival in this patient population.

Suggested Readings

1. Attal M, Harousseau JL, Facon T, et al. Single versus double autologous stem-cell transplantation for multiple myeloma. *N Engl J Med.* 2003;349:2495–2502.
2. Attal M, Harousseau JL, Leyvraz S, et al. Maintenance therapy with thalidomide improves survival in patients with multiple myeloma. *Blood.* 2006;108:3289–3294.
3. Attal M, Harousseau JL, Stoppa AM, et al. A prospective, randomized trial of autologous bone marrow transplantation and chemotherapy in multiple myeloma. Intergroupe Francais du Myelome. *N Engl J Med.* 1996;335:91–97.
4. Attal M, Lauwers-Cances V, Hulin C, et al. Lenalidomide, bortezomib, and dexamethasone with transplantation for myeloma. *N Engl J Med.* 2017;376(14):1311–1320.
5. Attal M, Lauwers-Cances V, Marit G, et al. Lenalidomide maintenance after stem-cell transplantation for multiple myeloma. *N Engl J Med.* 2012;366:1782–1791.
6. Barlogie B, Kyle RA, Anderson KC, et al. Standard chemotherapy compared with high-dose chemoradiotherapy for multiple myeloma: Final results of phase III US Intergroup trial S9321. *J Clin Oncol* 2006;24(6):929–936.
7. Benboubker L, Dimopoulos MA, Dispenzieri A, et al. Lenalidomide and dexamethasone in transplant-ineligible patients with myeloma. *N Engl J Med.* 2014;371(10):906–917.

8. Berenson JR, Lichtenstein A, Porter L, et al. Long-term pamidronate treatment of advanced multiple myeloma patients reduces skeletal events. Myeloma Aredia Study Group. *J Clin Oncol*. 1998;16:593–602.

9. Blade J, Rosinol L, Sureda A, et al. High-dose therapy intensification compared with continued standard chemotherapy in multiple myeloma patients responding to the initial chemotherapy: long-term results from a prospective randomized trial from the Spanish cooperative group PETHEMA. *Blood*. 2005;106:3755–3759.

10. Cavo M, Palumbo A, Zweegman S, et al. Upfront autologous stem cell transplantation (ASCT) versus novel agent-based therapy for multiple myeloma (MM): A randomized phase 3 study of the European Myeloma Network (EMN02/HO95 MM trial. *J Clin Oncol*. 2016;34(15 suppl): 8000–8000.

11. Cavo M, Tacchetti P, Patriarca F, et al. Bortezomib with thalidomide plus dexamethasone compared with thalidomide plus dexamethasone as induction therapy before, and consolidation therapy after, double autologous stem-cell transplantation in newly diagnosed multiple myeloma: a randomised phase 3 study. *Lancet*. 2010;376:2075–2085.

12. Cavo M, Tosi P, Zamagni E, et al. Prospective, randomized study of single compared with double autologous stem-cell transplantation for multiple myeloma: Bologna 96 clinical study. *J Clin Oncol*. 2007;25:2434–2441.

13. Child JA, Morgan GJ, Davies FE, et al. High-dose chemotherapy with hematopoietic stem-cell rescue for multiple myeloma. *N Engl J Med*. 2003;348:1875–1883.

14. Dimopoulos M, Siegel DS, Lonial S, et al.Vorinostat or placebo in combination with bortezomib in patients with multiple myeloma (VANTAGE 088): a multicentre, randomised, double-blind study. *Lancet Oncol*. 2013;14(11):1129–1140.

15. Dimopoulos M, Spencer A, Attal M, et al. Multiple Myeloma Study. Lenalidomide plus dexamethasone for relapsed or refractory multiple myeloma. *N Engl J Med*. 2007;357(21): 2123–2132.

16. Dimopoulos M, Terpos E, Comenzo RL, et al. International myeloma working group consensus statement and guidelines regarding the current role of imaging techniques in the diagnosis and monitoring of multiple myeloma. *Leukemia*. 2009;23:1545–1556.

17. Dimopoulos MA. Goldschmidt H, Niesvizky R, et al. Overall survival of patients with relapsed or refractory multiple myeloma treated with carfilzomib and dexamethasone versus bortezomib and dexamethasone in the randomized phase 3 ENDEAVOR trial. Annual meeting of European Hematology Association. Madrid, Spain:2017.

18. Dimopoulos MA, Lacy MQ, Moreau P, et al. Pomalidomide in combination with low-dose dexamethasone: demonstrates a significant progression free survival and overall survival advantage. In: *Relapsed/Refractory MM: A Phase 3, Multicenter, Randomized, Open-Label Study*. ASH Annual Meeting Abstracts 120:LBA-6-; 2012.

19. Dimopoulos MA, Lonial S, White D, et al. Elotuzumab plus lenalidomide/dexamethasone for relapsed or refractory multiple myeloma: ELOQUENT-2 follow-up and post-hoc analyses on progression-free survival and tumour growth. *Br J Haematol*. 2017;178(6): 896–905.

20. Dimopoulos MA, Moreau P, Palumbo A, et al. Investigators. Carfilzomib and dexamethasone versus bortezomib and dexamethasone for patients with relapsed or refractory multiple myeloma (ENDEAVOR): a randomised, phase 3, open-label, multicentre study. *Lancet Oncol*. 2016;17(1): 27–38.

21. Dimopoulos, MA, Oriol A, Nahi H, et al. Daratumumab, lenalidomide, and dexamethasone for multiple myeloma. *N Engl J Med*. 2016;375(14):1319–1331.

22. Dimopoulos MA, Palumbo A, Corradini P, et al. Safety and efficacy of pomalidomide plus low-dose dexamethasone in STRATUS (MM-010): a phase 3b study in refractory multiple myeloma. *Blood*. 2016;128(4):497–503.

23. Dimopoulos MA, Stewart AK, Masszi T, et al. Carfilzomib-lenalidomide-dexamethasone vs lenalidomide-dexamethasone in relapsed multiple myeloma by previous treatment. *Blood Cancer J*. 2017;7(4):e554.

24. Dingli D, Ailawadhi S, Bergsagel PL, et al. Therapy for relapsed multiple myeloma: guidelines from the Mayo Stratification for Myeloma and Risk-Adapted Therapy. *Mayo Clin Proc*. 92(4):578–598.

25. Durie BG, Harousseau JL, Miguel JS, et al. International uniform response criteria for multiple myeloma. *Leukemia*. 2006;20:1467–1473.

26. Durie BG, Hoering A, Abidi MH, et al. Bortezomib with lenalidomide and dexamethasone versus lenalidomide and dexamethasone alone in patients with newly diagnosed myeloma without intent for immediate autologous stem-cell transplant (SWOG S0777): a randomised, open-label, phase 3 trial. *Lancet*. 2017;389(10068):519–527.

27. Durie BG, Salmon SE. A clinical staging system for multiple myeloma. Correlation of measured myeloma cell mass with presenting clinical features, response to treatment, and survival. *Cancer*. 1975;36:842–854.

28. Dytfeld D, Jasielec J, Griffith KA, et al. Carfilzomib, lenalidomide, and low-dose dexamethasone in elderly patients with newly diagnosed multiple myeloma. *Haematologica*. 2014;99(9):e162–e164.

29. Einsele H, Liebisch P, Langer C, et al. Velcade, intravenous cyclophosphamide and dexamethasone (VCD) induction for previously untreated multiple myeloma (German DSMM XIa Trial). *Blood*. 2009;114(22):131.

30. Facon T, Lee JH, Moreau P, et al. Phase 3 Study (CLARION) of Carfilzomib, Melphalan, Prednisone (KMP) v Bortezomib, Melphalan, Prednisone (VMP) in Newly Diagnosed Multiple Myeloma (NDMM). *Clin Lymphoma, Myeloma Leuk*. 2017;17(1):e26–e27.

31. Facon T, Mary JY, Hulin C, et al. Melphalan and prednisone plus thalidomide versus melphalan and prednisone alone or reduced-intensity autologous stem cell transplantation in elderly patients with multiple myeloma (IFM 99-06): a randomised trial. *Lancet*. 2007;370:1209–1218.

32. Fermand J-P, Katsahian S, Divine M, et al. High-dose therapy and autologous blood stem-cell transplantation compared with conventional treatment in myeloma patients aged 55 to 65 years: Long-term results of a randomized control trial from the group myelome-autogreffe. *J Clin Oncol.* 2005;23(36):9227–9233.

33. Fermand JP, Ravaud P, Chevret S, et al. High-dose therapy and autologous peripheral blood stem cell transplantation in multiple myeloma: up-front or rescue treatment? Results of a multicenter sequential randomized clinical trial. *Blood.* 1998;92:3131–3136.

34. Garderet L, Iacobelli S, Moreau P, et al. Superiority of the triple combination of bortezomib-thalidomide-dexamethasone over the dual combination of thalidomide-dexamethasone in patients with multiple myeloma progressing or relapsing after autologous transplantation: the MMVAR/IFM 2005-04 Randomized Phase III Trial from the Chronic Leukemia Working Party of the European Group for Blood and Marrow Transplantation. *J Clin Oncol.* 2012;30(20):2475–2482.

35. Gay F, Oliva S, Petrucci MT, et al. Chemotherapy plus lenalidomide versus autologous transplantation, followed by lenalidomide plus prednisone versus lenalidomide maintenance, in patients with multiple myeloma: a randomised, multicentre, phase 3 trial. *Lancet Oncol.* 2015.16(16):1617–1629.

36. Greipp PR, San Miguel J, Durie BG, et al. International staging system for multiple myeloma. *J Clin Oncol.* 2005;23:3412–3420.

37. Harousseau JL, Attal M, Avet-Loiseau H, et al. Bortezomib plus dexamethasone is superior to vincristine plus doxorubicin plus dexamethasone as induction treatment prior to autologous stem-cell transplantation in newly diagnosed multiple myeloma: results of the IFM 2005-01 phase III trial. *J Clin Oncol.* 2010;28:4621–4629.

38. International Myeloma Working Group. Criteria for the classification of monoclonal gammopathies, multiple myeloma and related disorders: a report of the International Myeloma Working Group. *Br J Haematol.* 2003;121:749–757.

39. Jacobus S, Callander N, Siegel D, et al. Outcome of elderly patients 70 years and older with newly diagnosed myeloma in the ecog randomized trial of lenalidomide/high-dose dexamethasone (Rd) versus lenalidomide/low-dose dexamethasone (Rd). *Haematologica.* 2010;95:149,abs. 0370.

40. Jakubowiak AJ, Dytfeld D, Griffith KA, et al. A phase 1/2 study of carfilzomib in combination with lenalidomide and low-dose dexamethasone as a frontline treatment for multiple myeloma. *Blood.* 2012;120(9):1801–1809.

41. Jimenez Zepeda VH, Duggan P, Neri PE et al. Cyclophosphamide, bortezomib and dexamethasone (CyBORD) is a feasible and active regimen for non-transplant eligible multiple myeloma patients. *Blood.* 2014;124(21):5751–5751.

42. Kumar S, Flinn I, Richardson PG, et al. Randomized, multicenter, phase 2 study (EVOLUTION) of combinations of bortezomib, dexamethasone, cyclophosphamide, and lenalidomide in previously untreated multiple myeloma. *Blood.* 2012;119:4375–4382.

43. Kumar S, Paiva B, Anderson KC, et al. International Myeloma Working Group consensus criteria for response and minimal residual disease assessment in multiple myeloma. *Lancet Oncol.* 2016;17(8):e328–e346.

44. Kumar SK, Berdeja JG, Niesvizky R, et al. Safety and tolerability of ixazomib, an oral proteasome inhibitor, in combination with lenalidomide and dexamethasone in patients with previously untreated multiple myeloma: an open-label phase 1/2 study. *Lancet Oncol.* 2014;15(13):1503–1512.

45. Kumar SK, Lee JH, Lahuerta JJ, et al. Risk of progression and survival in multiple myeloma relapsing after therapy with IMiDs and bortezomib: a multicenter international myeloma working group study. *Leukemia.* 2012;26:149–157.

46. Kumar SK, Rajkumar SV, Kyle RA, et al. *Nat rev Dis Primers.* 2017;3:10746.

47. Kyle RA, Durie BG, Rajkumar SV, et al. Monoclonal gammopathy of undetermined significance (MGUS) and smoldering (asymptomatic) multiple myeloma: IMWG consensus perspectives risk factors for progression and guidelines for monitoring and management. *Leukemia.* 2010;24:1121–1127.

48. Kyle RA, Gertz MA, Witzig TE, et al. Review of 1027 patients with newly diagnosed multiple myeloma. *Mayo Clin Proc.* 2003;78:21–33.

49. Kyle RA, Rajkumar SV. Criteria for diagnosis, staging, risk stratification and response assessment of multiple myeloma. *Leukemia.* 2008;23:3–9.

50. Kyle RA, Remstein ED, Therneau TM, et al. Clinical course and prognosis of smoldering (asymptomatic) multiple myeloma. *N Engl J Med.* 2007;356:2582–2590.

51. Kyle RA, Therneau TM, Rajkumar SV, et al. A long-term study of prognosis in monoclonal gammopathy of undetermined significance. *N Engl J Med.* 2002;346:564–569.

52. Kyle RA, Therneau TM, Rajkumar SV, et al. Incidence of multiple myeloma in Olmsted County, Minnesota: trend over 6 decades. *Cancer.* 2004;101:2667–2674.

53. Kyle RA, Therneau TM, Rajkumar SV, et al. Prevalence of monoclonal gammopathy of undetermined significance. *N Engl J Med.* 2006;354:1362–1369.

54. Landgren O, Kyle RA, Pfeiffer RM, et al. Monoclonal gammopathy of undetermined significance (MGUS) consistently precedes multiple myeloma: a prospective study. *Blood.* 2009;113:5412–5417.

55. Landgren O, Weiss BM. Patterns of monoclonal gammopathy of undetermined significance and multiple myeloma in various ethnic/racial groups: support for genetic factors in pathogenesis. *Leukemia.* 2009;23:1691–1697.

56. Larocca A, Cavallo F, Bringhen S, et al. Aspirin or enoxaparin thromboprophylaxis for patients with newly diagnosed multiple myeloma treated with lenalidomide. *Blood.* 2012;119:933–939; quiz 1093.

57. Larsen JT, Kumar SK, Dispenzieri A, et al. Serum free light chain ratio as a biomarker for high-risk smoldering multiple myeloma. *Leukemia*. 2013;27:941–946.
58. Lonial S, Dimopoulos M, Palumbo A, et al. Elotuzumab therapy for relapsed or refractory multiple myeloma. *N Engl J Med*. 373(7):621–631.
59. Lynch HT, Ferrara K, Barlogie B, et al. Familial myeloma. *N Engl J Med*. 2008;359:152–157.
60. Lynch HT, Sanger WG, Pirruccello S, et al. Familial multiple myeloma: a family study and review of the literature. *J Natl Cancer Inst*. 2001;93:1479–1483.
61. Mai EK, Benner A, Bertsch U, et al. Single versus tandem high-dose melphalan followed by autologous blood stem cell transplantation in multiple myeloma: long-term results from the phase III GMMG-HD2 trial. *Br J Haematol*. 2016;173(5):731–741.
62. Mai EK, Bertsch U, Durig J, et al. Phase III trial of bortezomib, cyclophosphamide and dexamethasone (VCD) versus bortezomib, doxorubicin and dexamethasone (PAd) in newly diagnosed myeloma. *Leukemia*. 2015;29(8):1721–1729.
63. Mateos MV, Oriol A, Martinez-Lopez J, et al. Bortezomib, melphalan, and prednisone versus bortezomib, thalidomide, and prednisone as induction therapy followed by maintenance treatment with bortezomib and thalidomide versus bortezomib and prednisone in elderly patients with untreated multiple myeloma: a randomised trial. *Lancet Oncol*. 2010;11:934–941.
64. Mateos MV, Oriol A, Martinez-Lopez J, et al. Maintenance therapy with bortezomib plus thalidomide or bortezomib plus prednisone in elderly multiple myeloma patients included in the GEM2005MAS65 trial. *Blood*. 2012;120:2581–2588.
65. McCarthy PL, Owzar K, Hofmeister CC, et al. Lenalidomide after stem-cell transplantation for multiple myeloma. *N Engl J Med*. 2012;366:1770–1781.
66. Mikhael JR, Dingli D, Roy V, et al. Management of newly diagnosed symptomatic multiple myeloma: updated Mayo Stratification of Myeloma and Risk-Adapted Therapy (mSMART) consensus guidelines 2013. *Mayo Clin Proc*. 2013;88(4):360–376.
67. Moreau P, Avet-Loiseau H, Facon T, et al. Bortezomib plus dexamethasone versus reduced-dose bortezomib, thalidomide plus dexamethasone as induction treatment before autologous stem cell transplantation in newly diagnosed multiple myeloma. *Blood*. 2011;118(22):5752–5758.
68. Moreau P, Hulin C, Macro M, et al. VTD is superior to VCD prior to intensive therapy in multiple myeloma: results of the prospective IFM2013-04 trial. *Blood*. 2016;127(21):2569–2574.
69. Moreau P, Hulin C, Marit G, et al. Stem cell collection in patients with de novo multiple myeloma treated with the combination of bortezomib and dexamethasone before autologous stem cell transplantation according to IFM 2005-01 trial. *Leukemia*. 2010;24:1233–1235.
70. Moreau P, Masszi T, Grzasko N, et al. Oral Ixazomib, lenalidomide, and dexamethasone for multiple myeloma. *N Engl J Med*. 2016;374(17):1621–1634.
71. Moreau P, Pylypenko H, Grosicki S, et al. Subcutaneous versus intravenous administration of bortezomib in patients with relapsed multiple myeloma: a randomised, phase 3, non-inferiority study. *Lancet Oncol*. 2011;12:431–440.
72. Niesvizky R, Flinn IW, Rifkin R, et al. Community-based phase IIIB trial of three UPFRONT bortezomib-based myeloma regimens. *J Clin Oncol*. 2015;33(33): 3921–3929.
73. Orlowski RZ, Nagler A, Sonneveld P, et al. Randomized phase III study of pegylated liposomal doxorubicin plus bortezomib compared with bortezomib alone in relapsed or refractory multiple myeloma: combination therapy improves time to progression. *J Clin Oncol*. 2007;25(25):3892–3901.
74. Palumbo A, Bringhen S, Caravita T, et al. Oral melphalan and prednisone chemotherapy plus thalidomide compared with melphalan and prednisone alone in elderly patients with multiple myeloma: randomised controlled trial. *Lancet*. 2006;367:825–831.
75. Palumbo A, Bringhen S, Liberati AM, et al. Oral melphalan, prednisone, and thalidomide in elderly patients with multiple myeloma: updated results of a randomized controlled trial. *Blood* 2008;112(8):3107–3114.
76. Palumbo A, Chanan-Khan A, Weisel K, et al. Daratumumab, bortezomib, and dexamethasone for multiple myeloma. *N Engl J Med*. 2016;375(8):754–766.
77. Palumbo A, Falco P, Corradini P, et al. Melphalan, prednisone, and lenalidomide treatment for newly diagnosed myeloma: a report from the GIMEMA—Italian Multiple Myeloma Network. *J Clin Oncol*. 2007;25:4459–4465.
78. Palumbo A, Hajek R, Delforge M, et al. Continuous lenalidomide treatment for newly diagnosed multiple myeloma. *N Engl J Med*. 2012;366:1759–1769.
79. Palumbo A, Rajkumar SV, Dimopoulos MA, et al. Prevention of thalidomide- and lenalidomide-associated thrombosis in myeloma. *Leukemia*. 2008;22:414–423.
80. Palumbo AF, Cavallo F, Gay F, et al. Autologous transplantation and maintenance therapy in multiple myeloma. *N Engl J Med*. 2014;371(10): 895–905.
81. Rajkumar SV. Treatment of myeloma: cure vs control. *Mayo Clinic Proc*. 2008;83:1142–1145.
82. Rajkumar SV, Blood E, Vesole D, et al. Phase III clinical trial of thalidomide plus dexamethasone compared with dexamethasone alone in newly diagnosed multiple myeloma: a clinical trial coordinated by the Eastern Cooperative Oncology Group. *J Clin Oncol*. 2006;24:431–436.

83. Rajkumar SV, Dimopoulos MA, Palumbo A, et al. International Myeloma Working Group updated criteria for the diagnosis of multiple myeloma. *Lancet Oncol.* 2014;15(12):e538–e548.

84. Rajkumar SV, Hayman SR, Lacy MQ, et al. Combination therapy with lenalidomide plus dexamethasone (Rev/Dex) for newly diagnosed myeloma. *Blood.* 2005;106:4050–4053.

85. Rajkumar SV, Jacobus S, Callander NS, et al. Lenalidomide plus high-dose dexamethasone versus lenalidomide plus low-dose dexamethasone as initial therapy for newly diagnosed multiple myeloma: an open-label randomised controlled trial. *Lancet Oncol.* 2010;11:29–37.

86. Rajkumar SV, Kyle RA, Therneau TM, et al. Serum free light chain ratio is an independent risk factor for progression in monoclonal gammopathy of undetermined significance. *Blood.* 2005;106:812–817.

87. Rajkumar SV, Rosinol L, Hussein M, et al. Multicenter, randomized, double-blind, placebo-controlled study of thalidomide plus dexamethasone compared with dexamethasone as initial therapy for newly diagnosed multiple myeloma. *J Clin Oncol.* 2008;26:2171–2177.

88. Reeder CB, Reece DE, Kukreti V, et al. Cyclophosphamide, bortezomib and dexamethasone induction for newly diagnosed multiple myeloma: high response rates in a phase II clinical trial. *Leukemia.* 2009;23:1337–1341.

89. Richardson PG, Weller E, Lonial S, et al. Lenalidomide, bortezomib, and dexamethasone combination therapy in patients with newly diagnosed multiple myeloma. *Blood.* 2010;116:679–686.

90. Richardson PGP, Sonneveld MW, Schuster D, et al. Assessment of proteasome inhibition for extending remissions. Bortezomib or high-dose dexamethasone for relapsed multiple myeloma. *N Engl J Med.* 2005;352(24):2487–2498.

91. Rosen LS, Gordon D, Kaminski M, et al. Long-term efficacy and safety of zoledronic acid compared with pamidronate disodium in the treatment of skeletal complications in patients with advanced multiple myeloma or breast carcinoma: a randomized, double-blind, multicenter, comparative trial. *Cancer.* 2003;98:1735–1744.

92. Rosiñol LA, Oriol AI, Teruel D, et al. Superiority of bortezomib, thalidomide, and dexamethasone (VTD) as induction pretransplantation therapy in multiple myeloma: a randomized phase 3 PETHEMA/GEM study. *Blood.* 2012;120(8):1589–1596.

93. Roussel MV, Lauwers-Cances N, Robillard C, et al., Front-line transplantation program with lenalidomide, bortezomib, and dexamethasone combination as induction and consolidation followed by lenalidomide maintenance in patients with multiple myeloma: A Phase II Study by the Intergroupe Francophone du Myélome. *J Clin Oncol.* 2014;32(25):2712–2717.

94. San-Miguel JF, Hungria VT, Yoon SS, et al. Panobinostat plus bortezomib and dexamethasone versus placebo plus bortezomib and dexamethasone in patients with relapsed or relapsed and refractory multiple myeloma: a multicentre, randomised, double-blind phase 3 trial. *Lancet Oncol.* 2014;15(11):1195–1206.

95. San-Miguel JF, Hungria VTM, Yoon SS, et al. Overall survival of patients with relapsed multiple myeloma treated with panobinostat or placebo plus bortezomib and dexamethasone (the PANORAMA 1 trial): a randomised, placebo-controlled, phase 3 trial. *Lancet Haematol.* 2016;3(11):e506–e515.

96. San Miguel JF, Schlag R, Khuageva NK, et al. Bortezomib plus melphalan and prednisone for initial treatment of multiple myeloma. *N Engl J Med.* 2008;359:906–917.

97. San Miguel JK, Weisel P, Moreau M, et al. Pomalidomide plus low-dose dexamethasone versus high-dose dexamethasone alone for patients with relapsed and refractory multiple myeloma (MM-003): a randomised, open-label, phase 3 trial. *Lancet Oncol.* 2013;14(11):1055–1066.

98. Siegel DS, Martin T, Wang M, et al. A phase 2 study of single-agent carfilzomib (PX-171-003-A1) in patients with relapsed and refractory multiple myeloma. *Blood.* 2012;120:2817–2825.

99. Siegel R, Naishadham D, Jemal A. Cancer statistics, 2012. *CA Cancer J Clin.* 2012;62:10–29.

100. Sonneveld P, Schmidt-Wolf IG, van der Holt B, et al. Bortezomib induction and maintenance treatment in patients with newly diagnosed multiple myeloma: results of the randomized phase III HOVON-65/ GMMG-HD4 trial. *J Clin Oncol.* 2012;30 :2946–2955.

101. Stadtmauer EA, Pasquini MC, Blackwell B, et al. Comparison of autologous hematopoietic cell transplant (autoHCT), bortezomib, lenalidomide (Len) and dexamethasone (RVD) consolidation with len maintenance (ACM), tandem autohct with len maintenance (TAM) and autohct with len maintenance (AM) for up-front treatment of patients with multiple myeloma (MM): primary results from the randomized phase III trial of the blood and marrow transplant clinical trials network (BMT CTN 0702-StaMINA Trial), *Am Soc Hematology.* 2016.

102. Stewart AK, Rajkumar SV, Dimopoulos MA, et al. Carfilzomib, lenalidomide, and dexamethasone for relapsed multiple myeloma. *N Engl J Med.* 2015;372(2):142–152.

103. Stewart AK, Trudel S, Bahlis NJ, et al. A randomized phase 3 trial of thalidomide and prednisone as maintenance therapy after ASCT in patients with MM with a quality-of-life assessment: the National Cancer Institute of Canada Clinicals Trials Group Myeloma 10 Trial. *Blood.* 2013;121:1517–1523.

104. Tian E, Zhan F, Walker R, et al. The role of the Wnt-signaling antagonist DKK1 in the development of osteolytic lesions in multiple myeloma. *N Engl J Med.* 2003;349:2483–2494.

105. Weber DM, Chen C, Niesvizky R, et al. Lenalidomide plus dexamethasone for relapsed multiple myeloma in North America. *N Engl J Med.* 2007;357(21):2133–2142.

106. Zhou Y, Barlogie B, Shaughnessy JD, Jr. The molecular characterization and clinical management of multiple myeloma in the post-genome era. *Leukemia*. 2009;23:1941–1956.
107. Zingone A, Kwok ML, Manasanch EE, et al. Phase II clinical and correlative study of carfilzomib, lenalidomide, and dexamethasone followed by lenalidomide extended dosing (CRD-R) induces high rates of MRD negativity in newly diagnosed multiple myeloma (MM) patients. *Blood*. 2013;122(21):538–538.
108. Zonder JA, Crowley J, Hussein MA, et al. Lenalidomide and high-dose dexamethasone compared with dexamethasone as initial therapy for multiple myeloma: a randomized Southwest Oncology Group trial (S0232). *Blood*. 2010;116(26):5838–5841.

Non-Hodgkin's Lymphoma 28

Christopher Melani and Mark Roschewski

INTRODUCTION

The term *non-Hodgkin lymphoma* (NHL) encompasses a diverse group of lymphoproliferative disorders of B-cell, T-cell, and NK-cell origin that together account for approximately 90% of all lymphomas diagnosed in the United States. Although unified in their histopathologic distinction from Hodgkin lymphoma, these disorders vary considerably in morphologic appearance, clinical behavior, therapeutic options, and prognosis. The past two decades have seen significant therapeutic advancements as well as progress in our understanding of the genetic and molecular basis of the different NHL subtypes.

EPIDEMIOLOGY AND RISK FACTORS

NHL is the seventh most common adult malignancy in the United States, with 72,580 new cases expected to be diagnosed in 2016. The overall incidence of NHL has increased substantially over the past several decades, almost doubling between 1975 and 1995. Since the mid-1990s, however, this trend has become progressively less pronounced, with overall incidence rates stabilizing between 2005 and 2009. Although incompletely understood, these changes in NHL incidence have been attributed to a variety of factors such as the emergence of (and subsequent advancements in therapy for) HIV/AIDS, improvements in detection and reporting of NHL, and reduction in mortality rates from other causes.

The risk of developing NHL increases with each decade of adult life. Certain subtypes of NHL, however, such as primary mediastinal B-cell lymphoma (PMBL) and Burkitt lymphoma (BL), tend to occur in younger patients. Although NHL occurs within all ethnic groups, it is most common in the Caucasian population. There is also considerable geographic disparity in NHL incidence, with the highest rates seen in North America, Australia, and Western Europe, and the lowest rates seen in Asia, South America, and the Caribbean.

Disorders of the immune system, often in conjunction with chronic viral infection, are also associated with increased risk of NHL. Higher rates of NHL are seen in patients with congenital and acquired immunodeficiencies as well as diseases of immune dysregulation. Though most of these lymphomas are of B-cell lineage, there are notable exceptions such as enteropathy-associated T-cell lymphoma (EATL), which occurs most commonly in patients with gluten enteropathy, and hepatosplenic T-cell lymphoma (HSTCL), which often occurs in patients with inflammatory bowel disease or post–solid organ transplantation.

Epstein-Barr virus (EBV) is an oncogenic driver in multiple subtypes of NHL, including some that arise in the setting of immunosuppression. Among HIV-related lymphomas, EBV is virtually always associated with both primary CNS lymphoma (PCNSL) and plasmablastic lymphoma, oral type. It is also seen in primary effusion lymphoma (PEL), plasmablastic lymphoma, and posttransplant lymphoproliferative disorder (PTLD). EBV is also associated with a number of NHL subtypes in immunocompetent patients. One oncogenic mechanism of EBV in NHL involves constitutive activation of the NF-κB pathway, although the entire spectrum of oncogenic mechanisms remain unknown.

Other infections have also been associated with the development of NHL subtypes, such as HHV-8 and HTLV-1, which are found in all cases of PEL and adult T-cell lymphocytic leukemia (ATLL), respectively. Marginal zone lymphoma (MZL) is also frequently driven by both viral and bacterial antigens. Hepatitis C virus (HCV) is found in some cases of splenic and nodal MZL variants, *Helicobacter pylori* in most cases of gastric mucosa-associated lymphoid tissue (MALT) lymphoma, and *Chlamydia psittaci* in some cases of ocular adnexal MALT lymphoma (OAML) (see Table 28.1).

PATHOGENESIS AND MOLECULAR CHARACTERIZATION

The process of lymphomagenesis in NHL involves a complex array of genetic aberrations that disrupt normal cellular pathways of proliferation, differentiation, and apoptosis. These genetic events are most commonly acquired and functionally result in activation of proto-oncogenes and/or inactivation of tumor suppressor genes. Balanced chromosomal translocations are early genetic events that initiate

TABLE 28.1 Risk Factors Associated with NHL Development

Immunosuppression/ Immunodeficiencies	Drugs	Environmental/ Exposures	Infections	Other
Congenital	Immuno- suppressive agents	Radiation therapy	EBV	Advanced age
■ Ataxia telangiectasia			HTLV-1	Male gender
■ Wiskott-Aldrich syndrome	Phenytoin	Occupational exposures	*Helicobacter pylori*	Previous history of NHL
■ SCID	Methotrexate	■ Herbicides	HCV	
■ CVID	TNF inhibitors	■ Pesticides	HHV-8	Family history of NHL
■ Hyper- immunoglobulin M (Job syndrome)		■ Wood dust ■ Epoxy glue ■ Solvents	HIV *Borrelia burgdorferi*	
■ X-linked hypo- gammaglobulinemia		■ Agent orange	*Chlamydia psittaci*	
■ X-linked lymphoproliferative syndrome		■ Farming ■ Forestry ■ Painting ■ Carpentry	*Chlamydia trachomatis* *Chlamydia pneumonia*	
Acquired		■ Tanning	*Campylobacter jejuni*	
■ Solid organ transplantation		Silicone breast implants		
■ Stem cell transplantation				
■ AIDS				
■ Sjögren syndrome				
■ Rheumatoid arthritis				
■ Hashimoto thyroiditis				
■ IBD				
■ Celiac sprue				

SCID, severe combined immunodeficiency; CVID, common variable immunodeficiency; AIDS, acquired immunodeficiency syndrome; IBD, inflammatory bowel disease; TNF, tumor necrosis factor; EBV, Epstein-Barr virus; HTLV-1, human T-cell lymphotropic virus type I; HCV, hepatitis C virus; HHV-8, human herpesvirus 8; HIV, human immunodeficiency virus.

lymphomagenesis in certain types of NHL. As an example, up to 85% of patients with follicular lymphoma (FL) have a balanced translocation, t(14:18), while virtually every case of mantle cell lymphoma (MCL) is characterized by the t(11;14) translocation. Newer methods using high-throughput genetic sequencing have revealed a broad genomic landscape in NHL including a long tail distribution of somatic mutations and heterogeneity across subtypes. Further molecular characterization of lymphomagenesis with emerging technologies promises more precision in diagnosis, prognosis, and treatment selection.

CLASSIFICATION

Individual NHL subtypes are defined in the World Health Organization (WHO) classification system, most recently updated in 2016. Initially established in 2001, this system constituted the first international consensus on diagnosis and classification of lymphoma. Within this system, NHL is classified primarily by cell lineage and maturity (B- vs. T/NK cell, mature vs. precursor cell of origin) and then further subcategorized according to a combination of morphologic, immunophenotypic, genetic, molecular, and clinical features. It is expected that the current classification system for NHL will continue to evolve as our knowledge of the genetic and molecular basis of these diseases continues to improve.

DIAGNOSIS

A properly evaluated and technically adequate excisional lymph node biopsy remains the gold standard for diagnosis of suspected lymphoma. In recent years, some centers have adopted the practice of obtaining a combination of core-needle biopsy and fine-needle aspiration as an alternative to surgical lymph node excision, reserving surgical biopsies for nondiagnostic cases. Although this approach is relatively sensitive and cost-effective, a definitive diagnosis is unobtainable in approximately 20% to 25% of patients. Consequently, perioperative risk, institutional experience with core-needle biopsy, and the harm of diagnosis delay are considerations when deciding the diagnostic approach.

The pathologic classification of NHL subtype relies on a combination of morphologic appearance and immunophenotyping using immunohistochemistry (IHC) and flow cytometry. Additional studies that confirm clonality and further sub-classify tumor include cytogenetic analysis and molecular studies.

WORKUP AND STAGING

Initial workup and staging evaluation of NHL should include a complete history and physical examination and laboratory assessment of organ function. The following tests should be performed:

- Complete blood count with differential
- Complete metabolic panel including serum lactate dehydrogenase (LDH)
- Serologies for HIV, HBV, HCV (regardless of exposure history)
- CT scan of the chest, abdomen, and pelvis
- Whole-body FDG-PET scan
- Bone marrow (BM) aspirate and biopsy
- Lumbar puncture with CSF cytology and flow cytometry (in select cases only)

The Ann Arbor staging system, originally designed for Hodgkin lymphoma, also has prognostic and predictive utility in NHL, and its use is considered standard for newly diagnosed cases (see Table 28.2). Although this system has limited prognostic value due to the lack of contiguous orderly spread through lymph node regions, it nevertheless remains an integral component of the validated international prognostic indices for aggressive NHL (IPI) and FL (FLIPI).

TABLE 28.2 Staging Classification of Lymphoma

Stage	Ann Arbor Classification	Cotswold Modification
I	Involvement of a single lymph node region (I) or of a single extralymphatic organ or site (I_E)	Involvement of a single lymph node region or lymphoid structure
II	Involvement of two or more lymph node regions on the same side of the diaphragm alone (II) or with involvement of limited, contiguous extralymphatic organ or tissue (II_E)	Involvement of two or more lymph node regions on the same side of the diaphragm (the mediastinum is considered a single site, whereas the hilar lymph nodes are considered bilaterally); the number of anatomic sites should be indicated by a subscript (e.g., II_3)
III	Involvement of lymph node regions on both sides of the diaphragm (III), which may include the spleen (III_S); a limited contiguous extralymphatic organ or site (III_E); or both (III_{ES})	Involvement of lymph node regions on both sides of the diaphragm: III_1 (with or without involvement of splenic hilar, celiac, or portal nodes) and III_2 (with involvement of para-aortic, iliac, and mesenteric nodes)
IV	Multiple or disseminated foci of involvement of one or more extralymphatic organs or tissues, with or without lymphatic involvement	Involvement of one or more extranodal sites in addition to a site for which the designation E has been used

Note: All cases are subclassified to indicate the absence (A) or presence (B) of the systemic symptoms of significant fever (>38.0°C [100.4°F]), night sweats, and unexplained weight loss exceeding 10% of normal body weight within the previous 6 months. The clinical stage (CS) denotes the stage as determined by all diagnostic examinations and a single diagnostic biopsy only. In the Ann Arbor classification, the term pathologic stage (PS) is used if a second biopsy of any kind has been obtained, whether negative or positive. In the Cotswold modification, the PS is determined by laparotomy; X designates bulky disease (widening of the mediastinum by more than one-third or the presence of a nodal mass >10 cm), and E designates involvement of a single extranodal site that is contiguous or proximal to the known nodal site.

Restaging for Response Evaluation

Upon completion of therapy, CT scans should be repeated to categorize the response. Bone marrow biopsy is required for the determination of complete response if it was involved prior to therapy. In accordance with the Revised Response Criteria for Malignant Lymphoma, FDG-PET is mandatory for the evaluation of residual masses at the completion of therapy. Response to therapy is determined based on changes in the sum of the product of the diameters of the masses as well as resolution of hepatosplenomegaly and bone marrow involvement. FDG-PET was formally incorporated into staging and response assessment with the Lugano classification with responses being assessed by changes in the lesion(s) 5-point Deauville score, which standardizes the lesion(s) FDG-uptake in relation to the mediastinal blood pool and liver. This classification was also recently refined to incorporate changes, such as tumor flare or pseudoprogression, that can occur with modern immunotherapy treatments. In cases of suspected disease relapse or refractoriness to initial therapy, repeat biopsy should be strongly considered for confirmation.

PROGNOSTIC FEATURES

The International Prognostic Index (IPI) is a clinical prognostic index that has been validated in aggressive lymphoma. Five clinical factors comprise the IPI and 1 point is assigned to each factor:

- Age >60 years
- Eastern Cooperative Oncology Group (ECOG) performance status 2 or higher

■ LDH level greater than normal
■ Two or more extranodal sites
■ Ann Arbor stage III or IV disease

Scores of 0 to 1, 2, 3, and 4 to 5 correspond to 5-year survivals of 73%, 51%, 43%, and 26%, respectively, in diffuse large B-cell lymphoma (DLBCL). A validated clinical prognostic index has also been applied to patients with untreated FL. The Follicular Lymphoma International Prognostic Index (FLIPI) is scored according to the following:

■ Age >60 years
■ Ann Arbor stage III or IV disease
■ LDH level greater than normal
■ Hemoglobin <12 g/dL
■ 5 or more nodal areas involved

The FLIPI score has also been found to reliably predict survival in FL with scores of 0 to 1, 2, and 3 to 5 corresponding to 5-year survivals of 91%, 78%, and 53%, respectively. Gene expression profiling has emerged as a useful means of identifying molecularly distinct sub-classifications of NHL, and can be used to identify individuals who may benefit from treatment intensification or addition of novel agents given their poor prognosis with current standard therapies. Integration of somatic mutational profiles that correlate with individual subtypes has the potential to further refine these prognostic models. As an example, in FL patients receiving first-line chemoimmunotherapy, seven genes were incorporated into a clinico-genetic risk model, termed the m7-FLIPI, which identified a high-risk group more accurately than FLIPI or gene mutations alone. Such novel prognostic models that incorporate next-generation sequencing will undergo clinical validation in prospective trials before incorporation into clinical practice.

MANAGEMENT

Indolent B-Cell Non-Hodgkin Lymphoma

Follicular Lymphoma

FL is the most common indolent lymphoma, constituting approximately 70% of cases, and is considered incurable. Patients are typically older (median age of 60) with widespread disease at diagnosis. Constitutional symptoms and extra-nodal involvement can occur, but are uncommon. Many patients are asymptomatic at diagnosis despite involvement of multiple lymph node regions. FL is graded (1–3) according to the number of centroblasts per high power field. Therapeutic approaches to grades 1 to 3A are similar, whereas grade 3B is considered a variant of DLBCL for the purposes of treatment.

A wide range of clinical behavior is observed in FL. While the median survival is currently greater than 10 years, approximately 20% of patients will progress within 2 years of initial therapy, and these patients have a much poorer prognosis compared to those without early progression. Histologic transformation to a more aggressive NHL subtype (typically DLBCL) occurs at an approximate cumulative rate of 3% per year and is generally associated with an inferior prognosis.

Even though FL is incurable in most patients, those who present with truly limited stage disease (stage 1) can achieve prolonged remissions and long-term survival with radiotherapy alone to the involved regions. Multiple studies have reported a 15-year overall survival rate of approximately 50% in these patients, and only a few relapses reported after 10 years. For the majority of patients with FL, however, radiotherapy alone is not an option since the disease is in advanced stage. For asymptomatic patients with advanced stages of FL, immediate therapy is not mandatory. Multiple randomized trials that have tested early initiation of therapy in advanced stage FL compared to observation alone have not shown an improvement in overall survival (OS). The anti-CD20 monoclonal antibody, rituximab, has demonstrated both safety and efficacy in FL with an overall response rate (ORR) of 72% in previously untreated patients with advanced-stage, low-grade disease. A recent randomized trial compared rituximab monotherapy to observation alone in 379 patients with asymptomatic advanced stage FL. Treatment with rituximab monotherapy was associated with an improvement in progression-free survival, but did not decrease rates of histologic transformation or improve OS.

Patients who require first-line therapy for FL and have a high tumor burden are usually offered therapy with combination chemotherapy with rituximab since rituximab monotherapy is less effective in this setting (see Table 28.3). Although no one particular chemoimmunotherapy regimen has demonstrated superior OS or the ability to cure patients with advanced FL, regimens such as bendamustine and rituximab (BR) or rituximab with cyclophosphamide, doxorubicin, vincristine, prednisone (R-CHOP) are considered the current standard of care. Due to less overall toxicity and an improvement in progression-free survival (PFS), many physicians consider BR as the regimen of choice. A randomized study in Germany recently compared BR to R-CHOP in patients with indolent NHL, including FL, and BR demonstrated an improvement in PFS compared to R-CHOP with less overall toxicity. A similar study was conducted in the United States testing BR versus both R-CHOP or R-CVP and determined similar response rates across all regimens tested. A newer first-line treatment option is also emerging that incorporates the novel immunomodulatory agent, lenalidomide, in combination with rituximab. The lenalidomide-rituximab regimen was recently tested in 46 patients with untreated FL and demonstrated an overall response rate of 98% including 87% of patients achieving complete remission (CR). Given the promising activity of this novel regimen, lenalidomide-rituximab is now being compared to standard combination chemo-immunotherapy in an ongoing randomized multicenter international study.

TABLE 28.3 First-Line Treatment Regimens and Outcome for Follicular Lymphoma

First-Line Treatment Regimen	Number of Patients	Outcome	Study Reference
BR vs. R-CHOP	139	Median PFS NR	Rummel et al.
	140	Median PFS 40.9 months	
BR vs. R-CHOP/R-CVP	154	ORR 99% (CR 30%)	Flinn et al.
	160	ORR 94% (CR 25%)	
R-CHOP vs. CHOP	223	18-mo TTF 87%	Hiddemann et al.
	205	18-mo TTF 70%	
Rituximab induction	37	Median TTP 2.2 years	Witzig et al.
Watchful waiting vs.	187	3-y PFS 36%	Ardeshna et al.
rituximab induction vs.	84	3-y PFS 60%	
rituximab induction and maintenance	192	3-y PFS 82%	
Rituximab induction +	143	3-y PFS 50%	Kahl et al.
rituximab retreatment (RR) vs. maintenance rituximab (MR)	146	3-y PFS 78%	
Induction	513	3-y PFS 74.9%	Salles et al.
immunochemotherapy + observation vs. rituximab maintenance	505	3-y PFS 57.6%	
Lenalidomide + rituximab (R²)	50	3-y PFS 78.5%	Fowler et al.

BR, bendamustine and rituximab; R-CHOP, rituximab, cyclophosphamide, doxorubicin, vincristine, and prednisone; CHOP, cyclophosphamide, doxorubicin, vincristine, and prednisone; R-CVP, rituximab, cyclophosphamide, vincristine, and prednisone; R², rituximab and Revlimid (lenalidomide); PFS, progression free survival; NR, not reached; ORR, overall response rate; CR, complete response; TTP, time to progression; TTF, time to treatment failure.

Another important clinical decision with first line therapy for FL includes the option of extended duration or "maintenance" therapy with rituximab. The RESORT trial addressed this question in patients with low tumor burden FL who were considered good candidates for rituximab monotherapy. Patients who responded to induction therapy with rituximab were then randomized to a planned schedule of rituximab maintenance or a schedule that initiated rituximab only at the time of disease progression. No advantage was observed with scheduled rituximab maintenance in this trial compared to the strategy of rituximab re-treatment. The benefit of maintenance rituximab was also assessed following induction chemoimmunotherapy (R-CHOP, R-CVP, or R-FCM) for patients with high tumor burden FL in the randomized phase III PRIMA trial. Following induction therapy, responding patients were randomized to 2 years of rituximab maintenance or observation. Although there was improvement in median PFS with rituximab maintenance, this did not translate into an overall survival benefit and was associated with increased toxicity and infections.

Patients with relapsed/refractory FL can be treated with alternative chemoimmunotherapy regimens, single-agent rituximab, radioimmunotherapy (RIT), or novel agents that are currently under clinical development. RIT involves the delivery of targeted radiotherapy to tumor tissue by conjugating an anti-CD20 antibody to a radioactive isotope. In a randomized trial of relapsed or refractory follicular or transformed lymphoma, the ORR was better with ibritumomab tiuxetan than with rituximab (80% vs. 56%). However, a recently published phase III intergroup trial evaluating the role of RIT in newly diagnosed FL patients (R-CHOP vs. CHOP followed by [131]Iodine tositumomab) demonstrated similar PFS and OS in both groups at median 5 years of follow-up.

Novel targeted therapies have now been FDA-approved in FL (see Table 28.4), and numerous others are in clinical development for relapsed and refractory FL. The phosphatidylinositol-3-kinase delta (PI3Kδ) inhibitor, idelalisib, is approved as monotherapy for patients with FL who have received at least two prior systemic therapies. In a multicenter, single-arm trial in relapsed indolent NHL, idelalisib monotherapy resulted in an ORR of 54% with median duration of response (DOR) that was not reached. In the phase I study of previously treated indolent NHL patients who failed to respond or relapsed within 6 months of rituximab and an alkylating agent, idelalisib resulted in a similar ORR of 57% with CR in 6% of patients. Median time to response was 1.9 months with a median DOR of 12.5 months and median PFS of 12.5 months. The CALGB 50401 study randomized patients with recurrent FL to rituximab monotherapy, lenalidomide monotherapy, or combination therapy with both and showed statistically better ORR and CR rates (76% vs. 53% and 39% vs. 20%, respectively) as well as an improved median time to progression (2 years vs. 1.1 year) favoring combination therapy.

TABLE 28.4 Novel Targeted Treatment Regimens and Outcome for Follicular Lymphoma

Targeted Regimen	Number of Patients	Response Rate	Median TTR	Median DOR	Median PFS	Study Reference
Idelalisib	125 iNHL (72 FL)	ORR 57% CR 6%	1.9 mo	12.5 mo	11 mo	Gopal et al.
Lenalidomide vs.	45	ORR 53% CR 20%	N/A	N/A	1.1 years	Leonard et al.
R²	46	ORR 76% CR 39%	N/A	N/A	2 years	
Obinutuzumab + Bendamustine vs.	194 iNHL (150 FL)	ORR 69% CR 11%	N/A	NR	NR	Sehn et al.
Bendamustine monotherapy	202 iNHL (166 FL)	ORR 63% CR 12%	N/A	13.2 mo	14.9 mo	

R², rituximab and Revlimid (lenalidomide); iNHL, indolent non-Hodgkin lymphoma; FL, follicular lymphoma; ORR, overall response rate; CR, complete response; TTR, time to response; DOR, duration of response; PFS, progression free survival; NR, not reached; N/A, not available.

In rituximab refractory disease, the combination of obinutuzumab, a novel glycol-engineered type II anti-CD20 monoclonal antibody, was recently approved in combination with bendamustine followed by obinutuzumab maintenance. This approval was based on the GADOLIN study showing a significantly longer median PFS with combination therapy versus bendamustine alone (NR vs. 14.9 months). These targeted agents are currently being investigated in various combinations in the relapsed setting as well as front-line in combination with cytotoxic therapy.

Lymphoplasmacytoid Lymphoma/Waldenström Macroglobulinemia

LPL is an indolent lymphoma composed of mature plasmacytoid lymphocytes that typically involves the bone marrow but may also involve the lymph nodes and spleen. When LPL is associated with a monoclonal IgM production it is termed Waldenström macroglobulinemia (WM). LPL/WM primarily affects older patients and is most common in the Caucasian population. Patients typically present with symptoms of increased tumor burden (cytopenias due to marrow involvement, hepatosplenomegaly, lymphadenopathy, constitutional symptoms) and/or symptoms attributable to the secreted monoclonal immunoglobulin (hyperviscosity syndrome, autoimmune neuropathy, mucocutaneous bleeding). Asymptomatic patients are considered to have "smoldering" WM and can be safely managed with an initial period of observation. Symptomatic disease requiring treatment occurs in approximately 50% of patients within 3 years of diagnosis, although up to 10% of patients managed with watchful waiting will not require treatment for 10 years or longer.

First-line treatment options for WM include single-agent rituximab, chemoimmunotherapy regimens such as BR, and rituximab combined with novel agents such as bortezomib and dexamethasone. When rituximab is used, the patient must be observed carefully for hyperviscosity symptoms, as serum IgM levels can initially increase abruptly with rituximab. Plasmapheresis prior to rituximab-containing therapy should be strongly considered for any patient presenting with symptoms of hyperviscosity or high baseline serum IgM.

Over the past several years, whole-genome sequencing has identified pathogenic mutations, which have aided in the diagnosis of WM. MYD88 (L265P) mutations that result in IRAK-mediated NF-κB signaling have been identified as a key genetic alteration in over 90% of cases. Warts, hypogammaglobulinemia, infection, and myelokathexis syndrome (WHIM) mutations have also been identified in the CXCR4 gene in 27% of cases, with this mutation only previously being described in germline DNA. Familial cases of WM have recently been described using whole-exome sequencing, with LAPTM5 and HCLS1 as potential candidate genes predisposing to familial WM development.

MYD88 mutations with resultant increased NF-κB signaling provide the scientific rationale for the use of inhibitors of Bruton's tyrosine kinase (BTK) in treating this disease. In a prospective study of ibrutinib monotherapy in 63 patients with symptomatic WM who had received at least one prior therapy, ibrutinib was associated with an ORR of 90.5% with major responses in 73%. Higher responses were demonstrated in patients with mutated MYD88 (L265P) and wild-type CXCR4 with an ORR of 100% and major response rate of 91.2%. Based on this data, ibrutinib was granted breakthrough therapy designation by the FDA and approved for the treatment of patients with LPL/WM.

Marginal Zone Lymphomas

The spectrum of marginal zone lymphomas are all indolent lymphomas, comprising approximately 10% of NHL, that occur primarily in extranodal MALT (EMZL or MALT lymphomas), and to a lesser extent within the spleen (splenic MZL) and lymph nodes (nodal MZL). The majority of EMZL occurs within the gastrointestinal tract (most commonly the stomach), but can also occur in the parotid and salivary glands, thyroid, lungs, ocular adnexae, and breast, among others. Most patients present with localized disease, and 5-year survival is approximately 90%. EMZL is frequently antigen driven, and a history of chronic infection such as H.pylori-associated gastritis in gastric MALT lymphoma or Chlamydiphila psittaci in OAML is common. With current antibiotic regimens, approximately 62% of patients with early-stage gastric MALT lymphoma will achieve complete remission with bacterial eradication alone. Patients found to have a t(11;18) translocation detected by cytogenetics, FISH, or polymerase chain reaction (PCR) are less likely to respond to antibiotic therapy alone and should be considered for alternative treatment. In OAML, data indicate that eradication of C. psittaci with doxycycline can induce complete remission in approximately 22% of patients with partial remissions in another 22% and minimal responses (<50% regression) in 33%. For patients with advanced or antibiotic-refractory disease, or those with MALT subtypes not associated with known infectious agents, therapeutic options include rituximab, chemoimmunotherapy regimens similar to those used in FL, radiation, and surgical resection in sites amenable to complete resection.

Splenic MZL accounts for approximately 20% of MZL, and typically presents with splenomegaly and BM involvement. Five-year overall survival is approximately 80%. Splenectomy has been the historical standard of care; however, rituximab is increasingly being used as an alternative or adjunct to surgical therapy. In a retrospective trial of 43 patients with splenic MZL, rituximab monotherapy was as effective as combination chemoimmunotherapy with CR rates of 90% and 79%, respectively, and significantly less toxicity. Rituximab combined with splenectomy was associated with improved responses (CR 100% vs. 67%) compared to unsplenectomized patients and improved 3-year disease-free survival (DFS) was shown with rituximab therapy compared to splenectomy or chemotherapy alone (79% vs. 29% vs. 25%). Similar to EMZL, splenic MZL can also be antigen driven; approximately one-third of cases are associated with HCV, and many of these patients can enter remission with antiviral therapy alone.

Nodal MZL is the least common MZL, and is characterized by nodal disease in the absence of a mucosal component. The clinical course of nodal MZL tends to be more aggressive than its extranodal or splenic counterparts, and 5-year overall survival is slightly lower at approximately 76%. Although it can also be associated with HCV infection in up to 20% of cases, it is typically not associated with a known infectious etiology. A distinct pattern of genetic alterations was recently shown when comparing nodal MZL to its splenic counterpart, with a high prevalence of *MLL2* (aka *KMT2D*), *PTPRD, NOTCH2,* and *KLF2* mutations in nodal disease. Mutations in *PTPRD*, a receptor-type protein tyrosine phosphatase, resulted in cell-cycle deregulation and increased proliferation and was only seen in nodal MZL. This mutation provides further insight into the pathogenesis of disease and may serve as a novel marker in diagnosis. The therapeutic approach for nodal MZL generally follows that of FL.

Aggressive B-Cell Non-Hodgkin Lymphoma

Diffuse Large B-Cell Lymphoma

DLBCL is the most common NHL subtype, accounting for approximately 30% of all cases. Although it is most commonly diagnosed in the seventh decade of life, DLBCL can occur at any age. DLBCL can occur either *de novo* or as a histologic transformation from an indolent NHL. Gene expression profiling classifies DLBCL into two major molecular subtypes, germinal center B cell (GCB) and activated B cell (ABC), with the latter being less curable with standard therapies. ABC-DLBCL is always associated with constitutive activation of the NF-κB pathway through a variety of mechanisms. One important and well-characterized mechanism involves chronic active B-cell receptor (BCR) signaling via activating mutations in the BCR subunits, *CD79A* and *CD79B*, as well as mutations in *MYD88* and *CARD11*.

Patients with all stages of DLBCL are treated with systemic chemoimmunotherapy with curative intent (see Table 28.5). In multiple studies, R-CHOP given every 21 days (R-CHOP-21) has been shown to significantly improve response rates, PFS, and OS compared to CHOP alone in previously untreated patients with advanced disease, and consequently this regimen is now considered standard. The addition of Involved-field radiation therapy (IFRT) to an abbreviated course of systemic therapy is considered an option in patients with early-stage DLBCL, although such an approach introduces the risk of long-term complications of radiation treatment. The use of "dose-dense" R-CHOP every 14 days with myeloid growth factor support (R-CHOP-14) has failed to demonstrate superiority over standard R-CHOP-21. Dose intensity may still have a role in DLBCL, however, as the dose-intensive regimen of rituximab, doxorubicin, cyclophosphamide, vindesine, bleomycin, and prednisone (R-ACVBP) (full chemo regimens in the legend with the table below) demonstrated superior 3-year PFS and OS in untreated DLBCL patients aged 18 to 59 with low-intermediate IPI compared to R-CHOP. Although serious adverse events were more than twice as common with R-ACVBP, it nevertheless remains a promising regimen that can be considered for younger patients. Dose-adjusted (DA) EPOCH-R is another alternative regimen that has shown promising results in phase II trials and is currently being evaluated against R-CHOP-21 in a randomized phase 3 study. In a multicenter, phase 2 study conducted by the CALGB in untreated DLBCL, 5-year time to progression (TTP) and event free survival (EFS) were 100% and 94% for GCB and 67% and 58% for

TABLE 28.5 First-Line Treatment Regimens and Outcome for Diffuse Large B-Cell Lymphoma

First-Line Treatment Regimen	Number of Patients	Outcome	Study Reference
R-CHOP	202	2-y EFS 57%	Coiffier et al.
vs.		2-y OS 70%	
CHOP	197	2-y EFS 38%	
		2-y OS 57%	
R-CHOP-21	298	3-y EFS 60%	Delarue et al.
vs.		3-y PFS 62%	
R-CHOP-14		3-y OS 72%	
	304	3-y EFS 56%	
		3-y PFS 60%	
		3-y OS 69%	
R-ACVBP	196	3-y EFS 81%	Recher et al.
vs.		3-y PFS 87%	
R-CHOP		3-y OS 92%	
	183	3-y EFS 67%	
		3-y PFS 73%	
		3-y OS 84%	
DA-EPOCH-R	69	5-y EFS 75%	Wilson et al.
		(94% GCB, 58% non-GCB)	
		5-y PFS 81%	
		(100% GCB, 67% non-GCB)	
		5-y OS 84%	
		(94% GCB, 68% non-GCB)	

R-CHOP, rituximab, cyclophosphamide, doxorubicin, vincristine, and prednisone; CHOP, cyclophosphamide, doxorubicin, vincristine, and prednisone; DA-EPOCH-R, dose-adjusted etoposide, prednisone, vincristine, cyclophosphamide, doxorubicin, and rituximab; R-ACVBP, rituximab, doxorubicin, cyclophosphamide, vindesine, bleomycin, and prednisone; EFS, event free survival; OS, overall survival; PFS, progression free survival; GCB, germinal center B-cell; non-GCB, non-germinal center B-cell.

non-GCB, respectively. This regimen is also associated with a lower observed incidence of cardiac toxicity compared to R-CHOP and can be considered for patients in whom this is a concern.

Novel agents that target BCR signaling and reduce NF-κB activity are currently being tested as monotherapy in the relapsed/refractory setting as well as in combination with front-line cytotoxic therapy, especially in ABC-DLBCL. In a phase I/II study of 80 patients with relapsed or refractory DLBCL, a higher ORR was seen with ibrutinib monotherapy in ABC-DLBCL (37% vs. 5%) with a median response duration of approximately 5 months. Responses were enriched in patients with *CD79B* mutations compared to wild-type (ORR 55.5% vs. 31%) but were lower in those with isolated *MYD88, CARD11,* or *TNFAIP3* mutations, given these mutations provide an alternative mechanism of NF-κB activation. The highest responses were seen in those patients with concomitant *CD79B* and *MYD88* mutations with an ORR of 80%. When combined with R-CHOP in the front-line setting, all newly-diagnosed DLBCL patients who received the recommended phase II dose (560 mg daily) responded, with 100% CR rate in non-GCB subtype and 71% CR rate in GCB subtype.

The immunomodulatory agent, lenalidomide, through downregulation of IRF4 and SPIB, leads to decreased NF-κB activity and augmentation of INFβ production. Through these effects it has shown significant activity in ABC-DLBCL, both as monotherapy and in combination with cytotoxic therapy. In relapsed/refractory aggressive NHL, the majority DLBCL, lenalidomide monotherapy resulted in an

ORR of 35% with CR rate of 12% and a median DOR and PFS of 6.2 and 4 months, respectively. This response was confirmed in a large international phase II study demonstrating an ORR of 28% with 7% CR and median duration of remission and PFS of 4.6 and 2.7 months, respectively. A retrospective study investigated responses based on molecular subtype and found significantly higher responses in non-GCB compared to GCB subtype, with ORR and CR rates of 52.9% vs. 8.7% and 23.5% vs. 4.3%, respectively. Combination with standard-dose R-CHOP on days 1 to 10 of each cycle in untreated DLBCL patients resulted in an ORR of 98% with a CR rate of 80%. Compared to historic controls treated with conventional R-CHOP alone, lenalidomide overcame the negative impact of non-GCB DLBCL showing no difference in 24-month PFS or OS in the R^2-CHOP treated patients based on DLBCL subtype. These targeted therapies as well as other novel agents are currently being investigated in the front-line setting but are not yet commercially available for use outside of a clinical trial. Consequently, the GCB/ABC distinction cannot yet be used to guide choice of initial therapy for DLBCL.

Primary mediastinal B-cell lymphoma (PMBL) is a subtype of DLBCL that clinically and biologically more closely resembles classical Hodgkin lymphoma than other subtypes of DLBCL. Standard treatment approaches in the past have involved chemotherapy followed by mediastinal radiation. While combined modality therapy has been very effective in most patients, mediastinal radiation is associated with long-term sequelae and increased risks of cardiac disease and secondary tumors, particularly breast cancer in females. In a phase II study, DA-EPOCH-R demonstrated high efficacy in this disease with a 5-year EFS and OS of 93% and 97%, respectively, obviating the need for radiation in almost all patients.

Up to 10% of patients with DLBCL harbor t(8;14) with overexpression of *MYC*, and many of these patients are also positive for t(14;18) with overexpression of *BCL2* (so-called "double-hit" lymphoma). Many of these tumors may fit into the WHO category of "B-cell lymphoma unclassifiable with features intermediate between BL and DLBCL." In several retrospective studies, these patients have demonstrated inferior outcomes with standard therapies and benefit more from intensive treatment, similar to that used in Burkitt lymphoma. A multicenter study using DA-EPOCH-R in *MYC*-rearranged DLBCL is ongoing with encouraging preliminary results but at this time the optimal management of patients with "double-hit" lymphoma is unknown.

Primary CNS Lymphoma

PCNSL is a rare and aggressive lymphoma that is confined to the CNS (brain parenchyma, meninges, cranial nerves, eyes, spinal cord). It is of DLBCL histology in over 95% of cases, and can occur in both immunocompetent and immunocompromised patients. It most commonly affects the brain parenchyma, although there can be concomitant or isolated leptomeningeal involvement in approximately 20% of cases. Intraocular involvement is also common and in some cases can predate the development of brain lesions by months.

PCNSL is not effectively treated by standard DLBCL chemoimmunotherapy regimens due to inability of the component agents to penetrate effectively through the blood–brain barrier. High-dose methotrexate (up to 8 g/m^2) achieves therapeutic levels within the CSF and produces high response rates and 2-year OS of 50% to 70%. A randomized phase III study assessing the addition of whole brain radiation therapy (WBRT) to high-dose methotrexate failed to demonstrate an improvement in OS with the addition of WBRT. In a randomized phase II trial, the addition of high-dose cytarabine to high-dose methotrexate improved response rates (ORR 69% vs. 40%) and showed a trend toward improved OS (3-year OS of 46% vs. 32%, P=0.07). Consequently, this combination is now considered a standard first-line treatment option. The role of WBRT consolidation after chemotherapy remains controversial, as it is associated with significant and sometimes disabling neurotoxicity. Patients not achieving CR to chemotherapy have a poor prognosis and are generally offered WBRT. A study of salvage WBRT (median dose, 36 Gy) following initial high-dose methotrexate failure, resulted in a high ORR of 74% but median OS from initiation of WBRT was only 10.9 months. Relapsed and refractory PCNSL represents an unmet clinical need for effective salvage therapies and eligible patients should be considered for participation in clinical trials.

Approximately 96% of PCNSL tumors in immunocompetent individuals express an ABC immunophenotype by IHC. High-throughput sequencing has allowed for better characterization of the genomic landscape of PCNSL, leading to ongoing studies using novel targeted agents. Compared to systemic DLBCL, PCNSL has been shown to harbor more frequent mutations in the NF-κB pathway, including *MYD88* and *CD79B* mutations, with often concurrent mutations at multiple sites in the same pathway. These mutations provide the scientific rationale for targeting the BCR pathway and BTK, and current studies with ibrutinib monotherapy and in combination with cytotoxic chemotherapy are ongoing. Ibrutinib was combined with a novel chemotherapy regimen DA-TEDDI-R (dose-adjusted temozolomide, etoposide, doxil, dexamethasone, ibrutinib, and rituximab with intraventricular cytarabine) in untreated and relapsed/refractory PCNSL patients. In 18 PCNSL patients, 94% showed tumor reductions with ibrutinib alone during a 14 day lead-in window period with 86% of evaluable patients achieving CR with DA-TEDDI-R. Programmed death 1 (PD-1) and/or programmed death ligand 1 (PD-L1) has been shown to be expressed on tumor cells, tumor infiltrating lymphocytes, or tumor-associated macrophages in 90% of PCNSL specimens from immunocompetent individuals. Frequent copy gains in 9p24.1, resulting in increased expression of *PD-L1* and *PD-L2*, have been identified in 52% of EBV-negative PCNSL with 6% of PCNSL specimens having previously unidentified translocations involving the *PD-L1* or *PD-L2* loci. Studies using inhibitors of PD-1 in patients with PCNSL are currently ongoing.

Burkitt Lymphoma

BL is a highly aggressive but curable lymphoma, accounting for 1% to 2% of lymphomas in the United States. Most cases in the United States and Western countries are either sporadic or associated with immunodeficiency, typically affecting children and young adults and demonstrating EBV positivity in 30% to 50% of cases. Endemic BL, by contrast, is strongly associated with EBV infection and is highly prevalent in young children in equatorial Africa. Whereas endemic BL presents most commonly with jaw and facial bone disease, sporadic BL tends to present with bulky abdominal disease. Involvement of the BM, GI tract, and CNS are also common. All variants of BL are characterized by acute clinical onset and rapid disease progression without therapy.

Like DLBCL, the cell of origin for Burkitt lymphoma is presumed to be a normal germinal center B-cell. *MYC* is the most recurrently mutated gene in BL, found in up to 70% of the cases, but multiple other regulatory pathways are deregulated and cooperate with *MYC* in oncogenesis. Tonic BCR signaling is augmented through mutations in the transcription factor *TCF3* or *ID3*, its negative regulator, and can be seen in up to 70% of sporadic BL cases. Frequent mutations in *CCND3* stabilize cyclin D3 isoforms and drive cell cycle progression in approximately 38% of sporadic BL cases. These mutations provide insight into the underlying pathogenesis of disease as well as can serve as potential targets for novel therapies in the future.

Dose-intensive multiagent chemotherapy regimens incorporating high-dose methotrexate, high-dose cytarabine, and intrathecal chemotherapy (CODOX-M/IVAC, hyper-CVAD) are commonly used to treat BL, with approximately 60% to 80% of patients achieving long-term survival. The addition of rituximab to intensive chemotherapy was recently shown to improve EFS in a randomized phase III trial of 260 patients with untreated HIV-negative BL, and is now considered standard in most BL regimens. Additionally, treatment with DA-EPOCH-R appears to be an effective, less-toxic therapy for both HIV-negative and HIV-positive BL patients with freedom from progression (FFP) of 95% to 100% at the median follow-up. A confirmatory multicenter study of this regimen in BL and MYC+ DLBCL is ongoing.

Mantle Cell Lymphoma

MCL is an incurable and variably aggressive lymphoma. Median age at diagnosis is 60, and most those affected are men. Patients commonly present with advanced disease, splenomegaly, and involvement of the BM, peripheral blood, and GI tract. Virtually all cases of MCL harbor t(11;14) with resultant overexpression of cyclin D1, although a small minority of MCL can be negative for cyclin D1.

Although response rates to chemotherapy are high in MCL, remissions tend to be short-lived and historic median survival is approximately 3 to 6 years. The mantle cell IPI (MIPI) classifies patients into prognostic categories based upon age, performance status, LDH, and WBC count, and can aid in therapeutic decision making. Given that a subset of MCL behaves in an indolent manner, watchful waiting is a reasonable approach in asymptomatic patients with a low risk MIPI. For symptomatic patients or those with a high risk MIPI, therapeutic options include standard chemotherapy (R-CHOP, BR, DA-EPOCH-R) or dose-intensive chemotherapy such as R-hyper-CVAD/MA (see Table 28.6). Although the latter approach has recently yielded impressive results (median OS of 10.7 years), it has also been associated with considerable toxicity, especially in older patients. In younger patients, high-dose chemotherapy with autologous stem cell rescue (HDT/ASCR) in first remission after induction chemotherapy has been studied extensively and may extend PFS over chemotherapy alone, although it is not curative. A recent randomized study from the European MCL Network strongly suggested that induction regimens that utilize cytarabine during induction are superior to regimens without cytarabine in younger patients who undergo HDT in first remission. Such intensive regimens followed by HDT/ASCR are the standard of care in many regions, although this approach is not broadly applicable to all patients with MCL. Nonmyeloablative allogeneic stem cell transplantation (SCT) is still considered investigational, although currently it remains the only potentially curative option.

Since many patients with MCL are over the age of 65, a highly intensive treatment such as HDT/ASCR in first remission is associated with excessive toxicity. Thus, alternative strategies have been developed for patients considered unfit or those who wish to avoid dose intensive therapy in the front-line setting. In a randomized, non-inferiority trial of BR compared to R-CHOP in the first-line treatment of patients with MCL, BR was associated with improved PFS and less overall toxicity compared to R-CHOP in all histologic subtypes, including MCL (median PFS 35.4 vs. 22.1 months). The proteasome inhibitor, bortezomib, as well as the immunomodulatory agent, lenalidomide, have both shown activity in MCL and have been used as front-line therapy in combination with chemoimmunotherapy and rituximab, respectively. In a randomized, phase III study of R-CHOP vs. substitution of bortezomib for vincristine (VR-CAP), patients with newly-diagnosed MCL who received the bortezomib-containing regimen had improved PFS (median 24.7 vs. 14.4 months) with a trend toward improved OS (median NR vs. 56.3 months), but this was at the expense of increased hematotoxicity. Bortezomib was also

TABLE 28.6 First-Line Treatment Regimens (non-HDT/ASCR) and Outcome for Mantle Cell Lymphoma

First-Line Treatment Regimen	Number of Patients	Outcome	Study Reference
R-hyper-CVAD/MA	97	Median FFS 4.8 y Median OS 10.7 y	Chihara et al.
BR	46	Median PFS 35.4 mo	Rummel et al.
vs.			
R-CHOP	48	Median PFS 22.1 mo	
VR-CAP	243	Median PFS 24.7 mo	Robak et al.
vs.			
R-CHOP	244	Median PFS 14.4 mo	
R-CHOP + Bortezomib induction and maintenance	65	Median PFS 29.5 mo	Till et al.
R²	38	2-year PFS 85% 2-year OS 97%	Ruan et al.

R-hyper-CVAD/MA, rituximab, fractionated cyclophosphamide, vincristine, doxorubicin, and dexamethasone alternating with methotrexate and cytarabine; BR, bendamustine and rituximab; R-CHOP, rituximab, cyclophosphamide, doxorubicin, vincristine, and prednisone; VR-CAP, bortezomib, rituximab, cyclophosphamide, doxorubicin, and prednisone; R², rituximab and Revlimid (lenalidomide); FFS, failure free survival; OS, overall survival; PFS, progression-free survival.

combined with R-CHOP induction therapy followed by bortezomib maintenance in the phase II SWOG S0601 trial, and resulted in durable remissions in a subset of patients (5-year PFS 28% and OS 66%) with acceptable toxicity. In a multicenter, phase II study of lenalidomide and rituximab (R^2), an ORR of 92% with CR rate of 64% was demonstrated in the up-front setting along with a 2-year PFS and OS of 85% and 97%, respectively. This regimen represents a promising chemotherapy-free approach with significant activity and acceptable safety, especially in patients unable to tolerate more aggressive cytotoxic regimens (see Table 28.6).

Multiple novel agents have demonstrated significant activity in MCL and are approved for use in the relapsed and/or refractory setting (see Table 28.7). In a multicenter phase II study, bortezomib monotherapy resulted in an ORR of 33% with a median DOR of 9.2 months. The phase II MCL-001 (EMERGE) study demonstrated an ORR of 28% with CR/CRu in 7.5% and median DOR of 16.6 months with lenalidomide monotherapy in MCL patients who relapsed after or were refractory to bortezomib. The randomized, phase II MCL-002 (SPRINT) study compared lenalidomide to investigator's choice (rituximab, gemcitabine, fludarabine, chlorambucil, or cytarabine) and demonstrated a significantly improved PFS (8.7 vs. 5.2 months) in relapsed or refractory patients ineligible for intensive chemotherapy or stem-cell transplantation. In combination with rituximab, R^2 demonstrated an ORR of 57% with a median DOR of 18.9 months. Durable responses with the BTK inhibitor, ibrutinib, have also been shown in relapsed or refractory MCL patients with an ORR of 68% (no difference comparing patients with prior bortezomib treatment) and a median DOR of 17.5 months. Extended follow-up of this study revealed a 2-year PFS and OS of 31% and 47%, respectively. Ibrutinib combined with rituximab resulted in increased response rates with ORR and CR rates of 88% and 44%, respectively, with acceptable toxicity. A randomized phase III study compared ibrutinib to temsirolimus

TABLE 28.7 Novel Targeted Treatment Regimens and Outcome for Mantle Cell Lymphoma

Targeted Regimen	Number of Patients	Response Rate	Median TTR	Median DOR	Median PFS	Study Reference
Bortezomib	155	ORR 33% CR/CRu 8%	1.3 mo	9.2 mo	6.2 mo	Fisher et al.
Lenalidomide	134	ORR 28% CR/CRu 7.5%	2.2 mo	16.6 mo	4 mo	Goy et al.
Lenalidomide vs.	170	ORR 40% CR 5%	4.3 mo	16.1 mo	8.7 mo	Trneny et al.
single-agent investigator's choice	84	ORR 11% CR 0%	NR	10.4 mo	5.2 mo	
R^2	52	ORR 57% CR 36%	2 mo	18.9 mo	11.1 mo	Wang et al.
Ibrutinib	111	ORR 68% CR 21%	1.9 mo	17.5 mo	13.9 mo	Wang et al.
Ibrutinib + Rituximab	50	ORR 88% CR 44%	1.8 mo	NR	NR	Wang et al.
Ibrutinib vs.	139	ORR 72% CR 19%	N/A	NR	14.6 mo	Dreyling et al.
Temsirolimus	141	ORR 40% CR 1%	N/A	7 mo	6.2 mo	

R^2, rituximab and Revlimid (lenalidomide); ORR, overall response rate; CR, complete response; CRu, complete response unconfirmed; TTR, time to response; DOR, duration of response; PFS, progression free survival; NR, not reached; N/A, not available.

and demonstrated a significant improvement in PFS with ibrutinib (14.6 vs. 6.2 months) with less treatment-emergent adverse events (68% vs. 87%) and reduced need for study drug discontinuation (6% vs. 26%). Bortezomib and ibrutinib monotherapy are both currently FDA approved for treatment of patients with MCL who have received at least one prior therapy with lenalidomide approved after two prior therapies, at least one including bortezomib.

Peripheral T-Cell Lymphomas

The term "peripheral T-cell lymphoma" (PTCL) encompasses the various lymphomas derived from mature T and natural killer (NK) cells. T-cell lymphomas are less common than B-cell lymphomas, accounting for approximately 10% to 15% of NHL. Their behavior ranges from indolent to aggressive, although the majority are relatively aggressive lymphomas with poor response rates to chemotherapy and poor OS relative to B-cell lymphomas. There are notable exceptions, however, such as ALK-positive anaplastic large cell lymphoma (ALCL) and mycosis fungoides (MF) with limited skin disease, which have excellent prognoses. Although various distinct disease entities exist within the realm of PTCL, the most common subclassification remains "PTCL-not otherwise specified," underscoring the need for further elucidation of the genetic and molecular basis of these diseases.

Anaplastic Large Cell Lymphoma

ALCL is a CD30-positive subtype of PTCL that encompasses two biologically distinct diseases: ALCL that overexpresses anaplastic lymphoma kinase (ALK), usually due to t(2;5), and ALK-negative ALCL. The former is typically a disease of children and young adults, while the latter tends to affect older individuals. Patients with both forms typically present with diffuse lymphadenopathy, extranodal disease, and systemic symptoms. ALK-positive ALCL has an excellent prognosis compared to most PTCL subtypes, with a 5-year OS of approximately 70% after anthracycline-based chemotherapy. ALK-negative ALCL has poorer outcomes, and the approach to therapy generally follows that of PTCL-NOS. DA-EPOCH-R has shown promising efficacy in a prospective study of 24 patients with newly-diagnosed ALCL with EFS rates of 72% and 62.5% and OS rates of 78% and 87.5% for ALK-positive and ALK-negative patients, respectively, at a median follow-up of 14.4 years. Additionally, the anti-CD30 monoclonal antibody/cytotoxic conjugate, brentuximab vedotin, was FDA approved for relapsed/refractory ALCL after demonstrating an ORR of 86% with a CR rate of 57% and median duration of overall and complete response of 12.6 and 13.2 months, respectively. This promising agent is being further evaluated in combination with chemotherapy and in the first-line setting.

Primary cutaneous ALCL is a separate disease entity characterized by indolent behavior, predominantly dermatologic involvement, and excellent long-term survival. Additionally, a recent phenomenon of primary breast ALCL occurring in women with breast implants has been reported over the past decade. A recent FDA analysis concluded that breast implants are potentially associated with an increased relative risk, but still very low absolute risk, of primary breast ALCL. A study of 87 breast implant-associated ALCL (BI-ALCL) patients showed a 3- and 5-year OS rate of 93% and 89%, respectively, with superior EFS and OS in patients who underwent a complete surgical excision (total capsulectomy and breast implant removal) compared to patients who had a partial capsulectomy, systemic chemotherapy, or XRT.

Peripheral T-Cell Lymphoma, Not Otherwise Specified (PTCL-NOS)

This sub-classification includes all T-cell lymphomas not identified as clinicopathologically distinct by the WHO classification. They are generally aggressive lymphomas that affect men disproportionately, present with both nodal and extranodal disease, and respond poorly to CHOP-like chemotherapy, with 5-year OS of approximately 30% to 40%. Improved 3-year EFS (75.4% vs. 51.0%) was seen in younger (≤60 years old) T-cell lymphoma patients with normal LDH levels with the addition of etoposide (CHOEP) to CHOP in patients treated on trials of the German High-Grade NHL Study Group (DSHNHL). PTCL-NOS patients had the worst outcome regardless of the regimen received with 3-year EFS and OS of 41.1% and 53.9%, respectively. Dose-intensive regimens such as hyper-CVAD have not been shown to improve outcomes over CHOP. A phase II study by the Nordic Lymphoma Group (NLG) of upfront HDT/ASCT in PTCL demonstrated good results, with 5-year PFS and OS of 44% and

TABLE 28.8 Novel Targeted Treatment Regimens and Outcome for PTCL

Targeted Regimen	Number of Patients	Response Rate	Median TTR	Median DOR	Median PFS	Study Reference
Romidepsin	130	ORR 25% CR/CRu 15%	1.8 mo	16.6 mo	4 mo	Coiffier et al.
Belinostat	120	ORR 25.8% CR 10.8%	5.6 weeks	13.6 mo	1.6 mo	O'Connor et al.
Pralatrexate	111	ORR 29% CR 11%	46 days	10.1 mo	3.5 mo	O'Connor et al.
Brentuximab vedotin	34 All	ORR 41% CR 24%	N/A	7.6 mo	2.6 mo	Howitz et al.
(CD30+ PTCL)	13 AITL	ORR 54% CR 38%	N/A	5.5 mo	6.7 mo	
	22 PTCL-NOS	ORR 33% CR 14%	N/A	7.6 mo	1.6 mo	

CD30, cluster of differentiation 30; PTCL, peripheral T-cell lymphoma; AITL, angioimmunoblastic T-cell lymphoma; PTCL-NOS, peripheral T-cell lymphoma, not otherwise specified; ORR, overall response rate; CR, complete response; CRu, complete response unconfirmed; TTR, time to response; DOR, duration of response; PFS, progression free survival; NR, not reached; N/A, not available.

51%, respectively. Although this approach is promising, randomized studies to assess the true benefit of HDT/ASCR are needed.

Several novel agents have demonstrated activity in relapsed/refractory PTCL in recent years, and are currently being evaluated in combination with chemotherapy and in the front-line setting (see Table 28.8). These include the histone deacetylase inhibitors, romidepsin and belinostat, and the novel antifolate, pralatrexate, which have all been FDA approved for relapsed/refractory PTCL. Romidepsin was approved based on a phase II trial showing an ORR of 25% with median DOR of 17 months, with responses seen independent of number of prior therapies or ASCT. PTCL patients treated on the phase II BELIEF (CLN-19) study with belinostat monotherapy had an ORR of 25.8% with median DOR of 13.6 months. The PROPEL study with pralatrexate demonstrated an ORR of 29% and median DOR of 10.1 months and led to its approval for PTCL in the relapsed setting. Other agents being studied include brentuximab vedotin for patients with relapsed PTCL-NOS who are CD30 positive. A phase II study of BV in 35 patients with CD30-positive PTCL (22 patients with PTCL-NOS) revealed an ORR for the entire cohort and PTCL-NOS patients of 41% and 33%, respectively. Median PFS was worse in the PTCL-NOS patients compared to those with angioimmunoblastic T-cell lymphoma (AITL) (1.61 vs. 6.74 months). Given the currently poor outcomes with these agents in patients with relapsed and/or refractory PTCL-NOS, enrollment in a clinical trial is preferred for eligible patients.

Angioimmunoblastic T-cell Lymphoma

AITL is one of the more common subtypes of PTCL, accounting for 15% to 20% of cases. Median age at diagnosis is 65, and patients typically present with diffuse lymphadenopathy, hepatosplenomegaly, extranodal involvement, systemic symptoms, rash, and hypergammaglobulinemia. Autoimmune phenomena, both hematologic and nonhematologic, are also common. Response rates to anthracycline-based chemotherapy are relatively poor, and 5-year OS is approximately 30%. High-dose chemotherapy with autologous stem cell rescue as first-line therapy for AITL is being studied; however, currently the benefit of this approach remains unclear. The phase II study of brentuximab vedotin in relapsed/refractory PTCL showed a higher ORR of 54% and median PFS of 6.7 months in AITL patients compared to those with PTCL-NOS and represents an option for CD30-positive patients (see Table 28.8).

Immunosuppressive therapy with cyclosporine has shown promising early results, and can be considered in select cases. The efficacy of cyclosporin A (CsA) in patients with recurrent AITL is being evaluated in a prospective study (ECOG 2402). Otherwise, the approach to treatment of AITL largely follows that of PTCL-NOS.

Rare Extranodal NK/T-cell Lymphomas

The two main subclassifications of NK/T-cell lymphoma are extranodal NK/T-cell lymphoma, nasal type (ENKL), and aggressive NK-cell leukemia (ANKL). These diseases are almost always EBV positive, and are extremely rare in North America and Europe but prevalent in Asia and Central/South America. ENKL typically involves the nasopharynx and nasal cavity, palate, and can also affect the skin, gastrointestinal tract, and testis. EBV viral load serves as a useful biomarker of disease in the blood and should be measured at diagnosis and followed throughout the course of treatment as a marker of possible persistent disease. A separate prognostic system involving four parameters (serum LDH >normal, B symptoms, LN involvement, N1-N3, not M1 and Ann Arbor Stage IV) comprises the NK/T-cell lymphoma prognostic index and divides into risk groups based on 0, 1, 2, or 3 to 4 risk factors with 5-year OS of 80.9%, 64.2%, 34.4% and 6.6%, respectively. Newer models exist for patients treated with non-anthracycline-based chemotherapies with or without concurrent chemoradiation or radiotherapy, termed the prognostic index of natural killer lymphoma, and another newer model incorporates EBV viral load. Patients with disease confined to the nasal cavity can be successfully treated using IFRT with or without chemotherapy (DeVIC, VIPD, SMILE, or GELOX), while those with extranasal disease and ANKL have a very poor prognosis. Encouraging results have recently been seen with L-asparaginase-based chemotherapy regimens, and further studies evaluating this agent in ENKL and ANKL are ongoing. The SMILE regimen in patients with newly diagnosed stage IV or relapsed/refractory disease yielded an ORR and CR rate of 79% and 45%, respectively, after 2 cycles of therapy with a majority of patients who completed the protocol proceeding to HSCT. A retrospective study of another regimen using pegaspargase with gemcitabine and oxaliplatin (P-GEMOX) in patients with newly-diagnosed stage III/IV or relapsed/refractory disease, demonstrated an ORR and CR rate or 80% and 51.4%, respectively, and represents and alternative option for therapy. Both of these regimens have been utilized alone as well as have been tested with sequential or sandwich radiotherapy.

Gamma-Delta T-Cell Lymphomas

These are rare and aggressive T-cell lymphomas that originate from gamma-delta lymphocytes. The WHO 2008 classification divided these lymphomas into two separate entities: hepatosplenic gamma-delta T-cell lymphoma (HSGDTL) and primary cutaneous gamma-delta T-cell lymphoma (PCGDTL). HSGDTL typically affects young men and involves the liver, spleen, and BM. Histologic diagnosis can often be difficult to obtain. Prognosis is poor regardless of choice of therapy, with a median OS of approximately 2 years. There is no standard of care, although most patients are treated with CHOP-like regimens with or without HDT/ASCR. PCGDTL is extremely rare and accounts for <1% of primary cutaneous lymphomas. Cutaneous disease is variable and clinical course is typically aggressive with poor long-term survival. Small single-center studies indicate brentuximab vedotin as a potential treatment option for chemotherapy-refractory patients whose tumors express CD30.

Enteropathy-Associated T-Cell Lymphoma

This is a rare and aggressive PTCL of the small intestine that typically affects older individuals with celiac disease, although many patients are diagnosed with EATL who have no known history of enteropathy. Patients typically present with abdominal pain and anorexia. A large, multicenter cohort study of 61 EATL patients showed overall poor prognosis with 1 and 5-year OS rates of 40% and 11%, respectively. Patients receiving the most aggressive treatments, including surgical resection, chemotherapy, and ASCT, showed the best outcomes with 1- and 5-year OS of 100% and 33%, respectively. Combination therapy appears to result in superior outcomes but the benefit of consolidative ASCT needs to be confirmed in larger randomized studies.

Cutaneous T-Cell Lymphoma/Mycosis Fungoides

CTCLs are typically mature T-cell neoplasms that originate within, and often remain confined to, the skin, with variable spread to the lymph nodes, BM, and peripheral blood. MF constitutes the majority of CTCL. Sezary syndrome (SS) is the much less common leukemic manifestation of MF, accounting for 3% of CTCL. MF is considered an indolent lymphoma, although behavior and prognosis are highly variable; patients with limited patch or plaque disease of the skin have excellent long-term survival, while prognosis is poorer for those with erythrodermal skin involvement and extracutaneous disease.

MF is staged per the revised MFCG staging system, which incorporates extent of skin, nodal, visceral organ, and peripheral blood involvement. Patients with limited skin disease are typically treated with topical corticosteroids, topical retinoids, topical chemotherapy, phototherapy, or local radiation. Patients with more extensive skin involvement can be treated with the same modalities or with total skin electron beam therapy (TSEBT). Patients with more advanced disease are treated initially with systemic therapies such as extracorporeal photopheresis (ECP), oral retinoids, interferon, or HDAC inhibitors, with chemotherapy being reserved for patients who progress on these agents or for those with aggressive disease with visceral organ involvement. Systemic chemotherapy agents used include alemtuzumab, brentuximab, bortezomib, doxil, gemcitabine, low-dose methotrexate, pentostatin, and temozolomide. A recent phase II study of brentuximab vedotin showed an ORR of 54% in patients with MF/SS, with responses seen independent of CD30 expression. A large, single-center study of allogeneic HSCT in advanced CTCL, after failure of standard therapy, reported long-term remissions in a subset of patients with 4-year OS and PFS of 51% and 26%, respectively, but at the risk of a cumulative incidence of non-relapse mortality of 16.7% at 2 years. The current role of allogeneic HSCT in the treatment of advanced and relapsed/refractory disease remains unclear at this time.

Treatment Approaches for Relapsed Aggressive Lymphomas

Treatment for relapsed aggressive DLBCL generally involves salvage chemotherapy followed by HDT/ASCR in fit patients who demonstrate chemosensitive disease. Commonly used salvage chemotherapy regimens include R-ICE, R-DHAP, R-ESHAP, and EPOCH-R. Patients with chemoresistant disease do not benefit from HDT/ASCR and should be enrolled into clinical trials, considered for allogeneic HSCT, or treated palliatively. Additionally, the results of the CORAL study indicate that the benefit of HDT/ASCR may be significantly limited in the rituximab era, as patients in this trial who were previously treated with rituximab had a 3-year EFS of only 21% after HDT/ASCR. This study also demonstrated a similarly poor 3-year EFS in patients who relapsed less than 12 months after initial diagnosis. Consequently, careful consideration of disease factors, as well as a frank discussion of treatment and available trial options, should precede referral for HDT/ASCR. Nontransplant candidates who are not eligible for a clinical trial can be treated palliatively with any of the aforementioned salvage regimens or with BR or lenalidomide.

The other aggressive B-cell lymphomas (MCL, BL) and most aggressive T-cell lymphomas are rarely, if ever, cured with conventional salvage chemotherapy or HDT/ASCR, although studies of HDT/ASCR in relapsed PTCL have demonstrated a 5-year OS of approximately 40% and patients with ALK-positive ALCL can be cured with this approach. HDT/ASCR is considered an option in patients with PTCL who demonstrate chemosensitivity to salvage chemotherapy, although again careful consideration should be given to investigational therapies to include allogeneic HSCT.

Novel Treatment Approaches and Future Directions

Genetically modified T-cells expressing the anti-CD19 chimeric antigen receptor (CD19 CAR T-cells) can be used to treat patients with advanced B-cell malignancies that express CD19. A small, single-center study of 15 patients with advanced, chemotherapy refractory DLBCL, indolent B-cell lymphoma, and CLL, resulted in CR in 8 patients with 4 of the 7 DLBCL patients in CR ranging from 9 to 22 months duration. CD19 CAR T-cell therapy represents a promising approach to the treatment of patients with chemotherapy-refractory disease and is currently being tested using autologous and allogeneic cells, prior to and following allogenic HSCT, respectively.

Immune checkpoint inhibition, with inhibitors of programmed cell death 1 (PD-1) and programmed cell death ligand 1 (PD-L1), are currently being investigated in the treatment of NHL with promising safety and efficacy. The most robust data for PD-1 inhibition in hematologic malignancies is in the treatment of Hodgkin lymphoma, but several studies have indicated efficacy in NHL as well. Preliminary results of the phase I study with nivolumab, a humanized IgG4 PD-1 monoclonal antibody, in lymphoid malignancies demonstrated acceptable safety with an ORR of 28% and CR rate of 7% in B-cell NHL (ORR of 36% in DLBCL and 40% in FL) and an ORR of 17% in T-cell NHL (ORR of 40% in PTCL-NOS). The combination of pidilizumab, a humanized PD-1 monoclonal antibody, and rituximab was tested in a phase II study of rituximab-sensitive relapsed FL patients and was well tolerated with an ORR of 66% (CR 52% and PR 14%). Recent preclinical data suggest that ibrutinib, an inhibitor of both BTK and ITK, can enhance the effect of immune checkpoint inhibition through shifting from a Th2 to Th1 antitumor immune response. This provides scientific rationale for combination therapy and inhibitors of PD-1 and PD-L1 are currently being tested both as monotherapy and in combination with cytotoxic and targeted therapy in the treatment of NHL.

Novel methods have emerged over the past few years enabling the detection of small fragments of circulating-tumor DNA (ctDNA) in the peripheral blood. In a correlative biomarker study comparing ctDNA to CT scans in previously untreated DLBCL patients, interim monitoring of ctDNA revealed significantly improved 5-year TTP (80.2% vs. 41.7%) in patients with undetectable interim ctDNA and also detected early relapse 3.5 months prior to clinical disease when used in the surveillance setting. Beyond its use in interim and surveillance monitoring, ctDNA also has prognostic potential both at diagnosis and during MRD assessment following therapy. When used as a "liquid biopsy", ctDNA can aid in non-invasive diagnosis and may eventually guide selection of targeted therapy in a precision-directed fashion. Further validation of this novel technique is needed in prospective studies, but ctDNA has the potential to transform our current methods of diagnosis, response assessment, and relapse detection in NHL.

Suggested Readings

1. Ardeshna KM, Qian W, Smith P, et al. Rituximab versus a watch-and-wait approach in patients with advanced-stage, asymptomatic, non-bulky follicular lymphoma: an open-label randomised phase 3 trial. *The Lancet Oncology.* 2014;15(4):424–435.
2. Batchelor T, Carson K, O'Neill A, et al. Treatment of primary CNS lymphoma with methotrexate and deferred radiotherapy: a report of NABTT 96-07. *J Clin Oncol: official journal of the American Society of Clinical Oncology.* 2003;21(6):1044–1049.
3. Coiffier B, Lepage E, Briere J, et al. CHOP chemotherapy plus rituximab compared with CHOP alone in elderly patients with diffuse large-B-cell lymphoma. *New Engl J Med.* 2002;346(4):235–242.
4. Coiffier B, Pro B, Prince HM, et al. Results from a pivotal, open-label, phase II study of romidepsin in relapsed or refractory peripheral T-cell lymphoma after prior systemic therapy. *J Clin Oncol: official journal of the American Society of Clinical Oncology.* 2012;30(6):631–636.
5. Dreyling M, Jurczak W, Jerkeman M, et al. Ibrutinib versus temsirolimus in patients with relapsed or refractory mantle-cell lymphoma: an international, randomised, open-label, phase 3 study. *Lancet (London, England).* 2016;387(10020):770–778.
6. Dunleavy K, Pittaluga S, Maeda LS, et al. Dose-adjusted EPOCH-rituximab therapy in primary mediastinal B-cell lymphoma. *New Engl J Med.* 2013;368(15):1408–1416.
7. Dunleavy K, Pittaluga S, Shovlin M, et al. Low-intensity therapy in adults with Burkitt's lymphoma. *New Engl J Med.* 2013;369(20):1915–1925.
8. Ferreri AJ, Reni M, Foppoli M, et al. High-dose cytarabine plus high-dose methotrexate versus high-dose methotrexate alone in patients with primary CNS lymphoma: a randomised phase 2 trial. *Lancet.* 2009;374(9700):1512–1520.
9. Fisher RI, Bernstein SH, Kahl BS, et al. Multicenter phase II study of bortezomib in patients with relapsed or refractory mantle cell lymphoma. *J Clin Oncol: official journal of the American Society of Clinical Oncology.* 2006;24(30):4867–4874.
10. Flinn IW, van der Jagt R, Kahl BS, et al. Randomized trial of bendamustine-rituximab or R-CHOP/R-CVP in first-line treatment of indolent NHL or MCL: the BRIGHT study. *Blood.* 2014;123(19):2944–2952.
11. Fowler NH, Davis RE, Rawal S, et al. Safety and activity of lenalidomide and rituximab in untreated indolent lymphoma: an open-label, phase 2 trial. *The Lancet Oncology.* 2014;15(12):1311–1318.
12. Gisselbrecht C, Glass B, Mounier N, et al. Salvage regimens with autologous transplantation for relapsed large B-cell lymphoma in the rituximab era. *J Clin Oncol: official journal of the American Society of Clinical Oncology.* 2010;28(27):4184–4190.
13. Gopal AK, Kahl BS, de Vos S, et al. PI3Kdelta inhibition by idelalisib in patients with relapsed indolent lymphoma. *New Engl J Med.* 2014;370(11):1008–1018.
14. Goy A, Sinha R, Williams ME, et al. Single-agent lenalidomide in patients with mantle-cell lymphoma who relapsed or progressed after or were refractory to bortezomib: phase II MCL-001 (EMERGE) study. *J Clin Oncol: official journal of the American Society of Clinical Oncology.* 2013;31(29):3688–3695.

15. Hermine O, Hoster E, Walewski J, et al. Addition of high-dose cytarabine to immunochemotherapy before autologous stem-cell transplantation in patients aged 65 years or younger with mantle cell lymphoma (MCL Younger): a randomised, open-label, phase 3 trial of the European Mantle Cell Lymphoma Network. *Lancet* (London, England). 2016;388(10044):565–575.

16. Kahl BS, Hong F, Williams ME, et al. Rituximab extended schedule or re-treatment trial for low-tumor burden follicular lymphoma: eastern cooperative oncology group protocol e4402. *J clin oncol: official journal of the American Society of Clinical Oncology.* 2014;32(28):3096–3102.

17. O'Connor OA, Horwitz S, Masszi T, et al. Belinostat in patients with relapsed or refractory peripheral T-cell lymphoma: Results of the pivotal phase II BELIEF (CLN-19) Study. *J Clin Oncol: official journal of the American Society of Clinical Oncology.* 2015;33(23):2492–2499.

18. O'Connor OA, Pro B, Pinter-Brown L, et al. Pralatrexate in patients with relapsed or refractory peripheral T-cell lymphoma: results from the pivotal PROPEL study. *J Clin oncol: official journal of the American Society of Clinical Oncology.* 2011;29(9):1182–1189.

19. Recher C, Coiffier B, Haioun C, et al. Intensified chemotherapy with ACVBP plus rituximab versus standard CHOP plus rituximab for the treatment of diffuse large B-cell lymphoma (LNH03-2B): an open-label randomised phase 3 trial. *Lancet.* 2011;378(9806):1858–1867.

20. Ribrag V, Koscielny S, Bosq J, et al. Rituximab and dose-dense chemotherapy for adults with Burkitt's lymphoma: a randomised, controlled, open-label, phase 3 trial. *Lancet.* 2016;387(10036):2402–2411.

21. Robak T, Huang H, Jin J, et al. Bortezomib-Based Therapy for Newly Diagnosed Mantle-Cell Lymphoma. *New Engl J Med.* 2015;372(10):944–953.

22. Ruan J, Martin P, Shah B, et al. Lenalidomide plus Rituximab as Initial Treatment for Mantle-Cell Lymphoma. *New Engl J Med.* 2015;373(19):1835–1844.

23. Rummel MJ, Niederle N, Maschmeyer G, et al. Bendamustine plus rituximab versus CHOP plus rituximab as first-line treatment for patients with indolent and mantle-cell lymphomas: an open-label, multicentre, randomised, phase 3 non-inferiority trial. *Lancet.* 2013;381(9873):1203–1210.

24. Salles G, Seymour JF, Offner F, et al. Rituximab maintenance for 2 years in patients with high tumour burden follicular lymphoma responding to rituximab plus chemotherapy (PRIMA): a phase 3, randomised controlled trial. *Lancet.* 2011;377(9759):42–51.

25. Treon SP, Tripsas CK, Meid K, et al. Ibrutinib in previously treated Waldenstrom's macroglobulinemia. *New Engl J Med.* 2015;372(15):1430–1440.

26. Wang ML, Rule S, Martin P, et al. Targeting BTK with ibrutinib in relapsed or refractory mantle-cell lymphoma. *New Engl J Med.* 2013;369(6):507–516.

27. Wilson WH, Jung SH, Porcu P, et al. A Cancer and Leukemia Group B multi-center study of DA-EPOCH-rituximab in untreated diffuse large B-cell lymphoma with analysis of outcome by molecular subtype. *Haematologica.* 2012;97(5):758–765.

28. Witzig TE, Vose JM, Zinzani PL, et al. An international phase II trial of single-agent lenalidomide for relapsed or refractory aggressive B-cell non-Hodgkin's lymphoma. *Annf oncol: official journal of the European Society for Medical Oncology / ESMO.* 2011;22(7):1622–1627.

29. Yamaguchi M, Kwong YL, Kim WS, et al. Phase II study of SMILE chemotherapy for newly diagnosed stage IV, relapsed, or refractory extranodal natural killer (NK)/T-cell lymphoma, nasal type: the NK-Cell Tumor Study Group study. *J Clin Oncol : official journal of the American Society of Clinical Oncology.* 2011;29(33):4410–4416.

Hodgkin Lymphoma 29

Robert Dean and Matt Kalaycio

EPIDEMIOLOGY

Hodgkin lymphoma (HL) is a common lymphoid malignancy, representing 10% of all lymphomas. The National Cancer Institute SEER registry estimates that approximately 8,500 patients will be diagnosed with HL in 2016 in the United States. Median age at the time of diagnosis is 39 years, with a peak incidence at age 20 to 35 years. The age-adjusted incidence rate of HL is 2.6 per 100,000 individuals per year. Unlike non-Hodgkin lymphoma, HL incidence has not increased over the past decades. The male to female ratio is 1.3:1.0. In the United States, it affects African Americans slightly less commonly than Caucasians.

ETIOLOGY AND RISK FACTORS

The cause of HL remains unknown.

- Epstein-Barr virus (EBV) has been postulated to play a role in the pathogenesis of some cases of classical HL (CHL) (particularly mixed cellularity and lymphocyte-depleted subtypes).
- Loss of immune surveillance in immunodeficiency states (e.g., HIV infection, allogeneic stem cell transplantation, and solid organ transplantation) may predispose to development of HL.
- Two-fold increased risk of HL is seen in smokers.
- Family history of classical HL increases the risk to develop disease by 3-fold to 9-fold. Identical twin sibling of a HL patient has a 99-fold higher risk of developing HL.

PATHOLOGY

HL is a neoplastic disease of B-cell origin. Classical HL (CHL) is characterized by the presence of Reed-Sternberg (RS) cells and mononuclear variants, amidst an inflammatory background consisting of lymphocytes, eosinophils, monocytes, and histiocytes. Nodular lymphocyte predominant HL (NLPHL) is characterized by RS variants termed LP cells in a background of lymphocytes and histiocytes but without other inflammatory cells.

RS and LP cells are derived from follicular center B cells with clonally rearranged V heavy-chain genes. RS cells often exhibit symmetrical bilobed nuclei (owl's eyes appearance) (Fig. 29.1). RS cells are positive for CD30 and CD15 and typically negative for CD20 and CD45, whereas LP cells express B-cell markers including CD20, CD45, and CD79a but are negative for CD30 and CD15.

Pathologic Classification

The World Health Organization (WHO) classification divides HL into two main types (Table 29.1):

- Classical Hodgkin lymphoma (CHL)
  - CHL is characterized by the presence of RS cells in an inflammatory background and is divided into four histologic subtypes, based mainly on the characteristics of the non-neoplastic reactive infiltrate.

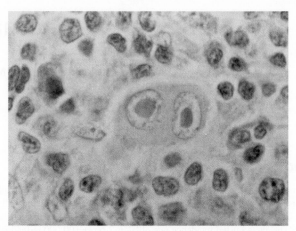

FIGURE 29.1 Diagnostic Reed-Sternberg (RS) cell, with Owl's Eye nucleus, seen in classic types of Hodgkin lymphomas (mixed cellularity, nodular sclerosis, lymphocyte depletion).

TABLE 29.1 Immunophenotypic Features of Hodgkin Lymphoma

	Classical Hodgkin Lymphoma	Nodular Lymphocyte Predominant Hodgkin Lymphoma
CD45	Negative	Positive
CD30	Positive	Negative[a]
CD15	Positive (80% of cases)	Negative
CD20	Variable[b]	Positive
CD79a	Negative[a]	Positive
EMA	Majority of cases positive	Negative

[a]Positive in rare cases.

[b]Present in up to 40% of the cases but usually expressed on minority of tumor cells with variable intensity.

- Nodular sclerosis HL
- Mixed cellularity HL
- Lymphocyte-rich HL
- Lymphocyte-depleted HL
■ NLPHL
  - NLPHL lacks RS cells but is characterized by LP cells, which are sometimes referred to as *popcorn cells.*

Table 29.2 summarizes the clinical and pathologic features of the disease subtypes.

CLINICAL FEATURES

■ Lymphadenopathy: Most commonly above the diaphragm (cervical, axillary, or mediastinal). Enlarged nodes are non-tender, with a characteristic firm rubbery consistency. Lymph node pain may occasionally be precipitated by alcohol intake.

TABLE 29.2 Classification of Hodgkin Lymphoma

Pathologic Type	Pathologic Features	Clinical Features
Classical Hodgkin lymphoma		
Nodular sclerosis	Nodular growth pattern with broad bands of fibrosis	Most common type; and has a better prognosis. Common in resource-rich countries. Peak incidence at ages 15–34 y
Mixed cellularity	Typical RS cells in a rich inflammatory background and fine reticular fibrosis; 70% are positive for Epstein-Barr virus	Second most common type; more common in patients with HIV infection and in developing countries. Median age is 38 y, with a male predominance
Lymphocyte-rich	Scattered RS cells in a usually nodular background consisting of small lymphocytes	Common in elderly; has good prognosis
Lymphocyte-depleted	Relative predominance of RS cells with depletion of background lymphocytes	Rare, often associated with HIV infection; has poor prognosis. Median age ranges from 30 to 37 y
Nodular lymphocyte predominant		
	No RS cells, but characterized by "popcorn" or LP cells (lobulated nucleus)	More common in adult males; often presents with early stage and has good prognosis, but late relapses are not uncommon. Peak incidence at ages 30–50 y

- Chronic pruritus.
- Most common extranodal sites of involvement are lung, bone marrow, liver, and bones.
- B symptoms.
  - Unexplained weight loss (>10% body weight over 6 months before diagnosis)
  - Fever of >38°C, intermittent with 1- to 2-week cycles
  - Drenching night sweats

Staging

The modified Ann Arbor staging of lymphoma is used to clinically stage HL (Table 29.3).

Diagnostic Evaluation

Excisional biopsy of an enlarged lymph node is strongly recommended for initial diagnosis. A core biopsy may be appropriate if adequate tissue can be obtained to avoid major surgery, but this may limit accurate classification among CHL subtypes. A fine-needle aspiration is *not* recommended for initial diagnosis.

Laboratory Tests

- Complete blood count (CBC), differential, and platelets.
- Erythrocyte sedimentation rate (ESR): Adverse prognostic biomarker, if elevated.
- Lactate dehydrogenase (LDH) and albumin.
- Liver function tests: If abnormal, may be associated with liver involvement.
- Alkaline phosphatase: May be nonspecifically high or associated with bone involvement.

TABLE 29.3 Cotswolds Modified Ann Arbor Staging of Lymphoma

Stage I   Single lymph node region, lymphoid structure (e.g., spleen, thymus, or Waldeyer ring), or a single extralymphatic site (IE)

Stage II   Two or more lymph node regions on the same side of the diaphragm, or localized extranodal extension (contagious to a nodal site) plus one or more nodal regions (IIE)

Stage III   Lymph node regions on both sides of the diaphragm. This may be accompanied by localized extranodal site (IIIE), or splenic involvement (IIIS), or both (IIIE+S)

Stage IV   Diffuse or disseminated involvement of one or more extranodal organs or tissue beyond that designated E, with or without associated lymph node involvement

Each stage is designated A or B, where B means presence and A means absence of B symptom

X: A mass >10 cm or a mediastinal mass larger than one-third of the thoracic diameter

E: Extranodal contiguous extension, which can be encompassed within an irradiation field appropriate for nodal disease of the same anatomic extent. More extensive extranodal disease is designated stage IV

- BUN, creatinine, electrolytes, and uric acid.
- Pregnancy test: Women of childbearing age.
- HIV testing in patients with risk factors for HIV.

Radiologic Studies

- Chest radiograph (PA and lateral views) for assessment of mediastinal disease bulk.
- Diagnostic computerized tomography (CT) scan of the chest, abdomen, and pelvis are recommended for staging. CT scan of the neck may be needed for objective assessment of palpable lymphadenopathy, or in obese patients.
- Positron emission tomography/computerized tomography (PET/CT) scan.

Unilateral Bone Marrow Biopsy and Aspiration

Recommended if PET/CT shows focal areas of skeletal uptake, or if unexplained cytopenias are present. Generally not needed in clinical stage III or IV.

Evaluation/Procedures for Specific Treatments and Counseling

- MUGA scan or echocardiography to evaluate left ventricular ejection fraction before anthracycline treatment.
- Pulmonary function tests (including DLCO) are recommended prior to bleomycin-containing treatment.
- Fertility counseling (to discuss sperm, ovarian tissue, and/or oocyte cryopreservation).
- Smoking cessation counseling.

MANAGEMENT

- HL is sensitive to radiation and many chemotherapeutic agents. All patients, regardless of stage, should be treated with a curative intent. Cure rates are high (>80%), thus limiting long-term toxicities is a major consideration of treatment.
- Early-stage disease may be treated with combined-modality chemotherapy and radiation treatment (RT), or chemotherapy alone.

TABLE 29.4 CALGB Study Comparing Different Regimens in Hodgkin Lymphoma

Regimen	Complete Response Rate (%)	5-y Overall Survival Rate (%)
MOPP	67	66
ABVD	82	73
Alternating MOPP/ABVD	83	75

- Advanced-stage disease is usually treated with chemotherapy alone.
- In advanced-stage disease, radiation consolidation can be considered for PET-positive areas following a full course of chemotherapy, particularly in patients who are poor candidates for intensive second-line therapy including autologous transplantation. Radiation consolidation should be omitted in patients with PET-negative residual masses. Based on pre-PET era studies, routine radiation consolidation in patients with bulky (≥10 cm or one-third the diameter of the chest on CXR) disease is widely practiced in North American centers; however, radiation consolidation may not be necessary in PET-negative bulky masses.

Principles of Chemotherapy

- The standard regimen for HL in North America is ABVD (doxorubicin, bleomycin, vinblastine, dacarbazine) since it superseded MOPP (mechlorethamine, vincristine, procarbazine, prednisone) regimen in the large randomized trial of the Cancer and Leukemia Group B (CALGB) in 1992 (Table 29.4). ABVD was associated with less myelosuppression and reduced risk of secondary leukemias and infertility compared to MOPP regimen. Prophylactic use of growth factors may increase the risk of pulmonary toxicity with ABVD and is therefore discouraged. Treatment delay and/or dose reduction due to uncomplicated leukopenia is not recommended, given that febrile neutropenia is uncommon with ABVD.
- The German Hodgkin Lymphoma Study Group (GHSG) developed the dose-escalated BEACOPP regimen and showed it to be superior to COPP-ABVD and standard-dose BEACOPP in advanced HL. However the significant associated toxicities of dose-escalated BEACOPP (3% rate of treatment-related death, 2% to 3% rate of secondary leukemias, and nearly universal infertility) have precluded its widespread use in North America. Dose-escalated BEACOPP is not recommended for older HL patients (≥60 years).
- Stanford V is a dose-intense 12-week regimen. Involved field radiation to macroscopic splenic disease and all lymph nodes measuring ≥5 cm in size is an integral part of Stanford V. The cumulative doses of doxorubicin and bleomycin in Stanford V are less than those in ABVD, with potentially less risk for cardiac and pulmonary toxicity. In the three randomized prospective trials (from Italy, United Kingdom, and United States) compared to ABVD, Stanford V had inferior complete remission rates and was associated with more hematologic and neurologic toxicity.

Chemotherapy regimens are described in Table 29.5.

Principles of Radiotherapy

- Radiation therapy for HL targets sites with radiographic disease (involved nodal or involved site). Historical approaches included involved areas alone (involved field), involved *plus* adjacent areas (extended field). Extended fields are either "mantle field" for the cervical, axillary, and mediastinal regions or "inverted Y field" for spleen, para-aortic, and pelvic regions. When inverted Y field radiation is given together with mantle field radiation, the combination is called total nodal radiation.

TABLE 29.5 Commonly Used Chemotherapy Regimens for Hodgkin Lymphoma

ABVD (every 28 d)	Doxorubicin 25 mg/m²/dose IV on days 1 and 15
	Bleomycin 10 units/m²/dose IV on days 1 and 15
	Vinblastine 6 mg/m²/dose IV on days 1 and 15
	Dacarbazine (DTIC) 375 mg/m²/dose IV
	on days 1 and 15
Dose-escalated BEACOPP	Bleomycin 10 international units/m² IV on day 8
(every 3 wk)	
	Etoposide (VP-16) 200 mg/m² IV on days 1–3
	Doxorubicin (driamycin) 35 mg/m² on day 1
	Cyclophosphamide (Cytoxan) 1,200 mg/m² on day 1
	Vincristine 1.4 mg/m² (max 2 mg) on day 8
	Procarbazine 100 mg/m² PO on days 1–7
	Prednisone 40 mg/m² PO on days 1–14
	Filgrastim (G-CSF) support is needed
Stanford V (every 4 wk) × three	Nitrogen mustard 6 mg/m² IV day 1
cycles (12 wk)	
	Doxorubicin (Adriamycin) 25 mg/m² IV days1 and 15
	Vinblastine 6 mg/m² IV days 1 and 15
	Vincristine 1.4 mg/m² IV days 8 and 22
	(maximum dose is 2 mg/dose).
	Bleomycin 5 units/m² IV days 8 and 22
	Etoposide (VP-16) 60 mg/m² IV days 15 and 16
	Prednisone 40 mg PO qod × 10 wk, then taper by 10 mg
	every other day between weeks 10 and 12
	For patients older than 50, reduce vinblastine to 4 mg/m²
	and vincristine to 1 mg/m² in cycle 3

- Dose of RT depends on the extent of the disease. In combined-modality therapy, RT is initiated ideally within 3 weeks of finishing chemotherapy.

Treatment Response Evaluation

All patients (early and late stages) should receive interim restaging with PET/CT after two cycles of chemotherapy to evaluate the response to treatment. Restaging may be repeated after four cycles of chemotherapy to evaluate ongoing response, where applicable. Restaging should be repeated 2 months after the end of treatment if complete remission is not achieved in the interim assessment.

TREATMENT OF EARLY DISEASE (STAGES I AND II)

Early-stage CHL is stratified as favorable or unfavorable disease, and treatment varies accordingly. Unfavorable risk factors in this subset of patients vary somewhat among international clinical trial groups and are also summarized in guidelines from the National Comprehensive Cancer Network (NCCN).

NCCN Unfavorable Prognostic Features for Early-Stage Disease (I and II)

Any of the following features:

- Bulky disease: A mass >10 cm in diameter, or mediastinal mass ratio exceeding one-third of maximum intrathoracic diameter
- ESR >50 or presence of B symptoms
- More than 3 nodal areas

Early-stage patients with unfavorable risk factors are best treated like advanced-stage (stage III/IV) disease. The remaining favorable-risk early-stage patients are managed as follows:

Favorable early-stage disease (by NCCN criteria): These patients may be treated with ABVD × two cycles followed by 20 Gy of involved nodal or involved site radiation. The cure rate of these patients is >90%.

- An alternative for favorable early-stage disease is chemotherapy with four to six cycles of ABVD alone without involved field radiation. This option is especially attractive for patients with abdomen only disease and in young patients where radiation to chest or axillae is associated with a high risk of subsequent second cancers (particularly breast cancer in young female patients) and premature coronary artery disease.
- Unfavorable early-stage disease (by NCCN criteria): Patients with bulky stage I or II disease without B symptoms are treated with ABVD × four cycles followed by 30 Gy of involved nodal or involved site radiation. Patients with stage IB or IIB disease, or with stage II disease encompassing more than 3 nodal areas, are treated with ABVD x six cycles, usually followed by 30 Gy of involved nodal or involved site radiation to sites of initial bulky disease.
- Rarely, in patients who are unfit for chemotherapy, treatment with subtotal nodal or mantle field radiation alone may be considered.

TREATMENT OF ADVANCED DISEASE (STAGES III AND IV)

Aggressive histology (e.g., mixed cellularity or lymphocyte-depleted) is more common among patients with advanced CHL.

Unfavorable Prognostic Features for Advanced Stages (III and IV)

Hasenclever index (also called international prognostic score [IPS]) identifies seven adverse prognostic factors:

- Stage IV disease
- Age >45 years
- Male gender
- WBC ≥15,000/mm³
- Lymphopenia (<600/mm³ or <8% of total WBC)
- Hemoglobin <10.5 g/dL
- Albumin level <4 g/dL

The 5-year overall survival decreases with higher IPS scores as follows: 0 factor (89%), 1 factor (90%), 2 factors (81%), 3 factors (78%), 4 factors (61%), and 5 or more factors (56%).

The primary treatment of advanced-stage CHL is chemotherapy. ABVD is the standard of care in North American centers. The recommended initial treatment is six cycles of ABVD. In a phase III trial, initial treatment of advanced-stage CHL with brentuximab vedotin, doxorubicin, vinblastine, and dacarbazine was associated with improved progression-free survival, decreased pulmonary toxicity, and a trend toward lower overall mortality compared with ABVD. Brentuximab vedotin is not currently approved for primary treatment of CHL. Initial therapy with dose-escalated BEACOPP does not improve survival and increases the risk of subsequent myelodysplastic syndrome. Stanford V is also not recommended as initial therapy outside the setting of a clinical trial.

Treatment decisions are increasingly being made on the basis of PET scans obtained after chemotherapy has begun (Interim PET).

- Evidence supports continuing ABVD if a PET or PET/CT scan is negative following two cycles of ABVD chemotherapy. Current data indicate that bleomycin may be discontinued in patients who achieve PET-negative response after two cycles of ABVD, continuing with AVD to complete six cycles with outcomes comparable to ABVD. This approach merits particular consideration in older adults, who are at higher risk for pulmonary toxicity and mortality with bleomycin-based therapy.
- If a PET or PET/CT scan is positive according to the Deauville criteria, then evidence supports intensification of treatment with either 1) 6 cycles of dose-escalated BEACOPP or 2) ifosfamide-based rescue chemotherapy followed by high-dose chemotherapy with autologous hematopoietic cell rescue.

Nonbulky advanced-stage patients with a negative PET/CT at the end of chemotherapy do not need radiotherapy consolidation, particularly if interim restaging with PET or PET/CT scan was negative following 2 cycles of chemotherapy. RT can also be omitted in bulky disease patients with a negative CT or PET/CT after finishing chemotherapy, but this is an area of significant controversy. Bulky HL patients with a positive PET/CT after finishing chemotherapy can be offered 36 Gy of involved field RT.

TREATMENT OF NODULAR LYMPHOCYTE–PREDOMINANT HODGKIN LYMPHOMA

The NLPHL subtype represents 5% of HL. Unlike CHL, NLPHL is strongly CD20 positive and typically behaves like an indolent non-Hodgkin lymphoma. While conventional HL approaches continue to be applied to NLPHL, as outlined below, there are compelling biologic and clinical arguments for a different therapeutic approach.

Conventional Treatment Approaches

- Stages IA and IIA can be treated with 30 to 36 Gy of involved field radiation alone.
- Stages IA, IB, IIA, and IIB can be managed with a combined-modality approach (e.g., two to four cycles of ABVD or R-CHOP followed by involved field radiation).
- Watchful waiting in patients with asymptomatic stage III/IV disease is reasonable. Patients with symptomatic advanced-stage disease are managed with systemic chemotherapy. The optimal chemotherapy regimen for NLPHL remains unknown. While ABVD is the "historical" standard, regimens designed for non-Hodgkin lymphomas such as CHOP, CVP, or dose-escalated EPOCH with rituximab (because of strong CD20 expression on LP Hodgkin cells) are also appropriate. Single-agent rituximab is also active in NLPHL and can be considered in patients with low bulk disease. It is important to recognize the "aggressive" presentations of NLPHL such as those with disseminated disease, including cases involving the bones and bone marrow and transformation to aggressive histologies. Such cases should be managed like aggressive non-Hodgkin lymphomas.

FOLLOW-UP AFTER COMPLETION OF TREATMENT

The purpose of follow-up is the detection of disease relapse and late treatment-related complications.

- Clinical evaluation with CBC, ESR, chemistry panel every 3 months for 2 years, then every 6 months for 5 years.

- There is no evidence to support routine radiographic surveillance following completion of treatment and confirmation of complete remission. Surveillance PET/CT imaging should be avoided because of frequent false-positive results.
- Annual influenza vaccination.
- Thyroid stimulating hormone (TSH) annually if neck RT was given (risk of hypothyroidism).
- Annual mammogram screening should start 8 to 10 years after RT or at age of 40 years, whichever is earlier, for patients who received RT above the diaphragm. Annual breast MRI is also recommended by the American Cancer Society in addition to mammogram in female patients who received radiation to chest or axillae between the ages 10 and 30 years. Breast self-exam should be encouraged.

LATE TREATMENT–RELATED COMPLICATIONS

- Hypothyroidism and thyroid cancer can occur after neck or mediastinal RT.
- Breast cancer can occur in females after chest or axillary RT. The risk is higher in patients who receive RT at younger age. It occurs after an average of 15 years after finishing treatment.
- Lung cancer: High risk is evident in patients who received RT to chest, received alkylating agents, and smoke cigarettes.
- Infertility risk is high after pelvic RT, MOPP regimen, BEACOPP regimen, and autologous transplantation.
- Leukemia and myelodysplastic syndromes (especially with MOPP, BEACOPP, RT, and autologous transplantation).
- Pulmonary toxicity after bleomycin treatment: Risk may be increased when G-CSF is used during treatment; hence G-CSF use is discouraged with ABVD. Supplemental oxygen should be used sparingly when needed, to minimize the risk of inducing pneumonitis.
- Cardiac toxicity secondary to anthracycline is uncommon (total cumulative anthracycline dose is not prohibitive). The risk for premature coronary artery disease and cerebrovascular accidents is increased after mediastinal and cervical RT, respectively.
- Lhermitte sign: It is an infrequent complication that can occur 6 to 12 weeks after neck RT and resolves spontaneously. Patients feel electric-like shock sensation radiating down the back and extremities when neck is flexed. This sign is attributed to transient spinal cord demyelinization.
- Encapsulated organism infection (pneumococcal, meningococcal, and hemophilus) can occur in patients not vaccinated after splenic RT or splenectomy (rarely used now).

TREATMENT OF RELAPSED HODGKIN LYMPHOMA

- Relapsed disease must be confirmed by repeat biopsy.
- CHL:
  - In rare cases where RT was the first-line treatment, conventional chemotherapy (ABVD) at the time of relapse without autologous transplantation can be curative.
  - If conventional chemotherapy (with or without RT) was the primary treatment, salvage chemotherapy such as ICE, DHAP, ESHAP, or GND (Table 29.6) followed by autologous transplantation is curative for about 50% of the patients.

TABLE 29.6 Salvage Chemotherapy Regimen for Hodgkin Lymphoma

ESHAP (etoposide, methylprednisolone, high-dose cytarabine, and cisplatin)
ICE (ifosfamide, carboplatin, and etoposide)
DHAP (dexamethasone, high-dose cytarabine, and cisplatin)
GND (gemcitabine, vinorelbine, and liposomal doxorubicin)
GCP (gemcitabine, cisplatin, and methylprednisolone)

- Brentuximab vedotin consists of an anti-CD30 chimeric monoclonal antibody; brentuximab, linked to the antimitotic agent monomethyl auristatin E (MMAE). The antibody portion of the drug attaches to CD30 on the surface of HL cells, delivering MMAE which exerts anti-HL activity. In patients with relapsed or refractory Hodgkin lymphoma after autologous transplant, brentuximab vedotin induces remission in 75% with estimated 3-year overall survival and progression-free survival rates of 73% (95% confidence interval [CI]: 57%, 88%) and 58% (95% CI: 41%, 76%), respectively.
- For brentuximab naïve HL patients, brentuximab vedotin added as maintenance therapy following autologous stem cell transplant improves progression-free survival compared to placebo, particularly in high-risk HL patients who do not achieve complete remission with rescue chemotherapy before autologous stem cell transplant.
- In patients with relapsed and refractory HL, the PD-1 inhibitor nivolumab induced remission in 87% resulting in a progression-free survival of 86% with 6 months of follow-up. Similarly, the PD-1 inhibitor pembrolizumab induced responses in 69% of patients with previously treated HL, with 63.4% progression-free survival at 9 months of follow-up.
- A small proportion of heavily pretreated, but otherwise healthy HL patients relapsing after an autologous transplant can be cured with an allogeneic stem cell transplant with better results obtained in those achieving remission first.
- NLPHL: Relapsed disease is best approached as an indolent lymphoma. Reasonable options include observation, rituximab alone or with chemotherapy, and/or RT.

Palliative Treatment

- Sequential single-agent chemotherapy such as gemcitabine, vinblastine, bendamustine, or lenalidomide.
- RT can be used to relieve pain or pressure symptoms of bulky masses.
- Investigational treatment is encouraged through enrollment in clinical trials.

Future Directions

- Phase III studies are underway or planned to combine standard chemotherapy with novel agents such as brentuximab vedotin and checkpoint inhibitors like nivolumab in the first-line setting to improve patient outcomes.

SUGGESTED READINGS

1. Aleman BM, Raemaekers JM, Tirelli U, et al. Involved-field radiotherapy for advanced Hodgkin's lymphoma. *N Engl J Med.* 2003;348:2396–2406.
2. Ansell SM, Lesokhin AM, Borrello I, et al. PD-1 blockade with nivolumab in relapsed or refractory Hodgkin's lymphoma. *N Engl J Med.* 2015;372:311–319.
3. Bonadonna G, Bonfante V, Viviani S, et al. ABVD plus subtotal nodal versus involved-field radiotherapy in early-stage Hodgkin's disease: long-term results. *J Clin Oncol.* 2004;22:2835–2841.
4. Canellos GP, Anderson JR, Propert KJ, et al. Chemotherapy of advanced Hodgkin's disease with MOPP, ABVD, or MOPP alternating with ABVD. *N Engl J Med.* 1992;327:1478–1484.
5. Chen R, Zinzani PL, Fanale MA, et al. Phase II study of the efficacy and safety of pembrolizumab for relapsed/refractory classic Hodgkin lymphoma. *J Clin Oncol.* 2017;35:2125–2132.
6. Chisesi T, Bellei M, Luminari S, et al. Long-term follow-up analysis of HD9601 trial comparing ABVD versus Stanford V versus MOPP/EBV/CAD in patients with newly diagnosed advanced-stage Hodgkin's lymphoma: a study from the Intergruppo Italiano Linfomi. *J Clin Oncol.* 2011;29:4227–4233.
7. Connors JM, Klimo P, Adams G, et al. Treatment of advanced Hodgkin's disease with chemotherapy—comparison of MOPP/ABV hybrid regimen with alternating courses of MOPP and ABVD: a report from the National Cancer Institute of Canada clinical trials group. *J Clin Oncol.* 1997;15:1638–1645.
8. Diehl V, Franklin J, Pfreundschuh M, et al. Standard and increased-dose BEACOPP chemotherapy compared with COPP-ABVD for advanced Hodgkin's disease. *N Engl J Med.* 2003;348:2386–2395.
9. Eberle FC, Mani H, Jaffe ES. Histopathology of Hodgkin's lymphoma. *Cancer J.* 2009;15(2):129–137.
10. Eich HT, Diehl V, Görgen H, et al. Intensified chemotherapy and dose-reduced involved-field radiotherapy in patients with early unfavorable Hodgkin's lymphoma: final analysis of the German Hodgkin Study Group HD11 trial. *J Clin Oncol.* 2010;28:4199–4206.

11. Engert A, Plütschow A, Eich HT, et al. Reduced treatment intensity in patients with early-stage Hodgkin's lymphoma. *N Engl J Med*. 2010;363:640–652.

12. Fabian CJ, Mansfield CM, Dahlberg S, et al. Low-dose involved field radiation after chemotherapy in advanced Hodgkin disease. A Southwest Oncology Group randomized study. *Ann Intern Med*. 1994;120:903–912.

13. Ferme C, Eghbali H, Meerwaldt JH, et al. Chemotherapy plus involved-field radiation in early-stage Hodgkin's disease. *N Engl J Med*. 2007;357:1916–1927.

14. Gopal AK, Chen R, Smith SE, et al. Durable remissions in a pivotal phase 2 study of brentuximab vedotin in relapsed or refractory Hodgkin lymphoma. *Blood*. 2015 125:1236–1243.

15. Harris NL. Hodgkin's disease: classification and differential diagnosis. *Mod Pathol*. 1999;12:159–175.

16. Hasenclever D, Diehl V. A prognostic score for advanced Hodgkin's disease. International Prognostic Factors Project on Advanced Hodgkin's Disease. *N Engl J Med*. 1998;339:1506–1514.

17. Hoskin PJ, Lowry L, Horwich A, et al. Randomized comparison of the stanford V regimen and ABVD in the treatment of advanced Hodgkin's lymphoma: United Kingdom National Cancer Research Institute Lymphoma Group Study ISRCTN 64141244. *J Clin Oncol*. 2009;27:5390–5396.

18. Kobe C, Dietlein M, Franklin J, et al. Positron emission tomography has a high negative predictive value for progression or early relapse for patients with residual disease after first-line chemotherapy in advanced-stage Hodgkin lymphoma. *Blood*. 2008;112:3989–3994.

19. Johnson P, Federico M, Kirkwood A, et al. Adapted treatment guided by interim PET/CT scan in advanced Hodgkin's Lymphoma. *N Engl J Med*. 2016; 374: 2420–2429.

20. Lister TA, Crowther D, Sutcliffe SB, et al. Report of a committee convened to discuss the evaluation and staging of patients with Hodgkin's disease: Cotswolds meeting. *J Clin Oncol*. 1989;7:1630–1636.

21. Meyer RM, Gospodarowicz MK, Connors JM, et al. ABVD alone versus radiation-based therapy in limited-stage Hodgkin's lymphoma. *N Engl J Med*. 2012;366:399–408.

22. Moskowitz CH, Nademanee A, Masszi T, et al. AETHERA Study Group. Brentuximab vedotin as consolidation therapy after autologous stem-cell transplantation in patients with Hodgkin's lymphoma at risk of relapse or progression (AETHERA): a randomised, double-blind, placebo-controlled, phase 3 trial. *Lancet*. 2015;385:1853–1862.

23. Noordijk EM, Carde P, Dupouy N, et al. Combined-modality therapy for clinical stage I or II Hodgkin's lymphoma: long-term results of the European Organisation for Research and Treatment of Cancer H7 randomized controlled trials. *J Clin Oncol*. 2006;24:3128–3135.

24. Press OW, Li H, Schoder H, et al. US Intergroup trial of response-adapted therapy for stage III to IV Hodgkin lymphoma using early interim flurodeoxyglucose-positron emission tomography imaging: Southwest Oncology Group S0816. *J Clin Oncol*. 2016;34:2020–2026.

25. Savage KJ, Skinnider B, Al-Mansour M, et al. Treating limited-stage nodular lymphocyte predominant Hodgkin lymphoma similarly to classical Hodgkin lymphoma with ABVD may improve outcome. *Blood*. 2011;118:4585–4590.

26. Schmitz N, Pfistner B, Sextro M, et al. Aggressive conventional chemotherapy compared with high-dose chemotherapy with autologous haemopoietic stem-cell transplantation for relapsed chemosensitive Hodgkin's disease: a randomised trial. *Lancet*. 2002;359:2065–2071.

27. Steidl C, Lee T, Shah SP, et al. Tumor-associated macrophages and survival in classic Hodgkin's lymphoma. *N Engl J Med*. 2010;362:875–885.

28 van Leeuwen FE, Klokman WJ, Hagenbeek A, et al. Second cancer risk following Hodgkin's disease: a 20-year follow-up study. *J Clin Oncol*. 1994;12:312–325.

29. Viviani S, Zinzani PL, Rambaldi A, et al. ABVD versus BEACOPP for Hodgkin's lymphoma when high-dose salvage is planned. *N Engl J Med*. 2011;365:203–212.

30. von Tresckow B, Plütschow A, Fuchs M, et al. Dose-intensification in early unfavorable Hodgkin's lymphoma: final analysis of the German Hodgkin study group HD14 trial. *J Clin Oncol*. 2012;30:907–913.

31. Younes A, Gopal AK, Smith SE, et al. Results of a pivotal phase II study of brentuximab vedotin for patients with relapsed or refractory Hodgkin's lymphoma. *J Clin Oncol*. 2012;30:2183–2189.

32. Zinzani PL, Broccoli A, Gioia DM, et al. Interim Positron Emission Tomography Response-Adapted Therapy in Advanced-Stage Hodgkin Lymphoma: Final Results of the Phase II Part of the HD0801 Study. *J Clin Oncol*. 2016;34:1376–1385.

30 Hematopoietic Cell Transplantation

Abraham S. Kanate, Michael Craig, and Mehdi Hamadani

INTRODUCTION

The effective therapeutic implementation of hematopoietic cell transplantation (HCT) took the concerted efforts of several prominent investigators spanning the 20th century. Seminal work done predominantly on murine models identified the cellular basis of hematopoiesis and raised the possibility of HCT in humans in the first half of the 20th century. The latter half witnessed the successful (albeit with early setbacks) therapeutic application of human HCT. For his pioneering efforts in the field, Dr. E. Donnall Thomas received the Nobel Prize in Physiology or Medicine in 1990. Currently, it is estimated that over 50,000 patients undergo HCT annually worldwide that includes both autologous (auto-HCT) and allogeneic (allo-HCT) transplantation.

Hematopoietic transplantation is an effective therapeutic option for patients with a wide range of malignant and benign conditions. While high dose therapy and auto-HCT, where the patient serves as the donor, are implemented chiefly in the management of multiple myeloma (MM) and lymphoma, allo-HCT is primarily used in the treatment of leukemia, myelodysplastic syndromes (MDS) and bone marrow failures states and involves the transfer of hematopoietic cells from a donor to the patient. Apart from matched related donor (MRD) allo-HCT, patients may be offered allografts from matched unrelated donors (MUD), mismatched unrelated donors (MMUD), haploidentical related donors or umbilical cord blood (UCB). In recent years the application of HCT has broadened to include older and frail patients with the advent of reduced intensity conditioning (RIC) regimens. Advances in supportive care, human leukocyte antigen (HLA) typing, prevention and treatment of graft-versus-host disease (GVHD) and better management of complications have led to improved survival and outcomes. A brief overview of autologous and allogeneic HCT is provided in this chapter, along with a discussion of the complications and their management.

HEMATOPOIETIC STEM CELLS

Hematopoietic stem cells (HSC) reside within the bone marrow space in close association with stromal cells and extracellular matrix proteins and are capable of producing progenitor cells that can reconstitute the hematopoietic system including lymphoid and myeloid cell lines. True HSC are characterized by their unlimited self-renewal capacity, pluripotency (ability to differentiate), quiescence and extensive proliferative capacity. While committed progenitor cells may retain some of the HSC properties and may repopulate the hematopoietic system, they lack self-renewal capacity. In humans, the HSC immunophenotype is characterized as $CD34^+$, $CD38^-$, Thy-1^{low} and lacking lineage-specific markers, although a population of $CD34^-$ stem cells has also been described. Considering the abundance of hematopoietic cells, true HSCs are relatively rare and constitute only 1 in 10,000 bone marrow cells. The HSC when infused to a recipient retains the ability to migrate and occupy bone marrow niches by virtue of surface adhesion molecules, chemokines and their receptors. The number of $CD34^+$ cells in the infused graft product has important ramifications on post-HCT outcomes as lower CD34⁺ cell dose may be associated with a higher risk of graft failure, delayed engraftment and hematopoietic recovery resulting in higher non-relapse mortality (NRM).

STEM CELL SOURCES

Bone Marrow

Originally bone marrow was considered the sole source of acquiring HSCs for both autologous and allogeneic transplantation and is obtained via repeated aspiration of the marrow from the posterior iliac crest usually under general anesthesia. The goal is to obtain ≥ 2 x 10^8/kg recipient body weight of total nucleated/mononuclear cells (TNC) to allow safe engraftment. The maximum volume of marrow that may safely be removed at a given time is 20 mL/kg donor weight. The harvesting procedure is very well tolerated with no long-term adverse effects. Common side effects include pain at the procedure site, neuropathy, infection, and rarely anemia. Transfusion of autologous red cells obtained from the harvested product is considered in many centers. Transplantation with peripheral blood progenitor cells (PBPC) has largely replaced marrow-derived HSCs as the choice of cells for almost all auto-HCT and majority of the allo-HCT in adult patients. However, marrow remains the chief source of HSCs in pediatric patients and in some adults with non-malignant hematological disorders such as aplastic anemia. Recent data have also led to resurgent use of marrow-derived products in unrelated and haploidentical-related donor HCT.

Peripheral Blood

Growth factors such as granulocyte colony-stimulating factor (G-CSF) are used to "mobilize" or increase the number of HSCs and progenitor cells in the peripheral blood, which are collected by apheresis. The minimum goal of PBPC collection is 2 x 10^6/kg recipient body weight of CD34⁺ cells. The PBPC collection is very safe with no long-term adverse effects to the donor. The administration of growth factors to healthy donors may produce minor bone pain, with splenic rupture and myocardial infraction being extremely rare but significant complications. Plerixafor is a chemokine receptor antagonist against CXCR4, which mobilizes HSC and is currently approved in combination with G-CSF prior to auto-HCT in lymphoma and myeloma patients. In the setting of auto-HCT, cytotoxic agents are sometimes used prior to G-CSF mobilization. The post-chemotherapy recovery phase improves the PBPC yield and may also in addition provide antineoplastic effects. PBPC grafts generally result in more rapid engraftment and hematopoietic recovery. Based on existing evidence, PBPC is preferred over marrow grafts in auto-HCT. It is more controversial in the setting of allo-HCT. Due to the 10 to 20 fold higher T-lymphocytes present in the PB product, there is concern for increased GVHD. Results of early comparative studies in MRD allo-HCT demonstrated earlier engraftment, similar acute GVHD and relapse rates, but increased chronic GVHD with the use of PBPC in some but not all studies. A randomized trial evaluating peripheral blood vs. bone marrow allo-HCT in the MUD setting showed increased chronic GVHD with the peripheral blood product, which was offset by delayed engraftment with marrow graft. Although graft source did not impact relapse rate or survival, long-term follow up suggest improved quality of life parameters with the use bone marrow allografts. Registry studies have shown increased chronic GVHD and poorer survival in patients receiving PBPC allo-HCT in severe aplastic anemia compared to those receiving bone marrow product, thus making it the graft source of choice in aplastic anemia. A risk-adapted approach, taking into account diagnosis, disease status, and donor type, is warranted in choosing the ideal graft source.

Umbilical Cord Blood

Umbilical cord blood (UCB) obtained from the umbilical cord and placenta after delivery of the baby is another source for HSC, which can be cryopreserved for later use. This represents an enriched source of HSC in a relative small volume of blood in comparison to bone marrow or PBPC and is readily available upon request but is expensive.

INDICATIONS FOR TRANSPLANTATION

Hematopoietic cell transplantation is considered a therapeutic option in the management of several disease entities. The National Marrow Donor Program (NMDP) website, http://www.bethematch.org, provides a more complete list. See table 30.1 for common indications in adults. Some of the salient features are as follows:

- In pediatric population (≤20 years), chief indications for auto-HCT are non-hematological malignancies and for allo-HCT they are benign hematological and immune system disorders (erythrocyte disorders, inherited immune system defects, congenital metabolic diseases).
- In the adult population, myeloma and lymphoma are common indications for auto-HCT, while acute and chronic leukemias, myeloid neoplasms, lymphomas, myelodysplastic syndrome, and aplastic anemia are common indications for allo-HCT.
- Trends in HCT have changed over time with therapeutic advances. An important example is allo-HCT used to be standard of care for chronic myeloid leukemia (CML) but not so in the era of *bcr-abl* tyrosine kinase inhibitors.

PRETRANSPLANT EVALUATION

Prior to treatment, a thorough discussion highlighting the transplantation procedure as well as risks and benefits associated with the procedure should take place between the physician and the patient.

1. HLA typing of the patient and a search for an HLA-matched donor is required if an allogeneic transplant is being considered. Donor search is initiated with matched siblings as first choice, followed by matched unrelated donors and alternative donors (haploidentical, UCB, and MMUD).

TABLE 30.1 Common Indications for Hematopoietic Cell Transplantation in Adults

Diagnosis	Autologous HCT	Allogeneic HCT
Aplastic anemia	No	Yes
Acute lymphoblastic leukemia	No	Yes; CR1, Ph+ CR1, ≥CR2, Rel/Ref[a]
Acute myeloid leukemia	Yes; CR1[a]	Yes; High risk CR1, ≥CR2, Rel/Ref
Chronic lymphoid leukemia	No	Yes
Chronic myeloid leukemia	No	Yes; TKI intolerance/resistance, >CP1
Diffuse large B-cell lymphoma	Yes; 1st relapse/CR2 (chemosensitive)	Yes; >CR2, >2nd relapse, Ref
Follicular lymphoma	Yes; 1st relapse/CR2 (chemosensitive)	Yes; >CR2, >2nd relapse, Ref
Germ cell tumor (testicular)	Yes; Rel[a]	No
Hodgkin lymphoma	Yes; 1st relapse/CR2 (chemosensitive)	Yes; >CR2, >2nd relapse, Ref
Mantle cell lymphoma	Yes; CR1 and >CR1	Yes; >CR1
Multiple myeloma	Yes	No[a]
Myelodysplastic syndrome	No	Yes
Myeloproliferative neoplasms	No	Yes
T-cell lymphoma	Yes; CR1 and >CR1	Yes; >CR1

[a]Either investigational or ideally considered as part of clinical trial.

HCT, hematopoietic cell transplantation; CR, complete remission; Ph, Philadelphia chromosome; Rel, relapsed; Ref, refractory; TKI, tyrosine kinase inhibitor; CP, chronic phase.

2. Medical history and evaluation.
   - Age—remains an important predictor of treatment-related morbidity and mortality. However, with improving supportive care, HLA typing, and use of RIC regimens, physiologic age is considered more important than chronological age.
   - Review of original diagnosis and previous treatments, including radiation.
   - Concomitant medical problems.
   - Current medications, important past medications, and allergies.
   - Determination of current disease remission status and restaging (by imaging studies, bone marrow biopsy, flow cytometry on blood or bone marrow, lumbar puncture, tissue biopsy as warranted).
   - Transfusion history and complications, as well as ABO typing and HLA antibody screening.
   - Psychosocial evaluation and delineation of a caregiver.
3. Physical examination.
   - Thorough physical examination including evaluation of oral cavity and dentition
   - Neurologic evaluation to rule out central nervous system involvement, if indicated
   - Performance status evaluation
4. Organ function analysis.
   - Complete blood count.
   - Renal function: Preferably a creatinine clearance >60 mL per minute, except in myeloma.
   - Hepatic function: Alanine aminotransferase (ALT) and aspartate aminotransferase (AST) less than twice the upper level of normal and bilirubin <2.00 μg/dL.
   - Cardiac evaluation: Electrocardiogram and echocardiography or multiple-gated acquisition imaging with ejection fraction.
   - Chest x-ray and pulmonary function testing, including diffusing capacity of lung for carbon monoxide and forced vital capacity.
   - The use of scoring schemes such as the hematopoietic cell transplantation specific-comorbidity index (HCT-CI) can predict NRM based on patient factors may be used to risk stratify patients.
5. Infectious disease evaluation.
   - Cytomegalovirus (CMV), human immunodeficiency virus (HIV), toxoplasmosis, and hepatitis serology
   - Serology for herpes simplex virus (HSV), Epstein-Barr virus (EBV), and varicella zoster virus (VZV)
   - Assess for prior history of invasive fungal (aspergillus) infection
6. Pregnancy testing for all women of child-bearing age and consideration of referral to reproductive center for sperm banking or in vitro fertilization.

AUTOLOGOUS HEMATOPOIETIC CELL TRANSPLANTATION

The principle behind high dose therapy (HDT) is the administration of maximal tolerated doses of cytotoxic agents and/or radiation to maximize tumor kill and overcome relative tumor resistance, which causes prolonged and lethal cytopenias from which the patient may be rescued with the infusion of autologous progenitor cells to reconstitute the hematopoietic system. HDT regimens typically use combinations of cytotoxic agents with non-overlapping organ toxicities. Commonly used regimens include (a) BEAM – carmustine + etoposide + cytarabine + melphalan (lymphoma), (b) CBV – cyclophosphamide + carmustine + etoposide (lymphoma), and (c) single agent melphalan 200 mg/m² (myeloma). HDT is considered in chemotherapy sensitive tumors or as consolidation therapy for patients in remission (Table 30.1). Overall it is well tolerated with a NRM of < 5%. Typically, the auto-HCT product is mobilized with G-CSF alone or in combination with either chemotherapy or the chemokine antagonist plerixafor. The mobilized PBPC is collected by apheresis and is cryopreserved viably in dimethyl sulfoxide (DMSO) and thawed just prior to infusion. Complications related to HDT and auto-HCT include:

- Rare infusion reactions may include bronchospasm, flushing, hypertension, or hypotension secondary to DMSO.
- Pancytopenia is universal, packed red cell (PRBC) and platelet transfusions maybe required. Neutrophil recovery takes 10-14 days with GCSF support.

- Infectious complications – bacterial, viral and fungal infections may manifest during the cytopenic phase but can be effectively prevented with antimicrobial prophylaxis. Late infections include *Pneumocystis jiroveci* and varicella reactivation require continued prophylaxis beyond engraftment.
- Regimen related toxicities may be (a) acute – infusion reaction (carmustine), hemorrhagic cystitis (cyclophosphamide), hypotension (etoposide) or (b) delayed – pulmonary toxicity (carmustine, total body irradiation (TBI)), sinusoidal obstruction syndrome or SOS (TBI or alkylating agents) and myelodysplasia (TBI, alkylating agents, etoposide).
- Relapse of the primary malignancy remains a major barrier to long-term survival.

ALLOGENEIC HEMATOPOIETIC CELL TRANSPLANTATION

Allo-HCT has progressed from an experimental treatment of last resort to standard of care therapy for several disease conditions (Table 30.1). Extensive planning and co-ordination of care is required for all transplant candidates, usually involving a network of physicians and support staff. For patients without a MRD, the NMDP is an invaluable resource for the purpose of MUD allo-HCT. All physicians may perform a free initial search for an HLA-matched unrelated donor in the NMDP, which maintains a registry of about 13.5 million potential donors and 225,000 UCB units. As of 2016, the NMDP can search over 27 million MUD and 680,000 UCB units as potential donors through its international networks.

Graft-versus-Tumor Effect

In the context of malignancies, the major therapeutic benefit of allo-HCT is the potential for the donor immune system to recognize and eradicate the malignant stem cell clone, the so called graft-versus-tumor (GVT) effect. This immune effect is largely mediated by transplanted donor lymphocytes and is evidenced by the lower relapse rate of hematological malignancies in patients who undergo allo-HCT than in those who undergo auto-HCT, as well as by an increased risk of relapse in syngeneic (identical twin) donor or T-cell depleted allo-HCT. Arguably the most important and direct evidence for GVT effect comes from the ability of therapeutic donor lymphocyte infusion (DLI) to induce remission in those that relapse after allo-HCT. CML, low-grade lymphomas, chronic lymphocytic leukemia (CLL), and acute myeloid leukemia (AML) are most susceptible to the GVT effects, whereas acute lymphoblastic leukemia and high-grade lymphomas are relatively resistant. Donor-derived T-lymphocytes predominantly mediate GVT reactions, although new evidence supports potential contribution from nonspecific cytokines (host and/or donor derived) and alloreactive natural killer (NK) cells (haploidentical allo-HCT).

Human Leukocyte Antigen Typing

The HLA system consists of a series of cell surface proteins and antigen-presenting cells encoded by the major histocompatibility complex located on chromosome 6 and play a vital role in immune recognition and function. A striking feature of the HLA system is its enormous diversity. HLA class-I molecules include HLA -A, -B, and -C antigens and class-II molecules are made up of more than 15 antigens (HLA -DP, -DQ, and -DR). The complexity of the HLA system was revealed with the advent of molecular-based HLA typing, which showed that matched HLA phenotypes by serologic testing (antigen level) were actually diverse when classified by DNA analysis (allele level). The importance of careful HLA matching prior to the selection of a donor cannot be over-emphasized and independently impacts graft failure, GVHD and overall survival (OS). High resolution HLA typing at the allele level is recommended for all recipients at HLA -A, -B, -C, and -DRB1 at the earliest as it avoids unnecessary delays in identifying a donor. The NMDP recommends rigorous matching at the allele level for HLA -A, -B, -C, and -DRB1 (8/8 match) for adult patients and donors and a less stringent match at HLA -A, -B (antigen level) and HLA -DRB1 (allele level) for UCB units.

Donor Types for Allogeneic Hematopoietic Cell Transplantation

1. Matched Related Donor (MRD)

    In the United States, approximately 30% of patients will have an HLA-matched sibling and is the preferred donor source. The probability that a sibling pair is HLA matched is about 25%. The risk of

GVHD is higher with increasing HLA disparity and therefore, most transplant centers prefer at least 6/6 HLA match (HLA -A, -B, -DRB1).

2. Syngeneic Donor

   Rarely, an identical twin may serve as the donor. As the donor and recipient are genetically identical, GVHD does not typically occur (rarely noted, when a parous female serves as the donor) and post-HCT immunosuppression is not required. By the same principle, such HCT lack GVT effects and malignancy relapse risk tend to be higher.

3. Matched Unrelated Donor (MUD)

   As discussed above the search for an appropriate MUD is performed through the NMDP. It typically takes 3 to 6 months from the time a suitable donor is located to obtaining the allograft, although this period may be shortened when expedited searches are requested. Seventy percent of Caucasians will have a suitable MUD, while it is more difficult for ethnic minorities owing to disparities in registered volunteers in the NMDP registry. High resolution (allele level) matching at HLA -A, B, C, and -DRB1 (8/8) is considered for MUD when possible additional matching at -DQ (10/10 match) and -DP (12/12 match) are considered. Recent data suggest high-resolution MUD allo-HCT have similar outcomes to MRD allo-HCT.

4. Alternative Donors

   In the absence of an HLA-matched sibling donor, a MUD is traditionally considered. When a MUD is not available alternative donors may be used.

   (i) Mismatched unrelated donors (MMUD)—MMUD are potential alternative donors. Studies have established that donor-recipient HLA mismatches decrease OS and increase the risk of GVHD and graft failure. Most centers consider a 7/8 match in this setting (at -A, -B, -C, and -DRB1) and the NMDP requires a minimum 6/8 match prior to approving a match. In MMUD it is important to look for (i) presence of recipient HLA antibodies against the donor HLA called donor-specific HLA antibodies (DSA) and (ii) matching at secondary HLA loci such as -DQB1, -DRB3/4/5, and -DP.

   (ii) Haploidentical Donor—Ready availability of an unrelated donor remains a major concern for patients who are not Caucasians. Haploidentical-related donors (defined as ≥2 antigen level mismatches) are a less expensive and readily available source for most patients across ethnic and racial barriers. Early reports utilizing haploidentical donors were associated with prohibitive GVHD in T-cell replete grafts. Extensive in vivo or ex vivo T-cell depletion used to mitigate this risk led to a higher risk disease relapse, delayed immune reconstitution, infectious complications resulting in a higher NRM. A relatively newer strategy using marrow derived T-cell replete haploidentical allografts with post-transplant administration of high dose cyclophosphamide selectively targets alloreactive T-cells (effector cells implicated in acute GVHD) rapidly proliferating early after an HLA-mismatched transplant, but relatively sparing regulatory T-cells and nondividing hematopoietic cells, has shown encouraging results with prompt engraftment, low GVHD, and favorable NRM. Although lacking prospective data, large observational studies have demonstrated comparable post-transplant outcomes with haploidentical transplantation compared to more traditional MUD and MRD allo-HCT in leukemia and lymphoma. Haploidentical donor HCT is potentially an attractive choice for ethnic minorities and resource restricted regions.

   (iii) Umbilical cord blood—Obtained and cryopreserved from a newborn's cord, the presence of immunologically naïve immune cells allows for HLA mismatches without increasing the risk of GVHD. Graft rejection and delayed engraftment occur more frequently owing to lower number of nucleated cells. However, the simultaneous use of two UCB (double UCB) units from different donors has shown to improve engraftment. Higher total nucleated cell doses and better degrees of HLA match are associated with improved transplant outcomes. Current goal is to maximize matching at the antigen level for HLA-A and -B, and at the allele-level for and the NMDP recommends at least ≥4/6 HLA-matched cord blood unit with adequate cell dose and also to consider evaluating for HLA antibodies, HLA-C matching and screening for non-inherited maternal antigens (NIMA). The ideal alternative donor source is unknown and mostly dependent of the specific center's expertise. An ongoing randomized trial (BMT CTN 1101) compares allo-HCT outcomes with double UCB versus haploidentical donors.

Donor Evaluation

Careful donor selection and evaluation is an integral part of the pretransplantation workup. The donor must be healthy and able to withstand the apheresis procedure or a bone marrow harvest.

1. HLA typing
2. ABO typing
3. History-relevant information of the donor:
   Any previous malignancy within 5 years, except non-melanoma skin cancer, is considered and absolute exclusion criteria. Age, sex, and parity of the donor impacts HCT outcomes and though are not exclusion criteria; younger men and nonparous women are preferred when available. Comorbidities like cardiac or coronary artery disease, lung diseases, back or spine disorders, medications, and complications to general anesthesia to be considered.
4. Infection exposure
   HIV, human T-lymphotropic virus (HTLV), hepatitis, CMV, HSV, and EBV serology
5. Pregnancy testing for women

PHASES OF ALLOGENEIC TRANSPLANT

Pre-transplant Phase—Conditioning ("The Preparative Regimen")

This phase of HCT precedes the graft infusion and is characterized by the administration of chemotherapeutic agents +/– radiation. In the conventional sense, the goals of the conditioning regimen include immunosuppression of the recipient to prevent graft rejection and to eradicate residual disease. Newer conditioning strategies such as RIC/NMA regimens preserve immunosuppressive effects to aid donor engraftment with minimal or no myelosuppression.

1. Myeloablative conditioning
   The most commonly used myeloablative conditioning regimens incorporate high-dose cyclophosphamide (120 mg/Kg) in combination with TBI (usually 12 Gy) or busulfan. The choice of regimen is guided by factors such as the sensitivity of the malignancy to drugs in the regimen, the toxicities inherent to individual conditioning agents, prior therapies, and age and performance status of the patient. Early regimen-related toxicity include mucositis, nausea, diarrhea, alopecia, pancytopenia, seizures, and SOS. Late effects include pulmonary toxicity, hypothyroidism, growth retardation, infertility, an increased risk of cardiovascular disease, and second malignancies (mostly related to TBI).
2. Nonmyeloablative (NMA)/Reduced intensity conditioning (RIC)
   RIC or NMA conditioning provides immunosuppression to aid donor engraftment and relies principally on the GVT reactions to eliminate residual malignancy. Cytopenias are limited requiring no or minimal transfusion support. Commonly used truly NMA regimens incorporate fludarabine combined with low-dose TBI ($\leq$2 Gy) or alkylating agent such as cyclophosphamide, busulfan, or melphalan. While the division is somewhat arbitrary, RIC is intermediate between myeloablative and NMA regimens and is usually associated with cytopenias needing transfusion support. The advent of RIC/NMA regimens has broadened the applicability of allo-HCT to include older patients (>60), and those with poor performance status and co-morbidities. Regimen-related toxicity and NRM tend to be less. Unique to RIC/NMA is the presence of assortment of donor and recipient hematopoietic cells in the initial months post-HCT (called mixed chimerism). Several reports indicate that persistent mixed chimerism may lead to higher relapse rates. Immunosuppression withdrawal and less commonly DLI are implemented to convert mixed chimerism by the gradual donor-immune mediated eradication of recipient hematopoietic cells. GVT effects have been observed in several hematologic malignancies, as well as in select metastatic solid tumors such as renal cell carcinoma and neuroblastoma.

Transplant Phase

The transplantation phase is characterized by the intravenous infusion of the graft and usually starts 24 to 48 hours after completing the preparative regimen. Infusion is usually well tolerated by the recipient. The day of transplantation is traditionally referred to as "day 0."

Post-transplant (pre-engraftment) Phase

Early post-transplant phase is characterized by marrow aplasia and pancytopenia. Regimen-related toxicity and infectious complications are common during this phase and usually require intensive support with aggressive hydration, antimicrobial prophylaxis and treatment, GVHD prophylaxis and transfusion support. All transfused products should be irradiated (to avoid transfusion associated GVHD) and leukoreduced (CMV safe). Engraftment is the term used to define hematopoietic recovery after HCT. Earliest to occur and sometimes used synonymously with the term engraftment is myeloid engraftment defined as sustained recovery of neutrophil count of >0.5x10^9/L. Platelet engraftment usually lags behind granulocyte recovery and is usually defined platelet counts of at least >20x10^9/L without transfusion for 7 days. Erythrocyte engraftment occurs much later and is characterized by independence from PRBC transfusions. Post-transplant cytopenias depend on conditioning regimen used, diagnosis and disease status, donor source, CD34$^+$ cell dose in the allograft, use of growth factors, and GVHD prophylaxis.

Post-transplant (post-engraftment) Phase

Even after myeloid engraftment occurs the recipient remains immunosuppressed due to GVHD prophylaxis/treatment and slow immune reconstitution, which may take up to 12 months to occur. Notable complications during this phase include infections and GVHD and require continued monitoring. Immunosuppression withdrawal in the absence of GVHD is employed at this stage to facilitate immune reconstitution.

COMPLICATIONS

Figure 30.1 highlights the timeline for some important post-transplant complications after allo-HCT. The following text elaborates the salient features of some key adverse effects and may not be considered comprehensive.

Graft Failure

Graft failure is a rare but serious complication characterized by the lack of engraftment and hematopoietic recovery after allo-HCT. Causes include HLA disparity, recipient alloimmunization, low CD34$^+$ dose, T cell depletion of the graft, inadequate immunosuppression, disease progression, infections, and medications. Graft failure may be primary (early) when no hematopoietic recovery is noted post-HCT by day +28 or secondary (late) when the initial hematopoietic recovery is lost. Host immune mediated graft rejection is an important cause of graft failure. Growth factor support, manipulating dosage of immunosuppressive agents, CD34$^+$ stem cell boost, DLI, and re-grafting represent approaches to the management of graft failure.

Infections

Infection remains a major cause of morbidity for patients undergoing HCT. Indwelling catheters and transmigration of intestinal flora are common sources of infections, and bacteremia and sepsis may occur during the pre-engraftment (neutropenic) phase of HCT. Current approaches to minimize the risk of life-threatening infections include the use of prophylactic antibacterial, antifungal, and antiviral agents, as well as aggressive screening and treatment for common transplantation-associated infections.

(i) Cytomegalovirus—CMV infection most commonly occurs due to reactivation in seropositive patients or very rarely because of the transfer of an infection from the donor. The infection usually occurs after engraftment and may coincide with GVHD and/or its treatment. The risk for reactivation is highest up to day +100. CMV pneumonia and colitis can cause significant morbidity and mortality. In addition, it can cause febrile disease, hepatitis, and marrow suppression. Screening for viral reactivation is performed weekly after transplantation by measuring the CMV antigen levels or by polymerase chain reaction (PCR). Initial treatment is with intravenous ganciclovir

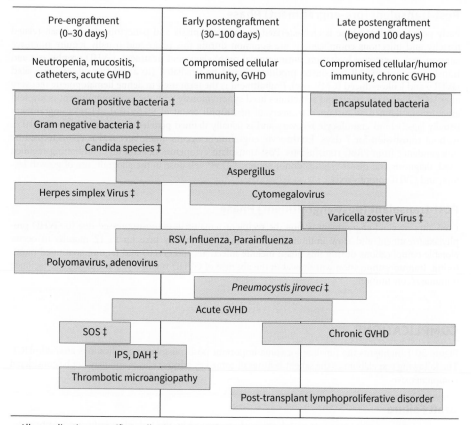

Pre-engraftment (0–30 days)	Early postengraftment (30–100 days)	Late postengraftment (beyond 100 days)
Neutropenia, mucositis, catheters, acute GVHD	Compromised cellular immunity, GVHD	Compromised cellular/humor immunity, chronic GVHD

All complications specific to allogeneic transplantation unless noted by symbol (‡), in which case also seen in auto-transplant recipients.

Abbreviation: GVHD – graft-versus-host disease; RSV – respiratory syncitial virus; SOS – sinusoidal obstruction syndrome; IPS – idiopathic pulmonary syndrome; DAH – diffuse alveolar hemorrhage

FIGURE 30.1 Timeline of complications after hematopoietic cell transplantation.

or oral valganciclovir ± intravenous immunoglobulin. Foscarnet and cidofovir are alternatives (especially in patients with cytopenias). The use of ganciclovir for the initial prophylaxis or pre-emptive therapy in patients who reactivate CMV post-transplant (i.e. become CMV-PCR +) can significantly prevent CMV disease and has resulted in a substantial reduction in CMV associated morbidity and mortality.

(ii) Invasive Fungal Infection—With the routine use of fluconazole prophylaxis in HCT patients, once lethal invasive *Candida* infections are relatively uncommon. Other important pathogens include *Aspergillus*, *Fusarium*, and *Zygomycetes*. Common presentations include pneumonia, rhinosinusitis, skin infections, or fungemia. Patients with GVHD on high dose steroids are especially at risk for invasive fungal infection and may benefit from expanded selection of antifungal prophylaxis.

(iii) Others—HSV and VZV reactivation is effectively prevented with acyclovir prophylaxis, but late VZV reactivation after cessation of prophylaxis has been noted. EBV reactivation and post-transplant lymphoproliferative disorders are seen more commonly with T-cell depleted transplants and in cord blood transplant recipients, especially those who receive anti-thymocyte globulin (ATG).

Sinusoidal Obstruction Syndrome (formerly veno-occlussive disease)

Hepatic SOS is characterized by jaundice, tender hepatomegaly, and unexplained weight gain or ascites and usually manifests in the first 2 weeks post-HCT. SOS is difficult to treat and typically involves supportive care measures focused on maintaining renal function, coagulation system, and fluid balance. The risk of SOS is higher in combination regimens containing alkylators with higher dose TBI or ablative doses of busulfan. The intravenous use and pharmacokinetic monitoring of busulfan drug levels has dramatically reduced the incidence of SOS. Defibrotide, a deoxyribonucleic acid derivative, which is an anticoagulant, was approved by the food and drug administration (FDA) in March 2016 for treatment of SOS.

Pulmonary Toxicity

Bacterial, viral, or fungal organisms may cause infectious pneumonia. Idiopathic pulmonary syndrome, characterized by fever, diffuse infiltrates, and hypoxia may occur in 10% of patients and has an abysmal prognosis in severe cases requiring ventilator support. A subset of patients with diffuse alveolar hemorrhage may respond to high-dose steroids. Other causes such as CMV pneumonitis, transfusion associated circulatory overload (TACO) and transfusion-associated lung injury (TRALI) must be excluded. Risk factors for pulmonary toxicity include ablative conditioning regimen (TBI), older age, prior radiation, a low DLCO, tobacco use, and GVHD.

Graft-versus-Host Disease

After allo-HCT, donor-derived T-lymphocytes may recognize recipient tissue as foreign and mount an immunologic attack resulting in GVHD. It is one of the main treatment-related toxicities and impacts NRM significantly. Conventionally acute GVHD was defined as occurring within day +100, and chronic GVHD beyond 100 days of transplant. It is no longer true and the classification should be based on clinical features rather than time of onset.

Acute GVHD: Up to 40% to 50% of MRD allo-HCT can be complicated by acute GVHD. Though varied in clinical presentation, it typically manifests in the first 2 to 6 weeks and affects the skin, liver, and the gastrointestinal system. The consensus criteria for staging/grading of acute GVHD is presented in Table 30.2. Risk factors for acute GVHD include degree of HLA mismatch, infections (CMV, VZV), unrelated donors, older patients, multiparous donor, older donors in MUD transplants, ABO-mismatches, sex-mismatched transplants (female donor → male recipients), and the use of intensive conditioning regimens.

- Prevention of acute GVHD

  Strategies to prevent acute GVHD have been established and are more effective than treating acute GVHD. Commonly employed strategies include the following:

  1. Pharmacologic therapy: Combination therapy of non-specific immunosuppressive agents (methotrexate, steroids) and T-cell–specific immunosuppressant (calcineurin inhibitors—cyclosporine and tacrolimus, mycophenolate mofetil) is preferred to single agent therapy. Methotrexate IV on days +1, +3, +6, and +11 with tacrolimus or cyclosporine IV/PO starting day −2 is most commonly used. Sirolimus and mycophenolate are sometimes used in lieu of methotrexate. Drug toxicities and interactions are extremely important to monitor and drug levels are followed closely for calcineurin inhibitors and sirolimus.

  2. T-cell depletion: Achieved by (a) ex vivo separation by CD34+ selection or the use of monoclonal antibodies to remove T cells or (b) in vivo T cell depletion with the use of monoclonal antibodies such as ATG or alemtuzumab or (c) the administration of post-transplant high cyclophosphamide. Though effective in reducing GVHD, these maneuvers may increase relapse rates and infections due to late immune reconstitution. In recent years the administration of post-transplantation cyclophosphamide, which mitigates the risk of GVHD by targeting alloreactive T-cells rapidly proliferating early after an HLA-mismatched transplant, has led to increased use of haploidentical-related donor transplants. The ongoing BMT CTN 1301 clinical trial is comparing this strategy to traditional GVHD prophylaxis and CD34+ selection in MRD and MUD allografts.

TABLE 30.2 Acute Graft-versus-Host Disease Staging by Consensus Criteria

Stage	Skin	Liver (bilirubin)	Gastrointestinal (GI)
0	No skin rash	<2 mg/dL	<50 mL/d or persistent nausea alone
1	Maculopapular rash <25% BSA	2.1–3 mg/dL	500–1,000 mL/d, or persistent nausea, vomiting, anorexia, or positive upper GI biopsy[a]
2	Maculopapular rash 25%–50% BSA	3.1–6 mg/dL	1,000–1,500 mL/d
3	Maculopapular rash >50% BSA	6.1–15 mg/dL	>1,500 mL/d
4	Generalized erythroderma, plus bullae, or desquamation	>15 mg/dL	> 2000 mL/d, severe abdomen-al pain +/− ileus

Clinical Grade	Skin	Liver	Gastrointestinal
I	Stages 1–2	None	None
II	Stage 3	Stage 1	Stage 1
III	–	Stages 2–3	Stages 2–4
IV	Stage 4	Stage 4	–

[a] milliliter/day of liquid stool.

BSA, body surface area.

Przepiorka D, Weisdorf D, Martin P, et al. 1994 Consensus conference on acute GVHD grading. *Bone Marrow Transplant.* 1995;15(6):825–828.

- Treatment of acute GVHD

  Frontline treatment for clinically significant (grades II–IV) acute GVHD is methylprednisolone at a dose of 2 mg/kg/day and calcineurin inhibitors should be continued or restarted. For those not responding or with partial response mycophenalate is usually added. Additional agents (azathioprine, daclizumab, photopheresis, ATG, infliximab) are used with variable success. Steroid refractory acute GVHD portends very poor prognosis. Prophylactic antifungal therapy against aspergillus should be considered in those on corticosteroid treatment.

  Chronic GVHD: Use of PBPC allografts, MUD, and prior history of acute GVHD are risk factors. Chronic GVHD thought to be mediated chiefly by donor B-lymphocytes, presents with variable and multisystem organ involvement, and clinical manifestations may resemble autoimmune disorders (i.e., lichenoid skin changes, sicca syndrome, scleroderma-like skin changes, chronic hepatitis, and bronchiolitis obliterans). Chronic GVHD is often accompanied by cytopenias and immunodeficiency. Treatment involves prolonged courses of steroids and other immunosuppressive agents as well as prophylactic antibiotics (e.g., penicillin) and antifungal agents. Other potentially useful agents include thalidomide, mycophenolate mofetil, imatinib mesylate, pentostatin, rituximab, photopheresis, and Psoralen ultraviolet radiation (skin GVHD). More recently, B-cell receptor antagonist, ibrutinib (Bruton tyrosine kinase inhibitor), has shown clinical activity in Phase I/II trial which has prompted FDA to grant breakthrough status for patients with chronic GVHD not responding to initial therapy.

Relapse

Relapses after allo-HCT is ominous, especially for aggressive malignancies such as AML and ALL. Most relapses occur within 2 years of transplantation and those that relapse within 6 months have a worse prognosis. Immunosuppression is typically withdrawn to enhance GVT effect and, in some cases, DLI is administered. DLI administration frequently results in GVHD. The most favorable responses to

DLI have been seen in patients with CML, especially those with molecular or chronic phase relapse. Second transplant for relapsed disease rarely results in long-term disease-free survival and is associated with a very high risk of NRM.

SURVIVORSHIP

It is estimated that there are over 125,000 patients who are long-term (>5 years) survivors after HCT. While survivors after auto-HCT lead near normal lives, studies have consistently shown that allograft recipients have lower life expectancy than age-matched population. Long-term complications depend on the conditioning regimen, age, and presence of chronic GVHD. Some key points are as follows:

1. Auto-HCT survivors are at risk for lung dysfunction, cardiovascular diseases, and secondary myelodysplasia/AML.
2. Major complications afflicting allo-HCT survivors include chronic GVHD, infections, organ dysfunction (pulmonary, cardiovascular, endocrine, and immune systems), secondary myelodysplasia/AML and solid organ malignancies. In addition, the pediatric population is at risk for growth retardation.
3. Immunizations are recommended for auto-HCT patients starting at 6 months and after withdrawal of immunosuppressive agents for allo-HCT. Long-term antibiotic prophylaxis is needed for patients receiving prolonged treatment for chronic GVHD.
4. Recommended screening and preventive measures for survivors have been established (see reference list). This include routine hemogram, hepatic, and renal function tests, endocrine screening (lipid panel, vitamin D, thyroid panel), immunological studies, and others studies (echocardiogram, pulmonary function tests, age appropriate cancer screening, ophthalmologic evaluation, bone densitometry)

CONCLUSION

Hematopoietic cell transplantation has evolved into an effective therapeutic option for a broad range of disease entities. The improved safety profile of the procedure and the increasing availability of donor sources have led to an increase in the number of transplants performed each year. There have been improvements in survival, less acute complications, and improved awareness and treatment of chronic complications. The number of patients who benefit from this procedure will likely increase as future transplantation strategies continue to evolve, minimizing adverse effects and expanding the stem cell source, while maximizing the beneficial effects donor immune-mediated GVT effects.

Suggested Readings

1. Alousi AM, Bolaños-Meade J, Lee SJ. Graft-versus-Host Disease: The State of the Science. *Biology of Blood and Marrow Transplantation*. (0). Available at: http://www.sciencedirect.com/science/article/pii/S1083879112004582.
2. Anasetti C, Logan BR, Lee SJ, et al. Peripheral-Blood Stem Cells versus Bone Marrow from Unrelated Donors. *N Engl J Med.* 2012;367(16):1487–1496.
3. Brunstein CG, Fuchs EJ, Carter SL, et al. Alternative donor transplantation after reduced intensity conditioning: results of parallel phase 2 trials using partially HLA-mismatched related bone marrow or unrelated double umbilical cord blood grafts. *Blood.* 2011;118(2):282–288.
4. Cantor AB, Lazarus HM, Laport G. Cellular basis of hematopoiesis and stem cell transplantation. In: *American Society of Hematology - Self Assessment Program*. 3rd ed. American Society of Hematology; 2010.
5. Copelan EA. Hematopoietic Stem-Cell Transplantation. *N Engl J Med.* 2006;354(17):1813–1826.
6. Hamadani M, Craig M, Awan FT, Devine SM. How we approach patient evaluation for hematopoietic stem cell transplantation. *Bone Marrow Transplant.* 2010;45(8):1259–1268.
7. Horowitz MM, Confer DL. Evaluation of hematopoietic stem cell donors. *ASH Education Program Book.* 2005;2005(1):469–475.

8. Invaluable web resources for further reading: www.bethematch.org (National Marrow Donor Program), www.cibmtr.org (Center for International Blood and Marrow Transplantation), www.asbmt.org (American Society of Blood and Marrow Evaluation of Hematopoietic Stem Cell Donors Transplantation).

9. Majhail NS, Rizzo JD, Lee SJ, et al. Recommended screening and preventive practices for long-term survivors after hematopoietic cell transplantation. *Biology of Blood and Marrow Transplantation*. 2012;18(3):348–371.

10. Rezvani A, Lowsky R, Negrin RS. Hematopoietic cell transplantation. In: Kaushansky K, Lichtman MA, Prchal JT, Levi M, Press O, Burns L, Caligiuri M, eds. *Williams Hematology*. 9th ed. The McGraw-Hill Companies; 2016.

Carcinoma of Unknown 31 Primary

F. Anthony Greco

DEFINITION

- Cancer of unknown primary (CUP) is a clinical pathologic syndrome defined by the presence of metastatic cancer in the absence of a clinically recognized anatomical primary site of origin.
- CUP represents a heterogeneous group of different cancers, most with a very small (occult) primary tumor site, but with the capacity to metastasize. The pathologic diagnosis is made by biopsy of a metastasis.
- Autopsy series of CUP patients revealed small invasive primary sites in 75% with more than 25 cancer types (mostly carcinomas) documented.

EPIDEMIOLOGY AND PATHOGENESIS

- CUP is relatively common being among the ten most frequently diagnosed advanced cancers worldwide; estimated 50,000 patients annually in the United States.
- The exact incidence is not known since many CUP patients are arbitrarily assigned a specific primary site/cancer type based on the physician's clinical opinion or pathology report despite the inability to detect an anatomical primary site and these cancers are not listed in tumor registries as CUP.
- Male to female ratio is about 1.2 to 1.
- The cause of the CUP syndrome remains an enigma. The clinically occult invasive primaries metastasize and metastases grow and become clinically detectable. Acquired genetic and/or epigenetic alterations are likely to be the basis of the syndrome. However, no specific unique nonrandom genetic alterations have yet been discovered.

CLINICAL FEATURES AND PROGNOSIS

- Nearly all patients have symptoms related to metastasis, which can be present at any site, but are most common in lymph nodes, liver, lungs, and bones.
- CUP is not a single cancer type, but many specific metastatic cancers, which have a common unique feature—an occult clinically undetectable invasive anatomical primary site.
- Most CUP patients (greater than 50%) present with multiple sites of metastasis but a minority have only 1 to 2 sites. Although metastatic sites are occasionally atypical for the primary, most CUP cancers metastasize to sites expected for the primary and are otherwise biologically similar to their counterparts with known primaries. The major difference in CUP cancers and metastasis from a known primary cancer appears to be the size of the primary site.
- In the past all patients were grouped together since the specific type or origin of the cancer was not definable; CUP was considered as a single entity assumed to be biologically similar; a minority (about

15%) of patients were eventually defined within several favorable subsets based on clinicopathologic features (discussed later).

- In general, when CUP patients are treated with nonspecific empiric chemotherapy their median survival time (excluding the favorable subsets) is about 9 months with a 1-year survival of 25% and 5-year survival less than 10%.
- Poor prognostic factors in the past were largely determined from untreated patients or those treated with empiric chemotherapy in the era when the specific cancer type was not possible to define.
- Historically poor prognostic factors included men, adenocarcinoma histology, increasing number of metastasis to multiple organ sites, hepatic or adrenal involvement, poor performance status, high serum LDH, and low serum albumin; many of these factors also apply to patients with many types of advanced cancer.
- Patients with more favorable prognostic factors included favorable clinical pathologic subsets (discussed later), predominant lymph node involvement without major visceral involvement.

DIAGNOSIS

- The initial diagnostic evaluation recommended is outlined in Table 31.1. If an anatomical primary site is identified the patient does not have CUP.
- Biopsy samples should be generous if possible, avoiding fine needle aspirations since several tests may be necessary. The first goal is confirming the diagnosis of cancer and second goal the specific type of cancer.
- Standard pathologic examination including immunohistochemical (IHC) staining is routinely done on CUP biopsies.
- Table 31.2 lists some of the useful IHC staining patterns, but the selection of stains is often based on the light microscopic histopathological appearance of the biopsy and clinical features; obtaining multiple stains indiscriminately exhausts the biopsy specimen and rarely improves the diagnostic ability.
- Additional evaluation recommended based on the initial findings is outlined in Table 31.3.
- The lineage of the cancer (carcinoma, sarcoma, melanoma, lymphoma) is usually diagnosed by light microscopic appearance and if necessary by IHC staining.
- Molecular cancer classifier assays have been developed based on gene expression profile patterns and are a major advance in the diagnosis of the cancer type in CUP patients. In the United States there are

---

TABLE 31.1 Initial Diagnostic Evaluation of a Possible CUP Patient

- Complete history and physical examination
- Laboratory Tests: urine analysis, CBC, CMP, LDH, PSA in men, others depending on clinicopathologic features
- Computerized tomographic (CT) scans of chest, abdomen, pelvis
- Positron emission tomography (PET) scan in selected patients (squamous carcinoma in cervical/inguinal nodes and those with a suspected single site of involvement)
- Mammography in women; MRI breasts if breast cancer highly suspected
- Biopsy should be generous specimen if feasible; avoid fine needle aspiration
- Pathology evaluation: screening IHC stains of the biopsy on carcinomas (CK7, CK20, TTF-1, CDX-2); other stains or specialized pathology depending on histology and clinicopathologic features (see Tables 31.2. and 31.3.)
- Additional clinical, laboratory, and pathologic evaluation based on details from history, physical examination, laboratory testing, and medical imaging
- If an anatomical primary site is not found the patient has CUP
- Molecular cancer classifier assay on very small biopsy/aspiration/cytology specimens or when a reasonable number of IHC stains is not diagnostic of a single cancer type or tissue of origin

TABLE 31.2 IHC Staining Patterns Characteristic of a Single Cancer or Tissue of Origin[a]

Prostate	CK7–, CK20–, PSA+
Breast	CK7+, CK20–, GCDFP-15+, mammoglobin+, ER+,PR+, GATA3+ Her-2-neu+
Lung-adenocarcinoma and large cell	CK7+, CK20– TTF-1+, Napsin A+
Colorectal	CK7–, CK20+, CDX2+
Germ cell	PLAP+,OCT4+, SALL4+
Lung-Neuroendocrine (small cell/large cell)	Chromogranin+, synaptophysin+, CD56+, TTF-1+
Thyroid carcinoma (papillary/follicular)	Thyroglobin+, TTF-1+
Melanoma	MelanA+, HMB45+, S100+
Adrenal carcinoma	Alpha-inhibin+, Melan-A+(A103)
Renal cell carcinoma	RCC+, PAX8+
Ovary carcinoma	CK7+, CK20–, WT-1+, PAX8+, ER+
Hepatocellular carcinoma	Hepar-1+, CD10+, CD13+

[a] In the appropriate clinical and pathologic setting the staining profiles may be diagnostic of the tissue of origin or cancer type. Stains frequently overlap and not all are always positive or negative as indicated above.

TABLE 31.3 Additional Evaluation Based on Findings from Initial Diagnostic Evaluation in CUP

Results of Initial Diagnostic Evaluation	Additional Evaluation	
	Clinical	IHC Staining/Other Testing
Features highly suggestive of colorectal carcinoma (peritoneal/liver metastasis; biopsy CK20+, CK7–, CDX2+)	Colonoscopy	KRAS mutation of biopsy
Features highly suggestive of lung carcinoma (mediastinal/hilar adenopathy; biopsy CK7+, CK20–, TTF-1+)	Consider bronchoscopy	Genomic analysis of biopsy for EGFR mutation and ALK/ROS1 rearrangement
Features suggestive of ovarian carcinoma (peritoneal/pelvic metastasis; biopsy CK7+)	Intravaginal/pelvic ultrasound	WT-1, PAX8, andER stains of biopsy
Features suggestive of breast carcinoma (axillary nodes, lung, bone, liver metastasis; CK7+)	Breast MRI	ER, GCDFP-15, mammoglobin, and GATA3 stains; Her-2-neu testing of biopsy
Mediastinal and/or retroperitoneal masses in young adults (usually men)	Testicular ultrasound, serum AFP, HCG, and LDH	PLAP,OCT4, SALL4 stains of biopsy; FISH for i(12)p of biopsy
Poorly differentiated carcinoma, with or without clear cell features	Serum AFP if liver involvement; octreotide scan if neuroendocrine stains+	Chromogranin, synaptophysin, RCC, PAX8, Hepar1, MelanA, and HMB-45 stains of biopsy
Liver lesions predominant (CK7–,CK20–)	Serum AFP	Hepar1 stain of biopsy
Any histology without a single cancer site or tissue of origin predicted by IHC or small amount of biopsy		Molecular cancer classifier assay of biopsy

three commercially available assays (BioTheranostics, Inc. Cancer TYPE ID, a 92 gene RT-PCR assay that provides a molecular classification of 50 cancer types/subtypes with an overall 87% accuracy; Cancer Genetics, Inc. Tissue of Origin test, a 2000 gene microarray assay that identifies 15 cancer types with an 89% accuracy; Rosetta Genomics (Cancer Origin Assay) which is a microarray, micro RNA assay with about a 90% accuracy which can identify 49 cancer types.)

- Data are accumulating for these three molecular cancer classifier assays as well as a new DNA-based epigenetic assay (EPICUP) also demonstrating about a 90% accuracy.
- The diagnostic ability of the combination of IHC and molecular cancer classifiers often provides critical information to plan appropriate treatment for each patient.

HISTOLOGIC/MORPHOLOGIC CELL TYPES

- The light microscopic classification of CUP includes several recognized histologic types including adenocarcinoma (60%), poorly differentiated carcinoma with some features of adenocarcinoma (30%), squamous cell carcinoma (5%), neuroendocrine carcinomas (3%), and poorly differentiated neoplasm with confusing or undefined lineage (2%). Occasionally, melanoma or sarcoma presents as CUP and generally are treated with site specific therapies and not further discussed in this brief review.
- Segregation of the above histologic types is important since various favorable subsets could be more easily recognized. Over the past four decades, several favorable subsets (15% of all CUP patients) are now treated with site-specific therapy based on their presumed tissue of origin (discussed later).
- The majority of CUP patients (85%) are not included in any of the favorable subsets, and there does not appear to be any prognostic significance of the light microscopic histology.
- Nonspecific empiric chemotherapy regimens were developed in large part from 1995 through 2006 and the 85% of CUP patients with unfavorable prognostic features were usually treated; the cancer type could not be determined in most patients and the same empiric chemotherapy regimens were used for all patients assuming all CUP cancers were biologically similar. Although these empiric regimens helped a minority of patients, the overall median survival in larger series (greater than 100 patients) has been only about 9 months.

FAVORABLE SUBSETS OF CUP PATIENTS

Clinical features including gender, metastatic sites, and histologic classification of these cancers and more recently IHC and molecular cancer classifier assays have provided the basis to presume a specific primary tumor or cancer type for selected patients. Treatment based upon these presumptive diagnoses has generally improved the overall outcome of these patient subsets (see Table 31.4.) Recent data reveal the cancer types of many of the favorable CUP subsets reported several years ago are as expected based on IHC staining and/or molecular cancer classifier assays.

A. Extragonadal germ cell cancer syndrome
- These patients represent a rare, but important subset, since they have very treatable and potentially curable advanced cancers if recognized and treated appropriately.
- Most commonly these tumors are found in young men, but also even more rarely in women. These carcinomas usually involve the midline location (mediastinum and/or retroperitoneum) and/or multiple lung nodules.
- The histology of the biopsy is usually a poorly differentiated carcinoma or poorly differentiated neoplasm.
- Elevated serum levels of beta HCG and/or alpha-fetoprotein (AFP) are commonly seen.
- IHC staining for germ cell tumors and/or a molecular cancer classifier assay or FISH testing for an isochromosome of 12 may be diagnostic.
- Therapy for germ cell carcinomas is indicated even if the histology is atypical which is characteristic in these patients.

TABLE 31.4 Favorable Subsets of CUP

Subset	Therapy
A. Young men (rarely women) retroperitoneal and/or mediastinal masses; serum B-HCG and/or AFP may be positive	Treat as germ cell carcinoma
B. Squamous cell carcinoma in cervical/neck nodes	Treat as head/neck carcinoma
C. Squamous cell carcinoma in inguinal/iliac nodes	Treat as anal, cervical, or vulvar carcinoma
D. Women (rarely men) with axillary carcinoma	Treat as breast carcinoma
E. Women (rarely men) with peritoneal carcinoma (usually serous adenocarcinoma)	Treat as ovarian carcinoma
F. Neuroendocrine carcinoma	
Well differentiated	Treat like carcinoid
Poorly differentiated	Treat like small cell lung carcinoma
G. Men with osteoblastic bone metastasis-PSA+	Treat like prostate carcinoma
H. CUP colorectal subset (IHC and/or molecular cancer classifier assay diagnosis of colorectal)	Treat like colorectal carcinoma.
I. Single small site of metastasis	Treat with surgery and/or RT; chemotherapy
J. Poorly differentiated neoplasms (linage unknown)	Many responsive neoplasms (further evaluation critical)
K. Isolated pleural effusion with carcinoma	Many responsive carcinomas (further evaluation critical)
L. Gestational carcinoma serum B-HCG elevated	Treat as gestational choriocarcinoma

B. Axillary carcinoma in women and rarely men
  • Most of these patients have occult breast carcinoma.
  • IHC stains are usually positive for breast markers, but some are triple negative; molecular classifiers assays usually predict breast carcinoma.
  • Mammography is negative; breast MRI and PET scans detect some small primaries.
  • If mastectomy is done, about 60% have documented small invasive primary breast carcinomas. It is possible that many others also have a very small primary, but are missed as it may take hundreds of tissue sections to find a very small clinically occult invasive primary.
  • Treatment guidelines should be similar to stage II or III breast carcinoma; primary radiotherapy of the ipsilateral breast is an acceptable alternative to surgery; neoadjuvant or adjuvant chemotherapy and/or hormone therapy as per breast cancer guidelines is indicated.
  • The prognosis of these patients appear similar to women with known stage II or III breast cancer when they are treated appropriately.
  • In patients with an axillary mass and other metastasis, the suspicion of occult breast cancer should remain high.
C. Squamous cell carcinoma in upper cervical/neck nodes
  • Highly suggests an occult head and neck carcinoma.
  • PET scanning reveals the primary site in more than one-third of these patients, despite the inability to find it by any other testing.
  • Human papillomavirus (HPV) association is common.
  • Treatment with combined modality chemotherapy and radiotherapy as per head and neck carcinoma and outcomes similar.
D. Squamous cell carcinoma in inguinal or pelvic lymph nodes
  • Most likely arising from an occult primary from the uterine cervix, anal canal, or more rarely the vulva or skin. HPV association is seen with both cervical and anal cell carcinomas.
  • Potentially curable cancers with combined modality therapy.

E. Peritoneal carcinoma in women and rarely men
  - They usually have serous adenocarcinoma but may be poorly differentiated carcinoma; these tumors are more common in BRCA1/2 germline mutation patients.
  - IHC staining and/or molecular classifier assays usually consistent with ovarian, fallopian tube or primary peritoneal carcinoma.
  - Serum CA 125 often elevated but not specific.
  - Treatment should be similar to stage III ovarian carcinoma and the outcomes are similar.

F. Neuroendocrine carcinoma
  - An important distinction is the grade of the tumor—well differentiated or poorly differentiated; some poorly differentiated carcinomas are not recognized as neuroendocrine unless specific IHC stains and/or a molecular cancer classifier assay are obtained.
  - Well-differentiated tumors have a similar biology to well-differentiated carcinoid or islet cell tumors.
  - Treatment for well-differentiated tumors is similar to advanced carcinoid tumors; overall prognosis fair to good in part due to the indolent nature of these cancers and the evolving improving therapies.
  - Treatment for high grade or poorly differentiated neuroendocrine tumor should be similar to small cell lung cancer or extra-pulmonary small cell carcinomas with cisplatin- or carboplatin-based chemotherapy; radiotherapy should be added in those with local regional involvement.
  - A small percentage (about 10%) of patients with poorly differentiated neuroendocrine tumors have long-term survival following combination chemotherapy including etoposide and platinum (most other patients have responses to chemotherapy with improvement in the quality and quantity of life).

G. Men with elevated prostate-specific antigen (PSA) or osteoblastic metastasis
  - Hormonal therapy for prostate carcinoma should be administered when the serum PSA is elevated (serum PSA recommended for all men with CUP) or tumor PSA stain is positive. Men with osteoblastic metastasis warrant a trial of hormone therapy in selected clinical settings regardless of the PSA level. A molecular cancer classifier assay may also help with the diagnosis.

H. Single small site of metastasis
  - Local therapy with surgical resection and/or radiotherapy.
  - Site specific therapy should be considered depending on the determination of the cancer type by immunostaining and/or a molecular cancer classifier assay.

I. Poorly differentiated neoplasms
  - About 2% of all CUP patients have a poorly differentiated neoplasm without a definitive lineage by light microscopic examination; after IHC staining only a small minority of these cancers remain undefined; in this group a molecular cancer classifier has been proven to be useful in the majority of patients.
  - Precise diagnosis in these patients is important by the appropriate use of IHC staining panels and if necessary a molecular cancer classifier assay (several of these patients have highly treatable neoplasms including germ cell tumors, lymphoma, melanomas, and others).

J. CUP colorectal subset
  - A subset of CUP patients with IHC stains and or a molecular cancer classifier assay diagnostic of a lower GI primary have improved outcomes with median survivals about 24 months similar to known colorectal adenocarcinomas when treated with colorectal site specific regimens.
  - These patients do not have their primary sites found at colonoscopy and most have metastasis typical for colorectal primaries (liver, peritoneal cavity, retroperitoneal nodes).
  - These CUP patients should be treated in a similar fashion as known metastatic colorectal adenocarcinoma since their outcome is improved.

K. Amelanotic melanoma
  - Melanoma has been known for decades by pathologists as the "great imitator"; the histology can be confusing, particularly when no melanin pigment is identified in the cancer cells; melanoma may appear as a poorly differentiated carcinoma or the lineage may not be recognized.
  - Appropriate IHC stains usually are diagnostic, but if there is a doubt a molecular cancer classifier assay is usually helpful.

- Treatment implications are obvious since BRAF inhibitors and immune checkpoint inhibitors often provide useful therapy.
L. Isolated pleural effusion
  - This subset is recognized with an overall better prognosis than those with multiple metastasis.
  - A small peripheral lung carcinoma obscured by fluid should be suspected but occult breast cancer, ovarian cancer, and other occult primaries may present with metastasis and isolated pleural effusion; nonspecific empiric chemotherapy has been useful for some of these patients in the past, but specialized pathology with appropriate IHC stains and if necessary a molecular cancer classifier assay is indicated to direct site specific therapy for these patients.
M. Unrecognized gestational choriocarcinoma
  - CUP in a young woman with poorly differentiated carcinoma or neoplasm particularly during pregnancy or in the postpartum period or after spontaneous abortion should be suspected of harboring gestational choriocarcinoma; examination of the placenta or other tissue is usually diagnostic.
  - A serum beta HCG is always elevated and chemotherapy for choriocarcinoma is usually curative; in the gestational setting choriocarcinoma is most likely but an elevated serum beta HCG may also be from a germ cell carcinoma.

GENERAL PRINCIPLES, EVALUATION, AND TREATMENT OF CUP PATIENTS

- The goal in any patient with metastatic cancer is to determine the primary site or cancer type.
- Therapy is based upon an accurate identification of the precise cancer type.
- In patients with CUP an anatomical primary site is not clinically identified after a reasonable evaluation; determination of the cancer type depends on considering all clinicopathologic data, but particularly IHC staining panels and if necessary a molecular cancer classifier assay performed on a biopsy of a metastatic lesion.
- Molecular cancer classifier assays have been proven to diagnose the cancer type in CUP in about 95% of patients.
- Data from several prospective and retrospective studies now support the use of molecular cancer classifier assays in the majority of patients (about 66%) who are not diagnosed with a single cancer type by IHC staining panels.
- Once the cancer type in CUP is diagnosed, site-specific therapy for that cancer should be administered since data shows an improved outcome for many patients compared to nonspecific empiric chemotherapy, which was the standard in the past.
- Precision or personalized therapy is now indicated for CUP patients based on the recognition of the cancer. CUP is not a single cancer and each patient has a specific cancer and therapy is indicated for their cancer type. For some cancer types (including breast, lung, colorectal, ovary renal, and others) several site-specific therapies, in some instances used sequentially, improve patient survival; the effectiveness and outcomes is variable and better for patients with cancers known to be responsive to therapies; the presence of genetic alterations which are successfully targeted by various drugs now also have proven survival benefit for some patients with lung, melanoma, breast, GE junction/gastric, colorectal, and other cancers. The recognition of the usefulness of immune checkpoint inhibitors in several patients with a number of advanced cancers also makes the precise diagnosis of the cancer type important.
- CUP patients have a large range of cancer types arising from many occult anatomically undetectable primaries and some, particularly with the more responsive cancers, may be treated effectively if recognized.
- A small minority of CUP patients (about 5%) cannot have their precise cancer type identified despite the use of appropriate IHC panels and molecular cancer classifier assays; nonspecific empiric chemotherapy is appropriate in these patients.
- Examples of four frequently used empiric regimens for CUP including high grade neuroendocrine carcinoma are illustrated in Table 31.5.
- The suggested algorithm for the management of a possible CUP patient is illustrated in Figure 31.1.

TABLE 31.5 Empiric Chemotherapy Commonly Used in the Past for Carcinoma of Unknown Primary

Adenocarcinoma or poorly differentiated carcinoma

Paclitaxel	200 mg/m² IV day 1
Carboplatin	AUC 6 IV day1
	Repeat cycle 3 weeks
	6 cycles
Gemcitibine,	1,250 mg/m² IV days 1,8
Cisplatin	80–100 mg/m² day 1 Repeat cycle 3 weeks
	6 cycles

High grade neuroendocrine carcinoma

Etoposide	100 mg/m² IV days 1,2,3
Carboplatin	AUC 5 IV day 1
	Repeat cycle 3 weeks
	4–6 cycles
Etoposide	100 mg/m² IV days 1,2,3
Cisplatin	80–100 mg/m² IV day 1
	Repeat cycle 3–4 weeks
	4–6 cycles

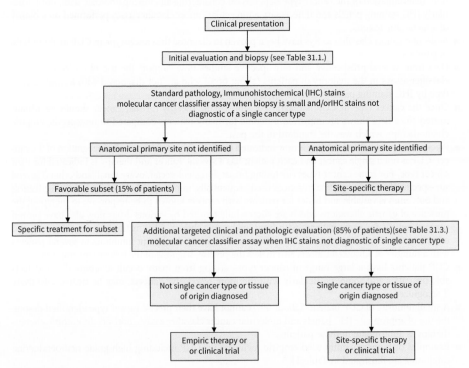

FIGURE 31.1 Suggested evaluation of a possible CUP patient.

Suggested Readings

1. Ettinger DS, Handorf CR, Agulnik M, et al. Occult primary, Version 3.2014. *J Natl Compr Canc Netw.* 2014;12:969–974.
2. Greco FA, Hainsworth JD. Cancer of unknown primary site. In: DeVita VT Jr., Lawrence TS, Rosenberg SA, eds. *Cancer: Principles and Practice of Oncology.*10th ed. Philadelphia, PA: Wolters Kluwer Publishers; 2015:1720–1737.
3. Greco FA, Lennington WJ, Spigel DR, Hainsworth JD. Molecular profiling diagnosis in unknown primary cancer: accuracy and ability to complement standard pathology. *J Natl Cancer Inst.* 2013;105:782–790.
4. Greco FA, Lennington WJ, Spigel DR, Hainsworth JD. Poorly differentiated neoplasms of unknown primary site; diagnostic usefulness of a molecular cancer classifier assay. *Mol Diagn Ther.* 2015;19:91–97.
5. Greco FA. Cancer of unknown primary site: still an entity, a biological mystery and a metastatic model. *Nat Rev Cancer.* 2014;14:3–4.
6. Greco FA. Molecular diagnosis of the tissue of origin in cancer of unknown primary site: useful in patient management. *Curr Treat Options Oncol.* 2013;14:634–642.
7. Greco FA. Gene expression profiling in patients with carcinoma of unknown primary site; from translational research to standard of care. *Virchows Arch.* 2014;464:393–402.
8. Hainsworth JD, Rubin MS, Spigel DR, et al. Molecular gene expression profiling to predict the tissue of origin and direct site-specific therapy in patients with carcinoma of unknown primary site: a prospective trial of the Sarah Cannon Research Institute. *J Clin Oncol.* 2013;31:217–223.
9. Moran S, Martinez-Cardus A, Sayols S, et al. Epigenetic profiling to classify cancer of unknown primary: a multicentre, retrospective analysis. *Lancet Oncol.* 2016;17:1386–1385.
10. Oien KA, Dennis JL. Diagnostic work-up of carcinoma of unknown primary: from immunohistochemistry to molecular profiling. *Ann. Oncol.* 2012;23:271–277.
11. Pentheroudakis G, Golfinopoulos V, Pavlidis N. Switching benchmarks in cancer of unknown primary from autopsy to microarray. *Eur J Cancer.* 2007;43:2026–2036.
12. Varadhachary GR, Karanth S, Qiao W, et al. Carcinoma of unknown primary with gastrointestinal profile: immunohistochemistry and survival data for this favorable subset. *Int J Clin Oncol.* 2014;19:479–484.
13. Varadhachary GR, Raber MN. Carcinoma of unknown primary site. *N Engl J Med.* 2014;371:757–765.
14. Yoon HH, Foster NR, Meyers JP, et al. Gene expression profiling identifies responsive patients with cancer of unknown primary treated with carboplatin, paclitaxel, and everolimus: NCCTG No871(alliance). *Ann Oncol.* 2016;27:339–344.

32 Central Nervous System Tumors

Emanuela Molinari and Mark R. Gilbert

INTRODUCTION

Tumor of the central nervous system (CNS) can be divided into primary, arising directly in the brain or spinal cord, or secondary, due to metastatic disease. This chapter will discuss both with emphasis on the former to provide a schematic and practical approach to their classification and management. Emphasis has been placed on the new classification of CNS tumors, which combine molecular and histologic features, as this is the way forward in neuro-oncology and it has significant implications in clinical management and clinical decisions.

Brain tumors account for approximately 88% of all primary CNS tumors, and concerns regarding the increasing incidence of brain tumors have been reported over the past three decades, likely due to the increase in life expectancy and increase in brain tumor identification with widespread use of CT and MR imaging. Additionally, this increase in incidence of brain tumor subtypes may partially be attributable to the recent shift in diagnostic categories, thus reflecting changes in diagnostic practice and criteria. Although recent advances in diagnostic and treatment approaches have improved the management, improvement in outcomes for patients with brain tumors has been modest and the survival rate continues to remain poor.

Most brain tumors are sporadic. However, about 5% of primary brain tumors have known hereditary factors, as neurofibromatosis type I and II, tuberous sclerosis, von Hippel-Lindau disease, Turcot's disease, familial polyposis, and Li-Fraumeni syndrome.

Brain tumors are often morphologically heterogeneous and many of them do progress over time, becoming more malignant due to the accumulation of genetic alterations, resulting in changes in the tumor biology. Although the initial differential diagnosis can be postulated by a combination of radiological findings, location and patient's age, and occasionally initial behavior of the lesion, the definite diagnosis of CNS tumors requires tissue sampling and is based on an integrated classification combining phenotypic and genotypic characteristics. Although the precision of diagnosis has markedly improved with the integration of histology and genetic markers, further research is needed to establish prognostic and predictive biomarkers thereby guiding individualized treatment and positively affecting the mortality and morbidity outcome of patients.

Metastatic brain tumors are more frequent than primary brain tumors and their incidence is rising due to a combination of factors including advanced screening programs, improved treatments, and consequent increased survival after initial cancer diagnosis, allowing the spread of cancer to the brain to occur as a late complication. It has been estimated that up to one-fourth of patients with a diagnosis of cancer have brain metastases before death with primary sources to be more frequently lung, breast, skin, kidney, and gastrointestinal tract.

Molecular Diagnosis of Primary Brain and CNS Tumors

In 2016 the World Health Organization (WHO) formulated a major reconstruction of CNS tumor diagnoses by combining histological features and molecular parameters. This dynamic pathogenetic classification improves diagnosis by grouping tumors that share similar prognostic markers, and increasingly guides patient management by enabling the use of therapies for entities with similar biological and genetic characteristics. The grading system (WHO) that determines the level of aggressiveness of each type of tumor has been maintained based on histological features with additional criteria for atypical meningioma that includes brain invasion. The malignancy grade divides tumors from 1 to 4, respectively, from less to more aggressive. The grade of malignancy is determined by the area of the most malignant features based on criteria of cellular atypia, mitotic activity, degree of cellularity, degree of necrosis, and/or microvascular proliferation. Low-grade tumors such as the pilocytic astrocytoma, designated as grade 1, are biologically distinct from the grade 2 to 4 as they typically are well circumscribed, rarely undergo malignant transformation and may be cured with surgical resection. Therefore, there are important differences between grade 1 and grade 2 gliomas, the latter are typically not curable with resection and can undergo malignant transformation to grade 3 or 4.

Clinical Diagnosis and Considerations

Brain tumors cause symptoms and signs through a combination of mechanisms. Clinical manifestations depend on location, size, and rapidity of growth. Direct effects of the tumor are related to invasion and compression of the tumor on the brain parenchyma. Secondary effects are mostly related to vasogenic edema. Symptoms may be focal, reflecting the location of the tumor (e.g., hemiparesis); generalized, which are nonlocalizing (e.g., headache); or false localizing, which are caused by raised intracranial pressure (e.g., tinnitus) (see Table 32.1). The most common symptoms are headache, which is usually nonspecific, seizures, mental status changes and behavioral changes, and unilateral weakness (paresis). Between 30% and 90% of patients with brain tumors experience seizures either at presentation or at some time during the disease trajectory, often with progression. Secondary epilepsy is always focal in origin although seizures can secondarily generalize; this is more common in primary tumors than metastases, and is more often associated with slow growing/low grade tumors. The most common signs are paresis, normal examination, and memory impairment. Quite commonly there could be involvement of cranial nerves, optic discs, and visual fields. In children, most frequently symptoms and signs are related to increased intracranial pressure, often associated with ataxia.

The time between the onset of symptoms and diagnosis varies and there seems to be a degree of inverse association between apparent delay in diagnosis and poorer outcome. This may be explained by the less specific symptomatology that slower growing tumors are more likely to have in comparison with more severe and localizing symptoms earlier in the disease course of more aggressive tumors.

Acute Complications

The brain and CSF are compressible components contained within a nonexpandable space due to rigid skull in adults. Mass occupying brain tumors cause displacement of the brain from one cranial compartment to another, following the path of least resistance. The most important clinical consequences are increased intracranial pressure and herniation syndromes, which are reflected by a depressed level of consciousness. Five common herniation syndromes can occur, either alone or in combination: subfalcine modification (cingulate), uncal (transtentorial), central, upward and downward cerebellar (tonsillar) herniation (Figure 32.1).

TABLE 32.1 Brain Tumor: Symptoms and Signs

Localizing	seizures, hemiparesis, diplopia, aphasia, vertigo, incoordination, sensory abnormalities and dysphagia
Generalized	headache, nausea, vomiting, dizziness, mental status changes, visual obscurations and seizures
False-localizing	tinnitus, diplopia, hearing and visual loss

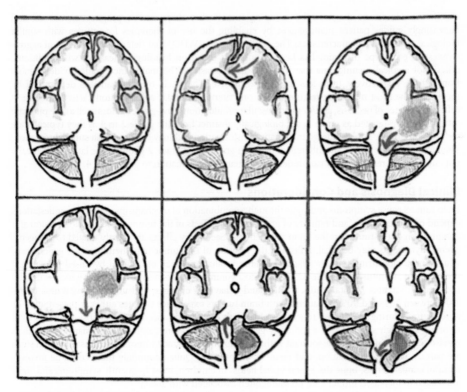

FIGURE 32.1 Herniation syndromes.

Legenda: top row, from left to right: normal brain, subfalcine herniation, uncal herniation. Bottom row, from left to right: central herniation, upward cerebellar, downward cerebellar

(edited from a figure courtesy of Heidi Maj)

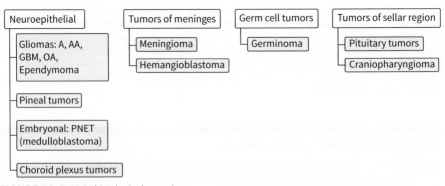

FIGURE 32.2 Main histological grouping.

Legenda: a= astrocytoma, aa= anaplastic astrocytoma, gbm= glioblastoma, oa=oligodendroglioma, pnet= primitive neuroectodermal tumors

TREATMENT CONSIDERATIONS

Therapeutic regimens typically encompass multiple treatment modalities. As previously described, patient prognosis remains poor; therefore, treatment should balance the quality of life of patients with the goal of prolonging survival. Experience from long-term follow-up has documented the early and late impact of the disease and treatment on both symptom burden and on the patient's quality of life (QoL).

Surgery

Surgery is the initial component of the management of CNS tumors. Although occasionally resection can be curative in grade 1 tumors, for higher grade tumors it frequently does not achieve complete tumor removal due to the infiltrative nature of the disease. Surgery is usually aimed at maximal safe debulking of the tumor burden, where the limit is often set by the vicinity of eloquent brain areas and the related surgical risk of neurologic deficits. Surgery helps in the management of acute symptoms, relieving deficits caused by mass effect, and maximizing the benefits of other therapies by providing less tumor burden to be treated and potentially reducing toxicity risks from increased intracranial pressure and improving seizure control in selected patients. In addition to direct damage to the surrounding normal brain tissue, surgery does carry other risks, such as infection and wound breakdown. Stereotactic biopsy is a minimally invasive procedure for diagnostic purposes with very limited morbidity and mortality estimated to be 4% and 0.9%, respectively. However, biopsy may not provide a diagnosis in up to 5% of cases and limited diagnostic accuracy due to the limited sampling. In one study, the diagnosis was changed in 38% of cases when tumor tissue from biopsy was compared to tumor obtained by surgical resection. This discrepancy in pathological diagnosis has significant repercussions in clinical practice, affecting treatment decisions and outcome.

Radiation Toxicity

The tolerance of normal brain parenchyma to radiation treatment is based on the total dose, the dose per fraction, and the volume of brain treated. Neurotoxicity due to radiation therapy (RT) can be acute, subacute, or delayed and late onset. Acute toxicity occurs during or soon after the treatment. It is thought to be due to edema and demyelination causing a clinical syndrome most commonly manifest as excessive somnolence and encephalopathy, and is usually self-limited. Subacute or delayed toxicity manifest up to 3 to 6 months after the completion of radiation but is most commonly seen with the first imaging study after completing radiation treatment, and has been termed pseudo-progression (see below). Late effects may occur month to years after the treatment and are often referred to as radiation necrosis (see below). These chronic complications are thought to be due to damage to the normal cellular component of brain parenchyma and alterations in the function and integrity of the cerebral vasculature. There are a wide range of clinical manifestations, including seizures and cognitive loss potentially leading to dementia. In children with an incompletely developed nervous system, radiation treatment can impair growth and development. A unique delayed radiation toxicity has recently been described as stroke-like migraine attacks after radiation therapy (SMART) syndrome. The disorder is characterized by complex migraine attacks associated with focal neurological deficits, and is associated with marked alterations in imaging that can be misinterpreted as tumor progression. Exposure to ionizing radiation can also increase the rate of other tumor occurrence, as meningiomas, and vascular abnormal formation typically cavernomas.

Chemotherapy Toxicity

Chemotherapy agents used for brain tumor treatment are typically administered systemically either by oral or intravenous routes. Therefore, typical systemic toxicities occur but in addition, patients with CNS cancers are at increased risk of neurologic effects, likely the consequence of disease and treatment-induced brain injury. Seizures, neurocognitive impairment, and worsening of focal neurologic function can follow both systemic as well as locally delivered treatment. For example, chemotherapy-induced cognitive changes may represent the effect of DNA damage, telomere shortening, cytokine deregulation, genetic predisposition to increased chemotherapy vulnerability, as well as potentiating effects on cognitive decline from other concomitant treatments.

Targeted Treatments

Treatments targeting molecular signaling pathways that are essential to tumor growth, such as angiogenesis and growth factors, may also impact neurologic function as well as impair the ability of the brain to repair after injury therefore impacting functional recovery. Most of the long-term side effects of the new treatments are unknown; therefore, it is crucial to systematically assess outcomes aimed to establish the impact of treatments on neurological functions both in the short and long term.

FOLLOW-UP AND MONITORING CHALLENGES

The evaluation and assessment of patients with brain tumors to determine treatment response, progression, and treatment side effects can be very challenging. The notion of treatment-induced changes in imaging characteristics complicate the interpretation of imaging studies. For example, treatment-induced inflammatory changes, often called pseudo-progression, will appear as a contrast enhancing mass with extensive edema. Conversely, some treatments, particularly anti-angiogenic therapies will decrease diffusion of contrast material leading to an improved imaging study but not necessarily indicating a decrease in tumor burden and has been termed pseudoresponse. Radiation can also cause damage to the brain tissue, in particular, the white matter, leading to change in appearances even years after treatment. This damage, referred to as radiation necrosis, can continue to increase further mimicking tumor progression, thus increasing the challenges of disease evaluation for the clinician.

- Postsurgery: MRI should be performed within 48 hours and not later than 72 hours to better detect residual tumor and minimizing postoperative changes that may mimic residual tumor.

During or soon after radiation treatment: Increases in MRI contrast enhancement can be induced by a variety of processes, such as treatment-related inflammation, postsurgical changes and ischemia, radiation necrosis, and subacute radiation effects. In the first three months (although this may occur later) after radiation treatment (particularly when combined with chemotherapy), pseudoprogression is a recognized event. This pseudoprogression can be seen in up to 25% of patients. Patients with MGMT-methylated tumors are thought to be in higher risks for pseudoprogression. Although the pathogenesis is not known, it is thought to reflect a transient and local reaction characterized by inflammatory response, demyelination and abnormal vessel permeability, due to increased sensitivity to radiation of oligodendrocytes and endothelial cells

The neuroimaging of pseudoprogression is characterized by increased enhancement on MRI caused by abnormal vessel permeability (breakdown of the blood–brain barrier (BBB)) and increased T2 and fluid-attenuated inversion recovery (FLAIR) weighted signal due to edema, and usually, but not always, the absence of increased perfusion. Certain imaging characteristics patterns are also more suggestive for pesudoprogression, as linear pattern of enhancement and periventricular white matter changes, but these findings can also be seen with tumor growth. In most patients, the increase in radiologic abnormalities is clinically asymptomatic. When symptomatic, it usually reflects general cognitive functioning or pre-existing symptoms. As it is partly due to transient demyelination, it may benefit from corticosteroids that decrease the inflammatory response and the BBB leakage.

Later in the disease trajectory, radiation necrosis is a known complication. It is a late delayed reaction, and usually occurs 18 to 24 months after radiation but as early as two months and up to 5 years. The incidence reports vary but has been reported to occur in 3% to 24% of brain tumors. The pathophysiology is thought to be the consequence of vascular change, edema and fibrinoid exudate. On imaging studies, radiation necrosis appears as space-occupying lesion with mass effect therefore very difficult to be distinguished from tumor recurrence. It often affects the area of maximum radiation dose and periventricular white matter appearing with an enhancing "soap bubble" appearance. Metabolic studies may be difficult to interpret due to inflammatory activity and MR spectroscopy may help in differentiating from tumor recurrence by showing increased Lactate/Creatine, decreased Choline/Creatine, and lack of the 2-hydroxyglutarate (2HG) in IDH-mutated tumors, although the sensitivity and specificity of MR spectroscopy remain too low to use this methodology as the exclusive means of differentiating tumor from necrosis.

Radiation necrosis can cause symptoms and decline in neurological function. In clinically symptomatic patients, management options include surgery that will confirm the underlying diagnosis and

TABLE 32.2 Main Groupings of 2016 WHO Classification of Glial CNS Tumors

Glial neoplasms	Main subtypes	Molecular profile	Grade
Diffuse Astrocytic and Oligodendroglial tumors	Diffuse Astrocytoma	IDH mutant	I
	Anaplastic Astrocytoma	IDH mutant	III
	Glioblastoma	IDH mutant and wild-type	IV
	Oligodendroglioma	IDH mutant	II
	Anaplastic Oligodendroglioma	1p/19q codeleted	III
	Diffuse midline glioma, H3 K27 mutant	IDH mutant 1p/19q codeleted H3K27M-mutated	IV
Other Astrocytic tumors	Pilocytic Astrocytoma	BRAF V600E mutationBRAF fusion	I
	Pleomorphic Astrocytoma (PXA)	BRAF V600E mutation	II
	Subependymal Giant cell Astrocytoma (SEGA)	TSC 1/ 2 mutation	I
Ependymal Tumors	Subepensymoma, maxillopapillary, ependymoma, ependymoma RELA fusion positive, anaplastic*	Allelic loss 22q NF2 mutation Combination of DNA methylation and genomic alterations for spine, infratentorial and supratentotial (CIMP, RELA; YAP)	I-III

* molecular and histopathology details of 9 ependymoma subgroups go beyond the scope of the chapter but the reader is suggested to refer to the 2016 WHO classification for details

resolve the mass-related complications and symptoms. Further options include addition of anti-VEGF treatment to reverse the effect of increased VEGF expression in the white matter following radiation therapy (RT) that correlates with BBB breakdown and brain edema. This treatment has been proven in a randomized, placebo-controlled clinical trial. A variety of other treatments have been tried, but most reports are anecdotal. These include hyperbaric oxygen therapy, oral vitamin E administration, and laser interstitial thermal therapy.

Conversely, pseudoresponse is a phenomenon that describes imaging changes of signal reduction that are possibly due to "normalization" of the BBB and are often associated with treatments as anti-VEGF therapies.

PRIMARY BRAIN AND CNS TUMORS

There are more than 130 types of primary brain and CNS tumors. The section will focus on the most common and those of particular scientific interest. Despite classification based on the appearance of the tumor cells, the cellular origin for most brain tumors is unknown and there are no recognized precursor lesions that define a premalignant status. Primary brain tumors are grouped accordingly to their histological appearances that most closely resemble normal CNS cell constituents. Neuroepithelial cells are thought to give rise to gliomas, pineal tumors, and embryonal tumors such as medulloblastoma), meninges, choroid plexus, germ cells, and sellar origin (including pituitary tumors and craniopharyngiomas) (Figure 32.2). Brain tumors are thought to arise from neural stem, progenitors cells, or de-differentiated mature neural cells that undergo malignant transformation. Glial tumors account for approximately two thirds of all intracranial tumors with age-related incidence by defined molecular and histological subtypes. Childhood tumors have different incidence, different localization preference (i.e., posterior fossa with main involvement of the cerebellum) and different molecular profiles; therefore, pediatric CNS cancers warrant consideration of the impact of age and site of origin as well as outcomes and treatment approaches.

Epidemiology

- Primary CNS tumors are relatively rare, accounting for 1.8% of all cancers
- US incidence rate for brain and CNS tumors in adults (>20 years old) is 22.36 cases per 100,000, and 5.47 cases per 100,000 in the pediatric population
- The population subgroups at higher risk for brain cancer are elderly, Caucasians, men and those living in metropolitan counties
- Incidence rate follows a bimodal distribution, with a small peak in early childhood and more pronounced peak in late middle age
- The higher incidence for older individuals suggests a possible role for bioaccumulation from environmental toxic exposure
- Established environmental causal factors for brain tumors are ionizing radiation and possibly prolonged exposure to hydrocarbons. Exogenous hormone use among women is an established risk factors for meningioma.
- Possible protective factors for glioma risk are allergy-related immune responses, elevated IgE, and previous history of chickenpox and/or positive VZV IgG
- According to the Central Brain Tumor Registry of the United States, 16,947 deaths are estimated to be attributed to primary malignant brain and other CNS tumors in the United States in 2017
- Five-year survival rates after diagnosis of primary brain tumor progressively decrease with age
- Meningiomas make up 36.4% of all primary brain tumors
- One third of tumors are malignant, with the most frequent being glioblastoma (WHO Grade 4)
- CNS tumor are the second largest category of cancer in the pediatric population, with more frequent localization in the posterior fossa for age between 4 and 10 years old
- Embryonal or primitive neuroectodermal tumors (PNET) as well as astrocytic lineage tumors are the most frequent before the age of 20
- In childhood, there is dichotomy distribution for site (infratentorial and supratentorial) as well as predominance of low-grade tumor with age-group peaks at 5 to 9 years and 15 to 19 years, while high-grade tumors often presents before the age of five and their incidence decrease with age.

Gliomas

Gliomas encompass a heterogeneous group of tumors that affect patients of different ages with often substantial differences in molecular profiles and behavior. Most gliomas in adults diffusely infiltrate the adjacent brain tissue and therefore are often referred as "diffuse gliomas" that encompass grade 2 to 4. Per the 2016 WHO classification, there are three main groups of glial neoplasms, categorized as diffuse astrocytic and oligodendroglial tumors, other astrocytic tumors and ependymal tumors (Table 32.2).

Diagnostic Approach and Clinico-genetic Considerations

Genomic alterations driving gliomagenesis pathways have been analyzed. For example, isocitrate dehydrogenase 1 or 2 mutation (IDH1 or IDH2 mutation) have been established as a common initiating event of carcinogenesis in lower-grade gliomas. Progression to more aggressive tumors is associated with additional genetic changes and more complex chromosomal and genetic alterations (Table 32.3).

Specific molecular signatures are now recognized as of crucial biological importance and underpin a new diagnostic approach with significant clinical repercussions and practical relevance in patient's management (Table 32.4). The major distinction for adult gliomas is based on IDH1 or IDH2 mutations compared with "wild-type" IDH status, which characterizes their distinctive biology and clinical behavior, with better outcomes with IDH mutant gliomas in comparison with IDH wild-type. IDH mutations are associated with specific pattern of methylation and DNA hypermethylation profile. Gliomas with IDH mutations, including glioblastomas, have a better prognosis. For lower grade gliomas (LGG), IDH mutated tumors with loss of one copy of chromosome arms 1p and 19q (1p/19q codeletion), are associated with longer median overall survival. The related strong practical clinical impact of such knowledge comes clear, for example, when identifying IDH-mutated gliomas with G-CIMP low profile. Conversely, the absence of IDH mutation (IDH wild-type) in low-grade tumors marks poor GBM-like prognosis. However, there is a very small subgroup of low-grade tumors (6%)

TABLE 32.3 Schematic Grading of Glioma by Combined Molecular Profile Subtype

No precursor	Diffuse gliomfas			Focal glioma
	IDH mutant		IDH wild-type	BRAF
EGFR amplification PTEN mutation LOH 10q	1p/19q codeletion	1p/19 q intact TP53 mutation ATRX loss	EGFR PTEN CKDN2A	
	OLIGODENDROGLIOMA WHO II-III	ATROCYTOMA WHO II-IV	ASTROCYTOMA WHO II-IV	PILOCYTIC ASTROCITOMA WHO GR I
		Additional alterations Often LOH 10q, DCC loss expression		
PRIMARY GBM MGMT methylation status Dismal prognosis Better with MGMT methylation (less frequent)	Good prognosis	SECONDARY GBM MGMT methylation status Intermediate prognosis Better with MGMT methylation (more frequent)	Poor prognosis	Excellent prognosis

TABLE 32.4 Practical Approach to Glioma Subgroups in the Adult Population: Clinical and Molecular Correlations

Primary brain tumor type		GLIOMAS						
Molecular subtype		IDH mutant			IDH wild type			
		Codel 1p/19q	G-CIMP high	G-CIMP low	Classic-like	Mesenchymal-like	LGm6-GBM	PA-like
Main molecular biomarkers	ainTERT up	√			√	√		
	ATRX loss		√	√				
	TP53 mut		√	√				
	EGFR amp				√	√		√
	Chr7gain/chr10del				√	√		
	Chr19amp/chr20 amp				√			
	CDK4 amp			√				√
	CDKN2A del			√				√
	BRAF mut							√
	NF1 mut							√

TABLE 32.4 (Continued)

		OD	A	GBM	GBM	GBM	GBM	A/OD
Main represented histopathology								
Clinical features	**Peak age yr**	30-50	30	30	60	60	60	30
	Main grade	2-3	2-3	3-4	4	4	4	2-3
	Survival prognosis	Favorable	Intermediate	Poor	Worse	Worse	Worse	Favorable

Adapted from Ceccarelli et al., 2016, Cell 164, 500-563

that do not harbor an IDH mutation but have some characteristics of pilocytic astrocytoma (BRAF mutation) that have a very low mortality rate.

New Classification: Histopathological and Genetic Considerations

The 2016 WHO classification defines both grades 2 and 3 oligodendroglioma by requiring the demonstration of IDH mutation and 1p/19q codeletion. The new classification also sees the delegation of oligoastrocytoma diagnosis to a rare finding of both 1p/19q codeletion and the combination of p53 mutation and ATRX loss. To date, there are only few biomarkers with diagnostic and risk stratification implications and predictive information that guide therapeutic decisions. In particular

- O⁶-methylguanine-DNA-methyltransferase (MGMT) promoter methylation
- 1p/19q codeletion
- IDH mutation
- BRAF duplication/fusion

Diffuse gliomas in adult and pediatric patients, although with similar histopathologic appearance, are molecularly distinct. Pediatric gliomas rarely have IDH mutations or 1p/19q codeletions. Instead, BRAF and H3K27M mutations are more common, particularly for low grade and midline tumors, respectively. These findings suggest a different pathogenesis and biology for pediatric brain tumors, mandating different treatment considerations, approaches, and eventually different outcomes.

Imaging: Advanced Techniques and Genetic Implications

Neuroimaging is used for diagnostic purposes and to monitor the effect of treatment of brain tumors. Brain computed tomography (CT) and magnetic resonance imaging (MRI), as well as structural and functional techniques, provide information regarding differential diagnoses (abscess, demyelinating plaques, stroke), features helpful in the grading of the tumor, evaluation and treatment planning, and monitoring of treatment response, disease progression and side effects of treatment (radiation necrosis and pseudoprogression). Advanced neuroimaging is increasingly being used to correlate findings with the genetic profile of the tumor, but this remains investigational.

Important aspects of imaging studies include

- CT imaging has a role in the detection of hemorrhage (e.g. postoperative), herniation, hydrocephalus.
- CT imaging is valuable to detect calcifications within the mass, suggesting brain tumor types as oligodendrogliomas or meningiomas.
- Contrast enhancement correlates with local breakdown of the blood brain barrier and is a key feature of high-grade tumor although there are some exceptions, including some low-grade tumor such as pilocytic astrocytomas in children that do enhance.
- T2/FLAIR signal abnormalities around the mass lesion correlates with peri-tumoral edema.
- Oligodendroglial tumors typically have a heterogeneous image by contrast-enhanced MRI.
- MRI spectroscopy is often used to help differentiate tumor from inflammation or radiation-induced injury, although the sensitivity and specificity are limited
  - MRI spectroscopy is not specific, detecting peaks of N-acetylaspartate (NAA) decrement because of processes that destroy or replace normal neurons and increased peak of Choline that correlates with increased cell turnover and can be seen with other processes such as demyelinating diseases.
  - MRI spectroscopy provides a diagnostic biomarker; detecting accumulation of 2-hydroxyglutarate (2HG) within the tumor as this is associated with IDH-mutated glioma.
- Perfusion MRI can help differentiating treatment-related changes from tumor recurrence, and can help plan tumor sampling when contemplating a biopsy.
- MRI with diffusion weighted imaging (DWI) can help distinguish a primary CNS lymphoma; an important consideration to avoid profound tumor reduction with corticosteroids leading to a nondiagnostic neurosurgical procedure.

Gliomas (MG)

Malignant gliomas (MG) account for more than 75% of newly diagnosed malignant primary brain tumors and carry a disproportionately high rate of morbidity and mortality despite treatment advances. Glioblastoma (GBM), grade 4 by WHO criteria, is the most aggressive tumor subtype and accounts for more than half MG. Anaplastic astrocytoma (AA), WHO grade 3, typically affects a younger adult population and although the prognosis is better than grade 4 tumors, it remains a highly malignant neoplasm. The only established risk factors for MG are exposure to ionizing radiation and rare familial syndromes, such as Lynch syndrome and Li-Fraumeni syndrome. Approximately 5% of patients with MG have a family history of gliomas. Clinically, patients may present with a combination of generalized and localizing symptoms and signs. Patients often complain of headache that does not have specific features, resembling tension-type headache, usually worse in the morning, and presentation with seizure onset is common. Imaging studies, most commonly MRI, reveals an irregular, enhancing mass with associated edema and mass effect. Metabolic imaging using fluorodeoxyglucose positron emission tomography (FDG PET) reveals increased glucose uptake, evidence of hypermetabolism. Evaluation of blood flow and tumor blood volume using either MRI with perfusion sequences or single-photon emission computed tomography (SPECT) demonstrates an increase compared to the contralateral uninvolved brain parenchyma.

Patients with MG present with a variety of neurological complications. These include the following:

- Seizures. These are typically focal with secondary generalization. Treatment is required and preferably utilizing the newer antiepileptic drugs (e.g., levetiracetam, lamotrigine, gabapentin) that do not affect the hepatic cytochrome P450 system, thereby avoiding altering the metabolism and clearance of many systemic cancer treatments.
- Nonlocalized signs such as confusion and mental status alteration. These are often due to peritumoral edema and increased intracranial pressure, although seizures may precipitate similar findings. Treatment is typically with corticosteroids, although in some situations, hyperosmotic agents such as mannitol or emergency tumor debulking may be required.
- Localized signs such as hemiparesis, language dysfunction, and visual field loss. The neurologic dysfunction is typically directly related to the location of the tumor. For example, involvement of the dominant cerebral hemisphere, particularly the posterior frontal lobe and temporal lobe may cause

aphasia, whereas involvement of the occipital lobe may result in contralateral hemianopia (visual field loss).

Standard treatment for newly diagnosed MG is maximal surgical resection, despite the infiltrative nature of gliomas. Advantages are as follows:

- Defining diagnosis that helps prognostication and drives further treatment options.
- Improvement of symptoms resulting from mass effect.
- Studies have demonstrated that the extent of resection correlates with outcome. This is particularly important for medulloblastoma and ependymoma.

Specific considerations for glioblastoma and anaplastic gliomas follow.

GLIOBLASTOMA (GBM)

- The median age is 54 years, although GBM can occur at any age. In adults, most current series have reported a median survival of 12 to 18 months even with standard of care treatment.
- Glioblastomas may occur de novo, also known as primary or after transformation from a lower-grade glioma. This latter category, called a secondary glioblastoma and which accounts for approximately 10% of all glioblastoma, is characterized by mutation in either the IDH 1 or 2 gene. These patients have a better prognosis than patients harboring the primary GBM.

Molecular Pathogenesis

- Primary GBM, defined arising as a de novo glioblastoma, presents with a genetic profile of IDH wild-type. Their characteristic molecular genetic profile includes epidermal growth factor receptor (EGFR) amplifications and mutations, LOH 10q (2/3 of cases), PTEN mutation (1/3 of cases), and p16 deletions.
- Secondary GBM, defined as the result of transformation from a lower-grade glioma, presents with IDH1 mutation, TP53 mutations, platelet-derived growth factor (PDGFR) overexpression, LOH 10q.
- MGMT methylation state is an epigenetic modification present in 35% to 75% of GBMs that ultimately determines less effective DNA repair and therefore increased chemotherapy sensitivity to alkylating agents such as temozolomide. Additionally, some studies suggest that tumors with MGMT methylation may be more prone to develop "pseudoprogression" after treatment with radiation and chemotherapy.

Imaging

- GBM characteristically enhance after contrast administration on both MRI and CT, often have a central necrotic cavity, and more peritumoral edema, and are more likely to cross the corpus callosum.

Treatment

Standard of care since 2005 EORTC-NCIC study for newly diagnosed GBM following resection is radiotherapy (RT 60Gy) with concomitant and adjuvant temozolomide (75 mg/m^2/d followed by 6 monthly cycles of 150 to 200 mg/m^2/d for 5 days per cycle. A recent study in elderly patients (age 65 and older) with GBM compared a short course of RT (40 Gy in 15 fractions) with this radiation schedule and concurrent temozolomide; demonstrating an improvement in survival with the combined treatment.

Although concurrent radiation and temozolomide chemotherapy followed by maintenance temozolomide improves survival, tumor recurrence is inevitable. A variety of second-line therapies are used, although none have clearly demonstrated a survival benefit. They include:

- Implantation of carmustine-containing wafers.
- Cytotoxic chemotherapy agents such as lomustine, procarbazine, irinotecan, carboplatin.
- Bevacizumab, a monoclonal antibody against circulating VEGF, has reported response rates in the 30% to 50% range and prolongation of progression-free survival (PFS) in recurrent disease but a recent phase III study did not show a survival benefit.
- Targeted molecular therapies against regulatory signaling pathways, such as EGFR, PDGF, and mammalian target of rapamycin (mTOR) have been tested; however, none have demonstrated clinical efficacy.
- Immunotherapies are under evaluation for glioblastoma. These treatments include checkpoint inhibitors, peptide and dendritic cell vaccines, and tumor injections with oncolytic virus.

Prognosis

- Established prognostic factors for GBM include patient age, performance status, extent of tumor resection, and tumor MGMT methylation status.
- Median survival with standard treatment in GBMs is 15 to 18 months with a 2-year survival of 26.5% to 35%.
- Prognosis is improved for patients with MGMT-methylated GBM that have median survival of 21 to 23 months and 2-year survival rate of 40% to 50%.
- Up to 10% of patients with GMBs may live 5 years or longer.
- Children with high-grade tumors (grade 3 to 4) tend to do better than adults, with 5-year survival of 25%.
- Diffuse midline gliomas, H3-K27M-mutant is a new recognized entity in 2016 WHO classification that distinguish pediatric GBM from adult GBM that look alike histologically but have a different molecular profile and unfavorable outcome.

Anaplastic Astrocytoma

- Anaplastic astrocytoma (AA) affect younger people than GBM with median age of 45 years old. The definition of the median survival is evolving. Patients with AA harboring an IDH mutation have a median survival of 8 to 10 years, whereas those without an IDH mutation have a median survival of 2 to 3 years with current treatments.
- The optimal treatment of AA remains controversial. There is increasing consensus that grade 3 tumors (anaplastic gliomas, AG) that do not have an IDH mutation are pre-GBM and should be treated with chemoradiation following the standard therapy for GBM. AG that are IDH mutated have a much better prognosis and it is unclear whether concurrent radiation and chemotherapy is optimal as this treatment is associated with greater risk of brain injury. Early results from the CATNON study demonstrated that radiation plus postradiation temozolomide was superior to radiation alone in anaplastic glioma without 1p/19q codeletion. The benefit of combined radiation and chemotherapy has not yet been determined. This issue is even more complicated in AG with IDH mutation and 1p/19q codeletion, now defined as anaplastic oligodendroglioma and discussed below.

Anaplastic Oligodendroglioma (AO)

- Oligodendroglial tumors represent 5% to 20% of all glial tumors, with typical age peak at 40 to 60 years and anaplastic tumors preferring older age of onset. Survival time is prolonged and striking differences in oligodendroglial tumors subgroups point to completely different biologic entities and stress the importance of genetic profiling to individualize treatment.
- AOs are more sensitive to chemotherapy than astrocytic tumors. Molecular subtype and patient characteristics provide the basis for patient management ramification following surgery and RT. Indeed, chemosensitivity relates to 1p/19q status, the response rate report to be almost 100% response rate in 1p 19q codeleted tumors.
- The management of patients with recurrent disease despite treatment is unclear, but patients failing an agent do still present some response rate for another chemotherapy regime or second-line treatment.

Low Grade Gliomas (LGG)

Low grade gliomas (LGG) encompass a heterogeneous group of tumors with astrocytic or oligodendroglial features that usually affects younger patient population and have longer survival. Because the prognosis is better, the long-term consequences of treatment are a critical aspect of determining optimal therapy.

Clinical presentation:

- Seizures are the presenting sign in over 50% cases, and more than 80% of patients have a seizure during the disease trajectory. Seizures often originate from the brain tissue adjacent to the brain tumor and some locations as the motor strip correlate with resistance to antiepileptic drugs (AEDs). Radiotherapy, chemotherapy, and tumor resection may improve seizure control.
- Other presenting symptoms include gradual loss of motor, sensory, language function or visual field loss, depending upon tumor location.

Grade 1 (Pilocytic Astrocytoma)

Although the designation of low grade astrocytomas encompass both grade 1 (pilocytic astrocytomas) and grade 2 diffuse astrocytomas, they are biologically very different and must be considered separately. Most pilocytic astrocytomas develop before the age of 20 with peak of age around the end of the first decade, and often occur as midline posterior fossa lesion involving the cerebellum, although could manifest in the optic-hypothalamic region and in the brainstem as dorsally exophytic lesions. Surgery is the primary treatment and can be curative. Characteristically, these tumors

- Are cystic and well demarcated.
- Almost always enhance on MRI with brightly enhancing mural nodule appearance.
- Complete surgical excision is typically curative accounting for the excellent prognosis with a 10-year survival rate of 95%.
- Malignant transformation is uncommon, but may be associated with radiation treatment.

Grade 2 (Diffuse Low-Grade Astrocytomas)

Diffuse low-grade astrocytomas are classified as WHO grade 2. These tumors are typically slow growing but local infiltration of surrounding brain parenchyma prevents cure with surgical resection alone. These tumors commonly occur in young-middle aged adults with median age at diagnosis at 35 to 45 years.

Molecular Pathogenesis

- Nearly all grade 2 gliomas have an IDH mutation; 1p19q co-deletion is diagnostic of a grade 2 oligodendroglioma whereas p53 and/or ATRX mutations define an astrocytic lineage.
- IDH wild-type has been reported, but increasingly this is associated with a misdiagnosis such as a pilocytic astrocytoma or other rare variants.

Imaging

- T2 hyperintense signal that follows the white matter distribution on MRI
- Typically, the tumor is nonenhancing MRI. When enhancement is seen, it may indicate that there has been malignant transformation to a higher grade.

Treatment

There are a wide variety of treatment options, ranging from observation to aggressive combined treatment.

Maximum safe tumor resection is often pursued as this has important diagnostic and prognostic impact. These tumors may harbor regions demonstrating more malignant cells, thereby altering the diagnosis, prognosis, and treatment. Additionally, there is increasing evidence that extent of resection impacts survival.

Increasingly, grade 2 astrocytomas are being treated with radiation therapy followed by chemotherapy with either temozolomide or the PCV combination regimen. The RTOG 9802 study compared radiation with radiation followed by PCV and demonstrated an almost doubling of survival with the combination regimen.

Prognosis

- Median survival of 8 to 10 years
- Potential to transform into higher grade, more aggressive tumors
- Size greater than 6 cm, crossing midline, presurgery neurological deficits, age >40 years at disease onset are poor prognostic factors

Oligodendrogliomas (O)

Low-grade oligodendrogliomas are three times more frequent than anaplastic tumors, accounting for 2% to 5% of primary brain tumors and up to 15% of all gliomas. They do occur more frequently in young adult males with a peak of incidence between 30 and 40 years, and although not common, may present with intracerebral hemorrhage due to thin-walled capillary network. They have better prognosis than astrocytomas as they are more chemosensitive.

Molecular Pathogenesis

- Oligodendrogliomas are defined by 1p/19q codeletion and IDH mutation
- Neither ATRX nor p53 are mutated

Imaging

- Occur more frequently commonly along the convexity in subcortical areas particularly in frontotemporal lobes
- Appear as partially calcified mass lesions, easily detected as hyperintense on CT imaging particularly along the cortical ribbon as a gyriform pattern
- On MRI demonstrate a high signal on T2 and T2/FLAIR sequences
- Contrast enhancement is not typical for grade 2 oligodendroglioma and suggests a higher-grade tumor
- Despite the grade 2 designation, leptomeningeal spread has been reported in 1% to 2% of cases

Treatment

Optimal treatment remains controversial, centered around when to perform a surgical procedure and when to initiate therapy after surgical resection. Gross total resection may provide prolongation of PFS but the impact on overall survival (OS) has not been proven. Patients with gross total resection who are under age 40 are often carefully monitored without additional treatment until progression. Patients over age 40 or with residual tumor after surgery are typically treated. Results from RTOG 9802 suggest that radiation followed by chemotherapy may be better than radiation alone. Grade 2 oligodendroglioma are chemotherapy sensitive, therefore early use of chemotherapy to delay radiation treatment has been used, but this has not been proven to be a comparable approach.

Prognosis

- Median survival of 15 years
- Presence of contrast enhancement on MRI reduces the median survival, likely as this finding indicates a higher-grade tumor.

Ependymomas

Ependymomas range from grade I tumors (subependymoma and myxopapillary ependymoma) to grade 3. They are frequent in children especially below the age of 3, representing 10% of all intracranial tumors in pediatric population, and although rare in adults they represent the most common adult tumor of the spinal cord.

- The commonest location is the fourth ventricle, especially in children
- There is positive association with neurofibromatosis type II
- On neuroimaging they have typically heterogeneous appearances in all modalities due to areas of necrosis, calcification, cystic change and hemorrhage
- Symptoms at presentation depends on tumor localization, with supratentorial ependymomas causing more frequently increased intracranial pressure symptoms, infratentorial location giving raise to cranioneuropathies, ataxia and hydrocephalus, and spinal ependymomas often manifesting with back/radicular pain.
- Incidence of spinal seeding, that is, subarachnoid dissemination along CSF pathways with metastases along the spine, ranges from 10% to 22% with higher rate from infratentorial tumors origin site and higher tumor grade.

Molecular Pathogenesis

The molecular classification stratifies patient risks better than histopathological grading and 2016 WHO classification describes nine molecular subgroups associated with specific age groups and risk stratification for both OS and PFS. This classification also incorporates a genetically defined variant characterized RELA fusion positive profile and accounting for the majority of supratentorial ependymomas in children with a worse prognosis than tumors not harboring the RELA fusion.

Treatment

Surgery is the standard treatment as a complete resection can be curative, particularly for grade 1 ependymomas.

Most of data relate to pediatric population. Current therapeutic strategy includes maximal safe surgical resection, followed by adjuvant radiotherapy with exception of selected cases of supratentorial tumors with no ventricular communication and undergoing gross total resection. Adjuvant chemotherapy has been pursued especially in young children in attempt to avoid or delay radiation therapy, but multiple clinical trials have failed to show a survival benefit.

In adults, surgery is the initial approach for low-grade ependymomas. This may be followed by radiation beam therapy depending on diagnostic findings, resection success, and determination of risk of recurrence. Clinical and neuroimaging monitoring including spine imaging are advised as follow up. In case of recurrence, radiotherapy has been utilized using photon or proton radiation, with focal or craniospinal approach depending on individual risks, previous treatment and response, and dissemination findings. There are few established chemotherapy regimens, although carboplatin, cisplatin, and temozolomide have reported responses. Recent combinations temozolomide with lapatinib and carboplatin with bevacizumab have shown activity in recent clinical trials.

Prognosis

- The 10-year OS is about 64% in pediatric patients, with older patients doing better than younger ones, and ranges from 70% to 89% in adult patients.
- Two molecular subgroups of ependymoma (posterior fossa EPN-A subgroup that is characterized by DNA hypermethylation and supratentorial RELA-fusion) have been associated with poor outcome with 10-year OS of 50% and PFS of 20%.
- Recurrence rate is variable, usually occurring between 18 and 45 months, and traditionally with local relapses.

Non Glial Tumors

Nonglial tumors of the brain are more commonly meningiomas and acoustic schwannomas, followed by embryonal tumors, pituitary tumors, primary CNS lymphoma as well as tumors of the pineal gland and choroid plexus tumors. Rare tumors are slightly more common in men than in women, occurring across age ranges depending on tumor types and being characterized by longer survival rates than glial tumors. Detailed discussion of rare tumors is beyond the scope of this chapter. The following section will focus on the most common and those of relevance for specific age group or population subgroup.

Meningiomas

Meningiomas are extra-axial tumors, that is, they belong to tumors that arise from structures and tissue adjacent to the brain, like meninges. They account for 33.8 % of all brain and CNS tumors and are the most common brain tumors diagnosed above the age of 34 years old. Although they are usually benign, they can be associated with significant morbidity. Female sex, age, inherited susceptibility in DNA repair genes, genetic condition as neurofibromatosis type II, breast cancer and ionizing radiation exposure are recognized factor risks. Other possible predisposing factors are hormones, increased body index, and immunological factors. Meningiomas are classified as benign (grade 1), atypical (grade 2), and anaplastic (grade 3). The 2016 WHO classification has defined brain invasion as criteria for the diagnosis of grade 2 atypical meningioma.

Molecular Pathogenesis

- Common feature in sporadic meningiomas is deletion and inactivation of NF2 on chromosome 22.
- Malignant meningiomas have more genomic instability with multiple chromosomal copy number alterations, including loss of 1p, 10q, and 14q, and less frequently 6q and 18q.
- Familial meningiomas usually have germline defect in NF2 and other predisposing mutations.

- Specific mutations have been recently defined in subsets of meningioma. These include SMO and AKT, representing potential therapeutic targets.
- Epigenetic aberration as DNA methylation events may be predominant in meningioma biology.

Diagnosis

They are usually benign and slow-growing tumors, with clinical insidious onset. Most often present with focal neurological signs, headache, visual field defects, and seizures (up to 50% of patients). In addition to symptoms caused by compression and increased intracranial pressure, parasagittal meningiomas can cause symptoms due to dural venous sinus obstruction. The most common locations in descending order are convexity, parasagittal, sphenoid, and middle cranial fossa.

Imaging

- Presence of broad dural base, dural tails, diffuse contrast enhancement, preservation of arachnoid plane
- Calcification of T2 signal iso or hypointensity may predict decreased growth potential
- X ray and CT can display hyperostosis or lytic lesions by direct invasion or primary intraosseous meningiomas
- Alanine peak, decreased N-acetylaspartate (NAA) and distinct peak of the chemical substance resonating at 3.8 ppm detected by MR spectroscopy are unique to meningiomas
- Cerebral angiography and MR venogram to assess patency of dural-based blood sinuses are useful in planning treatment timing and evaluation

Medical Management

Incidental finding of meningioma may only require observation until become symptomatic. In particular, observational management with no treatment intervention may be pertinent in asymptomatic tumors in elderly as they are exposed to increased morbidity risks from treatment. Careful evaluation and consideration should be given to women of child-bearing potential with meningiomas because it may lead to tumor growth as a consequence of excessive hormone production during pregnancy. In addition, conflicting data have been published regarding the link between meningioma and hormonal replacement therapy (HRT) use but larger studies seem to confirm this positive association raising questions on HRT use in women.

Treatment

- Treatment goal is complete surgical resection, as it has a main impact on preventing recurrence.
- Radiotherapy is typically performed for grade 3 meningiomas and incompletely resected grade 2 tumors. Radiation treatment for incompletely resected grade 1 and completely resected grade 2 meningiomas remains controversial.
- Chemotherapy is considered in recurrent meningiomas refractory to other treatment or when there are no other treatment options. Despite the presence of hormonal receptors, meningiomas are nonresponsive to hormonal therapy. Treatment regimens include α-interferon, somatostatin receptor agonists, and vascular endothelial growth factor (VEGF) signaling pathway inhibitors

Prognosis

- 95% of meningiomas are benign
- Deletion of 1p is associated with higher recurrence rate
- Recurrence rate varies from 5% to 20% within 10 years and increases with the length of follow-up
- Loss of 14q and loss of 9p with a specific CDKN2A impairment is associated with worse prognosis

Medulloblastomas

Medulloblastomas are the most common malignant brain tumor of childhood, accounting for up to 25% of all pediatric CNS tumors and 40% of pediatric posterior fossa tumors. Around 80% of patients present between the age of 1 and 10 years old. Most commonly they present as midline masses in the roof of the fourth ventricle. In the adult population, where they account for 0.4% to 1% of brain tumors, they present in the third or fourth decade in atypical location. Medulloblastomas are associated with a variety of genetic syndromes as Coffin-Siris, Cowden, Gardner, Gorlin, Li-Fraumeni, Turcot, and Rubinstein-Tyabi syndromes.

Molecular Pathogenesis

Medulloblastoma classification has undergone major reconstruction in the 2016 WHO revision. The combination of four histological groups and four genetic variants stratifies the prognostic risks and outcome of patients from low-risk tumors (WNT-activated) to high-risk tumors (SHH-activated/TP53 mutant, and non WNT/non-SHH).

- Up to 40% of medulloblastomas present abnormalities of chromosome 17
- P53 mutation has no prognostic implication on WNT subgroup while it does affect prognosis on SHH subgroup almost doubling 5-year OS in the p53 wild-type

Diagnosis

Half of the patients have a short symptomatic interval of 6 weeks prior to diagnosis and the main symptoms are linked to intracranial hypertension and hydrocephalus, with a combination of the most frequent symptoms and signs being papilledema, headache, recurrent vomiting, ataxia, nystagmus, and appendicular dysmetria. Risk stratification is based on localized disease at diagnosis and total or near-total resection for average risk group versus disseminated disease at diagnosis and/or partial resection for high risk group.

Imaging

Typically, CT and MRI reveal a contrast enhancing posterior fossa mass on the midline

- 94% of pediatric medulloblastomas localize in the cerebellum and three quarter in the vermis
- Adult medulloblastomas localize in the cerebellar hemispheres
- Iso to hyperintense to grey matter in T2/FLAIR sequences with heterogeneous appearance due to cystic formation and presence of calcification and necrosis

Treatment

Standard therapy consists of surgical resection followed by craniospinal irradiation (36 Gy or reduced 24 Gy in localized disease) with boost to the primary tumor site (32.4 Gy) and metastatic sites. Treatment in pediatric population with medulloblastoma is stratified on risk-adapted strategies and studies are being carried out to evaluate the risk/benefit ratio of reducing further radiation dose to the neuraxis in children to 18 Gy. Radiotherapy in children below 3 years of age is controversial because of the more severe neurodevelopmental effect of the treatment, and chemotherapy is often used to fill the interval gap before radiation therapy could be given with less long-term side effects burn.

- In average-risk patients with nondisseminated disease, reduced dose RT with adjuvant chemotherapy consisting in 8 cycles of lomustine (CCNU), vincristine, and cisplatin regimen, has been beneficial showing 3-year PFS rate of around 80%.
- In high risk patients, chemotherapeutic agents typically used are cisplatin, carboplatin, cyclophosphamide, and vincristine.
- In recurrent disease, attempts with high dose chemotherapy (cyclophosphamide) and with stem cell harvest for possible transplant has been tested, and treatments targeting molecular pathways such as SHH are under investigation.

There are few evidence-based guidelines for treatment in the adult population, and treatment considerations are modeled by data extrapolation from the pediatric experience. Surgery followed by craniospinal radiotherapy at 36 Gy with boost of 18.8 Gy to the origin tumor site in partial resection is the mainstream treatment approach. Proton beam RT of the neuraxis should always been considered as preferred option in adults as it significantly decreases the long-term side effects, spares the bone marrow reserve and ovary toxicity in women, and it is better tolerated. New therapies are evaluated in clinical trials based on subgroup molecular profiling of medulloblastomas.

Prognosis

- Disease-wide 5-year survival stands at 60% to 70%.
- 17p loss has been associated with poor outcome.
- MYC gene amplification and TP53 mutations are prognostic factors of poor outcome.
- Metastatic disease at diagnosis (seeding in one third of patients at diagnosis), age <3 years and disease relapse, are very poor prognostic factors.
- Staging evaluation is important and has been historically based on tumor size and extent of metastatic disease (spinal dissemination, bone marrow invasion) by Harisiadis and Chang in 1977.
- Despite 5-year survivorship with current therapies up to 80%, current treatment toxicity and long-term sequelae significantly impact the neurological and neurocognitive development of pediatric patients.

Primary CNS Lymphomas

Primary CNS Lymphomas (PCNLS) are extranodal high grade non-Hodgkin B-cell lymphomas (NHL) arising in the CNS (brain, eyes, leptomeninges, spinal cord) that are diagnosed in the absence of systemic lymphomas and that typically remains in the brain. They account for 3% to 5% of all brain tumors and 1% of NHL. After a steady increase in incidence since the end of the 20th century, over the past decade, there has been a plateau or even a decrease in incidence of PCNLS among immunodeficient patients, likely linked to improved treatment and outcome of HIV/AIDS patients. Nonetheless, the incidence among immunocompetent elderly population remains high, with median age at diagnosis of 60 years old.

Risk Factors

A prominent risk factor for the development of PCNSL is immunodeficiency, due to congenital disorders, iatrogenic immunosuppression, and most notably, HIV that historically increased the risk of developing PCNLS by 3600-fold. It is also strongly associated with Epstein-Barr virus (EBV) infection in immunosuppressed patients and immunocompetent elderly patients treated with mychopenolate mofetil, methotrexate, or azathioprine.

Diagnosis

Presentation is usually with focal neurologic symptoms and symptoms of increased intracranial pressure. Elderly patients more commonly present with change in behavior and personality. A profound steroid-induced response is classic but may prevent a tissue diagnosis; therefore, steroids should be withhold until tissue confirmation of diagnosis. CSF analysis highlights lymphomatous cells in 10% to 30% of patients. High suspicion is raised in HIV/AIDS patients with classic lesion on brain imaging and positive EBV DNA in the CSF. As systemic involvement is rare, staging is often achieved through neuroimaging, HIV testing, CSF analysis, ocular slit-lamp examination, and clinical assessment. In selected cases body CT scan and bone marrow biopsy are pursued. For occult lymphoma, FDG body PET is required.

Imaging

- CNS lymphoma is typically manifest on MRI or CT as homogeneously enhancing solitary (two third of cases) or multiple lesions in the periventricular areas.
- Ring enhancement is more commonly seen in immunodeficient patients.
- Rapid leakage of contrast medium is reflected by distinct signal-time intensity curves.
- Significant elevation of lipid resonance at spectroscopy studies.

Treatment

Despite poor overall prognosis, the treatment of primary brain lymphoma has made advances and 20% to 30 % of patients can achieve long-term remission. The standard of care for PCNSL is systemic chemotherapy with or without whole brain radiotherapy (WBRT) or intrathecal chemotherapy. Traditionally surgery has been discouraged apart from diagnostic biopsy but this paradigm has been recently challenged by a German PCNSL study group that showed increased PFS and OS in patients undergoing subtotal or gross total resection. WBRT usually at dosage of 40 to 50 Gy has several limitations including delayed neurotoxicity especially on neurocognitive functions, while low dose radiation (23.4 Gy) in patients older than 60 years old, the group most prone to late radiation effects does not seem to have comparable efficacy to the higher dose regimens. High dose methotrexate has been used as induction chemotherapeutic regimen, and it is usually coupled with preventive measures to limit its toxicity side effects as hydration, urine alkalization, and avoidance of interacting agents (penicillin derivatives). High-dose chemotherapeutic consolidation has been investigated in a further attempt to decrease the need for radiation. Although several regimens are in use, most centers incorporate high-dose cytarabine and etoposide. For newly diagnosed PCNSL patients, a novel program has evaluated immunochemotherapy combination regimen (induction consisting of methotrexate, temozolomide, and rituximab followed by consolidative infusional etoposide plus high-dose cytarabine), with promising results. In recurrent disease, a key consideration is whether the lymphoma is methotrexate-sensitive, while other salvage treatments including autologous stem-cell transplantation are under study.

Prognosis

The significant advances in PCNSL treatment lead to anticipate that between 40% to 50% of PCNSL patients will exhibit long-term survival and a significant proportion may be cured. Nonetheless, research stresses the importance of future developments as at least 40% to 50% of PCNSL patients will develop disease refractory to the current treatment agents

Pineal Region Tumors

Most pineal region masses are malignant cell tumors that occur in young male patients, the most frequent being germinoma. Given the location, these tumors can compress the aqueduct resulting in hydrocephalus. Symptoms are therefore related to increased intracranial pressure with headache, nausea and vomiting, and cranial nerve palsies. When tumor compress the superior colliculi, it leads to Parinaud syndrome characterized by impaired upgaze, convergence and retraction nystagmus, eyelid retraction also called Collier sign and pupillary light-near dissociation. Tumor markers may be increased as α-fetoprotein, α-human chorionic gonadotropin, and placental alkaline phosphatase.

Pineal region masses give rise of a wide differential due to the variety of cell types in the region. Several characteristics may help differentiating them, although biopsy is indicated for diagnosis confirmation:

- Germ cell tumors, half of which being germinoma, usually appear as homogeneous mass with signal intensity and attenuation similar to those of gray matter; engulfing a densely calcified pineal gland.
- Pineal parenchyma tumors are usually either pineocytomas (grade 1) or pineoblastomas (grade 4). Recently, a third category has been described, pineal parenchymal tumor of intermediate differentiation, graded as a WHO II-III depending upon cellular characteristics.
- Pineal parenchymal tumors demonstrate calcifications dispersed peripherally to the mass on neuroimaging.
- Pineal cysts often have a rim thin enhancement at contrast imaging.
- Tentorial meningioma tends to depress cerebral veins while intrinsic pineal tumors tend to cause upward displacement of the internal cerebral veins.
- Tectal astrocytoma are slightly hyperintense on T2 weighted images, can present cystic spaces and calcifications, and usually do not or minimally enhance.

Diagnostic evaluation should include craniospinal MRI and CSF analysis. Biopsy should be pursued depending on the suspected lesion with stereotactic or endoscopic approach in germinoma or tectal glioma and microsurgical techniques for open biopsy in other cases. Radiation therapy is first-line treatment for germinomas. Craniospinal radiotherapy associated with adjuvant chemotherapy is pursued when there is evidence of CSF seeding or malignant tumor.

METASTATIC CNS TUMORS

Tumour cells detaching from systemic tumours spread hematogenously into the CNS by producing and secreting angiogenic substances that enable them to open the BBB locally. Different cancers show different intracranial compartment tropism.

Brain Metastases

Brain metastases occur in 15% to 40% of patients with systemic cancer. Although the true incidence of metastatic brain tumors remains unknown, it is following an increasing trend likely due to better control of systemic cancer and prolonged survival. Still, it remains undetected in 15% of patients. Aging is a factor risk and the most frequent primary tumor origin is lung, breast, melanoma, and colorectal. Hematological tumors constitute 10% of brain metastases and primarily affect the leptomeninges. Presentation is usually with focal neurologic deficits related to mass compression, edema, and increased intracranial pressure. From a neuroimaging point of view lesions are characteristically localized at the grey/white matter junction and are surrounded by significant edema with higher edema/tumor size ratio. Most metastatic brain lesions are hypointense on T1 weighted images on MRI that could indicate haemorrhage and necrosis, and hyperintense on T2 weighted images.

Medical management usually comprise the use of oral steroids to decrease the edema at common dose range of dexamethasone 4 to 8 mg/day and up to 16mg/day for severe symptoms. One quarter of patients do present with seizure and antiepileptic treatment is indicated. There is no evidence based role for seizure prophylactic treatment, although short prophylactic treatment with a one week course and rapid tapering off scheme has been adopted for the perioperative period. Often there is an increased risk of venous thromboembolism partly due to chemotherapeutic agents use, and in high-risk patients, perioperative prophylaxis with heparin has reduced the related mortality without increasing the risk of intracranial haemorrhage.

The treatment of brain metastases is individualised and tailored in the context of the primary tumor and the patient's overall systemic options. Depending on the primary tumor staging and grading, brain metastases treatment may encompass surgery, radiotherapy and in certain cases chemotherapy for chemosensitive tumors as small cell lung carcinoma, germ cell tumors, and lymphoid neoplasms. The other predictive factor of chemotherapy response to be considered is the BBB permeability of the agent, although its importance is much less critical than chemotherapy agent choice based on primary tumor efficacy. The overall prognosis is often below a year of survival but there is a wide heterogeneity that can be stratified depending on primary disease control, age of the patient (>65 years old), functional status of the patients, Karnofsky performance score (KPS< 70), single or multiple brain metastases. Interestingly, there is now evidence that brain metastases can be prevented by targeted therapy of the primary brain tumor. In patients with good prognosis, emphasis is placed on balancing treatment effectiveness against neurotoxicity and the goal of therapy has shifted from short-term palliation to long-term survival and quality of life (QoL). Hence, whole-brain radiation therapy (WBRT) is less preferable in situations where stereotactic radiosurgery and systemic agents are reasonable options. Surgical treatment with removal of brain parenchyma adjacent to the metastatic lesion confers better local control than gross total resection. The pathologic confirmation of tumor-free resection margins provides rate of local recurrence comparable to standard gross total resection and adjuvant radiotherapy.

Spinal Metastases

Metastases of the spine most frequently involve vertebral elements and epidural space and arise from lung, breast, liver, skeletal, and prostate primary tumors. Management includes tailored approach depending on individual localization, clinical symptomatology, and previous treatments, and may include combination of steroids, surgery, radiation, and chemotherapies. Spinal cord compression because of these metastases to the spine with extension into the spinal canal represents a true oncologic emergency as neurologic deficits may not improve particularly if the compression results in vascular compromise to the spinal cord. Metastases that involve the subarachnoid space are leptomeningeal metastases. Intradural metastases are far less common but are typically referred to as drop metastases as they are extramedullary and either compress the cord or invade into the spinal cord parenchyma.

Neoplastic Meningitis

Meningeal involvement can occur by local infiltration or by dissemination of tumor cells by the cerebrospinal flow. Seeding of the leptomeninges by malignant cells may occur in primary brain tumor patients as well as in cancer patients for both hematological (more frequent) and solid (breast, lung, and melanoma) tumors in a percentage that is variable from 1% to 15%. Extensive investigations with contrast MRI of brain and spine, as well as repeated lumbar punctures for CSF analysis are needed as CSF cytology may be negative in almost half of the patients. Neoplastic meningitis causes progressive neurological dysfunction. Treatment with focal radiation to areas of bulk disease or neurologic symptoms from involvement of cranial or spinal nerves may improve function. In individual cases, intrathecal chemotherapy may be of benefit and more recently selected chemotherapy agents have been administered at high doses systemically to generate therapeutic concentrations within the CSF. The optimal treatment of patients with leptomeningeal cancer is based on consideration of the primary cancer type, patient's performance status, CSF disease burden, and extent of systemic disease.

SUMMARY

Treatment of cancer in the central nervous system is complicated. Primary brain tumors, while rarely spreading outside of the CNS, are typically invasive therefore not curable with surgery. Radiation and chemotherapy regimens have been developed for most primary brain tumors and are being increasing refined by tumor type and recently molecular subtypes, underscoring the importance of accurate histologic and molecular classification. Secondary CNS cancers (brain and leptomeningeal metastases) are often late complications of systemic cancer and optimal treatment is based on the cancer type and stage or extent of the systemic disease. In all patients, realistic appraisal of treatment outcomes in the context of both short- and long-term toxicities highlights the need for systematic evaluation of patient outcomes to provide patients with cancer information necessary for informed decision making.

Suggested Readings

1. Amirian ES, Scheurer ME, Zhou R, et al. History of chickenpox in glioma risk: a report from the glioma international case-control study (GICC). *Cancer Med.* 2016;5(6):1352–1358.
2. Blakeley JO, Grossman SA. Management of pineal region tumors. *Curr Treat Options Oncol.* 2006;7(6):505–516.
3. Blitshten, S, Crook JE, Jaeckle KA. Is there an association between meningioma and hormone replacement therapy? *J Clin Oncol.* 2008;26(2):279–282.
4. Bouffet E, Foreman N. Chemotherapy for intracranial ependymomas. *Childs Nerv Syst.* 1999;15(10):563–570.
5. *CBTRUS Statistical Report: Primary Brain and Central Nervous System Tumors diagnosed in the United States in 2004-2008.* Central Brain Tumor Registry of the United States; 2008.
6. Chamberlain MC. Treatment of meningioma, including in cases with no further surgical or radiotherapy options. *Oncology.* 2015;29(5):369–371.
7. Crocetti E, Trama A, Stiller C, et al. Epidemiology of glial and non-glial brain tumors in Europe. *Eur J Cancer.* 2012;48(10):1532–1542.
8. Demir MK, Iplikcioglu AC, Dincer A, et al. Single voxel proton MR spectroscopy findings of typical and atypical intracranial meningiomas. *Eur J Radiol.* 2006;60(1):48–55.
9. Fox BD, Cheung VJ, Patel AJ, et al. Epidemiology of metastatic brain tumors. *Neurosurg Clin N Am.* 2011;22(1):1–6.
10. Fraser E, Gruenberg K, Rubenstein JL, et al. New approaches in primary central nervous system lymphoma. *Chin Clin Oncol.* 2015;4(1):11.
11. Gottardo NG, Gajjar A. Chemotherapy for malignant brain tumors of childhood. *J Child Neurol.* 2008;23(10):1149–1159.
12. Jun P, Hong C, Wong JM, et al. Epigenetic silencing of the kinase tumor suppressor WNK2 is tumor-type and tumor-grade specific. *Neuro Oncol.* 2009;11(4):414–422.
13. Kleinschmidt-DeMasters BK, Damek DM, Lillehei K, et al. Epstein Barr virus-associated primary CNS lymphomas in elderly patients on immunosuppressive medications. *J Neuropathol Exp Neurol.* 2008;67(11):1103–1111.
14. Korshunov A, Ryzhova M, Hovestadt V, et al. Integrated analysis of pediatric glioblastoma reveals a subset of biologically favorable tumors with associated molecular prognostic markers. *Acta Neuropathol.* 2015;129(5):669–678.
15. Kousi E, Tsougos I, Fountas K, et al. Distinct peak at 3.8 ppm observed by 3T MR spectroscopy in meningiomas, while nearly absent in high-grade gliomas and cerebral metastases. *Mol Med Rep.* 2012;5(4):1011–1018.

16. Kuratsu J, Kochi M, Ushio Y. Incidence and clinical features of asymptomatic meningiomas. *J Neurosurg.* 2000;92(5):766–770.
17. Lafay-Cousin L, Mabbott DJ, Halliday W, et al. Use of ifosfamide, carboplatin, and etoposide chemotherapy in choroid plexus carcinoma. *J Neurosurg Pediatr.* 2010;5(6):615–621.
18. Louis, DN, Perry A, Reinfeberger G, et al. The 2016 World Health Organization Classification of Tumors of the Central Nervous System: a summary. *Acta Neurpathol.* 2016;131(6):803–820.
19. Ma C, Cao L, Zhao J, et al. Inverse association between Prediagnostic IgE Levels and the risk of brain tumors: A systematic review and meta-analysis. *BioMed Res Int.* 2015;2015:94213.
20. McCabe MG, Backlund LM, Leong HS, et al. Chromosome 17 alterations identify good-risk and poor-risk tumors independently of clinical factors in medulloblastoma. *Neuro Oncol.* 2011;13(4):376–383.
21. Metha M, Vogelbaum MA, Chang S, et al. Neoplasms of the central nervous system. In L. T. DeVita Jr, *Cancer: Principles and Practice of Oncology. 9th ed.* Philadelphia: Lippincott Williams & Wilkins; 2011:1700–1749.
22. Mohile NA, DeAngelis LM, Abrey LE. The utility of body FDG PET in staging primary central nervous system lymphoma. *Neuro Oncol.* 2008;10(2):223–228.
23. Ostrom QT, Gittleman H, Liao P, et al. CBTRUS statistical report: primary brain and central nervous system tumors diagnosed in the United States in 2007-2011. *Neuro Oncol.* 2014;16(4):iv1–63.
24. Pajtler KW, Witt H, Sill M, et al. Molecular classification of Ependymal Tumors across all CNS compartments, histopathological grades, and age groups. *Cancer Cel.* 2015;27(5):728–743.
25. Palma L, Celli P, Mariottini A, et al. The importance of surgery in supratentorial ependymomas. Long-term survival in a series of 23 cases. *Childs Nerv Syst.* 2000;16(3):170–175.
26. Perreault S, Ramaswamy V, Achrol AS, et al. MRI surrogates for molecular subgroups of medulloblastoma. *Am J Neuroradiol.* 2014;35(7):1263–1269.
27. Perry JR, Laperriere N, O'Callaghan CJ, et al. Short-course radiation plus temozolamide in elderly patients with glioblastoma. *N Engl J Med.* 2017;376:1027–1037.
28. Pizer BL, Clifford SC. The potential impact of tumour biology on improved clinical practice for medulloblastoma: progress towards biologically driven clinical trials. *Br J Neurosurg.* 2009;23(4):364–375.
29. Sjostrom S, Hjalmars U, Juto P, et al. Human immunoglobulin G levels of viruses and associated glioma risk. *Cancer Causes Control.* 2011;22(9):1259–1266.
30. Stupp R, Hegi ME, Mason WP, et al. Effects of radiotherapy with concomitant and adjuvant Temozolomide verusu radiotherapy alone on survival in glioblastoma in a randomised phase III study: 5-year analysis of the EORTC-NCIC study. *Lancet Oncol.* 2009;10(5):459–466.
31. Sundeep D, Lynch CF, Sidenaller ZA, et al. Trends in brain cancer incidence and survival in the United States: Surveillance, Epidemiology, and End Results Program, 1973 to 2001. *Neurosurg Focus.* 2006;20(4):E1.
32. Weller M, Martus P, Roth P, et al. Surgery for primary CNS lymphoma? Challenging a paradigm. *Neuro Oncol.* 2012;14(12):1481–1484.
33. Wiemesl J, Wrensch M, Claus EB. Epidemiology and etiology of meningioma. *J Neuro Oncol.* 2010;99(3):307–314.
34. Yew A, Trang A, Nagasawa DT, et al. Chromosomal alterations, prognostic factors, and targeted molecular therapies for malignant meningiomas. *J Clin Neurosci.* 2013;20(1):17–22.
35. Zhukova N, Ramaswamy V, Remke M, et al. Subgroup-specific prognostic implications of TP53 mutation in medulloblastoma. *J Clin Oncol.* 2013;31(23):2927–2935.

Endocrine Tumors 33

Jaydira Del Rivero and Ann W. Gramza

INTRODUCTION

Endocrine tumors arise from hormone-secreting glands. They may be sporadic or part of a familial cancer syndrome (Table 33.1), the most common being the multiple endocrine neoplasia syndromes. With the exception of thyroid cancer, endocrine tumors are often difficult to diagnose and treat effectively. They may cause morbidity and mortality through local and distant metastasis or through systemic effects caused by hormones produced by tumor cells. While relatively uncommon as a group, thyroid cancer has increased in incidence over the last decade more than any other malignancy. The most common endocrine tumors include

- Thyroid carcinoma
- Pheochromocytoma and Paraganglioma
- Carcinoid tumors
- Pancreatic neuroendocrine tumors (NETs)
- Adrenocortical carcinoma (ACC)
- Parathyroid carcinoma

THYROID CARCINOMA

General

Epidemiology

- Thyroid cancer is the most common endocrine malignancy, now over twice as common in the United States as it was 10 years ago, and it is now the fifth most common cancer in women in the United States.
- The National Cancer Institute has estimated that 62,450 new cases of thyroid carcinoma are diagnosed in the United States annually, accounting for approximately 1950 deaths. The incidence of thyroid carcinoma is now about 9 per 100,000, with approximately 2.7 to 3.1 times as many women as men affected (in women at a rate >5% per year). The ratio of female to male patients is approximately 3:1.
- Mortality has also been rising for the past two decades. The precise reasons for the increase in incidence and mortality are unknown.

Risk Factors

- The best-established risk factor for thyroid cancer is head and neck radiation exposure during childhood for diseases such as Hodgkin lymphoma; hereditary factors, family history of thyroid cancer and history of goiter or thyroid nodule, and/or preceding autoimmune thyroid disease are implicated in some patients as the cause of the increased risk of thyroid cancer.
- Autoimmune thyroid disease is more prevalent in women and this may explain why thyroid cancer is more common in women that in men.

TABLE 33.1 Hereditary Endocrine Cancer Syndromes

Familial Syndrome	Associated Malignancies	Gene Mutated
MEN 1 (Werner syndrome)	Pituitary adenomas Functioning pancreatic neuroendocrine tumors (insulinoma, gastrinoma) Nonfunctioning pancreatic neuroendocrine tumors Parathyroid hyperplasia/adenomas causing hyperparathyroidism Peptic ulcers (with Zollinger-Ellison syndrome) Bronchial, thymic, gastric carcinoid	MEN 1
MEN 2A (Sipple syndrome)	Medullary thyroid cancer Pheochromocytoma Primary hyperparathyroidism (parathyroid hyperplasia)	RET
MEN 2B	Medullary thyroid cancer Pheochromocytoma Marphanoid body habitus Multiple mucosal and digestive neurofibromas Megacolon	RET
Familial MTC	MTC in kindreds with 4 to 10 or more affected members	RET
Neurofibromatosis 1	Carcinoids Pheochromocytomas/paragangliomas Pancreatic neuroendocrine tumors Gastrointestinal stromal tumors (GIST),	NF1
von Hippel-Lindau	Pheochromocytomas Pancreatic neuroendocrine tumors Hemangioblastomas Retinal angiomas Renal cell carcinomas Endolymphatic sac tumors Epididymal papillary cystadenomas	VHL
Li-Fraumeni	Adrenocortical cancer Breast cancer Sarcoma Leukemia Brain tumors	TP53
Beckwith-Wiedemann	Adrenocortical carcinoma Wilms tumor Rhabdomyosarcoma Neuroblastoma Hepatoblastoma	Multiple in the 11p15 region
Carney complex	Adrenocortical tumors Thyroid follicular neoplasms Pituitary adenomas Myxomas Schwannomas Sertoli cell tumors Leydig cell tumors	PRKAR1A

TABLE 33.1 (Continued)

Familial Syndrome	Associated Malignancies	Gene Mutated
Familial polyposis coli	Thyroid carcinoma Sarcoma Hepatoblastoma Pancreatic carcinoma Medulloblastoma Adenomatous colon polyps	*APC*
Cowden	Follicular thyroid cancer Breast cancer Endometrial carcinoma	*PTEN*
Peutz-Jeghers	Thyroid cancer, benign ovarian sex cord tumors, calcifying Sertoli tumors of the testis, endometrial cancer, breast cancer, gastrointestinal cancer, pancreatic cancer, cervical cancer	*STK11/LKB1*
Hyperparathyroidism-jaw tumor	Parathyroid cancer, ossifying fibromas of the jaw, cystic and neoplastic renal lesions, uterine tumors	*HPRT2*

- Thyroid cancer has been observed 20 to 25 years after radiation exposure among atomic bomb survivors, and in some regions of Japan the incidence of thyroid cancer in screened populations is as high as 0.1%—10-fold greater than expected based on US incidence rates.

Prognosis

- Prognosis varies by thyroid cancer subtype, but the overall 5-year relative survival is nearly 98%. This is because more than 80% of cases are papillary thyroid cancer (PTC), the subtype with the best survival.

Differentiated Thyroid Cancer: Papillary, Follicular, Hurthle Cell

- More than 90% of all thyroid cancers are a subtype of differentiated thyroid cancer (DTC) with papillary thyroid cancer (PTC) the most common subtype (80% to 85%).
- PTC is generally unilateral, but may be multifocal within a lobe. Histologic subtypes of PTC that have a worse prognosis include tall cell variant, columnar cell variant, and diffuse sclerosing variant. A worse prognosis is also seen with highly invasive variants of follicular cancer, which is characterized by extensive vascular invasion and invasion into extrathyroidal tissues or extensive tumor necrosis with many mitoses. PTC metastasizes primarily via lymphatic invasion; vascular invasion is uncommon.
- DTCs are derived from thyroglobulin-producing follicular cells (thyrocytes), often secrete thyroglobulin (TG) and are typically initially radioiodine (RAI) responsive. TG can be used as a tumor marker in antithyroglobulin antibody–negative patients.
- Genetic alterations involved in the mitogen-activated protein kinase (MAPK) signaling pathway are found in at least 75% of PTC cases. $BRAF^{V600E}$ mutation is found in approximately 45% of PTCs, while rearranged during transfection (*RET*) are found in approximately 25%. Activating point mutations in the *RAS* oncogenes occur in approximately 10% of cases. RET rearrangements are found in approximately 25% and upregulation of vascular endothelial growth factor (VEGF) signaling is also common in metastatic disease.
- Follicular thyroid cancer (FTC) is the second most common type of thyroid carcinoma, comprising 10% to 15% of thyroid cancers. FTC typically disseminates hematogenously, with metastases to bone and lung being most common in advanced disease.
- *RAS* point mutations and the *PAX8/PPARγ* translocation are the most common genetic alterations in FTC.

■ Hurthle cell cancer (HCC) is also referred to as oxyphilic or oncocytic thyroid cancer, and represents approximately 5% of all DTCs. It is often considered a variant of FTC with less sensitivity to radioiodine and a more aggressive clinical course.

Clinical Presentation

■ Most patients present with an asymptomatic thyroid nodule. Clinical symptoms may include the following:
  * Hoarseness caused by invasion of the recurrent laryngeal nerve or by direct compression of the larynx
  * Cervical lymphadenopathy
  * Dysphagia
  * Horner syndrome (miosis, partial ptosis, hemifacial anhidrosis)

Diagnosis

■ Evaluation of any suspected thyroid nodule >1 cm should include a serum thyroid stimulating hormone (TSH) and thyroid ultrasound. Occasionally, thyroid nodules <1 cm require evaluation because of suspicious ultrasound findings, associated with lymphadenopathy, head and neck irradiation, or a family history of thyroid cancer.
■ If a nodule is seen on ultrasound
  * If TSH is normal or high, a fine-needle aspirate (FNA) should be done.
  * If the TSH is low, the nodule should be evaluated by radionuclide thyroid scan with either a ^{99m}Tc pertechnetate or ^{123}I to see if it is hyperfunctioning. Hyperfunctioning nodules are benign and patients with them should be treated for hyperthyroidism.
■ Up to 30% of FNAs are indeterminate; therefore, a definitive diagnosis is often not made until the nodule is resected. A new gene expression classification assay was able to predict benign pathology when FNA cytology was indeterminate (e.g., BRAF, NRAS, HRAS, KRAS, RET/PTC1, RET/PTC3, PAX8-PPARγ) and may allow a more conservative approach for those who would otherwise undergo a diagnostic surgical procedure. If the cytology reading reports follicular neoplasm, a lobectomy or total thyroidectomy should be considered.
■ Carcinoma is suggested by the following clinical findings: a history of head and neck radiation, family history of thyroid cancer, exposure to ionizing radiation, rapid growth of the nodule, hoarseness, vocal cord paralysis, and lymphadenopathy. There may also be specific features on ultrasound that are suggestive of possible malignancy.
■ Staging for DTC incorporates age. For patients ≤45 years old, the most advanced they can be is stage II given their excellent prognosis.

Treatment

Surgery

■ Total thyroidectomy is recommended for a DTC lesion >1 cm, a lesion that extends beyond the thyroid, or for patients with history of prior exposure to ionizing radiation to head/neck.
■ Unilateral lobectomy with en bloc resection of tumor may be considered for a DTC lesion <1 cm or for follicular lesion with no evidence of multicentric disease.
■ Total thyroidectomy with modified radical neck dissection should be done for regional lymph node metastases.
■ Thyroidectomy should be performed in patients with distant metastases to permit treatment with radioiodine, which can still be curative.
■ Mortality consequent to thyroidectomy in DTC is extremely low. Complications include recurrent laryngeal nerve damage in 2% of patients and hypoparathyroidism that is lifelong in 1% to 2% of patients.

TSH suppression

■ TSH suppression via administration of "supra-therapeutic" levothyroxine is an essential component in the treatment of high-risk DTC, as residual cancer cells are usually initially responsive to TSH growth stimulation. Levothyroxine (T_4, usual dosage range 125 to 200 μg by mouth daily) is administered to keep the TSH level suppressed below 0.1 mIU/L in high-risk (macroscopic tumor invasion, incomplete tumor resection, distant metastases) to intermediated risk patients (microscopic invasion of tumor into the perithyroidal soft tissues, cervical lymph nodes metastases, tumor with aggressive histology, or vascular invasion).

- For low risk patients, the goal is to maintain TSH below the lower limit of normal 0.1 to 0.5 mIU/L.
- Suppression of TSH below 0.1 mIU/L imposes long-term adverse effects on bone and can negatively impact quality of life, sometimes producing symptoms of thyrotoxicosis.

Adjuvant Therapy

- Treatment with radioiodine (I-131, RAI) is used to ablate normal residual thyroid tissue, treat micrometastases, and decrease cancer-related death, tumor recurrence, and development of distant metastases. Table 33.2 outlines indications for iodine-131 treatment after surgery.
- Adjuvant external beam radiotherapy is sometimes recommended for those patients with gross or microscopic residual disease or those with high-risk histology and visible extrathyroidal extension. Locally recurrent disease not amenable to surgery or radioiodine therapy can also be treated with external beam radiotherapy.

Targeted Therapy/Chemotherapy

- Several VEGFR inhibitors have been shown to have activity in well-differentiated thyroid cancers and two—sorafenib and lenvatinib—have received FDA approval on the basis of randomized phase III trials for patients with advanced disease that is refractory to iodine-131.
- Sorafenib is an inhibitor of several protein tyrosine kinases (VEGFR and PDGFR) and some intracellular serine/threonine kinases (e.g., C-Raf, wild-type and mutant B-Raf). Safety and effectiveness were established in a randomized trial involving 417 participants with locally recurrent or metastatic, progressive differentiated thyroid cancer that had not responded to radioactive iodine treatment. The sorafenib dose was 400 mg twice a day. The median progression-free survival (PFS) was 10.8 months with sorafenib compared to 5.8 months with placebo ($P < 0.0001$). Partial responses were observed in 12.2% of patients receiving sorafenib compared with 0.5% in the placebo arm ($P < 0.0001$). The most common side effects with sorafenib were diarrhea, fatigue, alopecia, hand-foot skin reaction, rash, weight loss, anorexia, nausea, gastrointestinal and abdominal pains, and hypertension (see Table 33.3).

TABLE 33.2 Indications for Postsurgical Treatment with Iodine-131 in Patients with Thyroid Cancer

| | Iodine-131 | |
Finding	Indicated	Not Indicated
Low risk of cancer-specific mortality or relapse		X
Incomplete excision of tumor	X	
Complete excision of tumor but high risk of mortality	X	
Complete excision of tumor but high risk of relapse due to	X	
Age (<16 y or >45 y)		
Histologic subtype (tall cell, columnar cell, diffuse sclerosing papillary variants; widely invasive or poorly differentiated follicular subtypes; Hurthle cell carcinomas)		
Extent of tumor (large tumor mass, extension beyond thyroid capsule, lymph node metastases)		
Distant metastases	X	
Elevated serum thyroglobulin >3 mo postsurgery	X	

TABLE 33.3 Systemic Therapy Regimens for Advanced or Metastatic Endocrine Cancers

Regimen	Malignancy
Sorafenib 400 mg orally twice daily	Radioactive iodine refractory differentiated thyroid cancer
Lenvatinib 14 mg orally daily	Radioactive iodine refractory differentiated thyroid cancer
Vandetanib 300 mg orally daily	Medullary thyroid cancer
Cabozantinib 140 mg orally daily	Medullary thyroid cancer
Cyclophosphamide 750 mg/m^2 day 1,Vincristine 1.4 mg/m^2 day 1,Dacarbazine 600 mg/m^2 day 1, and Dacarbazine 600 mg/m^2 day 2, every 21–28 d	Malignant pheochromocytoma[a]
Sunitinib 37.5 mg orally daily	Pancreatic neuroendocrine tumors, malignant pheochromocytoma[a]
Everolimus 10 mg orally daily	Pancreatic neuroendocrine tumors, carcinoid
Octreotide 150–250 µg SC TID or depot 20 mg IM every 4 weeks	Pancreatic neuroendocrine tumors, carcinoid
Depot octreotide 30 mg IM every 28 d and Everolimus 10 mg daily	Pancreatic neuroendocrine tumors, carcinoid
Streptozocin 500 mg/m^2/d IV days 1–5 and5-Fluoruracil 400 mg/m^2/d IV days 1–5 every 6 weeks	Pancreatic neuroendocrine tumors, carcinoid[a]
Streptozocin 500 mg/m^2/d IV days 1–5 and Doxorubicin 50 mg/m^2 IV days 1, 22 every 6 weeks	Pancreatic neuroendocrine tumors, carcinoid[a]
Capecitabine 750 mg/m^2 twice daily on days 1–14 plus temozolomide 200 mg/m^2 daily on days 10–14	Pancreatic neuroendocrine tumors, carcinoid[a]
Mitotane orally continuously (starting dose = 1–2 g/d, increase to mitotane level of 14–20 mg/L or toxicity)	Adrenocortical carcinoma
Mitotane orally continuously (starting dose = 1–2 g/d, increase to mitotane level of 14–20 mg/L or toxicity) andStreptozotocin (1 g on days 1–5 in cycle 1; 2 g on day 1 in subsequent cycles every 3 weeks)	Adrenocortical carcinoma
Mitotane orally continuously (starting dose = 1–2 g/d, increase to mitotane level of 14–20 mg/L or toxicity) and Etoposide (100 mg /m^2 IV days 2, 3, and 4), Doxorubicin (40 mg/m^2 IV day 1), and Cisplatin (40 mg/m^2 IV days 3 and 4) every 4 weeks	Adrenocortical carcinoma

[a] Limited phase II data.

- Lenvatinib is an inhibitor of the vascular endothelial growth factor receptor 2 (VEGFR2). The approval of lenvatinib was based on a multicenter, double blind, placebo-controlled trial that enrolled 392 patients with locally recurrent or metastatic radioactive iodine-refractory differentiated thyroid cancer and radiographic evidence of progression within 12 months prior to randomization. Patients received lenvatinib 24 mg orally per day. Median PFS was 18.3 months in the lenvatinib arm and 3.6 months in the placebo arm (P <0.0001). Objective response rates were 65% and 2% in the lenvatinib and placebo arms, respectively. No statistically significant difference in overall survival between the two arms was demonstrated. The most common adverse reactions were hypertension, fatigue, diarrhea, arthralgia/myalgia, anorexia, weight loss, nausea, stomatitis, headache, vomiting, proteinuria, palmar-plantar erythrodysesthesia (PPE) syndrome, abdominal pain, and dysphonia. Adverse reactions led to dose reductions in 68% of patients receiving lenvatinib and 18% of patients discontinued lenvatinib for adverse reactions (see Table 33.3).

Medullary Thyroid Cancer

- Medullary thyroid cancer (MTC) is a neuroendocrine tumor of the parafollicular or C cells of the thyroid gland. MTC accounts for approximately 4% of thyroid carcinomas. Its estimated incidence in the United States for 2010 is about 1,300 to 2,200 patients. Sporadic MTC accounts for about 80% of all cases of the disease. The typical age of presentation is in the fifth or sixth decade, and there may be a slight female preponderance.
- Hereditary MTC is divided into three distinct clinical subtypes. Multiple endocrine neoplasia (MEN) 2A, or Sipple's syndrome, is the most common subtype, accounting for approximately 70% to 80% of patients with hereditary MTC. MEN 2A is characterized by MTC in 100% of affected individuals, by pheochromocytoma in 50%, and by primary hyperparathyroidism in 20%. MTC is usually the first manifestation of the syndrome. Patients typically present with a thyroid nodule or neck mass by 15 to 20 years of age, but MTC can appear as early as 5 years of age. Sporadic tumors tend to be solitary, whereas familial tumors tend to be bilateral and multifocal.
- MEN 2B is less common than MEN 2A, accounting for approximately 5% of MTC cases. It is characterized by a clinically more aggressive form of MTC that is manifest at a younger age (second decade) and that occurs in 100% of affected individuals, by pheochromocytoma in 50%, and by characteristic dysmorphic features including distinctive mucosal neuromas on the tongue, lips, and subconjunctival areas, diffuse ganglioneuromas of the gastrointestinal tract, and marfanoid habitus. Hyperparathyroidism is not associated with MEN 2B (see Table 33.1).
- Familial MTC is the third clinical subtype of inherited MTC. It accounts for 10% to 20% of hereditary MTC cases and is defined by the presence of MTC in kindreds with four to 10 or more affected members and with objective evidence of the absence of adrenal and parathyroid gland involvement. This form of hereditary MTC is less aggressive and has an older age at onset, usually between 20 and 40 years, compared to MEN 2A and 2B

Clinical Presentation

- Patients typically present with an asymptomatic thyroid mass. Some may also have local symptoms such as dysphagia, dyspnea, or hoarseness.
- Approximately 10% will present with systemic symptoms usually consisting of bone pain, flushing, and/or diarrhea.
- Approximately 50% of patients present with regional lymphadenopathy.
- Distant metastases typically occur in late-stage disease and usually involve lung, liver, bones, and adrenal glands.

Diagnosis

- Guidelines for evaluation of thyroid nodules should be followed as described for DTC.
- If the FNA is suggestive of MTC, further evaluation should consist of calcitonin and CEA measurement and genetic testing for germline *RET* mutations.

Treatment

- Total thyroidectomy with central lymph node dissection is the appropriate surgery.
- Surgery and/or external beam radiotherapy can be used for residual or recurrent disease treatment; however, the survival benefit for either modality is unclear.
- Metastatic MTC is the most common cause of death in patients with MEN 2a, MEN 2b, or FMTC, and the tumor is relatively unresponsive to conventional doses of radiation therapy and to standard or novel chemotherapeutic regimens. Until recently, doxorubicin was the only US Food and Drug Administration (FDA)–approved treatment for patients with advanced thyroid cancer. Doxorubicin has resulted in transient tumor response rates in up to 20% of patients with MTC and is associated with significant toxicity. There is no treatment (apart from complete surgical removal) that has been shown to be effective for recurrent or persistent MTC.
- Vandetanib, an oral inhibitor of VEGFR, RET, and epidermal growth factor receptor (EGFR) has been approved in April 2011 by the U.S. Food and Drug Administration (FDA) for the treatment of advanced (metastatic or unresectable locally advanced) medullary thyroid cancer based

on an international randomized phase III trial. In a preliminary report of results (median follow-up 24 months), median PFS was improved in patients randomly assigned to vandetanib versus placebo (hazard ratio 0.45, 95% CI, 0.30 to 0.69). The overall response rate was 45%. Objective responses were durable on the basis of the median duration of response not being reached at 24 months of follow-up. Its toxicity profile is extensive including diarrhea, rash, nausea, hypertension, headache, fatigue, decreased appetite; Grade 3 toxicities reported are diarrhea, hypertension, and fatigue. Therefore, toxicity can limit its use in patients with small volume, asymptomatic or indolent disease.

- Cabozantinib, a tyrosine kinase inhibitor (TKI) of hepatocyte growth factor receptor (MET), VEGFR2, and RET, demonstrated clinical activity in patients with medullary thyroid cancer (MTC). A double-blind, phase III trial comparing cabozantinib with placebo in 330 patients with documented radiographic progression of metastatic MTC was performed. The estimated median PFS was 11.2 months for cabozantinib versus 4.0 months for placebo (hazard ratio, 0.28; 95% CI, 0.19 to 0.40; $P < 0.001$). Prolonged PFS with cabozantinib was observed across all subgroups including by age, prior TKI treatment, and RET mutation status (hereditary or sporadic). Response rate was 28% for cabozantinib and 0% for placebo; responses were seen regardless of RET mutation status. Kaplan-Meier estimated of patients alive and progression-free at 1 year are 47.3% for cabozantinib and 7.2% for placebo. Common cabozantinib-associated adverse events included diarrhea, PPE, decreased weight and appetite, nausea, and fatigue and resulted in dose reductions in 79% and holds in 65% of patients. Adverse events led to treatment discontinuation in 16% of cabozantinib-treated patients. See Table 33.3 for vandetanib and cabozantinib dosing.
- Both vandetanib and cabozantinib have recently been approved by the US FDA for the treatment of advanced MTC based on improvement in PFS in phase III trials. No improvement in overall survival has been demonstrated; therefore, patients with indolent disease should consider observation until their disease becomes necessary to treat.

Anaplastic Thyroid Cancer

- Anaplastic thyroid cancer (ATC) is a rare, high-grade, aggressive malignancy that accounts for 2% to 5% of all thyroid carcinomas. Up to 50% of patients have antecedent or concurrent history of DTC. Disease-specific mortality is nearly 100%.
- Patients typically present with a rapidly enlarging neck mass.
- Approximately 90% will have locoregional or distant metastases at the time of diagnosis.
- Treatment is primarily palliative and often aimed at preventing asphyxiation, the most common cause of death in these patients. It can consist of surgery, radiation, chemotherapy, or a combination of these modalities.
- Surgical resection does not improve local control or survival in patients. If surgery is performed, it should be followed by locoregional radiotherapy usually within 2 to 3 weeks after surgery. Local control is desirable in patients with ATC because of the likelihood of asphyxia from the rapidly enlarging tumor.
- Treatment with external beam radiotherapy with systemic therapy appears to achieve local control in two-thirds of patients with ATC, however, almost all subsequently die of distant metastases.
- A number of novel agents have been preliminarily studied in ATC such as fosbretabulin assessed in phase II trial with increased overall survival in some patients. TKIs such as sorafenib, axitinib, gefitinib has been studied with no evidence of RECIST response; however, a limited number of patients were reported to have stable disease.

Other Thyroid Cancers

- Primary thyroid lymphoma
- Metastasis to the thyroid
- Thyroid sarcoma

PHEOCHROMOCYTOMA

Epidemiology

▪ Pheochromocytomas (PHEOs) and paragangliomas (PGLs) are rare rine tumors NETs that arise from chromaffin cells. Pheochromocytomas account for 90% of cases and arise in the adrenal glands, whereas paragangliomas, the extra-adrenal counterpart of pheochromocytomas, arise from ganglia along the sympathethic and parasympathetic chain (e.g., carotid body/skull base, urinary bladder, heart, organ of Zuckerkandl).

▪ Most PHEOs represent sporadic tumors and 15% of these are associated with somatic mutations. However, about 35% are familial in origin and patients are found to harbor germline mutations in susceptibility genes.

▪ The number of genes associated with susceptibility to PHEOs/PGLs was recently increased to 19, and includes the von Hippel-Lindau (*VHL*) tumor suppressor gene, the *RET* proto-oncogene, the neurofibromatosis type 1 (*NF1*) tumor suppressor gene, the genes encoding the four succinate dehydrogenase complex (*SDH*) subunits (*SDHA, -B, -C, -D*), and the gene encoding the enzyme responsible for flavination of the SDHA subunit (*SDHAF2*). Additionally, new susceptibility genes, transmembrane protein 127 (*TMEM127*), MYC-associated factor X (*MAX*), and hypoxia-inducible factor 2α (*HIF2A*), have been identified. Others include the kinesin family member 1B, transcript variant β (*KIF1Bβ*), prolyl hydroxylase 1 and 2 (*PHD1/EGLN2* and *PHD2/EGLN1*), Harvey Ras sarcoma viral oncogene (*H-RAS*), Kirsten Ras sarcoma viral oncogene (*K-RAS*), isocitrate dehydrogenase 1 (IDH1), fumarate hydratase (*FH*) and BRCA1-associated protein-1 (*BAP1*). Finally, germline mutations in malate dehydrogenase 2 (*MDH2*) and somatic mutations in alpha thalassemia/mental retardation syndrome X-linked (*ATRX*) genes were identified in PHEOs/PGLs (see Table 33.5)

Clinical Presentation

▪ Clinical manifestations of PHEO/PGL are diverse, with similar symptoms occurring in other disease conditions. Most of the signs and symptoms are attributed to the direct actions of the over production of catecholamines. These include hypertension, headache, palpitations, and anxiety. Hypertension can be paroxysmal or sustained. Some patients may present with orthostatic hypotension. Biochemically silent tumors may be suspected from tumor mass effect or may be found incidentally on imaging studies (see Table 33.4).

TABLE 33.4 Potential Clinical Manifestations of Pheochromocytomas

Mild labile hypertension to hypertensive crisis; sustained hypertension also common
Myocardial infarction
Cerebral infarction
Classic pattern of paroxysmal hypertension (30%–50% of cases)
Spells of paroxysmal headache
Pallor or flushing
Tremor
Apprehension
Palpitation
Orthostasis
Mild weight loss
Diaphoresis

TABLE 33.5 Clinical Characteristics of Genetic Mutations Associated with PHEO/PGL

Gene	Syndrome	Germline/ somatic	Common PHEO/PGL sites	Malignancy	Other associated clinical characteristics/ tumors
SDHA		AD	Adrenal PHEOs or extra-adrenal PGLs	0%–14%	Homozygous patients: Leigh syndrome Renal cell carcinoma Gastrointestinal stromal tumors Pituitary adenomas
SDHB	PGL4	AD	Sympathetic PGLs (rarely adrenal PHEOs and head and neck PGLs)	31%–71%	Renal cell carcinoma Gastrointestinal stromal tumors Pituitary adenomas Possibly breast carcinoma
SDHC	PGL3	AD	Head and neck PGLs, sometimes multiple (rarely sympathetic PGLs or adrenal PHEOs)	Rare	Possible papillary thyroid carcinoma Renal cell carcinoma Gastrointestinal stromal tumors Pituitary adenomas
SDHD	PGL1	AD	Head and neck PGLs, commonly multiple (rarely extra-adrenal abdominal PGLs or adrenal PHEOs)	<5%	Renal cell carcinoma Gastrointestinal stromal tumors Pituitary adenomas
SDHAF2	PGL2	AD	Head and neck PGLs, sometimes multiple	Further study needed	
VHL	VHL	AD	Adrenal PHEOs (rarely sympathetic or head and neck PGLs)	<5%	Hemangioblastomas Pheochromocytoma Renal cell carcinoma Pancreatic serous cystadenoma Endolymphatic sac tumor Pancreatic neuroendocrine tumors Epididymal papillary cystadenomas Retinal angiomas

NF1	NF1	AD	Adrenal PHEOs (rarely sympathetic PGLs)	~12%	Café-au-lait spots Neurofibromas Freckles Benign iris hamartomas Optic-nerve gliomas Sphenoid bone dysplasia/pseudoarthritis
RET	MEN2	AD	Adrenal	Rare	MEN2A: Medullary thyroid cancer, pheochromocytoma, hyperparathyroidism MEN2B: Medullary thyroid cancer, pheochromocytoma, marphanoid habitus and mucosal ganglioneuromas
MAX		AD PI	Adrenal	20–25%	Possibly linked to breast carcinoma
TMEM127		AD	Adrenal	<5%	Possibly linked to papillary thyroid carcinoma
HIF2A	Pacak-Zhuang	Somatic	Extra-adrenal PGLs, usually multiple PHEOs	None reported	Multiple somatostatinomas Polycythemia
KIF1β		Somatic	Further study needed	None reported	
PHD2	Yes	Germline	Multple PGLs	None reported	
IDH		Somatic	Carotid PGL	None reported	
FH		Germline	Adrenal PHEO	None reported	Glioblastoma multiforme
H-RAS		Somatic	Both PHEO and PGL	None reported	Polycythemia

- The incidence of malignancy is about 10%, with metastases the only definite proof of malignancy, as there are no definitive histopathologic criteria for malignancy. Oncologists must read the literature carefully given that descriptions of benign and malignant are often combined.
- The overall 5-year survival rate for patients with malignant pheochromocytoma is 36% to 44%. About 50% or more of SDHB mutation carriers will develop malignant paragangliomas, and up to 60% of patients with a malignant paraganglioma harbor a SDHB mutation.

Diagnosis

- Measurement of 24-hour urinary-fractionated metanephrines is the most specific tool for diagnosis of pheochromocytoma.
- Plasma-fractionated metanephrines measurement is the most sensitive test, but has a high rate of false positives.
- Clonidine suppression test is recommended for indeterminate plasma catecholamine or metanephrine levels, both of which will not be suppressed in patients with pheochromocytoma.
- CT and MRI are equally sensitive diagnostic tools for pheochromocytoma.
- Labeled metaiodobenzylguanidine (^{131}I-MIBG), which is structurally similar to norepinephrine, is taken up and concentrated in adrenergic tissue. It is highly sensitive and specific for malignant tumors and familial syndromes, but is inferior to bone scan for detecting bone metastases.
- Vascular invasion and extension into the cortex may be seen with both benign and malignant tumors.

Treatment

Surgery

- Surgery, remains the only curative treatment option with pheochromocytoma/paraganglioma. Minimally invasive adrenalectomy is recommended for most adrenal pheochromocytomas and open resection for large or invasive tumors to ensure complete resection and avoid local recurrence.
- Patients with hormone secreting tumors should undergo preoperative blockade for 7 to 14 days with α-adrenergic receptor blockers such as phenoxybenzamine or doxazosin to prevent perioperative cardiovascular complications.
- Many patients require the addition of β-blockers, which are indicated for persistent tachycardia; however, to prevent hypertensive crisis secondary to unopposed vasoconstriction, β-blockers should not be given before α-antagonists. In patients in whom elevated blood pressure and arrhythmia cannot be controlled with α- and β-blockade, α-methyl-para-tyrosine (metyrosine, Demser) a competitive inhibitor of tyrosine hydroxylase can be used.
- Importantly, normal postoperative biochemical test results do not exclude microscopic disease. Long-term periodic follow-up is recommended especially important if the tumors harbor mutations of disease-causing genes.

Radiation

- Radiation has a limited role in the treatment of pheochromocytoma, but may be used for bone and soft-tissue metastases.
- Therapeutic doses of ^{131}I-MIBG in patients showing evidence of radiotracer uptake on MIBG scans have provided both radiographic and symptomatic responses.

Chemotherapy/Targeted Therapy

- Combined chemotherapy with cyclophosphamide, vincristine and dacarbazine (CVD) has emerged as a standard option. Results of a nonrandomized, single-arm trial included fourteen patients with confirmed malignant PHEO with metastatic disease and elevated urinary catecholamine secretion. After optimization of antihypertensive therapy, patients received cyclophosphamide, 750 mg/m^2 on day 1; vincristine, 1.4 mg/m2 on day 1, and dacarbazine, 600 mg/m^2 on days 1 and 2, every 21 days. Combination chemotherapy with cyclophosphamide, vincristine, and dacarbazine produced a complete plus partial response rate of 57% (median duration, 21 months; range, 7 to more than 34). Complete and partial biochemical responses were seen in 79% of patients (median duration, more than 22 months; range, 6 to more than 35). All responding patients had objective improvement in performance status and blood pressure.

- A long-term follow-up study was conducted in 18 patients treated with CVD at the National Institutes of Health. Combination chemotherapy with CVD produced a complete response rate of 11% and a partial response rate of 44%. Median survival was 3.8 years for patients whose tumors responded to therapy and 1.8 years for patients whose tumors did not respond ($P = 0.65$). All patients with tumors scored as responding reported improvement in their symptoms related to excessive catecholamine release and all had objective improvements in blood pressure. In this 22-year follow-up there was no difference in OS between patients whose tumors objectively shrank and those with stable or progressive disease. However, patients reported improvement in symptoms, had objective improvements in blood pressure, and had tumor shrinkage that made surgical resection possible. CVD therapy is not indicated in every patient with metastatic PHEOs/PGLs, but should be considered in the management of patients with symptoms and where tumor shrinkage might be beneficial.
- Anecdotal reports suggest that the efficacy of chemotherapy may be high in patients with mutations in *SDHB*. Although the CVD regimen led to an overall response of approximately 50%, it is not clear if the administration of CVD impacts overall survival, as nearly all patients develop progressive and ultimately fatal disease.
- Responses have also been reported with the targeted agent sunitinib.
- See Table 33.3 for detailed chemotherapy regimens.

NEUROENDOCRINE TUMORS

NETs are cancers of the interface between the endocrine system and the nervous system. These rare tumors are distinguished from most other solid tumors by their ability to secrete biologically active molecules that can produce systemic syndromes. The 2010 WHO classification separates NETs into well-differentiated and poorly differentiated based on tumor grade, mitotic count, and Ki-67 proliferation index. The most common types of NETs are carcinoid tumors and pancreatic NETs, both of which are typically well differentiated.

Carcinoid Tumors

- Incidence in the United States is approximately 2 per 100,000 individuals.
- Carcinoids are slow-growing malignant tumors that arise from enterochromaffin cells of the aerodigestive tract.
- They are traditionally categorized by their embryonic origin and are most commonly found in the foregut (bronchial) and small intestine.
- The typical carcinoid syndrome consists of flushing and diarrhea and is seen most often with small intestine carcinoid tumors.
- Carcinoid syndrome is observed in 10% of patients, especially those with liver metastases, retroperitoneal disease, or disease outside of the GI tract where excessive hormones can bypass metabolism in liver.
- Features of foregut, midgut, and hindgut carcinoids are outlined in Table 33.6.

Treatment

- Abdominal and rectal carcinoids tend to be small (2 cm). Surgery involves segmental resection with mesenteric lymphadenectomy.
- Appendiceal carcinoid is often discovered incidentally. If it is >2 cm or there is invasion or positive margins, right hemicolectomy is recommended. Right hemicolectomy is more controversial for tumors that are <2 cm and confined to the appendix.
- Liver metastases can be treated locally with surgical debulking, hepatic arterial embolization, chemoembolization, cryotherapy, or radiofrequency ablation.

TABLE 33.6 Carcinoid Features

Origin	Common Sites	Symptoms	Secretory Products
Foregut	Stomach, duodenum	Abdominal pain, anemia, bleeding, atypical carcinoid syndrome uncommon	5-HTP, histamine, tachykinins, other hormones, and peptides
	Bronchus	Pulmonary symptoms, atypical carcinoid syndrome uncommon	
Midgut	Small bowel	Abdominal pain, carcinoid syndrome with liver metastases	Serotonin, other hormones, and peptides
	Appendix	Asymptomatic, usually found incidentally, carcinoid syndrome with liver metastases	
Hindgut	Distal colon, rectum	Bowel habit changes, pain, obstruction, bleeding, carcinoid syndrome rare	Rare

- Patients with carcinoid syndrome should be treated with a somatostatin analog (SSA) such as octreotide. Octreotide has also demonstrated antitumor activity, potentially improving time to progression.
- The U.S. Food and Drug Administration (FDA) has recently approved telotristat ethyl (targets tryptophan hydroxylase, an enzyme that mediates the excess serotonin production within NET cells), an orally administered therapy for the treatment of carcinoid syndrome diarrhea in combination with SSA therapy in adults inadequately controlled by SSA therapy.
- Carcinoids are resistant to most chemotherapeutic agents. Active agents include 5-fluorouracil, capecitabine, streptozocin, doxorubicin, and interferon. Chemotherapy is typically reserved for patients who are progressing with no other treatment options. See Table 33.3 for detailed systemic therapy regimens.
- Radiation therapy is for palliation only.

Pancreatic Neuroendocrine Tumors

Pancreatic NETs, also known as islet cell tumors, arise from the hormone-secreting cells of the pancreas. Up to 75% are nonfunctioning and not associated with clinical syndromes. The functioning pancreatic NETs and are categorized by the hormone and clinical syndrome they produce. Pancreatic NETs comprise approximately 3% of all pancreatic tumors, are generally well differentiated, and are malignant. They are associated with familial syndromes in up to 25% of cases (see Table 33.1).

Gastrinoma (Zollinger-ellison Syndrome)

Gastrinoma is a tumor that secretes gastrin. Primary tumors predominate in the pancreatic head but may also develop in the small intestine or stomach.

Epidemiology

- Gastrinoma occurs in 0.1% to 1% of patients with peptic ulcer disease.
- They are usually diagnosed between the third and sixth decades but can occur at any age.
- Approximately 20% of gastrinomas are associated with the familial syndrome MEN 1, and 80% are sporadic. Sporadic tumors often have somatic mutations in the *MEN1* gene.
- Approximately one-third of patients with gastrinoma have metastatic disease at diagnosis.

Diagnosis and Clinical Presentation

▪ Patients typically present with severe, often refractory peptic ulcer disease accompanied by abdominal pain and diarrhea.
▪ Diagnosis is made by a fasting gastrin level: >1,000 pg/mL with a gastric acid pH <5.0 or gastrin level that increases by ≥200 pg/mL within 15 minutes of intravenous infusion of secretin.
▪ Other common diagnostic procedures include ultrasonography, CT scan, MRI, endoscopic ultrasonography, angiography, and octreotide scan.

Treatment

▪ Medical therapy is standard for gastrinoma associated with MEN 1, given that tumors are often multifocal and incurable. Some surgeons will offer resection with the intent of reducing future morbidity from metastatic disease.
▪ Surgical resection with exploratory laparotomy is curative in up to 50% of patients with sporadic gastrinoma without metastatic disease.
▪ The goal of medical therapy is to control gastrin secretion and acid production. Therapies include proton pump inhibitors, somatostatin analogs (e.g., octreotide), and tumor embolization.
▪ Both sunitinib and everolimus were approved for the treatment of progressive, well-differentiated pancreatic NETs. Approval was based on improved PFS.
▪ Cytotoxic chemotherapy can also be used for metastatic disease. Active chemotherapeutic agents include streptozotocin, doxorubicin, temozolomide, 5-fluorouracil, and dacarbazine.
▪ See Table 33.3 for detailed chemotherapy regimens.
▪ For those patients with liver metastases, liver-directed therapies such as embolization, radiofrequency ablation, and cryosurgery are options.

Insulinoma

Epidemiology

▪ Insulinoma is the most common type of functioning pancreatic NET.
▪ It occurs most commonly in the fifth decade of life, with a slight female predominance.
▪ Most insulinomas are solitary and approximately 10% are malignant, as defined by the presence of metastases.

Diagnosis and Clinical Presentation

▪ Three criteria, known as Whipple triad, suggest insulinoma:
  ● Symptoms known or likely to be caused by hypoglycemia (confusion, personality change, palpitations, diaphoresis, tremulousness)
  ● Hypoglycemia during symptoms
  ● Relief of hypoglycemia symptoms when glucose is raised to normal
▪ An inappropriately high level of insulin during an episode of hypoglycemia establishes the presence of insulinoma.
▪ Asymptomatic patients may be diagnosed after prolonged fasting by testing levels of serum glucose, insulin, and C-peptide every 6 to 12 hours.

Treatment

▪ Surgery is the treatment of choice for insulinoma and is most often curative.
▪ Patients with recurrent disease that includes liver metastases can be treated with surgical resection (when possible) or liver-directed therapy such as chemoembolization or radiofrequency ablation.
▪ Refractory hypoglycemia can be treated with oral diazoxide, which inhibits pancreatic secretion of insulin and stimulates release of catecholamine and glucose from the liver.
▪ Both sunitinib and everolimus have been approved for the treatment of progressive, well-differentiated pancreatic NETs. Approval was based on improved PFS.

- Cytotoxic chemotherapy can also be used for metastatic disease. Active chemotherapeutic agents include streptozotocin, doxorubicin, temozolomide, 5-fluoruracil, and dacarbazine.
- See Table 33.3 for detailed chemotherapy regimens.

VIPoma (Verner-morrison Syndrome)

- VIPoma is a rare NET that usually originates in the pancreas and produces vasoactive intestinal peptide (VIP).
- Elevated serum VIP establishes the presence of VIPoma.
- Patients present with watery diarrhea, hypokalemia, and hypo- or achlorhydria.
- Diarrhea may be treated effectively with somatostatin analogs, which decrease VIP secretion. Interferon-α can also be used.
- Patients with recurrent disease that includes liver metastases can be treated with surgical resection (when possible) or liver-directed therapy such as chemoembolization or radiofrequency ablation.
- Both sunitinib and everolimus have been approved for the treatment of progressive, well-differentiated pancreatic NETs. Approval was based on improved PFS. See Table 33.3 for detailed chemotherapy regimens.

Glucagonoma

- Glucagonoma is a rare tumor of the pancreas that results in overproduction of the hormone glucagon.
- Serum levels of glucagon >500 pg/mL are diagnostic of glucagonoma.
- Glucagonoma leads to diabetes, weight loss, anemia, and increased risk of thromboembolism.
- Patients commonly present with necrolytic migratory erythema, which may be treated with zinc supplements and amino acid infusion.
- Surgery, somatostatin analogs, anticoagulants, and targeted therapy/chemotherapy (as described for the other pancreatic NETs) are therapeutic options for glucagonomas.

Somatostatinoma

- Somatostatinoma is a tumor of the endocrine pancreas that secretes excess somatostatin. The tumor inhibits secretion of insulin, other pancreatic hormones, pancreatic enzymes, and gastric acid production.
- Surgery is the treatment of choice, but targeted therapy/chemotherapy (as described for the other pancreatic NETs) is indicated for unresectable disease.

ADRENOCORTICAL CARCINOMA

Epidemiology

- ACC is a rare malignancy arising from the adrenal cortex, with 1.5 to 2 cases per million population per year.
- It has a bimodal age distribution, with a first peak in children younger than 5 years and a second peak in adults in their fourth to fifth decade.
- ACC remains a difficult to treat disease, with a 5-year survival of 10% to 25% and an average survival from diagnosis of ≈14.5 months.
- Most cases are sporadic, but it can be a component of a hereditary syndrome (Li-Fraumeni syndrome, Beckwith-Wiedemann syndrome, MEN-1) (see Table 33.1).

Clinical Presentation

Symptoms may arise from the effects of local mass or distant metastases. Approximately 50% of patients present with evidence of hormonal excess consisting of

- Hypercortisolism (Cushing syndrome)
- Virilization/feminization
- Mineralocorticoid excess

Diagnosis

- Imaging studies can usually distinguish benign adenomas from ACC. Because ACC have lower lipid content than benign adenomas they usually have higher density values on CT scans; while on MRI they are usually iso-intense with liver on T1 images, and have intermediate to high intensity on T2 images.
- Biochemical evaluation (urinary steroids and suppression tests) should be conducted if clinically warranted.
- FNA cannot differentiate an adrenal adenoma from ACC, and should only be done if the adrenal mass is suspected to be a metastasis from another malignancy.
- Diagnosis is often confirmed upon surgical resection; however, histologic differentiation of adrenocortical adenomas and carcinomas is challenging.
- Carcinomas tend to display mitotic activity, aneuploidy, and venous invasion. Carcinomas may also secrete abnormal amounts of androgens and 11-deoxysteroids.

Treatment

Surgery

- A tumor with local invasion and nodal involvement, tumor invading adjacent organs, or any tumor with distant metastases constitutes stage IV disease.
- En bloc resection is initially appropriate for stages I to III.
- Debulking of unresectable or stage IV disease should be considered, particularly for symptom relief from hormone-secreting tumors; local recurrence and metastatic disease require further resection when feasible.
- In general, adrenal tumors >6 cm (or <6 cm but suspected of being malignant) should be resected via open adrenalectomy. Because surgery remains the only proven curative option for a patient with ACC it must always be aggressively pursued at presentation and at relapse and a laparoscopic approach should never be used.

Adjuvant Therapy

- Adjuvant mitotane may improve survival for patients with stage I to III disease who have undergone a complete resection.
- Several small and one large retrospective studies suggest mitotane given as an adjuvant therapy and continued indefinitely can at a minimum delay and possibly prevent a recurrence of disease.
- Replacement steroids can be started with the initiation of mitotane or when clinical and laboratory parameters indicate adrenal insufficiency. Both fludrocortisone and hydrocortisone should be given.
- An international prospective randomized trial comparing mitotane to placebo in this patient population is currently ongoing.

Advanced Disease

- For advanced disease, mitotane monotherapy induces hormonal response rates in up to 75% of patients with functional tumors, with no change in OS.
- Combination chemotherapy with mitotane plus etoposide, doxorubicin, and cisplatin (EDP) demonstrated better rates of response and disease-free survival (DFS) than mitotane plus streptozotocin in patients with advanced disease based on the FIRM-ACT trial (**F**irst **I**nternational **R**andomized trial in locally advanced and **M**etastatic **A**drenocortical **C**arcinoma **T**reatment). The study found a significantly better response rate (23.2% vs. 9.2%, $P<0.001$) and PFS (5.0 months vs. 2.1 months; hazard ratio, 0.55; $P<0.001$) with EDP plus mitotane than with streptozocin plus mitotane as first-line therapy, with similar rates of toxic events.
- Radiofrequency ablation may also be implemented for local control or metastases in patients with unresectable disease.
- See Table 33.4 for detailed chemotherapy regimens.

PARATHYROID CARCINOMA

Clinically, it is important to distinguish this disease from other benign disorders that cause hyperparathyroidism. Parathyroid carcinoma accounts for less than 1% of cases of hyperparathyroidism.

Epidemiology and Natural History

- Parathyroid carcinoma occurs in <1 per million individuals per year, predominantly diagnosed in the fifth or sixth decade of life.
- Germline or somatic mutations of the *HRPT2* tumor suppressor gene are detected in the majority of cases.
- Ten-year survival rate is approximately 70%; however, 40% to 60% will recur after initial surgery.
- Morbidity and mortality are usually related to hypercalcemia rather than complications of metastases.

Clinical Presentation

Patients typically present with the following:

- Symptoms of hypercalcemia, with calcium levels usually >14 mg/dL
- Elevated parathyroid hormone levels
- Palpable neck mass in up to 70%
- Metastases to cervical lymph nodes, lungs bone, or liver in approximately 10%

Diagnosis

- Parathyroid carcinoma is difficult to diagnose preoperatively; differential includes parathyroid adenoma and hyperplasia.
- Most parathyroid carcinomas are diagnosed at surgery; however, some are not diagnosed until local recurrence or metastases. This is because there are no definitive histopathologic features to differentiate carcinoma from adenoma.
- FNA is inappropriate for diagnosis.

Treatment

Surgery

- Treatment consists of parathyroidectomy with en bloc resection of tumor and involved structures. This may include the ipsilateral lobe of thyroid. Radical lymph node dissection is not recommended.
- Recurrent tumor and oligometastases should also be resected.

Radiation

- Parathyroid tumors are generally not radiosensitive.
- Small retrospective studies suggest there may be improved local control with postoperative radiotherapy for high-risk patients.
- Radiation may have palliative benefit.

Medical Therapy

- Chemotherapy efficacy is limited to case reports, and there is no standard regimen.
- Management of hypercalcemia is essential while treating parathyroid carcinoma.

Suggested Readings

1. Abeloff M, Armitage J, Niederhuber J, Kastan M, McKenna W, eds. *Abeloff: Clinical Oncology.* 4th ed. Philadelphia, PA: Elsevier; 2008.
2. Amar L, Bertherat J, Baudin E, et al. Genetic testing in pheochromocytoma or functional paraganglioma. *J Clin Oncol.* 2005; 23:8812–8818.
3. Cooper DS, Doherty GM, Haugen BR, et al. Revised American Thyroid Association management guidelines for patients with thyroid nodules and differentiated thyroid cancer. *Thyroid.* 2009;19(11):1167–1214.

4. Falconi M, Bartsch DK, Eriksson B, et al. ENETS Consensus Guidelines for the management of patients with diges-tive neuroendocrine neoplasms of the digestive system: well-differentiated pancreatic non-functioning tumors. *Neuroendocrinology*. 2012;95(2):120–134.

5. Fassnacht M, Terzolo M, Allolio B, et al. Combination chemotherapy in advanced adrenocortical carcinoma. *N Engl J Med*. 2012;366:2189–2197.

6. Goldstein RE, O'Neill JA Jr., Holcomb GW 3rd, et al. Clinical experience over 48 years with pheochromocytoma. *Ann Surg*. 1999;229(6):755.

7. Haugen BR, Alexander EK, Bible KC, et al. 2015 American Thyroid Association management guidelines for adult patients with thyroid nodules and differentiated thyroid cancer: The American Thyroid Association guidelines task force on thy-roid nodules and differentiated thyroid cancer. *Thyroid*. 2016 Jan;26(1):1–133.

8. Hemminki K, Li X. Incidence trends and risk factors of carcinoid tumors: a nationwide epidemiologic study from Sweden. *Cancer*. 2001;92(8):2204.

9. Hundahl SA, Fleming ID, Fremgen AM, Menck HR. A National Cancer Data Base report on 53,856 cases of thyroid car-cinoma treated in the U.S., 1985–1995. *Cancer*. 1998;83:2638–2648.

10. Kloos RT, Eng C, Evans DB, et al. Medullary thyroid cancer: management guidelines of the American Thyroid Association. *Thyroid*. 2009;19:565–612.

11. Kulke MH, Hörsch D, Caplin ME, et al. Telotristat ethyl, a tryptophan hydroxylase inhibitor for the treatment of carcinoid syndrome. *J Clin Oncol*. 2017 Jan;35(1):14–23.

12. Kurzrock R, Sherman SI, Ball DW, et al. Activity of XL184 (Cabozantinib), an oral tyrosine kinase inhibitor, in patients with medullary thyroid cancer. *J Clin Oncol*. 2011;29:2660–2666.

13. Lodish MB, Stratakis CA. Rare and unusual endocrine cancer syndromes with mutated genes. *Semin Oncol*. 2010;37(6):680–690.

14. Luton JP, Cerdas S, Billaud L, et al. Clinical features of adrenocortical carcinoma, prognostic factors, and the effect of mitotane therapy. *N Engl J Med*. 1990;322:1195–1201.

15. Martucci V, Pacak K. Pheochormoyctoma and paragnglioma: Diagnosis, genetics, management and treatment. *Current Problems in Cancer*. 2014; 38:7–41.

16. Moertel CG, Lefkopoulo M, Lipsits S, et al. Streptozocin-doxorubicin, streptozocin-fluorouracil or chlorozotocin in the treatment of advanced islet-cell carcinoma. *N Engl J Med*. 1992;326(8):519–523.

17. Nikiforov YE, Nikiforova MN. Molecular genetics and diagnosis of thyroid cancer. *Nat Rev Endocrinol*. 2011;7(10):569–580.

18. Pacak K, Del Rivero J. Pheochromocytoma. Endotext [Internet]. South Dartmouth (MA): MDText.com, Inc.; 2000–2013 Jun 10.

19. Raymond E, Dahan L, Raoul JL, et al. Sunitinib malate for the treatment of pancreatic neuroendocrine tumors. *N Engl J Med*. 2011;364(6):501–513.

20. Schlumberger MJ. Papillary and follicular thyroid carcinoma. *N Engl J Med*. 1998;338:297–308.

21. Schlumberger M, Tahara M, Wirth LJ, et al. Lenvatinib versus placebo in radioiodine-refractory thyroid cancer. *N Engl J Med*. 2015 Feb 12;372(7):621–630.

22. Sherman SI. Thyroid carcinoma. *Lancet*. 2003;231:501–511.

23. Strosberg JR. Update on the management of unusual neuroendocrine tumors: pheochromocytoma and paraganglioma, medullary thyroid cancer and adrenocortical carcinoma. *Semin Oncol*. 2013;40(1):120–133.

24. Strosberg JR, Fine RL, Choi J, et al. First-line chemotherapy with capecitabine and temozolomide in patients with meta-static pancreatic endocrine carcinomas. *Cancer*. 2011;117(2):268–275.

25. Veytsman I, Nieman L, Fojo T. Management of endocrine manifestations and the use of mitotane as a chemotherapeutic agent for adrenocortical carcinoma. *J Clin Oncol*. 2009;27(27):4619–4629.

26. Wells SA, Robinson BG, Gagel RF, et al. Vandetanib in patients with locally advanced or metastatic medullary thyroid cancer: a randomized, double-blind phase III trial. *J Clin Oncol*. 2012; 30:134–141.

27. Wells SA Jr, Asa SL, Dralle H, et al. American Thyroid Association Guidelines task force on medullary thyroid carcinoma. Revised American Thyroid Association guidelines for the management of medullary thyroid carcinoma. *Thyroid*. 2015; 25:567–610.

28. Worden F, Fassnacht M, Shi Y, et al. Safety and tolerability of sorafenib in patients with radioiodine-refractory thyroid cancer. *Endocr Relat Cancer*. 2015

29. Yao JC, Hassan M, Phan A, et al. One hundred years after "carcinoid": epidemiology of and prognostic factors for neuro-endocrine tumors in 35,825 cases in the United States. *J Clin Oncol*. 2008;26(18):3063.

30. Yao JC, Shah MH, Ito T, et al. Everolimus for advanced pancreatic neuroendocrine tumors. *N Engl J Med*. 2011;364(6):514–523.

34 Hematopoietic Growth Factors

Philip M. Arlen and Andreas Niethammer

BACKGROUND

- Hematologic toxicity (leukopenia, anemia, and thrombocytopenia) is the most common side effect of chemotherapy and large field radiotherapy. Further, cytopenia is inherent to stem cell transplantation. It can lead to serious complications, such as neutropenic fever, which may require hospitalization.
- Hematopoietic growth factors are the regulatory molecules that stimulate the proliferation, differentiation, and survival of hematopoietic progenitor and stem cells. They were originally called colony-stimulating factors (CSFs) because of their role in colony formation in bone marrow cell cultures.
- Several hematopoietic growth factors are currently available for clinical use and are synthesized mainly by DNA recombinant technology.
- Recommendations in this chapter come primarily from the evidence-based clinical practice guidelines of the American Society of Clinical Oncology (ASCO), National Comprehensive Cancer Network (NCCN), and the American Society of Hematology (ASH).

MYELOID GROWTH FACTORS

- Currently, two myeloid growth factors, filgrastim and pegfilgrastim, both of which are granulocyte-colony stimulating factors (G-CSF), have been approved by the U.S. Food and Drug Administration (FDA) for use in prevention of chemotherapy-induced neutropenia. Filgrastim is specific for production of neutrophils, but has immunomodulatory effects on lymphocytes, monocytes, and macrophages. Anti-inflammatory effects have also been described for G-CSF. Pegfilgrastim is a pegylated form of filgrastim and has a longer half-life ranging from 15 to 80 hours.
- Sargramostim is a granulocyte-macrophage colony-stimulating factor (GM-CSF) that stimulates the production of monocytes and eosinophils, in addition to neutrophils, and prolongs their half-lives. It also enhances their function through activation of chemotaxis, phagocytosis, oxidative activity, and antibody-dependent cellular cytotoxicity. The labeled clinical indication is for use to shorten the time to neutrophil recovery following induction chemotherapy in older adult patients with acute myelogenous leukemia and other various stem cell transplantation settings.

INDICATIONS

Primary Prophylaxis

CSFs are recommended for use with first- and subsequent-cycle chemotherapy to prevent febrile neutropenia (FN) when risk of FN is high (>20%). Although no nomogram exists to calculate this risk, factors to consider determining a patient's risk of FN include type of chemotherapy regimen (dose-dense therapy, high-dose therapy, standard-dose therapy), goal of therapy (palliative or curative), and patient's risk factors including the following:

- Age above 65
- Poor performance status

- Extensive prior treatments, including large-port radiation
- Previous episodes of FN
- Cytopenia due to bone marrow involvement by tumor
- Advanced cancer
- Active infections or presence of open wounds
- Poor nutritional status
- Other serious comorbidities, or renal or liver dysfunction
- Neutropenia
- HIV-infected patient

Several placebo-controlled randomized controlled trials have shown that the prophylactic use of G-CSFs has been shown to reduce the incidence, length, and severity of chemotherapy-related neutropenia in various solid tumor types. Dose-dense chemotherapy regimens supported by G-CSF had shown superior clinical outcome compared to conventional chemotherapy in adjuvant treatment of node-positive breast cancer, and in elderly patients with aggressive lymphoma. Cochrane meta-analyses of 2607 randomized lymphoma patients from 13 trials reported that G-CSF and GM-CSF as a prophylaxis reduced the risk of neutropenia, FN, and infection. However, there was no evidence that either G-CSF or GM-CSF provide a significant benefit in terms of tumor response, freedom from treatment failure, or overall survival.

Secondary Prophylaxis

The guidelines recommend administering CSFs to patients who experienced febrile neutropenia or dose-limiting neutropenic event in a prior cycle of chemotherapy when no CSFs were given and a repeat of which episode could impact the next planned dose of chemotherapy . Dose reduction and treatment delay, however, are reasonable alternatives, especially in the palliative setting.

Neutropenic Fever

Routine adjunctive use of CSFs for FN is not recommended. CSFs should be considered in patients with FN who are at high risk for infection-associated complications, or who have prognostic factors that are predictive of poor clinical outcomes. High-risk features include the following:

- Age above 65
- Expected prolonged (more than 10 days)
- Profound (<100/mcl) neutropenia
- Sepsis syndrome
- Being hospitalized at the time of the development of fever
- Pneumonia
- Invasive fungal infection
- Uncontrolled primary disease

A multicenter randomized trial demonstrated that therapeutic G-CSF shortens hospital stay (median, 5 days versus 7 days; $P = 0.015$), antibiotic therapy (median, 5 days versus 6 days; $P = 0.013$), duration of grade 4 neutropenia (median, 2 days versus 3 days; $P = 0.0004$) in 210 solid tumor patients with febrile neutropenia, and at least one high-risk feature. Cochrane meta-analysis of 1518 patients from 13 trials reported that therapeutic CSF was associated with shorter hospital stay, duration of neutropenia, but no improvement in overall survival.

Hematopoietic Stem Cell Transplantation

CSFs are used routinely to mobilize peripheral blood stem cell (PBSC) and to shorten the duration of neutropenia after cytoreduction and autologous PBSC transplantation. Post auto-transplantation use of CSFs has been associated with shorter duration of neutropenia and hospitalization, and reduced medical costs. In contrast, CSFs used after allogeneic transplantation have been reported to increase the risk of severe graft-versus-host disease and to reduce survival.

For mobilization of stem cells before harvesting from the healthy donor or the patient before autologous stem cell transplant, different protocols exist.

Mobilizing stem cells typically involves daily injections of filgrastim with the most common adverse events being bone pain and allergic reactions. While initially there was a concern about secondary leukemia in subjects having received G-CSF, large studies show no increase in incidence. Severe side effects are rare with less than 1% of donors experiencing such toxicity. In a review by the National Marrow Donor Program, among >23,000 subjects having donated peripheral stem cells, 4 fatalities were observed and 37 severe adverse events. The incidence of hematologic malignancies in follow up (n=12) did not exceed the expected incidence in the adjusted general population. (Halter et al).

Leukemia and Myelodysplastic Syndromes

- In patients with acute myeloid leukemia (AML), CSFs can be used in two settings: (1) after completion of induction chemotherapy, and (2) after completion of consolidation chemotherapy. Use of G-CSF shortly after completion of induction chemotherapy can lead to a modest decrease in neutropenia duration, but has not shown to have favorable effect on remission rate, duration, or survival. Use of G-CSF after completion of consolidation chemotherapy seems to have a more profound beneficial effect on the duration of neutropenia and the rate of serious infections. However, no effect on complete response duration or overall survival can be observed. Indeed, a recent Cochrane meta-analysis including 5256 AML patients in 19 trials reported that the addition of CSFs did not alter all-cause mortality in the short and long term. In this meta-analysis, the administration of CSFs did not affect the occurrence of episodes of neutropenic fever, bacteremias, or invasive fungal infections. Thus, currently, there are insufficient data to support the use of CSF for leukemia priming effects. Likewise, insufficient data exist to support the use of long-acting CSF (pegfilgrastim) in AML.
- In myelodysplastic syndrome (MDS), intermittent use of CSFs may be considered in patients with severe neutropenia complicated by recurrent infections. There are no data on the safety of long-term use.
- In acute lymphoblastic leukemia (ALL), CSFs are recommended after the completion of the initial induction or first post-remission chemotherapy course to shorten the duration of neutropenia. Their effect on duration of hospitalization and acquisition of serious infections are less consistent.

SIDE EFFECTS

Bone pain is frequently encountered with the use of myeloid growth factors. Rarely, splenic rupture and severe thrombocytopenia have been reported. CSFs may cause a transient acute respiratory distress syndrome or inflammatory pleuritis and pericarditis, which are thought to be secondary to neutrophil influx or capillary leak syndrome. In patients with sickle cell disease, use of CSFs has led to severe sickle cell crisis, resulting in death in some cases. Concurrent use of CSFs with chemotherapy and radiation therapy should be avoided because of the potential sensitivity of rapidly dividing myeloid cells to cytotoxic chemotherapy. In addition, CSFs should be avoided in patients receiving concomitant chemoradiotherapy, particularly involving the mediastinum. This is because of observation that patients receiving CSF support while being treated with concurrent chemoradiotherapy for lung cancers had more significant thrombocytopenia and increased pulmonary toxicities compared to patients in placebo arms. These findings suggested potential for an adverse interaction between mediastinal radiotherapy and CSF administration.

GM-CSF

- May cause flulike symptoms, fever, and rash.
- There is in vitro evidence that GM-CSF may stimulate HIV replication; however, clinical studies have not shown adverse effects on viral load among patients on antiretroviral therapy.
- The liquid form of sargramostim was withdrawn from the market in January 2008 because of the increased reports of syncope, which was not seen with the lyophilized formulation.

G-CSF

- In general, G-CSF is better tolerated than GM-CSF and is used more commonly.
- May rarely cause pathologic neutrophil infiltration (sweet syndrome).
- Antibodies to growth factors have been detected with some preparations, but are not neutralizing.
- Fragmentary evidence has raised concerns for increased risk of late monosomy 7-associated MDS and AML in patients with aplastic anemia treated with long-term G-CSF.

DOSING

- Recommended dosing of CSFs is listed in Table 34.1.
- In chemotherapy patients, transient increase in neutrophil count is typically observed in the first 1 to 2 days after initiation of CSFs. Treatment should continue until post-nadir ANC reaches 10,000/ mm^3. Check complete blood count twice weekly.
- Pegfilgrastim should not be administered from 14 days before to 24 hours after myelosuppressive chemotherapy.
- Sargramostim is licensed for use after autologous or allogeneic bone marrow transplant and for AML.

2015 American Society of Clinical Oncology (ASCO) Clinical Practice Guidelines on the Use of Hematopoietic Colony-stimulating Factors (CSFs)

Key points include the following:

- Patients with a greater than 20% risk of febrile neutropenia, primary prophylaxis with CSF with first and subsequent cycles of chemotherapy is recommended. Regimens that do not require CSF and are equally effective should be considered as well.
- Patients with a neutropenic complication from a previous cycle of chemotherapy (without primary prophylaxis) and reduction or delay in treatment would alter outcome/survival, CSF is recommended for secondary prophylaxis. However, a reduction/delay may be reasonable in many.
- Adjunctive treatment of CSFs with antibiotics should not be routinely used for patients with febrile neutropenia. However, patients with febrile neutropenia who are considered at risk for poor outcomes or infection-related complications may be considered for adjunctive treatment with CSFs.
- In order to mobilize peripheral-blood progenitor cells, CSFs may be used with plerixafor, after chemotherapy, or alone.
- To lessen the duration of severe neutropenia, CSFs should be given after autologous stem-cell transplants.
- To lessen the duration of severe neutropenia, CSFs may be given after allogeneic stem-cell transplants. Since the 2006 update, reports of increased risk of grade 2 to 4 graft-versus-host disease with CSF use after allogeneic transplantation have not been confirmed.
- Patients aged 65 or older, particularly those with comorbidities, with aggressive forms of diffuse lymphoma treated with curative chemotherapy should be considered for CSF prophylaxis.
- Pediatric patients—CSFs for primary prophylaxis is considered reasonable in patients at high risk for febrile neutropenia. Secondary prophylaxis should be limited to patients who are at high risk.
- CSFs should be used in pediatric patients to facilitate dose-intense chemotherapy regimens that are known to have survival benefits (Ewing sarcoma).
- The guidelines do not recommend using CSFs in nonrelapsed acute myeloid leukemia or nonrelapsed acute lymphocytic leukemia in pediatric patients without infection.

ERYTHROPOIESIS-STIMULATING AGENTS

Erythropoiesis-stimulating agents (ESAs) are semisynthetic agents that simulate the effects of erythropoietin (EPO), an endogenous hormone produced by the kidneys. By binding to EPO receptors, ESAs stimulate the division and differentiation of committed erythroid progenitors in bone marrow. ESAs are

TABLE 34.1 Growth Factors for Transplant or Nonmyeloid Cancer Patients Only: FDA-approved Dosing and Indications

Drug	Dosing	Indications
Filgrastim (Neupogen)	5 µg/kg SC daily 24 h after completion of chemotherapy until ANC reaches 2,000 to 3,000/mm³ 10 µg/kg SC daily at least 4 d before the first leukapheresis; continue until the last leukapheresis	Myelosuppressive chemotherapy PBSC mobilization
Pegfilgrastim (Neulasta)	Single 6-mg fixed dose SC 24 h after completion of chemotherapy	Myelosuppressive chemotherapy
Sargramostim (Leukine)	250 µg/mm² i.v. daily until ANC reaches 1,500/mm³ for 3 consecutive days; reduce dose by 50% if ANC increases to >20,000/mm³	Auto/allo BMT, after AML induction chemotherapy
Epoetin alfa (Epogen; Procrit)	Start at 150 U/kg SC TIW or 40,000 U SC weekly	Chemotherapy-induced anemia
	Escalate dose to 300 U/kg TIW or 60,000 U SC weekly if Hb rises <1 gm/dL in 4 wks and remains below 10 gm/dl, no reduction in transfusion requirements or rise in Hb after 8 wk (for TIW dosing) Reduce dose by 25% when Hb reaches level needed to avoid transfusion or Hb rises >1 g/dL in 2 wk ▪ Hold when Hb rises to a level where transfusions may be required; resume at 25% below previous dose when Hb reaches level where transfusion may be required	
Darbepoetin alfa (Aranesp)	Start at 2.25 mcg/kg SC weekly or 500 mcg SC Q3W Escalate dose to 4.5 mcg/kg if Hb rises >1 g/dL after 6 wk Reduce dose by 40% of previous dose when Hb reaches level needed to avoid transfusion or Hb rises >1 g/dL in 2 wk Hold if Hb exceeds a level needed to avoid a blood transfusion. Resume at 40% below previous dose.	Chemotherapy-induced anemia
Oprelvekin (Neumega)	50 mcg/kg SC daily; start 6 to 24 h after completion of chemotherapy and continue until post-nadir platelet count is >50,000/mm³	Nonmyeloablative chemotherapy-induced thrombocytopenia

AML, acute myeloid leukemia; ANC, absolute neutrophil count; auto/allo BMT, autologous/allogeneic bone marrow transplant; d, days; ESA, erythropoiesis-stimulating agent; FDA, U.S. Food and Drug Administration; h, hours; Hb, hemoglobin; i.v., intravenously; PBSC, peripheral blood stem cell; Q3W, every 3 weeks; SC, subcutaneously; TIW, three times per week; wk, weeks.

manufactured by recombinant DNA technology and are available as epoetin alfa and darbepoetin alfa. Darbepoetin alfa has a half-life around three times longer than that of epoetin alfa; however, they are considered equivalent in terms of effectiveness and safety.

EFFECTS

▪ ESAs were first used to manage anemia in patients with chronic renal failure (CRF). Several randomized clinical trials have demonstrated that ESAs decrease blood transfusion requirements and improve the quality of life in patients on hemodialysis.

- In cancer patients undergoing chemotherapy, ESAs have been shown to reduce the need for transfusions, but their effects on anemia symptoms and quality of life have not been proven.
- A growing body of evidence has raised serious concerns about the safety of ESAs.

Transfusion Requirements and Quality of Life

A recent systematic review summarized the results of 57 trials involving 9,353 cancer patients randomly assigned to receive ESA plus RBC transfusion or transfusion alone. This meta-analysis included patients who did and patients who did not receive concurrent antineoplastic therapy. Results showed a 36% reduction in transfusion requirement in those receiving ESA. Although there was a positive overall effect on quality of life, the report could not draw definite conclusions because of the differing parameters used by the various studies.

Survival, Mortality, and Disease Control

- Observational studies have suggested that anemia in cancer patients is associated with shorter survival and that increasing hemoglobin (Hb) levels may improve survival and tumor response in some cancers. Because radiation and some chemotherapy agents are dependent on tissue oxygenation for their effect, it was speculated that improving oxygen delivery by increasing Hb levels may optimize the effects of antineoplastic treatments. Based on this hypothesis, several randomized trials in head and neck, breast, non-small cell lung, lymphoid, and cervical cancers were conducted to evaluate the effect of ESAs on survival and disease control. Most of these studies were terminated prematurely because of disease progression and increased mortality. A preliminary report of a study using ESAs in cancer patients not receiving chemotherapy showed no reduced need for blood transfusions; it did, however, show increased mortality. Based on this report, the FDA released a black box safety alert in February 2007 warning against the use of ESAs for anemia in cancer patients not receiving chemotherapy. The FDA also recommended a minimum effective dose of ESAs that would gradually increase Hb levels sufficient to avoid transfusion, but not to exceed 12 g/dL. Most of the ESA trials had set a goal of Hb >12 g/dL; however, the risks of shortened survival and TTP have persisted even when ESAs are dosed to achieve Hb levels >12 g/dL. An updated meta-analysis of 53 RCTs and 13,933 cancer patients looked for mortality as the primary end point and found ESAs to be associated with significantly greater overall on-study mortality. In those with chemotherapy-induced anemia (n = 10,441), a statistically significant mortality change could not be demonstrated. Poor outcomes could not be consistently attributed to a single mechanism.
- It has been suggested that shorter TTP could be attributed to EPO receptor-positive tumors. However, currently available assays to detect EPO receptors are nonspecific and their validity has not been determined.
- In July 2007, the Centers for Medicare and Medicaid Services revised their national coverage guidelines to limit reimbursement of ESAs. Coverage of ESAs in cancer patients is now restricted to those receiving chemotherapy whose Hb level is 10 g/dL or lower prior to initiation of ESA treatment.
- Increased mortality and adverse events have also been observed in CRF patients, which have led to lower Hb targets in this patient population.

INDICATIONS
ASCO and ASH Guidelines

In non-myeloid cancers, ESAs should be considered as one of the many options in patients receiving chemotherapy whose anemia is symptomatic and chemotherapy related. The goals are avoidance of blood transfusions and possible symptomatic benefit. ESAs can be initiated if Hb falls below 10. For Hb levels between 10 and 12, use of ESAs should only be based on symptoms, clinical circumstances, and patient preference. If there is no response after 6 to 8 weeks with appropriate dose modification, treatment should be discontinued. Blood transfusion is a therapeutic option.

FDA-approved Indications

ESAs are approved for chemotherapy-related anemia in non-myeloid malignancies treated with palliative intent, CRF, HIV (zidovudine) therapy, and to reduce the need for blood transfusion in elective non-cardiac and nonvascular surgeries.

Off-Label/Investigational Use

- There is evidence supporting the use of ESAs for anemia related to MDS. However, patients may require higher doses and response may be delayed. Predictors of response include low-risk MDS and low EPO levels (200 U/L). Combining ESAs and G-CSF in MDS patients has resulted in improved response rates.
- Other indications include multiple myeloma, non-Hodgkin's lymphoma, chronic lymphocytic leukemia, beta thalassemia, radiation therapy, rheumatoid arthritis, paroxysmal nocturnal hemoglobinuria, Castleman's disease, congestive heart failure, critical illnesses, hepatitis C (in patients treated with interferon-alfa and ribavirin), and blood-unit collection for auto-transfusion.

DOSING

Recommended dosing and dose adjustments of ESAs in chemotherapy-induced anemia are listed in Table 34.1. After initiation or dose modification of ESAs, Hb should be monitored weekly until it stabilizes.

SIDE EFFECTS

- The most serious side effects of ESAs are thromboembolic events, defined as transient ischemic attack, stroke, pulmonary emboli, deep vein thrombosis, and myocardial infarction. A meta-analysis showed that thromboembolic events increased 67% in cancer patients; for a population with baseline risk of 20%, the number needed to harm would be 7.5 patients (95% CI, 3.1 to 15.6). There is evidence for increased risk of thromboembolic events in CRF and surgical patients, especially with higher Hb targets. Preliminary analysis of a trial in spinal surgery patients given ESAs to decrease post-surgery transfusion requirements showed increased incidence of thromboembolic events in the ESA arm. Notably, patients received no prophylactic anticoagulants postoperatively.
- ESAs are contraindicated in uncontrolled hypertension, more commonly seen in CRF patients who receive i.v. ESAs.
- Other side effects include headache, fatigue, fever, rash, pruritus, hypersensitivity reactions, arthralgia and myalgia, nausea, seizures, and pure red-cell aplasia due to neutralizing antibodies to native EPO.

OTHER CONSIDERATIONS

- Iron supplementation should be considered in patients receiving ESAs, especially those with borderline iron stores, because iron deficiency can develop soon after initiation of ESAs and can adversely affect response to ESAs. Data from multiple controlled trials have shown that I.V. iron can enhance ESA efficacy and can reduce the required dose in cancer patients.
- Measuring serum EPO levels may help to identify patients more likely to respond to ESAs. Patients with baseline EPO levels 100 U/L are more likely to respond to ESAs than those with levels 100 U/L.

PLATELET GROWTH FACTORS

- Thrombocytopenia can be a life-threatening consequence of antineoplastic treatments. Platelet transfusions are required to prevent or mitigate hemorrhagic complications. Due to the short life span of

thrombocytes, transfusion necessity may arise as frequently as on a weekly bases. Patients at high risk for bleeding or who experience delays in receiving planned chemotherapy include the following:
- Patients with poor bone marrow reserve or a history of bleeding
- Patients on treatment regimens highly toxic to bone marrow
- Patients with a potential bleeding site (e.g., necrotic tumor)

- Fortunately, iatrogenic thrombocytopenia that requires platelet transfusion or causes major bleeding is relatively uncommon, although occurrence tends to increase with cumulative cycles of chemotherapy that are toxic to hematopoietic progenitor cells. At present, formal guidelines for the use of thrombopoietic growth factors are under development.

- Although several thrombopoietic agents are in clinical development, oprelvekin is the only thrombocytopoietic agent FDA-approved for clinical use in non-myeloid malignancies with chemotherapy-induced anemia. Oprelvekin is a product of recombinant DNA technology and is nearly homologous with native IL-11. Oprelvekin stimulates megakaryocytopoiesis and thrombopoiesis, and has been shown to modestly shorten the duration of thrombocytopenia and reduce the need for platelet transfusions in patients who develop platelet counts <20 X103 per mcL after prior antineoplastic treatments. Oprelvekin is not indicated following myeloablative chemotherapy.

Major side effects include fluid retention and atrial arrhythmias. Hypersensitivity reactions, including anaphylaxis, have also been reported. Table 34.1 provides the recommended dose of oprelvekin.

Recombinant thrombopoietins (TPOs) are no longer being developed because of antibody production. TPO mimetics (TPO receptor agonists) are currently under investigation.

Suggested Readings

1. American Society of Clinical Oncology. Cancer.Net. Donating Bone Marrow. 02/2015. http://www.cancer.net/navigating-cancer-care/diagnosing-cancer/tests-and-procedures/donating-bone-marrow
2. Bohlius J, Herbst C, Reiser M, Schwarzer G, Engert A. Granulopoiesis-stimulating factors to prevent adverse effects in the treatment of malignant lymphoma. *Cochrane Database Syst Rev.* 2008;(4):CD003189
3. Bohlius J, Schmidlin K, Brillant C, et al. Erythropoietin or darbepoetin for patients with cancer: Meta-analysis based on individual patient data. *Cochrane Database Syst Rev.* 2009;3:CD007303.
4. Boneberg EM, Hareng L, Gantner F, Wendel A, Hartung T. Human monocytes express functional receptors for granulocyte colony-stimulating factor that mediate suppression of monokines and interferon-gamma. *Blood.* 2000;95(1):270–276.
5. Caro JJ, Salas M, Ward A, Goss G. Anemia as an independent prognostic factor for survival in patients with cancer: a systemic, quantitative review. *Cancer* 2001;91(12):2214–2221.
6. Citron ML, Berry DA, Cirrincione C, et al. Randomized trial of dose-dense versus conventionally scheduled and sequential versus concurrent combination chemotherapy as postoperative adjuvant treatment of node-positive primary breast cancer: first report of Intergroup Trial C9741/Cancer and Leukemia Group B Trial 9741. *J Clin Oncol.* 2003;21(8):1431–1439.
7. Clark OA, Lyman GH, Castro AA, Clark LG, Djulbegovic B. Colony-stimulating factors for chemotherapy-induced febrile neutropenia: a meta-analysis of randomized controlled trials. *J Clin Oncol.* Jun 20 2005;23(18):4198–4214.
8. Cwirla SE, Balasubramanian P, Duffin DJ, et al. Peptide agonist of the thrombopoietin receptor as potent as the natural cytokine. *Science* 1997;276(5319):1696–1699.
9. Elliott S, Busse L, Bass MB, et al. Anti-Epo receptor antibodies do not predict Epo receptor expression. *Blood.* 2006;107(5):1892–1895.
10. Gribben JG, Devereux S, Thomas NS, et al. Development of antibodies to unprotected glycosylation sites on recombinant human GM-CSF. *Lancet.* 1990;335(8687):434–437.
11. Gurion R, Belnik-Plitman Y, Gafter-Gvili A, et al. Colony-stimulating factors for prevention and treatment of infectious complications in patients with acute myelogenous leukemia. *Cochrane Database Syst Rev.* 2012;6:CD008238.
12. Halter, J., Kodera, Y., Ispizua, A. et al. Severe events in donors after allogeneic hematopoietic stem cell donation. *Haematologica.* 2009;94(1):94–101.
13. Henke M, Mattern D, Pepe M, et al. Do erythropoietin receptors on cancer cells explain unexpected clinical findings? *J Clin Oncol.* 2006;24(29):4708–4713.
14. Henry DH, Dahl NV, Auerbach M, Tchekmedyian S, Laufman LR. Intravenous ferric gluconate significantly improves response to epoetin alfa versus oral iron or no iron in anemic patients with cancer receiving chemotherapy. *Oncologist.* 2007;12(2):231–242.
15. Koyanagi Y, O'Brien WA, Zhao JQ, Golde DW, Gasson JC, Chen IS. Cytokines alter production of HIV-1 from primary mononuclear phagocytes. *Science.* 1988;241(4873):1673–1675.

16. Kuderer NM, Dale DC, Crawford J, Lyman GH. Impact of primary prophylaxis with granulocyte colony-stimulating factor on febrile neutropenia and mortality in adult cancer patients receiving chemotherapy: a systematic review. *J Clin Oncol.* 2007;25(21):3158–3167.

17. Ludwig H, Fritz E, Leitgeb C, Pecherstorfer M, Samonigg H, Schuster J. Prediction of response to erythropoietin treatment in chronic anemia of cancer. *Blood.* 1994;84(4):1056–1063.

18. Miller, J., Perry, E., Price, T. et al. Recovery and safety profiles of marrow and PBSC donors: experience of the National Marrow Donor Program. *Biol. Bone Marrow Transplant.* 2008;14(9 Suppl):29–36.

19. Osterborg A, Brandberg Y, Molostova V, et al. Randomized, double-blind, placebo-controlled trial of recombinant human erythropoietin, epoetin Beta, in hematologic malignancies. *J Clin Oncol.* 2002;20(10):2486–2494.

20. Pajkrt D, Manten A, van der Poll T, et al. Modulation of cytokine release and neutrophil function by granulocyte colony-stimulating factor during endotoxemia in humans. *Blood.* 1997;90(4):1415–1424.

21. Ringden O, Labopin M, Gorin NC, et al. Treatment with granulocyte colony-stimulating factor after allogeneic bone marrow transplantation for acute leukemia increases the risk of graft-versus-host disease and death: a study from the Acute Leukemia Working Party of the European Group for Blood and Marrow Transplantation. *J Clin Oncol.* 2004;22(3):416–423.

22. Rizzo JD, Brouwers M, Hurley P, et al. American Society of Hematology/American Society of Clinical Oncology clinical practice guideline update on the use of epoetin and darbepoetin in adult patients with cancer. *Blood.* 2010;116(20):4045–4059.

23. Singh AK, Szczech L, Tang KL, et al. Correction of anemia with epoetin alfa in chronic kidney disease. *N Engl J Med.* 2006;355(20):2085–2098.

24. Smith T, Bohlke K, Lyman G, et al. Recommendations for the use of WBC growth factors: American Society of Clinical Oncology Clinical Practice Guideline Update. *J Clin Oncol.* July 13, 2015. [epub ahead of print] doi: 10.1200/JCO.2015.62.3488.

25. Smith RE Jr, Aapro MS, Ludwig H, et al. Darbepoetin alfa for the treatment of anemia in patients with active cancer not receiving chemotherapy or radiotherapy: results of a phase III, multicenter, randomized, double-blind, placebo-controlled study. *J Clin Oncol.* 2008;26(7):1040–1050.

26. Smith TJ, Khatcheressian J, Lyman GH, et al. 2006 update of recommendations for the use of white blood cell growth factors: an evidence-based clinical practice guideline. *J Clin Oncol.* 2006;24(19):3187–3205.

27. Stasi R, Abruzzese E, Lanzetta G, Terzoli E, Amadori S. Darbepoetin alfa for the treatment of anemic patients with low- and intermediate-1-risk myelodysplastic syndromes. *Ann Oncol.* 2005;16(12): 1921–1927.

28. Tepler I, Elias L, Smith JW II, et al. A randomized placebo-controlled trial of recombinant human interleukin-11 in cancer patients with severe thrombocytopenia due to chemotherapy. *Blood.* 1996;87(9):3607–3614.

29. Wright JR, Ung YC, Julian JA, et al. Randomized, double-blind, placebo-controlled trial of erythropoietin in non-small-cell lung cancer with disease-related anemia. *J Clin Oncol.* 2007;25(9):1027–1032.

Infectious Complications 35 in Oncology

Lekha Mikkilineni and Juan C. Gea-Banacloche

FEVER

- Fever is the most common sign of infection, and a common problem in patients with cancer.
- Fever is conventionally defined as one oral temperature greater than 38.3°C or two oral temperatures greater than 38°C measured 1 hour apart.
- Old age, malnutrition, and corticosteroids may blunt the febrile response. From the practical management standpoint one must separate between fever in the neutropenic cancer patient ("neutropenic fever") and fever in the absence of neutropenia.
- Fever is a very common manifestation of cytokine release syndrome (CRS), which is frequently seen following many current forms of immunotherapy (cellular therapies, monoclonal antibodies like blinatumomab). Management of fever during immunotherapy may be particularly challenging, but the general rules of neutropenic fever should apply when the absolute neutrophil count (ANC) is <500/ mm^3.

FEVER IN THE NEUTROPENIC CANCER PATIENT (NEUTROPENIC FEVER)

- Neutropenia, the most important risk factor for bacterial infection in cancer patients, is defined as an ANC <500/mm^3, or ANC ≤1,000/mm^3, with a predicted decline to <500/mm^3 within 48 hours.
- Fever during neutropenia is always considered to be of infectious origin, and managed accordingly.
- The risk of infection increases with the rapidity of onset, degree, and duration of neutropenia.
- Febrile neutropenic patients require immediate evaluation and prompt initiation of empirical broad-spectrum antibiotics with activity against *Pseudomonas aeruginosa* (Fig. 35.1). Antibiotics are usually administered intravenously, but oral administration may be acceptable when patients are determined to be at low risk of severe morbidity and mortality based on biological features and access to care (see below).
- Three distinct syndromes of fever during neutropenia are of practical importance.
  - **First fever:** In 20% to 25% of patients with fever and neutropenia an infection is documented microbiologically (most commonly bacteremia). In 20% to 30% of patients an infection is documented only clinically, without microbiologic confirmation (e.g., typhlitis with negative blood cultures). In 50% of patients with fever and neutropenia no infection is found. The response to empirical management with antibiotics is similarly favorable in these three subgroups. Gram-positive and gram-negative bacteria are isolated with roughly similar frequency. Treatment emphasizes coverage of gram-negative bacteria because these infections tend to progress faster and have higher mortality.
  - **Persistent fever:** The average time to defervescence for the first episode of neutropenic fever is 3 to 4 days. When fever persists for 5 days or more, (4 to 7, depending on the study) the frequency of invasive fungal infection is high enough that it is standard practice to add empirical antifungal

therapy. *Candida* and *Aspergillus* species are the most common causes of fungal infections in neutropenic patients and increase in frequency with longer duration of neutropenia. The antifungal agent of choice may vary with the clinical situation and the preexistent use of antifungal prophylaxis. In the absence of antifungal prophylaxis, the most common fungal pathogen causing persistent fever is *Candida albicans*. If antifungal prophylaxis was being administered, *Aspergillus* and non-*albicans* Candida become more likely. Randomized controlled trials support the empirical addition of amphotericin B (deoxycholate or liposomal), voriconazole, and caspofungin for persistent fever. The choice varies based on what (whether) antifungal prophylaxis was being used and an estimate of the risk. It is appropriate to look for invasive fungal infection by blood cultures and computed tomography (CT) of chest and possibly sinuses.

- **Recrudescent fever (new fever after resolution of the first episode):** This term refers to the reappearance of fever after the patient has been afebrile for more than 48 hours following the administration of broad-spectrum antibiotics for an episode of neutropenic fever. In this situation an infectious cause is identified in most cases (as opposed to the initial fever, in which most frequently no cause is found) and both breakthrough bacterial and fungal infections are possible. Management includes changing (or adding, if antifungals were not part of the regimen) **both** antibiotics **and** antifungals plus diagnostic studies (CTs as outlined above). Drug-resistant bacteria are increasing (e.g., extended-spectrum beta-lactamase-producing (ESBL) gram-negative bacilli, carbapenem-resistant *Enterobacteriaceae* (CRE), vancomycin-resistant enterococcus (VRE)), so the antibiotic choice should be guided by local prevalence. In institutions where CRE are common, early addition of colistin or substitution of ceftazidime-avibactam may be appropriate. Conversely, in an institution with high frequency of ESBLs early switch to imipenem or meropenem may be the best antibacterial strategy for recrudescent fever.
- The importance of fever during neutropenia is that it is a good surrogate marker for infection. It is not the only one, however, and other signs or symptoms suggestive of infection (e.g., abdominal pain, erythema, hypotension, hypothermia) should be similarly treated empirically with antibiotics as well.

EVALUATION

- History and physical examination should be performed with special attention to potential sites of infection: skin, mouth, perianal region, and intravenous catheter exit site.
- Routine complete blood count with differential, chemistries, including liver enzymes and creatinine, urinalysis, blood and urine cultures should be obtained. Evidence suggests a chest X-ray adds little information unless there are respiratory signs or symptoms, but we routinely recommend it as adding potentially useful baseline information.
- Blood cultures: Two sets of blood cultures are more sensitive than a single set for the diagnosis of bacteremia. There are data supporting the practice of drawing all cultures from the central line (sampling all lumens) in cancer patients to simply diagnose bacteremia. However, to determine if a bacteremic episode is related to the catheter, it is advisable to draw blood from the intravenous catheter and a peripheral vein simultaneously. A differential time to positivity of 2 hours or more (i.e., the cultures obtained from the catheter become positive earlier than the peripheral stick) has good predictive value for catheter-related bacteremia.
- Any accessible sites of possible infection should be sampled for gram stain and culture (catheter site, sputum, etc.).
- Ideally, blood cultures should be obtained prior to starting antibiotics, but failure to do so should not delay antibiotic administration.

EMPIRICAL ANTIBIOTIC THERAPY

- A summary of the initial management of the patient with fever and neutropenia and no localizing signs or symptoms is provided in Figure 35.1.

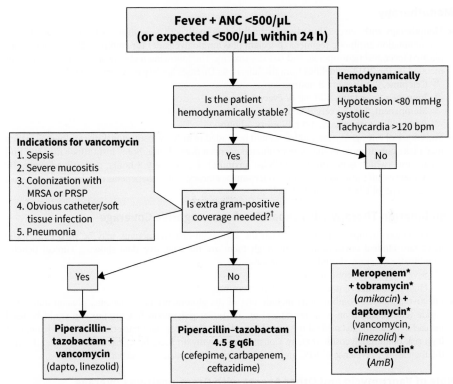

FIGURE 35.1 Approach to patients with fever and neutropenia without clinically or microbiologically documented infection. The choice between piperacillin–tazobactam (shown here emphasizing the higher dose required in neutropenic patients), cefepime, imipenem, meropenem, and ceftazidime will vary between institutions based on local resistance patterns. For specific infections, see the text and Table 35.1. * This antibacterial regimen for the neutropenic patient with sepsis will vary between institutions, depending on the local patterns of antibiotic resistance. Carbapenem + fluoroquinolone (or aminoglycoside or colistin) + vancomycin (or daptomycin or linezolid) + echinocandin is typical. We prefer meropenem and daptomycin because both can be "pushed" intravenously in a few minutes. The antifungal of choice will vary depending on previous antifungal prophylaxis.† The empirical gram-positive coverage should usually be discontinued after 48 to 72 hours if there is no bacteriologic documentation of a pathogen requiring its use, except in soft tissue or tunnel infections. Linezolid or daptomycin may be substituted for vancomycin if there is suspicion or high endemicity of VRE. For a detailed discussion of antifungal therapy options, as well as for the role of oral antibiotics in low-risk patients, see the text. AmB, amphotericin B; MRSA, methicillin (oxacillin)-resistant *Staphylococcus aureus*; PRSP, penicillin-resistant *Streptococcus pneumoniae*.

- The goal of treatment is to provide broad antibiotic coverage with minimal toxicity, *not* to initially cover any and all conceivable pathogens.
- Most bacterial infections during neutropenia are caused by microorganisms that colonize the oral mucosa, the bowel, and the skin of the patient. *P. aeruginosa* is particularly prevalent during neutropenia. Due to their potential for faster progression and higher morbidity, the emphasis is on coverage of gram-negative bacilli including *Pseudomonas*. This may be achieved by using single agents ("monotherapy") or by combining several antibiotics.

Monotherapy

■ Monotherapy with selected broad-spectrum β-lactams with activity against *P. aeruginosa* is as effective as combination antibiotic regimens (β-lactam plus aminoglycoside) for empirical therapy of uncomplicated fever and neutropenia, and has less toxicity. The following regimens are the options recommended by the 2011 guidelines from the Infectious Diseases Society of America (IDSA):
  ● Cefepime, 2 g IV every 8 hours
  ● Imipenem–cilastatin, 500 mg IV every 6 hours
  ● Meropenem, 1 g IV every 8 hours
  ● Piperacillin–tazobactam, 4.5 g IV every 6 hours
■ The choice of one agent over another should be guided mainly by institutional susceptibilities, which may make one or more of the aforementioned agents a poor choice. Some institutions may still find ceftazidime (which is not on the IDSA's list anymore), 2 g IV every 8 hours, perfectly adequate. By meta-analysis, all these agents seem to offer similar efficacy, but carbapenems may be associated with increased risk of *Clostridium difficile* colitis.

Combination Therapy with Expanded Gram-negative Coverage

■ Combination therapy aiming to broaden the anti–gram-negative activity may be used empirically in certain clinical circumstances, although there are no definitive data showing clinical benefit. Combination therapy should be used in cases of
  ● Severe sepsis or septic shock
  ● High prevalence of multidrug-resistant gram-negative bacilli (see Table 35.1)
■ Effective antibiotic combinations include one of the aforementioned β-lactams plus an aminoglycoside (choice based on local resistance) or colistin or polymyxin B. Ciprofloxacin could be used instead of an aminoglycoside if the prevalence of quinolone-resistant bacteria is low or in patients at high risk of aminoglycoside toxicity. Colistin and polymyxin B are being used more frequently with the increasing prevalence of KPC and multiresistant *Acinetobacter baumannii*.

Role of Vancomycin and Other Agents with Gram-positive Coverage

Gram-positive coverage with vancomycin should be part of the **initial empirical regimen** under the following circumstances:

■ **Severe sepsis or septic shock** (to ensure coverage of methicillin-resistant *Staphylococcus aureus* (MRSA), penicillin-resistant *Streptococcus pneumoniae* and *Streptococcus mitis*)
■ **Pneumonia** (consider it "healthcare-associated pneumonia")
■ **Soft tissue infection** (cellulitis, necrotizing fasciitis)
■ **Clinically suspected catheter-related infections** (e.g., because of tenderness or purulent drainage at the exit site; NOT the mere presence of an intravascular device)
■ **Severe mucositis** or other risk factors for infection with *Streptococcus mitis* **(oral infection, use of prophylaxis with fluoroquinolones or TMP/SMX, high-dose Ara-C, use of H$_2$ blockers)**
■ **Known colonization** with methicillin-resistant *Staphylococcus aureus* (MRSA) or penicillin-resistant *Streptococcus pneumoniae* (PRSP) (this is important, and frequently forgotten)

Addition of vancomycin to the initial regimen:

■ Persistent fever is NOT an indication for adding vancomycin, because a randomized controlled trial showed that adding vancomycin in this setting was not better than adding placebo.
■ Blood cultures that grow gram-positive bacteria are an indication for the addition of agents with gram-positive activity. Pending identification, the choice between vancomycin, linezolid, and daptomycin should be informed by the local prevalence of VRE and preliminary morphologic information from the gram stain as follows (see Table 35.2):
  ● Gram positive cocci in clusters: usually *Staphylococcus* (it may be *Staphylococcus aureus* or coagulase-negative *Staphylococcus*)—vancomycin provides adequate coverage. Rarely (typically in acute leukemia patients already on broad Gram-negative coverage) it may mean *Rothia mucilaginosa* (previously *Stomatococcus mucilaginosus*) a dangerous cause of bacteremia and meningitis best treated by the combination vancomycin + meropenem.

TABLE 35.1 Resistant Bacteria: What Everybody Should Know

	Resistant to	Treat With	Things to Remember
Gram positive			
Methicillin-resistant staphylococcus aureus (MRSA)	Semi-synthetic penicillins, first-, second- and third-generation cephalosporins, carbapenems	Vancomycin, daptomycin, ceftaroline	Community-acquired MRSA is frequently susceptible to clindamycin, doxycycline, and TMP/SMX
Vancomycin-resistant enterococcus (VRE)	Vancomycin and all beta-lactams	Linezolid, daptomycin, quinupristin/dalfopristin. Maybe tigecycline and oritavancin	Microbiological success is no higher than 40%, there is no clinical evidence to prefer one agent over another
Mycobacterium abscessus	Almost everything	*Infectious Diseases support required.* Combination therapy required, usually with meropenem + amikacin + azithromycin ± linezolid	Respiratory colonizer AND potential pathogen, particularly in patients with abnormal airways/lungs
Gram negative			
SPICE *Enterobacteriaceae* (*Serratia, Providentia,* Indole-positive *Proteus, Citrobacter,* and *Enterobacter*)	They may seem susceptible, then become resistant to third-generation cephalosporins (like ceftriaxone and ceftazidime) during treatment	Carbapenems, fluoroquinolones (ciprofloxacin, levofloxacin), maybe cefepime	Your Micro lab should add a note saying that **even if it looks susceptible by antibiogram**, the isolate may become resistant during treatment
ESBL-producing Enterobacteriaceae (most commonly *E. coli* and *Klebsiella*)	All cephalosporins	Carbapenems (use of piperacillin-tazobactam when the antibiogram shows the isolate is susceptible may be considered, but is discouraged by most authorities)	The antibiogram will show the resistance to third generation cephalosporins
CRE (Carbapenem-Resistant *Enterobacteriaceae*) Any *Enterobacteriaceae* may carry a gene conferring resistance to carbapenems through carbapenemases like KPC, OXA, MBLs)	All cephalosporins and carbapenems	*Infectious Diseases support required.* Some may respond to ceftazidime-avibactam, many will require combination therapy with amikacin and/or colistin	It is important to be familiar with the methodology of the Micro lab and ask for help interpreting the antibiogram. CRE produce carbapenemases, and these are of great epidemiological (as well as clinical) significance. Other mechanisms of resistance to carbapenems (e.g., porin genes) are less severe.

(continued)

TABLE 35.1 (Continued)

	Resistant to	Treat With	Things to Remember
MDR *Acinetobacter baumannii*	All commonly used antibiotics	*Infectious Diseases support required.* Combination of colistin + tigecycline + gentamicin ± doripenem has been used	Inhaled colistin has been used in cases of MDR Acinetobacter or Pseudomonas, but its efficacy is far from clear
MDR *Pseudomonas aeruginosa*	All commonly used antibiotics	*Infectious Diseases support required.* Combination of colistin (or polymixin B) and other agents may be required	
Stenotrophomonas maltophilia	Intrinsically resistant to carbapenems and aminoglycosides	TMP/SMX is the treatment of choice, levofloxacin and moxifloxacin and ceftazidime (if susceptible in vitro) are other options. Tigecycline and colistin have been used with variable results	Think of it when a patient on meropenem develops breakthrough gram-negative bacteremia

- Gram positive cocci in pairs and short chains: This may be *Enterococcus* or *Streptococcus pneumoniae*—the clinical setting should support one or the other (hospitalized patient, neutropenic, on a third generation cephalosporin: *Enterococcus*; outpatient with pneumonia at risk for encapsulated bacteria—e.g., multiple myeloma—*Streptococcus pneumoniae*). In an institution with high frequency of VRE, daptomycin or linezolid are adequate first line empirical agents here.
- Gram-positive cocci in long chains: *Streptococcus viridans*, it may be *Streptococcus mitis* associated with mucositis—vancomycin is appropriate.
- There is no good-quality evidence to suggest that patients known to be colonized with VRE should initially receive empirical coverage for it with linezolid or daptomycin.
- In the case of documented VRE infection, the choice between daptomycin, linezolid, quinupristn-dalfopristin, and tigecycline is not based on clinical outcome data, but on theoretical considerations and local resistance patterns.
- Daptomycin is inactivated by surfactant in the lungs and should not be used to treat pneumonia. There is good evidence, however, that it is as effective as vancomycin or oxacillin to treat staphylococcal bacteremia.

Oral Therapy

- Empirical oral antibiotics may be acceptable for neutropenic patients who are not at high risk of severe morbidity or death.
- High-risk patients are those who received chemotherapy associated with prolonged and profound neutropenia (e.g., AML induction therapy), as well as patients with symptoms or signs of clinical instability, significant comorbidities (e.g., COPD, heart failure) or with expected prolonged neutropenia. Low-risk patients do not exhibit any high-risk factors and their neutropenia is expected to be short lived (< 7 days). These patients may be considered for outpatient antibiotic treatment.

TABLE 35.2 How to Interpret Preliminary Information from Blood Culture Reports

Micro report	What it means	What to Do	Caveats
Blood culture positive for Gram-positive cocci in clusters	Coagulase-negative *Staphylococcus, Staphylococcus aureus* (In a patient with acute leukemia and prolonged neutropenia you may worry about *Rothia mucilaginosa*)	Repeat blood cultures from the line AND a peripheral stick (the peripheral is to check time to positivity and decide whether the line is the source of infection) and start vancomycin	Coagulase-negative *Staphylococcus* and *Staphylococcus aureus* are very different: *S. aureus* can kill your patient in hours, but almost no one dies of coagulase-negative Staph. bacteremia
Blood culture positive for Gram-positive cocci in pairs	*Enterococcus* (including VRE) *Streptococcus pneumoniae* Rarely, *Streptococcus agalactiae* (Group B Streptococcus)	Repeat blood cultures and start either 1) vancomycin if *Streptococcus pneumoniae* is more likely or the prevalence of VRE is low OR 2) daptomycin if *Enterococcus* is more likely and there is high prevalence of VRE OR 3) linezolid if you can't tell and are too tired to think	*Enterococcus* and pneumococcus may be indistinguishable by Gram stain, but patients are usually very different (e.g., a post allo-HCT with chronic GVHD and pneumonia is likely to have *S. pneumoniae* whereas a neutropenic patient on cefepime with abdominal pain is likely to have *Enterococcus*). Daptomycin should not be used for pulmonary infections
Blood culture positive for Gram-positive cocci in chains	*Streptococcus* If there is severe mucositis, think *S. mitis*; if there are abscesses around, think of *S. anginosus*, *S. constellatus* or *S. intermedius* (the trio called *S. milleri* in the UK) Remember *Streptococcus pyogenes* (Group A *Streptococcus*) and *Streptococcus agalactiae* (Group B), particularly in patients with soft tissue infection and at risk for infection with encapsulated bacteria (e.g., multiple myeloma)	Add vancomycin	Two oncology scenarios worth remembering: *Streptococcus mitis* bacteremia in neutropenic patients with severe mucositis and other risk factors (it can cause ARDS and septic shock, *see* text) and *Streptococcus gallolyticus,* formerly *Streptococcus bovis* in patients with colon cancer (sometimes not previously known).

(*continued*)

TABLE 35.2 (Continued)

Micro report	What it means	What to Do	Caveats
Blood culture positive for Gram-positive rods	Diphtheroids (skin contaminant) *Corynebacterium JK* (line infection) *Listeria monocytogenes* (bacteremia and meningitis in immuno-compromised) *Clostridium* (typhlitis or metastatic gangrene with *C. septicum*) *Bacillus* (catheter-related bacteremia) *Lactobacillus* *Propionibacterium acnes* (contaminant) Mycobacteria (line infection)	*Infectious Diseases support required.* The possibilities are too many and with too different clinical implications	As you can see by the possible etiologies, there is no way to give a simple, straightforward recommendation. Vancomycin would be "the right answer" most of the time, but it does not cover *Listeria, Lactobacillus* or mycobacteria and treatment is probably not needed for "diphtheroids" and *P. acnes.* Just call for help.
Blood culture positive for Gram-negative rods, "enteric-like" or "lactose-fermenting"	Enterobacteriaceae (e.g., *E.coli, Klebsiella, Enterobacter*)	If your institution does not have CREs, imipenem or meropenem will cover 100% of these. If CREs are highly prevalent, add colistin or switch to ceftazidime-avibactam	The important information from Micro is that this SHOULD NOT BE *Pseudomonas, Acinetobacter* or *Stenotrophomonas* (remember, preliminary means NOT definitive).
Blood culture positive for "Pseudomonas-like" gram-negative rods	*Pseudomonas aeruginosa,* much less likely *Stenotrophomonas maltophilia* or *Burkholderia*	Two antibiotics with activity against your institution's *P. aeruginosa* (e.g., ceftazidime + tobramycin or colistin)	*Pseudomonas aeruginosa* should be covered empirically with two antibiotics until final susceptibilities are known.
Blood culture positive for "non-fermenting Gram-negative rods"	This includes *Pseudomonas, Acinetobacter, Stenotrophomonas, Burkholderia* and a long-list of not very pathogenic bacteria that commonly cause catheter infection in immuno-compromised cancer patients (*Alcaligenes, Chryseobacterium, Comomonas, Sphingomonas, Elizabethkingia* among others)	*Infectious Diseases support required.* The general concept is that you should consider empirical addition of TMP/SMX or levofloxacin (depending what antibiotic the patient was on), as some of the possibilities are resistant to beta-lactams	No easy answer. Meropenem is the treatment of choice for *Burkholderia,* and completely ineffective against *Stenotrophomonas.* Just call for help.

TABLE 35.2 (Continued)

Micro report	What it means	What to Do	Caveats
Blood culture positive for Gram-negative coccobacilli	In the cancer patient, *Acinetobacter* should come to mind first	Institutional pattern of resistance dictates the choice	*Acinetobacter* may be difficult to identify on Gram stain. "Coccobacilli" is a term that should be avoided
Blood culture positive for Gram-negative cocci	*Neisseria meningitidis* and *Neisseria gonorrheae* are uncommon in the cancer patient. *Moraxella* is a possibility. If it is the anaerobic bottle only *Veillonella* should be considered	A carbapenem is the easy answer, but this is uncommon and it would be better to call Infectious Diseases	

- A quantitative risk assessment, the Multinational Association for Supportive Care in Cancer (MASCC) scoring system, has been validated. Points are allocated for burden of illness (no or mild symptoms 5, severe symptoms 3), absence of hypotension (5), no chronic obstructive pulmonary disease (4), solid tumor *or* no previous fungal infection (4), absence of dehydration (3), outpatient status (3), and age <60 years (2) and the points are added up. Patients with a score of ≥21 points (of 26 possible) are at "low risk," and can be considered for oral therapy.
- The two recommended oral regimens are
  - Ciprofloxacin, 750 mg PO every 12 hours, plus amoxicillin/clavulanate, 875 mg (amoxicillin component) PO every 12 hours
  - Ciprofloxacin, 750 mg PO every 12 hours, plus clindamycin 450 mg PO every 6 hours

We recommend starting oral antibiotics on an inpatient basis, and then consider discharge after 24 hours of observation and documentation that the blood cultures remain negative. Following discharge, patients should be seen daily and instructed to call or come in to clinic for new or worsening symptoms or persistent high fever. Approximately 20% of patients will need readmission to the hospital (factors associated with need for admission: >70 years old, poor performance, ANC <100/mm^3).

Low-risk patients with no documented infection who respond to empirical IV antibiotics can be switched to oral antibiotics until their neutropenia resolves based on clinical judgment. We recommend observing these patients on oral therapy as inpatients for at least 24 hours before discharge.

Modifications of the Initial Antibiotic Regimen

- After patients are started on empirical antibiotics for fever and neutropenia, their course must be monitored closely for the development of new signs or symptoms of infection; antibiotic therapy should be modified based on clinical findings.
- Therapy modification is necessary in 30% to 50% of cases during the course of neutropenia.
- Specific modifications are dictated by specific clinical syndromes or by microbiologic isolates.
- Persistent fever with no other clinical findings is not an indication for modification of the antibacterial regimen.
- If there is no documented gram-positive infection, gram-positive coverage may be stopped after 48h if it had been initiated.
- After 4 to 7 days of persistent fever, it is accepted practice to start some antifungal agent.

■ In the case of recrudescent fever the antibacterial and antifungal agents should be changed and imaging studies performed

Empirical Antifungal Therapy

Candida and *Aspergillus* infections are most common and increase in frequency with increased duration of neutropenia. An antifungal agent (see Table 35.3) should be added empirically for neutropenic patients in the following circumstances:

■ Severe sepsis or septic shock: it may be caused by *Candida*; amphotericin or an echinocandin should be added. Mould infections seldom cause septic shock.
■ Persistent fever after 4 to 7 days of broad-spectrum antibiotic therapy.
■ Recrudescent fever.
■ *Candida* colonization: candiduria, thrush.

Treatment options include

■ Amphotericin B deoxycholate, 0.6 to 1 mg/kg/day IV.
■ A lipid formulation of amphotericin B such as liposomal amphotericin B (Ambisome) or amphotericin B lipid complex (Abelcet), 3 to 5 mg/kg/day IV.
■ Voriconazole, 6 mg/kg IV every 12 hours for 24 hours followed by 4 mg/kg IV every 12 hours, aiming for a serum concentration >2 mcg/mL.
■ Caspofungin, 70 mg IV loading dose followed by 50 mg IV daily.
■ Posaconazole, 300 mg IV every 12 hours twice loading dose followed by 300 mg IV daily (no data on empirical treatment as opposed to the treatment of documented infection).
■ Isavuconazole, 200 mg IV every 8 hours for six doses loading followed by 200 mg IV daily (no data on empirical treatment as opposed to treatment of documented infection).

For persistent fever, amphotericin, caspofungin, and possibly voriconazole (not-FDA approved for this indication) are well validated as empirical additions. Of note, an effort should be made to rule out the presence of active invasive fungal infection by performing a thorough physical examination and obtaining CT studies as clinically indicated (CT chest, possibly CT sinus, CT of abdomen and pelvis if there are signs of intraabdominal infection or abnormal liver enzymes). A different approach suggests to start antifungal agents only when there is ancillary evidence of fungal infection besides the fever (e.g., positive serologic tests like galactomannan and/or ß-D-glucan). The role of this so-called "preemptive" antifungal therapy as opposed to the traditional "empirical" addition of antifungal agents in persistent fever has not been clearly defined.

The IV formulation of posaconazole allows loading and obtaining therapeutic levels early, so it may be now considered another alternative for treatment of suspected or proven fungal infections (the previous oral formulation did not achieve therapeutic levels for 5 to 7 days) but clinical evidence supporting is use as treatment (as opposed to prophylaxis) is still scant. Isavuconazole has shown to be non-inferior to voriconazole in a randomized controlled trial and similar to amphotericin for the treatment of mucormycosis in a case-control study.

Duration of Antibiotic Therapy

■ **Documented bacterial infection:** Antibiotics should be continued for the amount of time standard for that infection or until resolution of neutropenia, whichever is longer.
■ **Uncomplicated fever and neutropenia of uncertain etiology:** Antibiotics should be continued until the fever has resolved and the ANC is above 500 for 24 hours.
■ **If no infection was documented and the patient became afebrile on antibiotics, but the neutropenia persists, we recommend to complete 2 weeks of treatment.** At that point one may discontinue the antibiotics and observe. Alternatively, it is acceptable to resume fluoroquinolone prophylaxis until marrow recovery.
■ Limited evidence suggests that if no infection is found and the patient becomes afebrile it is possible to discountinue antibiotics after 48 hours without fever, being aware that some patients will become febrile again and require restarting the antibiotics.
■ If there is no documented fungal infection, antifungal agents can also be discontinued at the time of resolution of neutropenia.

FEVER IN THE NONNEUTROPENIC CANCER PATIENT

- Noninfectious causes of fever in cancer patients include, among others, the underlying malignancy, deep venous thrombosis and pulmonary embolism, medications, blood products, and, in allogeneic stem cell transplant, graft-versus-host disease.
- Infections, however, are common in patients with all types of malignancies in all stages of treatment. In addition to neutropenia, there are several other factors that contribute to increased susceptibility to infection and should be considered when trying to diagnose an episode of fever and formulate a treatment plan.
- Local factors: Breakdown of barriers (mucositis, surgery) that provide a portal of entry for bacteria; obstruction (biliary, ureteral, bronchial) that facilitates local infection (cholangitis, pyelonephritis, postobstructive pneumonia).
- Intravascular devices, drainage tubes, or stents may become colonized and lead to local infection, bacteremia, or fungemia.
- Splenectomy increases susceptibility to infection due to *S. pneumoniae* and other encapsulated bacteria
- Deficiencies of humoral immunity (multiple myeloma, chronic lymphocytic leukemia) lead to increased susceptibility to encapsulated organisms such as *S. pneumoniae* and *Haemophilus influenzae.*
- Defects in cell-mediated immunity (lymphoma, hairy cell leukemia, treatment with **steroids,** fludarabine, and other drugs, hematopoietic stem cell transplant [HSCT]) increase susceptibility to opportunistic infections caused by *Legionella pneumophila*, Mycobacteria, *Cryptococcus neoformans*, *Pneumocystis jirovecii*, cytomegalovirus (CMV), varicella zoster virus (VZV), and other pathogens.

Antibiotic Therapy in the Nonneutropenic Cancer Patient

- Antibiotics should be administered empirically in the setting of fever only when a bacterial infection is considered likely.
- Ideally one should formulate a "working hypothesis" as a fundamental basis to choose the appropriate regimen. For example, pneumonia, cholecystitis, and urinary tract infection would likely require different antibiotics.
- In the absence of localizing signs and symptoms, consider bacteremia, particularly in patients with intravascular devices. Many authorities recommend empirical antibiotics (levofloxacin, ceftriaxone) until bacteremia is ruled out.
- Clinically documented infections and sepsis should be treated with antibiotics as warranted by the clinical scenario.
- Whenever antibiotics are started, a plan with specific endpoints should be formulated to avoid unnecessary toxicity, superinfection, and the development of resistance.

SPECIFIC INFECTIOUS DISEASE SYNDROMES

If a patient presents with clinical signs and symptoms of a specific infection, with or without neutropenia, the workup and therapy are guided by the clinical suspicion (see Table 35.4).

Bacteremia/Fungemia

- A positive blood culture should prompt immediate initiation of appropriate antibiotics in a neutropenic patient or in a nonneutropenic patient who is febrile or clinically unstable.
- If the isolated organism is one that is commonly pathogenic, such as *S. aureus* or gram-negative bacilli, antibiotics should be started even if the patient is afebrile and clinically stable.
- If the isolate is a common contaminant, such as a coagulase-negative *Staphylococcus*, and the patient is afebrile, clinically stable, and nonneutropenic, it may be appropriate to repeat the cultures and observe before starting antibiotics.
- In every case of bacteremia, follow-up blood cultures should be obtained to document the effectiveness of therapy, and the source of the infection should be sought.

TABLE 35.3 Basic Information about Commonly Used Systemic Antifungal Agents

Antifungal	Spectrum	Notable resistant fungi*	When to use	Special concerns
Polyene				
Amphotericin B (deoxycholate and lipid formulations)	Most candida, aspergillus and agents of mucormycosis	Candida lusitaniae, Aspergillus terreus, Paecilomyces lilacinus	Treatment of choice for mucormycosis. Treatment of choice for cryptococcosis. As effective as echinocandins for candidiasis. Effective in persistent fever. Inferior to voriconazole for aspergillosis.	Nephrotoxicity. Loss of glomerular filtration rate may be minimized by "salt loading," but tubulopathy with loss of Mg and K cannot be prevented.
Echinocandins Different trials have used different echinocandins in different ettings, but they are considered essentially interchangeable for practical purposes	Candida and Aspergillus	Cryptococcus and all moulds other than Aspergillus	Treatment of choice for candidiasis.	Poor penetration in eye, CSF and urine
Caspofungin			Good data for persistent fever	
Micafungin			Weak (but some) data for aspergillosis. Good data for prophylaxis during neutropenia.	
Anidulafungin			Weak (but some) data for aspergillosis. Good data for combination therapy with voriconazole in aspergillosis	
Azoles				All the azoles interfere with the hepatic metabolism of multiple drugs used in Oncology (e.g., corticosteroids, vincristine, cyclophosphamide, calcineurin inhibitors) and have the potential for significant drug interactions.

Drug	Active against	Resistant/Less active	Comments	Toxicity
Fluconazole	Candida albicans	Candida krusei. All moulds	Best evidence for prophylaxis during neutropenia and for Candidiasis. Cryptococcosis. Coccidioidomycosis.	Hepatotoxicity
Voriconazole	Candida, Cryptococcus, Aspergillus, most hyaline moulds	Agents of mucormycosis Paecilomyces variotii	Treatment of choice for aspergillosis	Significant individual variability on serum levels achieved makes therapeutic drug monitoring advisable. Hallucinations, visual disturbances and hepatotoxicity. Photosensitivity and possibly fluorosis with long-term use
Posaconazole	Candida, aspergillus, most moulds including some agents of mucormycosis		Best data for antifungal prophylaxis during prolonged neutropenia. Probably as effective as voriconazole for aspergillosis (but no RCT yet). Active against some agents of mucormycosis.	Hepatotoxicity may be less than with voriconazole
Isavuconazole	Candida, Aspergillus, most moulds including some agents of mucormycosis		Equivalent to voriconazole for aspergillosis in a RCT. FDA-approved for mucormycosis based on comparison with registry controls.	Less variability in levels than voriconazole or posaconazole. Less hepatotoxicity than voriconazole. No prolongation of Q-T interval. Activity against mucormycosis still questionable

TABLE 35.4 Specific Infectious Disease Syndromes in Oncology Patients and Approach to Diagnosis and Management

Clinical Syndrome	Diagnostic Considerations	Management
Intravascular catheter-associated infections	Infections can be local involving the exit site or subcutaneous tunnel, or systemic causing bacteremia For local infections, check culture of exit-site discharge as well as blood cultures	For tunnel and systemic infections, empirical therapy should include vancomycin as well as gram-negative coverage (e.g., ceftazidime, cefepime, ciprofloxacin) Temporary intravascular catheters should always be removed. Permanent catheters should be removed in most cases, and we always remove them in the following situations: Tunnel infections Persistently positive blood cultures after 72 h of adequate therapy regardless of pathogen Specific pathogens: *Mycobacteria* spp, *Bacillus* spp, *S. aureus*, fungi; case-by-case decision for *Corynebacterium jeikeium,* VRE, and gram-negative organisms Consider antibiotic lock if feasible
Skin/soft tissue infections	Prompt biopsy with histologic staining and culture for bacteria, mycobacteria, viruses, and fungi Pathogens: *S. aureus*, *S. pyogenes*, gram-negative bacilli (e.g., *Pseudomonas*), VZV, HSV, *Candida* For vesicular lesions, scrape base for DFA or PCR for VZV and HSV	Ecthyma gangrenosum: coverage of *Pseudomonas* (e.g., ceftazidime, cefepime, ciprofloxacin) Infections with *S. pyogenes*: treat aggressively with penicillin G, clindamycin, IVIG, and surgical debridement Perianal cellulitis: broad-spectrum coverage including anaerobes (e.g., imipenem) VZV, HSV: acyclovir
Sinusitis	Evaluate with CT scan and examination by otolaryngologist Tissue should be biopsied if there is suspicion of fungal infection or no response to antibiotic therapy after 72 h Pathogens: *S. pneumoniae*, *H. influenzae*, *M. catarrhalis*, *S. aureus*, gram-negative bacilli (e.g., *Pseudomonas*), fungi including agents of mucormycosis (Mucorales)	Nonneutropenic: levofloxacin or amoxicillin/clavulanate Neutropenic: broad-spectrum coverage including *Pseudomonas* (e.g., carbapenem, cefepime) and MRSA and consider fungal coverage (e.g., amphotericin B, voriconazole)
Pulmonary infections	CT scan and BAL should be performed early Pneumonias in any cancer patient are often caused by	For all patients, ensure adequate coverage of community-acquired pneumonia including *Legionella* (e.g., levofloxacin)

TABLE 35.4 (Continued)

Clinical Syndrome	Diagnostic Considerations	Management
	gram-negative bacilli and *S. aureus* as well as community-acquired pneumonia pathogens: *S. pneumoniae*, *H. influenzae*, *Legionella* spp, and *Chlamydia pneumoniae*	Neutropenic: coverage of *S. pneumoniae*, *S. aureus*, and *Pseudomonas* (e.g., levofloxacin and ceftazidime and vancomycin); add antifungal coverage empirically (e.g., amphotericin B, voriconazole) if pneumonia develops while on antibiotics
	Neutropenic patients are at risk for invasive fungal infections, particularly aspergillosis	Cell-mediated immunodeficiency: consider coverage of *Pneumocystis* with TMP/SMX, CMV with ganciclovir, and *Nocardia* with TMP/SMX
	Patients with cell-mediated defects are at risk for infections with PCP, viruses (CMV, VZV, HSV), *Nocardia* spp, and *Legionella*	
	Mycobacteria should also be considered, particularly in patients with previous exposure	
Gastrointestinal tract infections	Lesions associated with mucositis can be superinfected with HSV or *Candida*	Mucositis or esophagitis: acyclovir and fluconazole
	Esophagitis can be caused by *Candida*, HSV, CMV	*C. difficile*: metronidazole or vancomycin if refractory
	Diarrhea is most commonly caused by *C. difficile* (send toxin assay) but can also be caused by *Salmonella*, *Shigella*, *Aeromonas*, *E. coli*, *Campylobacter*, viruses, parasites, etc.	Neutropenic enterocolitis: broad-spectrum coverage including *Pseudomonas* and anaerobes (e.g., carbapenem, piperacillin–tazobactam, cefepime + metronidazole)
	Enterocolitis in neutropenic patients is most commonly caused by a mix of organisms including *Clostridium* spp and *Pseudomonas*	
Urinary tract infections	Pathogens: gram-negative bacilli, *Candida*	Remove catheter to clear colonization
	Consider whether candiduria may represent disseminated candidiasis	Neutropenic patient: treat bacteriuria/candiduria regardless of symptoms
		Nonneutropenic patient: reserve treatment for symptomatic episodes
		Antibiotic treatment should be tailored to organism

(continued)

TABLE 35.4 (Continued)

Clinical Syndrome	Diagnostic Considerations	Management
CNS infections	Bacteria cause most cases of meningitis (*S. pneumoniae*, *Listeria*, *N. meningitidis*) In patients with cell-mediated immunodeficiency, also consider *Listeria* or *Cryptococcus* Encephalitis is most commonly caused by HSV but consider other viruses (HHV-6, JC virus) Brain abscesses may be confused with tumor	Bacterial meningitis: ceftriaxone, vancomycin, and ampicillin Cryptococcal meningitis: amphotericin B with flucytosine Encephalitis: treat *Listeria* and start ganciclovir, foscarnet, or both to cover both HSV and HHV-6

BAL, bronchoalveolar lavage; CMV, cytomegalovirus; HHV-6, human herpesvirus-6; HSV, herpes simplex virus; IVIG, intravenous immunoglobulin; VZV, varicella zoster virus.

Gram-positive Bacteremia

Gram-positive Cocci

- Coagulase-negative *Staphylococcus* species is the most common cause of bacteremia. The intravenous catheter is usually the source. In the setting of neutropenia or clinical instability, the patient should be treated with vancomycin.
- *S. aureus* bacteremia is associated with a high likelihood of metastatic complications if not treated adequately. Complicated *S. aureus* bacteremia (persistently positive blood cultures, prolonged fever, metastatic infection, and endocarditis) requires 4 to 6 weeks of treatment. Many authorities recommend that transesophageal echocardiogram should be performed in every case of *S. aureus* bacteremia to rule out endocarditis.
- Oxacillin and nafcillin are the drugs of choice for treating methicillin-susceptible *S. aureus*; vancomycin should be reserved for MRSA or the treatment of penicillin-allergic patients. Daptomycin may also be an alternative as long as there is no pulmonary involvement.
- Bacteremia with viridans group streptococci (*Streptococcus mitis*) may cause overwhelming infection with sepsis and acute respiratory distress syndrome (ARDS) in the neutropenic patient; vancomycin therapy should be used until susceptibility results are known (most, but not all, isolates are susceptible to ceftriaxone and carbapenems). Early information from the microbiology lab would likely be "gram-positive cocci in long chains."
- Risk factors for *Streptococcus mitis* bacteremia include severe mucositis (particularly following treatment with cytarabine), active oral infection, prophylaxis with trimethoprim/sulfamethoxazole (TMP/SMX) or a fluoroquinolone and H2-blockers.
- Enterococci (intrinsically resistant to all cephalosporins) often cause bacteremia in debilitated patients who have had prolonged hospitalization and have been on broad-spectrum antibiotics.
- VRE is an increasingly common cause of bacteremia and should be treated with linezolid (600 mg every 12 hours IV), daptomycin (6 mg/kg every 12 hours IV), or quinupristin–dalfopristin (7.5 mg/kg every 8 hours IV). Tigecycline (100 mg IV loading followed by 50 mg IV every 12 hours) has also been used. The overall success rate of treatment for VRE bacteremia is only around 40%.

Gram-positive Bacilli

- *Clostridium septicum* is associated with sepsis and metastatic myonecrosis during neutropenia. Treat with high-dose penicillin or a carbapenem.

- *Listeria monocytogenes* may cause bacteremia with or without encephalitis/meningitis in patients with defects in cell-mediated immunity. Ampicillin plus gentamicin is the treatment of choice. TMP/SMX can be used in penicillin-allergic patients.
- Other gram-positive bacilli such as *Bacillus*, *Corynebacterium*, and *Lactobacillus* species are common contaminants of blood cultures, but in the setting of neutropenia can cause true infection that is usually catheter related. *Propionibacterium* is almost always a contaminant, but it can cause infection of Ommaya reservoirs and other neurosurgical devices.

Gram-negative Bacteremia

- Gram-negative bacteria in the blood should never be considered contaminants and must be treated immediately.
- Depending on the preliminary result from the Microbiology lab (variable from one laboratory to another), preliminary information may be nonexistent or may be specific enough (e.g., "enteric-like" or "*Pseudomonas*-like" gram-negative bacillus) to guide antibiotic choice (See Table 35.2). Depending on institutional patterns and preliminary information it may be safer to initiate therapy with two antimicrobials to ensure adequate coverage until susceptibility results are available. Combination therapy offers no convincing benefit over single agent once susceptibilities are known.
- *Escherichia coli* and *Klebsiella* species are the most prevalent gram-negative pathogens in neutropenic patients; however, the use of prophylactic antibiotics such as ciprofloxacin or TMP/SMX may increase the prevalence of more resistant enteric organisms such as *Enterobacter*, *Citrobacter*, and *Serratia* species, some of which may carry an inducible β-lactamase (AmpC) that may result in treatment failure with third-generation cephalosporins like ceftazidime. Carbapenems, fluoroquinolones, and piperacillin–tazobactam may be used in this setting.
- The prevalence of strains of *Klebsiella* and *E. coli* that produce ESBL is increasing; carbepenems are the drugs of choice for these organisms.
- Klebsiella pneumoniae carrying the KPC carbapenemase and other CRE are becoming more prevalent and have caused institutional outbreaks with high mortality. There are no comparative data, and the treatment usually involves combination or several drugs including colistin, tigecycline, and gentamicin. In vitro data suggest that the addition of doripenem may result in synergistic antibacterial activity of the combination. Some CRE may be successfully treated with ceftazidime-avibactam 2.5 grams (ceftazidime 2 grams and avibactam 0.5 grams) every 8 hours IV.
- *P. aeruginosa* is one of the most lethal agents of gram-negative bacteremia in the neutropenic patient. Pending susceptibility results, combination therapy should be started to broaden the antimicrobial spectrum and ensure the patient is receiving at least one agent to which the isolate is susceptible.
- *Stenotrophomonas maltophilia* causes infection in patients who have been on broad-spectrum antibiotics (frequently carbapenems) or who have intravascular catheters; TMP/SMX is the treatment of choice. For the allergic patient, ceftazidime or moxifloxacin may be effective. S. *maltophilia* may show in vitro susceptibility to tigecyline and colistin, but the clinical efficacy of these agents is unknown.
- *Acinetobacter baumannii* bacteremia is frequently associated with infected intravascular catheters in cancer patients and is often resistant to multiple antibiotics, including imipenem–cilastatin. Ampicillin–sulbactam, tigecyclin, or colistin may be effective, but consultation with an infectious diseases specialist should be sought.

Fungemia

- *Candida* species cause most cases of fungemia in cancer patients. The frequency of non-*albicans* candidemia is increasing, probably as a consequence of the widespread use of fluconazole prophylaxis.
- The treatment of choice for candidemia is an echinocandin or amphotericin B.
- Fluconazole is reliably effective against *Candida albicans*. **Non-*albicans* species are likely to be resistant to fluconazole and should be treated with caspofungin, anidulafungin, micafungin, amphotericin B, or a lipid formulation of amphotericin B**
- All patients with candidemia should undergo ophthalmologic evaluation with fundoscopic examination. In most cases, intravascular catheters should be removed.

- Although *Candida* is the most common yeast found in blood cultures, other fungi with different susceptibility patterns may also cause fungemia: in patients with defects in cell-mediated immunity (e.g., AIDS, alemtuzumab use) *C. neoformans*, always resistant to echinocandins, should be considered. In neutropenic patients, *Fusarium*, *Scedosporium*, and *Trichosporon* species may also cause fungemia. Treatment for these relatively uncommon fungal isolates should be chosen in consultation with infectious diseases.

Intravascular Catheter-associated Infections

Definitions

- Exit-site infections are diagnosed clinically by the presence of erythema, induration, and tenderness within 2 cm of the catheter exit site.
- A tunnel infection is characterized by erythema along the subcutaneous tract of a tunneled catheter that extends 2 cm beyond the exit site.
- Catheter-associated bloodstream infection requires positive peripheral blood cultures (or a positive catheter-tip culture) *and* evidence that the catheter is the source of the bacteremia. **The most readily available evidence is a differential time to positivity of ≥2 hours between the peripheral blood culture and the culture drawn through the catheter.** The blood drawn through the catheter grows faster because the bacterial inoculum in the blood drawn through the catheter (where the bacteria-colonized biofilm lays) is higher. **Of note, this definition makes necessary to draw blood cultures from the catheter as well as directly from a vein via a peripheral stick to make the diagnosis of catheter-related bacteremia.**

Management

- If a local infection is suspected, a swab of exit-site discharge should be sent for culture, in addition to blood cultures.
- Uncomplicated catheter-site infections (no signs of systemic infection or bacteremia) can be managed with local care and oral antibiotics such as dicloxacillin.
- If the patient has fever or there is significant cellulitis around the catheter site, vancomycin should be used empirically while awaiting culture results.
- Tunnel infections require IV antibiotics and removal of the catheter; empirical therapy should include vancomycin, as well as coverage of gram-negative bacilli such as ceftazidime, cefepime, or ciprofloxacin. Therapy can then be modified if an organism is identified.
- Septic thrombophlebitis also necessitates catheter removal, and anticoagulation should be considered. Surgical drainage is occasionally necessary.
- Catheter-related bloodstream infections caused by coagulase-negative *Staphylococcus* or gram-negative bacilli should be treated for 14 days with antibiotics. After the cultures are negative, therapy may be completed with oral antibiotics (linezolid or a fluoroquinolone) in stable nonneutropenic patients.

Indications for Removal of Intravascular Catheters

- Infected temporary catheters must be removed. Removal of permanent (e.g., tunneled lines and implanted ports) catheters should always be considered, and we remove them in the following situations:
  - Tunnel (or pocket, in the case of implanted ports) infections.
  - Persistently positive blood cultures after 48 to 72 hours of appropriate therapy, regardless of the pathogen.
  - Septic thrombophlebitis.
  - Blood cultures positive for
  - *S. aureus*
  - *Bacillus* spp.
  - *Mycobacteria* spp.
  - *Candida* spp.
  - For other pathogens, including VRE, *Corynebacterium jeikeium*, and gram-negative pathogens like *Pseudomonas* and *Stenotrophomonas*, we occasionally attempt salvage therapy with systemic antibiotics and antibiotic lock. This approach should be considered only when the global risk of removing the catheter (refractory thrombocytopenia, paucity of IV access) is considered too high.

Skin and Soft Tissue Infections

- Soft tissue infections may represent local or disseminated infection.
- A biopsy for staining and culture for bacteria, mycobacteria, viruses, and fungi should be considered early in the evaluation of skin and soft tissue infections.
- Ecthyma gangrenosum often presents in neutropenic patients as a dark, necrotic lesion but can be quite variable in appearance. Typically a manifestation of *P. aeruginosa* bacteremia, it may also be caused by bacteremia due to other gram-negative bacilli. Antibiotic therapy with coverage of *Pseudomonas* should be initiated and early surgical involvement for possible debridement is imperative.
- VZV and herpes simplex virus (HSV) generally present as vesicular lesions and may be indistinguishable. Scrapings from the base of vesicles should be sent for direct fluorescent antibody (DFA) testing to diagnose VZV and for shell–vial culture or PCR to diagnose VZV or HSV. Treatment of VZV in the immunocompromised host is acyclovir 10 mg/kg IV every 8 hours, and for HSV acyclovir 5 mg/kg IV every 8 hours. We prefer to use IV acyclovir in immunocompromised hosts. In immunocompetent patients, oral acyclovir, valacyclovir, and famciclovir have been used successfully.
- Cancer patients are at increased risk for streptococcal toxic shock syndrome and severe soft tissue infections caused by *Streptococcus pyogenes*. Treatment is aggressive surgical debridement as needed and antibiotic therapy with penicillin G and clindamycin, as well as, in the case of shock, IV immunoglobulin (IVIG). The addition of clindamycin to penicillin G or ampicillin results in improved outcome, possibly because its action inhibiting protein (hence toxin) synthesis.
- Perianal cellulitis may develop in neutropenic patients. Antibiotic therapy should include gramnegative and anaerobic coverage (e.g., imipenem–cilastatin or meropenem or piperacillin-tazobactam as single agents or ceftazidime + metronidazole). A CT scan should be obtained to rule out a perirectal abscess. Incision and drainage may also be required in the setting of abscess or unremitting infection, but if possible should be delayed until resolution of neutropenia.
- Rash, including skin breakdown, is a common side effect of many new targeted therapies. Patients should have a detailed skin examination at each visit to evaluate for superinfections of their rash, as well as dermatology consultation as needed. Drugs commonly implicated include mAb like cetuximab (head and neck cancer, CRC) and tyrosine kinase inhibitor (TKI) like erlotinib (lung cancer) and sorafenib (renal cancer, HCC).
- Sweet syndrome can present with fever and cutaneous lesions that may resemble cellulitis, and should be considered in the differential diagnosis of fever and rash, particularly in patients with myeloid malignancies.

Sinusitis

- In immunocompetent patients, acute sinusitis is usually caused by *S. pneumoniae*, *H. influenzae*, and *Moraxella catarrhalis*, as well as *S. aureus*. Treatment is levofloxacin 500 mg daily or amoxicillin–clavulanate 875 mg twice daily.
- In immunocompromised hosts, sinusitis can also be caused by aerobic gram-negative bacilli, including *Pseudomonas*. Neutropenic patients are at high risk for fungal sinusitis.
- During neutropenia, sinusitis should be treated with broad-spectrum antibiotics, including coverage of *Pseudomonas*, and sinus CT scan and otolaryngology consult are appropriate. Biopsy should be obtained if there is any suspicion of fungal infection (e.g., bony erosion on CT scan, necrotic eschar of nasal turbinates) or if there is no response to antibiotic therapy within 72 hours.
- *Aspergillus* is the most common cause of invasive fungal sinusitis, but other molds such as *Mucor* and *Rhizopus* (which are resistant to voriconazole, the treatment of choice for aspergillosis) as well as *Fusarium* and, occasionally, dematiaceous molds like *Alternaria*, are increasingly recognized. When patients have been receiving voriconazole prophylaxis, the relative frequency of mucormycosis increases.
- If fungal sinusitis is confirmed, treatment is with surgical debridement and antifungal treatment, which should be started at maximum dosing:
  - Amphotericin B 1 to 1.5 mg/kg/day.
  - Lipid formulation of amphotericin B 5 to 7.5 mg/kg/day.
  - Voriconazole may be substituted only after it is certain that the infection is not caused by Zygomycetes (*Mucor*, *Rhizopus*), which are not susceptible to voriconazole.

- Posaconazole or isavuconazole given IV, with a very broad antifungal spectrum that covers most agents of fungal sinusitis, may be an alternative. If there is suspicion of mucormycosis we consider amphotericin the treatment of choice.

Pneumonia

- Pulmonary infiltrates in the immunocompromised host can be due to infectious or noninfectious causes. It is important to obtain an etiologic diagnosis. We recommend early use of bronchoalveolar lavage (BAL) if a diagnostic sputum specimen cannot be obtained.

Pulmonary Infiltrates in the Neutropenic Patient

- Most cases of pneumonia during neutropenia are caused by gram-negative bacilli, including *P. aeruginosa*.
- The treatment should include the standard regimen for fever and neutropenia plus vancomycin for *S. aureus* and some antibiotic active against *Legionella* and other agents of community-acquired pneumonia (e.g., newer generation fluoroquinolone like levofloxacin or moxifloxacin, or macrolide like azithromycin in addition to cefepime).
- CT scan and bronchoscopy for BAL should be performed early, particularly if there is no prompt improvement.
- If pulmonary infiltrates appear while the patient is on broad-spectrum antibiotic therapy, the likelihood of fungal pneumonia is high. Empirical antifungal coverage with voriconazole, liposomal amphotericin B, or amphotericin B should be started immediately. **Echinocandins should not be used for empirical fungal therapy for pulmonary infiltrates in neutropenic patients, as they have no activity against non-*Aspergillus* moulds and their activity against Aspergillus is not known to be equivalent to voriconazole or amphotericin B.**

Fungal Pneumonia

- Fungal pneumonia is rare in the absence of neutropenia or corticosteroids.
- *Aspergillus* species are the most common disease-causing molds in cancer patients.
- Lack of systemic toxicity is characteristic. Clinical presentation includes the following:
  - Persistent or recurrent fever
  - Development of pulmonary infiltrates while on antibiotics
  - Chest pain, hemoptysis, or pleural rub
- In the setting of allogeneic HSCT, most cases of *Aspergillus* pneumonia occur after engraftment, when the patient is no longer neutropenic. The most important risk factors in this setting are graft-versus-host disease, corticosteroid use, and CMV disease.
- Demonstration of fungal elements in biopsy tissue is necessary for definitive diagnosis. When a biopsy is not possible, positive respiratory cultures (sputum or BAL fluid) are highly predictive of invasive disease in a high-risk patient.
- Galactomannan (*Aspergillus*) and ß-D-glucan are serologic assays used to diagnose invasive fungal infections. **Galactomannan can also be determined in the BAL, where it has high sensitivity and specificity for aspergillosis.**
- There are molds that do not produce either galactomannan or ß-D-glucan (e.g., mucor, rhizopus). This means that a negative test *cannot* rule out invasive fungal infection.
- Positive serum galactomannan and ß-D-glucan (usually defined as two consecutive rising values when the tests are obtained twice weekly or every other day) can be helpful to identify fungal infections early.
- The treatment of choice for invasive aspergillosis is voriconazole 6 mg/kg IV every 12 hours for 24 hours, then 4 mg/kg IV. We routinely add an echinocandin to voriconazole until we document a therapeutic serum voriconazole level.
- Other options include
  - Isavuconazole, 200 mg IV every 8h for six doses loading followed by 200 mg IV daily
  - High-dose lipid formulation of amphotericin B (5 mg/kg/day)

- Amphotericin B (1 to 1.5 mg/kg/day)
- Caspofungin (70 mg loading dose followed by 50 mg/day IV) has been approved for patients with invasive aspergillosis who are unresponsive to or intolerant of amphotericin B
- Mucorales (previously known as zygomycetes) such as *Rhizopus*, *Mucor*, and *Cunninghamella* species are less common causes of pulmonary infection in neutropenic patients. They are voriconazole resistant but have variable susceptibility to posaconazole and isavuconazole. Treatment should include high-dose amphotericin B (deoxycholate or lipid formulation). Early consideration should be given to surgical excision where feasible.
- *Fusarium* is a less common cause of pulmonary infection in neutropenic patients. Voriconazole, isavuconazole, or high-dose amphotericin can be tried. Response is usually contingent on neutrophil recovery.
- Dematiaceous fungi such as *Scedosporium*, *Alternaria*, *Bipolaris*, *Cladosporium*, and *Wangiella* species are rare causes of pneumonia in neutropenic patients. The best treatment is not well established, and consultation with infectious diseases is strongly advised.

Pulmonary Infiltrates in Patients on High-dose Corticosteroids or with Other Defects in Cell-mediated Immunity

- In addition to the common bacterial causes of pneumonia, patients with defects in cell-mediated immunity are at risk for infections with *P. jirovecii*, *Nocardia* species, and viruses (see below), as well as *Legionella*, mycobacteria, and fungi.
- Bronchoscopy for BAL should be performed to aid in diagnosis.
- Empirical antibiotics should include newer generation fluoroquinolone for coverage of bacterial pathogens including *Legionella* and TMP/SMX for coverage of *Pneumocystis* and *Nocardia*. Consideration should also be given to antifungal and antiviral agents, depending on the clinical presentation.

Pneumocystis Pneumonia

- Patients with pneumonia from *P. jirovecii* usually present with rapid onset of dyspnea, nonproductive cough, hypoxemia, and fever. *Pneumocystis* pneumonia (PCP) may have a more indolent presentation in HIV-infected patients, stem cell transplant recipients, and patients on ibrutinib.
- Radiologic studies generally show diffuse bilateral interstitial infiltrates but can show focal infiltrates. The initial plain radiograph may be normal, but CT will almost always show characteristic groundglass opacities. Pleural effusions are uncommon.
- Treatment should be started based on clinical suspicion: TMP/SMX 5 mg/kg IV every 8 hours (**prednisone should be added if the pO$_2$ is <70 mm Hg or there is an A-a gradient >35 mm Hg**).
- In TMP/SMX-allergic/intolerant patients, alternatives for serious disease include IV pentamidine, and for moderate disease dapsone–trimethoprim, atovaquone, or clindamycin–primaquine. The combination clindamycin–primaquine may be the treatment of choice in cases of TMP/SMX failure.

Nocardia

- Pneumonia from *Nocardia* species can cause a dense lobar infiltrate or multiple pulmonary nodules with or without cavitation. Radiologically it may be indistinguishable from aspergillosis.
- Diagnosis is made from material obtained at bronchoscopy, either by pathology or culture. Culture may take 4 to 7 days.
- Antibiotic susceptibility varies with the species, although most are susceptible to TMP/SMX. Imipenem–cilastatin or meropenem and amikacin are also effective against the majority of isolate. Treatment is usually given for 6 months to 1 year. Depending on the species, Nocardia frequently causes disseminated infection involving the CNS. We recommend obtaining MRI with gadolinium in any patient with nocardiosis.

Viral Pneumonia

- Pneumonia due to respiratory viruses (respiratory syncytial virus [RSV], influenza, parainfluenza, adenovirus, and metapneumovirus) is more common in patients with defects in cell-mediated immunity like stem cell transplant recipients. In immunocompromised patients respiratory virus have been associated sometimes with high fever, and once pneumonia is established there is risk of progression to respiratory failure and death.

- The effect of antiviral treatment on the outcome of these viral respiratory infections is unclear. Anecdotal successes reported in case reports and case series have not been reproduced in controlled trials. Results seem to be better when treatment is initiated at the time of upper respiratory tract infection before progression to pneumonia.
- Influenza should be treated with neuraminidase inhibitors (most experience is with oral oseltamivir, 75 mg PO twice daily).
- RSV may be treated with aerosolized ribavirin 6 g daily delivered at a concentration of 20 mg/mL for 18 hours per day by a small particle aerosol generator unit (SPAG-2) via a face mask, ideally inside a scavenging tent to prevent environmental contamination or intermittently (2 g inhaled every 8 hours). The unproven efficacy and high cost of inhaled ribavirin have resulted in an increase of the use of oral ribavirin 600 to 800 mg PO bid for RSV infectio. Some experts recommend adding intravenous immunoglobulin (IVIG) or even the monoclonal antibody palivizumab, although there is no evidence that any of these interventions result in better outcome.
- Metapneumovirus and parainfluenza are also inhibited in vitro by ribavirin, but there is even less evidence than for RSV.
- Many strains of adenovirus are susceptible to cidofovir and some to ribavirin. Control of this infection, however, seems to be mainly related to the recovery of adenovirus-specific immunity.
- CMV pneumonia is a significant complication of allogeneic stem cell transplants that typically develops between 40 and 100 days posttransplant and presents with fever, dyspnea, hypoxemia, and diffuse interstitial infiltrates. Late CMV pneumonia (after day 100) may be becoming more common and should be considered in patients with a history of previous CMV infection.
- CMV infection and disease, typically restricted to allogeneic stem cell transplant recipients and AIDS patients, have also been rarely observed in patients with HTLV-I associated adult T-cell leukemia/lymphoma and patients treated with alemtuzumab.
- After allogeneic stem cell transplant, the detection by culture of CMV in the BAL is considered sufficient to establish the diagnosis. In other settings, tissue is required. Of note, identifying CMV in the BAL only by PCR is not diagnostic of CMV pneumonia (the test is too sensitive, quantitative PCR may help).
- Treatment of CMV pneumonia is with ganciclovir 5 mg/kg IV every 12 hours. The addition of IVIG 500 mg/kg every 48 hours for 3 weeks may be considered, but there is little evidence IVIG helps . Foscarnet (90 mg/kg every 12 hours) may be substituted for ganciclovir.

Gastrointestinal Infections

Mucositis

- The shallow, painful ulcerations of the tongue and buccal mucosa caused by chemotherapy can become superinfected with HSV or *Candida*.
- If severe, HSV infection is treated with acyclovir 5 mg/kg IV every 8 hours for 7 days. Milder infection may be treated with valaciclovir 1,000 mg PO every 12 hours or famciclovir 500 mg PO every 12 hours.
- Candidiasis can be treated locally with clotrimazole troches 10 mg dissolved in the mouth 5x/day, nystatin "swish and swallow" or systemically with fluconazole 200 mg PO/IV once, then 100 mg daily.
- Patients with fever and neutropenia with thrush should be covered empirically with systemic antifungals with activity against *Candida* species.

Esophagitis

- Odynophagia, dysphagia, and substernal chest discomfort can be a result of chemotherapy but may also be due to herpes or candidal infections.
- Endoscopy with biopsy should be performed when possible.

- If endoscopy and biopsy are not possible, empirical therapy with fluconazole for *Candida* and acyclovir for HSV is recommended. In neutropenic patients with fever and clinical symptoms of esophagitis, antibacterial therapy appropriate for upper GI flora should be added (e.g., ceftazidime + vancomycin or piperacillin–tazobactam or imipenem or meropenem).
- CMV can also cause esophagitis.

Diarrhea

- *Clostridium difficile* is the most common pathogen to cause diarrhea in cancer patients.
- Diagnosis can be made by detecting *C. difficile* toxin in the stool by immunoassay (EIA) or the toxin gene by PCR. Less commonly used tests include cytotoxicity assay and stool culture. It is important to be familiar with the diagnostic test used, as some toxin immunoassays are not sensitive enough to rule out the infection with certainty. Conversely, some tests like PCR are sensitive enough that repeating them is not associated with increased yield. In fact, PCR cannot differentiate between a patient colonized with *C. difficile* and diarrhea caused by some other reason and a patient with true *C. difficile*–associated disease (CDAD).
- Treatment for mild/moderate cases is with metronidazole 250 mg PO four times a day or 500 mg PO three times a day. The antiparasitic agent itazoxanide (500 mg PO twice a day) may offer similar efficacy. In severe and/or refractory cases, vancomycin 125 to 250 mg PO four times a day should be used. Fidaxomicin 200 mg PO twice daily was as effective as oral vancomycin in a randomized clinical trial. Metronidazole can be given IV if patients are unable to tolerate oral therapy or have ileus. Treatment is continued for 10 to 14 days. The stool should not be retested for *C. difficile* toxin, as many patients may remain asymptomatic carriers.
- Recurrent infection after metronidazole therapy should be treated with a longer course of metronidazole before oral vancomycin therapy is initiated.
- Recalcitrant CDAD has been successfully treated by fecal microbiota transplantation.
- Bacteria such as *E. coli, Salmonella, Shigella, Aeromonas,* and *Campylobacter* species, as well as parasites like *Giardia* and *Cryptosporidium* and viruses like norovirus and rotavirus are less common causes of diarrhea in cancer patients. Defects in cell-mediated immunity increase the likelihood of some of these pathogens. Stool should be sent for culture of bacterial pathogens. Stool should be sent for ova and parasites (O & P) on three consecutive days. Multiplex PCR in the stool is available and can detect more than 20 different pathogens.

Neutropenic Enterocolitis (Typhlitis)

- Typhlitis typically presents as abdominal pain, rebound tenderness, bloody diarrhea, and fever in the setting of neutropenia. The diagnosis should be entertained in every case of abdominal pain during neutropenia, although it is most common during prolonged, profound neutropenia during the treatment of acute leukemia.
- Characteristic CT scan findings include a fluid-filled, dilated, and distended cecum, often with diffuse cecal-wall edema and possibly air in the bowel wall (pneumatosis intestinalis). However, the CT may be unremarkable in the early stages; it has a reported sensitivity of only 80%.
- Pathogens are typically mixed aerobic and anaerobic gram-negative bacilli (including *Pseudomonas*) and *Clostridium* species.
- Treatment is with broad-spectrum antibiotics including coverage of *Pseudomonas* (e.g., imipenem or meropenem or the combination ceftazidime or cefepime plus metronidazole plus vancomycin) and anaerobes.
- Patients should be monitored closely for complications that may require surgical intervention, such as bowel perforation, bowel necrosis, or abscess formation.

Perforations/Fistulas

- Bevacizumab, a monoclonal antibody to vascular endothelial growth factor, has been associated with a gastrointestinal perforation/fistula rate of 1% to 5%.
- Patients with colon cancer and ovarian cancer have been found to be at greatest risk.

- Other risk factors may include prior abdominal/pelvic irradiation, bowel involvement by tumor, or unresected colon cancer.
- Any patient on bevacizumab with abdominal pain or new rectal bleeding should have prompt evaluation for perforation/fistula with imaging, as well as broad-spectrum antibiotic therapy covering gram-negative bacteria and anaerobes.

Hepatosplenic candidiasis

- Hepatosplenic candidiasis typically presents as fever during neutropenia (sometimes after resolution of neutropenia) without localizing signs or symptoms.
- When neutropenia resolves, the patient may continue to have fever, develop right upper quadrant pain and hepatosplenomegaly, and have significant elevation in alkaline phosphatase.
- CT scan, ultrasound, or MRI will show hypoechoic and/or bulls-eye lesions in the liver and spleen and sometimes the kidneys.
- Blood cultures are typically negative. A liver biopsy is recommended, since other fungal infections, tuberculosis and lymphoma may show similar findings. The diagnosis will be established by pathology showing granulomatous inflammation and yeast, as biopsy culture results are usually negative.
- Treatment consists of a prolonged course of fluconazole 400 to 800 mg daily. Caspofungin has also been effective.

Hepatitis B

- Hepatitis B virus (HBV) reactivation can occur in chronic carriers who are undergoing cytotoxic chemotherapy, with lymphoma patients being at highest risk especially with rituximab administration.
- Risk factors include positive hepatitis B DNA, HBsAg, HBeAg, and young age.
- Entecavir prophylaxis (0.5 mg/d) is recommended for patients with serological evidence consistent with past Hepatitis B, including those with undetectable HBV DNA, beginning 1 week before chemotherapy and for several months after completion of treatment. Entecavir has shown to be superior to lamivudine in randomized trials.

Urinary Tract Infections

- In the presence of neutropenia, it is reasonable to treat bacteriuria even in the absence of symptoms. In the nonneutropenic patient, treatment should be reserved for symptomatic episodes.
- Patients with indwelling stents may have persistent microbial colonization and pyuria. Treatment should be initiated in neutropenic patients with pyuria even with a history of chronic asymptomatic pyuria.
- Candiduria may represent colonization in a patient with an indwelling urinary catheter, particularly in the setting of broad-spectrum antibiotics. Removal of the catheter is frequently sufficient to clear it.
- Persistent candiduria can occasionally cause infections such as pyelonephritis or disseminated candidiasis in immunocompromised patients. Additionally, candiduria can be indicative of disseminated candidiasis. However, treatment of asymptomatic candiduria with systemic antifungals has not been associated with improved outcomes overall.
- If a decision is made to treat, fluconazole 400 mg per day for 1 to 2 weeks is the treatment of choice. In the case of non-*albicans* candiduria, another azole or amphotericin should be used. Caspofungin is minimally present in the urine, and there is no clinical experience in this setting.

Central Nervous System Infections

- Changes in mentation or level of consciousness, headache, or photophobia should be evaluated promptly with MRI and lumbar puncture.
- In addition to the usual bacterial causes of meningitis (*S. pneumoniae*, *Neisseria meningitidis*), *Listeria* and *Cryptococcus* should be considered, particularly when a defect in cell-mediated immunity is present.
- For *Listeria*, the treatment of choice is ampicillin 2 mg IV every 4 hours in combination with gentamicin.

- For *Cryptococcus*, treatment is with liposomal amphotericin B 3 mg/kg/day or amphotericin B 0.5 to 0.7 mg/kg/day in combination with flucytosine 37.5 mg/kg every 6 hours for 2 weeks. If the patient improves (afebrile, cultures negative), therapy can be subsequently changed to fluconazole 400 mg daily.
- Encephalitis in patients with cancer is most commonly caused by HSV. Diagnosis is made by the presence of viral DNA in CSF and should be treated with acyclovir 10 mg/kg IV every 8 hours. Potential clinical indications for empirical HSV treatment include predominance of altered mentation symptoms and focal changes on EEG or MRI, especially in the temporal lobes.
- VZV, CMV, and HHV-6 are other less common causes of encephalitis.
- Progressive multifocal leukoencephalopathy (PML), caused by JC virus, presents with multiple nonenhancing white matter lesions and has been associated with rituximab and mycophenolate mofetil (MMF).
- Brain abscesses that develop during neutropenia are typically caused by fungi (most commonly *Aspergillus* and *Candida*). Bacterial abscesses may also be a local extension of infection (sinusitis, odontogenic infection), caused by mixed aerobic and anaerobic flora (streptococci, *Staphylococcus*, *Bacteroides*). Pending results from biopsy and cultures, we recommend empirical treatment with ceftazidime plus vancomycin plus metronidazole plus voriconazole.
- Toxoplasmosis may present with multiple intracranial ring-enhancing lesions, frequently involving the basal ganglia. It is mainly an early complication of allogeneic stem cell transplant, but it has also been described after alemtuzumab.
- Nocardia (discussed above under pulmonary infections) may present as single of multiple brain abscess, usually on patients who are receiving corticosteroids.

Infectious Issues Secondary to Monoclonal Antibody Therapy

- The increased use of monoclonal antibodies, in particular those targeting leukocytes, has important implications for infectious disease.
- Alemtuzumab, an anti-CD52 antibody approved for chronic lymphocytic leukemia, results in profound depletion of cell-mediated immunity and places patients at risk for viral reactivation and infection with intracellular pathogens. *Pneumocystis*, HSV, and EBV infection, as well as CMV reactivation, are being seen regularly.
- Rituximab, a monoclonal antibody against CD20 used in lymphoma and leukemia treatment, causes B-cell depletion from 6 to 9 months and can also result in prolonged hypogammaglobulinemia and reactivation of viral hepatitis.
- Perforation and fistula are rare but serious side effects of bevacizumab.
- Cetuximab (anti-EGFR) is associated with acneiform rash and secondary bacterial infection.

PROPHYLAXIS
Antibacterial Prophylaxis

- Fluoroquinolones are the most commonly used antibiotics for prophylaxis against bacterial infections in neutropenic patients and can significantly reduce the frequency of gram-negative infections. However, they could conceivably result in the emergence of resistance among enteric gram-negative bacteria. Meta-analyses suggest fluoroquinolone prophylaxis may be associated with improved overall survival in patients with prolonged neutropenia. This approach is currently recommended for high-risk patients who are expected to remain neutropenic for more than 7 to 10 days. We start levofloxacin 500 mg PO the first day of neutropenia and continue until the ANC is ≥ 500/μL.

Antiviral Prophylaxis
HSV and VZV

- Prophylaxis against HSV should be considered in patients who are seropositive or have a history of herpetic stomatitis and are undergoing allogeneic stem cell transplant or highly immunosuppressive chemotherapy, including high-dose steroids and alemtuzumab. Patients treated with bortezomib are at high risk for VZV reactivation and should be considered for prophylaxis.

- In allogeneic transplant recipients we institute acyclovir prophylaxis at the beginning of the conditioning chemotherapy prior to transplant and continue for 1 year. This approach is effective for VZV prophylaxis, although a significant fraction of patients will develop shingles in the first few months after discontinuing acyclovir. In general, it is not considered necessary to routinely administer prophylaxis for HSV beyond the immediate peritransplant period.
- The drugs of choice are acyclovir 250 mg/m^2 IV every 12 hours or 800 mg PO twice daily or valaciclovir 500 mg PO once or twice daily.

CMV

- Prophylactic ganciclovir can reduce the incidence of CMV disease, but its use is limited by myelosuppressive toxicity. Valganciclovir (the prodrug of ganciclovir) is also effective, but it may result in a higher frequency of myelosuppression if the dose is not adjusted for weight and renal function.
- Patients who have undergone allogeneic stem cell transplant should be monitored for CMV replication by following CMV antigenemia or PCR weekly.
- If positive, patients should be treated with ganciclovir 5 mg/kg IV every 12 hours for 14 days followed by 5 mg/kg IV daily until CMV antigenemia or PCR results are negative 1 week apart.
- Alternative treatments include (a) foscarnet 60 to 90 mg/kg IV every 12 hours for 14 days followed by 90 mg/kg daily, (b) valganciclovir 900 mg IV every 12 hours for 14 days followed by 900 mg daily, or (c) cidofovir 5 mg/kg IV weekly for 2 weeks followed by 5 mg/kg IV every other week (very limited evidence is available regarding use of cidofovir for this indication).

Pneumocystis jirovecii Pneumonia Prophylaxis

- Prophylaxis against *Pneumocystis* is generally administered to patients during the 6-month poststem cell transplant period or after being treated with alemtuzumab. Patients with a history of PCP or with brain tumors on high-dose steroids should also receive prophylaxis.
- The regimen of choice is 160 mg TMP/800 mg SMX PO daily 3 days a week.
- Alternative prophylaxis options include (a) dapsone 100 mg PO daily (rule out G6PDH deficiency before using dapsone and monitor for methemoglobinemia), (b) inhaled pentamidine 300 mg every 4 weeks, or (c) atovaquone 1,500 mg daily with a fatty meal.

Antifungal Prophylaxis

- Fluconazole 400 mg PO/IV daily has been the regimen of choice. Of note, fluconazole has no activity against molds like *Aspergillus*.
- Posaconazole 200 mg PO three times a day (older liquid formulation) proved to be more effective than fluconazole/itraconazole in patients with prolonged neutropenia, and it also resulted in less cases of aspergillosis in patients receiving corticosteroids for GVHD. With the newer oral and IV forms of posaconazole it is appropriate to consider it the antifungal prophylactic agent of choice when the risk of mould infection is considered significant.
- Prophylaxis should be continued until 100 days posttransplant and until immunosuppressants have been discontinued.
- Use of fluconazole has led to increased frequency of fluconazole-resistant infections such as *Candida glabrata* and *C. krusei*.

Suggested Readings

1. Debast SB, Bauer MP, Kuijper EJ, The Committee. European society of clinical microbiology and infectious diseases (ESCMID): Update of the treatment guidance document for clostridium difficile infection (CDI). *Clin Microbiol Infect*. 2013, Oct 5;20 Suppl 2:1–26.
2. Freifeld AG, Bow EJ, Sepkowitz KA, et al. Clinical practice guideline for the use of antimicrobial agents in neutropenic patients with cancer: 2010 update by the infectious diseases society of america. *Clin Infect Dis*. 2011, Feb 15;52(4):e56–93.
3. Gea-Banacloche J. Evidence-based approach to treatment of febrile neutropenia in hematologic malignancies. *Hematology Am Soc Hematol Educ Program*. 2013;2013:414–422.

4. Kalil AC, Metersky ML, Klompas M, et al. Management of adults with hospital-acquired and ventilator-associated pneumonia: 2016 clinical practice guidelines by the infectious diseases society of america and the american thoracic society. *Clin Infect Dis.* 2016, Sep 1;63(5):e61–e111.
5. Lehrnbecher T, Phillips R, Alexander S, et al. Guideline for the management of fever and neutropenia in children with cancer and/or undergoing hematopoietic stem-cell transplantation. *J Clin Oncol.* 2012, Dec 10;30(35):4427–4438.
6. Mermel LA, Allon M, Bouza E, et al. Clinical practice guidelines for the diagnosis and management of intravascular catheter-related infection: 2009 update by the infectious diseases society of America. *Clin Infect Dis.* 2009, Jul 1;49(1):1–45.
7. Pappas PG, Kauffman CA, Andes DR, et al. Clinical practice guideline for the management of candidiasis: 2016 update by the infectious diseases society of america. *Clin Infect Dis.* 2016, Feb 15;62(4):e1–e50.
8. Patterson TF, Thompson GR, Denning DW, et al. Practice guidelines for the diagnosis and management of aspergillosis: 2016 update by the infectious diseases society of america. *Clin Infect Dis.* 2016, Aug 15;63(4):e1–e60.
9. Reddy KR, Beavers KL, Hammond SP, Lim JK, Falck-Ytter YT. American gastroenterological association institute guideline on the prevention and treatment of hepatitis B virus reactivation during immunosuppressive drug therapy. *Gastroenterology.* 2015, Jan;148(1):215–219.
10. Tunkel AR, Glaser CA, Bloch KC, et al. The management of encephalitis: Clinical practice guidelines by the infectious diseases society of America. *Clin Infect Dis.* 2008, Aug 1;47(3):303–327.

36 Oncologic Emergencies and Paraneoplastic Syndromes

Meena Sadaps and James P. Stevenson

INTRODUCTION

While statistics show that the number of new cancer diagnoses in recent years has been climbing, the 5-year relative survival rate has now increased to 69%. This translates to the prevention of more than 1.7 million cancer deaths. These improvements in survival are a reflection of both patients being diagnosed at earlier stages and the introduction of novel agents into standard care. Because of these notable advances in oncology and the subsequent expanding population of cancer survivors, it is pertinent to gain familiarity with the diagnosis of and initial treatment for common oncological emergencies. Cancer patients are at increased risk of developing unique complications that can require emergent evaluation and treatment, often by frontline providers such as primary care and emergency department practitioners. The most common emergencies we encounter can be classified into metabolic, hematologic, cardiovascular, neurologic, infectious, and chemotherapy-related side effects. In this chapter, we will discuss each emergency in detail to facilitate their prompt recognition and management.

SUPERIOR VENA CAVA (SVC) SYNDROME

SVC syndrome occurs when blood flow through the thin-walled vessel becomes obstructed due to external compression by a tumor or internal occlusion by tumor invasion, fibrosis, or an intraluminal thrombus. This subsequently impairs venous drainage from the head, neck, upper extremities, and thorax. Decreased venous return to the heart, in turn, causes decreased cardiac output, increased venous congestion, and edema.

Etiology

The causes of SVC syndrome can be classified into two main categories: malignant (>90% of cases) and benign. The most common malignancies associated with SVC syndrome include lung cancer (primarily small cell and squamous cell), lymphoma (primarily non-Hodgkin's including diffuse large cell lymphoma (DLCL) or lymphoblastic lymphoma), and metastatic disease (breast cancer being the most common). Other mediastinal tumors, such as thymomas and germ cell tumors, account for <2% of cases. The most common benign etiology is an intravascular device (indwelling central venous catheter or pacemaker), and in these cases the findings are predominantly unilateral. Other benign causes include retrosternal goiter, sarcoidosis, TB, and postradiation or idiopathic fibrosis.

Clinical Signs/Symptoms

The severity of symptoms (see Table 36.1) depends on the acuity of the obstruction/occlusion. Gradual progression allows for the development of collateral circulation in the azygous venous system and thus

TABLE 36.1 Clinical Presentation of SVC Syndrome

Dyspnea	63%	Arm swelling	18%
Facial plethora	50%	Chest pain	15%
Cough	24%	Dysphagia	9%

a more benign presentation. However, sudden obstruction is a true emergency that can lead to airway compromise, increased intracranial pressure, and cerebral edema.

Common symptoms include dyspnea (63%) and facial swelling/sensation of head fullness (50%). Cough, chest pain, and dysphagia are less frequently encountered. Characteristic physical exam findings include venous distention of neck (66%), venous distention of chest wall (54%), and facial edema (46%). Other exam findings may include cyanosis, arm swelling, facial plethora, and edema of arms. Symptoms are generally exacerbated by bending forward, stooping, or lying down.

Diagnosis

Although SVC syndrome is a clinical diagnosis, imaging studies may be obtained for further confirmation. Common abnormalities seen on CXR include superior mediastinal widening and pleural effusion. CT scan +/– venography, however, remains the most useful study for imaging the mediastinum, through identification of the site of obstruction, and, if warranted, to guide percutaneous biopsy. More invasive methods such as bronchoscopy, thoracotomy, and mediastinoscopy represent alternative methods to obtain diagnostic tissue if needed in these patients.

Treatment

The treatment and prognosis of SVC syndrome is driven by the underlying pathological process, and its management has shifted over the years from empiric radiotherapy to a more methodological and individualized approach. It has been shown that radiation prior to obtaining tissue diagnosis impedes accurate interpretation of the biopsy sample in >50% of cases. Exceptions to this rule, however, may include those with impending airway obstruction and/or a severe increase in intracranial pressure.

Symptomatic treatment with supplemental oxygen, diuretics, bedrest with head of bed elevation (>45 degrees), and corticosteroids can help provide initial relief. Once a histologic diagnosis has been made, treatment should be tailored accordingly. Chemotherapy alone or in combination with radiotherapy is effective in patients with SCLC. In patients with recurrent disease, it has actually been shown that additional chemotherapy +/– radiotherapy is still likely to provide further alleviation.

Radiotherapy or chemotherapy can also be used in patients with NSCLC; however, the percentage of patients who have been reported to have experienced relief were less than that of the SCLC population. The obstruction was also found to recur in approximately 20% of patients. Thus, the general recommendation for these patients consists primarily of radiation therapy, endovascular stenting, or a combination of both modalities. Some studies have shown that the presence of SVCS in patients with NSCLC foreshadows a shorter median survival of only 6 months as compared to 9 months in those without.

No treatment modality (chemo, chemo + XRT, XRT alone) has proven superior in the treatment for NHL. Relapse, however, remains common in this population and median survival has been approximated at 21 months.

When the goals of therapy are palliative or when urgent intervention is required (significant cerebral edema, laryngeal edema with stridor, or significant hemodynamic compromise), direct opening of the occlusion by endovascular stenting, angioplasty, and/or possible thrombolysis should be considered. Complete occlusion of the SVC is not a contraindication to stent placement.

If SVC syndrome is detected early in patients with an indwelling venous catheter, fibrinolytic therapy can be used without removal of the catheter. Otherwise, these patients should have the catheter removed and be placed on anticoagulation to prevent embolization. The role for SVC bypass surgery in patients with SVC syndrome secondary to other benign causes (e.g., mediastinal granuloma, fibrosing mediastinitis) has been one of great debate. While the overall good prognosis of these patients sways physicians away from surgical methods, many have advocated surgical consideration in patients where the syndrome develops suddenly or progresses/persists after 6 to 12 months of observation.

INCREASED INTRACRANIAL PRESSURE

The contents of our skull and dura can be divided into three main compartments: brain parenchyma (which occupies a volume of approximately 1.4 L), spinal fluid (52 to 160 ml), and blood (150 ml). An increase in any of these three compartments, as per the Monro-Kellie hypothesis, will occur at the expense of the remaining two. In addition, intracranial compliance has been noted to decrease with rising pressure, thus causing further compromise in cerebral perfusion. The normal range of ICP has been reported to be 5 to 15 mm Hg.

Etiology

In cancer patients, volume changes in brain parenchyma can be the result of primary or secondary brain tumors +/– intratumoral hemorrhage, vasogenic (peritumoral) or cytotoxic (in the setting of cytotoxic chemotherapy) edema, extra-axial mass lesions (dural tumors, infection, or hemorrhage), or indirect neurologic complications. Brain metastases are, in fact, the most common cause of increased ICP in this population. Lung cancer and melanoma, specifically, are most commonly associated with central nervous system (CNS) metastasis.

An imbalance between cerebral spinal fluid (CSF) production and reabsorption may also contribute to increased intracranial pressure (ICP). Mass lesions located at or near "bottleneck regions" (foramen of Monro, cerebral aqueduct, medullary foramina, basilar subarachnoid cisterns) cause obstruction. Some examples of primary brain tumors that favor these locations include subependymal giant cell astrocytoma, lymphoma, choroid plexus papilloma, ependymoma, and meningioma. Carcinomatosis and meningitis impede CSF reabsorption at the arachnoid granulations. Fibrosis of arachnoid granulations can be seen in patients that have received whole-brain or less commonly, partial-brain irradiation. Retinoic acid, an agent used for the treatment of promyelocytic leukemia, has also been associated with decreased CSF reabsorption. Increased production of CSF, on the other hand, is a rare cause of increased ICP. It can sometimes be seen in patients with choroid plexus papilloma, especially if the disease is multifocal in nature.

The third and last compartment within the skull is blood. Cerebral perfusion pressures are normally maintained over a wide range (50 to 160 mmHg), however, passive increases in ICP are seen when this autoregulatory mechanism fails. Venous outflow obstruction can be thrombotic or non-thrombotic. Patients receiving L-asparaginase therapy are at increased risk of developing dural venous sinus thrombosis. Nonthrombotic causes may include dural mass lesions such as meningioma, metastases from breast or prostate cancer, non-Hodgkin's lymphoma, Ewing sarcoma, plasmacytoma, or neuroblastoma.

Intrathoracic pressure changes reflect on ICP as well, as demonstrated by coughing, sneezing, and straining. While these minimal fluctuations may not seem significant alone, patients with decreased compliance may experience transient decompensation.

Clinical Signs/Symptoms

The presentation of elevated ICP largely depends on the acuity of the underlying cause, with rapid progression often indicating hemorrhage. Slow, progressive changes may be accompanied by little to no symptoms, whereas dynamic changes can cause clinical deterioration. The Cushing response details the body's response to a rise in intracranial pressures. First, the systolic blood pressure rises. In response, pulse pressure widens and bradycardia and irregular breathing ensue. Without correction, the heart rate will begin to rise, breathing will become shallow with episodes of apnea, and blood pressure will fall. With herniation and eventual cessation of brain stem activity, the patient goes into cardiac and respiratory arrest.

In the vast majority of cancer patients, the onset of symptoms occurs over days to weeks. Headache is the most common presenting symptom. Due to decreased venous drainage while in the supine position, patients generally report that their pain is most severe in the morning. Common analgesics rarely provide relief, however, patients have been noted to experience immediate relief with emesis. Fundoscopic examination may be revealing, with absence of venous pulsations in the center of the optic disc being an early findings and papilledema with blurring of disc margins and/or small hemorrhages being a later finding. Elevated ICP in the setting of mass-effect can present with focal neurologic deficits based on the location of the mass. Patients with chronic disturbance of spinal fluid reabsorption can present with a triad of cognitive decline, incontinence, and ataxic gait. Hyponatremia may also be noted on laboratory testing as SIADH is a common metabolic complication seen with elevated ICP.

Diagnosis

While imaging is critical in the determination of the underlying etiology, thorough clinical history and physical examination are most pertinent for diagnosis of increased ICP. Lumbar puncture is used to directly measure CSF pressure; however, CT should be obtained prior in order to rule out mass lesions of the posterior fossa and/or compartmentalization, as these would be contraindications due to the risk of herniation. CT scan without contrast is generally the initial preferred imaging study as it can identify the presence of CSF obstruction, herniation, hemorrhage, or neoplastic/infectious mass lesions. MRI with gadolinium can further be used to differentiate between neoplastic, infectious, inflammatory, and ischemic process. Obstruction or infiltration of the dural venous sinuses is best visualized with magnetic resonance venography.

Treatment

Few patients present emergently, such as those with obstructive hydrocephalus, and in these cases immediate neurosurgical intervention will be necessary. In non-emergent cases, certain measures can be taken initially to help decrease intracranial pressure. These include elevation of the head of the bed above 30 degrees, antipyretic use when the patient is febrile, and maintenance of high-normal serum osmolality with osmotic diuresis as needed. The most commonly used hyperosmolar agent used is 20% to 25% mannitol solution given at 0.75 to 1 g/kg body weight followed by 0.25 to 0.5 g/kg body weight every 3 to 6 hours. While moderate to high dose dexamethasone (6 to 10 mg every 6 hours up to 100 mg/day) can be effective in patients with vasogenic edema, they should be avoided in patients suspected to have CNS lymphoma prior to tissue diagnosis. Steroids are known to induce lymphocytic apoptosis and can therefore obscure the diagnosis. The most rapid, but transient, method to decreasing ICP is mechanical hyperventilation with goal PCO2 25 to 30 mmHg.

In addition to symptomatic management in these patients, it is crucial to treat the underlying disease process, whether that includes surgical resection/decompression, systemic/intrathecal chemotherapy, and/or whole brain irradiation.

SPINAL CORD COMPRESSION

Spinal cord compression (SCC) is a true oncologic emergency as delays in diagnosis can cause severe, irreversible neurologic compromise, decline in functional status, and impaired quality of life. Spinal cord compression affects roughly 5% to 10% of all patients with cancer; an estimated 20,000 patients are diagnosed each year in the United States. The majority of cases result from spine metastases with extension into the epidural space. It is the second most frequent neurologic complication of cancer after brain metastases. The median overall survival of patients with spinal cord compression ranges from 3 to 16 months and most die of systemic tumor progression.

Etiology

Although all cancers capable of hematogenous spread can cause malignant spinal cord compression, the most common underlying cancer diagnoses associated with this complication are breast, prostate, lung, multiple myeloma, and lymphoma.

Hematogenous seeding of tumor to the vertebral bodies is the most common cause of spinal metastases, followed by direct extension and cerebrospinal fluid spread. Nearly 66% of spinal cord compression involves the thoracic spine and 20% involves the lumbar spine. Colon and prostate malignancies more commonly spread to the lumbosacral spine while lung and breast cancers frequently affect the thoracic spine. The cervical and sacral spines are rarely involved (less than 10% for each region).

The median time interval between cancer diagnosis and manifestation of SCC is approximately 6 to 12.5 months. Malignant spinal cord compression is rarely the primary manifestation of a malignancy.

Clinical Signs/Symptoms

The most common presenting symptom of malignant spinal cord compression is back pain. The complaint of back pain in a cancer patient, specifically with a malignancy that frequently seeds the spine, should be considered metastatic in origin until proven otherwise. The characteristic back pain that is described is often worst in the recumbent position, thus resulting in maximal intensity upon morning awakening. As time progresses, the back pain can become radicular in nature.

Other symptoms of malignant SCC are primarily dependent on the region of the spine that is affected.

Cervical spine involvement generally presents with headache, arm/shoulder/neck pain, breathing difficulties, loss of sensation, and weakness/paralysis in the upper extremities. Thoracic and lumbosacral spine involvement can present with pain in the back or chest, loss of sensation below the level of tumor, increased sensation above the level of tumor, positive Babinski sign, bladder/bowel retention, and/or sexual dysfunction.

A thorough physical exam should be performed including percussion of the spinal column, evaluation for motor and sensory deficits including pinprick testing, straight-leg raise, and a rectal examination to assess sphincter tone.

The most important prognostic factor for regaining ambulatory function after treatment of SCC is pretreatment neurologic status, making the physical exam a vital component of overall prognosis. Generally speaking, the quicker the neurologic deficit evolves, the lower the chance of recovery after treatment.

Diagnosis

Despite the availability of diagnostic testing, there remains a lag between onset of symptoms and diagnosis (approximately 3 months). This delay can be primarily attributed to a delay in obtaining the diagnostic imaging by health-care professionals. As back pain is a common complaint and the differential remains broad, having a high clinical suspicion is crucial. Red flags for SCC should include pain in the thoracic spine, persistence of symptoms despite conservative measures, and exacerbation of pain in the supine position.

Magnetic resonance imaging (MRI) with contrast of the spine is the most sensitive diagnostic test. Its advantages include the ability to accurately identify the level of the metastatic lesion, define soft tissue from bone, and separate metastatic cord compression from other pathologic processes involving the axial skeleton, epi- or intradural space, and spinal cord. It avoids the need for lumbar or cervical puncture that is required with CT myelography and can be safely performed in most patients.

CT myelography after intrathecal injection of contrast was the study of choice in the pre-MRI era but is now used much less frequently. It remains useful, however, for patients in whom MRI is contraindicated.

If SCC is the initial presentation for a malignancy, a biopsy is mandatory prior to initiation of treatment.

Treatment

Primary goals of treatment include pain control, preservation/recovery of neurologic function, and prevention of complications secondary to tumor growth.

Treatment with corticosteroids should be initiated immediately when spinal cord compression is suspected. This begins with an initial loading dose of 10 mg IV dexamethasone followed by 4 mg

IV dexamethasone every 6 hours afterwards. Corticosteroids facilitate pain management but also reduce swelling around the cord and may prevent additional spinal cord damage from decreased blood perfusion.

Immediate consultations to surgery and radiation oncology are required after diagnosis. Further therapy is then decided based on the clinical picture, availability of histologic diagnosis, spinal stability, and previous treatment. Patients with spinal instability, even in the absence of clinical signs/symptoms, should undergo surgery unless otherwise contraindicated.

At the time of diagnosis, 66% of patients receive radiation, 16% to 20% undergo surgical decompression, and the remainder are provided with comfort care measures. In a study of symptomatic patients with SCC with metastatic tumors other than lymphoma, debulking surgery followed by radiation resulted in four times longer duration of maintained ambulation after treatment and three times higher chance of regaining ambulation for non-ambulatory patients than radiation alone. Combined-modality approaches help to achieve better pain control and bladder continence. This can also reduce steroid and narcotic use.

Radiation therapy is the most commonly used treatment modality. It is typically applied in asymptomatic individuals or symptomatic patients who are poor surgical candidates. Patients with radiosensitive tumors (breast, lymphoma, myeloma, prostate cancer) have a higher chance of regaining/preserving motor function than those with less radiosensitive tumors (non-small cell lung cancer, melanoma, and renal cell carcinoma). Standard radiation doses consist of 3000 to 4000 cGy in 5 to 10 fractions. It can also be used for palliative purposes with one fraction of 8 Gy. Stereotactic radiation therapy is becoming a more frequent modality for spine metastases. It provides the ability to deliver a higher radiation dose without exceeding the tolerance of the spinal cord.

Systemic chemotherapy is most appropriate as a primary treatment modality only for patients with SCC caused by highly chemosensitive tumors such as Hodgkin and non-Hodgkin lymphoma, small cell lung cancer, breast, and prostate cancers. It can also be used in those who are not candidates for radiation or surgery.

TUMOR LYSIS SYNDROME

Tumor lysis syndrome (TLS) refers to a constellation of metabolic imbalances that occurs when malignant cells rapidly undergo lysis and empty their intracellular contents into the bloodstream at a rate that far exceeds the kidney's clearance capacity. The overwhelming release of nucleic acid products results in hyperuricemia, which can then contribute to crystallization and subsequent obstruction within the renal tubules. Hyperkalemia and hyperphosphatemia with secondary hypocalcemia can also be seen in these patients. Without appropriate time-sensitive treatment (see Table 36.2), TLS can lead to lactic acidosis, acute renal failure, and even death.

Etiology

While TLS is most commonly seen in patients with high-grade lymphomas (particularly Burkitt lymphoma) or acute leukemias, it can also be seen in those with kinetically active solid tumors and, at times, may even occur spontaneously. Factors that increase the risk of TLS include high baseline urate levels, large tumor burden (white blood cell count >50 x 10^9/L, high low-density lipoprotein, large tumor size), and chemo-sensitive disease. Generally speaking, many of the patients that develop TLS are patients that have recently started chemotherapy. TLS most commonly occurs within hours to 3 days following chemotherapy. Additional incidences, though fewer, have been reported following other treatment modalities including ionizing radiation, embolization, radiofrequency ablation, monoclonal antibody therapy, glucocorticoids, interferon, and hematopoietic stem cell transplantation.

Clinical Signs/Symptoms

The presentation of patients with TLS is fairly non-specific and depends on the electrolyte abnormalities that are present. Although symptoms may precede initiation of chemotherapy, they are most often noted within 12 to 72 hours after initiation of cytoreductive treatment. Hyperkalemia can manifest with arrhythmias, muscle cramps, weakness, paresthesia, nausea/vomiting, and diarrhea. Hyperphosphatemia and hyperuricemia contribute to acute renal failure, which is evidenced by decreased urine output (UOP) and/or volume overload. Hyperphosphatemia also leads to secondary hypocalcemia. Hypocalcemic signs include muscle twitches, cramps, carpopedal spasm, paresthesia, tetany, mental status changes, nephrocalcinosis and rarely, seizures.

Diagnosis

Of all the metabolic abnormalities seen with TLS, hyperkalemia poses the most immediate threat and is often the first sign of the disease. Hyperuricemia, on the other hand, is the most common lab abnormality noted in these patients. Additional labs may be notable for elevated phosphorus, elevated lactate

TABLE 36.2 Management of Electrolyte Abnormalities in TLS

Metabolic Derangement	Severity	Treatment
Hyperkalemia	Moderate (≥6 mmol/L) and asymptomatic	■ Limit intake ■ ECG/Telemetry ■ Sodium polystyrene sulfonate 15-30 g PO
	Severe (>7 mmol/L) and/or symptomatic	As above, plus any of the following: ■ If ECG changes present, calcium gluconate 1g slow infusion ■ Regular insulin 10U IV + 100 mL D50 IV ■ Sodium bicarbonate 45-50 mEq slow IV infusion over 5–10 mins ■ Albuterol 10–20 in 4mL nebulized saline over 20 mins ■ Dialysis
Hypocalcemia (≤7 mg/dL)	Asymptomatic	No treatment necessary
	Symptomatic	■ Hyperphosphatemia should be corrected first, if present, unless the patient develops tetany or an arrhythmia ■ Calcium gluconate 1 g, administered slowly with ECG monitoring
Hyperphosphatemia	Moderate (≥6.5 mg/dL)	■ Limit intake ■ Phosphate binders (Calcium acetate, calcium carbonate, sevelamer, lanthanum carbonate, or aluminum hydroxide)
	Severe	■ Hemodialysis
Hyperuricemia (≥8 mg/dL)	Low risk	■ IV normal saline 150–200 cc/hour +/–Allopurinol 300 mg PO daily (100 mg/m² every 8 hr)
	Intermediate risk	-IV normal saline 150–200 cc/hr -Allopurinol 300 mg PO daily (100 mg/m² every 8 hr) +/–Rasburicase 0.15 mg/kg IV daily for 5–7 days
	High risk	■ IV normal saline 150–200 cc/hr ■ Rasburicase 0.2 mg/kg IV daily for 5–7 days +/–Dialysis

dehydrogenase, and low calcium levels. Clinical and laboratory TLS is defined by the Cairo and Bishop classification and grading system. Laboratory TLS is diagnosed when levels of two or more serum values of urate, potassium, phosphate, or calcium are abnormal at presentation or if there is a 25% change within 3 days before or 7 days after the initiation of treatment. Clinical TLS is diagnosed when laboratory TLS is present and one or more of the following complications are present: renal insufficiency, cardiac arrhythmias/sudden death, and seizures. Laboratory TLS is either present or absent, whereas, clinical TLS is graded on a scale of 0 to 5 based on the severity of the clinical manifestation.

Treatment

Prevention is key in the management of TLS. Patients at low risk can be closely monitored while patients at intermediate or high risk should be treated prophylactically to reduce incidence of TLS. The recommended prophylactic treatment for intermediate risk patients is allopurinol (100 mg/m^2 every 8 hours) for 2 to 3 days prior to administration of chemotherapy and continued for 3 to 7 days afterward until normalization of serum urate levels. Severe cutaneous adverse events have been reported with allopurinol in patients with inheritance of the HLA-B*58:01 allele; screening is advised in high risk patients (Han Chinese, Thai, Korean populations). Patients should also undergo aggressive hydration (in order to maintain urine output of atleast 100 cc/m^2/hr) and be given oral phosphate binders. Metabolites should be vigilantly monitored in intervals of 3 to 4 hours after initiation of treatment.

Uric acid levels are generally not expected to decrease until 48 to 72 hours of treatment as the mechanism of allopurinol is through the inhibition of xanthine oxidase. The medication, therefore, only affects further uric acid synthesis and not pre-existing uric acid. Rasburicase can be considered in patients at intermediate or high risk of TLS and with pre-existing hyperuricemia (>= 7.5 mg/dl) and should be administered within four hours of presentation. This medication, in contrast, acts on the degradation of uric acid. There has only been one phase III clinical trial to compare allopurinol with rasburicase in adults. While rasburicase was proven superior in time to control serum uric acid levels, there was a lack of evidence to determine whether clinical outcomes were improved. At this time, the evidence remains stronger for rasburicase use in children with high-risk conditions than in adults, however, the medication has been approved for use in both populations, with the recommended dose of 0.2 mg/kg/day for 5 to 7 days. In patients at intermediate risk, a single dose of 0.15 mg/kg may be sufficient and can minimize cost. In a retrospective study utilizing patient data from over 400 U.S. hospitals from 2005 to 2009, it was noted that rasburicase administration compared to allopurinol was associated with a significant reduction in uric acid levels, ICU length of stay (LOS), overall LOS, overall cost. In patients receiving single dose rasburicase, it is recommended that they receive allopurinol following the rasburicase treatment. G6PD deficiency is a contraindication for rasburicase treatment because hydrogen peroxide can cause severe hemolysis; therefore patients should undergo screening prior to use.

In patients in whom allopurinol and rasburicase are not an option, febuxostat can be cautiously considered as an alternative. Febuxostat was compared with allopurinol in the FLORENCE trial. The decrease in mean serum urate levels observed with febuxostat did not translate to improvement in laboratory or clinical TLS following chemotherapy. In addition, the arm that received febuxostat was noted to have a higher incidence of liver dysfunction, nausea, joint pain, and rash.

Patients diagnosed with TLS require hospitalization for further monitoring and treatment. An ECG should be obtained in these patients to evaluate for serious arrhythmias and conduction abnormalities. Hyperkalemia can be treated with any combination of calcium gluconate, sodium bicarbonate, insulin with hypertonic dextrose, loop diuretics, and kayexalate (sodium polystyrene sulfonate). Patients may require hemodialysis depending on the severity of the hyperkalemia, renal dysfunction, and volume status. With the exception of hyperkalemia management, calcium administration is generally avoided as it can promote metastatic calcifications. Hyperphosphatemia is treated with phosphate binders (i.e. aluminum hydroxide) or hypertonic dextrose with insulin. As hypocalcemia resolves with management of the underlying hyperphosphatemia, treatment with calcium gluconate is only needed if the patient is symptomatic. Urine alkalinization is no longer common practice as there is a lack of data to demonstrate its efficacy and it poses the risk of calcium phosphate deposition in the kidneys, heart, and other organs.

HYPONATREMIA

Cancer patients may develop hyponatremia due to imbalances in water and sodium homeostasis. The reported incidence is 3.7%.

Etiology

The differential for hyponatremia is quite extensive, including pulmonary infections, intracranial lesions, recent radiation therapy, gastrointestinal (GI) losses, heart failure, hypothyroidism, diabetes, and offending medications. In cancer patients specifically, the leading causes remain dehydration, GI or renal losses, and syndrome of inappropriate secretion of antidiuretic hormone (SIADH). SIADH generally occurs as either a paraneoplastic syndrome or as a complication of chemotherapy. The excess production of antidiuretic hormone (ADH) may originate from the hypothalamus or be ectopic, arising from cancer cells. Ectopic ADH is most commonly associated with small cell lung cancer, indicating a poor prognosis. Other associated malignancies include head and neck carcinomas, hematological malignancies, and non-small cell lung cancer. Chemotherapy agents that can cause SIADH include cyclophosphamide, ifosfamide, vincristine, vinblastine, vinorelbine, bortezomib, carboplatin, and cisplatin.

Ectopic production of a peptide similar to ADH, known as atrial natriuretic peptide (ANP), has also been described in patients with small cell lung cancer (SCLC). ANP is released from atrial myocytes and works by increasing renal sodium excretion and possibly by suppressing an aldosterone response.

"Pseudohyponatremia" is a condition frequently seen in patients with multiple myeloma and hyperproteinemia as a way for the body to preserve electrical neutrality. Lastly, hyponatremia can also occur with cerebral salt wasting syndrome (CSWS) in patients with cerebral malignancies or metastases.

Clinical Signs/Symptoms

The clinical manifestations of hyponatremia largely depend on the severity. If the imbalance develops over a prolonged time period and/or the hyponatremia is not significant, patients may be asymptomatic. The most common symptoms reported in patients with mild hyponatremia have been nausea and weakness. Other symptoms may include anorexia, constipation, myalgia, polyuria, and polydipsia. With severe hyponatremia, patients may experience altered mentation, seizures, and even coma or death from the resultant cerebral edema and increased intracranial pressure. Physical exam findings, if present, may be notable for papilledema and hypoactive reflexes.

Diagnosis

Hyponatremia is defined as serum sodium level less than 130 mEq/L. The essential features for diagnosis of SIADH, in particular, include decreased effective osmolality, urine osmolality >100 mOsm/kg of water, clinical euvolemia, urine sodium >40 mmol/L in the setting of normal salt intake, normal thyroid and adrenal function, and no recent diuretic use. The major criteria for CSWS include the presence of a cerebral lesion and high urinary excretion of sodium and chloride in a patient with contraction of extracellular fluid volume.

Treatment

The initial step in the treatment of hyponatremia should be to determine the underlying cause. Any offending medications should immediately be stopped. The cornerstone of therapy consists of free water restriction (500 to 1000 ml per day) and furosemide. As a general rule, the rapidity of correction of serum sodium is determined by its acuity, so as to prevent patients from developing an osmotic demyelination syndrome. Patients with acute presentations are likely to be more symptomatic and can tolerate more rapid correction. For asymptomatic patients who developed hyponatremia over weeks with serum sodium less than 125 mmol/L, the goal should be to increase serum sodium by 0.5 to 2 mmol/L/hr. For symptomatic patients or patients with a serum sodium level below 115 mmol/L, sodium should be increased by 2 mmol/L/hr, with the initial use of hypertonic saline. If the hyponatremia does not improve or worsen after 72 to 96 hours of free water restriction, IV fluids, and lasix, plasma levels of AVP and ANP should be measured to evaluate for SIADH and SIANP. Patients with

SIADH should be treated with demeclocycline 300 to 600 mg twice daily and ADH-receptor antagonists such as IV conivaptan or oral tolvaptan may also be considered. Patients with SIANP will continue to have worsening hyponatremia, despite free water restriction, if they do not increase their salt intake. Management of cerebral salt wasting includes aggressive fluid and electrolyte replacement as well as mineralocorticoid supplementation with fludrocortisone 100 to 400 mg/day.

HYPERCALCEMIA

Of all paraneoplastic syndromes, hypercalcemia is the most common, seen in 10% to 30% of cancer patients at some time during their disease. Severe hypercalcemia, especially if combined with elevated parathyroid hormone-related protein, indicates a poor prognosis. Survival is often less than 6 months following diagnosis of hypercalcemia.

Etiology

The etiology of hypercalcemia in cancer patients can be divided into two distinct groups: the first being a humoral paraneoplastic syndrome (most common cause of hypercalcemia in cancer patients) and second, the result of bone destruction. Humoral hypercalcemia is most frequently seen with malignancies of the breast, lung, kidney, and head and neck whereas hypercalcemia in the setting of osteolytic metastases is most frequently seen with multiple myeloma. In the latter group, tumor cells have been found to release local factors such as cytokines and growth factors that activate osteoclasts, either directly or indirectly via osteoblast-related up-regulation of osteoclast-activating factors (OAFs). In the former group, tumor cells release systemic factors that affect bone resorption and calcium reabsorption at the level of the kidney. Parathyroid hormone-related protein (PTHrP) is the most commonly secreted systemic factor, found in about 80% of hypercalcemic cancer patients. PTHrP further exacerbates hypercalcemia via its synergistic activity with local factors such as interleukin-1, interleukin-6, and tumor necrosis factor alpha. As a third mechanism, some lymphomas cause hypercalcemia by releasing 1,25 dihydroxyvitamin D, which then promotes intestinal calcium absorption and bone resorption.

Clinical Signs/Symptoms

Patients will generally present with nonspecific findings such as nausea, vomiting, constipation, polyuria, dehydration, and/or confusion. These patients are also at high risk for bradycardia, arrhythmias, shortened QT interval, prolonged PR interval, and cardiac arrest.

Diagnosis

The diagnosis of hypercalcemia is determined by measuring the serum ionized calcium level. If total serum calcium is obtained, it must be appropriately adjusted for albumin levels. Corrected calcium = measured total calcium + [0.8 x (4 − serum albumin concentration)]. A low chloride level should raise suspicion for malignancy-related hypercalcemia.

Treatment

Patients who are asymptomatic with calcium levels less than 13 mg/dl only require conservative management with hydration. Symptomatic patients with calcium levels greater than 13 mg/dl require hydration in addition to more aggressive treatment. Hemodialysis should be considered when calcium levels exceed 18 to 20 mg/dl and/or the patient develops neurological symptoms. Once adequate hydration has been attained, small doses of furosemide can be utilized to enhance calcium excretion. Bisphosphonates remain the most effective treatment for malignancy-related hypercalcemia, with zoledronate being the current best choice. Pamidronate may also be used. Normalization of serum calcium levels is achieved in 4 to 10 days and the effects last for about 4 to 6 weeks in 90% of patients. Bisphosphonates have a complex mechanism of action that ultimately leads to a decrease in bone resorption. As they have no effect on humorally mediated calcium reabsorption, they are less effective in patients with humoral-mediated hypercalcemia. Osteonecrosis of the jaw may be a potentially devastating adverse effect of bisphosphonate use, with myeloma patients at higher risk. Depending on the clinical urgency of bisphosphonate use, patients should undergo dental evaluation prior, if able, as poor dentition also places patients at increased risk.

Novel agents in the pipeline include osteoprotegerin (OPG), a decoy receptor that acts to inhibit bone resorption. The cytokine system of which OPG is a part of also consists of the receptor RANK and its ligand RANKL. When RANKL binds to RANK, osteoclast formation is increased and osteoclast apoptosis is inhibited. This process is counterbalanced by OPG. Denosumab is a monoclonal antibody with high affinity for RANKL and has been approved for treatment of hypercalcemia of malignancy refractory to bisphosphonate therapy as well as for treatment of bone metastases. In three randomized, phase III clinical trials, denosumab has proven to be superior than zoledronic acid by a median of 8.21 months for prevention of skeletal-related events in patients with bone metastases from advanced disease. Denosumab also does not require the close monitoring and renal dosing that is needed with zoledronic acid.

Hypercalcemia that is refractory to bisphosphonates may be treated with gallium nitrate, plicamycin, or calcitonin. Calcitonin can quickly lower calcium levels, however, the effect is often transient. Plicamycin and gallium nitrate are associated with serious adverse effects and therefore, infrequently used. Glucocorticoids are effective in hypercalcemia secondary to elevated levels of vitamin D and can also be useful for relief of other symptoms related to metastatic disease. Long-term treatment and prevention of recurrence will ultimately require treatment of the underlying malignancy. Comfort care should be considered for truly refractory cases.

FEBRILE NEUTROPENIA

Infection can be a significant source of morbidity and mortality in cancer patients, especially in patients who are immunosuppressed from chemotherapy or who have low neutrophil counts secondary to their disease.

Etiology

While febrile neutropenia most frequently occurs in patients undergoing chemotherapy, it can also be seen in patients with acute leukemia, myelodysplatic syndrome, or in other diseases with leukopenias. In general, patients' neutrophil counts tend to be at their lowest 510 days following the last dose of chemotherapy with recovery of counts within 5 days of this nadir. Common pathogens that cause febrile neutropenia include gram negative bacteria (E.coli, pseudomonas aeruginosa, and klebsiella pneumoniae), gram positive bacteria (staphylococcus species, streptococcus species, and enterococcus species) or polymicrobial infections. In about 75–80% of cases, however, no organism is able to be identified.

Clinical Signs/Symptoms

Fever is commonly the only symptom that these patients present with as other typical signs of infection can be masked in the setting of neutropenia. Other possible symptoms may include chills, diarrhea, rash, nausea, vomiting, cough, and shortness of breath. A thorough physical exam, including inspection of the oral cavity and perianal region, should be performed on these patients.

Diagnosis

Neutropenia is defined as an absolute neutrophil count (ANC) less than 1500 cells/microL and severe neutropenia is defined as an ANC less than 500 cells/microL or an ANC that is expected to decrease to less than 500 cells/microL in the next 48 hours. Risk of infection is higher in patients with severe neutropenia, especially when the neutropenia is prolonged (>7 days). Fever is defined as a temperature greater than 100.4°F that is sustained for more than an hour or a single temperature greater than 101.3°F. All patients who have received chemotherapy within 6 weeks of presentation and meet criteria for a systemic inflammatory response syndrome (SIRS) are assumed to have a neutropenic sepsis syndrome, unless proven otherwise.

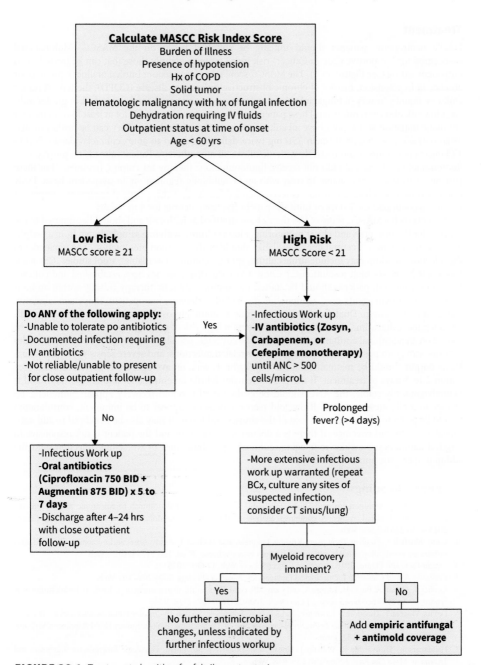

FIGURE 36.1 Treatment algorithm for febrile neutropenia.

Treatment

Febrile neutropenic patients should initially be stratified based on the MASCC (Multinational Association for Supportive Care in Cancer) risk index score to identify those that can be treated in an outpatient setting (see Figure 36.1). The MASCC score takes into account burden of illness, presence or absence of hypotension, history of chronic obstructive pulmonary disease (COPD), the type of tumor (solid vs. liquid), history of fungal infections, volume status, and age. A total score of 21 or greater indicates low risk of serious infection. These patients can be monitored in the ED for at least four hours after antibiotic initiation and should have all cultures drawn prior to discharge. They can be further treated as an outpatient with ciprofloxacin 750 mg twice daily in addition to amoxicillin/clavulanate 500 to 125 mg every 8 hours or alternatively with moxifloxacin monotherapy. Patients already on prophylactic fluoroquinolone therapy should not receive fluoroquinolone therapy for empiric treatment. For these patients, it would be reasonable to treat with an IV antibiotic regimen on an outpatient basis. Daily evaluation by a health-care provider is recommended for the first three days of treatment. Outpatient therapy is continued for 7 days or until the patient has been afebrile for 4 to 5 days.

Patients with a MASCC score of less than 21 are stratified as high-risk and should be admitted to the hospital for IV antibiotics and closer monitoring. Blood cultures, with one sample drawn from a peripheral vein and one from a central line, if available, should be drawn upon presentation. The remainder of the infectious workup may include urine culture, sputum culture (if available), stool studies, CSF analysis, chest X-ray +/– high resolution CT Chest. Once the diagnosis has been established and cultures have been collected, patients should be started on empiric antibiotic therapy (ideally within an hour of triage). Common agents used as monotherapy include cefepime, meropenem, imipenem-cilastatin, ceftazidime, and zosyn. Dual therapy agents include an aminoglycoside in addition to either piperacillin, cefepime, ceftazidime, or a carbapenem. Patients at high risk of gram-positive bacteremia should be started on an additional antibiotic with appropriate coverage, usually vancomycin. This group includes patients with gram positive colonization, catheter-related infections, and severe sepsis +/– hypotension. Urine output should be maintained at >0.5 ml/kg/hr. Fevers, on average, are expected to defervesce within 2 to 5 days of treatment. If the patient remains febrile on empiric antibiotics (>4 days) and is hemodynamically stable, the ANC should be evaluated. If myeloid recovery appears imminent, no change in antibiotics is needed. If myeloid recovery does not appear to be imminent, consideration should be given to obtaining a CT scan of the sinuses and lungs. It may also be beneficial to add antifungal +/– antimold coverage. If there is a documented infection and the patient is not responsive to targeted antibiotics, consider re-imaging, culture/biopsy/drain sites of worsening infection, and the addition of empiric antifungal therapy.

Suggested Readings

1. Araki, Kazuhiro, Yoshinori Ito, and Shunji Takahashi. Re: Superiority of denosumab to zoledronic acid for prevention of skeletal-related events: A combined analysis of three pivotal, randomised, phase 3 trials. *Eur J Cancer.* 2013;49(9):2264–2265. Web.
2. Cairo, Mitchell S, Stephen Thompson, Krishna Tangirala, and Michael T. Eaddy. Costs and outcomes associated with rasburicase versus allopurinol in patients with tumor lysis syndrome. *Blood.* 120.3175 (2012): Web.
3. Cancer Facts and Figures 2016. American Cancer Society. Web. 17 Oct. 2016.
4. Cervantes A, and Chirivella I. Oncological Emergencies. *Annals of Oncology.* 2004:299–306. Web.
5. Coiffier B, Altman A, Pui C-H, Younes A, and Cairo MS. Guidelines for the management of pediatric and adult tumor lysis syndrome: An evidence-based review. *J Clin Oncol.* 2008;26(16):2767–2778. Web.
6. DeVita, Vincent T, Theodore S. Lawrence, and Steven A. Rosenberg. Section 16 Oncologic Emergencies. *DeVita, Hellman, and Rosenberg's Cancer: Principles & Practice of Oncology.* 9th ed. Philadelphia: Wolters Kluwer Health/Lippincott Williams & Wilkins, 2011:2123–2152. Print.
7. Halfdanarson, Thorvardur R, William J. Hogan, and Timothy J. Moynihan. Oncologic Emergencies: Diagnosis and Treatment. *Mayo Clin Proc.* 2006;81(6):835–848. Web.
8. Higdon, Mark L, and Jennifer A. Higdon. Treatment of oncologic emergencies. *American Family Physician.* 2006;74(11): 873–880. Web.
9. Larson, Richard A., and Ching-Hon Pui. Tumor Lysis Syndrome: Prevention and treatment. UpToDate, Oct. 2016. Web. Oct.17, 2016.
10. Nagaiah, Govardhanan, Quoc Truong, and Manish Monga. Chapter 36 oncologic emergencies and paraneoplastic syndromes. *The Bethesda Handbook of Clinical Oncology.* 4th ed. Philadelphia: Wolters Kluwer Health/Lippincott Williams & Wilkins, 2014. 468-79. Print.

Psychopharmacologic **37** Management in Oncology

Donald L. Rosenstein, Maryland Pao, Sheryl B. Fleisch, and Daniel E. Elswick

INTRODUCTION

Psychiatric syndromes, predominantly depression and anxiety, occur commonly in patients with cancer, and, if misdiagnosed or poorly managed, can have profoundly negative effects on optimal oncologic care. The comprehensive psychiatric care of patients with cancer includes psychosocial, behavioral, and psychoeducational interventions as well as appropriate pharmacologic and psychotherapeutic treatment. This chapter focuses on the psychopharmacologic management of the major psychiatric syndromes encountered in the oncology setting and includes information on specialist referral. The chapter concludes with specific recommendations for psychopharmacologic management in pediatric oncology.

CONSIDERATIONS PRIOR TO PRESCRIBING PSYCHOPHARMACOLOGIC AGENTS

- Psychiatric symptoms are often manifestations of an underlying medical disorder or complications of its treatment (Table 37.1). For example, specific malignancies (e.g., lung, breast, renal, melanoma) are prone to metastasize to the central nervous system (CNS). In addition, advanced cancer can result in metabolic CNS insults that precipitate psychiatric symptoms. For those patients whose psychiatric symptoms fail to respond to psychopharmacologic treatment, CNS involvement should be reconsidered, even in malignancies that do not commonly metastasize to the brain.
- Medically ill patients are particularly susceptible to CNS adverse effects of medications. Specific examples of medications associated with mood, cognitive, and behavioral symptoms include the following: corticosteroids, interleukin-2, interferon-α, opiates, benzodiazepines (BZDs), and dopamine-blocking antiemetics (e.g., prochlorperazine, metoclopramide, and promethazine). For patients who develop psychiatric symptoms after treatment with such agents, it is often more prudent to lower the dose or discontinue the use of a currently prescribed medication than introduce yet another agent (i.e., a psychotropic) in an attempt to combat the adverse effect as it may exacerbate the psychiatric symptoms.
- Polypharmacy is unavoidable in patients with cancer; however, most clinically significant interactions with psychotropic agents are predictable and can be avoided by choosing alternative agents or by making dose adjustments. The use of monoamine oxidase inhibitors (MAOIs) with either meperidine (Demerol) or selective serotonin reuptake inhibitors (SSRIs) can be life-threatening by causing serotonin syndrome. Serotonin syndrome classically includes mental status changes, autonomic hyperactivity, and neuromuscular abnormalities, but patients can also demonstrate a broad range of clinical signs and symptoms. Supportive care remains the mainstay of treatment. Up-to-date drug interaction resources can be found at several internet websites (e.g., http://medicine.iupui.edu/flockhart/).

TABLE 37.1 Medical Conditions Associated with Anxiety and Depression

Neoplasms	Cardiovascular
Brain tumors	Ischemic heart disease
Head/neck cancer	Arrhythmias
Pancreatic cancer	Congestive heart failure Stroke
Lung cancer	
Lymphoma	Metabolic
Leukemia	
Insulinoma	Electrolyte disturbances
	Uremia
Endocrinologic	Vitamin B_{12} or folate deficiency
Thyroid ↑↓	
Cushing syndrome	
Adrenal ↑↓	Other
Hypopituitarism	Substance abuse and withdrawal
Pheochromocytoma	Pain (uncontrolled)
	Hematologic (e.g., anemia)
Medication related	Sexual dysfunction
Interferon-α	
Corticosteroids	
Interleukin-2	
Dopamine-blocking antiemetics	

- Inadequate pain control frequently induces symptoms of anxiety, irritability, or depression. It is essential to have pain well controlled so that the appropriate psychiatric diagnosis and treatment can proceed (see Chapter 00). One note of caution in this regard concerns the use of SSRIs and tricyclic antidepressants (TCAs), which are occasionally used in combination to treat neuropathic pain. Some SSRIs (e.g., fluoxetine, paroxetine) inhibit the metabolism of TCAs, which can in turn prolong the corrected QT (QTc) interval.

COMMON PSYCHIATRIC SYNDROMES IN THE ONCOLOGY SETTING

Adjustment Disorder

This is a time-limited, maladaptive reaction to a specific stressor that typically involves symptoms of depression, anxiety, or behavioral changes and impairs psychosocial functioning. The diagnostic criteria include the onset of symptoms within 3 months of the stressor but the duration of symptoms is no more than 6 months.

Management

The initial treatment approach includes crisis intervention and brief psychotherapy. Time-limited symptom management with medications may be indicated. For example, anxiety, tearfulness, and insomnia are frequent reactions to the diagnosis of a new or recurrent malignancy. Short-term treatment of these symptoms with BZDs (e.g., lorazepam and clonazepam) is appropriate, effective, and rarely associated with the development of abuse or dependence. Short-term use of non-BZD sleep agents (e.g., zolpidem, eszopiclone) is also commonplace in clinical practice (Table 37.2).

Major Depression

Major depression and subsyndromal depressive disorders are common in patients with cancer. Prevalence rates vary between 5% and 50% depending on how depression is defined, whether study samples are drawn from outpatient clinics or hospital wards and the type of cancer involved. Untreated

TABLE 37.2 Commonly Used Hypnotic Agents

Generic	Brand	Dose Range	Half-Life
Eszopiclone	Lunesta	1–3 PO	Short
Zalepon	Sonata	5–20 PO	Short
Zolpidem	Ambien	2.5–10 PO	Short
	Ambien CR	6.25–12.5 PO	Extended Release

TABLE 37.3 Risk Factors for Suicide

Historical Considerations	Clinical Descriptors
Prior suicide attempts	Elderly men
Family history of suicide	Recent loss and poor social support
Prior psychiatric illness	Current depression, anxiety, substance abuse
History of substance abuse	Advanced cancer, pain, poor prognosis
Impulsive behavior	Delirium, psychosis, illogical thoughts

depression has been correlated with poor adherence with medical care, increased pain and disability, and a greater likelihood of considering euthanasia and physician-assisted suicide. Recent studies suggest that depression is also associated with increased mortality in patients with cancer.

A frequent diagnostic task in the oncology setting is differentiating symptoms of major depression from those symptoms that are caused by the underlying cancer or its treatment. Patients with cancer, especially those with advanced disease who are undergoing chemotherapy, are more likely to experience fatigue, anorexia, weight loss, and insomnia, whether a major depression is present or absent. Our practice is to institute empiric trials of antidepressants using a targeted symptom-reduction approach. In questionable cases, a personal or family history of depression and the presence of symptoms of excessive guilt, poor self-esteem, anhedonia, and ruminative thinking strengthen the argument for a medication trial. Furthermore, because the number of well-tolerated, safe, and effective antidepressants has grown, we have lowered our threshold for treating subsyndromal depression in the oncology setting.

Because patients with cancer have an increased risk of suicide compared with the general population, particular attention should be paid to symptoms of hopelessness, helplessness, suicidal ideation, and intense anxiety (Table 37.3). Cancer at certain sites, including lung, gastrointestinal tract, and head and neck cancers, is associated with an even greater risk of suicide. Risk of suicide appears to be highest immediately after diagnosis and decreases thereafter but remains increased for years as compared to suicide rates in the general population. Suicide rates are higher among patients with advanced disease at diagnosis but not among patients with multiple primary tumors. Other risk factors for suicide include male sex, white race, and being unmarried, similar risk factors for suicide in the general population. In addition, adult survivors of childhood cancers are at increased risk for suicidal ideation related to cancer diagnosis as well as posttreatment mental and physical health problems, even many years after completion of therapy.

Management

Treatment modalities include pharmacotherapy (Table 37.4) and psychotherapy. Electroconvulsive therapy (ECT) is highly effectivef in the treatment of major depressive disorder resistant to pharmaco- and psychotherapy. Selection of an antidepressant in major depression should be based on a number of considerations such as active medical problems, the potential for drug interactions, prior treatment response, and an optimal match between the patient's target symptoms and the side-effect profile of the antidepressant (e.g., using a sedating agent for the patient with anxiety and insomnia).

TABLE 37.4 Commonly Used Antidepressants in Patients with Cancer

Generic Names* (Brand Names)	Dose Range (mg)	Class and Common Adverse Effects
SSRIs		**Class effects:** GI symptoms, weight changes, sleep disruption, sexual dysfunction, agitation, anxiety
Fluoxetine (Prozac, Sarafem)[a,b,c]	5–80	Long T1/2, weekly dosing available
Sertraline (Zoloft)[a,c]	12.5–200	GI symptoms common
Paroxetine (Paxil CR)[b,c]	10–60	Anticholinergic effects, withdrawal syndrome
Citalopram (Celexa)[c]	10–40	Doses above 40 mg/d are not recommended due to the increased risk for QT prolongation. Patients over the age of 60 or those with hepatic or renal dysfunction should not exceed doses of 20 mg/d.
Escitalopram (Lexapro)[a]	5–20	Structurally similar to citalopram
Fluvoxamine (Luvox CR)[a]	25–300	Commonly used for obsessive-compulsive disorder.
		Many drug interactions. Contraindicated with pimozide, thioridazine, mesoridazine, CYP1A2, 2B6, 2C19, and 3A4 inhibitors
Novel antidepressants		
Venlafaxine (Effexor XR)[b]	18.75–300	GI symptoms, sexual dysfunction, anticholinergic effects, hypertension at dose >225 mg/d, reduces hot flashes
Mirtazapine (Remeron, (SolTab))[d]	7.5–45	Sedation, dry mouth, increased appetite and weight gain, constipation, dizziness common. Low incidence of sexual dysfunction
Bupropion (Wellbutrin (XL/SR), Forfivo XL, Zyban)[b]	37.5–450	Zyban approved for smoking cessation. GI symptoms, tremor, increased risk for seizures at high dose or with CNS lesions. May treat sexual side effects of other antidepressants
Trazodone	25–400	Sedation, orthostatic hypotension, priapism, some weight gain
Duloxetine (Cymbalta)	20–60	GI symptoms, headache, dizziness; also indicated for generalized anxiety disorder, diabetic neuropathy, and fibromyalgia
CNS stimulants		**Class effects:** Insomnia, agitation, GI symptoms, headache, tics. Can affect blood pressure and heart rate
Methylphenidate[a] Concerta, Metadate (CD/ER), Methylin, Quillivant XR, Ritalin (LA/SR)[b]	2.5–72	
Dextroamphetamine (Dexedrine)[a,b]	2.5–60	Has been associated with serious cardiovascular events

(continued)

TABLE 37.4 (Continued)

Generic Names* (Brand Names)	Dose Range (mg)	Class and Common Adverse Effects
Tricyclic antidepressants		**Class effects:** Dry mouth, sedation, GI symptoms, headache, ECG changes, orthostatic hypotension, anticholinergic effects
Amitriptyline (Elavil)[a]	25–150	
Desipramine (Norpramin)	25–150	
Nortriptyline (Pamelor)[a,c]	25–150	Tremor
Doxepin (Sinequan)[a,c]	10–300	Potent antihistamine, used for itching

* Drugs with sedating effects are listed in italics.

[a] FDA approval for use in children/adolescents.

[b] Sustained-release and extended-release formulations available.

[c] Liquid formulation available.

[d] Orally disintegrating tablets or wafers available.

CNS, central nervous system; ECG, electrocardiogram; GI, gastrointestinal; SSRI, selective serotonin reuptake inhibitor.

Potential interactions with cancer therapeutics should also be considered. For example, several antidepressants are inhibitors of cytochrome P-450 2D6. This inhibition reduces the metabolism of tamoxifen to its active metabolite, endoxifen. Venlafaxine (Effexor) has the least inhibitory effect at 2D6 and thus is preferred in breast cancer patients taking tamoxifen (Table 37.5).

An antidepressant frequently used in patients with cancer is mirtazapine (Remeron) as it is sedating, causes weight gain, has few significant drug interactions, and is a 5HT-3 receptor antagonist (i.e., has antiemetic properties). Mirtazapine may also be used as an augmentation agent for depression treatment in conjunction with SSRIs. Elderly patients or patients with medical comorbidities (especially hepatic impairment) generally require smaller dose of antidepressants.

Anxiety Disorders

Many medical conditions seen in the oncology setting, such as heart failure, respiratory compromise, seizure disorders, pheochromocytoma, and chemotherapy-induced ovarian failure, may cause anxiety. Additional conditions that may cause both anxiety and depression are listed in Table 37.1. Similarly, anxiety is an adverse effect of numerous medications such as high-dose corticosteroids. In particular, dopamine-blocking antiemetics may cause akathisia, an adverse effect characterized by subjective restlessness and increased motor activity, which is commonly misdiagnosed as anxiety. Initiation of treatment with an antidepressant may also induce a transient anxiety state. It is important to inform patients of this potential side effect in order to improve adherence.

Management

In addition to behavioral therapy and psychotherapy, BZDs are the medications that are most frequently used for the short-term treatment of anxiety (Table 37.6). For anxiety that persists beyond a few weeks, treatment with an antidepressant (see Table 37.4) is indicated. BZDs are often started concurrently with an antidepressant as a "bridge therapy" as there is a typical delay in therapeutic effect for antidepressants of up to several weeks. If the patient has already been taking an SSRI, it is important not to discontinue it (with the exception of fluoxetine because of its long half-life) abruptly to avoid a withdrawal syndrome that may include gastrointestinal distress, flu-like symptoms, insomnia, agitation, and irritability. Low-dose second-generation antipsychotics are often useful for severe and persistent anxiety or for conditions such as anxiety secondary to steroids and delirium (Table 37.7).

TABLE 37.5 Antidepressant Inhibitors: CYP2D6

Strong	Fluoxetine, paroxetine, bupropion
Moderate	Duloxetine, sertraline, and fluvoxamine
Mild	Citalopram and escitalopram
Minimal	Venlafaxine, mirtazapine,[a] and desvenlafaxine[a]

[a] Based on limited data.

Adapted from: Desmarais JE, Looper KJ. Interactions between tamoxifen and antidepressants via cytochrome P450 2D6. J Clin Psychiatry. 2009;70(12):1688–1697.

TABLE 37.6 Preferred BZDs in the Oncology Setting

	Lorazepam (Ativan)	Clonazepam (Klonopin)
Dose equivalency	1 mg	0.25 mg
Dose range	0.25–2 mg PO, sublingual, IM or IV routes, every 1–6 h based on clinical need (maximum daily dose, 8 mg)	0.25–1 mg PO route, every 8–12 h
Advantages	Fast onset of action	Less frequent dosing than with Lorazepam
	Multiple routes of administration (oral, IV, IM) liquid available	Longer half-life orally disintegrating wafer available

BZD, benzodiazepines; IM, intramuscularly; IV, intravenously; PO, orally.

TABLE 37.7 Commonly Used Neuroleptics in the Oncology Setting

	Initial Dose (mg)	Administrative Routes and Schedules	Maximum Daily Dose (mg)
haloperidol[a,b] (Haldol)	0.25–1 PO, or IV	Every 2–12 h SC, IM,	20
Chlorpromazine[a] (Thorazine)	12.5–50 PO, IM or IV	Every 4–12 h	300
Risperidone[a,b,c,d] (Risperdal [M-Tab])	0.25–2 PO	Every 12 h	6
Olanzapine[a,c] (Zyprexa [Zydis])	2.5–10 PO	Every 12–24 h	20
Quetiapine[a] (Seroquel)	25–50 PO	Every 12–24 h	800

[a] FDA approval for use in children/adolescents.

[b] Liquid formulation available.

[c] Orally disintegrating tablets or wafers available.

[d] Sustained release and extended release formulations available.

EPS, extrapyramidal symptoms; IM, intramuscularly; IV, intravenously; PO, orally; SC, subcutaneously.

The following issues associated with BZD use require attention:

- BZDs are the treatment of choice for delirium caused by alcohol or sedative–hypnotic withdrawal but predictably worsen other types of delirium.
- In patients with hepatic failure, lorazepam, temazepam, or oxazepam are the preferred BZDs as they do not require oxidation for metabolism.
- BZDs may result in "disinhibition," especially in delirium, substance abuse, "organic" disorders, and preexisting personality disorders. Disinhibition is more common in children and elderly patients.
- The abrupt discontinuation of BZDs with short half-lives (e.g., alprazolam [Xanax]) can cause rebound anxiety and precipitate a withdrawal syndrome.
- Long-term use of BZDs may lead to cognitive problems, tolerance, and dependence. Time-limited use is recommended.

Delirium

Delirium is an acute confusional state characterized by fluctuating cognitive impairment, perceptual disturbances, mood changes, delusions, and sleep–wake cycle disruption. Patients can have a hyperactive (agitated), hypoactive (quiet), or mixed (alternating hyper/hypoactive) delirium. Virtually any psychiatric symptom can be a manifestation of delirium. Anxiety and/or labile mood are common presentations often misdiagnosed as "depression." Patients who are elderly, on multiple medications, or who have underlying brain pathology are more prone to delirium. Surgical patients who undergo prolonged, extremely invasive, or multiple surgeries with repeated anesthesia are also at higher risk for delirium. Delirium in terminally ill patients is very common and often underdiagnosed. Several cancer-related therapies can induce delirium including methotrexate, ifosfamide, cytosine arabinoside, interferon-α, and interleukin-2. Total brain radiation may also cause cognitive changes and delirium.

Management

The first step in the management of delirium is making sure the patient is safe by attending to environmental cues including reorienting the patient and providing a personal nursing assistant (sitter) to prevent falls. Identifying and treating precipitating factors (including medical conditions such as infection) and discontinuing nonessential medications that may be deliriogenic (such as BZDs, anticholinergics, or opioids) will be important to the treatment of the delirium. Haloperidol (Haldol) continues to be the prototypical first-generation antipsychotic agent most frequently used in delirium because of its ease of administration (oral, IM, or IV) and many clinical trials proving its efficacy. Common adverse effects of the first-generation antipsychotics include sedation and hypotension. Newer second-generation antipsychotics such as olanzapine (Zyprexa) and risperidone (Risperdal) may also be used in the treatment of delirium and are associated with sedation, weight gain, and metabolic syndrome. Recent concerns have been raised about an increased risk of sudden death associated with antipsychotic use in elderly patients. These data suggest a small increase in the relative risk of death, which must be weighed against the substantial mortality risks of untreated delirium.

ADDITIONAL CONSIDERATIONS FOR PSYCHOPHARMACOLOGIC MANAGEMENT IN PEDIATRIC ONCOLOGY

Cancer is a leading cause of death among 10- to 24-year-olds and the leading cause of nonacute death among youth. As the 5-year survival rate for all childhood cancers combined has increased, more children are surviving into adulthood. Life-threatening illness in a child or an adolescent can be traumatic and is often associated with anxiety and depression. Although many patients cope well with and adapt to the trauma, symptoms of depression such as fatigue, cognitive impairment, decreased social interaction and exploration, and anorexia may occur as part of a cytokine or immunologic response to cancer and its treatments. Psychotropic medications targeted at specific symptoms may improve quality of life for children with cancer. These medications do not replace comprehensive, multimodal, multidisciplinary care but are adjuncts to decrease discomfort and improve functioning of medically ill children.

Assessment and Diagnosis in Pediatric Oncology

A thorough psychiatric assessment is needed to make a correct diagnosis and to institute treatment. Typically, this assessment is based on multiple brief examinations of the child and information gathered from additional sources including family, staff, and teachers. A patient's biologic vulnerability to depression and anxiety may be further exposed if there is (a) a family history of a mood or anxiety disorder, or other psychiatric disorder, and (b) previous psychiatric symptoms or psychiatric treatment.

Common complaints in medically ill children include

- Anxiety
- Pain
- Difficulty sleeping
- Fatigue
- Feeling "bored"

Adult psychiatric syndromes of adjustment disorder, major depression, anxiety, and delirium apply to children as well, but anxiety, rather than depression, is the most frequent diagnosis. Important determining factors for pharmacologic intervention are severity and duration of psychiatric symptoms.

Psychopharmacologic Treatment of Pediatric Patients

In 1994, manufacturers and federally funded researchers were mandated to study medications such as antidepressants in children. Although there have been no randomized, controlled antidepressant trials in depressed medically ill children, and the dose of psychiatric medications for children with cancer has not been systematically studied, antidepressants have been useful for treating anxiety and depression. Body weight, Tanner staging, clinical status, and potential for medications to interact are considered in deciding doses. See Tables 37.4 and 37.7 for psychotropics with U.S. Food and Drug Administration (FDA) approval for use in children and adolescents.

BZDs, such as lorazepam and clonazepam, used in low doses in conjunction with nonpharmacologic distraction techniques, may be appropriate for procedures that induce considerable anxiety in children. Clonazepam is longer acting and may be helpful with more pervasive and prolonged anxiety symptoms. BZDs can cause sedation, confusion, and behavioral disinhibition. Their use should be carefully monitored, especially in those patients with CNS dysfunction. BZD withdrawal precipitated by abrupt discontinuation occurs most frequently on transferring the patient from intensive care settings.

Antihistamines have been used to sedate anxious children. Diphenhydramine, hydroxyzine, and promethazine may be helpful for occasional insomnia. However, antihistamines are not helpful for persistent anxiety and their anticholinergic properties can precipitate or worsen delirium. Intravenous diphenhydramine may be misused because it can induce euphoria when given by IV push. Very high doses of IV diphenhydramine can also provoke seizures.

Fluoxetine is the only FDA-approved SSRI for depression in children older than 6 years. Fluoxetine and sertraline are approved for obsessive-compulsive disorder in children older than 6 years while fluvoxamine is approved for those who are 8 years and older. Fluoxetine, with its active metabolite norfluoxetine, and fluvoxamine are potent inhibitors of cytochrome P-450 (CYP) 3A3 and 3A4. They are contraindicated with macrolide antibiotics, azole antifungal agents, and several other medications. Escitalopram is approved for depression in those 12 years and older, while citalopram is not approved for use in those under 18. As with adults, use of SSRIs suggest monitoring of QTc and risk of bleeding in complicated post-transplant patients is warranted. Amitriptyline is approved for depression in children who are 12 years or older. TCAs are useful for treating insomnia, weight loss, anxiety, and some pain syndromes.

Some antidepressants may contribute to suicidal thinking in children and young adults through age 24 years as noted in FDA black box warnings. This possibility warrants careful monitoring of suicidality in all children treated with antidepressants. Use of non-FDA-approved psychopharmacologic agents in children with cancer may be considered for extreme or prolonged distress and poor functioning but must be monitored closely.

Children and adolescents who cannot tolerate antidepressants may benefit from stimulants for depression and apathy. Psychostimulants are generally well tolerated and have a rapid onset of action.

Children with delirium, hallucinations, severe agitation, or aggression may be safely treated with low-dose first-generation antipsychotics such as haloperidol or second-generation antipsychotics such as risperidone and olanzapine.

Although there is a dearth of research in pediatric cancer psychopharmacology, child psychiatry consultation may considerably improve the quality of life for children undergoing cancer treatment and dealing with cancer survival. Routine psychological screening of children with cancer and survivors can detect ongoing distress. Psychopharmacologic consultation may also help children with postradiation or postchemotherapy conditions related to attention, mood, and anxiety disorders.

SPECIALIST REFERRAL

Many psychiatric symptoms can be readily addressed by the primary oncologist or oncology service through counseling and pharmacotherapy. Sometimes it is helpful to involve a psychiatric specialist to assist with psychopharmacology and other supportive interventions. There are a growing number of practitioners working within oncology centers who focus on issues associated with cancer diagnosis, treatment, and survivorship. The subspecialty of psychosocial oncology (or psycho-oncology) has existed in some centers since the 1970s. There is a great deal of variability of access to psychosocial specialists at cancer centers and in the community. Some centers have dedicated services, while others utilize practitioners from palliative, general psychiatric, or psychosomatic medicine services. It may be beneficial for oncologists to establish relationships with local community mental health providers in settings where a dedicated service is not available.

Determining the appropriateness of a referral to assist with psychopharmacology can be difficult for some oncology providers. The National Comprehensive Cancer Network (NCCN) has established guidelines for management and referral for psychosocial issues in the Clinical Practice Guidelines in Oncology. There is a section on Distress Management (current version 2.2017) that includes referral and treatment algorithms for psychiatric, social, pastoral, and substance-related issues. A simple screening tool called the "Distress Thermometer" exists to help determine the need for referral to supportive services including referral to psychiatric care. A valid adapted pediatric version of the Distress Thermometer is available for outpatient clinic use. The NCCN guidelines are available online at https://www.nccn.org/professionals/physician_gls/pdf/distress.pdf. Additionally, fifteen evidence-based standards for psychosocial care were developed for children with cancer and their families and published in 2015.

SUMMARY

Psychiatric syndromes are frequently misdiagnosed and poorly treated in patients with cancer. Before initiating psychopharmacologic therapy, underlying medical disorders and adverse effects of medication must be addressed and potential drug interactions anticipated. Psychiatric symptoms should then be treated promptly and aggressively. Consultation from a psychiatrist is indicated in the following circumstances when the patient (a) has a complex psychiatric history and is taking multiple psychotropic medications; (b) exhibits depressive symptoms associated with extreme guilt, anxiety, and/or suicidal thoughts; (c) is confused, hallucinating, agitated, or violent; and/or (d) is nonadherent with care or rejects treatment and seeks physician-assisted suicide.

Suggested Readings

1. Academy of Psychosomatic Medicine. Psychiatric aspects of excellent end-of-life care: a position statement of the Academy of Psychosomatic Medicine. Available at: http://www.apm.org/papers/eol-care.shtml. Accessed February 4, 2013.
2. American Psychiatric Association. *Diagnostic and Statistical Manual of Mental Disorders*. 5th ed. 2013.
3. Cassem EH. Depressive disorders in the medically ill: an overview. *Psychosomatics*. 1995;36:S2–S10.
4. Cleeland CS, Bennett GJ, Dantzer R, et al. Are the symptoms of cancer and cancer treatment due to a shared biologic mechanism? A cytokine-immunologic model of cancer symptoms. *Cancer*. 2003;97:2919.

5. Coyle N, Adelhardt J, Foley KM, et al. Character of terminal illness in the advanced patient with cancer: pain and other symptoms during the last four weeks of life. *J Pain Symptom Manage*. 1990;5:83.
6. Desmarais JE, Looper KJ. Interactions between tamoxifen and antidepressants via cytochrome P450 2D6. *J Clin Psychiatry*. 2009;70(12):1688–1697.
7. Emanuel EJ, Fairclough DL, Daniels ER, et al. Euthanasia and physician-assisted suicide: attitudes and experiences of oncology patients, oncologists, and the public. *Lancet*. 1996;347:1805.
8. Endicott J. Measurement of depression in patients with cancer. *Cancer*. 1984;53:2243.
9. Fang F, Fall K, Mittleman MA, et al. Suicide and cardiovascular death after a cancer diagnosis. *N Engl J Med*. 2012;366(14):1310–1318.
10. Gothelf D, Rubinstein M, Shemesh E, et al. (2005). Pilot study: fluvoxamine treatment for depression and anxiety disorders in children and adolescents with cancer. *J Am Acad Child Adolesc Psychiatry*. 2005;44:1258–1262.
11. Holland J, Breitbart WS, Butow PN, Jacobsen PB et al. *Psycho-Oncology*. 3rd ed. New York: Oxford University Press; 2015.
12. Holland J, Greenberg D, Hughes M, et al. *Quick Reference for Oncology Clinicians: The Psychiatric and Psychological Dimensions of Cancer Symptom Management*. Charlottesville, VA: IPOS Press; 2006.
13. http://www.cancer.gov/research/progress/snapshots/pediatric (accessed 8/6/2016)
14. http://www.cdc.gov/injury/images/lc-charts/leading_causes_of_death_age_group_2014_1050w760h.gif (accessed 8/6/2016)
15. Kersun LS, Shemesh E. Depression and anxiety in children at the end of life. *Pediatr Clin N Am*. 2007;54:691–708.
16. Lipsett DR, Payne EC, Cassem NH. On death and dying. Discussion. *J Geriatr Psychiatry*. 1974;7:108.
17. Lynch ME. The assessment and prevalence of affective disorders in advanced cancer. *J Palliat Care*. 1995;11:10.
18. Miller AH, Raison CL. The role of inflammation in depression: from evolutionary imperative to modern treatment target. *Nat Rev Immunol*. 2016 Jan;16(1):22–34. doi: 10.1038/nri.2015.5.
19. Misono S, Weiss NS, Fann JR, Redman M, Yueh B. Incidence of suicide in persons with cancer. *J Clin Oncol*. 2008;26(29):4731–4738.
20. Pao M, Ballard E, Rosenstein DL, Wiener L, Wayne AS. Psychotropic medication use in pediatric patients with cancer. *Arch Pediatr Adolesc Med*. 2006;160:818–822.
21. Portteus A, Ahmad N, Tobey D, Leavey P, et al. The prevalence and use of antidepressant medication in pediatric cancer patients. *J Child Adolesc Psychopharmacol*. 2006;16:467–473.
22. Recklitis C, Diller LR, Li X, Najita J, Robison LL, Zeltzer L. Suicide ideation in adult survivors of childhood cancer: a report from the Childhood Cancer Survivor Study. *J Clin Oncol*. 2010;28:655.
23. Rodin G, Lloyd N, Katz M, et al. The treatment of depression in cancer patients: a systematic review. *Support Care Cancer*. 2007;15:123.
24. Rosenstein DL. Depression and end-of-life care for patients with cancer. *Dialogues Clin Neurosci*. 2011;13(1):101–108.
25. Spiegel D, Sands S, Koopman C. Pain and depression in patients with cancer. *Cancer*. 1994;74:2570.
26. Turkel SB, Hanft A. The pharmacologic management of delirium in children and adolescents. *Paediatr Drugs*. 2014;16(4):267–274pmid:24898718
27. Wiener L, Battles H, Zadeh S, Widemann BC, Pao M. Validity, specificity, feasibility and acceptability of a brief pediatric distress thermometer in outpatient clinics. *Psychooncology*. 2015 Nov 30. doi: 10.1002/pon.4038. [Epub ahead of print]
28. Wiener L, Kazak AE, Noll RB, Patenaude AF, Kupst MJ. Standards for the psychosocial care of children with cancer and their families: An introduction to the special issue. *Pediatr Blood Cancer*. 2015 Dec;62 Suppl 5:S419-24. doi: 10.1002/pbc.25675. Epub 2015 Sep 23.
29. Wiener L, Pao M, Kazak A, Kupst MJ, Patenaude A (eds.) *Quick Reference for Pediatric Oncology Clinicians: The Psychiatric and Psychological Dimensions of Pediatric Cancer Symptom Management*. 2nd ed. Oxford University Press: Oxford; 2015.
30. Wise TN. The physician and his patient with cancer. *Prim Care*. 1974;1:407.
31. Zadeh S, Pao M, Wiener L. Opening end-of-life discussions: how to introduce Voicing My CHOiCES™, an advance care planning guide for adolescents and young adults. *Palliat Support Care*. 2015 Jun;13(3):591-9. doi: 10.1017/S1478951514000054. Epub 2014 Mar 13.

Management of Emesis 38

David R. Kohler

RADIATION- AND CHEMOTHERAPY-ASSOCIATED EMETIC SYMPTOMS

Radiation- and chemotherapy-associated emetic symptoms are labeled as "acute" or "delayed" by their temporal relationship with the start of emetogenic treatments (Fig. 38.1). Although the terms are useful for describing clinical events and approaches to symptom management, the assignment of symptoms onset and duration to fixed periods predated identification of principal neural mechanisms that elicit acute- and delayed-phase symptoms, and remain an oversimplification of physiological events that occur when emetogenic treatments are repeated within the span of a single day or on two or more consecutive days.

Acute-phase Symptoms

Emetic symptoms that occur within 24 hours after treatment are identified as acute-phase symptoms (Table 38.1). Acute-phase symptoms have been shown to correlate with serotonin (5-hydroxytryptamine, 5-HT) release from enterochromaffin cells. Emetic signals are propagated at local serotonin (5-HT$_3$ subtype) receptors and transmitted along afferent vagus nerve fibers. They activate a diffuse series of effector nuclei in the medulla oblongata (the so-called "vomiting center"), which integrates afferent emetic signals and subsequently activates and coordinates motor nuclei that produce the physiologic changes associated with vomiting.

- In general, the greatest incidence of acute symptoms occurs within 2 to 6 hours after treatment.
- Onset is generally within 1 to 3 hours after commencing chemotherapy. Notable exceptions include the following:
  - Mechlorethamine (nitrogen mustard), which generally induces rapid symptom onset (≤1 hour)
  - Cyclophosphamide, after intravenous administration, and carboplatin have long latency periods before acute-phase onset, and symptoms may persist or intermittently recur for ≥12 hours after treatment.

Delayed-Phase Symptoms

Delayed-phase symptoms are defined as those that occur >24 hours after treatment (Table 38.1) and are associated with central activation of neurokinin type 1 (NK$_1$) receptors, for which substance P is the natural ligand. Drugs with high emetogenic potential and, in some cases, drugs with moderate emetic risk may cause delayed-phase symptoms (Table 38.2). Symptoms may commence as early as 16 to 18 hours after emetogenic treatment, with a period of greatest incidence between 24 and 96 hours after treatment. Delayed emesis may occur in patients who do not experience symptoms acutely, but incidence characteristically decreases in patients who achieve complete emetic control during the acute phase. Although emesis is typically less severe during the delayed phase than during the acute phase, the reported severity of nausea is similar during both phases.

Anticipatory Events

Anticipatory nausea or vomiting describes emetic symptoms occurring before repeated exposure to emetogenic treatment that develop as an aversive conditioned response as a consequence of poor

527

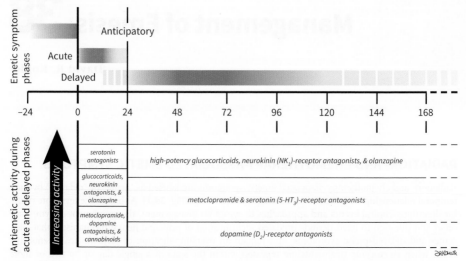

FIGURE 38.1 Comparison of emetic symptom phases and antiemetic activity. Top: Temporal relation between the start of emetogenic treatment (hour 0) and emetic symptom phases. For each phase, shaded bars indicate generally when nausea and emesis occur before and after emetogenic treatment; greater intensity of shading approximates the incidence of symptoms. Bottom: The most highly active antiemetic categories ranked by relative effectiveness against acute-phase (0 – 24 h) and delayed-phase (>24 h) emetic symptoms.

emetic control during prior therapy with nausea reported to occur more commonly than anticipatory vomiting. The risk of developing anticipatory symptoms has been shown to increase with repeated courses of emetogenic treatment, particularly in patients who experience incomplete emetic control during treatments they previously received, but emetic symptoms during pregnancy and motion sickness have been identified as contributing risk factors. Although anxiolytic amnestic drugs are helpful in preventing and delaying anticipatory symptoms, complete control throughout all antineoplastic treatments is the best preventive strategy against developing symptoms. Behavioral therapies such as relaxation techniques and systematic desensitization may be useful if symptoms occur. After symptoms develop, medical interventions for anticipatory symptoms during subsequent emetogenic treatment are limited to preventing the reinforcement of conditioned stimulae, which may exacerbate symptoms.

EMETOGENIC (EMETIC) POTENTIAL

Emetic potential or risk and symptom patterns vary among medications used in antineoplastic chemotherapy and radiation therapy techniques.

Chemotherapy

Intrinsic emetogenicity (Table 38.3) is an antineoplastic drug's propensity for causing emetic symptoms. Drug dose or dosage is often the second most significant factor affecting emetogenic potential and the duration for which symptoms persist.

The number of emetogenic drugs used in combination, administration schedule, treatment duration, and route of administration are also mitigating factors. Emetic potential may be lessened or eliminated by protracted drug delivery over hours or days, and increased by rapid drug administration, repeated emetogenic treatments, and brief intervals between repeated doses (Table 38.3). When emetogenic treatment is given on more than one day, physiological processes associated with acute and delayed phase symptoms may overlap and both should be considered in designing effective antiemetic

TABLE 38.1 Onset and Duration of Emesis with Selected Chemotherapy Agents

Drug	Onset of Emesis (h)	Duration of Emesis (h)
Aldesleukin	0–6	—
Altretamine	3–6	—
Asparaginase	1–3	—
Bleomycin	3–6	—
Carboplatin	6–8	>24
Carmustine	2–6	4–24
Chlorambucil	48–72	—
Cisplatin	1–6	24–48+
Cyclophosphamide	6–18	6–24+
Cytarabine	6–12	3–5
Dacarbazine	1–5	1–24
Dactinomycin	2–6	12–24
Daunorubicin	2–6	24
Doxorubicin	4–6	6–24+
Etoposide	3–8	6–12
Fluorouracil	3–6	3–4
Hydroxyurea	6–12	—
Ifosfamide	1–6	6–12
Irinotecan	2–6	6–12
Lomustine	2–6	4–12
Mechlorethamine	0.5–2	1–24
Melphalan	6–12	—
Mercaptopurine	4–8	—
Methotrexate	4–12	3–12
Mitomycin	1–6	3–12
Mitotane	Long latency	Persistent
Paclitaxel	3–8	3–8
Pentostatin	Long latency	Persistent (>24)
Plicamycin	4–6	12–24
Procarbazine	24–27	Variable
Streptozocin	1–4	12–24
Teniposide	3–8	6–12
Thioguanine	4–8	—
Thiotepa	6–12	Variable
Vinblastine	4–8	—
Vincristine	4–8	—
Vinorelbine	4–8	—

Adapted from: Borison HL, McCarthy LE. Neuropharmacology of chemotherapy-induced emesis. *Drugs.* 1983;25(Suppl 1):8–17; and Aapro M. Methodological issues in antiemetic studies. *Invest New Drugs.* 1993;11(4):243–253.

prophylaxis. The potential and duration for delayed symptoms depends upon the sequence in which emetogenic drugs are administered and the emetogenic risk each drug presents.

Radiation

The emetic potential of ionizing radiation correlates directly with the amount of radiation given per dose or fraction, the total dose administered, and the rate at which it is administered. Large

TABLE 38.2 Antineoplastic Drugs Implicated in Delayed Emesis

Drug	Dosages	Combinations that Exacerbate Developing Symptoms
Carboplatin	≥300 mg/m^2	± other cytotoxic agents
Cisplatin	≥50 mg/m^2	
Cyclophosphamide	≥600 mg/m^2	+ anthracycline combinations ± other cytotoxic agents
Doxorubicin	≥50 mg/m^2	
Oxaliplatin	≥85 mg/m^2	± other cytotoxic agents

TABLE 38.3 Emetic Risk for Single Agents as a Function of Drug, Dosage or Dose, and Route of Administration

	Acute Phase Emetic Potential (incidence^a)			
	High (>90%), Moderate (30%–90%), Low (10%–30%), Minimal (<10%)			
Drugs and Drug Combinations	MASCC/ESMO	NCCN	ASCO	Current Product Labeling
ado-Trastuzumab emtansine	Low^b	Low^c		
Afatenib (orally)	Low^b	Minimal–low^c		
Aldesleukin		Moderate^c (>12–15 million international units/ m^2); Low^c (≤12 million international units/ m^2)		
Alectinib (orally)		Minimal–low^c		
Alemtuzumab	Moderate^b	Minimal^c	Moderate^d	
Altretamine (orally)	High^b	Moderate–high^c		
Amifostine		Moderate^c (>300 mg/m^2); Low^c (≤300 mg/m^2)		
Arsenic trioxide		Moderate^c		
Asparaginase		Minimal^c		
Atezolizumab		Low^c		
Avelumab				Low^{e,f}
Axitinib (orally)	Low^b	Minimal–low^c		
Azacitidine	Moderate^b	Moderate^c	Moderate^d	
Belinostat	Low^b	Low^c		
Bendamustine	Moderate^b	Moderate^c	Moderate^d	
Bevacizumab	Minimal^b	Minimal^c	Minimal^d	
Bexarotene (orally)		Minimal–low^c		
Bleomycin	Minimal^b	Minimal^c	Minimal^d	
Blinatumomab	Low^b	Low^c		
Bortezomib	Low^b	Minimal^c	Low^d	
Bosutinib (orally)	Moderate^b	Minimal–low^c		

TABLE 38.3 (Continued)

Drugs and Drug Combinations	MASCC/ESMO	NCCN	ASCO	Current Product Labeling
Brentuximab vedotin	Low[b]	Low[c]		
Busulfan	Minimal[b]	Moderate[c]	Minimal[d]	
Busulfan (orally)		Moderate-high[c] (≥4 mg/d); Minimal-low[c] (<4 mg/d)		
Cabazitaxel	Low[b]	Low[c]	Low[d]	
Cabozantinib (orally)		Minimal-low[c]		
Capecitabine (orally)	Low[b]	Minimal-low[c]		
Carboplatin	Moderate[b]	High (AUC ≥4 mg/ mL·min)[c]; Moderate (AUC <4 mg/ mL·min)[c,j]	Moderate[d]	
Carfilzomib	Low[b]	Low[c]		
Carmustine	High[b]	High (>250 mg/m²)[c]; Moderate (≤250 mg/ m²)[c,j]	High[d]	
Catumaxomab[h]	Low[b]		Low[d]	Moderate[e,g]
Ceritinib (orally)	Moderate[b]	Moderate-high[c]		
Cetuximab	Low[b]	Minimal[c]	Minimal[d]	
Chlorambucil (orally)	Minimal[b]	Minimal-low[c]		
Cisplatin	High[b]	High[c]	High[d]	
Cladribine	Minimal[b]	Minimal[c]	Minimal[d]	
Clofarabine	Moderate[b]	Moderate[c]	Moderate[d]	
Cobimetinib (orally)		Minimal-low[c]		
Crizotinib (orally)	Moderate[b]	Moderate-high[c]		
Cyclophosphamide	High (≥1,500 mg/m²)[b]; Moderate (<1,500 mg/ m²)[b]	High (>1,500 mg/m²)[c]; Moderate[c] (≤1,500 mg/m²)	High[d] (≥1,500 mg/m²); Moderate[d] (<1,500 mg/m²)	
Cyclophosphamide (orally)	Moderate[b]	Moderate-high[c] (≥100 mg/m² per d); Minimal-low[c] (<100 mg/m² per d)		
Cyclophosphamide + an Anthracycline, including: daunorubicin, doxorubicin, epirubicin, or idarubicin; an "AC" regimen	High[b]	High[c] (only doxorubicin and epirubicin are included in the definition of an "AC" regimen)	High[d]	

(continued)

TABLE 38.3 (Continued)

Drugs and Drug Combinations	MASCC/ESMO	NCCN	ASCO	Current Product Labeling
Cytarabine	Moderate (>1,000 mg/m²)[b]; Low (≤1,000 mg/m²)[b]	Moderate[c] (>200 mg/m²); Low[c] (100–200 mg/m²); Minimal[c] (<100 mg/m²)	Moderate[d] (>1,000 mg/m²); Low[d] (≤1,000 mg/m²)	
Dabrafenib (orally)	Low[b]	Minimal–low[c]		
Dacarbazine	High[b]	High[c]	High[d]	
Dactinomycin		Moderate[c,i]	High[d]	
Daratumumab		Minimal[c]		
Dasatinib (orally)	Low[b]	Minimal–low[c]		
Daunorubicin	Moderate[b]	Moderate[c,i]	Moderate[d]	
Daunorubicin, liposomal[h]				Low[e,j]
Decitabine		Minimal[c]		
Denileukin diftitox		Minimal[c]		
Dexrazoxane		Minimal[c]		
Dinutuximab		Moderate[c]		
Docetaxel	Low[b]	Low[c]	Low[d]	
Doxorubicin	Moderate[b]	High (≥60 mg/m²)[c]; Moderate[c,i] (<60 mg/m²)	Moderate[d]	
Doxorubicin, liposomal	Low[b]	Low[c]	Low[d]	
Elotuzumab		Minimal[c]		
Epirubicin	Moderate[b]	High (>90 mg/m²)[c]; Moderate[c,i] (≤90 mg/m²)	Moderate[d]	
Eribulin mesylate	Low[b]	Low[c]		
Erlotinib (orally)	Minimal[b]	Minimal–low[c]		
Estramustine		Moderate–high[c]		
Etoposide	Low[b]	Low[c]	Low[d]	
Etoposide (orally)	Low[b]	Moderate–high[c]		
Everolimus (orally)	Low[b]	Minimal–low[c]		
Fludarabine	Minimal[b]	Minimal[c]	Minimal[d]	
Fludarabine (orally)[k]	Low[b]	Minimal–low[c]		
Floxuridine		Low[c]		
Fluorouracil	Low[b]	Low[c]	Low[d]	
Gefitinib (orally)[l]	Minimal[b]	Minimal–low[c]		
Gemcitabine	Low[b]	Low[c]	Low[d]	
Hydroxyurea (orally)	Minimal[b]	Minimal–low[c]		
Ibrutinib (orally)	Low[b]	Minimal–low[c]		
Idarubicin	Moderate[b]	Moderate[c]	Moderate[d]	
Idelalisib (orally)	Low[b]	Minimal–low[c]		
Ifosfamide	Moderate[b]	High (≥2,000 mg/m² per dose)[c]; Moderate[c,i] (<2,000 mg/m² per dose)	Moderate[d]	
Imatinib (orally)	Moderate[b]	Minimal–low[c]		

TABLE 38.3 (Continued)

Drugs and Drug Combinations	MASCC/ESMO	NCCN	ASCO	Current Product Labeling
Interferon alfa		Moderate[c] (≥10 million international units/m²); Low[c] (>5 to <10 million international units/m²); Minimal[c] (≤5 million international units/m²)		
Ipilimumab	Low[b]	Minimal[c]		
Irinotecan	Moderate[b]	Moderate[c,i]	Moderate[d]	
Irinotecan, liposomal		Low[c]		
Ixabepilone	Low[b]	Low[c]	Low[d]	
Ixazomib (orally)		Minimal–low[c]		
Lapatinib (orally)	Low[b]	Minimal–low[c]		
Lenalidomide (orally)	Low[b]	Minimal–low[c]		
Lenvatinib (orally)		Moderate–high[c]		
Lomustine (orally)		Moderate–high[c] (single day)		
Mechlorethamine	High[b]	High[c]	High[d]	
Melphalan		Moderate[c]		
Melphalan (orally)	Minimal[b]	Minimal–low[c]		
Mercaptopurine (orally)		Minimal–low[c]		
Methotrexate	Low[b]	Moderate[c,i] (≥250 mg/m²); Low[c] (>50 to <250 mg/m²); Minimal[c] (≤50 mg/m²)	Low[d]	
Methotrexate (orally)	Minimal[b]	Minimal–low[c]		
Mitomycin	Low[b]	Low[c]	Low[d]	
Mitotane (orally)		Moderate–high[c]		
Mitoxantrone	Low[b]	Low[c]	Low[d]	
Necitumumab		Low[c]		
Nelarabine		Minimal[c]		
Nilotinib (orally)	Low[b]	Minimal–low[c]		
Niraparib (orally)				Low[e,m]
Nivolumab	Minimal[b]	Minimal[c]		
Obinutuzumab		Minimal[c]		
Ofatumumab	Minimal[b]	Minimal[c]		
Olaparib (orally)	Low[b]	Moderate–high[c]		
Omacetaxine mepesuccinate		Low[c]		
Osimertinib (orally)		Minimal–low[c]		
Oxaliplatin	Moderate[b]	Moderate[c,i]	Moderate[d]	
Paclitaxel	Low[b]	Low[c]	Low[d]	

(continued)

TABLE 38.3 (Continued)

Drugs and Drug Combinations	MASCC/ESMO	NCCN	ASCO	Current Product Labeling
Paclitaxel protein (albumin-)-bound particles (*nab*-paclitaxel)	Low[b]	Low[c]		
Palbociclib (orally)		Minimal–low[c]		
Panitumumab	Low[b]	Minimal[c]	Low[d]	
Panobinostat (orally)		Moderate–high[c]		
Pazopanib (orally)	Low[b]	Minimal–low[c]		
Pegaspargase		Minimal[c]		
Peginterferon alfa		Minimal[c]		
Pembrolizumab	Minimal[b]	Minimal[c]		
Pemetrexed	Low[b]	Low[c]	Low[d]	
Pentostatin		Low[c]		
Pertuzumab	Low[b]	Minimal[c]		
Pixantrone dimaleate[h]	Minimal[b]			
Plicamycin[h]				Low–moderate[e,n,o]
Pomalidomide (orally)	Minimal[b]	Minimal–low[c]		
Ponatinib (orally)	Low[b]	Minimal–low[c]		
Pralatrexate	Minimal[b]	Low[c]	Minimal[d]	
Procarbazine (orally)	High[b]	Moderate–high[c]		
Ramucirumab		Minimal[c]		
Regorafenib (orally)	Low[b]	Minimal–low[c]		
Ribociclib (orally)				Low[e,p]
Rituximab	Minimal[b]	Minimal[c]	Minimal[d]	
Romidepsin	Moderate[b]	Low[c]		
Rucaparib (orally)		Moderate–high[c]		
Ruxolitinib (orally)	Minimal[b]	Minimal–low[c]		
Siltuximab		Minimal[c]		
Sonidegib (orally)		Minimal–low[c]		
Sorafenib (orally)	Minimal[b]	Minimal–low[c]		
Streptozocin	High[b]	High[c]	High[d]	
Sunitinib (orally)	Low[b]	Minimal–low[c]		
Talimogene laherparepvec		Low[c]		
Tegafur uracil[h] (orally)	Low[b]			
Temozolomide (injection)	Moderate[b]	Moderate[c]		
Temozolomide (orally)	Moderate[b]	Moderate – high[c] (>75 mg/m²·day); Moderate[c] (≤75 mg/m²·day if given concurrently with radiation therapy); Minimal – low[c] (≤75 mg/m²·day)		
Temsirolimus	Low[b]	Minimal[c]	Low[d]	

TABLE 38.3 (Continued)

Drugs and Drug Combinations	MASCC/ESMO	NCCN	ASCO	Current Product Labeling
Teniposide				Low–moderate[e,q]
Thalidomide (orally)	Low[b]	Minimal–low[c]		
Thioguanine (orally)	Minimal[b]	Minimal–low[c]		
Thiotepa	Moderate[b]	Low[c]		
Topotecan	Low[b]	Low[c]	Low[d]	
Topotecan (orally)		Minimal–low[c]		
Trabectedin	Moderate[b]	Moderate[c,i]		
Trametinib (orally)		Minimal–low[c]		
Trastuzumab	Minimal[b]	Minimal[c]	Low[d]	
Tretinoin (orally)		Minimal–low[c]		
Trifluridine/tipiracil (orally)		Moderate–high[c]		
Valrubicin		Minimal[c]		
Vandetanib (orally)	Low[b]	Minimal–low[c]		
Vemurafenib (orally)	Minimal[b]	Minimal–low[c]		
Venetoclax (orally)		Minimal–low[c]		
Vinblastine	Minimal[b]	Minimal[c]	Minimal[d]	
Vincristine	Minimal[b]	Minimal[c]	Minimal[d]	
Vincristine, liposomal		Minimal[c]		
Vinflunine ditartrate[h]	Low[b]			
Vinorelbine	Minimal[b]	Minimal[c]	Minimal[d]	
Vinorelbine (orally)[h]	Moderate[b]			
Vismodegib (orally)	Minimal[b]	Minimal–low[c]		
Vorinostat (orally)	Low[b]	Minimal–low[c]		
ziv-Aflibercept	Low[b]	Low[c]		

[a] Assignment to emetic risk categorizes (*high, moderate, low, minimal*) follows guidelines published by oncology professional organizations. Emetic potential for drugs not yet categorized by one of the listed organizations are estimated from product labeling for the drug given as a single agent at a dosage, schedule, and route of administration approved by the U.S. FDA, or, in the case of drugs marketed outside the USA, from product-specific summaries of product characteristics.

[b] Roila F, Molassiotis A, Herrstedt J, et al. 2016 MASCC and ESMO guideline update for the prevention of chemotherapy- and radiotherapy-induced nausea and vomiting and of nausea and vomiting in advanced cancer patients. *Ann Oncol.* 2016;27(Suppl 5):v119–v33.

[c] NCCN Clinical Practice Guidelines in Oncology (NCCN Guidelines®), Antiemesis, Version 1.2017 — February 22, 2017. National Comprehensive Cancer Network, Inc. URL: https://www.nccn.org/ [Accessed 10. March, 2017]

[d] Basch E, Prestrud AA, Hesketh PJ, et al. Antiemetics: American Society of Clinical Oncology clinical practice guideline update. *J Clin Oncol.* 2011;29(31):4189–4198.

[e] Categorization of emetic risk reported in product labeling may be inaccurate, because the data from which it is derived may represent:

- Inconsistent characterization and selective reporting or underreported emetic symptoms during antineoplastic drug development.

- Inconsistent methods for reporting adverse drug events; e.g., events reported after a single dose of an emetogenic drug, after repeated doses within a cycle, after repeated cycles.

- Unregulated antiemetic use during emetogenic drug development prior to establishing an agent's emetogenic risk.

- A predisposition for developing emetic symptoms due to personal risk factors and/or history of poor emetic control during previously administered emetogenic treatment among subjects who received the emetogenic drug during its clinical development.

(continued)

TABLE 38.3 (Continued)

[f] BAVENCIO® (avelumab) injection, for intravenous use; product label, March 2017. EMD Serono, Inc. and Pfizer Inc., NY, NY

[g] ASSESSMENT REPORT FOR Removab. European Medicines Agency. EMEA/CHMP/100434/2009 At: http//:www.emea.europa.eu Accessed: 9 March 2017

[h] The product is not currently commercially available in the USA.

[i] The agent may be highly emetogenic in some patients. NCCN Guidelines®, Antiemesis, Version 1.2017 — February 22, 2017

[j] DaunoXome® (daunorubicin citrate liposome injection); product label, December 2011. Galen US Inc., Souderton, PA

[k] The indicated drug has not received FDA approval for oral administration; i.e., product formulations for oral administration are not commercially available in the USA.

[l] In the USA, gefitinib is only available to patients already enrolled on the Iressa Access Program (restricted distribution program) administered by AstraZeneca Pharmaceuticals, LP.

[m] ZEJULA™ (niraparib) capsules, for oral use; product label, March 2017. TESARO, Inc., Waltham, MA

[n] The agent may be less emetogenic when given by continuous (protracted) administration.

[o] Mithracin® (plicamycin) FOR INTRAVENOUS USE; product label, September 1987. Miles Pharmaceuticals, Division of Miles Laboratories, Inc., West Haven CT

[p] KISQALI® (ribociclib) tablets, for oral use; product label, March 2017. Novartis Pharmaceuticals Corporation East Hanover, NJ

[q] Teniposide Injection; product label, March 2015. WG Critical Care, LLC, Paramus, NJ

treatment volumes (>400 cm^2); fields including the upper abdomen, upper hemithorax, and whole body; and a history of poor emetic control with chemotherapy are risk factors for severe emesis. Emetic potential increases when radiation and chemotherapy are administered concomitantly ("radiochemotherapy").

PATIENT RISK FACTORS

Patients at greatest risk for emetic symptoms include the following:

- Female sex, particularly women with a history of persistent and/or severe emetic symptoms during pregnancy
- Children and young adults
- Patients with a history of acute- and/or delayed-phase emetic symptoms during prior treatments are at great risk for poor emetic control during subsequent treatments
- Patients with low performance status and a predisposition to motion sickness.
- Nondrinkers are at greater risk than patients with a history of chronic alcohol consumption (>100 g ethanol daily for several years)
- Patients with intercurrent pathologies, such as gastrointestinal (GI) inflammation, compromised GI motility or obstruction, constipation, brain metastases, metabolic abnormalities (hypovolemia, hypercalcemia, hypoadrenalism, uremia), visceral organs invaded by tumor, and concurrent medical treatment (opioids, bronchodilators, aspirin, nonsteroidal anti-inflammatory drugs), may predispose and exacerbate emetic symptoms during treatment and complicate good emetic control

PRIMARY ANTIEMETIC PROPHYLAXIS

Primary prophylaxis is indicated for all patients whose antineoplastic treatment presents at least a low risk of producing emetic symptoms; that is, when >10% of persons receiving similar chemotherapy or radiation therapy without antiemetic prophylaxis are predicted to experience emetic symptoms (Table 38.3).

▪ Planning effective antiemetic primary prophylaxis
- Evaluate the emetic potential for each drug included in treatment, which includes the severity, onset, and duration of symptoms associated with individual drugs (Table 38.1), and how drug dose or dosage, schedule, and route of administration may affect those factors.
- Patients who receive combination chemotherapy should receive antiemetic prophylaxis based on the most emetogenic component of treatment.
  - Include primary prophylaxis against acute-phase symptoms for all treatments with low, moderate, or high emetic potential, and delayed-phase prophylaxis for treatments with moderate or high emetic potential.
  - For patients who receive antineoplastic chemotherapy and radiation concomitantly, antiemetic prophylaxis is selected based on the chemotherapy component that presents the greatest emetogenic potential, *unless* the emetic risk from radiation is greater.
- Patients who receive moderately or highly emetogenic treatment for more than one day should receive antiemetic prophylaxis appropriate for the drug with greatest emetogenic potential on each day of treatment.
- If antineoplastic treatment is associated with delayed emetic symptoms, continue antiemetic prophylaxis:
  - For at least three days after highly emetogenic treatment is completed.
  - For at least two days after moderately emetogenic treatment is completed.
- Treatment-appropriate antiemetic prophylaxis should precede each emetogenic treatment and proceed on a fixed schedule. Patients should not be expected to recognize symptom prodromes and to rely on unscheduled (i.e., *as needed*) antiemetics.
- Antiemetics should be given at the lowest effective doses.
- Patients' responses to antiemetic prophylaxis and treatment should be serially monitored and documented with standardized validated tools.
  - Health care providers historically underestimate the incidence and severity of emetic symptoms associated with chemotherapy and radiation therapy, particularly nausea.
  - Patient input is essential to capture information about
    - Events that health-care providers cannot observe due to patient location and the subjective nature of nausea.
    - Conditions and interventions that modulate a patient's emetic symptoms.
    - Changes in a patient's response to antiemetic prophylaxis through a succession of treatment cycles or courses.
  - The MASCC has developed and makes available online a standardized eight-item questionnaire that can be used to document the number of vomiting episodes and the number and severity of episodes of nausea both acutely and within the four days (24 to 120 hours) following the day on which emetogenic treatment was given.
    - The MASCC Antiemesis Tool (MAT), a guide for using the tool, and Patient Outcomes Score Sheets are available in 17 languages in digital formats for downloading, and in an application for handheld devices.
    - Non-profit entities may use the MAT without incurring charges. Commercial companies are required to obtain written approval from MASCC, and will incur a nominal fee prior to using the MAT.
    - Information about gaining approval for using the MAT is available online at http://www.mascc.org/index.php?option=com_content&view=article&id=352:MAT&catid=24:guidelines-and-assessment-tools [Accessed 4 December 2017].

Figure 38.2 integrates evidence-based guidelines for treatment-appropriate antiemetic prophylaxis recommended by the National Comprehensive Cancer Network, the Multinational Association of Supportive Care in Cancer and European Society for Medical Oncology, the American Society of Clinical Oncology, current labeling for medications that have received U.S. Food and Drug Administration (FDA) approval for commercial use, and the consensus of experts in oncology. Recommendations are based on the assessment of emetic risk and generally apply to adult patients, but may not be appropriate

HIGH Risk PARENTERALLY administered chemotherapy

The order in which the following SIX primary antiemetic prophylaxis options appear does not indicate preference.
Start antiemetics before administering emetogenic treatment; continue daily with scheduled doses (not "as needed").

Day 1

A 5-HT₃-receptor antagonist (select from the following):
- **Palonosetron** 0.25 mg IV once, OR
- **Granisetron** 10 mg SQ once[a], or
  2 mg PO once, or
  0.01 mg/kg (maximum dose = 1 mg) IV once, or
  3.1-mg/24 h transdermal patch applied
  topically 24–48 h before chemotherapy, OR
- **Ondansetron** 16–24 mg PO once, or
  8–16 mg IV once, OR
- **Dolasetron** 100 mg PO once

PLUS one of the following:
- **Aprepitant** 125 mg PO once
- **Dexamethasone** 12 mg PO or 12 mg IV once[b,c]

OR

- **Fosaprepitant** 150 mg IV once
- **Dexamethasone** 12 mg PO or 12 mg IV once[b,c]

OR

- **Rolapitant** 180 mg PO once[e]
- **Dexamethasone** 20 mg PO or 20 mg IV once[c,f,g]

OR

- **Aprepitant** 125 mg PO once, OR
  Fosaprepitant 150 mg IV once[h]
- **Dexamethasone** 12 mg PO or 12 mg IV once[b,c]
- **Olanzapine** 10 mg PO once[i]

Days 2, 3, & 4

Followed by:
- **Aprepitant** 80 mg PO daily on days 2 and 3
- **Dexamethasone** 8 mg PO or 8 mg[b,c] IV daily
  on days 2, 3, and 4[d]

- **Dexamethasone** 8 mg PO or 8 mg[b,c] IV
  on day 2, *then:*
- **Dexamethasone** 8 mg PO or 8 mg[b,c] IV twice
  daily on days 3 and 4[d]

- **Dexamethasone** 8 mg PO or 8 mg[c,f] IV twice
  daily on days 2, 3, and 4[d]

- **Dexamethasone** 8 mg PO or 8 mg[b,c] IV once
  daily on days 2, 3, and 4
- **Aprepitant** 80 mg PO once daily on days 2 and 3
  (if aprepitant was given on day 1)
- **Olanzapine** 10 mg PO once daily on days 2, 3,
  and 4[d,i]

OR

- **Netupitant** 300 mg + **Palonosetron** 0.5 mg PO once[j]
- **Dexamethasone** 12 mg PO, or 12 mg IV once[b,c]

- **Dexamethasone** 8 mg[b,c] PO once daily
  on days 2, 3, and 4

OR

- **Palonosetron** 0.25 mg IV once
- **Dexamethasone** 20 mg IV once[c]
- **Olanzapine** 10 mg PO once[i]

- **Olanzapine** 10 mg PO once daily
  on days 2, 3, and 4[i]

± **Lorazepam** 0.5–2 mg PO, IV, or sublingually every 6 hours as needed on days 1–4

± A histamine (**H₂**)-receptor antagonist *or* **proton pump inhibitor**[k]

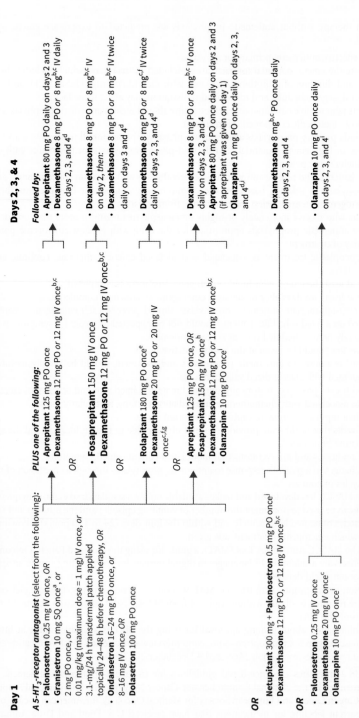

FIGURE 38.2 Algorithms for antiemetic prophylaxis and treatment for parenterally and orally administered emetogenic drugs and ionizing radiation (external beam).

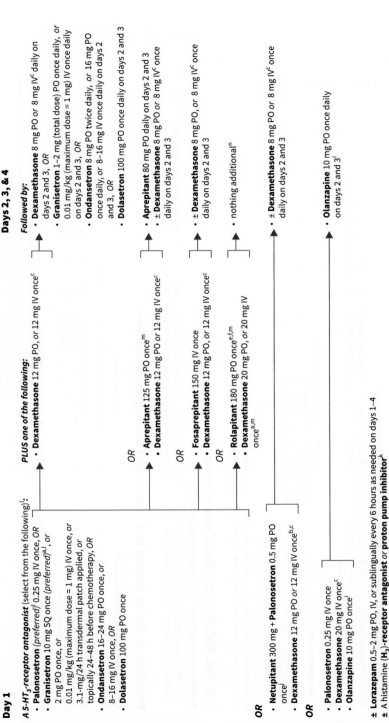

MODERATE Risk PARENTERALLY administered chemotherapy

The order in which the following SIX primary antiemetic prophylaxis options appear does not indicate preference.

Day 1

A 5-HT₃-receptor antagonist (select from the following[l]):
- **Palonosetron** (preferred)[l] 0.25 mg IV once, OR
- **Granisetron** 10 mg SQ once (preferred)[a,l], or 2 mg PO once, or 0.01 mg/kg (maximum dose = 1 mg) IV once, or 3.1-mg/24 h transdermal patch applied, or topically 24–48 h before chemotherapy, OR
- **Ondansetron** 16–24 mg PO once, or 8–16 mg IV once, OR
- **Dolasetron** 100 mg PO once

PLUS one of the following:
- **Dexamethasone** 12 mg PO, or 12 mg IV once[c]

OR

- **Aprepitant** 125 mg PO once[m]
- **Dexamethasone** 12 mg PO or 12 mg IV once[c]

OR

- **Fosaprepitant** 150 mg IV once
- **Dexamethasone** 12 mg PO or 12 mg IV once[c]

OR

- **Rolapitant** 180 mg PO once[e,f,m]
- **Dexamethasone** 20 mg PO, or 20 mg IV once[a,m]

OR

- **Netupitant** 300 mg + **Palonosetron** 0.5 mg PO once[j]
- **Dexamethasone** 12 mg PO or 12 mg IV once[b,c]

OR

- **Palonosetron** 0.25 mg IV once
- **Dexamethasone** 20 mg IV once[c]
- **Olanzapine** 10 mg PO once[i]

Days 2, 3, & 4

Followed by:
- **Dexamethasone** 8 mg PO or 8 mg IV[c] daily on days 2 and 3, OR
- **Granisetron** 1–2 mg (total dose) PO once daily, or 0.01 mg/kg (maximum dose = 1 mg) IV once daily on days 2 and 3, OR
- **Ondansetron** 8 mg PO twice daily, or 16 mg PO once daily, or 8–16 mg IV once daily on days 2 and 3, OR
- **Dolasetron** 100 mg PO once daily on days 2 and 3

- **Aprepitant** 80 mg PO daily on days 2 and 3
- ± **Dexamethasone** 8 mg PO or 8 mg IV once daily on days 2 and 3

- ± **Dexamethasone** 8 mg PO, or 8 mg IV[c] once daily on days 2 and 3

- nothing additional[n]

- ± **Dexamethasone** 8 mg PO or 8 mg IV[c] once daily on days 2 and 3

- **Olanzapine** 10 mg PO once daily on days 2 and 3[i]

± **Lorazepam** 0.5–2 mg PO, IV, or sublingually every 6 hours as needed on days 1–4
± A histamine (H₂)-receptor antagonist or proton pump inhibitor[k]

FIGURE 38.2 (Continued)

LOW Risk PARENTERALLY administered chemotherapy

The order in which the following FOUR primary antiemetic prophylaxis options appear does not indicate preference. Start antiemetics before administering emetogenic treatment and repeat each day on which multi-day emetogenic medications are given with scheduled doses (not "as needed").

One of the following:

- **Dexamethasone** 12 mg PO, or 12 mg IV once
  OR
- **Metoclopramide** 10 mg PO, or 10 mg IV once
  OR
- **Prochlorperazine** 10 mg PO, or 10 mg IV once

OR a 5-HT$_3$-receptor antagonist (select from):
- **Dolasetron** 100 mg PO once, OR
- **Granisetron** 1–2 mg PO once, OR
- **Ondansetron** 8–16 mg PO once

± **Lorazepam** 0.5–2 mg PO, IV, or sublingually every 6 hours as needed on days of emetogenic treatment
± A histamine (**H$_2$**)-receptor antagonist or proton pump inhibitor[k]

MINIMAL Risk PARENTERALLY administered chemotherapy

Routine primary antiemetic prophylaxis is not indicated.

- If emetic symptoms occur, follow the guidelines for breakthrough symptoms, and continue antiemetic treatment for at least the duration of emetogenic treatment.
- Consider using antiemetic prophylaxis appropriate for LOW emetic risk during subsequent emetogenic treatments.[o]

Prophylaxis during Second and Subsequent Emetogenic Treatments

Control achieved during previous cycle

No emetic symptoms

Nausea without emesis

Emetic symptoms controlled by rescue ("breakthrough") medications

Uncontrolled emetic symptoms

Interventions

No change in initial antiemetic regimen

Include in prophylaxis for repeated emetogenic treatment medications that were effective in treating breakthrough symptoms during the previous cycle.
- Antiemetic prophylaxis should be given around-the-clock at scheduled intervals.

Acute management:
- Implement fluids and electrolytes support.
- Escalate antiemetic doses or shorten administration intervals with agents currently in use, or add agents from other pharmacological classes.
- Add nonpharmacological interventions.
Management during repeated treatments:
- Escalate antiemetic primary prophylaxis to the next greater emetic potential risk level.

FIGURE 38.2 (Continued)

HIGH to MODERATE Risk ORALLY administered chemotherapy

Initial Prophylaxis[o,p,q]

The order in which the following options for primary antiemetic prophylaxis appear does not indicate preference.

Start antiemetics before emetogenic treatment; continue daily with scheduled doses (not 'as needed'):

A 5-HT₃-receptor antagonist (select from the following)**:**
- **Dolasetron** 100 mg PO daily; *OR*
- **Granisetron** 1–2 mg (total dose) PO daily, *or* 1 mg PO q.12 h, *or* 3.1-mg/24 h transdermal patch for 7 days, applied topically 24–48 h before chemotherapy; *OR*
- **Ondansetron** 8–16 mg PO daily

± **Lorazepam** 0.5–2 mg PO *or* SL q.4–6 h

LOW to MINIMAL Risk ORALLY administered chemotherapy

Initial Prophylaxis[o,p,q]

Start antiemetics if/as needed.

If antiemetics are needed, give a dose before subsequent emetogenic treatment and continue daily.

The order in which the following options for primary antiemetic prophylaxis appear does not indicate preference.

Select one of the following:
- **Metoclopramide** 10–20 mg PO, and then q.6 h PRN (maximum 40 mg/day)[r]; *OR*
- **Prochlorperazine** 10 mg PO, and then q.6 h PRN; *OR* (a 5-HT₃-receptor antagonist; select one of the following:)
- **Dolasetron** 100 mg PO daily, PRN; *OR*
- **Granisetron** 1–2 mg (total dose) PO daily, PRN; *OR*
- **Ondansetron** 8–16 mg (total dose) PO daily, PRN

± **Lorazepam** 0.5–2 mg PO *or* SL q.4 – 6 h

FIGURE 38.2 (Continued)

Breakthrough Symptoms

Add one or more antiemetics for breakthrough symptoms.

Breakthrough Symptoms

Add one or more antiemetics for breakthrough symptoms. Include in prophylaxis for repeated emetogenic treatment medications that were previously effective in treating breakthrough symptoms.

Primary Antiemetic Prophylaxis for RADIATION THERAPY

Emetic Potential	Primary Prophylaxis[f,o,p]	Treatment for Breakthrough Symptoms
High Risk Total Body Irradiation (TBI)	A 5-HT3 receptor antagonist before each RT fraction; e.g.: **Granisetron** 2 mg PO daily or 1 mg PO q.12 h; *or* 0.01 mg/kg IV q.12 h; *OR* **Ondansetron** 8 mg PO or 0.15 mg/kg IV (maximum single dose ≤16 mg) q.8–12 h; *OR* **Palonosetron** 0.25 mg IV every second day of RT • Continue for at least 24 h after RT is completed ± **Dexamethasone** 4 mg PO or 4 mg IV before the first 5 RT fractions[k]	Add agents from other pharmacological classes (see guidance for "Treatment for Breakthrough Symptoms with Emetogenic Treatment")
Moderate Risk Fields including: Craniospinal; Upper abdomen (includes fields formerly described as "hemi-body" & "upper body", both of which included the upper abdomen)	A 5-HT₃ receptor antagonist as above • An optimal duration for prophylaxis after RT has not been identified ± **Dexamethasone** 4 mg PO or 4 mg IV before the first 5 RT fractions[k]	
Low Risk Fields including: Cranium Head and neck; thorax region (includes the fields formerly identified as "upper thoracic" and "lower thoracic" regions); pelvis	Primary prophylaxis or rescue with Dexamethasone. Primary prophylaxis or rescue with Dexamethasone, a D₂-receptor antagonist, or any of the 5-HT₃-receptor antagonists identified above	Add an agent not used in primary prophylaxis; e.g., Dexamethasone, a D₂-receptor antagonist, or a 5-HT₃-receptor antagonist • Continue use before each remaining RT fraction
Minimal Risk Fields limited to the breast or extremities	Rescue with Dexamethasone, a Dopamine (D₂)-receptor antagonist, or any of the 5-HT₃-receptor antagonists identified above	Rescue with an agent not used in primary prophylaxis; e.g., Dexamethasone, a D₂-receptor antagonist, or a 5-HT₃-receptor antagonist • Continue use before each remaining RT fraction
RT + Chemotherapy	Give antiemetic prophylaxis appropriate for the chemotherapy in use unless the emetic risk of radiation is greater than that for chemotherapy	

Prophylaxis and Treatment for ANTICIPATORY SYMPTOMS

Prevention
Complete protection against emetic symptoms preempts or delays developing anticipatory symptoms

Behavior modification and relaxation techniques for prevention and treatment
Systematic desensitization, distraction, biofeedback, relaxation, guided imagery, hypnosis

Acupuncture or acupressure for prevention and treatment

Adjunctive pharmacotherapy[o]
lorazepam 0.5–2 mg PO or sublingually
• The night before and morning of single-day treatment, repeated every 6–12 h on days of emetogenic treatment; *OR*
alprazolam 0.5–2 mg PO
• The night before and morning of single-day treatment, repeated four times daily on days of emetogenic treatment

FIGURE 38.2 (Continued)

Treatment for BREAKTHROUGH SYMPTOMS associated with Emetogenic Treatment[o,p,s,z]

- Add to the current regimen a drug that is pharmacologically different from drugs already in use:

Category	Drug	Dose
Glucocorticoids	Dexamethasone	12 mg PO daily, or 12 mg IV daily[b]; OR [k]
	Methylprednisolone	125 mg IV daily
Serotonin (5-HT₃) Receptor Antagonists	Dolasetron	100 mg PO daily; OR
	Granisetron	0.01 mg/kg IV (maximum dose 1 mg) daily, or 2 mg PO daily; or 1 mg PO every 12 h, or 3.1-mg/24 h transdermal patch[t] applied topically every 7 days; OR
	Ondansetron	8–16 mg IV daily, or 0.15 mg/kg IV daily (maximum single dose ≤16 mg)[u] or 16–24 mg PO daily; OR
	Palonosetron	0.25 mg IV x1 dose, or 0.25 mg IV every second day for emetogenic treatment on multiple consecutive days
Cannabinoids	Dronabinol	5–10 mg PO every 4–6 h; OR
	Nabilone	1–2 mg PO twice daily
Benzodiazepines	Lorazepam	0.5–2 mg PO, SL, or IV, every 4–12 h; OR
	Alprazolam	0.5–2 mg PO or SL, every 6–12 h; OR
	Midazolam	0.04 mg/kg slow IV over 3–5 minutes
Dopamine Receptor Antagonists[w]	Metoclopramide	10–20 mg IV every 6 h[r], or 0.5–2 mg/kg IV every 6 h[r], or 10–20 mg PO every 6 h[r]; OR
	Haloperidol	0.5–2 mg IV every 4–6 h, or 1–5 mg PO every 4–6 h; OR
	Prochlorperazine	10–30 mg IV every 6 h, or 25 mg PR every 4–6 h, or 10 mg PO every 4–6 h; OR
	Thiethylperazine	10–20 mg IV every 6 h, or 10–20 mg PO every 4–6 h; OR
	Perphenazine	2–4 mg IV every 8 h, or 2–4 mg PO every 8 h; OR
Antimuscarinic & Histamine Receptor Antagonists	Promethazine	12.5–25 mg IV every 4–6 h, or 25 mg PR every 4–6 h, or 12.5–25 mg PO every 4–6 h; OR
	Scopolamine transdermal system[t]	1.5 mg/patch topically, (delivers 1 mg) every 72 h; OR
	Meclizine	12.5–50 mg PO every 12 h (maximum 100 mg/24 h); OR
	Dimenhydrinate	50–100 mg PO every 4–6 h (maximum 400 mg/24 h); OR
	Cyclizine	50 mg PO every 4–6 h (maximum 200 mg/24 h)
Mechanism of Action Not Categorized	Olanzapine	5–10 mg PO daily[x]

FIGURE 38.2 (Continued)

FIGURE 38.2 (Continued)

a Granisetron extended-release injection is a unique formulation of granisetron incorporated into a polymer-based drug delivery system. The formulation is administered only by SUBCUTaneous injection and is not interchangeable with granisetron formulated for intraVENous or intraMUSCular administration. Granisetron extended-release injection has an extended elimination half-life (~24 h) and should not be administered at intervals <1 wk.

b If NK_1-receptor antagonists are not given on day 1, recommend dexamethasone 20 mg either PO or IV once on day 1, followed by 8 mg twice daily either PO or IV on days 2, 3, and 4.

c Dexamethasone dose and schedule recommendations are based on those used in clinical trials or in FDA-approved product labeling; however, dexamethasone doses may be individualized: lower doses, frequency of use, and omission on the second and subsequent days after starting emetogenic treatment may be acceptable based on patient characteristics.

d NCCN Guidelines® indicate some NCCN member institutions use a $5-HT_3$-receptor antagonist on days 2, 3, and 4 in addition to a steroid and a NK_1-receptor antagonist except when palonosetron, granisetron extended-release injection, or granisetron transdermal patch were given on day 1 (Antiemesis, V.1.2017—February 22, 2017. National Comprehensive Cancer Network, Inc., 2017. Accessed March 9, 2017, at http://www.nccn.org).

e Rolapitant has an extended elimination half-life (169–183 h) and should not be administered at intervals <2 wk.

f VARUBI™ (rolapitant) tablets, for oral use; September 2015, product label. TESARO Inc., Waltham MA.

g The recommendation for dexamethasone dose and schedule is contrary to the recommendation that appears in NCCN Guidelines®. Dexamethasone bioavailability is not increased by concomitant use with rolapitant; thus, FDA approved product labeling for VARUBI™ stipulates a 20-mg dexamethasone dose on day 1 and dexamethasone 8 mg twice daily on days 2–4.

h Consider escalating to this option when emesis occurred during a previous cycle of chemotherapy using an olanzapine regimen without a NK_1-receptor antagonist or a NK_1-receptor antagonist-containing regimen without olanzapine.

i Consider decreasing the olanzapine dose to 5 mg/day for elderly or overly sedated patients.

j Available in the USA only as a fixed-dose combination product containing netupitant 300 mg and palonosetron 0.5 mg per capsule for oral administration.

k Consider administering a histamine (H_2 subtype)-receptor antagonist (other than cimetidine) OR a proton pump inhibitor concurrently with dexamethasone to mitigate gastrointestinal irritation.

l When used in combination with a NK_1-receptor antagonist, there is no preferred $5-HT_3$-receptor antagonist.

m Consider adding a NK_1-receptor antagonist to dexamethasone and a $5-HT_3$-receptor antagonist as with prophylaxis for high emetic risk regimens for select patients with additional risk factors, or those who previously experienced suboptimal emetic control with the combination of a steroid and $5-HT_3$-receptor antagonist.

n No additional primary prophylaxis is recommended if palonosetron or granisetron extended-release injection was given, or granisetron transdermal system (patch) was applied 24–48 h prior to starting emetogenic treatment.

o Antiemetic prophylaxis should be repeated each day emetogenic treatment is administered.

p Oral prophylaxis should begin one hour before commencing cytotoxic treatment. IV prophylaxis may be given minutes before emetogenic treatment.

q When ≥2 orally administered emetogenic drugs are used concomitantly, the emetic risk potential may be increased and require more aggressive prophylaxis.

r In July 2013, the European Medicines Agency's Committee on Medicinal Products for Human Use recommended changes to the use of metoclopramide-containing medicines in the European Union, including restricting the dose and duration of metoclopramide use to minimize known risks of potentially serious neurological adverse effects. For adults and children the maximum recommended dose during a 24-hour period is 0.5 mg/kg body weight; in adults, the recommended dose is 10 mg given up to three times daily (i.e., a maximum daily dose of 30 mg) by all routes of administration. References: European Medicines Agency recommends changes to the use of metoclopramide; 26 July 2013, EMA/443003/2013 and *ibid*. Changes aim mainly to reduce the risk of neurological side effects; 20 December 2013, EMA/13239/2014 Corr. 1. At: www.ema.europa.eu Last accessed 17 March 2017

[s] Medications are not listed in order of preference. Groups of pharmacologically similar alternatives are circumscribed by a broken line.

[t] Avoid using sustained-, delayed- and extended-release formulations (oral, transdermal patches, and injectable products) to establish control of ongoing symptoms.

[u] Product labeling for ondansetron hydrochloride injection approved by the U.S. FDA recommends single intravenously administered doses should not exceed 16 mg. [ZOFRAN® (ondansetron hydrochloride) injection, for intravenous or intramuscular use; March 2017 product label. GlaxoSmithKline, Research Triangle Park, NC]

[v] Dexamethasone 12 mg is the only dexamethasone dose tested in combination with aprepitant in large randomized trials.

[w] Generally, regimens containing D_2-receptor antagonists and metoclopramide doses ≥20 mg should include primary prophylaxis with anticholinergic agents against acute dystonic extrapyramidal reactions; e.g., diphenhydramine 25 – 50 mg PO or IV every 6 hours. Benztropine and trihexyphenidyl are alternatives. Parenteral administration is preferred for prompt treatment of extrapyramidal symptoms, as well as interrupting or discontinuing the drug which provoked the adverse reaction.

[x] When olanzapine is not part of antiemetic prophylaxis already in use.

[y] When administered IV, phenothiazines should be given over 30 minutes to prevent hypotension.

[z] Medications identified for breakthrough symptoms should be added to a patient's primary antiemetic prophylaxis regimen without replacing drugs used in primary prophylaxis unless drugs used to treat breakthrough symptoms duplicate mechanistically those used in primary prophylaxis or a patient has experienced unacceptable adverse effects attributable to a component of primary prophylaxis.

5-HT$_3$, serotonin receptor [5-HT$_3$ subtype], ASCO, American Society of Clinical Oncology, D$_2$, dopamine receptor [D$_2$ subtype], IM, intramuscularly, IV, intravenously, NCCN, National Comprehensive Cancer Network®, MASCC/ESMO (Multinational Association of Supportive Care in Cancer/European Society for Medical Oncology), PO (orally), PR (rectally), q: (every), RT (radiation therapy), SL (sublingually), SQ (SUBCUTaneously).

in all clinical situations. Drug selection and utilization should be tempered by professional judgment, including an assessment of patient-specific risk factors and circumstances, and recognition of available resources.

Clinicians may expect to encounter a minority of patients who do not respond to treatment-appropriate antiemetic prophylaxis recommended by oncology specialty organizations' guidelines. Suboptimal antiemetic prophylaxis places patients at risk for breakthrough and refractory emetic symptoms and debilitating morbidity, which may adversely affect patient safety, comfort, and quality of life, and complicate their care.

For patients who respond sub-optimally to initial antiemetic prophylaxis, re-evaluate factors that may cause or contribute to emetic symptoms, and those that may compromise the effectiveness of pharmacological prophylaxis, including

- The emetogenic risk associated with treatment.
  - The appropriateness of initial antiemetic prophylaxis for the emetogenic challenge presented by treatment.
    - Selection of drugs, doses/dosages, and administration routes and schedules for use.
- Healthcare provider adherence in prescribing and patient compliance in using planned antiemetic prophylaxis.
- Disease status.
- Co-morbid conditions (electrolyte abnormalities, renal failure, sepsis, constipation, tumor infiltrating or obstructing the gastrointestinal tract, intracranial disease, vestibular dysfunction).
- Whether medications concomitantly administered with emetogenic drugs and antiemetics may potentially compromise antiemetic effectiveness:
  - Using medications with intrinsic emetogenic potential unrelated to antineoplastic treatment that nevertheless increase the cumulative emetogenic burden.
  - By altering the pharmacokinetics of emetogenic drugs that result in exposures greater in magnitude or duration than would otherwise occur.
  - By altering the pharmacokinetics of agents used in antiemetic prophylaxis or treatment.

Empiric secondary prophylaxis and treatment for patients who demonstrate sub-optimal antiemetic control should follow a rational approach. In general, pharmacological interventions typically include drugs presumed to mediate antiemetic effects through an interaction with one or more neurotransmitter receptors implicated in either provoking or mitigating emesis, and through mechanisms not exploited by antiemetics already in use. Unfortunately, drugs used empirically often are less safe at effective or clinically useful doses and schedules (e.g., dopaminergic and cannabinoid receptor antagonists) than agents recommended for primary prophylaxis. Whether used adjunctively or as replacement for initial prophylaxis, second-line alternatives may increase treatment costs and the risk of overtreatment and adverse effects.

BREAKTHROUGH SYMPTOMS

Primary antiemetic prophylaxis recommended by oncology specialty organizations' guidelines are associated with complete control (no emesis) during the acute phase in ≥80% of patients who receive highly emetogenic treatments and even greater complete control rates in the setting of moderately emetogenic treatment; however, more than 50% of patients who receive moderately or highly emetogenic therapy still may experience delayed or breakthrough nausea or emesis in spite of good control achieved acutely. In general, it is more difficult to arrest emetic symptoms after they develop than it is to prevent them from occurring. Breakthrough symptoms require rapid intervention. All patients who receive moderately or highly emetogenic treatment should from the outset of treatment have access to antiemetic medications for treating breakthrough symptoms, whether through orders for treatment during a visit or admission to a healthcare facility, or, for outpatients, a supply of antiemetic medication and clear instructions about how to use it in supplementing or modifying their initial antiemetic regimen. If needed and once begun, breakthrough treatment should be administered at scheduled intervals and continued at least until after emetogenic treatment is completed and symptoms abate.

In general, nausea may still occur and often is more prevalent than vomiting in patients who achieve overall good or better control of emesis during the acute and delayed symptoms phases.

Sub-optimal Control

Sub-optimal control of emetic symptoms with antiemetic prophylaxis raises the following questions:

- Was the prophylactic strategy given an adequate trial (time of initiation relative to the start of emetogenic treatment and duration of use)?
- Were the antiemetics selected and the doses and administration schedules prescribed appropriate for the emetogenic challenge?
- Did the patient understand and comply with instructions for antiemetic use?
- Would increased doses or shorter administration intervals improve antiemetic effectiveness without causing or exacerbating adverse effects associated with the antiemetics utilized?

Rescue Interventions

If it becomes necessary to "rescue" a patient from a suboptimal response

- Assess a symptomatic patient's state of hydration and serum/plasma electrolytes for abnormal results.
  - Replace fluids and electrolytes as needed.
- Add antiemetic agents that act through mechanisms different from antiemetics already in use.
  - It may be necessary to use more than one additional drug to establish antiemetic control.
- Give scheduled doses *around-the-clock* at least until emetogenic treatment is completed, and at doses and on a schedule appropriate for the medication.
  - Do not rely on *as needed* administration to achieve or maintain control of emetic symptoms.
- Consider replacing ineffective drugs with a more potent or longer-acting agent from the same pharmacologic class.
- Consider replacing an antiemetic medication that requires ingestion and absorption from the gastrointestinal tract or percutaneous absorption with the same or a different drug given by a different administration route (disintegrating tablets and soluble films for oral administration, injectable formulations).
  - Emetic symptoms may impair GI motility and drug absorption from the gut.
  - Some patients may be too ill to swallow and retain oral medications.
  - Rectal suppositories are a practical alternative for patients who cannot ingest medications, but the rate and extent of absorption varies among drugs and patients.
    - Clinicians should query and ascertain patients' willingness to comply with rectal administration.
  - Sustained- and extended-release formulations (oral, transdermal patches, and injectable sustained- or extended-release products) should not be used to initially bring ongoing symptoms under control.
- Replace drugs associated with unacceptable adverse effects with one or more drugs from the same or a different pharmacologic class without a potential for the same toxicity, or for which particular adverse effects are less likely to occur.

These strategies may be utilized during cyclical treatment or to intervene when response to prophylaxis is unsatisfactory.

Secondary Antiemetic Prophylaxis and Treatment

When antiemetic treatment is needed for breakthrough symptoms, re-evaluate the prophylactic regimen that failed to provide adequate antiemetic control before repeating cycles of emetogenic treatment. Consider alternative antiemetic prophylaxis strategies during subsequent emetogenic treatments, including

- Consider escalating antiemetic prophylaxis to a regimen appropriate for the next greater level of emetic risk.
- Add additional scheduled antiemetics at appropriate doses and administration intervals.
  - Consider drugs that previously proved of value in controlling breakthrough symptoms or another drug that acts through the same pharmacological mechanism.
- For regimens that included a 5-HT$_3$ antagonist, consider switching to a different 5-HT$_3$ antagonist.
  - Not all patients achieve the same measure of antiemetic control with every 5-HT$_3$ antagonist.
- Consider adding an anxiolytic drug to the patient's regimen.
- Consider adding a NK$_1$-receptor antagonist to antiemetic prophylaxis if its potential for pharmacokinetic interactions will not adversely affect concomitantly administered medications.
- If alternative treatment for a patient's neoplastic disease exists, consider a different regimen with which similar therapeutic benefit may be achieved without greater adverse outcomes.
  - Perhaps worth considering only if the goal of treatment is not curative.

NON-PHARMACOLOGICAL INTERVENTIONS

- Guidance for patients that may preserve nutritional status and alleviate emetic symptoms, include
  - Eat small frequent meals low in fat content, especially for patients with anorexia or early satiety.
  - Choose healthful foods.
  - Eat soft, bland, easily digested foods served at room temperature.
    - Eat dry foods; for example, crackers, toasted bread, and dry cereals.
    - Avoid foods and beverages known or found to produce nausea.
    - Advise patients to avoid favorite foods to prevent developing conditioned aversions to those foods, particularly at times when emetic symptoms are anticipated to occur.
    - Avoid sweet, fatty, highly salted and spicy foods, dairy products, and foods with strong odors.
  - For patients who are nauseated by the smell of food:
    - Let someone else do the cooking. Leave areas when and where cooking smells are present.
    - Avoid foods and beverages that provoke nausea.
      - Patients may experience sensitivities to food odors, appearance, taste, textures ("mouth feel").
      - Greasy and fried foods and brewing coffee may provoke symptoms.
    - Suggest prepared foods that can be warmed at a low temperature or a meal that does not need to be cooked.
- Acupressure or acupuncture
  - Stimulation of the ventral side of the wrist where the median nerve is closest to the surface of the skin, an acupuncture point referred to as pericardium-6 (P-6) or Neiguan point may be of benefit in some patients.

ANTIEMETIC DRUGS

Serotonin (5-HT$_3$ subtype)-Receptor Antagonists

- Among 5-HT$_3$-receptor antagonists that have received FDA approval for commercial use, dolasetron, granisetron, and ondansetron comprise the first-generation agent, palonosetron is a second-generation agent.

Acute Phase

- 5-HT$_3$-receptor antagonists are safer and more effective against acute-phase symptoms than other pharmacological classes of medications with clinically useful antiemetic activity.
- Administering 5-HT$_3$-receptor antagonists at doses/dosages greater than those shown to be maximally effective do not substantially improve emetic control.

■ Single-dose prophylaxis is preferred for acute-phase symptoms.
  ● After administration of a single maximally effective dose, additional doses of 5-HT$_3$-receptor antagonists within the first 24 hours after emetogenic treatment have not been shown to improve emetic control.
■ Dolasetron, granisetron, ondansetron, and palonosetron have excellent oral bioavailability, and, when given at maximally effective doses, each agent provides equivalent antiemetic protection whether given orally or parenterally.

Delayed Phase

■ Metoclopramide and prochlorperazine are less expensive, and as effective as dolasetron, granisetron, and ondansetron at controlling emetic symptoms.
■ Palonosetron has the longest half-life among 5-HT$_3$-receptor antagonists currently marketed in the USA, and has additional pharmacological characteristics not shared by first-generation 5-HT$_3$-receptor antagonists.
  ● A single dose of palonosetron 0.5 mg orally, or 0.25 mg intravenously, is recommended before starting chemotherapy, but other doses and schedules have proven safe (see below).

Potential Side Effects

■ Side effects common to all 5-HT$_3$-receptor antagonists include
  ● Headache
  ● Constipation
  ● Diarrhea
  ● Transiently increased hepatic transaminase concentrations
  ● Transient effects on cardiac electrophysiology, decreased cardiac rate, and cardiovascular adverse effects (see drug-specific comments below)
  ● Serotonin syndrome, most often associated with concomitant use of drugs that affect serotonin neurotransmission and/or reuptake

5-HT3-Receptor Antagonists and Pharmacogenomics

■ Pharmacogenomic evaluation may help to identify patients at risk for sub-optimal and adverse responses to 5-HT$_3$-receptor antagonists that are substrates for catabolism by cytochrome P450 (CYP) enzymes (Table 38.4).
■ CYP2D6 is polymorphically expressed among human populations.
  ● Persons with >2 functionally competent (wild type) *CYP2D6* alleles may have increased metabolic capacity (characterized as ultra-rapid metabolizers), which has been associated with diminished emetic control in patients who received 5-HT$_3$-receptor antagonists for which CYP2D6 metabolism predominates.
  ● Patients who lack one or both *CYP2D6* alleles or express one or more variant alleles with reduced function generally have altered functional capacity for CYP2D6 substrates (poor and intermediate metabolizers) and may have high concentrations and attenuated elimination of 5-HT$_3$-receptor antagonist substrates for which CYP2D6 metabolism predominates.
■ Patients who express genetic polymorphism for 5-HT$_3$ receptors or the ABCB1 (P-glycoprotein, MDR1) transporter may experience suboptimal antiemetic responses with 5-HT$_3$-receptor antagonists.

Dolasetron

■ The oral tablet formulation is approved for use in antiemetic prophylaxis in initial and repeat courses of moderately emetogenic chemotherapy in patients ≥2 years of age.
■ The frequency and magnitude of adverse effects associated with dolasetron use are related to serum concentrations of hydrodolasetron, its active metabolite.

TABLE 38.4 Catabolism of 5-HT$_3$-receptor antagonists by cytochrome P450 (CYP) enzymes.

5-HT$_3$-receptor antagonists	Catalysts for metabolism	Metabolites (activity vs. parent drug)
Dolasetron	Stereoselectively by carbonyl reductase	Reduction to hydrodolasetron (~50-times more active than dolasetron)
Hydrodolasetron	Primarily CYP2D6, also CYP3A subfamily and flavin monooxygenase	Hydroxylation (inactive)
Granisetron	Primarily CYP3A subfamily. Also, CYP1A1	Oxidation, then conjugation (inactive)
Ondansetron	Primarily CYP3A4. Also, CYP2D6 and CYP1A2	Hydroxylation, then conjugation (inactive)
Palonosetron	Primarily CYP2D6, also CYP3A4 and CYP1A2	N-oxide-palonosetron (<1% parent drug activity), 6-S-hydroxypalonosetron (<1% parent drug activity)

- On December 17, 2010, the U.S. FDA announced the removal of the indication for dolasetron mesylate injection for preventing nausea and vomiting associated with initial and repeated courses of emetogenic chemotherapy, and the addition to product labeling of a contraindication against this use in pediatric and adult patients. The FDA Communication explained dolasetron mesylate causes a dose-dependent prolongation in cardiac QT, PR, and QRS intervals that can increase the risk of developing torsade de pointes, which may be fatal [FDA Drug Safety Communication: Abnormal heart rhythms associated with the use of Anzemet (dolasetron mesylate). URL: https://www.fda.gov/drugs/drugsafety/ucm237081.htm [Accessed 4 December 2017].
- Risk factors for serious abnormal arrhythmias include
  - Underlying structural heart disease and preexisting conduction system abnormalities; for example, patients with congenital long-QT syndrome, complete heart block, or those at risk for complete heart block
  - Elderly individuals
  - Sick sinus syndrome, atrial fibrillation with slow ventricular response, myocardial ischemia, persons receiving drugs known to prolong the PR interval (e.g., verapamil) and QRS interval (e.g., flecainide, quinidine)
  - Hypokalemia or hypomagnesemia
    - Serum potassium and magnesium concentrations should be evaluated, and, if abnormal, corrected before initiating treatment with dolasetron.
    - Potassium and magnesium concentrations should be monitored after dolasetron administration as clinically indicated.
    - Patients at risk for developing hypokalemia or hypomagnesemia while receiving dolasetron should be monitored with ECG.
- The FDA also recommended ECG monitoring in patients with congestive heart failure, bradycardia, underlying heart disease, and in the elderly and patients with renal impairment who receive dolasetron.
- Dolasetron mesylate tablets may still be used in antiemetic prophylaxis for emetogenic chemotherapy, because the risk of developing aberrant cardiac conduction with the oral formulation is considered less than what has been observed with the dolasetron injection.
- Dolasetron mesylate injection also retained FDA approval for the prevention and treatment of postoperative nausea and vomiting patients whose age is ≥2 y, because dosages for that indication

(intravenously, a single dose of 0.35 mg/kg up to a maximum of 12.5 mg/dose) are less than those used in antiemetic prophylaxis for chemotherapy (1.8 mg/kg·dose up to a maximum of 100 mg/dose), and therefore, are less likely to adversely affect cardiac electrophysiology.

Granisetron

▪ Indicated for use in antiemetic prophylaxis in initial and repeated courses of emetogenic cancer therapies, including high-dose cisplatin and radiation therapy.
  • Granisetron Injection has received FDA approval for use in patients ≥2 years of age.
    • Injectable products may contain benzyl alcohol, which has been associated with serious adverse reactions, including death in neonates.
      • Injectable formulations without preservatives are currently marketed.
  • Oral formulations (tablets and solution) have not received FDA approval for use in pediatric patients.
    • Product labeling for granisetron tablets and solution for oral administration include descriptions of use in patients 2–16 years of age, but, in contrast with labeling for injectable formulations, stipulate safety and effectiveness in pediatric patients have not been established.
▪ Granisetron transdermal patch (Sancuso®; Kyowa Kirin, Inc., Bedminster, NJ), an adhesive-backed patch (52 cm²), contains 34.3 mg of granisetron and delivers an average daily dose of 3.1 mg granisetron for up to 7 days.
  • The patch is indicated for the prevention of nausea and vomiting in patients receiving moderately and/or highly emetogenic chemotherapy regimens of up to 5 consecutive days duration.
    • Safety and effectiveness in pediatric patients have not been established.
  • A patch is applied to clean, dry, intact skin on the outer upper arm a minimum of 24 hours (up to 48 hours) before emetogenic chemotherapy administration and remains in place ≥24 hours after chemotherapy is completed.
  • The duration of application should not exceed 7 days.
    • Patches should not be cut into pieces.
    • Patches should not be reapplied or reused after being removed from an application site.
  • During clinical development, patients who received granisetron 3.1 mg/day transdermally for up to 7 days experienced a comparatively greater incidence of constipation than patients who received granisetron 2 mg/day orally for 1–5 days (5.4% vs. 3%, respectively) and a lesser incidence of headache (0.7% vs. 3%, respectively).
    • Continuous transdermal administration of granisetron may increase the potential for 5-HT₃-receptor antagonists to mask progressive ileus and gastric distention attributable to malignancy or another pathology.
  • Granisetron may degrade with exposure to natural or artificial sunlight (e.g., sun lamps, tanning beds), and results of an in vitro study suggested a potential for photogenotoxicity. Patients must be instructed to keep the transdermal patch covered with clothing at all times, and to keep the application site protected from light exposure for 10 days after a patch is removed.
  • Application of a heating pad (average temperature 42°C [107.6°]) over a granisetron transdermal patch for four hours daily during five consecutive days of wear resulted in increased concentrations of granisetron in plasma during the period when heat was applied. Heating pads and other heat sources should not be applied over or near a site where a granisetron transdermal patch is applied.
  • Adverse effects unique to the product and associated with the route of administration, such as
    • Skin reactions at or around the site of patch application, including the following:
      • Patch non-adhesion
      • Erythema
      • Irritation, pain
      • Hypersensitivity reactions (erythematous macular or papular rashes, pruritis, urticaria)
      • Vesicle formation, burn
▪ Granisetron extended-release injection for subcutaneous use (SUSTOL®; Heron Therapeutics, Redwood City, CA). Each prefilled syringe contains 10 mg granisetron incorporated in an extended-release polymer vehicle comprising one dose.

- Indicated in combination with other antiemetics for prophylaxis against acute and delayed emetic symptoms during initial and repeated courses of moderately emetogenic cancer therapies or anthracycline + cyclophosphamide-containing regimens.
- Each subcutaneously administered dose continuously delivers granisetron for an extended period of time.
  - Measurable granisetron levels can be detected in serum for up to seven days after administration.
  - Safety and effectiveness in patients <18 years of age have not been established.
  - Preparation and administration
    - SUSTOL® is intended ONLY for subcutaneous injection administered by a health care provider.
    - The product is supplied as a kit stored under refrigeration (2°–8°C [35.6°–46.4°F]) and protected from light.
    - Each kit contains a single-use, amber, glass syringe pre-filled with the granisetron/polymer matrix product, a special thin-walled administration needle, two pouches for warming the syringe, and a needle protection device.
- None of the kit components should be substituted with other materials or devices.
  - Preparation for use entails:
  - Kit removal from refrigeration at least 60 minutes before administration.
  - Warming the kit contents to room temperature.
  - Activating a syringe warming pouch and wrapping the syringe pre-filled with medication in the pouch for 5–6 minutes.
  - After warming the product syringe to body temperature, the drug is administered as a single subcutaneous injection in the skin of the back of the upper arm or the abdomen at least one inch from the umbilicus, avoiding sites where skin is burned, hardened, inflamed, swollen, or otherwise compromised.
  - A topical anesthetic may be used at the injection site prior to administration.
  - The drug product is a viscous liquid and should be administered subcutaneously, slowly by sustained pressure over 20 to 30 seconds.
- Health care providers are advised depressing the syringe plunger forcefully will NOT hasten administration.
  - Initial and repeated administration is constrained by renal function:
    - Not more frequently than every 7 days in patients whose creatinine clearance (Clcr) is ≥60 mL/min (≥1 mL/s)
    - Not more frequently than every 14 days in patients with Clcr = 30 to 59 mL/min (0.5–0.98 mL/s)
    - AVOID use in patients with Clcr <30 mL/min (<0.5 mL/s)
- Adverse effects unique to the product and associated with the route of administration, include
  - Infections at the injection site.
  - Bleeding at the injection site.
  - Bruising/hematomas at the injection site with median onset of 2 days; delayed onset ≥5 days in 15% of patients.
  - Pain and tenderness at the injection site with median duration of 5 days, but persisting for >7 days in 6% of patients.
  - Nodule formation at the injection site that may persist for >3 weeks after administration.
- ECG abnormalities are rare with granisetron use at FDA-approved dosages and schedules.

Ondansetron

- Used in antiemetic prophylaxis in initial and repeat courses of emetogenic cancer therapies:
  - Ondansetron injection has received FDA approval for use in patients ≥6 months of age for the prevention of emetic symptoms associated with highly emetogenic chemotherapy.
  - Oral formulations (tablets, orally disintegrating tablets, film, and solution) have received FDA approval for use in patients ≥4 years of age receiving moderately emetogenic chemotherapy.

- The safety and effectiveness of ondansetron formulations for oral administration have not received FDA approval for use in pediatric patients for the prevention of emetic symptoms associated with highly emetogenic cancer chemotherapy or radiation therapy.
- The risk of adverse effects is low at FDA-approved dosages and schedules.
  - The risk of ECG abnormalities associated with use has been shown to vary directly with the dose administered.
- On June 29 2012, the FDA announced preliminary results from a clinical study conducted by GlaxoSmithKline showed ondansetron prolongs the cardiac QT interval in a dose-dependent manner, which could pre-dispose patients to develop an abnormal and potentially fatal ventricular tachyarrhythmia known as torsades de pointes [FDA Drug Safety Communication: New information regarding QT prolongation with ondansetron (Zofran) at https://www.fda.gov/drugs/drugsafety/ucm310190.htm Last accessed 4 December 2017].
  - Risk factors for developing QT prolongation with ondansetron include the following:
    - Underlying heart conditions, such as congenital long QT syndrome, congestive heart failure, or bradyarrhythmias
    - Hypokalemia and hypomagnesemia
    - Concomitant use of medications that also are associated with QT prolongation
  - A comparison between single intravenous doses of ondansetron 32 mg and 8 mg revealed the maximum mean difference in QTcF (the QT interval measurement corrected by the Fridericia formula) from placebo after baseline-correction was 20 msec and 6 msec, respectively.
  - Consequently, product labeling was amended to state ondansetron 0.15 mg/kg administered intravenously over 15 minutes every 4 hours for three doses may continue to be used in adults and children with chemotherapy-induced nausea and vomiting, but no single intravenous dose should exceed 16 mg.
    - Ondansetron product labeling includes warnings against using the drug in patients with congenital long QT syndrome and recommends ECG monitoring in patients with uncorrected electrolyte abnormalities such as hypokalemia or hypomagnesemia, congestive heart failure, bradyarrhythmias, and in patients concomitantly using other medications that can prolong the QT interval.
    - Patients should be advised to contact a healthcare professional immediately if they experience signs and symptoms of an abnormal heart rate or rhythm while they are taking ondansetron.
  - Recommendations for a single, oral, 24-mg ondansetron dose in prophylaxis against chemotherapy-induced nausea and vomiting were not affected.

Palonosetron

- Palonosetron is a second-generation 5-HT$_3$-receptor antagonist with a substantially longer elimination half-life (approximately 40 hours) than dolasetron, granisetron, or ondansetron, and additional characteristics that, in contrast with first-generation 5-HT$_3$-receptor antagonists, suggest pharmacological advantages, including
  - Allosteric binding that produces a conformational change in 5-HT$_3$ receptors with increased binding affinity between the receptor and palonosetron, which may be the result of at least one more molecule binding to the same receptor (suggests positive cooperativity).
    - In contrast, granisetron and ondansetron exhibit simple competitive binding with 5-HT$_3$ receptors.
  - Binding to 5-HT$_3$-receptor that results in receptor internalization, and, consequently, a persistent inhibition of receptor function.
  - Evidence indicating palonosetron bound to internalized NK$_1$-receptors diminishes signalling (crosstalk) between NK$_1$ and substance P receptors.
- Palonostron is currently available as an injectable product, and in a product for oral administration formulated in combination with the NK$_1$-receptor antagonist, netupitant.
  - Palonosetron injection received FDA approval for use in adult patients in antiemetic prophylaxis for
    - Acute and delayed nausea and vomiting in initial and repeat courses of moderately emetogenic chemotherapy.

- Acute nausea and vomiting in initial and repeat courses of highly emetogenic chemotherapy.
- Palonosetron injection also received FDA approval for use in pediatric patients from 1 month to 17 years of age in antiemetic prophylaxis for initial and repeat courses of emetogenic chemotherapy including highly emetogenic chemotherapy.
- Palonosetron is one among 5-HT$_3$-receptor antagonists, or the only drug preferentially recommended for antiemetic prophylaxis by the following:
  - National Comprehensive Cancer Network® guidelines for patients who receive moderately emetogenic intravenously administered chemotherapy without concomitant use of a NK$_1$-receptor antagonist antiemetic
  - Multinational Association of Supportive Care in Cancer/European Society for Medical Oncology guidelines for patients treated with chemotherapy regimens containing an anthracycline and cyclophosphamide (an "AC" regimen) when a NK$_1$-receptor antagonist cannot be used in combination with dexamethasone and a 5-HT$_3$-receptor antagonist.
- There is a low risk of adverse effects at dosages and schedules currently approved by the U.S. Food and Drug Administration.
  - The risk of ECG abnormalities associated with palonosetron use, including QTc prolongation, has been shown less than that associated with dolasetron and ondansetron.
    - FDA-approved product labeling indicates single doses of palonosetron 0.25, 0.75, or 2.25 mg in 221 healthy adult men and women in a double blind, randomized, parallel, placebo, and positive (moxifloxacin) controlled trial demonstrated no significant effect on any ECG interval including QTc interval duration.
  - Product labeling for palonosetron injection indicates a single dose before starting chemotherapy, but safety has been demonstrated with other doses and schedules:
    - 10 mcg/kg single dose (healthy subjects)
    - 0.75 mg single dose before chemotherapy
    - 0.25 mg/dose every second day for 3 doses with dexamethasone before chemotherapy
    - 0.25 mg/day for 3 consecutive days (healthy subjects)
    - 0.25 mg/day for 1, 2, or 3 consecutive days (prior to high-dose chemotherapy)
      - No differences were observed in control of vomiting over a 7-day evaluation period among patients who received 1, 2, or 3 doses.
      - Only about 8% of patients who received one dose and about 20% of patients who received two or three doses were without emesis and did not receive rescue medications.
    - Palonosetron 0.25 mg IV followed at least 72 h after the initial dose by a second 0.25 mg dose for breakthrough symptoms was effective in 67% of patients who experienced nausea or vomiting.

Neurokinin (NK$_1$ Subtype)-Receptor Antagonists

- NK$_1$-receptor antagonists have demonstrated activity against acute phase emetic symptoms, but are more effective against delayed phase emesis than other pharmacological classes of antiemetics currently available.
- International guidelines recommend using a 5-HT$_3$-receptor antagonist, dexamethasone, and a NK$_1$-receptor antagonist in antiemetic primary prophylaxis for patients receiving highly emetogenic and high-dose chemotherapy regimens, and as an option for moderately emetogenic chemotherapy.
- Currently, three NK$_1$-receptor antagonists in formulations for oral administration have received FDA approval for commercial use in the USA, including aprepitant, rolapitant, and netupitant. Fosaprepitant dimeglumine is a pro-drug for aprepitant formulated for intravenous administration.
- Safe use of NK$_1$-receptor antagonists with other medications prudently requires health care providers to recognize the potential for drug-drug interactions during concomitant use.
  - Table 38.5 identifies pharmacokinetic characteristics that become important when NK$_1$-receptor antagonists are used concomitantly with other medications.

TABLE 38.5 Selected Pharmacokinetic Characteristics for NK$_1$-Receptor Antagonists

Drug	Half-life[a]	Plasma protein binding	Metabolic Catalysts Substrate for	Inhibits	Induces	Transporters Substrate for	Inhibits	Induces
Aprepitant	9–13 h	95%	CYP3A4 > CYP1A2 & CYP2C19	CYP3A4, weakly (40-mg dose) to moderately (125/80-mg doses)	CYP3A4, CYP2C9 (moderately)	P-gp (unlikely to interact with other P-gp substrates)		
Fosaprepitant dimeglumine	approximately 11 h (for aprepitant)			CYP3A4, weakly	—[b]			
Rolapitant	169–183 h	99.8%	CYP3A4	CYP2D6, moderately (may persist for ≥7 days after a single dose)			BCRP P-gp	
M19 (active C4-pyrrolidine-hydroxylated rolapitant)	158 h							
Netupitant (formulated with palonosetron)	80 ±29 h	>99.5%	CYP3A4 > CYP2C9 & CYP2D6	CYP3A4, moderately[c,d]			BCRP[c] P-gp[c]	
Netupitant active metabolites: M1 (N-demethyl netupitant) M2 (netupitant N-oxide) M3 (monohydroxy netupitant)		>97% (concentrations 100–2000 ng/mL)		CYP3A4[c]		P-gp		

Abbreviations: BCRP, Breast Cancer Resistance Protein efflux transporter (ABCG2, MXR1); CYP. . . , prefix designating a cytochrome P450 enzyme superfamily; P-gp, P-glycoprotein efflux transporter (ABCB1, MDR1).

[a] Mean terminal half-life, except were noted.

[b] Fosaprepitant 150 mg given as a single dose weakly inhibits CYP3A4, an effect that persists for two days after administration. Unlike CYP enzyme inhibition, induction is a result of repeated or continual exposure to an inducing stimulus. Thus, a single dose of fosaprepitant does not induce CYP3A4 as does aprepitant, when the latter is given repeatedly for 3–5 days.

[c] Based on in vitro observations.

[d] Based on in vivo observations.

Aprepitant and Fosaprepitant

- Aprepitant is currently FDA approved for use in preventing acute and delayed nausea and vomiting associated with initial and repeat courses of moderately or highly emetogenic cancer chemotherapy in patients ≥6 months of age (≥6 kg).
- Commercially available products for oral administration include the following:
  - Aprepitant capsules for patients ≥12 years of age.
  - Aprepitant liquid (suspension) for patients ≥6 months of age (≥6 kg) who are not able to swallow capsules.
  - Fosaprepitant for injection (lyophilized powder): safety and effectiveness is not established in pediatric patients.
- Approval was based on studies with emetogenic chemotherapy given on a single day.
  - Aprepitant and fosaprepitant utilization in prophylaxis for emetogenic chemotherapy given on a single day (Day 1)[a]:

Regimen	Day 1	Days 2 and 3[b]
Oral only	Aprepitant 125 mg orally, 1 hour before starting chemotherapy	Aprepitant 80 mg/day orally in the morning for 2 days[b]
IV only	Fosaprepitant 150 mg intravenously, 30 min before starting chemotherapy	No additional doses

[a] Use with multiple-day chemotherapy regimens and daily use for >5 consecutive days has not been adequately studied.

[b] Aprepitant has been safely given for up to 5 days: an initial dose of 125 mg orally (day 1), followed by doses of 80 mg orally given daily for 4 consecutive days (days 2–5). Evidence in support of safety and effectiveness for longer durations of use (up to 12 days) is limited.

- Potential drug interactions with aprepitant and fosaprepitant
  - Both aprepitant and fosaprepitant share the liability of potential interactions with concomitantly administered medications
    - Aprepitant is a substrate and moderate inhibitor of the cytochrome P450 (CYP) enzyme CYP3A4, and a moderate inducer of CYP3A4 and CYP2C9. Inhibition may occur after a single dose; induction occurs after repeated doses.
    - Aprepitant inhibits CYP3A4 in the gut and liver.
    - The potential for interaction with many CYP3A4 substrates is unknown.
- Aprepitant increases the bioavailability of concomitantly administered dexamethasone and methylprednisolone.
  - When either dexamethasone or methylprednisolone is used in combination with aprepitant 125- or 80-mg doses for antiemetic prophylaxis, decrease orally administered glucocorticoid doses by 50% and intravenously administered glucocorticoid doses by 25%.
  - Do not modify the doses of steroids used as components of a chemotherapy regimen.
- Aprepitant metabolism and elimination may be adversely affected by drugs that inhibit or induce CYP3A4.
  - Common side effects of aprepitant in combination with a 5-HT$_3$-receptor antagonist and high-potency glucocorticoids include the following:
    - Abdominal pain, epigastric discomfort
    - Dyspepsia
    - Hiccups
    - Anorexia
    - Dizziness
    - Fatigue, asthenia

Netupitant

- Netupitant received FDA approval for commercial use, but only in combination with palonosetron in a product formulated for oral administration with a fixed strength ratio of netupitant 300 mg with

0.5 mg palonosetron (AKYNZEO® capsules; Distributed and marketed by Eisai Inc., Woodcliff Lake, NJ, under license of Helsinn Healthcare SA, Switzerland).
- AKYNZEO® is indicated for the prevention of acute and delayed nausea and vomiting associated with initial and repeat courses of cancer chemotherapy, including, but not limited to, highly emetogenic chemotherapy.
▪ Recommendations for AKYNZEO® (netupitant with palonosetron) use in antiemetic primary prophylaxis with emetogenic chemotherapy given on a single day (Day 1) for patients ≥18 years of age:

Day 1	Days 2–4
Highly emetogenic chemotherapy: AKYNZEO® one capsule orally, approximately 1 h before starting chemotherapy, *plus* Dexamethasone 12 mg orally, 30 min before starting chemotherapy	Dexamethasone 8 mg orally, once daily for 4 consecutive days
Chemotherapy not considered highly emetogenic, including anthracyclines and cyclophosphamide-based chemotherapies: AKYNZEO® one capsule orally, approximately 1 h before starting chemotherapy, *plus* Dexamethasone 12 mg orally, 30 min before starting chemotherapy	No additional prophylaxis necessary

▪ Potential drug interactions with netupitant
  - Netupitant is a substrate for metabolism and a moderate inhibitor of CYP3A4.
    - Avoid concomitant use of CYP3A4 substrates for one week, if feasible. If concomitant use of CYP3A4 substrates during 7 days after Akynzeo® use is not avoidable, consider reducing the doses of CYP3A4 substrates.
    - The potential for interaction with many CYP3A4 substrates is unknown.
    - Netupitant increases the bioavailability of concomitantly administered dexamethasone.
      - Dexamethasone doses should be decreased when used in combination with netupitant for antiemetic prophylaxis.
      - Do not modify the doses of steroids used as components of a chemotherapy regimen.
▪ Adverse reactions associated with the use of netupitant-plus-palonosetron fixed combination product:
  - Headache
  - Asthenia
  - Fatigue
  - Dyspepsia
  - Constipation

Rolapitant

▪ Rolapitant is indicated for use in patients ages ≥18 years in prevention against acute and delayed nausea and vomiting associated with initial and repeat courses of cancer chemotherapy, including, but not limited to, highly emetogenic chemotherapy.
▪ Rolapitant is administered orally, one-to-two hours before emetogenic chemotherapy.
▪ Adverse reactions associated with the use of rolapitant in combination with dexamethasone and a 5-HT$_3$-receptor antagonist as antiemetic prophylaxis for highly or moderately emetogenic chemotherapy regimens, include:
  - Fatigue
  - Constipation
  - Headache
  - Hiccups

- Abdominal pain
- Dizziness
- Dyspepsia
■ Potential drug interactions with rolapitant:
  - There is no drug interaction between rolapitant and dexamethasone. No dose adjustment for dexamethasone is required when used concomitantly with rolapitant.
  - After a single dose or rolapitant CYP2D6 inhibition lasts at least 7 days and may last longer.
    - Avoid concomitant use of rolapitant and pimozide (CYP2D6 substrate). The resulting increase in concentrations of pimozide in plasma may result in QT/QTc prolongation.
    - Monitor for adverse reactions if rolapitant use concomitant with other CYP2D6 substrates with a low or narrow therapeutic index cannot be avoided.
    - Rolapitant had no significant effects on the pharmacokinetics of ondansetron, a CYP2D6 substrate.
  - Rolapitant inhibits intracellular efflux transport of substrates for efflux transport by the Breast Cancer Resistance Protein (BCRP, ABCG2, MXR1) transport.
    - Be wary of concomitant use of rolapitant and BCRP substrates that have a low or narrow therapeutic index (e.g., daunorubicin, doxorubicin, epirubicin, irinotecan, methotrexate, mitoxantrone, rosuvastatin, topotecan).
    - Monitor for adverse reactions related to BCRP substrates if concomitant use with rolapitant cannot be avoided.
    - Use the lowest effective dose of rosuvastatin if it is used concomitantly with rolapitant.
  - Rolapitant inhibits intracellular efflux transport of P-glycoprotein (P-gp, MDR1, ABCB1) substrates.
    - Monitor for adverse reactions related to P-gp substrates if concomitant use with rolapitant cannot be avoided.

Glucocorticoids

■ High-potency glucocorticoids such as dexamethasone and methylprednisolone are effective as single agents against mild to moderate acute-phase symptoms.
■ Dexamethasone and methylprednisolone are active against both acute- and delayed-phase symptoms.
  - At clinically useful doses, dexamethasone and methylprednisolone are equally effective after either intravenous or oral administration.
  - Both dexamethasone and methylprednisolone enhance the antiemetic effectiveness of 5-HT$_3$ and NK$_1$-receptor antagonists when used concomitantly.
■ Prophylaxis and treatment are empirically based; safety and efficacy comparisons are lacking.
■ In antiemetic prophylaxis for emetogenic treatment given on a single day, single doses of dexamethasone and methylprednisolone are as effective as multiple-dose schedules.
  - Optimal dosages and schedules have not been determined, but there is no evidence that single doses of dexamethasone >20 mg improves antiemetic response.
■ Potential for adverse effects after a single dose is generally low and limited to GI upset and activating psychogenic effects such as anxiety, insomnia, and sleep disturbances.
  - Co-administration with drugs that decrease gastric acid production (histamine H$_2$-receptor antagonists or proton pump inhibitors) is recommended to prevent GI irritation.
  - Administering steroids early in a patient's waking cycle may minimize adverse effects on sleep.
■ Adrenocortical suppression is generally not a problem when high-potency glucocorticoids are used for brief periods.
■ Glycemic control may be a problem in patients with incipient or frank diabetes.

Dopamine (D$_2$ subtype)-Receptor Antagonists

■ Optimal doses and schedules have not been established.
■ Overall, antiemetic activity varies directly with D$_2$-receptor antagonism.
■ Adverse effects correlate with dose and frequency of administration, and include the following:
  - Sedation
  - Extrapyramidal reactions (dystonias, akathisia, dyskinesia)
  - Anticholinergic effects
  - ECG changes (haloperidol, droperidol)

- Hypotension with rapid intravenous administration (phenothiazines)
▪ Anecdotal evidence supports the use of D_2-receptor antagonists with 5-HT$_3$ antagonists ± steroids for acute-phase symptoms, and with steroids, metoclopramide, or lorazepam for delayed-phase symptoms.

Metoclopramide

▪ Metoclopramide has affinity for several neurotransmitter receptors associated with antiemetic activity, but is often categorized among D_2-receptor antagonists, and, at high doses, becomes a competitive antagonist at vagal and central 5-HT$_3$ receptors.
▪ Activity against delayed-phase symptoms is equivalent to that of ondansetron.
▪ Gastrointestinal prokinetic effects may benefit patients with intercurrent GI motility disorders or gastroesophageal reflux disease.
▪ Long-term use has been associated with developing dyskinesias, tardive dyskinesia may be irreversible.

Benzodiazepines

▪ Benzodiazepines are important adjuncts to antiemetics for their anxiolytic and anterograde amnestic effects.
  - Irrespective of its cause, anxiety may be a factor in developing or exacerbating emetic symptoms prior, during, and after completing emetogenic treatments.
  - Benzodiazepines are clinically useful for mitigating akathisias associated with D_2-receptor antagonists.
▪ Available products:
  - Lorazepam, midazolam, diazepam are available in oral and injectable formulations.
  - Alprazolam is available in solid formulations for oral administration.
    - Lorazepam and alprazolam tablets are rapidly absorbed after sublingual administration.
▪ Primary liability is dose-related sedation.
▪ Pharmacodynamic effects are exaggerated in elderly patients.

Cannabinoids

▪ Commercially available cannabinoids are agonists at endocannabinoid (CB$_1$ subtype) receptors.
  - Dronabinol is an oral formulation of Δ^9-tetrahydrocannabinol (Δ^9-THC) with antiemetic activity similar to low doses of prochlorperazine.
  - Nabilone is a synthetic CB$_1$-receptor agonist formulated for oral administration.
  - Both dronabinol and nabilone are controlled substances (Schedule II) in the United States
▪ Antiemetic benefit may be achieved without producing psychotropic effects. Cannabinoid use is empiric since optimal doses and administration schedules have not been determined.
▪ The incidence of adverse effects associated with dronabinol and nabilone is greater than with phenothiazines at doses and schedules that produce comparable antiemetic effects.
▪ Adverse effects occur within the range of clinically useful doses; incidence and severity vary with dose and correlate inversely with the interval between successive doses. Potential adverse effects include the following:
  - Sedation
  - Confusion/decreased cognition
  - Dizziness
  - Short-term memory loss
  - Euphoria/dysphoria
  - Ataxia
  - Dry mouth
  - Orthostatic hypotension ± increased heart rate

Anticholinergic (Antimuscarinic) Agents and Histamine (H$_1$)-Receptor Antagonists

▪ Utility in preventing and treating emetic symptoms is not defined.
▪ Anticholinergics may be most effective in prophylaxis; less effective after emetic symptoms develop.

- Anticholinergics are useful in prophylaxis and treatment for patients whose emetic symptoms are referable to movement.
- Individual agents have in different proportions affinities for histaminic and cholinergic neuronal receptors, and, in some cases, agonistic and antagonistic activities at adrenergic, dopaminergic, and other neuroreceptors.
- Adverse effects correlate directly with dose and frequency of administration, and include the following:
  - Sedation
  - Dry mouth
  - Loss of visual accommodation/blurred vision
  - Deceased GI motility with constipation or diarrhea
  - Urinary retention or frequency
  - Mydriasis ± photophobia
  - Increased heart rate

Olanzapine

- Olanzapine, an atypical neuroleptic or antipsychotic, is a potent antagonist at multiple neurotransmitter receptors, including muscarinic ($m_1 > m_{2-4}$), serotonergic ($5\text{-}HT_{2A}$, $5\text{-}HT_{2C}$, $5\text{-}HT_3$, $5\text{-}HT_6$), alpha adrenergic (α_1), dopaminergic (D_1, D_2, D_4), and histaminergic receptors (H_1).
- Olanzapine 10 mg/day orally for four consecutive days or placebo in combination with dexamethasone, aprepitant or fosaprepitant, and a $5\text{-}HT_3$-receptor antagonist demonstrated significantly better control of nausea than the comparator arm during the acute, delayed, and overall (0–120 h) periods after treatment-naïve patients' initial cycle of cisplatin ≥70 mg/m^2 ± other antineoplastics or cyclophosphamide 600 mg/m^2 + doxorubicin 60 mg/m^2 regimens.
  - Olanzapine is a substrate for direct glucuronidation catalyzed by uridine diphosphate glucuronosyltransferase (UGT) enzymes, UGT1A4 and UGT2B10, and for oxidation catalyzed primarily by CYP1A2 and flavin-containing monooxygenase-3, and to a lesser extent by CYP2D6 and CYP3A4.
    - Olanzapine's pharmacokinetic behavior is susceptible to drugs and substances that induce and inhibit CYP1A2 (e.g., carbamazepine, fluvoxamine, tobacco)
  - Olanzapine is a substrate with moderate affinity for P-glycoprotein (P-gp, MDR1, ABCB1), and has been shown to inhibit P-gp at concentrations achieved during therapeutic use
- Adverse effects associated with olanzapine include the following:
  - Sedation, insomnia, fatigue
  - Nervousness, agitation, cognitive impairment
  - Headache
  - Dizziness and orthostatic hypotension
  - Increased appetite
  - Weight gain, new-onset diabetes, hyperlipidemia, and increased serum alanine aminotransferase with prolonged use
  - CAUTION: Product labeling for olanzapine includes a boxed warning about its use in elderly patients. In clinical trials, elderly patients (≥65 y) with dementia-related psychosis experienced an increased incidence of death and adverse cerebrovascular events including stroke.
    - Olanzapine shares with other atypical neuroleptics a potential for inhibiting human ether à go-go-related (hERG) gene-encoded potassium channels, but has demonstrated a low potential for inhibiting ventricular repolarization, and, therefore, for causing torsades de pointes; however, effects on cardiac electrophysiological similar to class III anti-arrhythmic drugs were observed at concentrations that can be measured under conditions of impaired olanzapine elimination, during concomitant use of CYP1A2 competitive substrates or inhibitors, and under conditions of overdose.

STRATEGIES FOR COMBINING ANTIEMETICS

Antiemetics in combination can be more effective than single agents by targeting two or more operative neural pathways.

▪ Numerous studies have demonstrated control of acute-phase emetic symptoms improves significantly with the combination of 5-HT$_3$-receptor antagonists and high-potency glucocorticoids. Acute-phase symptom control is further augmented when aprepitant is used in combination with a 5-HT$_3$-receptor antagonist and a glucocorticoid.

▪ Delayed-phase symptom control is improved by the combination of high-potency glucocorticoids and NK$_1$-receptor antagonists. However, NK$_1$-receptor antagonists may compromise the safety of concomitantly administered medications due to potential inhibition or inductive effects on cytochrome P450 metabolizing enzymes.

　● In cases where prophylaxis against delayed-phase symptoms is indicated but concurrent medications make the use of a NK$_1$-receptor antagonist problematic, glucocorticoids alone or in combination with either metoclopramide or a 5-HT$_3$ or D$_2$-receptor antagonist may improve control of symptoms.

Suggested Readings

1. Aapro M. Methodological issues in antiemetic studies. *Invest New Drugs.* 1993;11(4):243–253.
2. Aapro MS, Grunberg SM, Manikhas GM, et al. A phase III, double-blind, randomized trial of palonosetron compared with ondansetron in preventing chemotherapy-induced nausea and vomiting following highly emetogenic chemotherapy. *Ann Oncol.* 2006;17(9):1441–1449.
3. Aapro MS, Molassiotis A, Olver I. Anticipatory nausea and vomiting. *Support Care Cancer.* 2005;13(2):117–121.
4. Antiemesis, V.1.2017 — February 22, 2017. National Comprehensive Cancer Network, Inc., 2017. Available at: http://www.nccn.org [Accessed March 9, 2017]
5. Basch E, Prestrud AA, Hesketh PJ, et al. Antiemetics: American Society of Clinical Oncology clinical practice guideline update. *J Clin Oncol.* 2011;29(31):4189–4198.
6. Borison HL, McCarthy LE. Neuropharmacology of chemotherapy-induced emesis. *Drugs.* 1983;25(Suppl 1):8–17.
7. Botrel TE, Clark OA, Clark L, Paladini L, Faleiros E, Pegoretti B. Efficacy of palonosetron (PAL) compared to other serotonin inhibitors (5-HT3R) in preventing chemotherapy-induced nausea and vomiting (CINV) in patients receiving moderately or highly emetogenic (MoHE) treatment: systematic review and meta-analysis. *Support Care Cancer.* 2011;19(6):823–832.
8. Bubalo JS, Cherala G, McCune JS, Munar MY, Tse S, Maziarz R. Aprepitant pharmacokinetics and assessing the impact of aprepitant on cyclophosphamide metabolism in cancer patients undergoing hematopoietic stem cell transplantation. *J Clin Pharmacol.* 2012;52(4):586–594.
9. Celio L, Frustaci S, Denaro A, et al. Palonosetron in combination with 1-day versus 3-day dexamethasone for prevention of nausea and vomiting following moderately emetogenic chemotherapy: a randomized, multicenter, phase III trial. *Support Care Cancer.* 2011;19(8):1217–1225.
10. D'Acquisto R, Tyson LB, Gralla RJ, et al. The influence of a chronic high alcohol intake on chemotherapy-induced nausea and vomiting [abstract]. *Proc Am Soc Clin Oncol.* 1986;5:257.
11. de Wit R, Herrstedt J, Rapoport B, et al. Addition of the oral NK1 antagonist aprepitant to standard antiemetics provides protection against nausea and vomiting during multiple cycles of cisplatin-based chemotherapy [see comments]. *J Clin Oncol.* 2003;21(22):4105–4111. Comment in: *J Clin Oncol.* 2003;21:4077–4080.
12. Feyer PC, Maranzano E, Molassiotis A, Roila F, Clark-Snow RA, Jordan K. Radiotherapy-induced nausea and vomiting (RINV): MASCC/ESMO guideline for antiemetics in radiotherapy: update 2009. *Support Care Cancer.* 2011;(19 Suppl 1):S5–14.
13. Gralla R, Lichinitser M, Van Der Vegt S, et al. Palonosetron improves prevention of chemotherapy-induced nausea and vomiting following moderately emetogenic chemotherapy: results of a double-blind randomized phase III trial comparing single doses of palonosetron with ondansetron. *Ann Oncol.* 2003;14(10):1570–1577.
14. Hesketh PJ, Bohlke K, Lyman GH, et al. Antiemetics: American Society of Clinical Oncology focused guideline update. *J Clin Oncol.* 2015;34:381–386.
15. Hesketh PJ, Rossi G, Rizzi G, et al. A randomized phase III study evaluating the efficacy and safety of NEPA, a fixed-dose combination of netupitant and palonosetron, for prevention of chemotherapy-induced nausea and vomiting following moderately emetogenic chemotherapy. *Ann Oncol.* 2014;25:1340–1346.
16. Hickok JT, Roscoe JA, Morrow GR, et al. 5-Hydroxytryptamine-receptor antagonists versus prochlorperazine for control of delayed nausea caused by doxorubicin: a URCC CCOP randomised controlled trial. *Lancet Oncol.* 2005;6(10):765–772.
17. Hunt TL, Gallagher SC, Cullen MR Jr, Shah AK. Evaluation of safety and pharmacokinetics of consecutive multiple-day dosing of palonosetron in healthy subjects. *J Clin Pharmacol.* 2005;45(5):589–596.
18. Italian Group for Antiemetic Research. Cisplatin-induced delayed emesis: pattern and prognostic factors during three subsequent cycles. *Ann Oncol.* 1994;5(7):585–589.
19. Kaiser R, Sezer O, Papies A, et al. Patient-tailored antiemetic treatment with 5-hydroxytryptamine type 3 receptor antagonists according to cytochrome P-450 2D6 genotypes [see comments]. *J Clin Oncol.* 2002;20(12):2805–2811. Comment in: *J Clin Oncol.* 2002;20:2765–2767.

20. Kris MG, Gralla RJ, Clark RA, et al. Incidence, course, and severity of delayed nausea and vomiting following the administration of high-dose cisplatin. *J Clin Oncol.* 1985;3(10):1379–1384.

21. Kris MG, Roila F, De Mulder PH, Marty M. Delayed emesis following anticancer chemotherapy. *Support Care Cancer.* 1998;6(3):228–232.

22. Molassiotis A, Coventry PA, Stricker CT, et al. Validation and psychometric assessment of a short clinical scale to measure chemotherapy-induced nausea and vomiting: the MASCC antiemesis tool. *J Pain Symptom Manage.* 2007;34(2):148–159.

23. Morrow GR, Hickok JT, Burish TG, Rosenthal SN. Frequency and clinical implications of delayed nausea and delayed emesis. *Am J Clin Oncol.* 1996;19(2):199–203.

24. Navari RM, Gray SE, Kerr AC. Olanzapine versus aprepitant for the prevention of chemotherapy-induced nausea and vomiting: a randomized phase Ill trial. *J Support Oncol.* 2011;9(5):188–195.

25. Navari RM, Qin R, Ruddy KJ, et al. Olanzapine for the prevention of chemotherapy-induced nausea and vomiting [see comment]. *N Engl J Med.* 2016;375(2):134–142. Comment in: *N Engl J Med.* 2016;375(14):1395–1396.

26. Rapoport BL, Chasen MR, Gridelli C, et al. Safety and efficacy of rolapitant for prevention of chemotherapy-induced nausea and vomiting after administration of cisplatin-based highly emetogenic chemotherapy in patients with cancer: two randomised, active-controlled, double-blind, phase 3 trials. *Lancet Oncol.* 2015;16(9):1079–1089.

27. Roila F, Herrstedt J, Aapro M, et al. Guideline update for MASCC and ESMO in the prevention of chemotherapy- and radiotherapy-induced nausea and vomiting: results of the Perugia consensus conference. *Ann Oncol.* 2010;21(Suppl 5):v232–43.

28. Roila F, Molassiotis A, Herrstedt J, et al. 2016 MASCC and ESMO guideline update for the prevention of chemotherapy- and radiotherapy-induced nausea and vomiting and of nausea and vomiting in advanced cancer patients. *Ann Oncol.* 2016;27(Suppl 5):v119–v33.

29. Rojas C, Slusher BS. Mechanisms and latest clinical studies of new NK_1 receptor antagonists for chemotherapy-induced nausea and vomiting: rolapitant and NEPA (netupitant/palonosetron). *Cancer Treat Rev.* 2015;41(10):904–913.

30. Rojas C, Slusher BS. Pharmacological mechanisms of $5-HT_3$ and tachykinin NK_1 receptor antagonism to prevent chemotherapy-induced nausea and vomiting. *Eur J Pharmacol.* 2012;684(1–3):1–7.

31. Roscoe JA, Morrow GR, Aapro MS, Molassiotis A, Olver I. Anticipatory nausea and vomiting. *Support Care Cancer.* 2011;19(10):1533–1538.

32. Ruhlmann C, Herrstedt J. Palonosetron hydrochloride for the prevention of chemotherapy-induced nausea and vomiting. *Expert Rev Anticancer Ther.* 2010;10(2):137–148.

33. Saito M, Aogi K, Sekine I, et al. Palonosetron plus dexamethasone versus granisetron plus dexamethasone for prevention of nausea and vomiting during chemotherapy: a double-blind, double-dummy, randomised, comparative phase III trial. *Lancet Oncol.* 2009;10(2):115–124.

34. Schwartzberg LS, Modiano MR, Rapoport BL, et al. Safety and efficacy of rolapitant for prevention of chemotherapy-induced nausea and vomiting after administration of moderately emetogenic chemotherapy or anthracycline and cyclophosphamide regimens in patients with cancer: a randomised, active-controlled, double-blind, phase 3 trial. *Lancet Oncol.* 2015;16(9):1071–1079.

35. Sullivan JR, Leyden MJ, Bell R. Decreased cisplatin-induced nausea and vomiting with chronic alcohol ingestion. *N Engl J Med.* 1983;309(13):796.

36. Tremblay PB, Kaiser R, Sezer O, et al. Variations in the 5-hydroxytryptamine type 3B receptor gene as predictors of the efficacy of antiemetic treatment in cancer patients. *J Clin Oncol.* 2003;21(11):2147–2155.

Nutrition **39**

Marnie Grant Dobbin

INTRODUCTION

While only effective cancer treatment can reverse the symptoms of cancer cachexia, nutritional deficits and weight loss in patients with cancer can be minimized with timely nutritional intervention and pharmacologic management.

INCIDENCE AND IMPACT OF MALNUTRITION

- More than 40% of oncology patients develop signs of malnutrition during treatment.
- Malnourished patients incur higher costs for their care, have impaired responses to treatment, greater risk of drug toxicity, and increased rates of morbidity and mortality compared to patients with normal nutritional status.
- As many as 20% of oncology patients die from nutritional complications rather than from their primary diagnosis.
- When malnutrition is identified, diagnosed, and treated, reimbursement to cover the increased cost of care can also be increased—if the physician includes the diagnosis and degree of malnutrition in his documentation, using the currently accepted criteria for diagnosing adult malnutrition. See Table 39.1.

CANCER CACHEXIA

- Nearly two-thirds of patients with cancer develop cancer cachexia characterized by systemic inflammation, anorexia, immunosuppression, and metabolic derangements. These can lead to unintentional weight loss and failure to preserve muscle and fat mass.
- There is no consistent relationship between tumor type, tumor burden, anatomic site of involvement, and cancer cachexia.
- Hypermetabolism is not uniformly present.
- Tumor-induced changes in host production of proinflammatory cytokines (TNF, IL-1, IL-6, and IFN) can lead to hypermetabolism and to anorexia due to changes in gherlin, seratonin, and leptin production. Tumor production of proteolysis-inducing factor and lipid-mobilizing factor contribute to loss of muscle and fat mass—even in the presence of adequate nutrition intake. Inefficient energy metabolism and insulin resistance lead to further depletion of lean body mass.
- Identification of patients with muscle loss has become increasingly difficult as 40% to 60% of patients with cancer are overweight or obese, with fat mass masking muscle loss.
- Overfeeding is likely to worsen metabolic dysregulation and will not result in weight gain.

SCREENING FOR NUTRITIONAL RISK

- Nutritional deterioration can be minimized if patients are screened at each visit, so that problems can be identified and interventions provided when they can have the most impact. The Joint Commission

TABLE 39.1 Clinical Characteristics to Support a Diagnosis of Malnutrition in Adults

Clinical Characteristic	Related to Acute Illness/Injury	Related to Chronic Illness	Related to Social or Environmental Circumstance
Moderate Protein-Calorie Malnutrition ICD-10 Code: E44.0			
Weight Loss	1–2% in 1 week 5% in 1 month 7.5% in 3 months	5% in 1 month 7.5% in 3 months 10% in 6 months 20% in 12 months	5% in 1 month 7.5% in 3 months 10% in 6 months 20% in 12 months
Energy Intake (* per registered dietitian assessment)	< 75% of estimated needs* for > 7 days	< 75% of estimated needs* for ≥ 1 month	< 75% of estimated needs* for ≥ 3 months
Physical Findings: Mild fat and muscle loss, mild fluid accumulation			
Severe Protein-Calorie Malnutrition ICD-10 Code: E43.0			
Weight Loss	> 2% in 1 week > 5% in 1 month > 7.5% in 3 months	> 5% in 1 month > 7.5% in 3 months > 10% in 6 months > 20% in 12 months	> 5% in 1 month > 7.5% in 3 months > 10% in 6 months > 20% in 12 months
Energy Intake	≤ 50% of estimated needs for ≥5 days	< 75% for ≥ 1 month	≤ 50% for ≥1 month
Fat Loss (e.g. of orbital fat pads, triceps, biceps, ribs, lower back)	Moderate depletion (e.g. iliac crest prominent)	Severe depletion (e.g. loss of orbital fat pads)	Severe depletion (e.g. depression between ribs very apparent)
Muscle Mass Loss (e.g. of the temporalis, clavicle, scapular and patella region, dorsal hand, posterior calf)	Moderate depletion (e.g. visible clavicle bone in male; clavicle protruding in female)	Severe depletion (e.g. wasting of the temporalis muscle)	Severe depletion (e.g. flattening of interosseous muscle between thumb and forefinger)
Fluid Accumulation	Moderate to severe (e.g. slight swelling of extremity)	Severe (e.g. 3+ edema)	Severe (e.g. deep pitting)
Functional Assessment	Grip strength has decreased	Grip strength below normative values	Grip strength below normative values

Adapted from White JV, Guenter P, Jensen G, et al, "Consensus Statement: Academy of Nutrition and Dietetics and American Society for Parenteral Nutrition: Characteristics Recommended for the Identification and Documentation of Adult Malnutrition, *J Parenteral Enteral Nutr.* 2012:36:275–283

on Healthcare Accreditation standards state that inpatients are to be screened for nutritional risk within 1 day of admission. Validated screening tools such as the Subjective Global Assessment (SGA) form (https://www.accc-cancer.org/oncology_issues/supplements/Scored-Patient-Generated-Subjective-Global-Assessment-PG-SGA.pdf), may be especially helpful in the outpatient setting. Parameters include weight change, symptoms impacting nutrition, changes in diet, functional status, changes in metabolism and in muscle, fat and fluid status. Use of the form also serves to demonstrate to the patient that nutrition is a priority of the medical team.

- The Pediatric Subjective Global Nutritional Assessment (SGNA) rating form has been validated for use in children. The tool combines clinical judgment and objective criteria to determine a global rating of nutritional status and for identifying those at higher risk of nutrition-related complications (https://www.ncbi.nlm.nih.gov/pubmed/22717202). Parameters include appropriateness of current

TABLE 39.2 To Address Patients' Questions about Nutrition or Dietary Supplements

Refer to a registered dietitian nutritionist (RD or RDN) for individualized nutrition counseling	The registered dietitian nutritionist is the only professional with standardized education, clinical training, continuing education, and national credentialing necessary to be directly reimbursed as a provider of nutrition therapy. RD requirements include: a bachelor's degree or higher (>40% have a master's or doctoral degree), 1200 hr. supervised internship, a national credentialing exam and continuing education. Other nutrition credentials, degrees or titles do not meet these standards. http://www.eatright.org/find-an-expert
For free, responsible nutrition/ cancer guidelines	"Heal Well" from the American Institute for Cancer Research, LIVESTRONG, and Meals to Heal addresses common nutrition concerns and myths such as "Does sugar feed cancer?" http://www.aicr.org/assets/docs/pdf/education/heal-well-guide.pdf "Eating Hints" from the National Cancer Institute—provides nutrition suggestions for patients undergoing treatment https://www.cancer.gov/publications/patient-education/eatinghints.pdf
For vitamin and other dietary supplement information	The NIH Office of Dietary Supplements provides evidence-based, responsible professional and consumer level handouts https://ods.od.nih.gov/factsheets/list-all/ The Natural Medicines Comprehensive Database (published by the Therapeutic Research Faculty) provides thorough, frequently updated, well-referenced information including potential drug interactions and has consumer level information available. http://naturaldatabase.therapeuticresearch.com/home.aspx?cs=cepda&s=ND

height for age (stunting), current weight for height (wasting), and unintentional changes in body weight, adequacy of dietary intake, gastrointestinal symptoms, functional capacity and metabolic stress of disease, loss of subcutaneous fat, muscle wasting and nutrition-related edema.

NUTRITIONAL ASSESSMENT

▪ Registered dietitian nutritionists (RD or RDN) use anthropometric data, biochemical indices, nutrition-focused physical assessment, diet and medical histories to assess the nutritional status of patients and to determine appropriate intervention. See Table 39.2 for RD referral information and suggestions for faddressing nutrition and dietary supplement questions from patients.

BODY COMPOSITION

▪ Obtaining baseline measurements of body composition and comparing these measurements over time can be helpful for monitoring nutritional status.
▪ Body composition is an important predictor of anti-cancer drug efficacy and toxicity. The use of body surface area (BSA) for dosing chemotherapy is being questioned as cytotoxic drugs are largely metabolized and excreted by the liver and kidney, which does not correlate with BSA. There is literature to suggest that lean body mass or fat free mass may be a better basis for normalizing drug dosages in patients with cancer, especially for hydrophilic drugs.
▪ The recommended measurement for diagnosing sarcopenia (muscle loss) is by direct measurement of lean body mass by either DXA (dual energy x-ray absorptiometry) or computed tomography (CT). The DXA, however, does not distinguish between lean and adipose tissue sub-compartments.
▪ The third lumbar vertebra has been validated as the standard landmark for body composition analysis (via CT) because in this region, the percentage of skeletal muscle and adipose tissue has been found to accurately reflect the percentage of skeletal muscle and fat in the entire body.

- Especially as patients with cancer frequently have routine CT monitoring, the use of the third lumbar CT slice to monitor changes in body composition may become routine in the future.
- Measures of muscle mass can include the use of skin calipers to measure mid-arm circumference (MAC) and mid-arm muscle circumference (MAMC). Triceps skinfold measurements can be used to estimate fat stores. There is evidence that ultrasound may also become a useful tool for monitoring muscle mass (e.g., used at bedside to measure the quadriceps).
- Body mass index (BMI) correlates well with body fat, morbidity, and mortality. However, BMI could incorrectly categorize highly muscled patients or those with edema or ascites as having excess fat stores. The BMI is a reasonable means of estimating recommended weights. See Table 39.3.
- Ideal body weight is not appropriate for setting weight goals as it does not reflect standard heights and weights.

PROTEIN

- If energy intake is inadequate, catabolism of protein will occur, especially as tumors preferentially metabolize protein. Limiting protein intake has not been shown to interfere with tumor growth and may lead to protein malnutrition and impaired immunity.
- Protein turnover in patients with cancer is similar to that of patients with infection or injury; their protein requirements are 50% above those of healthy individuals.
- Transport proteins (such as albumin and thyroxin-binding prealbumin) are negative acute-phase proteins that decrease in the presence of inflammation, regardless of a patient's protein status. Earlier

TABLE 39.3 IBW and BMI

IBW Ideal body weight	IBW Men (metric) = 48 kg. for first 152.4 cm of height + 1.1 kg for each additional cm. IBW Men (US) = 106# for first 5 feet of height + 6 # for each additional inch IBW Women (metric) = 45 kg. for first 152.4 cm of height + 0.9 kg for each additional cm. IBW Women (US) = 100# for first 5 feet of height + 5# for each additional inch Derived from 1943 standard height/weight insurance tables—IBW included a component of frame size and height was measured while wearing 1" heels. IBW came to represent fat-free mass—useful for pharmaceutical and other equations. IBW is not recommended for setting target weight goals as it does not represent current standards for height or weight.	
BMI Body Mass Index	BMI = Weight(kg)/Height (meter)^2 BMI <18.5 kg/m^2 = Underweight BMI 18.5–24.9 kg/m^2 = reference range BMI 25–29.9 kg/m^2 = Overweight BMI 30–34.9 kg/m^2 = Obesity 1 BMI 35–39.9 kg/m^2 = Obesity II BMI >40 kg/m^2 = Obesity III	BMI may overestimate body fat in taller individuals, athletes, or those with muscular builds. BMI may underestimate body fat in those who are shorter or have low muscle mass.
Maximum recommended weight	Maximum recommended weight (BMI = 24.9 kg/m^2) To find corresponding weight: Weight = 24.9 x height (meter)^2 Example—for patient 160 cm tall: Recommended maximum weight = Height (meter)^2 x 24.9 Recommended maximum weight = (1.60 m)^2 x 24.9 = 63.7 kg	
Minimum recommended weight	Minimum recommended weight (BMI = 18.5 kg/m^2) To find corresponding weight: Weight (kg) = 18.5 x height (meter)^2 Example—for patient 160 cm tall: Recommended minimum weight = Height (meter)^2 x 18.5 Recommended minimum weight = (1.60 m)^2 x 18.5 = 47.4 kg	

studies incorrectly correlated these proteins with nutritional status, not accounting for their role as inflammatory markers. Dietary history and nitrogen balance measurements are more reliable measures of protein adequacy.

▪ The Society for Critical Care Medicine and the American Society for Parenteral and Enteral Nutrition published guidelines for nutrition support of the critically ill patient in 2016, which includes the recommendation that visceral proteins (such as prealbumin and albumin) not be used as markers of nutrition status.[10]

NUTRITIONAL REQUIREMENTS

▪ Indirect calorimetry, the preferred method for estimating resting energy expenditure, measures O_2 consumed (VO_2) and volume of carbon dioxide produced (VCO_2) to determine respiratory quotient (RQ). This can be done with a portable metabolic cart operated by a respiratory therapist, or by a handheld device recently approved by the FDA.

▪ There are a variety of recommended calculations for estimating energy, fluid, and protein requirements (Tables 39.4, 39.5, and 39.6). However, formulas that rely on stress and activity factors, or calculations such as >45 kcal/kg "for stress," have been shown to overestimate requirements. It is important not to overfeed patients with cancer. Overfeeding can increase risk of infection and induce respiratory distress, hyperglycemia, and fatty liver.

▪ The initial calorie goal for critically ill patients should be to meet their estimated resting energy expenditure only.

NUTRITIONAL INTERVENTION

▪ Nutritional counseling by an RD is associated with improvement in the quality of life scores and nutritional parameters, and with success of oral nutritional intervention for oncology patients. Continual reassessment, pharmacologic management, and nutritional counseling can often help avoid costly, risky nutritional support options. See Table 39.7 for nutrition recommendations appropriate for patients who are able to tolerate oral or enteral feedings.

NUTRITIONAL SUPPORT

Although tumor growth is stimulated by a variety of nutrients, limiting the nutrients preferred by tumors can be detrimental to the patient. If patients have moderate to severe malnutrition and are unable to meet

TABLE 39.4 Estimates of Energy Requirements

Patient/Condition	Kilocalories/kg[a]
Acutely ill; obese (BMI 30–50)	11–14 (use actual weight)
Cancer	25–30
Hypermetabolism; malabsorption	35
Stem cell transplant	30–35

[a] Fever increases energy needs by ~14%/°F.

TABLE 39.5 Mifflin-St. Jeor Formula for Estimating Resting Energy Expenditure

Males	REE = 10W + 6.25H – 5A + 5
Females	REE = 10W + 6.25H – 5A – 161

A, age (y); H, height (cm); REE, resting energy expenditure; W, weight (kg).

TABLE 39.6 Recommended Protein Intake for Adults

Disease State	Grams of Protein per Kilogram Body Weight
Cancer	1–1.2
Cancer cachexia	1.2–1.5
Hematopoietic stem cell transplant	1.5
Renal disease:	
Obese patient	1.2 (using actual, not adjusted weight)
Predialysis GFR 26–55 mL/min	0.8
GFR 10–25 mL/min	0.6
Hemodialysis	1.1–1.4
Peritoneal dialysis	1.2–1.5
CVVHD	1.5–2
Liver disease:	1–1.5
Hepatitis chronic or acute	
Encephalopathy grade 1 or 2	0.5–1.2
Encephalopathy grade 3 or 4	0.5

GFR, glomerular filtration rate.

their nutritional needs with oral intake alone, specialized nutrition support such as parenteral or enteral nutrition is indicated (Figure 39.1). Sample parenteral nutrition recommendations are shown in Table 39.8.

Enteral Nutrition

- Reviews of nutritional support practices indicate that parenteral nutrition (PN) is often instituted even when safer, more physiologic enteral nutritional (EN) support could have been provided. The benefits of EN over PN have been well demonstrated, including fewer infections, decreased catabolic hormones, improved wound healing, shorter hospital stay, and maintenance of gut integrity. In other words, if the gut works, use it.
- To be successful, EN should be implemented as soon as possible. Surgeons may approve of enteral feeding within 4 hours of placement of gastrostomy tubes and immediately after Jejunostomy (because bowel sounds are not needed). Prophylactic placement of gastrointestinal tubes can considerably reduce weight loss during radiotherapy and may reduce the need for hospitalization due to dehydration, weight loss, or other complications of mucositis.
- Many long accepted practices for initiating and monitoring enteral and parenteral nutrition have been overturned recently. See with the 2016 SCCM and ASPEN guidelines for the nutrition support of critically ill patients for the most current recommendations.

Parenteral Nutrition

- PN can be beneficial to cancer patients when response to treatment is good but associated nutritional morbidity is high, and when the GI tract is unavailable to support nutrition. Perioperative PN should be limited to patients who are severely malnourished, with surgery expected to prevent oral intake for more than 10 days after surgery.
- For the families of cancer patients, feeding is often synonymous with caring. However, end-stage patients who are encouraged to eat and drink as desired may have better quality of life than if specialized nutrition support is provided (which could contribute to incontinence, fluid imbalance, and respiratory compromise). The risks and benefits of PN must be addressed individually and evaluated for each case with patient and family input. In general, PN is not usually indicated in patients with an expected survival of less than 3 months.

TABLE 39.7 Oral Nutrition Recommendations for Patients (by Condition)

Condition	Recommendations
Diabetes/ hyperglycemia	Begin by familiarizing patients with the carbohydrate content of foods. Most men need 45 to 75 g of carbohydrate per meal; most women need 45 to 60 g per meal. If a snack is taken, 15 to 30 g of carbohydrate is usually recommended. (One ounce of bread product, ½ cup cooked starch, ½ cup fruit or juice, and 8 oz. milk each provide ~15 g of carbohydrate)
Diarrhea	↓ Lactose, ↓ fat, ↓ insoluble fiber (wheat bran, skin, and seeds of produce), ↑ soluble fiber (peeled fruit, oat bran, guar gum products). Cheese has insignificant carbohydrate/lactose content (<2 g/100 g of cheese) and yogurt is naturally low in lactose
Early satiety	Calorically dense foods/nutrition products (e.g., medical nutrition beverages with >1.5 kcal/mL); foods such as nuts, cheese, seeds, modular kcal, or protein supplements that can be added to foods without significantly altering the flavor or volume of foods
Fat malabsorption	↓ Fat diet and MCT–oil fortified foods/products. A diet with <30% of kcal from fat or <40 g of fat/d may be unrealistic long-term. A trial of pancreatic enzymes and bile acid sequestrants may significantly improve symptoms
Hypercalcemia of malignancy	Does not respond to low-calcium diet. Often, crucial sources of protein and kcal are limited by such a diet
Magnesium and potassium status	Refractory hypokalemia is often related to limited Mg stores, even when serum Mg levels are within normal range. Repletion of Mg may help normalize K levels. Increased intake of dietary Mg, K, and P can reduce reliance on supplements without the gastrointestinal side effects associated with supplementation
Malabsorption	Semi elemental palatable products, trials of pancreatic enzymes, bile acid sequestrants, and medium-chain triglycerides (MCT) may reduce symptoms
Neutropenia	Many hematopoietic transplant centers emphasize prevention of food-borne illness (verifying temperatures of cooked foods/meats with a thermometer, avoiding unpasteurized dairy products and juices, etc.) rather than strict diets that limit fresh produce, have poor compliance rates, and have no proven benefit in reducing infection rates
Poor appetite/ fatigue	Recommend >5 scheduled feedings/day to lessen dependence on appetite, with use of nutritious liquids for high % of kcal (milk, lactose-treated milk, soup, soy milk, fruit smoothies made with nut butters, or meal replacement beverages). Discourage patients from relying on water alone to meet fluid requirement, as nutritious beverages such as milk contain >90% water and could provide significant nutrition; excess water intake may blunt appetite
Diet Advancement	Based on expert consensus, clear liquids are not required as the first meal postoperatively. Patients should be allowed solid foods as tolerated.

COMPLICATIONS OF NUTRITIONAL SUPPORT

Refeeding Syndrome

Feeding after starvation is associated with increased intravascular volume, cardiopulmonary compromise, and plummeting levels of phosphorus, magnesium, and potassium due to the intracellular movement of electrolytes during anabolism. Malnourished individuals with severe weight loss, negligible intake for >7 days, a history of alcoholism, recent surgery, electrolyte losses due to diarrhea, high-output fistulas, or vomiting are especially vulnerable. Initially, no more than 50% of estimated needs (~15 kcal/kg/day and no more than 150 g dextrose/day) are recommended. Because thiamin is an important coenzyme for carbohydrate metabolism, the addition of 100 mg of thiamin for at least the first week of feeding is warranted.

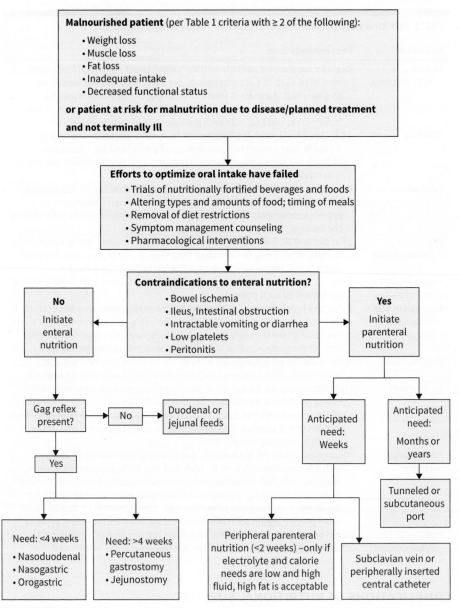

FIGURE 39.1 Nutrition support algorithm.

Hypertriglyceridemia

For individuals receiving PN who have preexisting hyperlipidemia and obesity, or for those taking sirolimus, cyclosporine, and other medications associated with increased triglyceride (TG) levels, the goal is to keep TG <400 mg/dL. Ensure that blood is drawn 4 hours after lipid infusion or before lipids are hung, to avoid falsely elevated TG. Lipid dose should be reduced if TG is between 300 mg/dL and 600 mg/dL; however, stopping lipid altogether can worsen liver dysfunction. Five hundred milliliters per week of 20% IVFE can prevent essential fatty acid deficiency in adults.

TABLE 39.8 Sample Parenteral Nutrition Recommendations

	Infants/Children (3–30 kg)	Adolescents (≥30 kg)	Adults
Water	1,500–1,800 mL/m²/d 1,500 mL/kg for first 20 kg and 25 mL/kg for remaining weight	1,500 mL/m²/d	1,500 mL/m²/d 35 mL/kg or 1 mL/kcal
Energy	70–110 cal/kg/d	40–60 cal/kg/d	20–35 cal/kg/d
Dextrose (3.4 kcal/g for the hydrated form)			
Initial	5%–10% (50–100 g/L)	5%–10% (50–100 g/L)	10%–15% (100–150 g/L)
Advance	5% (50 g/L)	5% (50 g/L)	5%–10% (50–100 g/L)
Max dextrose oxidation rate	12–15 mg/kg/min	5–13 mg/kg/min	4–5 mg/kg/min
Max dextrose concentration	20–35% (200–350 g/L)	20%–35% (200–350 g/L)	20%–35% (200–350 g/L) for central access; 10% for peripheral
Protein			
Initial	1 g/kg/d	1 g/kg/d	At goal
Advance	0.5–1 g/kg/d	1 g/kg/d	—
Max	2–3 g/kg/d	1.5–2 g/kg/d	2 g/kg/d
IVFE	20% lipid provides 2 kcal/mL. Due to glycerol in fat emulsions, 1 g of fat in 20% emulsions = 10 kcal; ~1 g of fat per 5 mL of 20% IVFE		
Initial	1 g/kg/d	1 g/kg/d	At goal; usually ≥250 mL 20% IVFE for ~30% of total kcal
Advance	1 g/kg/d	1 g/kg/d	—
Max	2–3 g/kg/d	2 g/kg/d	2 g/kg/d (60% of total kcal)
Minerals			
Sodium	2–4 mEq/kg/d	2–3 mEq/kg/d	1–2 mEq/kg 60–150 mEq/d max 155 mEq/L
Potassium	2–3 mEq/kg/d	1.5–3 mEq/kg/d	1–2 mEq/kg 40–240 mEq/d max 80 mEq/L
Magnesium	0.3–0.5 mEq/kg/d	0.2–0.3 mEq/kg/d	8–24 mEq/d
Calcium	0.5–2.5 mEq/kg/d	0.5–1 mEq/kg/d	10–40 mEq/d max 30 mEq/L
Phosphorus	0.5–2 mM/kg/d	0.5–1.3 mM/kg/d	20–40 mM/d max 30 mM/L
Selenium	2 mcg/kg/d (40 mcg/max)	2 mcg/kg/d (40 mcg/max)	40 mcg
Trace metals and multivitamins	Daily	Daily	Daily

IVFE, intravenous fat emulsion.

Parenteral Nutrition–Associated Liver Disease

Hepatic fat accumulation is most common in adults and usually resolves within 2 weeks, even if PN continues. It typically presents within 2 weeks of PN with moderate elevations in serum aminotransferase concentrations. Parenteral nutrition–associated liver disease (PNALD) is usually a complication of overfeeding; it has become less common in the past 10 years, since calories provided via PN have become more appropriate.

Parenteral Nutrition–Associated Cholestasis

- Parenteral nutrition–associated cholestasis (PNAC) is primarily a result of excess calories in PN. Overfeeding contributes to fat deposition in the liver by stimulating insulin release, which promotes lipogenesis and inhibits fatty acid oxidation. PNAC occurs most often in children. It is associated with elevated serum conjugated bilirubin (>2 mg/dL) and may progress to cirrhosis and liver failure. Factors unrelated to PN that have been misattributed to PNAC include bacterial and fungal infections.
- Fat-free PN formulations have also been implicated in the development of fatty liver, since a high percentage of calories from carbohydrates can lead to fat deposition in the liver. Providing a balance of calories from dextrose and fat seems to decrease the incidence of steatosis, possibly by decreasing hepatic TG uptake and promoting fatty oxidation.

Suggested Readings

1. August DA, Huhmann MB. A.S.P.E.N. clinical guidelines: nutrition support therapy during adult anticancer treatment and in hematopoietic cell transplantation. *J Parenter Enteral Nutr.* 2009;33(5):472–500.
2. Bischoff-Ferrari HA. Optimal serum 25-hydroxyvitamin D levels for multiple health outcomes. *Adv Exp Med Biol.* 2008;624:55–71.
3. Boateng AA, Sriram K, Meguid MM, Crook M. Refeeding syndrome: treatment considerations based on collective analysis of literature case reports. *Nutrition.* 2010;26:156–167.
4. Elliott L, Molseed LL, McCallum PD, Grant B, eds. The Clinical Guide to Oncology Nutrition. 2nd ed. Oncology Nutrition Dietetic Practice Group. Chicago, IL: American Dietetic Association; 2006.
5. Gariballa S. Refeeding syndrome: a potentially fatal condition but remains underdiagnosed and undertreated. *Nutrition.* 2008;24:604–606.
6. Heaney RP. The vitamin D requirement in health and disease. *J Steroid Biochem Mol Biol.* 2005;97:13–19.
7. Johnson G, Salle A, Lorimier G, et al. Cancer cachexia: measured and predicted resting energy expenditures for nutritional needs evaluation. *Nutrition.* 2008;24:443–450.
8. Leser M, Ledesma N, Bergerson S et al *Oncology Nutrition for Clinical Practice.* Chicago, IL: Academy of Nutrition and Dietetics; 2013.
9. Marian M, Robert S. Clinical Nutrition for Oncology Patients. Sudberry, MA (USA, 01776). Jones & Bartlett Publishers; 2010.
10. McClave SA[1], Martindale RG, Vanek VW et al, Guidelines for the Provision and Assessment of Nutrition Support Therapy in the Adult Critically Ill Patient: Society of Critical Care Medicine (SCCM) and American Society for Parenteral and Enteral Nutrition (A.S.P.E.N.).*JPEN J Parenter Enteral Nutr.* 2009 May-Jun;33(3):277–316.
11. Mehta NM, Corkins, MR, Lyman B et al Defining Pediatric Malnutrition: A paradigm shift toward etiology-related definitions, *JPEN* 2013 Jul; 37 (4):460–481.
12. Moutzakis M, Prado CMM, Lieffers JR et al A practical and precise approach to quantification of body composition in cancer patients using computed tomography images acquired during routine care, *Applied Physiology,Nutrition and Metabolism,* 2008; 33(5):997–1006.
13. Mueller CM. The A.S.P.E.N. Adult Nutrition Support Core Curriculum. 2nd ed. Silver Spring, ML: American Society for Parenteral and Enteral Nutrition; 2012.
14. National Cancer Institute: PDQ Hypercalcemia. Bethesda, MD: National Cancer Institute; 2011. Available at: http://cancer.gov/cancertopics/pdq/supportivecare/hypercalcemia/Health Professional. Accessed September 29,2016 .
15. *Philips W,* Coding for Malnutritionin the Adult Patient: What the Physician Needs to Know. *Practical Gastroenterology,* Sep 2014. Available at: https://med.virginia.edu/ginutrition/wp-content/uploads/sites/199/2014/06/Parrish-Sept-14.pdf.
16. Ryan, AM, Power DG, Daly L et al Cancer-associated malnutrition, cachexia and sarcopenia: the skeleton in the hospital closet 40 years later, *Proceedings of the Nutrition Society* 2016;75(2):199–211.
17. Schlein KM, Coulter SP, Best practices for determining resting energy expenditure in critically ill adults. *Nutr Clin Pract.* 2014 Feb;29(1):44–55.
18. White JV, Guenter P, Jensen G et al, Consensus statement: Academy of Nutrition and Dietetics and American Society for Parenteral and Enteral Nutrition: characteristics recommended for the identification and documentation of adult malnutrition (undernutrition) JPEN *J Parenter Enteral Nutr.* 2012 May;36(3):275–283.

Pain and Palliative Care **40**

Christina Tafe, Jean-Paul Pinzon, and Ann Berger

DEFINITIONS

- Palliative care is based on a holistic model of symptom management. It concerns improving the quality of life for patients and their families facing life-threatening or terminal illnesses by preventing, identifying, and relieving suffering associated with physical, psychosocial, and spiritual problems.
- Concurrent palliative care involvement adds benefit to the oncology patient by managing symptoms of disease and treatment early to promote compliance of treatment and maintain quality of life while disease modifying treatments are rendered.
- A breakthrough study published in 2010 looked at early integration of palliative care in the treatment of metastatic nonsmall cell lung cancer patients and found that patients receiving early palliative care, as compared with those receiving standard care alone, had improved survival (Temel et al., 2010).
- Pain is a common referral for palliative care consultation and is usually, but not always, associated with tissue damage. It is always subjective and may be influenced by emotional, psychological, social, and spiritual factors, as well as financial concerns and fear of death. This is referred to as "total pain" and is best treated with an interdisciplinary approach to address all areas of suffering for patient and family.
- Acute pain is the predictable physiologic response to an adverse chemical, thermal, or mechanical stimulus. It is normally associated with surgery, trauma, and acute illness. It is generally time limited and responsive to a variety of pharmacologic and nonpharmacologic therapies.
- When acute pain persists over time, it is classified as chronic pain.

EPIDEMIOLOGY

- Most cancer patients experience some degree of pain, especially in the advanced and metastatic phases of disease. In advanced cancer, the prevalence of pain is about 70%, but varies with the type and stage of disease.
- There are several published guidelines for cancer pain management recommended by the World Health Organization (WHO), and effective treatments are available for 70% to 90% of cases.
- Nevertheless, an estimated 40% of cancer patients remain undertreated for reasons related to the health care provider, the patient and family, or cultural mores. The most frequent cause of under treatment is misconceptions about the use of opioids.

ASSESSMENT

- Proper pain assessment can help to establish a good doctor/patient relationship, guide the therapeutic regimen, improve pain management, maximize patient comfort and function, and increase patient satisfaction with therapy. Failure to fully assess pain in the cancer patient may result in adverse pain outcomes, regardless of the amount or type of analgesia and adjuvants used.

573

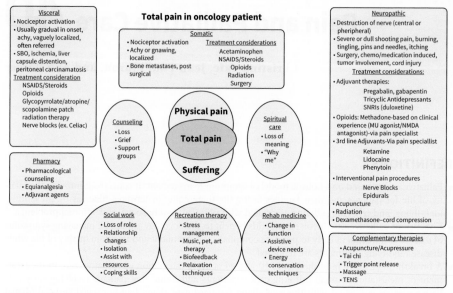

FIGURE 40.1 Total pain in oncology patient.

- Patients' self-reports should be the main source of pain assessment. For infants and the cognitively impaired, physicians can utilize nonverbal pain scales (PAIN-AD, Wong-Baker Faces, CNVI) (Quill et al., 2010).
- Patients should be reassessed frequently by inquiring how much their pain has been relieved after each treatment. A consistent disparity between patients' self-report of pain and their ability to function necessitates further assessment to ascertain the reason for the disparity.
- When addressing total pain, it is important to look at other forms of suffering and appropriate treatments in addition to physical suffering to ensure that medication management such as opioids are not over or underutilized for management of the oncology patient. (Fig. 40.1)

TREATMENT

- Treatment of physical pain should be tailored to each patient, based on the type of pain and duration of expected pain. (Somatic, visceral, neuropathic, and acute vs. chronic).
- Use an interdisciplinary team to assist with suffering to improve management of the patient's total pain (i.e. social work, chaplain, recreation therapist, physical therapist, pharmacist), thus helping to limit the use of prescription medications for nonphysical pain.
- No maximal therapeutic dose for analgesia has been established. Immediate-release opioids (mu receptor agonists) are short-acting and may be appropriate for acute incidental pain, breakthrough pain, or to initiate and titrate opioid therapy. Long-acting opioids are used around the clock for baseline pain and to maintain analgesia.
- Titration of opioids: Start at lower doses and titrate as tolerance to side effects develops. If pain persists, titration upward by dose increments of 30% to 50% may be necessary to achieve adequate analgesia. For severe uncontrolled pain (extremis), increase the dose by up to 100% and reassess at peak effect. Also adjust based on kidney function when titrating opioids, and stop escalation at adequate pain control or dose limiting side effects (Table 40.1).

TABLE 40.1 Opioid Doses Equianalgesic to Morphine 10 mg Parenteral (IV/IM) for Treatment of Chronic Pain in Cancer Patients (Derby, Chin, Portenoy, 1998)[1]

Drug	mg Oral	mg IV/IM	Duration (h)	Considerations
Morphine	30	10	2–4 (IV) 2–4 (IR) 8–24 (SR/CR)	▪ Most toxic metabolites in renal failure should be avoided ▪ Various formulations of long acting agents with different duration
Oxycodone	20		3–4 (IR) 8–12 (SR)	▪ As with all SR/CR tablets, do not crush ▪ IR opioids can be crushed Use cautiously in renal failure
Hydromorphone	7.5	1.5	2–4(IV) 2–4 (IR)	
Methadone	—	—	—	▪ Complex pharmacodynamics and highly recommend management per pain or palliative care specialists ▪ Based on clinical experience, helpful with somatic and neuropathic pain ▪ Can prolong QTc interval and requires monitor with EKG with use ▪ Can be used in renal dysfunction
Oxymorphone	10		2–4	
Fentanyl		0.1 (100 mcg)	30–60 min	▪ Can be administered as continuous IV or SC. infusion; based on clinical experience, 10 mcg IV = 1 mg IV morphine ▪ Can be used in renal dysfunction, cautious use in liver dysfunction.
Fentanyl Transdermal			48–72	▪ Based on clinical experience, 25 mcg/h is roughly equianalgesic to morphine 50mg PO per day ▪ Adequate adipose tissue required for absorption so would not recommend in cachexia ▪ Fevers and diaphoresis can affect absorption

IR(Immediate release) SR (Sustained Released) CR (Controlled Release)

[1]Adapted from Derby S, Chin J, Portenoy RK. Systemic opioid therapy for chronic cancer pain: practical guidelines for converting drugs and routes of administration. *CNS Drugs.* 1998;9(2):99–109

▪ Common adverse effects of opioids include constipation, sedation, nausea/vomiting, pruritus, sweating, dry mouth, and weakness.
▪ With the exception of constipation, tolerance often develops rapidly to most of the common opioid-related adverse effects. Start bowel regimen when initiating opioids unless contraindicated.
▪ Uncommon adverse effects of opioids include dyspnea, urinary retention, confusion, hallucinations, nightmares, myoclonus, dizziness, dysphoria, and hypersensitivity/anaphylaxis.

SAFE AND RESPONSIBLE PRESCRIBING

- Physicians have an ethical and regulatory duty to inform the patient of the risks and benefits of long-term opioid use, particularly when initiating treatment in patients at high risk for misuse of opioids (utilize random urine drug tests, referrals to pain management physicians and pain contracts in high-risk patients).
- Opioid therapy should be tailored to each patient, based on the type and expected duration of pain, as it is difficult to predict which patients will achieve adequate analgesia or develop intolerable adverse effects from a given opioid.
- Certain factors, such as personal or family history of substance abuse, risk of diversion of opioids, or lack of compliance, dictate a multidisciplinary approach, including the involvement of a pain specialist.
- Long-term use of opioids should always be supported by maximal use of co-analgesics and adjuvants, psychological therapy, spiritual counseling, and appropriate follow-up.
- The CDC has published guidelines for the management of chronic pain to help minimize the harms associated with opioids including overdose and opioid use disorders. These guidelines are useful to help focus on effective treatments available for chronic pain such as adjuvants and non-pharmacological approaches to pain control.
- Key recommendations include the following:
  - Nonopioid therapy is preferred for chronic pain outside of active cancer, palliative, and end-of-life care.
  - When opioids are used, the lowest possible effective dosage should be prescribed to reduce risks of opioid use disorder and overdose.
  - Providers should always exercise caution when prescribing opioids and monitor all patients closely.

Risks of Long-Term Opioid Use

- Addiction: Extremely rare in cancer patients but all patients should be assessed for risk factors and continuously reassessed.
  - Risk Factors: Personal and family history of substance abuse; age; history of preadolescent sexual abuse; certain psychiatric disorders: Attention deficit disorder, obsessive-compulsive disorder, bipolar, schizophrenia, and depression (Webster & Webster, 2005).
- Physical dependence: Manifested by withdrawal syndrome at cessation or dose reduction.
- Tolerance: Diminution of one or more of the opioid's effects over time often related to disease progression in the oncology patient.
- Pseudoaddiction: Iatrogenic syndrome that develops in response to inadequate pain management.

Termination of Opioid Therapy

- When opioids are no longer required for pain management, appropriate tapering is essential to reduce the risk of withdrawal syndromes from physical dependence. The recommended regimen involves reducing dosage by 10% to 20% daily, or more slowly if symptoms such as anxiety, tachycardia, sweating, or other autonomic symptoms arise.
- Symptoms may be relieved by clonidine 0.1 to 0.2 mg per day PO up to tid or low-dose transdermal patch every third day.

Suggested Readings

1. Berger A, Shuster J, Von Roenn H. Principles and practice of palliative care & supportive oncology. 4th ed. Philadelphia, PA: Lippincott Williams & Wilkins, 2013.
2. Cherny N. The management of cancer pain. *Cancer J Clin.* 2000;50:70–116.
3. Cohen MZ, Easley MK, Ellis C, et al. Cancer pain management and the JCAHO's pain standards: an institutional challenge. *J Pain Symptom Manage.* 2003;25:519–527.
4. Dalal S, Bruera E. Assessing cancer pain. *Curr Pain Headache Rep.* 2012;16(4):314–324.

5. Dowwell D, Haegerich TM, Chou R. CDC Guidelines for Prescribing Opioids for Chronic Pain - United States, 2016. *MMWR Recomm Rep* 2016;65(No.RR-1):1–49. DOI: http://dx.doi.org/10.15585/mmwr.rr6501e1

6. Hearn J, Higginson IJ. Cancer pain epidemiology: a systematic review. In: Bruera ED, Portenoy RK, eds. *Cancer Pain, Assessment and Management.* New York: Cambridge University Press; 2003.

7. Jennings AL, Davies A, Higgins JP, Broadley K. Opioids for the palliation of breathlessness in terminal illness. *Cochrane Database Syst Rev.* 2001;4:CDE002066.

8. Koller A, Miaskowski C, De Geest S, Opitz O, Spichiger E. A systematic evaluation of content, structure, and efficacy of interventions to improve patients' self-management of cancer pain. *J Pain Symptom Manage.* 2012;44(2):264–284.

9. Paley CA, Johnson MI, Tashani OA, Bagnall AM. Acupuncture for cancer pain in adults. *Cochrane Database Syst Rev.* 2011;19(1):CD007753. doi:10.1002/14651858.CD007753.pub2.

10. Qaseem A, Snow V, Shekelle P, Casey Jr. D, Cross Jr. T, Owens D. Evidence-based interventions to improve the palliative care of pain, dyspnea, and depression at the end of life: a clinical practice guideline from the American College of Physicians. *Ann Intern Med.* 2008;148(2):141–146.

11. Quill T, Bower K, Holloway R, et al. Primer of palliative care. 6th ed. Glenview, IL: American Academy of Hospice and Palliative Medicine, 2014.

12. Temel J, Greer J, Muzikansky A, et al. Early palliative care for patients with metastatic non–small-cell lung cancer. *N Engl J Med.* 2010;363:733–742.

13. von Gunten CF. Evolution and effectiveness of palliative care. *Am J Geriatr Psychiatry.* 2012;20(4):291–297.

14. Webster L, Webster R. Predicting aberrant behaviors in opioid-treated patients: preliminary validation of the opioid risk tool. *Pain Med.* 2005;6(6):432–442.

15. Zeppetella G. Opioids for the management of breakthrough cancer pain in adults: a systematic review undertaken as part of an EPCRC opioid guidelines project. *Palliat Med.* 2011;25(5):516–524.

41 Central Venous Access Device

Peter A. Zmijewski and Hannah W. Hazard-Jenkins

INTRODUCTION

Once the diagnosis of cancer has been made, the patient will go through a rigorous staging process resulting in the development of a plan of care for the newly diagnosed. Typically, blood tests are drawn to help facilitate the staging and treatment of the patient's disease. Additionally, tests are performed to document the patient's clinical well-being and monitor the progress of his or her treatment. Added to this is the potential for a rigorous venous sampling schedule and the use of contrast agents during radiologic imaging studies performed for staging purposes. Most of these studies can be instituted without establishment of a long-term venous access device; however, it is prudent to assess the need for central venous access early in treatment to avoid any delays. Chemotherapy administration for the cancer patient may be delivered over a more prolonged schedule with the placement of a long-term, central venous access device (CVAD). Moreover, these devices have facilitated the implementation of increasingly complex treatment regimens at home.

The rationale for placing CVADs is derived from the caustic properties of chemotherapeutic agents and the consequences of repeated venipuncture on the peripheral veins. The innermost layer of a vein is known as the tunica intima. It is this layer that becomes damaged with the repeated trauma associated with peripheral venipuncture. This damaged endothelium results in exposure of the underlying thrombogenic layer, the tunica media, which results in platelet aggregation and subsequent thrombosis. Implanted venous access devices are either tunneled through the periphery or bypass the periphery altogether and are directly implanted in the central venous system. In both circumstances, trauma to the peripheral veins is reduced. The instillation of potentially damaging substances is more tolerable in the central veins, as they have a much larger volume of blood flow and thicker vein walls. Once the decision has been made to place a CVAD, various factors must be taken into consideration. These factors may include specific patient characteristics and preferences, patient history and associated comorbidities, and specific infusion needs. The many options for venous access can then be considered in a cooperative fashion.

The initial interaction with the patient should be used to evaluate the level of care they will be capable of providing for whichever vascular device is ultimately selected. Moreover, lifestyle, habits, and activities should be taken into account during the selection process. Patients may prefer to have devices placed on their nondominant side to facilitate care. Devices implanted in the chest may be positioned low to assist in hiding them under garments and to provide for easy visualization without the need of a mirror. Consideration should be given in females to the position of bra straps and modifying placement accordingly. Additionally, patients who partake in certain recreational activities such as firearm shooting may prefer to have an implanted port positioned away from the shoulder in which the firearm rests.

A history of previous venous device placement also must be assessed as this could modify the preferred site of catheter insertion. Preoperative ultrasound evaluation of the upper extremities, jugular, and central veins may be beneficial in patients with a history of multiple central venous accesses. Moreover, any surgical interventions or currently placed devices such as automated implantable cardioverter defibrillators and pacemakers should be noted. The presence of inferior vena cava (IVC) filter devices should also be noted as this may require the use of an alternate type of access wire (i.e., straight wires instead of J-curved wires). Patient allergies need to be documented as well and the device and surgical equipment modified accordingly. Finally, the physical examination is also a key part of the preoperative patient assessment. The skin at the insertion and final placement sites should be assessed for adequacy. Patients with underlying skin conditions or prior surgical sites may dictate location of implantable device. Moreover, evidence of dilated superficial veins may herald an undisclosed central venous stenosis that may complicate catheter placement and initiate further evaluation before operative intervention.

Ultimately, the type of infusion agent and the frequency needed may dictate the type of access device used. Patients in need of chronic and continuous infusion may best benefit from tunneled devices, whereas subcutaneous ports are ideal devices for patients who will only need accessed intermittently. The type of infusates used and their relative compatibilities may also be a consideration in deciding the number of lumens that may be needed in a particular device.

INDICATIONS

Indications for venous access placement in the oncology patient are guided by complex factors that evolve during the transition from diagnosis to treatment and finally into remission. Consideration is given to the composition of the infusates being administered, the frequency of treatment (monthly, weekly, and daily), the size or number of lumens required, the patient's ability to provide self-care of the device, and patient's preference (which may be influenced by vanity, an appropriate consideration in the decision-making process). Additional factors to consider are the potential for daily maintenance needs such as flushes and dressing changes that may or may not be covered by insurance and patients may not be able to do on their own. For example, a bone marrow transplant patient may require a large-bore multichannel catheter for stem cell collection initially, but will also need a long-term catheter for the remainder of the transplant process.

CONTRAINDICATIONS

The placement of various CVADs is associated with very few contraindications. Patients with uncontrolled coagulopathy are at risk for developing hematomas at sites of surgical dissection (port pocket sites, cephalic vein cut-down) and around percutaneous catheter insertion sites. Every effort should be made to correct coagulopathy before a CVAD is placed. It is also important to realize that the subclavian vein is essentially non-compressible due to the overlying clavicle and direct pressure may not work to control catheter site bleeding. For coagulopathy patients, a more compressible vessel, such as the internal jugular may be preferable for access. Attempted access in specific vessels with known thrombosis, diagnosed by ultrasound or contrasted imaging, is a contraindication and only patent vessels should be attempted to be accessed. A bloodstream infection, as demonstrated by positive blood cultures, is also a contraindication for long-term CVADs due to the high colonization rates and thus requiring subsequent removal. The CVAD may be placed once the infection has been adequately treated and negative blood cultures are documented.

Certain CVADs require the positioning of a device in the subcutaneous tissue of the chest, may not be appropriate options in some situations or certain types of tumors. Moreover, certain patients, such as those with cystic fibrosis, may require constant chest percussive therapy making a secondary site of placement a more viable option. These sites include the upper arm or a part of the abdomen. In addition to port placement, it is also necessary to understand the position of the catheter. For instance, in patients with head and neck cancer, presence of an internal jugular catheter may interfere with radiation and future surgical exploration. For these patients, subclavian or contralateral internal jugular access may be more appropriate.

INFUSION DEVICES

Venous access devices can be categorized into five groups based on the mechanism of insertion and catheter dwell potentials. These categories include peripheral angiocatheters, peripherally inserted central catheters (PICCs), percutaneous non-tunneled central catheters, tunneled central catheters, and implanted ports. Each category is then further defined by device-specific characteristics such as flow rates, lumen size, catheter tip location, and dwell time. In utilizing this process, it is easier to identify which catheter meets the specific needs of the patient in Table 41.1.

While not a CVAD, it is worth mentioning the peripheral intravenous angiocatheter (PIV), as it is simplest access to utilize. The angiocatheters are relatively easy to insert and remove, specialized

TABLE 41.1 Venous Access Devices

Type of Catheter	Indications	Limitations
Peripheral angiocatheters	Hydration, PPN, short-term access	Frequent infiltration/phlebitis, easily dislodged, short dwell time (up to 72 hours) cannot be used for solutions with extreme pH or osmolarity, not for at home patients
Midline catheters	Hydration, PPN, short-term access	Less frequent infiltration/phlebitis than angiocatheters, 2–4 week dwell time, cannot be used for solutions with extreme pH or osmolarity, not for at home patients
Peripherally inserted central catheters (PICCs)	Hydration, antibiotic, blood transfusions, venous sampling, chemotherapy, medication administration	Requires weekly dressing change and flushing, must keep dry at all times, limited flow rates, visible, potential for easily dislodgement, higher occlusion rate, avoid placement if potential dialysis in future, up to 12 month dwell time
Nontunneled central venous catheters: a. Central lines b. Temporary dialysis or pheresis catheters	a. Acute-care medication, large-bore access, hydration, all IV medication, CVP measurements b. Hemodialysis, stem cell collection and transplant requiring only double-lumen access, plasmapheresis treatment	Short dwell time: 7–14 days for central lines, 1–4 weeks for pheresis catheters, higher risk of infection than tunneled catheter, increased risk of dislodgement, highly visible, increased risk for pneumothorax, not typically used for at home patients
Tunneled central venous catheters: a. Traditional tunneled catheter b. Tunneled dialysis catheters c. Hybrid triple-lumen tunneled catheters	a. Long-term IV medication, hydration, chemotherapy b. Hemodialysis, plasmapheresis, stem cell collection/double-lumen transplant access c. Stem cell collection, transplantation requiring triple lumen	Requires routine dressing changes and flushing, must keep site dry at all times, may be visible to others, lower risk of infection than non-tunneled catheters
Implantable ports a. Chest ports b. Arm ports	Intermittent IV access, chemotherapy, hydration, antibiotics, lab draws	Requires needle stick to access, difficult to access in obese patients, port may rotate and become difficult to access, typically requires OR procedure for placement and removal

training or certification is not required for insertions and most practitioners are qualified to place a PIV. These catheters come in a variety of gauges and lengths to accommodate patients as well as large-bore peripheral catheters preferred for rapid infusion of large volumes such as venous contrast or blood products. Intermittent nonvesicant chemotherapy can be administered via peripheral access. However, reliability of obtaining access during each treatment session may be unpredictable and if unsuccessful, may delay treatment. Therapeutic agents with extremes of pH (normal pH = 7.35 to 7.45) or osmolarity (normal 280 to 295 mOsm/L) should not be administered through peripheral access as the concentration of material infused can lead to patient discomfort, infiltration, clotting, and infection. One exception is parenteral nutrition in which dextrose contents are under 10% and the osmolarities >500 mOsm/L (INS). In this case, it is considered safe to administer this therapy peripherally. Limitations of PIV catheters include short dwell time (1 to 3 days), high thrombophlebitis rates, thrombosis and shear of the vessel, infiltration into the surrounding tissue, cellulitis, and pain with infusions. As a result of these limitations, PIVs are reserved primarily for hospital/clinic use and management by health-care professionals.

One subclass of peripheral angiocatheters is the *midline catheter*. With the guidance of a handheld ultrasound device, these catheters are usually inserted at the antecubital fossa or into the brachial veins. The catheter is approximately 20 cm in length and typically is placed with the tip near or in the axillary vein. In this position, the catheter is not considered central and should be treated as a peripheral angiocatheter with regard to infusates. However, since the catheter tip is in a larger vessel with increased blood flow, the risk of phlebitis and infiltration is decreased as compared to peripheral angiocatheters. Typical dwell time for midline catheters is 2 to 4 weeks with careful monitoring for complications. In addition to extended dwell time, the midline catheter, unlike the PICC, does not need radiographic verification for tip placement, since it is not advanced centrally. As a result, this is a less costly means of access and simplifies positioning. Phlebitis and thrombosis are also less likely to occur with midline catheters as compared to central venous lines. Midlines are particularly beneficial in patients who would otherwise

TABLE 41.2 **Complication of Central Venous Access Devices**

Complication	PICC	Non-tunneled Catheter	Tunneled Catheter	Implantable Port
Arterial puncture	Rare	Internal jugular: 6.3%–9.4% Subclavian: 3.1%–4.9% Femoral: 9.0%–15.0%	Internal jugular: 6.3%–9.4% Subclavian:3.1%–4.9% Femoral: 9.0%–15.0%	Internal jugular: 6.3%–9.4% Subclavian: 3.1%–4.9% Femoral: 9.0%–15.0%
Malposition	10%	Right IJ: 4.3% Left IJ: 12% Right subclavian: 9.3% Left subclavian: 7.3%	Right IJ: 4.3% Left IJ: 12% Right subclavian: 9.3% Left subclavian: 7.3%	Right IJ: 4.3% Left IJ: 12% Right subclavian: 9.3% Left subclavian: 7.3%
Pneumothorax	NA	Internal jugular: 0.1%–0.2% Subclavian: 1.5%–3.1%	Internal jugular: 0.1%–0.2% Subclavian:1.5%–3.1%	Internal jugular: 0.1%–0.2% Subclavian: 1.5%–3.1%
Bacteremia	2.1/1,000 catheter days	2.7/1,000 catheter days	1.6/1,000 catheter days	0.1/1,000 catheter days
Pocket infection	NA	NA	NA	0.7%
References	17, 24, 26	17, 23, 25	17, 23	17, 18, 23

require serial placements of short PIVs and do not need the long-term access or a PICC line. Midline catheters can also be used when there is a relative contraindication to PICC access such as in patients with end-stage renal disease where the central veins should be accessed as minimally as possible.

Midline catheters do have limitations. First, their tips do not reside centrally so infusates are limited to those that are safe for PIVs. Since the axillary vein lies deep in the axillary region, it may be difficult to identify early phlebitis, infiltration, or infection. Frequently, a blood return is not achieved for confirmation of vascular patency or specimen collection. The short intravenous catheter length compared to the external component yields increased risk of dislodgement. Midline catheters require daily flushing to maintain patency and dressing changes at least weekly, which may require home health services. Moreover, catheter-related bloodstream infection rates are similar to those of PICCs.

Peripherally Inserted Central Catheters (PICC)

Hoshal first described the peripherally inserted central venous catheter (CVC) in 1975. In a case series, he described threading 61 cm silicone catheters into the SVC through the basilic or cephalic veins. Thirty of 36 catheters lasted the entire duration of treatment (up to 56 days) of total parenteral nutrition and thus successful application of the concept of central access. In current practice, a PICC is a long, flexible catheter inserted into a peripheral vein and advanced into the central circulation, typically placed in a vein of the upper arm. Alternative access sites can include the internal or external jugular veins, the long or short saphenous veins, the temporal vein, or the posterior auricular veins. The saphenous, temporal, and posterior auricular veins are typically reserved for pediatric patients. Once the vein is cannulated, the catheter is advanced until its distal tip resides in the superior vena cava (SVC) or the IVC, depending on originating vein. The tip location of the PICC is desired in the lower third of the SVC, preferably at the junction of the right atrium with either the SVC or the IVC. The external component is secured to skin, preferably with a removable locking device or sutures. One advantage of a PICC line is there is minimal risk to chest organs as compared to catheters placed directly in the central venous system.

PICCs come in single, dual, or triple lumens and a variety of luminal sizes. The catheters have a small outer diameter allowing for initial insertion into smaller vessels prior to advancement centrally and are radio-opaque for visualization of catheter tip placement on chest radiograph. The length of these devices can be modified to accommodate different patient body habitus.

PICCs are used for patients with poor venous access that need infusions of solutions with extreme pH or osmolarity, extended intravenous medications use (1 week to several months in duration), intermittent blood sampling, and as a respite from long-term catheters. For these purposes, PICCs are associated with greater ease and safety with insertion when compared with conventional CVCs. Moreover, PICCs also help minimize the pain associated with repeated venipuncture whether for replacement IVs or lab draws. Power-injectable PICCs may be utilized in patients where frequent contrasted imaging studies are likely. Certified nurses can perform insertions during inpatient hospitalization, in outpatient settings, and in the home.

There are a few potentially negative factors to take into consideration when contemplating the placement of a PICC line. PICC lines have relatively small lumen(s) and the long length of the catheter results in decreased flow rates. This is especially so with infusions of viscous solutions such as blood products and intravenous nutrition therapy. PICC lines often cannot be used for gravity-driven infusions as is frequently used in a home settings. Frequent flushing of the catheter with normal saline and/ or heparin lock, and dressing changes weekly or more frequently may be challenging for some patients. In addition, careful attention is required to protect the exposed catheter exit site from contamination or damage and a patient's modesty may be compromised due to visibility of the external component. There are activity limitations with PICC catheters that include but are not limited to any straining maneuvers such as heavy lifting or straining that could elevate the intra-thoracic pressure leading to catheter malposition. Malpositioning can even occur with physiologic pressure changes during cough or forceful emesis. Submersion of the extremity in water when bathing in pools or hot tubs is forbidden secondary to increased infection risks. Patients may not be candidates for PICCs if they have had surgical alteration of vascular anatomy, lymphedema, ipsilateral radiation to the chest or arm, loss of skin integrity at the anticipated insertion site, or anticipate future dialysis access needs. Finally, due to their small caliber, these lines are not considered adequate intravenous access for resuscitation in the setting of hemodynamic compromise.

However minimal, PICC-related complications should be recognized. These include infection, phlebitis, vein thrombosis, catheter occlusion, catheter fracture and leak, and inadvertent removal prior to completion of therapy (Table 41.2). At a baseline, oncology patients are at increased risk for venous thrombus formation secondary to their malignancy, treatment regimen, and the trauma of catheter insertion. Improper final tip positioning and subclavian access as opposed internal jugular access may also contribute to thrombosis. However, in cancer patients, PICCs have been shown to have less incidence of deep venous thrombosis than tunneled catheters used for the same purpose.

Percutaneous Central Venous Catheters

Aubaniac was the first to describe cannulation of a central vein (the subclavian) for venous access. These CVCs, either the thin flexible or the larger rigid variety, are inserted directly into the central circulation via the subclavian vein, the external jugular vein, the internal jugular vein, or the femoral vein. Catheters included in this category include the standard CVC or temporary rigid hemodialysis/apheresis catheters. CVCs are typically used for rapid infusion, when multiple infusates are needed simultaneously or for hemodynamic monitoring (central venous pressure measurement). Thus, CVCs are for use in hospitalized patients in acute care settings only with typical dwell times of 7 to 14 days.

The rigid, non-tunneled, central catheters are typically used for acute hemodialysis, access after removal of an infected tunneled dialysis catheter, stem cell collection for autologous transplant, healthy donor collection, or for therapeutic apheresis. Certified nurse practitioners, physician assistants, or physicians can place these catheters, in a surgical suite, or in interventional radiology. Image guidance is essential. Catheter exchange at the same venous site can indefinitely maintain a single access site, which may be limited in hemodialysis patients or oncology patients due to prior access and thrombosis of other central access points, however this practice should be reserved for the patient with truly limited central venous access.

Complications related to these devices include infection, bleeding, inadvertent arterial access, air embolism, pneumothorax, hemothorax, cardiac perforation with tamponade, and cardiac dysrhythmia. The cancer patient with cachexia is at increased risk for insertion complications as are patients with large body habitus or coagulopathies. Utilization of image-guided placement with ultrasound technology for venipuncture and modified Seldinger approach helps to minimize these risks. While the catheter is in place, infections, thrombosis of the accessed vein, loss of catheter lumen patency, and dislodgment can occur and consideration should be made for removal of the device if this occurs. Frequent assessment of the catheter for integrity, dislodgment, and site evaluation is required. Flushing of each catheter lumen is performed frequently for patency. The catheter exit site must be kept dry with an intact occlusive dressing and changed biweekly to minimize infection risks. The lumens are usually given a high-dose heparin lock to maintain patency. Accidental dislodgment of the rigid catheter can occur even though sutures are placed and due to the large caliber of these devices, unrecognized dislodgement can lead to life-threatening hemorrhage. Usage of these catheters and dressing changes are typically reserved for certified technicians or nurses to provide consistent management.

Tunneled Catheters

A tunneled catheter is a larger bore catheter inserted into the central circulation followed by tunneling through the subcutaneous tissue to an exit site remote from the access site. After tunneling, the catheter is advanced into the central circulation via the jugular veins, subclavian vein, femoral vein, or lumbar vein access (only in vein-compromised patients). The tip of the catheter should terminate in the SVC/right atrial junction or IVC/right atrial junction, depending on venous access origin. A retention cuff, which causes inflammation and ingrowth into the cuff, is integrated on the catheter and the cuff is positioned approximately 1 to 2 cm within the skin insertion point. The cuff serves as a barrier to bacteria migration along the tract into the central circulation. Additionally, the cuff helps prevent inadvertent catheter dislodgement.

Tunneled catheters can be further divided into three types: traditional tunneled catheters, dialysis catheters, and hybrid tunneled catheters. The traditional tunneled catheters are best known as the Hickman or Broviac catheter. These are intended for patients requiring long-term central venous access use in instances such as total parenteral nutrition, chemotherapy, chronic medication administration, transfusions, and blood sampling. The second are the dialysis catheters. These are typically used for hemodialysis but they are also utilized for stem cell collection and posttransplant venous access. The final catheter type, the hybrid tunneled catheters, are most often used in transplant patients for stem cell collection, transplant access, or photophoresis treatments in graft-versus-host disease. All three of these catheters are available in single, double, or triple lumens, with a variety of lumen sizes and catheter lengths. These catheters are known for lower infection rate as compared to nontunneled catheters.

Management of tunneled catheters requires flushing protocols, weekly dressing changes, and protection from inadvertent dislodgment. In addition, the patient is restricted from submersion of the catheter during bathing or swimming. Tunneled catheters with high-dose heparin lock solution require removal of the lock prior to catheter use to prevent inadvertent systemic heparinization. Catheters containing valve devices may only require saline flushes, thus simplifying this regimen.

Complications of tunneled catheters include those associated with the insertion procedure (i.e., bleeding, air embolus, pneumothorax, hemothorax, and cardiac dysrhythmia) as well as long-term issues (i.e., infection, migration, thrombosis, and catheter shear). Most medical centers will stock catheter repair kits that allow for the salvage of cracked or leaking catheters. Extrusion of the cuff from the subcutaneous position is an indication for replacement or removal of the tunneled catheter.

Implanted Ports

Implanted ports are CVC attached to a reservoir with a self-sealing septum. The reservoir is surgically implanted into a pocket in subcutaneous tissue and the attached catheter is tunneled subcutaneously before advancement into the central venous circulation. The implanted port is ideal for patients undergoing intermittent or cyclic therapy when daily access is not required. Ports are also suited to chemotherapy administration or venous access for lab draws in vein-compromised patients requiring chronic venous access. Early identification of patients who will need ports helps to facilitate placement prior to the anticipated neutropenia, weakness, and wound healing difficulties often associated with chemotherapy. Newer models of implanted ports allow power injections of contrast material for radiologic imaging. Medical device companies also promote ports with differing flow patterns or characteristics within the reservoir chamber (i.e., "the port") that claim to improve infusion, blood draws, and lower thrombosis rates. Compared to tunneled catheters, studies have also demonstrated up to a 10-fold advantage in long term infection rates due to the completely implanted nature of the catheter. Nevertheless, continuous access of the port will certainly defeat this advantage. Ports provide patients with improved modesty as it is not visible, especially if the port pocket is located in a discrete location. In addition, active patients may find more freedom during de-accessed periods. These catheters have an extended dwell time of several years or longer depending on number of punctures into the septum and the needs of the patient. Consideration should be given to retaining the port for a period of time after completion of therapy for use in surveillance blood testing purposes.

Patients with uncontrolled coagulopathy, bacteremia, or sepsis should have those conditions addressed prior to the placement of a new indwelling device, as with other CVADs. Some individuals with severe malnutrition or cachexia may have an extremely poor healing capacity and may be at undue risk for port erosion through the skin. These patients should undergo therapy with a PICC or other alternative until such a time when a port may be better tolerated.

As mentioned previously, the port is placed in a subcutaneous pocket most commonly in a location on the anterior chest wall, the arm, or thigh with the catheter advanced into the corresponding vein. Use of the port requires sterile preparation of the site and access with a non-coring, Huber needle, to prevent damage to the reservoir. As the entire system is subcutaneous, the patient may feel a needle stick as the port is being accessed, but applying topical anesthetics to the skin over the port prior to the needle stick may minimize the discomfort. While the port is accessed, it requires daily flushing and it must be flushed after each use as well. When the port is not actively being used, monthly flushes are required to help maintain patency. Complications associated with ports are rare and are divided into early and late events. Early complications in oncology patients include hematomas, malpositioning, and iatrogenic pneumothoraces. Late complications are dominated by catheter thrombosis and infection, however catheter facture and embolization can also occur.

SPECIAL CONSIDERATIONS

Power Injection Catheters

Traditional catheters have been studied in the past for safety when power injections are done for radiographic studies with mixed results. The studies found efficacy depends on the gauge, length, and material of the catheter. Incidence of inadequate flow rates and catheter rupture due to limited pounds per square inch (PSI) restrictions outlined by the manufacturers limits the use of most catheters for power injection. However, more recent products over come these limitations. Optimal contrast imaging requires uniform contrast delivery, which is best achieved by power injection at 2 mL/s. In fact, these limitations have led to current trends in catheter manufacturing resulting in some catheters capable of tolerating 300 PSI. One should consider power injection catheters for patients anticipated to have recurring contrast medium injection studies. Special equipment may be required for accessing power injection ports so as to prevent rupture or extravasation. In addition, the more rigid catheter required for power injection may lead to increased complications such as phlebitis or thrombosis.

Herts et al. studied a variety of CVCs including standard CVC, tunneled catheters, and implanted ports and found power injections are possible without harm to the patients or the catheters. Their findings suggest usage of central lines as a possible alternative to peripheral angiocatheters. Before using standard central access devices for power injection, institutional policies should be in place to address the practice as there may be additional training required of the staff prior to utilizing such devices to minimize complications.

Valve Technology

Ongoing clinical presentation of heparin allergies, specifically heparin-induced thrombocytopenia has led to the development of catheters with valve technology. The valve remains closed unless acted upon by negative (aspiration) or positive (infusion) pressure. By opposing central venous pressure and preventing the reflux of blood into the catheter tip during the cardiac cycle or changes in intrathoracic pressure that naturally occurs in everyday life, valvular technology is designed to improve patency and minimize exposure and/or need for regular flushing of the device. Additionally, removal of a syringe after flushing or de-accessing the port can facilitate negative pressure drawing blood into the catheter. Without blood in the catheter tip, the risk of catheter occlusion related to internal clotting is thought to be eliminated. Lamont et al. found the PASV (Boston Scientific Corporation, Natick, Mass) valved implanted port had a lower incidence of difficulty in obtaining a blood return than the Groshong (Bard Access System, Salt Lake City, Utah), which resulted in less nursing time trouble shooting malfunctioning or poorly functioning catheters. Valve technology has been incorporated into some catheters at the distal tip or in the proximal end piece. This technology is also available as an "add-on" device for catheters. A saline-only flush is recommended; however, heparin flushes are not a contraindication.

CONCLUSION

The diagnosis of a malignancy and the subsequent rigorous treatment regime(s) are overwhelming for most patients. If venous access for administration of treatment becomes difficult, it adds to a patients stress and anxiety during an already difficult time of their life. Central venous access devices can and often do minimize that one aspect of a patients care. However, care must be taken to ensure the device selected and placed is optimal for the type of treatment regime selected. Treatment factors to consider (but not limited to) include frequency of therapy administration, pH and osmolality of the medication, location of treatment (home vs. hospital) and duration of therapy. Patient characteristics to take into account include comorbidities, prior line placement, history of thrombosis or thrombophlebitis, and the ability and resources to care for a device. Finally, and most importantly, the patient should be able to help select the device that is most appropriate for them based on their lifestyle and personal preferences. When selected and used appropriately, central venous devices are extremely useful to the patient and the provider as they allow for adherence to treatment regimes while minimizing patient discomfort.

Suggested Readings

1. Alexandrou E, Spencer TR, et al. Central venous catheter placement by advanced practice nurses demonstrates a low procedural complication and infection rates - a report from 13 years of service. *Crit Care med.* 2014;42(3):536–543.
2. Aubaniac R. Subclavian intravenous injection: advantages and tehnic. *Presse Med.* 1952;60(68):1456.
3. Chemaly RF, de Parres JB, Rehm SJ. Venous thrombosis associated with peripherally inserted central catheters: a retrospective analysis of the Cleveland clinic experience. *Clin Infect Dis.* 2002;34:1179–1183.
4. Chopra V, Anand S, Krein SL, Chenoweth C, Saint S. Bloodstream infection, venous thrombosis, and peripherally inserted central catheters: reappraising the evidence. *Am J Med.* 2012 Aug;125(8):733–741.
5. Gallieni M, Pittiruti M, Biffi R. Vascular access in oncology patients. *CA Cancer J Clin.* 2008;58:323–34.
6. Graham A, Ozment C, Tegtmeyer K, et al. Central venous catheterization. *N Engl J Med.* 2007;356:e21.
7. Herts B, O'Malley C, Wirht S, Lieber M, Pohlman B. Power injection of contrast media using central venous catheters. *Am J Roentgenol.* 2001;176:447–453.
8. Hoffer E, Borsa J, Santulli P, Bloch R, Fontaine A. Prospective randomized comparison of valved versus nonvalved peripherally inserted central vein catheters. *Am J Roentgeno.* 1999;173:1393–1398.
9. Hoshal VL Jr. Total intravenous nutrition with peripherally inserted silicone elastomer central venous catheters. *Arch Surg.* 1975;110(5):644–646.
10. Kim JT, Oh TY, Chang WH, Jeong YK. Clinical review and analysis of complications of totally implantable venous access devices for chemotherapy. *Med Oncol.* 2012;29:1361–1364.
11. Lamont J, McCarty T, Stephens J, et al. A randomized trial of valved vs nonvalved implantable ports for vascular access. *BUMC Proc.* 2003;16:384–387.
12. Maki D, Kluger D, Crnich C. The risk of bloodstream infection in adults with different intravascular devices: a systematic review of 200 published prospective studies. *May Clin Proc.* 2006;81:1159–1171.
13. Marcy P. Central venous access: techniques and indications in osncology. *Eur Radiol.* 2008;18(10):2333–2344.
14. McGee D, Gould M. Preventing complications of central venous catheterization. *N Engl J Med.* 2003;348:1123–1133.
15. Randolph A, Cook D, Gonzales C, et al. Tunneling short-term central venous catheters to prevent catheter-related infection: a meta-analysis of randomized, controlled trials. *Crit Care Med.* 1998;26(8):1452–1457.
16. Saber W, Moua T, Williams E, et al. Risk factors for catheter-related thrombosis (CRT) in cancer patients: a patient-level data (IPD) meta-analysis of clinical trials and prospective studies. *J Thromb Haemost.* 2011;9:312–319.
17. Sansivero G. Features and selection of vascular access devices. *Semin Oncol Nurs.* 2010;26(2):88–101.
18. Schummer W, Schummer C, Rose N, et al. Mechanical complications and malpositions of central venous cannulations by experienced operators. A prospective study of 1794 catheterizations in critically ill patients. *Intensive Care Med.* 2007;33(6):1055–1059.
19. Schwengel D, McGready J, Berenholtz S, Kozlowski L, Nichols D, Yaster M. Peripherally inserted central catheters: a randomized, controlled, prospective trial in pediatric surgical patients. *Anesth Analg.* 2004;99:1038–1043.
20. Scott E, Hudson K, Trerotola S, Smith H, Porter D, Sood S. Risk factors for venous thromboembolism in hospitalized cancer patients with central catheters. *ASH Annu Meet Abstr.* 2010;116:810–855.
21. Todd J, Hammond P. Choice and use of peripherally inserted central catheters by nurses. *Prof Nurse.* 2004;19:493–497.
22. Trerotola SO, Thompson S, Chittams J, et al. Analysis of tip malposition and correction in peripherally inserted central catheters placed at bedside by a dedicated nursing team. *J Vasc Interv Radiol.* 2007;18:513–518.
23. Vanek V. The ins and outs of venous access: part I. *Nutr Clin Pract.* 2002;17(2):85–98.
24. Verso M, Agnelli G. Venous thromboembolism associated with long-term use of central venous catheters in cancer patients. *J Clin Oncol.* 2003;21(19):3665–3675.
25. Walser E. Venous access ports: indications, implantation technique, follow-up, and complications. *Cardiovasc Intervent Radiol.* 2012;35(4):751–764.
26. Williamson E, McKinnley J. Assessing the adequacy of peripherally inserted central catheters for power injection of intravenous contrast agents for CT. *J Comput Assist Tomogr.* 2001;25(6):932–937.

Procedures in Medical Oncology 42

Kerry Ryan and George Carter

Procedures performed in oncology patients may serve both diagnosis and treatment. This chapter describes common procedures performed in medical oncology, along with special considerations and techniques to assist in performing them rapidly and confidently, and to keep the patient comfortable and well informed.

INFORMED CONSENT AND UNIVERSAL PROTOCOL

Written informed consent, or a legally sufficient substitute, must be obtained before every procedure described here and filed in the patient's medical record. If appropriate for the planned procedure, mark the procedure side and perform a "time out" to verify correct patient, correct site, and correct procedure.

ANESTHESIA

All procedures are typically performed under local anesthesia. For certain patients and procedures, premedication with a narcotic (fentanyl) and a benzodiazepine (midazolam) should be considered. Lidocaine (1% mixed in a 3:1 or 5:1 ratio with $NaHCO_3$ to prevent the usual lidocaine sting) or alternative anesthetic will ensure proper anesthetic effect.

INSTRUMENTS

Most medical facilities are equipped with sterile trays or self-contained disposable kits specific to each procedure. Additional instruments may be used at the operator's discretion or preference.

PROCEDURES

Bone Marrow Aspiration and Biopsy

Indications

- Diagnosis
- Analysis of abnormal blood cell production
- Staging of hematologic and non-hematologic malignancies

Contraindications

- Only absolute contraindication is the presence of hemophilia, severe disseminated intravascular coagulopathy, or other severe bleeding disorder.
- Severe thrombocytopenia is not a contraindication. However, depending on the circumstances may transfuse for platelets <20,000.
- Skin infection at proposed site of biopsy; consider alternative site.
- Biopsy at previously radiated site may cause fibrosis; consider alternative site.
- Avoid sternal aspirate in patients under the age of 12, with thoracic aortic aneurysm, or with lytic bone disease of ribs or sternum.
- Determine if the patient is taking an anticoagulation agent or clopidogrel. If the patient is on these medications, consider stopping them if the risk of bleeding outweighs the risk of thrombosis in the patient. Bone Marrow Biopsy is considered a low risk bleeding for bleeding.

Anatomy

- Sternal aspiration (not recommended as a site of biopsy due to risk of fatal hemorrhage, if it is a chosen site then a skilled and experienced clinician should perform procedure).
  - Patient is supine; head is not elevated.
  - Landmarks: sternal angle of Louis and lateral borders of sternum in second intercostal space.
- Posterior superior iliac spine aspiration and biopsy (Fig. 42.1) (this is the preferred site of biopsy and aspiration).
  - Patient is prone or in lateral decubitus position.
- Anterior iliac crest aspiration and biopsy (consider for patients with history of radiation to pelvis or extremely obese patients).
  - Patient is supine.

Imaging Guidance

Some institutions have started performing bone marrow biopsy and aspiration of the posterior iliac crest with the use of CT guidance. Imaging guidance should be considered, particularly, in obese patients where surface anatomical landmarks may prove unreliable.

Procedure

- Posterior superior iliac spine aspiration and biopsy
  1. The technique described here is for the Jamshidi bone marrow needle. Other available needles, such as the HS Trapsystem Set, Goldenberg Snarecoil, T-Lok bone marrow biopsy system, are variations of the Jamshidi with their own specific instructions. Also available is the OnControl

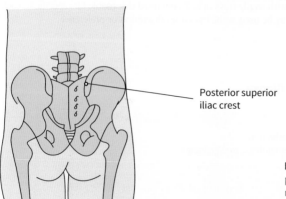

Posterior superior iliac crest

FIGURE 42.1 Biopsy site in the posterior superior iliac spine. The needle should be directed toward the anterior superior iliac spine.

Bone Marrow Biopsy System that utilizes a battery-powered drill to insert the needle into the iliac bone.

2. The patient may be prone, but the lateral decubitus position is more comfortable for the patient and better for identifying anatomic sites. These positions are suitable for all but the most obese patients. For extremely obese patients or for those who have had radiation to the pelvis, aspirate and biopsy may be taken from the anterior iliac crest.

3. Once the site has been prepared and anesthetized, make a small incision at the site of insertion, and advance the needle into the bone cortex until it is fixed. Attempt to aspirate 0.2 to 0.5 mL of marrow contents. If unsuccessful, advance the needle slightly and try again. Failure to obtain aspirate, known as a "dry tap," is often due to alterations within the marrow associated with myeloproliferative or leukemic disorders and less commonly due to faulty technique. In such case, a touch preparation of the biopsy often provides sufficient cellular material for diagnostic evaluation.

4. Biopsy can be performed directly after aspiration without repositioning to a different site on the posterior iliac crest. Advance the needle using a twisting motion, without the obturator in place, to obtain the recommended 1.5 to 2 cm biopsy specimen. To ensure successful specimen collection, rotate the needle briskly in one direction and then the other, then gently rock the needle in four directions by exerting pressure perpendicular to the shaft with the needle capped. Gently remove the needle while rotating it in a corkscrew manner. Remove the specimen from the needle by pushing it up through the hub with a stylet, taking care to avoid needle stick injuries. Jamshidi needle kits include a small, clear plastic guide to facilitate this process.

Aftercare

▪ Place a pressure dressing over the site and apply direct external pressure for 5 to 10 minutes to avoid prolonged bleeding and hematoma formation.

▪ The pressure dressing should remain in place for 24 hours.

▪ The patient may shower after the pressure dressing is removed, but should avoid immersion in water for 1 week after the procedure to avoid infection.

Complications

Infection and hematoma are the most common complications of bone marrow biopsy and aspiration. Careful technique during and after the procedure can minimize these effects.

Lumbar Puncture

Indications

▪ Analysis of cerebrospinal fluid (CSF), including pressure measurement, for diagnosis and to assess adequacy of treatment

▪ Administration of intrathecal chemotherapy

Contraindications

▪ Increased intracranial pressure

▪ Coagulopathy or thrombocytopenia. There is not significant data regarding the optimum platelet count at which a lumbar puncture can be performed. American National Red Cross transfusion guidelines suggested a minimum of 40,000

▪ Infection near planned site of lumbar puncture (LP)

▪ Anticoagulation agents and clopidogrel should be discontinued before procedure and may be resumed after hemostasis is achieved.

Anatomy

▪ Avoid interspaces above L3 (Fig. 42.2), as the conus medullaris rarely ends below L3 (L1–L2 in adults, L2–L3 in children).

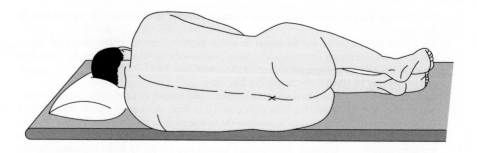

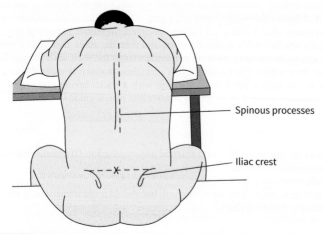

Spinous processes

Iliac crest

FIGURE 42.2 Anatomy of the lumbar spine. Ideal needle insertion is between L3 and L4 interspace, which can be found where the line joining the superior iliac crests intersects the spinous process of L4. Positioning of patient for lumbar puncture: in lateral decubitis or sitting positon. (From Zuber TJ, Mayeaux EF. *Atlas of Primary Care Procedures*. Philadelphia, PA: Lippincott Williams & Wilkins; 1994:13.)

- The L4 spinous process or L4 to L5 interspace lies in the center of the supracristal plane (a line drawn between the posterior and superior iliac crests).
- There are eight layers from the skin to the subarachnoid space: skin, supraspinous ligament, interspinous ligament, ligamentum flava, epidural space, dura, subarachnoid membrane, and subarachnoid space.

Imaging Guidance

The fluoroscopic guidance for a LP should be considered if multiple attempts without imaging were performed and were unsuccessful. Also, could be considered if the patient is obese or has a difficult anatomy due to prior surgery.

Procedure

1. Describe the procedure to the patient, with assurances that you will explain what you are about to do before you do it.
2. Patient should be in a lateral decubitus or sitting position. The prone position is usually used for LPs performed under fluoroscopic guidance and will not be discussed here. The lateral decubitus

position is preferable for obtaining opening pressures. The seated position may be used if the patient is obese or has difficulty remaining in the lateral decubitus position. Either seated or lying on one side, the patient should curl into a fetal position with the spine flexed to widen the gap between spinous processes (Fig. 42.2).

3. Identify anatomic landmarks and the interspace to be used for the procedure.
4. Using sterile technique, prepare the area and one interspace above or below it with povidone-iodine solution. Drape the patient, establishing a sterile field.
5. Using 1% lidocaine/bicarb mixture, anesthetize the skin and deeper tissues, carefully avoiding epidural or spinal anesthesia.
6. Insert the spinal needle through the skin into the spinous ligament, keeping the needle parallel to the bed or table. Immediately angle the needle 30 to 45 degrees cephalad. The bevel of the spinal needle should be positioned facing the patient's flank, allowing the needle to spread rather than cut the dural sac. Advance the needle through the eight layers in small increments. With practice, an experienced operator can identify the "pop" as the needle penetrates the dura into the subarachnoid space. Even so, it is wise to remove the stylet to check for CSF before each advance of the needle.
7. When the presence of CSF is confirmed, attach a manometer (either traditional manometer or digital pressure transducer device) to the hub of the needle to measure opening pressure. Collect the minimum amount of CSF required to perform the tests being ordered, typically 8 to 15 mL of CSF is required. If special studies are required, up to 40 mL of CSF may be safely removed. Confirm with your laboratory the order of the tests that should be done on each tube, as different laboratories have different preferences.
8. Replace the stylet, withdraw the needle, observe the site for CSF leak or hemorrhage, and bandage appropriately.
9. Ease the patient into a recumbent position. Bedrest is often still done for a period of time following a LP; however, it has been established that bed rest does not decrease the incidence of headache after lumbar puncture.

Complications

▪ Spinal headache occurs in approximately 20% of patients after LP. Incidence appears to be related to needle size and CSF leak and not to post-procedure positioning. There is no evidence that increased fluid intake prevents spinal headache. It is characterized by pounding pain in the occipital region when the patient is upright. Incidence is highest in female patients, younger patients (peak 20 to 40), and patients with a history of headache prior to LP. Patients should remain recumbent if possible and take over-the-counter analgesics. For severe and/or persistent spinal headache, stronger medication, caffeine, or an epidural blood patch may be indicated. Data indicate that a Sprotte ("pencil-tipped") needle reduces the risk of post-LP headache.
▪ Nerve root trauma is possible but rare. A low interspace entry site reduces the risk of this complication.
▪ Cerebellar or medullary herniation occurs rarely in patients with increased intracranial pressure. If recognized early, this process can be reversed.
▪ Infection, including meningitis.
▪ Bleeding. A small number of red blood cells in the CSF is common. In approximately 1% to 2% of patients, serious bleeding can result in neurologic compromise from spinal hematoma. Risk is highest in patients with thrombocytopenia or serious bleeding disorders, or patients given anticoagulants immediately before or after LP.

Paracentesis

Indications

▪ To confirm diagnosis or assess diagnostic markers
▪ As treatment for ascites resulting from tumor metastasis or obstruction

Contraindications

▪ The complication rate for this procedure is about 1%.

- The potential benefit of therapeutic paracentesis outweighs the risk of coagulopathy. However, they should be avoided in patients with disseminated intravascular coagulation.
- Perform with caution in patients that have organomegaly, bowel obstruction, distended bladder, or intra-abdominal adhesions. Consider ultrasound guidance in these patients. Also, a nasogastric tube should be placed first in patients with bowel obstruction and a urinary catheter should be inserted in patients with urinary retention.
- Modify site location to avoid surgical scars. Surgical scars have been associated with tethering of the bowel to the abdominal wall.

Anatomy

- Identify the area of greatest abdominal dullness by percussion, or mark the area of ascites via ultrasound. Take care to avoid abdominal vasculature and viscera.

Procedure

1. Place the patient in a comfortable supine position at the edge of a bed or table.
2. Identify the area of the abdomen to be accessed (Fig. 42.3). Ultrasound can be used to confirm the presence of fluid and the absence of bowel or spleen in the selected site.
3. Prepare the area with povidone-iodine solution and establish a sterile field by draping the patient.
4. Anesthetize the area with a 1% lidocaine/bicarb mixture.
5. For diagnostic paracentesis, insert a 22- to 25-gauge needle attached to a sterile syringe into the skin, then pull the skin laterally and advance the needle into the abdomen. Release the tension on the skin and withdraw an appropriate amount of fluid for testing. This skin-retraction method creates a "z" track into the peritoneal cavity, which minimizes the risk of ascitic leak after the procedure (Fig. 42.4).
6. For therapeutic paracentesis, use the z-track method with a multiple-port flexible catheter over a guide needle. When the catheter is in place, the ascites may be evacuated into multiple containers. Make sure that the patient remains hemodynamically stable while removing large amounts of ascites.

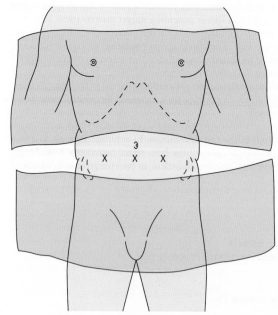

FIGURE 42.3 Sites for diagnostic paracentesis. (From Zuber TJ, Mayeaux EF. *Atlas of Primary Care Procedures.* Philadelphia, PA: Lippincott Williams & Wilkins; 1994:46.)

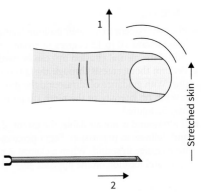

FIGURE 42.4 "Z"-track technique for inserting needle into peritoneal cavity. (From Zuber TJ, Mayeaux EF. *Atlas of Primary Care Procedures*. Philadelphia, PA: Lippincott Williams & Wilkins; 1994:47.)

7. When the procedure is completed, withdraw the needle or catheter and, if there is no bleeding or ascitic leakage, place a pressure bandage over the site.
8. Following therapeutic paracentesis, the patient should remain supine until all vital signs are stable. Offer the patient assistance getting down from the bed or table.
9. If necessary, standard medical procedures should be used to reverse orthostasis. The patient should be hemodynamically stable before being allowed to leave the operating area.

Complications

- Hemorrhage, ascitic leak, infection, and perforated abdominal viscus have been reported. Properly siting paracentesis virtually eliminates these complications.

Thoracentesis

Indications

- Diagnostic or therapeutic removal of pleural fluid.

Contraindications

There are no absolute contraindications to diagnostic thoracentesis. Relative contraindications include the following:

- Coagulopathy and thrombocytopenia (platelets less than 50,000/uL). A decision to reverse the coagulopathy or correct the thrombocytopenia needs to be individualized, weighing the risks and benefits, as a thoracentesis is considered a low-risk bleeding procedure.
- Bullous emphysema (increased risk of pneumothorax)
- Pleural effusion less than 1 cm at its maximum depth adjacent to the parietal pleura (when ultrasound guidance is used).
- Patients on mechanical ventilation with positive end expiratory pressure (PEEP) have no greater risk of developing a pneumothorax than non-ventilated patients. However, mechanically ventilated patients are at greater risk of developing tension physiology or persistent air leak if a pneumothorax does occur.
- Patients unable to cooperate.
- Cellulitis, if thoracentesis would require penetrating the inflamed tissue.

Imaging Guidance

Ultrasound-guided thoracentesis has become a standard of practice in most institutions for performing a thoracentesis, as it decreases the risk of pneumothorax and has a higher sensitivity for identifying pleural effusions. An ultrasound should be used to identify the puncture site either while the procedure is being done or before the procedure is done to mark the site. If a pleural effusion is complex or loculated, CT imaging may be required.

Anatomy

- Place the patient in a seated position facing a table, arms resting on a raised pillow. Have the patient lean forward 10 to 15 degrees to create intercostal spaces. The lateral recumbent position (with the side of the pleural effusion up) can be used if the patient is unable to sit up.
- Perform thoracentesis through the seventh or eighth intercostal space, along the posterior axillary line. With guidance of ultrasound the procedure may be performed below the fifth rib anteriorly, the seventh rib laterally, or the ninth rib posteriorly. Without radiographic guidance, underlying organs may be injured.
- If ultrasound is not available, the extent of pleural effusion is indicated by decreased tactile fremitus and dullness to percussion. Begin percussion at the top of the chest and move downward, listening for a change in sound. When a change is noted, compare to the percussive sound in the same interspace and location on the opposite side. This will denote the upper extent of pleural effusion.

Procedure

1. After the appropriate site has been identified either by ultrasound or physical exam, position the patient and clean the site with antiseptic. Initially, infiltrate the epidermis using a 25-gauge needle and 1% or 2% lidocaine. Next, with a syringe attached to a 22-guage-needle advance toward the rib and then "walk" over the superior edge of the rib (Fig. 42.5). This decreases the risk of injury to the neurovascular bundle. Aspirate frequently to ensure that no vessel has been pierced and to determine the distance from the skin to the pleural fluid. When pleural fluid is aspirated, remove the anesthesia needle and note the depth of penetration.
2. A small incision may be needed to pass a larger gauge thoracentesis needle into the pleural space. Generally, a 16- to 19-gauge needle with intracath is inserted just far enough to obtain pleural fluid. Fluid that is bloody or different in appearance from the fluid obtained with the anesthesia needle may be an indication of vessel injury. In this case, the procedure must be stopped. If there is no

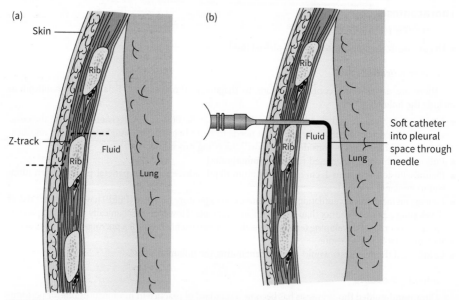

FIGURE 42.5 Thoracentesis. (a) "Z"-track technique for anesthetizing to prevent injury to neurovascular bundle. (b) Advancement of soft plastic catheter through the needle into pleural space. (Zuber TJ, Mayeaux EF. *Atlas of Primary Care Procedures*. Philadelphia, PA: Lippincott Williams & Wilkins; 1994:26, 27.)

apparent change in the pleural fluid aspirated, advance the flexible intracath and withdraw the needle to avoid puncturing the lung as the fluid is drained. Using a flexible intracath with a three-way stopcock allows for removal of a large volume of fluid with less risk of pneumothorax. If only a small sample of pleural fluid is needed, a 22-gauge needle connected to an airtight three-way stopcock is sufficient. Attach tubing to the three-way stopcock and drain fluid manually or by vacutainer. Withdrawing more than 1,000 mL per procedure requires careful monitoring of the patient's hemodynamic status. As the needle is withdrawn, have the patient hum or do the Valsalva maneuver to increase intrathoracic pressure and lower the risk of pneumothorax.

3. After the procedure, obtain a chest radiograph to determine the amount of remaining fluid, to assess lung parenchyma, and to check for pneumothorax. Small pneumothoraces do not require treatment; pneumothoraces involving >50% lung collapse do.

Complications

▪ Pneumothorax
▪ Air embolism (rare)
▪ Infection
▪ Pain at puncture site
▪ Bleeding
▪ Splenic or liver puncture

Suggested Readings

1. Avery RA, Mistry RD, Shah SS, et al. Patient position during lumbar puncture has no meaningful effect on cerebrospinal opening pressure on children. *J Child Neurol.* 2010 Feb 22 [Medicine].
2. Desalpine M, Bragga PK, Gupta PK, Kataria AS. To evaluate the role of bone marrow aspiration and bone marrow biopsy in pancytopenia. *J Clin Diagn Res.* 2014 Nov;8(11):FC 11-5[Medicine]. [Full Text].
3. Duncan DR, Morgenthaler TI, Ryu JH, Daniels CE. Reducing iatrogenic risk in thoracentesis: establishing best practice via experimental training in a new-risk environment. *Chest.* 2009 May;135(5):1315–1320 [Medicine].
4. Ellenby MS, Tegtmeyer K, Lai S, Braner DA. Videos in clinical medicine. Lumbar puncture. *N Engl J Med.* 2006;355(13):e12.
5. Evans RW, Armon C, Frohman EM, Goodin DS. Assessment: prevention of post-lumbar puncture headaches: report of the Therapeutics and Technology Assessment Subcommittee of the American Academy of Neurology. *Neurology.* 2000;55(7):909–914.
6. Fend F, Tzankov A, Bink K, et al. Modern techniques for the diagnostic evaluation of trepine bone marrow biopsy: methodological aspects and application. *Prog Histochem Cytochem.* 2008;42(4):203–252.[Medicine].
7. Hooper C, Maskel N, BTS audit team. British Thoracic Society national pleural procedures audit 2010. *Thorax.* 2011: 66(7):636–637.
8. Humphries JE. Dry tap bone marrow aspiration: clinical significance. *Am J Hematol.* 1990;35(4):247–250.
9. Kuntz KM, Kokmen E, Stevens JC, Miller P, Offord KP, Ho MM. Post-lumbar puncture headaches: experience in 501 consecutive procedures. *Neurology.* 1992;42(10):1884–1887.
10. LeMense GP, Sahn SA. Safety and value of thoracentesis in medical ICU patients. *J Intensive Care Med.* 1998;13:144.
11. Malempati S, Joshi S, Lai S, Braner D, Tegtmeyer K. Bone marrow aspiraiton and biopsy. *N Engl J Med.* 2009; 361:e28.
12. Mc Gibbon A, Chen GI, Peltekian KM, van Zanten SV. An evidence base manual for abdominal paracentesis. *Dig Dis Sci.* 2007 Dec;52(12):3307–3315.[Medicine].
13. McCartney JP, Adams JW II, Hazard PB. Safety of thoracentesis in mechanically ventilated patients. *Chest.* 1993;103(6);1920–1921.
14. Quesada AE, Tholpady A, Wanger A, Nguyen AN, Chen L. Utility of bone marrow examination for workup of fever of unknown origin in patients with HIV/AIDS. *J Clin Pathol.* 2015 Mar;68(3):241–245. [Medicine].
15. Runyon BA. Paracentesis of ascitic fluid. A safe procedure. *Arch Intern Med.* 1986;146(11):2259–2261.
16. Spyropoulos AC, Douketis JD. How I treat anticoagulated patients undergoing an elective procedure or surgery. *Blood* 2012;120:2954.
17. Strupp M, Schueler O, Straube A, Von Stuckrad-Barre S, Brandt T. "Atraumatic" Sprotte needle reduces the incidence of post-lumbar puncture headaches. *Neurology.* 2001;57(12):2310–2312.
18. Swords A, Anguita J, Higgins RA, et al. A new rotary powered device for bone marrow aspiration and biopsy yields superior specimens with less pain: results of a randomized clinical study. *Blood* 2010;116(21):650–651.
19. Thomsen T, DeLaPena J, Setnik G. Thoracentesis. *N Engl J Med.* 2006; 255:e16.

20. Thomsen TW, Shaffer RW, White B, Setnik GS. Videos in clinical medicine. Paracentesis. *N Engl J Med.* 2006 Nov 9;355(19):e21.[Medicine].
21. Tung CE, So YT, Lansberg MG. Cost comparison between the atraumatic and cutting lumbar puncture needles. *Neurology.* 2012 Jan 10;78(2):109–113. Epub 2011 Dec 28.
22. Van Veen JJ, Nokes TJ, Markis M. The risk of spinal haematoma following neuraxial anaesthesia or lumbar puncture in thrombocytopenia invividuals. *Br J Haemetol.* 2009;148:15–25.
23. Wickbom A, Cha SO, Ahlisson A. Thoracentesis in cardiac surgery patients. *Multimed Man Cardiothoracic Surg.* 2015. [Medicine].
24. Williams J, Lyle S, Umpathi T. Diagnostic lumbar puncture minimizing complications. *Intern Med J.* 2008;38:587–591.
25. Wolff SN, Katzenstein AL, Phillips GL, Herzig GP. Aspiration does not influence interpretation of bone marrow biopsy cellularity. *Am J Clin Pathol.* 1983;80(1):60–62.
26. Zuber TJ, Mayeaux EF. *Atlas of Primary Care Procedures.* Philadelphia, PA: Lippincott Williams & Wildins, 1994:26, 27.

Basic Principles of **43** Radiation Oncology

Chirag Shah, Nikhil P. Joshi, and Bindu Manyam

INTRODUCTION

Radiation therapy represents an essential modality in the treatment of patients with many different types of malignancy and differs significantly from other commonly used modalities such as surgery and systemic therapy in its delivery and mechanism of action. The purpose of this chapter is to provide a review of the basics of radiation oncology, including an introduction to radiation biology and radiation physics, a summary of patient workflow and treatment delivery and finally, an evaluation of alternative radiation techniques beyond conventional external beam radiation therapy.

RADIATION BIOLOGY AND PHYSICS

Radiation therapy is primarily delivered using external beam radiation therapy via a linear accelerator with the predominant treatment mode being high-energy photons or x-rays. These photons represent ionizing radiation and are part of the electromagnetic spectrum. Alternatives to photons exist including electrons (available on linear accelerators) and to a lesser degree protons and neutrons (seperate devices). Photon-based radiation therapy is considered indirectly ionizing, in that it does not produce damage directly for the most part but instead has its energy transferred to secondary particles (usually electrons), which produce DNA damage. This primarily occurs through the Compton process for photons. Heavy charged particles, though less frequently used, are directly ionizing and can cause damage without secondary particles. Radiation therapy causes biologic effects through DNA damage, in particular double stranded DNA breaks. DNA damage occurs through interactions between particles and DNA, which can occur directly or indirectly. Direct action occurs when the photon transfers energy to an electron, which subsequently interacts with the DNA. Indirect action occurs when the secondary electron interacts to produce free radicals, which can then damage DNA. Photon-based radiation therapy works primarily through indirect action while heavy charged particles work primarily through direct action. Radiation therapy is typically delivered via fractionation, with multiple small radiation doses delivered, allowing for a higher total dose to be delivered, increasing tumor control probability while reducing the risk of normal tissue toxicity. It should be noted that with improvements in treatment planning, treatment delivery, and image guidance, there is a renewed interest in hypofractionation (larger doses per fraction); further the development of stereotactic body radiotherapy (SBRT) allows for the delivery of radiation therapy in five fractions or less using large doses per fraction.

The four fundamental radiobiologic principles guiding standard fractionation and clinical radiation oncology are 1) repair, 2) re-assortment, 3) repopulation, and 4) reoxygenation. Repair is essential and one of the key reasons for fractionation. After receiving photon-based radiation therapy, normal tissue cells are able to repair sublethal damage, limiting toxicity while cancer cells are limited in their abilities to repair sublethal damage, allowing for an improvement in the therapeutic ratio with fractionation. Re-assortment is important because cancer cells have varying degrees of radiosensitivity based on the stage of the cell cycle they are in, with the G2-M phase being the most radiosensitive and the S phase being the least sensitive. As such, fractionation allows for re-assortment of cells into more radiosensitive phases of the cell cycle, enhancing cell kill. Repopulation is important for two reasons; repopulation with fractionation allows for normal tissues to recover if an adequate time interval is introduced. More importantly, some malignancies have been shown to clinically demonstrate repopulation (e.g., head and neck cancer, cervical cancer) during treatment requiring clinicians to complete treatment within a certain duration of time or risk suboptimal local control and outcomes. Finally, reoxygenation represents a key principle of radiation sensitivity and damage. As most radiation is delivered with photons, the primary mechanism of DNA damage is indirect action via free radicals. The presence of oxygen allows "fixation" of the DNA damage caused by free radicals enhancing the impact of the radiation. Fractionation enhances reoxygenation, increasing radiation sensitivity of tumors.

TREATMENT WORKFLOW AND DELIVERY

Regardless of treatment location, radiation oncology workflows are fairly consistent. Patients are initially seen in consultation to discuss the role of radiation therapy and inform patients regarding the potential benefits of treatment as well as acute, sub-acute, and chronic toxicities associated with treatment to allow for informed decision making. This is followed by radiation therapy planning, which begins with a simulation or planning scan. The simulation typically consists of some form of imaging; traditionally, this was done with 2-D films or fluoroscopy but this has been replaced primarily with a CT simulator. At the time of simulation, immobilization is created to achieve reproducible patient positioning, depending on location (e.g., mask for CNS and head and neck cases). Immobilization can also be dependent on the type of treatment; for example, more rigid immobilization may be used when high dose treatments (e.g., SBRT) are performed. At the time of simulation, contrast can be used to enhance assessment of vasculature and lymph nodes and 4D scans are performed to assess the impact of respiratory motion on target and organ at risk volumes. The patient is scanned and an isocenter is placed; additionally, tattoos are commonly placed to facilitate patient setup daily.

Once simulation is complete, the images obtained are transferred to a treatment planning computer. The physician will then draw in contours or volumes for the target including the gross tumor volume (GTV), the clinical target volume (CTV), and the planning target volume (PTV) based on physical exam, imaging, and any other procedures (e.g., Colonoscopy, EGD, nasopharyngoscopy). Additionally, if a 4D scan is performed, an internal target volume (ITV) can be created to account for organ motion. Contours are also made for all critical normal tissue structures in the treatment field. A radiation plan is then created by a dosimetrist and reviewed by the physician. Once approved by the physician, a medical physicist reviews the treatment plan and it undergoes quality assurance checks which are dependent on the technique utilized.

Modern radiation therapy is typically delivered with a linear accelerator. A linear accelerator generates high-energy photons by accelerating electrons and having them approach a target. The x-rays/photons are primarily produced when the electrons are deflected (Bremsstrahlung radiation); additionally, electrons can be used as the therapeutic particle when the target is removed. Inside the head of the linear accelerator are several structures designed to allow to for safe and efficient treatment delivery. In patients treated with photons, beyond the x-ray target is a flattening filter, which creates a more uniform radiation field as well as ion chambers, which measure radiation dose, and subsequently jaws, which can shape the beam. There is a light field to visualize the treatment field as well as an optical distance indicator to measure the source to surface distance. Modern linear accelerators also include a multileaf collimator, which can be used to shape the beam. A similar set of structures is used for electron treatments with the exception of the target being removed and the use of scattering foils rather than flattening filter. Radiation therapists perform treatment delivery; treatment plans created in the treatment planning system are sent to information systems that communicate with the linear accelerator while also serving as an electronic medical record to document daily treatment.

Multiple treatment techniques can be utilized to deliver external beam radiation therapy. Modern radiation therapy primarily utilizes a CT simulator for treatment planning and therefore a three-dimensional approach. Beams can then be shaped using the jaws in the linear accelerator or with leaves within a multi-leaf collimator. Such approaches are known as three-dimensional conformal radiotherapy (3D-CRT). Over the past two decades, an alternative technique to 3D-CRT has emerged known as intensity modulated radiation therapy (IMRT). IMRT allows for the modulation of the intensity of the beam, providing clinicians the ability to preferentially give dose to one area while sparing another. This is accomplished primarily through inverse treatment planning algorithms where the treatment planning system is provided dose constraints for the target and normal tissue structures (with weighting for each objective provided), as well as beam angles. IMRT is routinely performed in the treatment of many different malignancies including CNS malignancies, head and neck cancers, cancers of the thorax and abdomen, sarcomas, and genitourinary as well as gynecologic malignancies.

External beam radiation therapy can be utilized in many different scenarios. Definitive radiation therapy can be utilized in the management of some CNS tumors, lymphomas, and prostate cancers. Definitive radiation in conjunction with chemotherapy can also be utilized in the treatment of some CNS malignancies, head and neck cancers, inoperable lung cancers, esophageal cancers, pancreas cancers, gynecologic malignancies, and bladder cancers allowing for organ preservation and the potential for improved toxicity and quality of life. Radiation therapy can also be delivered post-operatively for patients at high risk for recurrence or residual microscopic disease following surgery; this is most commonly seen in breast cancers but is also used in CNS malignancies, head and neck cancers, pancreatic cancer, sarcomas, genitourinary, and gynecologic malignancies. Finally, radiation therapy can be utilized for palliation, most commonly for bone metastases, brain metastases, lung masses, and bleeding. Common oncologic emergencies where radiation therapy is utilized include spinal cord compression, airway compromise, superior vena cava syndrome, and symptomatic brain metastases not amenable to surgery. Radiosensitizers can be used with radiation therapy to increase the response to treatment. Clinically, this is most commonly done with the addition of concurrent chemotherapy. However, alternatives have been studied including halogenated pyridmidines and hypoxic radiosensitizers, though both are used sparingly in the clinic at this time. Radioprotectors, compounds that protect the body from radiation, have also been explored. At this time, the only clinically utilized radioprotector is amifostine, which is utilized to prevent xerostomia with data demonstrating no difference in clinical oncologic outcomes when using amifostine in head and neck cancers.

Radiation therapy can be associated with acute, subacute, and chronic toxicities. The most common toxicities noted during treatment are fatigue and skin erythema/irritation. Additional acute toxicities are typically dependent on the area of the body being irradiated. Common acute and subacute side effects are listed based on treatment site: CNS (headache, nausea, alopecia, tinnitus), head and neck (mucositis, xerostomia, altered taste, dysphagia), thorax (esophagitis, pneumonitis), gastrointestinal (nausea, vomiting, diarrhea), genitourinary/gynecologic (urinary frequency/urgency, dysuria, diarrhea, vaginal irritation). Acute and subacute side effects tend to resolve within weeks to months of the completion of treatment. Chronic toxicities can be long-lasting; however, use of normal tissue toxicity constraints can limit the risk of chronic toxicities based on treatment site.

ADDITIONAL TECHNIQUES

As noted above, stereotactic radiation therapy is a technique that allows for the delivery of highly conformal radiation treatments, allowing for large doses per fraction. With respect to terminology, stereotactic radiosurgery (SRS) is usually associated with a single fraction while stereotactic body radiation therapy (SBRT) typically is more than one fraction and usually up to five fractions. SRS is best known for its use in the central nervous system and can be performed with a linear accelerator or more specialized treatment machines (e.g., Gamma Knife). While most commonly associated with the treatment of brain metastases, SRS can also be used for pituitary adenomas, trigeminal neuralgia, acoustic neuromas, meningiomas, and arteriovenous malformations as well. More recently, SRS has been incorporated into the management of spine metastases as well, replacing standard radiation therapy in some cases and offering the potential for improved local control and pain control.

SBRT is most commonly associated with the treatment of inoperable early stage non-small cell lung cancers. Promising initial data from Indiana University led to a multi-institutional study, which confirmed excellent rates of local control and an acceptable toxicity profile. Moving forward, current trials are evaluating optimal dose and fractionation schemes for peripheral and central tumors as well as comparing SBRT to surgery in operable patients. SBRT is also being utilized in the management of prostate cancer with trials evaluating five fraction regimens with promising results leading to comparisons to standard and hypofractionated radiation therapy. More recently, SBRT has been utilized to treat liver metastases and HCC's with encouraging preliminary outcomes with respect to local control and liver toxicity as well as pancreatic cancers. Additionally, SBRT is being evaluated in a number treatment sites including soft tissue sarcoma and head and neck cancers.

Brachytherapy is a radiation therapy technique where radioactive sources are implanted on or inside a patient. Brachytherapy can be performed with low dose rate (LDR) implants typically associated with prostate seed implants, or high dose rate (HDR) implants typically associated with temporary gynecologic or breast implants. Brachytherapy is a commonly utilized treatment in the management of prostate cancer. As noted above, many are familiar with LDR brachytherapy for prostate cancer with excellent clinical outcomes and toxicity profiles reported. Additionally, increasing data are available supporting HDR brachytherapy in prostate cancer, which, unlike LDR, allows for modulation of dose once catheters are in place and the potential for improved toxicity profiles. While treatment with brachytherapy in prostate cancer is primarily monotherapy, recent data are available on the use brachytherapy boost in patients with higher-risk prostate cancer.

Brachytherapy (placing radioactive material inside or on the surface of the body) has also emerged as a standard of care treatment option in appropriately selected women with early stage breast cancer via accelerated partial breast irradiation (APBI), which treats the lumpectomy cavity with a margin. Initial studies evaluated APBI using multi-catheter interstitial HDR; however, more recent studies have evaluated single entry applicators, increasing the ability for patients to receive this treatment. At this time, multiple randomized trials comparing brachytherapy with standard whole breast irradiation have been performed, with no difference in local recurrence noted. Intraoperative radiation therapy (IORT) represents a form of partial breast irradiation different from APBI and can be delivered with multiple techniques at the time of surgery; however, two randomized trials evaluating the technique have demonstrated increased rates of local recurrence compared with whole breast irradiation and as such this technique should not be considered off-protocol at this time. Brachytherapy remains an essential component in the management of gynecologic cancers; in patients with endometrial cancer, post-operative vaginal cylinder brachytherapy is routinely used based on clinical and pathologic factors while brachytherapy remains essential in the management of cervical cancers. Brachytherapy can also be utilized in head and neck cancers, as well as soft tissue sarcomas.

Traditionally, radiation therapy was delivered with photons (high energy x-rays) or electrons for superficial treatments. Photons, which are the most commonly utilized form of radiation therapy, are uncharged and are known for characteristics including the need for a build up region and dose deposition over several centimeters. Protons, on the other hand, are different than photons in that the majority of dose is deposited within a small range (few millimeters) known as the Bragg peak, which can be modulated by changing the energy of the protons. It should be noted however, this range is typically too small for clinical utilization and as such, a spread out Bragg peak is used. The biology of protons is considered similar to photons with the advantage being primarily improved dose distribution rather than greater biologic effect as seen with neutrons for example. While previously limited to a few centers throughout the United States, the past two decades has seen a significant expansion in the number of proton centers. One of the challenges associated with proton therapy is the amount of resources required to deliver treatment and therefore, the cost of treatment. However, proton therapy is particularly attractive for pediatric malignancies with data available supporting the utilization of protons in pediatric cancers, particularly CNS malignancies. With respect to other malignancies, much has been made of the role of protons in the management of prostate cancer. However, at this time, the data does not consistently support the utilization of protons in the management of prostate cancer and should be only performed on-protocol. Similarly, there is limited data supporting the role of protons in breast cancer; while recent data suggests protons can be used for APBI and may be cost-effective, the limited number of patients treated with this technique mandates further study before patients are routinely treated off-protocol. Moving forward, further technological advances including intensity modulated proton therapy and advanced image guidance may allow for further improvement in outcomes with proton therapy; in the interim, in light of the limited data suggesting comparable or improved outcomes and the lack of data demonstrating cost-effectiveness, outside of accepted indications (e.g., pediatric cancers), proton therapy should be limited to use on-protocol primarily.

Suggested Readings

1. Bush DA, Do S, Lum S, et al. Partial breast radiation therapy with proton beam: 5-year results with cosmetic outcomes. *Int J Radiat Oncol Biol Phys.* 2014;90:501–505.
2. Grills IS, Martinez AA, Hollander M, et al. High dose rate brachytherapy as prostate cancer monotherapy reduces toxicity compared to low dose rate palladium seeds. *J Urol.* 2004;171:1098–1104.
3. Hall EJ, Giaccia AJ. Dose-response relationships for model normal tissues. In: Hall EJ, Giaccia AJ, ed. *Radiobiology for the Radiologist*, 6th ed. Philadelphia, PA: Lippincott Williams & Wilkins; 2006:303–326.
4. Hall EJ, Giaccia AJ. Oxygen effect and reoxygenation. In: Hall EJ, Giaccia AJ, ed. *Radiobiology for the Radiologist*, 6th ed. Philadelphia, PA: Lippincott Williams & Wilkins; 2006:85–105.
5. Hall EJ, Giaccia AJ. Physics and chemistry of radiation absorption. In: Hall EJ, Giaccia AJ, ed. *Radiobiology for the Radiologist*, 6th ed. Philadelphia, PA: Lippincott Williams & Wilkins; 2006:5–15.
6. Hall EJ, Giaccia AJ. Radioprotectors. In: Hall EJ, Giaccia AJ, ed. *Radiobiology for the Radiologist*, 6th ed. Philadelphia, PA: Lippincott Williams & Wilkins; 2006:129–134.
7. Hall EJ, Giaccia AJ. Radiosensitizers and bioreductive drugs. In: Hall EJ, Giaccia AJ, ed. *Radiobiology for the Radiologist*, 6th ed. Philadelphia, PA: Lippincott Williams & Wilkins; 2006:419–431.
8. Hall EJ, Giaccia AJ. Time, dose, and fractionation in radiotherapy. In: Hall EJ, Giaccia AJ, ed. *Radiobiology for the Radiologist*, 6th ed. Philadelphia, PA: Lippincott Williams & Wilkins; 2006:378–397.
9. Harkenrider MM, Block AM, Alektiar KM. American Brachytherapy Task Group Report: adjuvant vaginal brachytherapy for early-stage endometrial cancer. A comprehensive review. *Brachytherapy.* 2016 May 3 [Epub ahead of print].
10. Holloway CL, Delaney TF, Alektiar KM, et al. American Brachytherapy Society (ABS) consensus statement for sarcoma brachytherapy. *Brachytherapy.* 2013;12:179–190.
11. Jawad MS, Dilworth JT, Gustafson GS, et al. Outcomes associated with 3 treatment schedules of high-dose-rate brachytherapy monotherapy for favorable-risk prostate cancer. *Int J Radiat Oncol Biol Phys.* 2016;94:657–666.
12. Johnstone PA, Kerstiens J. Reconciling reimbursement for proton therapy. *Int J Radiat Oncol Biol Phys.* 2016;95:9–10.
13. Kotecha R, Vogel S, Suh JH, et al. A cure is possible: a study of 10-year survivors of brainmetastases. *J Neurooncol.* 2016;129:545–555.
14. Lanciano RM, Pajak TF, Martz K, Hanks GE. The influence of treatment time on outcome for squamous cell cancer of the uterine cervix treated with radiation: a patterns-of-care study. *Int J Radiat Oncol Biol Phys.* 1993;25:391–397.
15. Leroy R, Benahmed N, Hulstaert F, et al. Proton therapy in children: a systematic review of clinical effectiveness in 15 pediatric cancers. *Int J Radiat Oncol Biol Phys.* 206;95:267–278.
16. Ling DC, Vargo JA, Heron DE. Stereotactic body radiation therapy for recurrent head and neck cancer. *Cancer J.* 2015;22:302–306.
17. Marks LB, Yorke ED, Jackson A, et al. Use of normal tissue complication probability models in the clinic. *Int J Radiat Oncol Biol Phys.* 2010;76:S10–S9.
18. Martinez AA, Shah C, Mohammed N, et al. Ten-year outcomes for prostate cancer patients with Gleason 8 through 10 treated with external beam radiation and high-dose-rate brachytherapy boost in the PSA era. *J Radiat Oncol.* 2016;5:87–93.
19. McDermott PN, Orton CG. Brachytherapy. In: McDermott PN, Orton CG, ed. *The Physics of & Technology of Radiation Therapy.* 1st ed. Madison, WI: Medical Physics Publishing; 2010:16:1–16:45.
20. McDermott PN, Orton CG. External beam radiation therapy units. In: McDermott PN, Orton CG, ed. *The Physics of & Technology of Radiation Therapy.* 1st ed. Madison, WI: Medical Physics Publishing; 2010:9:1–9:45.
21. McDermott PN, Orton CG. Imaging in radiation therapy. In: McDermott PN, Orton CG, ed. *The Physics of & Technology of Radiation Therapy.* 1st ed. Madison, WI: Medical Physics Publishing; 2010:19:1–19:50.
22. McDermott PN, Orton CG. Review of basic physics. In: McDermott PN, Orton CG, ed. *The Physics of & Technology of Radiation Therapy.* 1st ed. Madison, WI: Medical Physics Publishing; 2010:2:1–2:30.
23. McDermott PN, Orton CG. Special modalities in radiation therapy. In: McDermott PN, Orton CG, ed. *The Physics of & Technology of Radiation Therapy.* 1st ed. Madison, WI: Medical Physics Publishing; 2010:10:1–20:73.
24. McDermott PN, Orton CG. X-ray production II: basic physics and properties of resulting x-rays. In: McDermott PN, Orton CG, ed. *The Physics of & Technology of Radiation Therapy.* 1st ed. Madison, WI: Medical Physics Publishing; 2010:5:1–5:29.
25. McGarry RC, Papiez L, Williams M, et al. Stereotactic body radiation therapy of early-stage non-small-cell lung carcinoma: phase I study. *Int J Radiat Oncol Biol Phys.* 2005;63:1010–1015.
26. Miller JA, Balagamwala EH, Angelov Li, et al. Stereotactic radiosurgery for the treatment of primary and metastatic spinal sarcomas. *Technol Cancer Res Treat.* Apr 12 [Epub ahead of print].
27. Morris JW, Tyldesley S, Pai HH, et al. ASCENDE-RT: a multicenter randomized trial of dose-escalated external beam radiation therapy (EBRT-B) versus low-dose-rate brachytherapy (LDR-B) for men with unfavorable-risk localized prostate cancer. *J Clin Oncol.* 2015;33:s7:3.
28. Myrehaug S, Sahgal A, Russo SM, et al. Stereotactic body radiotherapy for pancreatic cancer: recent progress and future directions. *Expert Rev Anticancer Ther.* 2016;16:523–530.

29. Ovalle V, Strom EA, Godby J, et al. Proton partial-breast irradiation for early-stage cancer: Is it really so costly? *Int J Radiat Oncol Biol Phys.* 2016;95:49–51.

30. RTOG 0618: a phase II trial of stereotactic body radiation therapy (SBRT) in the treatment of patients with operable stage I/II non-small cell lung cancer. https://www.rtog.org/ClinicalTrials/ProtocolTable/StudyDetails.aspx?study=0618. Accessed August 20, 2016.

31. RTOG 0631: a phase II/III study of image-guided radiosurgery/SBRT for localized spine metastasis. https://www.rtog.org/ClinicalTrials/ProtocolTable/StudyDetails.aspx?study=0631. Accessed August 20, 2016.

32. RTOG 0813: seamless phase I/II study of stereotactic lung radiotherapy (SBRT) for early stage, centrally located, non-small cell lung cancer (NSCLC) in medically inoperable patients. https://www.rtog.org/ClinicalTrials/ProtocolTable/StudyDetails.aspx?study=0813. Accessed August 20, 2016.

33. RTOG 0915: a randomized phase II study comparing 2 stereotactic body radiation therapy (SBRT) schedules for medically inoperable patients with stage I peripheral non-small cell lung cancer. https://www.rtog.org/ClinicalTrials/ProtocolTable/StudyDetails.aspx?study=0915. Accessed August 20, 2016.

34. Rusthoven KE, Kavanagh BD, Cardenes H, et al. Multi-institutional phase I/II trial of stereotactic body radiation therapy for liver metastases. *J Clin Oncol.* 2009;27:1572–1578.

35. Sands SA. Proton beam radiation therapy: the future may prove brighter for pediatric patients with brain tumors. *J Clin Oncol.* 2016;34:1024–1026.

36. Schiff PB, Harrison LB, Strong EW, et al. Impact of time interval between surgery and postoperative radiation therapy on locoregional control in advanced head and neck cancer. *J Surg Oncol.* 1990;43:203–208.

37. Sheets NC, Goldin GH, Meyer AM, et al. Intensity-modulated radiation therapy, proton therapy, and conformal radiation therapy and morbidity and disease control in localized prostate cancer. *JAMA.* 2012;307:1611–1620.

38. Stone NN, Stock RG. 15-Year cause specific and all-cause survival following brachytherapy for prostate cancer: negative impact of long-term hormonal therapy. *J Urol.* 2014;192:754–759.

39. Takacsi-Nagy Z, Martinez-Mongue R, Mazeron JJ, et al. American Brachytherapy Society Task Group Report: combined external beam irradiation and interstitial brachytherapy for base of tongue tumors and other head and neck sites in the era of new technologies. *Brachytherapy.* 2016 Aug 31 [Epub ahead of print].

40. Timmerman R, Paulus R, Galvin J, et al. Stereotactic body radiation therapy for inoperable early stage lung cancer. *JAMA.* 2010;303:1070–1076.

41. Verma V, Shah C, Mehta MP. Clinical outcomes and toxicity of proton radiotherapy for breast cancer. *Clin Breast Cancer.* 2016;16:145–154.

42. Vicini F, Shah C, Tendulkar R, et al. Accelerated partial breast irradiation: An update on published Level I evidence. *Brachytherapy.* 2016;15:607–615.

43. Viswanthan AN, Thomadsen B. American Brachytherapy Society consensus guidelines for locally advanced carcinoma of the cervix. Part 1: general principles. *Brachytherapy.* 2012;11:33–46.

44. Weiner AA, Olsen J, Ma d, et al. Stereotactic body radiotherapy for primary hepatic malignancies-report of a phase I/II institutional study. *Radiother Oncol.* 2016 Aug 23 [Epub ahead of print].

45. Zaorsky NG, Shaikh T, Murphy CT, et al. Comparison of outcomes and toxicities among radiation therapy treatment options for prostate cancer. *Cancer Treat Rev.* 2016;48:50–60.

Clinical Genetics 44

Holly Jane Pederson and Brandie Heald

INTRODUCTION

Clinical genetics is the specialty that involves the diagnosis and management of hereditary disorders. As an oncology healthcare provider, recognition of these syndromes is critical in order to provide proper care related to cancer therapy decisions, to identify other risks for that patient, and to counsel family members about risks and options. Hereditary cancers are important to detect because the age of onset is early, multiple primary cancers can develop, and cancer predisposition may be inherited. Hereditary syndromes account for only a minority of cases of cancer, but those who are affected have extremely high risks. Patients at increased risk may benefit from enhanced surveillance, chemopreventive strategies, or risk-reducing surgeries.

If a hereditary cancer syndrome is suspected (Table 44.1), a focused exam specific to the syndrome (i.e., dermatologic and head circumference for *PTEN*-hamartoma tumor syndrome), and genetic counseling with an expanded pedigree detailing the types of cancer, bilaterality, age at diagnosis, ethnicity, and medical record documentation as needed (i.e., pathology reports of primary cancers or carcinogen exposure) should be done. Prior to genetic testing, patients must give informed consent with an understanding of the benefits, risks, and limitations of testing as well as the goals for cancer family risk assessment in alignment with the American Society of Clinical Oncology policy statement on genetic testing. Options exist for family planning including pre-implantation genetic testing and prenatal diagnosis. Patients should be made aware of the Genetic Information Nondiscrimination Act (GINA) of 2008, which prohibits employment and health insurance discrimination based on genetic information.

The tenets of genetic counseling are relevant to hereditary cancer syndromes. A detailed, four generation family tree is elicited, and this information, together with the personal history of the patient, allows the counselor to determine if the presentation is most suggestive of sporadic, familial, or hereditary cancer. This comprehensive risk assessment ensures that the correct genetic testing is offered to the most appropriate patients, with personalized interpretation of results and provision of future management recommendations. Guideline driven management recommendations are available for many syndromes.

In this chapter we will review the most commonly seen and tested hereditary cancer syndromes in adults.

HEREDITARY BREAST CANCER SYNDROMES

Hereditary Breast and Ovarian Cancer Syndrome

Hereditary breast cancer accounts for 5% to 10% of all breast cancers. The most common hereditary breast cancer syndrome involves pathogenic variants in the *BRCA1/2* genes, tumor suppressor genes that play a role in double-stranded DNA repair. These mutations account for 65% of hereditary breast cancer and have an autosomal dominant pattern of inheritance. The incidence is 1 in 400 for the general population and 1 in 40 in the Ashkenazi Jewish population.

TABLE 44.1 Hereditary Cancer Syndromes

Syndrome	Gene	Associated Cancers/Tumors
Birt-Hogg-Dube	*FLCN*	**RCC**
Familial adenomatous polyposis	*APC*	Colon, gastric, small bowel, thyroid, brain
Familial medullary thyroid cancer	*RET*	Medullary thyroid
Familial papillary renal cancer	*MET*	Type 1 papillary RCC
Fanconi anemia	Multiple genes including biallelic *BRCA2* mutations; diagnosis is made by increased chromosomal breakage in lymphocytes cultured in the presence of DNA cross-linking agents	AML, MDS, solid tumor especially squamous cell carcinoma of the head and neck or vulva. Breast cancer if associated with biallelic *BRCA2* mutations
Gorlin syndrome	*PTCH*	Basal cell, medulloblastoma
Hereditary breast and ovarian cancer syndrome	*BRCA1, BRCA2*	Breast, ovarian, prostate, pancreatic, melanoma, male breast cancer
Hereditary diffuse gastric cancer	*CDH1*	Diffuse gastric cancer, lobular breast cancer
Hereditary leiomyomatosis	*FH*	Type 2 papillary RCC
Hereditary melanoma	*CDKN2A, CDK4*	Melanoma, pancreas
Juvenile polyposis syndrome	*BMPR1A, SMAD4*	Juvenile/hamartomatous gastrointestinal polyposis, colorectal, gastric, hereditary hemorrhagic telangiectasia (*SMAD4* only)
Li–Fraumeni syndrome	*TP53*	Breast, sarcoma, leukemia, brain tumors, adrenocorticoid, lung bronchoalveolar
Lynch syndrome	*MLH1, MSH2, MSH6, PMS2, EPCAM*	Colon, endometrial, ovarian, gastric, small bowel, biliary, pancreatic, upper urinary tract, skin, brain
Multiple endocrine neoplasia type 1	*MEN1*	Parathyroid, pituitary, pancreatic, or extrapancreatic
Multiple endocrine neoplasia type 2A	*RET*	Medullary thyroid, pheochromocytoma, parathyroid
Multiple endocrina neoplasia type 2B	*RET*	Medullary thyroid, pheochromocytoma, mucosal neuromas, intestinal ganglioneuromas
MUTYH-associated polyposis	*MUTYH*	Similar to FAP
Peutz–Jeghers syndrome	*STK11*	Colon/rectum, breast, stomach, small bowel, pancreas, lung, cervix, ovaries, testicles
PTEN-hamartoma tumor syndrome	*PTEN*	Breast, endometrial, thyroid, kidney, melanoma, and colorectal
Von Hippel–Lindau disease	*VHL*	Clear cell RCC, pheochromocytomas, neuroendocrine

Pathogenic variants in these genes are associated with significantly elevated risks of both breast cancer (up to 87%) and ovarian cancer (up to 54%) and earlier age of onset of both cancers. The *BRCA1* gene can frequently be associated with triple-negative breast cancer histology and both genes are associated with serous ovarian cancer. Other cancers such as pancreatic cancer, prostate cancer, male breast cancer, and melanoma can also be seen, particularly in patients with *BRCA2* gene mutations. *BRCA1/2* testing is recommended per guidelines set forth by the National Comprehensive Cancer Network (NCCN) in individuals:

- from a family with a known pathogenic variant in *BRCA1* or *BRCA2*
- with a personal history of breast cancer and one of the following:
  - diagnosed at 45 years of age or younger
  - diagnosed at 50 years of age or younger with:
    - an additional breast cancer primary
    - a close blood relative with breast cancer at any age
    - a relative with pancreatic cancer
    - a relative with prostate cancer (Gleason score greater than or equal to 7)
    - an unknown or limited family history
  - diagnosed at 60 years of age or younger with triple negative breast cancer
  - diagnosed at any age with:
    - one or more close blood relatives with breast cancer diagnosed at the age of 50 or younger
    - two or more blood relatives with breast cancer diagnosed at any age
    - one or more close blood relatives with ovarian cancer
    - two or more blood relatives with pancreatic cancer and/or prostate cancer (Gleason score greater than or equal to 7) at any age
    - a close male blood relative with breast cancer
    - Ashkenazi Jewish ancestry
- with a personal history of ovarian cancer
- with a personal history of male breast cancer
- with a personal history of metastatic prostate cancer
- with a personal history of a somatic BRCA mutation

As with all hereditary syndromes, testing of unaffected individuals should only be considered when an affected family member is unavailable or unwilling to test and family history reveals a first- or second-degree relative meeting the above criteria. In this circumstance, the significant limitations of interpreting results should be discussed since negative test results in an unaffected individual are uninformative.

If a *BRCA* pathogenic variant is found, general options for risk management include enhanced surveillance, chemoprevention, and risk reducing surgery. Breast self-awareness is recommended starting at the age of 18. Women should be familiar with their breasts and report changes to their healthcare provider. Periodic, consistent breast self-exam (BSE) may facilitate breast self-awareness. Clinical breast examination is recommended every 6 to 12 months starting at age 25. Annual MRI screening is recommended beginning at the age of 25 until the age of 75 and annual screening mammograms should begin at 30. MRI has been shown to be more sensitive for cancer detection in this population. Risk-reducing mastectomy can reduce the risk of breast cancer by 90%. Counseling should include a discussion regarding the degree of protection, reconstructive options, and surgical risks. Data with tamoxifen for prevention in this population is limited but suggestive of reduction of ER+ disease, particularly in patients with a BRCA2 mutation. Given the elevated risk for ovarian cancer and the lack of effective screening, risk-reducing salpingo-oophorectomy (RRSO) is recommended between the ages of 35 and 40, or upon completion of childbearing, and may reduce breast cancer risk, particularly in BRCA2 carriers. This has been the only intervention thus far shown to reduce overall mortality. Because ovarian cancers occur in patients with *BRCA2* mutations an average of 8 to 10 years later than in patients with *BRCA1* mutations, it is reasonable to delay RRSO until age 40 to 45 in patients with *BRCA2* mutations who have already maximized their breast cancer risk reduction (have undergone RRM). Counseling includes a discussion of reproductive desires, extent of cancer risk, degree of protection for breast and ovarian cancer, management of menopausal symptoms, possible short-term hormone replacement therapy to a recommended maximum age of natural menopause, and related medical issues. Salpingectomy alone is not the standard of care for risk reduction although clinical trials are ongoing as the majority of serous ovarian cancers are felt to originate in the fallopian tubes. The concern for risk-reducing salpingectomy alone is that women may still be at risk for developing ovarian cancer, and that risk is of yet undefined. In addition, in premenopausal women, oophorectomy reduces the risk of developing breast cancer in *BRCA2* carriers by up to 50% depending upon age of procedure. For those patients who have not elected RRSO, while there may be circumstances where clinicians find screening helpful, data do not support routine ovarian screening. Transvaginal ultrasound for ovarian cancer screening has not been shown to be sufficiently sensitive or specific to support a positive recommendation, but may be considered at the clinician's discretion starting at the age of 30 to 35. Serum CA125 is an additional ovarian screening test with caveats similar to transvaginal ultrasound.

For men, the risk of breast cancer is 7% and more common in *BRCA2* carriers. Breast self-examination should start at the age of 35. Clinical examination should begin annually at 35, and prostate cancer screening is recommended starting at the age of 45. No specific screening guidelines exist for pancreatic cancer and melanoma, but screening may be individualized based on cancers observed in the family. There is only limited data to support breast imaging in men.

PTEN-Hamartoma Tumor Syndrome

PTEN-hamartoma tumor syndrome (PHTS) is a genetic diagnosis that encompasses the conditions Cowden syndrome and Bannayan-Riley-Ruvalcaba syndrome. It is an autosomal dominant syndrome with an incidence of 1 in 200,000. It is caused by a loss of function in the tumor suppressor *PTEN* gene and is associated with multiple hamartomas in a variety of tissues, characteristic dermatologic manifestations, and an increased risk of breast, endometrial, thyroid, kidney, melanoma, and colorectal cancers. The lifetime risk of breast cancer may be as high as 85% in patients with documented pathogenic variants in the *PTEN* gene. Thyroid cancer, typically follicular and rarely papillary, develops in two-third of carriers and can occur in childhood. Renal cell carcinoma can be seen in 13% to 34% of carriers. The prevalence of colon polyps is 66% to 93%. While hamartomatous polyps have predominantly been reported, patients with PHTS often develop a mix of ganglioneuromas, hamartomatous, adenomatous, serrated, and inflammatory polyps. This lifetime risk of developing colorectal cancer is as high as 16%. Neurologic manifestations include dysplastic gangliocytoma of the cerebellar cortex, macrocephaly, intellectual disability, and autism. Women commonly have benign abnormalities such as significant fibrocystic breast changes, breast hamartomas, uterine fibroids, and ovarian cysts. Men often have lipomatosis of the testes. Both men and women frequently have benign thyroid lesions, such as adenomas and multinodular goiter. Benign glycogenic acanthosis and lipomas can also be seen.

Genetic testing criteria are divided into major and minor criteria. The major criteria include breast cancer, follicular thyroid cancer, multiple gastrointestinal hamartomas or ganglioneuromas, macrocephaly, endometrial cancer, penile freckling, and characteristic mucocutaneous lesions. The minor criteria include Autism spectrum disorder, colon cancer, ≥3 esophageal glycogenic acanthuses, lipomas, intellectual disability, papillary or follicular variant of papillary thyroid cancer, structural thyroid lesions, renal cell carcinoma, single gastrointestinal hamartoma or ganglioneuroma, testicular lipomatosis, and vascular anomalies. PTEN testing should be offered to individuals with the following:

- two or more major criteria (one must be macrocephaly)
- three major criteria, without macrocephaly
- one major and three or more minor criteria
- four or more minor criteria
- adult Lhermitte-Duclos disease
- autism spectrum disorder and macrocephaly
- two or more biopsy-proven trichilemmomas

For those with a family member with a clinical diagnosis of Cowden syndrome or PHTS, genetic testing should be offered when any major criterion or two minor criteria are present. Clinical diagnostic Cowden syndrome criteria, which vary slightly from the testing criteria, have been established by the NCCN and International Consortium Cowden Consortium. The estimated lifetime risk of developing breast cancer in a patient with Clinical Cowden Syndrome is felt to be 25% to 50%. *PTEN* testing includes sequencing of the entire coding region and deletion/duplication analysis. Pathogenic variants have also been reported in the *PTEN* promoter region. Other candidate genes for Cowden syndrome are actively being investigated. De novo mutations are not uncommon.

The NCCN management guidelines for women with PHTS include breast self-examination training and education starting at age 18, clinical breast examination every 6 to 12 months starting at age 25, and annual mammography and breast MRI starting at age 30 to 35 or individualized based on the earliest age of onset in family. For endometrial cancer screening, consideration can be given to annual random endometrial biopsies and/or transvaginal ultrasound beginning at age 30 to 35. Risk-reducing mastectomies and hysterectomy can be considered. Men and women should have an annual physical examination starting at age 18 or 5 years prior to the youngest age of diagnosis of cancer in their family with emphasis on thyroid examination. Baseline thyroid ultrasound should be done at the time of diagnosis and annually thereafter. Screening colonoscopies should begin at age 35 with follow-up every 5 years. Consider renal ultrasound every 1 to 2 years beginning at age 40 years.

Li–Fraumeni Syndrome

Li–Fraumeni syndrome is a hereditary syndrome associated with a wide range of cancers that appear at an unusually young age. LFS has an autosomal dominant pattern of inheritance and is associated with pathogenic variants in the *TP53* tumor suppressor gene, which plays a major role in DNA repair. The lifetime risk of cancer is nearly 100%, with 90% of individuals diagnosed with cancer by age 60. The classic tumors seen in this syndrome are sarcoma, breast cancer, leukemia, brain tumors, and adrenal gland cancers.

Classic Li–Fraumeni criteria include a proband with sarcoma before the age of 45, a first-degree relative with cancer before the age of 45, and a first- or second-degree relative with cancer before the age of 45 or sarcoma at any age. Chompret criteria include one of the following:

- a proband who has a tumor belonging to the LFS spectrum (sarcoma, premenopausal breast cancer, brain tumor, adrenocorticoid tumor, leukemia, or lung bronchoalveolar cancer) before age 46 *and* at least one first- or second-degree relative with a tumor in the LFS spectrum before age 56 or with multiple tumors.
- a proband with multiple tumors (except multiple breast tumors), two of which belong to the LFS spectrum and the first of which occurred before age 46.
- a proband who is diagnosed with adrenocortical tumor or choroid plexus tumor regardless of age irrespective of family history.

Testing of individuals who meet either of these criteria or women with breast cancer before age 35 who have tested negative for the *BRCA1/2* variants is recommended. De novo mutations occur in 7% to 20% of patients.

The management guidelines for women with LFS include breast self-examination training and education starting at age 18 and clinical breast examination every 6 to 12 months starting at age 20 to 25. In the 20s, annual breast MRI is recommended or mammogram, if MRI is not available. Beginning at age 30, annual breast MRI alternating with low dose digital mammography is recommended. Risk-reducing mastectomies should be offered as an option. All carriers should have an annual physical examination, including dermatologic and neurologic examinations. Colonoscopy screening should be considered starting at age 25 with follow-up every 2 to 5 years. Other options for screening should be discussed with the patient such as whole-body MRI, and brain MRI. Targeted surveillance should be based on family history. Therapeutic radiation should be avoided if possible.

HEREDITARY GASTROINTESTINAL SYNDROMES

Lynch Syndrome

Lynch syndrome is an autosomal dominant disorder characterized by germline pathogenic variants in the DNA mismatch repair (MMR) genes or *EPCAM*. Lynch syndrome accounts for 2% to 3% of all colorectal cancers and is associated with a 15% to 74% lifetime risk of developing colorectal cancer. Lifetime risk of colorectal cancer can be further stratified by gender and MMR gene, with male *MLH1* carriers being at the highest risk. Compared to those with sporadic colorectal cancer, Lynch syndrome–associated colorectal cancers are usually younger at time of diagnosis (44–61 vs. 69 years old in the general population) and have more poorly differentiated, mucinous tumors found in the right colon. Despite these more aggressive histologic features, affected patients have better 5-year survival rates compared to those with common sporadic colorectal cancer. For those diagnosed with one colorectal cancer, treated with limited resection, the risk of developing another colorectal cancer 10 years after an initial diagnosis is 16% to 19%. At 20 years, this risk is 41% to 47%, and by 30 years, this risk reaches as high as 69%.

Endometrial carcinoma is the most common extra-colonic tumor in Lynch syndrome, accounting for about 2% of all endometrial cancers, with a lifetime risk ranging from 14% to 71% in female carriers. Similar to colorectal cancer in Lynch syndrome, women are typically younger in age at diagnosis (50s vs. 65 years old in the general population). Other organs at increased risk of cancer include the ovaries (4% to 20% lifetime risk), stomach (0.2% to 13%), small bowel (0.4% to 12%), pancreas/hepatobiliary tract (0.02% to 4%), upper urinary tract (0.2% to 25%), skin (1% to 9%), and brain (1% to 4%). In many families, breast and/or prostate cancers are seen, though risk has not been clearly defined.

Defects in the MMR system, which identifies base-pair mismatches and repairs them, is the hallmark characteristic of Lynch syndrome. The MMR genes affected in Lynch syndrome include *MLH1*, *MSH2*, *MSH6*, and *PMS2*. A germline deletion in *EPCAM*, which inactivates *MSH2*, has also been associated with Lynch syndrome. MMR and *EPCAM* mutations are inherited in an autosomal dominant manner. For an individual with Lynch syndrome, if the second allele is inactivated through one of several mechanisms (acquired somatic mutation, loss of heterozygosity, promoter hypermethylation), a defective MMR system ensues, resulting in a failure to repair DNA mismatches and an increased rate of mutations (genomic instability). DNA mismatches tend to occur in areas of repeated nucleotide sequences called microsatellites. An accumulation of mutations in these regions leads to expansion or contraction of the microsatellites, termed microsatellite instability (MSI). Approximately 90% to 95% of Lynch syndrome–associated colorectal cancers will display high levels of microsatellite instability (MSI-H).

Biallelic inheritance of mutations in one of the MMR genes causes constitutional mismatch repair-deficiency syndrome (CMMRD) and is associated with the development of Lynch syndrome–associated cancers, as well as childhood cancers, hematologic malignancies, polyposis, brain tumors, and neurofibromatosis features such as café-au-lait spots.

Patients with colorectal or endometrial cancer suspected of having Lynch syndrome can be screened through the detection of MSI by polymerase chain reaction (PCR) or the absence of the MMR protein product by immunohistochemistry (IHC). PCR detects MSI by identifying expansion or contraction of the microsatellite regions. If 30% or more of the microsatellites show instability, then the tumor is considered to have high levels of microsatellite instability (i.e., MSI-H), suggesting a defect in a DNA MMR gene. IHC uses antibodies to detect MMR proteins. Unlike MSI testing, IHC has the advantage of identifying the missing protein product, and by proxy, implicating the potentially mutated gene. An estimated 88% of colorectal cancers caused by Lynch syndrome will have abnormal IHC results. Confirmation of Lynch syndrome requires germline testing of the MMR gene(s).

Microsatellite instability is sensitive but not specific for Lynch syndrome. MSI-H can be found in up to 15% of sporadic colorectal cancers, most commonly due to the loss of MLH1 via hypermethylation of the *MLH1* promoter region. Approximately 50% of colorectal cancers with *MLH1* promoter hypermethylation will have a somatic *BRAF* V600E mutation, which is rarely seen in Lynch syndrome tumors. Endometrial cancers with *MLH1* promoter hypermethylation do not have somatic *BRAF* mutations, so *BRAF* testing is not a useful tool for testing endometrial cancers. In patients who have MSI-H colorectal tumors with loss of MLH1, testing for the *BRAF* V600E mutation (colorectal cancer only) or *MLH1* promoter hypermethylation (colorectal or endometrial cancers) should be done to rule out sporadic cases. If these tests are negative, then patients should be offered germline *MLH1* testing. The loss of other MMR proteins in colorectal or endometrial cancers should proceed directly to MMR gene testing and genetic counseling. An estimated 50% of individuals with abnormal MSI/IHC results will have a germline MMR mutation. Approximately 40% of patients with abnormal MSI/IHC results will have acquired somatic MMR mutations, which is not Lynch syndrome. If an MMR mutation is not detected on germline testing then consideration should be given to MMR gene testing on the tumor DNA.

Identifying patients who have Lynch syndrome remains a challenging task. The Amsterdam I criteria were originally developed to identify individuals appropriate for hereditary colorectal cancer research. The Amsterdam II Criteria were later broadened to include other cancers observed in these families. The Amsterdam Criteria are useful for identifying patients appropriate for genetic counseling and testing. Those families that meet the Amsterdam Criteria are given a clinical diagnosis of hereditary non-polyposis colorectal cancer (HNPCC). An estimated 50% of families with HNPCC will actually have Lynch syndrome. The Revised Bethesda guidelines were created to help identify colorectal cancers appropriate for MSI/IHC testing.

Amsterdam II Criteria

1. Three or more relatives with HNPCC-associated cancers (colorectal, endometrial, small bowel, ureter, or renal pelvis) cancer, one of whom is a first-degree relative of the other two.
2. Two or more generations with the above cancer(s).
3. At least one individual with the above cancer(s) in the family who was diagnosed before age 50.
4. The family does not have a different inherited colorectal cancer genetic condition called "familial adenomatous polyposis."

Revised Bethesda Guidelines:

▪ Colorectal cancer in a patient younger than 50 years.
▪ Colorectal cancer with MSI-H histology in a patient younger than 60 years.
▪ Presence of synchronous, metachronous colorectal, or other HNPCC-associated tumors, regardless of age.
▪ A patient with colorectal cancer who has one or more first-degree relatives with an HNPCC-associated tumor, with one of the cancers diagnosed under the age of 50.
▪ A patient with colorectal cancer who has two or more first- or second-degree relatives with HNPCC-related tumors, regardless of age.

Given the reduced sensitivity and specificity of the Amsterdam Criteria and Bethesda Guidelines, in 2009 the Evaluation of Genomic Application in Practice and Prevention (EGAPP) endorsed universally screening all newly diagnosed colorectal cancer with MSI and/or IHC.

For patients with Lynch Syndrome, colorectal cancer surveillance with colonoscopies should begin at the age of 20 to 25 with follow up every 1 to 2 years until age 40 when annual colonoscopy should commence. Patients must be aware that dysfunctional uterine bleeding warrants evaluation. There is no clear evidence to support screening for endometrial cancer for Lynch syndrome. However, annual office endometrial sampling is an option. While there may be circumstances where clinicians find screening helpful, data do not support routine ovarian screening for Lynch syndrome. Controversy exists surrounding the screening of other extracolonic cancers. No firm recommendations have been established except for annual skin surveillance. Upper endoscopy with visualization of the duodenum can be considered every 3–5 years starting at age 30–35 years. Primary prophylactic colectomy is generally not recommended. An annual urinalysis can be considered starting at age 30 to 35. Prophylactic hysterectomy and bilateral salpingo-oophorectomy should be considered in high-risk patients who are 35 years or older or have finished childbearing.

Familial Adenomatous Polyposis

Familial adenomatous polyposis (FAP) is an autosomal dominant disorder characterized by the presence of colorectal adenomatous polyposis. FAP is caused by germline pathogenic variants in the tumor suppressor adenomatous polyposis coli (*APC*) gene located on chromosome 5. FAP has a number of associated extracolonic carcinomas, but unlike colorectal cancer which has near complete penetrance, the penetrance for extracolonic tumors is variable.

FAP accounts for less than 1% of all colorectal cancers. Seventy-five percent of FAP cases inherit a germline *APC* mutation, whereas the remaining 25% of patients are de novo cases. Among patients with >1,000 adenomas, *APC* pathogenic variants are identified in 80%. The mutation detection rate drops to 56% (100 to 999 colorectal adenomas), 10% (20 to 99 adenomas), and 5% (10 to 19 adenomas).

Based on the colorectal adenoma burden, two classes of FAP have been described: classic/profuse FAP and attenuated FAP (AFAP). Patients with classic or profuse FAP have greater than 100 adenomatous polyps. Adenomas typically begin to develop around puberty, and, without surgical intervention the risk of colorectal cancer is 100%. The average age of colorectal cancer diagnosis is in the third decade of life. AFAP is characterized by less than 100 adenomas, which typically begin to develop in the late teenage years or early 20s. A lower, yet still significant, risk of colorectal cancer development is seen (up to 80%) with a later age of cancer diagnosis, often in the fifth decade of life.

Patients with FAP can also develop upper gastrointestinal tracts polyps. Fundic gland polyps and gastric adenomas develop in 12% to 84% of patients. The gastric cancer risk is low but increased over the general population. Duodenal adenomas develop in 50% to 90% of patients. The risk of duodenal cancer ranges from 4% to 12% is based on the Spigelman score.

Extraintestinal manifestations, both malignant and benign, are observed in individuals with FAP. Malignant extraintestinal tumors are rare and include papillary thyroid cancer, pancreatic cancer, childhood hepatoblastoma, and central nervous system (CNS) tumors. Benign findings include desmoid tumors, sebaceous or epidermoid cysts, lipomas, osteomas, fibromas, dental abnormalities, adrenal adenomas, and congenital hypertrophy of the retinal pigment epithelium (CHRPE). Turcot syndrome was previously used to refer to the association of familial colon cancer with CNS tumors. This includes medulloblastomas observed in FAP kindred. Gardner syndrome refers to families with FAP who also have osteomas and soft tissue tumors. Turcot syndrome associated with adenomatous polyposis and Gardner's syndrome are both forms of FAP caused by *APC* variants.

FAP should be suspected in any patient with 10 or more colorectal adenomas, and genetic counseling and testing for germline mutation of the *APC* gene should be offered to these patients. Testing for *MUTYH*-associated polyposis (see below) should also be considered in those who test negative for a mutation in the *APC* gene. Unlike most other hereditary cancer syndromes, genetic counseling and predictive genetic testing should be offered to children, generally around the age of 8 to 10 years.

Per the NCCN guidelines, screening flexible sigmoidoscopy or full colonoscopy should begin around puberty for classic/profuse type FAP with annual follow-up. Those with AFAP patients should begin screening colonoscopy in the late teenage years with follow-up every 2 to 3 years. Patients found to have profuse polyposis, multiple large (>1 cm) adenomas, or adenomas with villous histology or high-grade dysplasia should be treated with colectomy followed by routine surveillance of the ileal pouch. AFAP patients with less disease burden can undergo polypectomy followed by continued annual surveillance. Upper endoscopy with visualization of the ampulla should begin around age 20 to 25. Those with no duodenal polyposis should repeat endoscopy in 4 years. Those with Spigelman stage I (minimal polyposis; 1 to 4 tubular adenomas, size 1 to 4 mm) need repeat endoscopy in 2 to 3 years, those with stage II (mild polyposis; 5 to 19 tubular adenomas, size 5 to 9 mm) follow-up every 1 to 3 years, and those with stage III (moderate polyposis; 20 more lesions, or size 1cm or greater) every 6 to 12 months. Patients with stage IV duodenal disease (dense polyposis or high-grade dysplasia) should have surveillance every 3 to 6 months and be sent for surgical evaluation to consider mucosectomy, duodenectomy, or a Whipple procedure. Annual examination of the thyroid should commence in the late teenage years; thyroid ultrasound can be considered. For families with desmoid tumors, abdominal MRI or CT could be considered 1 to 3 years post-colectomy and every 5 to 10 years thereafter. Data are presently insufficient to support any additional screening or surveillance.

MUTYH-associated Polyposis

MUTYH-associated polyposis (MAP) is an autosomal recessive hereditary cancer syndrome characterized by adenomatous polyposis and early onset colorectal cancer. *MUTYH* is a base excision repair protein that plays a major role correcting in G:C>T:A transversions in the DNA. Among those of a northern European background, two common pathogenic variants c.536A>G (p.Tyr179Cys) and c.1187G>A (p.Gly396Asp) have been reported to account for up to 80% of *MUTYH* mutations. An estimated 1% to 2% of individuals from this ethnic group carry one of these mutations. Different founder mutations have been reported in those of Dutch, Italian, British Indian, Pakistani, Spanish, Portuguese, Tunisian, Brazilian, French, Japanese, and Korean backgrounds.

The majority of patients develop ten to hundreds of colorectal adenomas; profuse polyposis is typically not observed. Some individuals will also develop serrated polyps (hyperplastic polyps, sessile serrated adenomas/polyps, and serrated adenomas). The average age of diagnosis is around age 50 years.

A rare subset of patients will present with early onset colorectal cancer in the absence of polyposis. The lifetime risk of developing colorectal cancer for individuals with MAP ranges from 43% to 100%.

Patients with MAP also develop upper gastrointestinal tract neoplasms. Approximately 10% to 15% of patients will develop fundic gland polyps and/or gastric adenomas. It is unclear if MAP is associated with an increased risk of gastric cancer. Approximately 17% to 25% of patients will develop duodenal adenomas, with an estimated 4% lifetime risk of developing duodenal cancer.

Other cancers, including thyroid, skin, endometrial, ovarian, breast, and bladder, have been reported at an increased incidence in MAP patients. Additionally, patients have been reported to have benign thyroid disease, dermatologic findings, dental abnormalities, and CHRPE.

There is speculation that *MUTYH* carriers may have an increased risk of developing colorectal cancer. Odd ratios among carriers have been reported between 1.1 to 1.2 and 2 to 3.

The NCCN recommends beginning colonoscopy at age 25 to 30 for those with biallelic *MUTYH* mutations. If negative, the exam should be repeated every 2 to 3 years. If polyps are identified, colonoscopy and polypectomy should be repeated every 1 to 2 years. Colectomy should be considered when the polyp burden is >20 on a single exam, when polyps have been previously ablated, when some polyps reach >1 cm, or when advanced histology is encountered. The adenoma distribution and polyp burden should inform the extent of colectomy. Upper endoscopy with visualization of the ampulla could be considered beginning at age 30 to 35. Follow-up is based on Spigelman score, as discussed in the FAP section. For monoallelic *MUTYH* carriers the NCCN currently endorses beginning colonoscopy at age 40, or 10 years earlier than the age of a first degree relative with colorectal cancer, whichever is younger, with follow-up at least every 5 years.

Hereditary Diffuse Gastric Cancer

Hereditary diffuse gastric cancer is an autosomal dominant disorder caused by germline pathogenic variants in the *CDH1* gene that codes for E-cadherin, a cell-adhesion protein that allows cells to interact with each other and is critical for cell development, differentiation, and architecture. Individuals who harbor these germline mutations have a greater than 70% lifetime risk of developing diffuse gastric cancer by age 80 with a median age of onset of 38. These gastric cancers form beneath an intact mucosal surface, causing gastric wall thickening rather than the formation of a discrete mass. Because they are only visible late in the disease process, early detection is extremely challenging. Therefore, screening of high-risk individuals via EGD with random biopsies should begin in the late teenage years. Prophylactic gastrectomy should be offered to all *CDH1* mutation carriers between the ages of 18 and 40.

Like diffuse gastric cancer, the absence of E-cadherin expression is also the key underlying defect in lobular breast carcinoma. Female carriers therefore have a 42% lifetime risk of developing lobular breast carcinoma by age 80. Given this considerable risk for breast cancer, annual MRI screening in addition to annual screening mammography is recommended generally 10 years earlier than the first affected relative, or beginning at age 30. Risk reducing mastectomy is considered in patients with compelling family history.

Expert opinion clinical criteria for HDGC are as follows:

- two cases of gastric cancer regardless of age, at least one confirmed diffuse gastric cancer
- one case of diffuse gastric cancer <40 years
- personal or family history of diffuse gastric cancer and lobular breast cancer, one diagnosed <50 years

In 2015 experts also suggested that *CDH1* genetic testing could be considered for those with the following:

- bilateral lobular breast cancer or family history of two or more cases of lobular breast cancer <50
- a personal or family history of cleft lip/palate in a patient with diffuse gastric cancer
- in situ signet ring cells and/or pagetoid spread of signet ring cells

CDH1 mutation detection rates were previously reported to be 25% to 50% for those who met clinical criteria. With the expansion of the above testing criteria, the mutation detection rate has decreased to 10% to 18%.

Peutz–Jeghers Syndrome

Peutz–Jeghers syndrome (PJS) is a rare, autosomal dominant disorder characterized by multiple gastro-intestinal hamartomatous polyps, mucocutaneous pigmentation, and an increased risk of malignancies. Approximately 88% of patients with PJS will develop Peutz-Jeghers polyps. Peutz-Jeghers polyps are characterized by a cerebriform appearance due to smooth muscle arborization within the polyps. These polyps often begin to develop in the first decade of life and are most common in the small bowel but can be observed in the colon, rectum, and stomach. An estimated 50% of patients will present with intussception by age 20. PJS is often recognized by characteristic mucocutaneous pigmentation. The lesions are small (1 to 5 mm in size), flat, blue-gray to brown spots, and are commonly found around the mouth and nose, in the buccal mucosa, hands and feet, perianal areas, and genitals. Over time this pigmentation can fade. Malignancies are also commonly seen in PJS and affected patients carry up to an 80% to 90% lifetime risk of developing cancer. The most common malignancies occur in the colon and rectum, but an increased risk is also seen in the breast, stomach, small bowel, pancreas, lung, cervix, ovaries, and testicles.

The World Health Organization (WHO) established clinical criteria for PJS:

- three or more histologically confirmed Peutz-Jeghers polyps
- any number of Peutz-Jeghers polyps and a family history of PJS
- characteristic mucocutaneous pigmentation and a family history of PJS
- any number of Peutz-Jeghers polyps in an individual with characteristic mucocutaneous pigmentation

Germline mutations in *STK11* cause PJS. *STK11* mutations are found in 60% to 99% of patients who meet the WHO criteria. Annual screening breast MRI beginning at 25 in addition to annual screening mammography beginning at 30 is recommended. Individuals with PJS should receive a colonoscopy every 2 to 3 years, beginning in the late teens. Additional guidelines for screening of the stomach, small bowel, pancreas, uterus, ovaries, and testes are outlined in NCCN guidelines.

Juvenile Polyposis Syndrome

Juvenile polyposis syndrome (JPS) is caused by mutations in the genes *BMPR1A* and *SMAD4*. This syndrome is characterized by gastrointestinal hamartomatous polyps and increased malignancy risk. Juvenile describes the hamartomatous polyps observed in this syndrome. Polyps often begin to develop in the teenage years and are most common in the colon and rectum. Patients with *SMAD4* patho-genic variants can also develop massive gastric polyposis, which is more rarely observed in those with *BMPR1A* pathogenic variants. Small bowel polyps have been reported but are rare. The lifetime risk of developing cancer ranges from 17% to 68%, with a 50% lifetime risk of developing colorectal cancer. The risk of gastric or duodenal cancer is 15% to 21%. Germline *SMAD4* mutations have also been asso-ciated with hereditary hemorrhagic telangiectasia (HHT) and aortopathy. Clinical criteria have been established for JPS:

- more than three to five juvenile polyps of the colon or rectum
- juvenile polyps throughout the gastrointestinal tract
- any number of juvenile polyps and a positive family history of JPS

Among those that meet clinical criteria, *SMAD4* and *BMPR1A* mutations are identified in approxi-mately 40% to 50% of patients.

Colonoscopy and upper endoscopy should begin around age 15 years with follow-up every 1 to 3 years. Colectomy and/or gastrectomy may be considered in cases where polyp burden is endoscopi-cally unmanageable. Individuals with *SMAD4* mutations should undergo screening for HHT.

Testing Considerations

There is a shifting paradigm to move from single syndrome testing to performing next generation sequencing of multiple genes (panel testing). Gene panels include highly penetrant genes with estab-lished clinical utility; these panels also contain genes for which clinical validity or significance is less certain at this time. Since 2014, NCCN guidelines have recognized the impact that multi-gene panel testing has in changing the clinical approach to testing at-risk individuals. Panel testing may be a cost effective and efficient option, especially for individuals who have personal or family histories that are suspicious for more than one hereditary cancer syndrome, or for those who previously tested negative on single syndrome testing. In patients referred for *BRCA1* and *BRCA2* testing, for example, use of a 25-gene panel test in one study resulted in identification of genes other than *BRCA1* and *BRCA2* in 4.3% of patients. In another large prospective study of a sequential series of breast cancer patients, 10.7% were found to have a germline pathogenic variants in a gene that predisposes women to breast or ovarian cancer, using a panel of 25 predisposition genes, including 6.1% in *BRCA1* and *BRCA2*, and 4.6% in other breast/ovarian predisposition genes. Whereas young age ($P < 0.01$), Ashkenazi Jewish ancestry ($P < 0.01$), triple negative breast cancer ($P = 0.01$) and family history of breast/ovarian cancer ($P = 0.01$) predicted for *BRCA1* and *BRCA2* mutations, no factors predicted for mutations in other breast cancer predisposition genes. Approximately one-third of patients had at least one variant of uncertain significance (VUS) in this study, as has been reported in other series evaluating next generation sequencing panels. Most of these variants will eventually be reclassified, primarily as benign, but some will likely be pathogenic. VUSs should not be used to make clinical decisions.

NCCN continues to update medical management guidelines for highly penetrant genes and notably now include guidelines for moderate risk genes. For example, breast MRI screening is recommended for individuals with pathogenic variants in *ATM* and *CHEK2*. Although multigene panels can significantly aid in cancer risk management and expedite clinical translation of new genes, they equally have the potential to provide clinical misinformation and harm at the individual level if the data are not interpreted cautiously. Given the potential issues for patients and their families, gene panel testing for inherited cancer risk is recommended to be offered in conjunction with consultation with an experienced cancer genetic specialist (counselor or geneticist) as part of the testing process.

Suggested Readings

1. Aaltonen LA, Jarvin H, Gruber SB, Billaud M, Jass JR. Peutz-Jeghers syndrome. In: Hamilton SR, Aaltonen LA, eds. *Tumors of the Digestive System*. Lyon, France: World Health Organization; 2000:74–76.
2. Aretz S, Uhlhaas S, Goergens H, et al. MUTYH-associated polyposis: 70 of 71 patients with biallelic mutations present with an attenuated or atypical phenotype. *Int J Cancer*. 2006;119:807–814.
3. Bisgaard ML, Fenger K, Bulow S, Niebuhr E, Mohr J. Familial adenomatous polyposis (FAP): frequency, penetrance, and mutation rate. *Hum Mutat*. 1994;3:121–125.
4. Burt RW. Gastric fundic gland polyps. *Gastroenterology*. 2003;125:1462–1469.
5. Byrski T, Huzarski T, Dent R, et al. Pathologic complete response to neoadjuvant cisplatin in BRCA1-positive breast cancer patients. *Breast Cancer Res Treat*. 2014;147:401–405.
6. Canto MI, Harinck F, Hruban RH, et al. International Cancer of the Pancreas Screening (CAPS) Consortium summit on the management of patients with increased risk for familial pancreatic cancer. *Gut*. 2013;62:339–347.
7. Chen S, Parmigiani G. Meta-analysis of BRCA1 and BRCA2 penetrance. *J Clin Oncol*. 2007;25:1329–1333.
8. Chompret A, Abel A, Stoppa-Lyonnet D, et al. Sensitivity and predictive value of criteria for p53 germline mutation screening. *J Med Genet*. 2001;38:43–47.
9. Couch FJ, Hart SN, Sharma P, et al. Inherited mutations in 17 breast cancer susceptibility genes among a large triple-negative breast cancer cohort unselected for family history of breast cancer. *J Clin Oncol*. 2015;33:304–311.
10. Domchek SM, Friebel TM, Singer CF, et al. Association of risk-reducing surgery in BRCA1 or BRCA2 mutation carriers with cancer risk and mortality. *JAMA*. 2010;304:967–975.
11. Durno CA, Sherman PM, Aronson M, et al. Phenotypic and genotypic characterisation of biallelic mismatch repair deficiency (BMMR-D) syndrome. *Eur J Cancer*. 2015;51:977–983.
12. Easton DF, Pharoah PD, Antoniou AC, et al. Gene-panel sequencing and the prediction of breast-cancer risk. *N Engl J Med*. 2015;372:2243–2257.
13. Eggington JM, Bowles KR, Moyes K, et al. A comprehensive laboratory-based program for classification of variants of uncertain significance in hereditary cancer genes. *Clin Genet*. 2014;86:229–237.
14. Evaluation of Genomic Applications in P, Prevention Working G. Recommendations from the EGAPP Working Group: genetic testing strategies in newly diagnosed individuals with colorectal cancer aimed at reducing morbidity and mortality from Lynch syndrome in relatives. *Genet Med*. 2009;11:35–41.
15. Fackenthal JD, Olopade OI. Breast cancer risk associated with BRCA1 and BRCA2 in diverse populations. *Nat Rev Cancer*. 2007;7:937–948.
16. Farrington SM, Tenesa A, Barnetson R, et al. Germline susceptibility to colorectal cancer due to base-excision repair gene defects. *Am J Hum Genet*. 2005;77:112–119.

17. Ford D, Easton DF, Stratton M, et al. Genetic heterogeneity and penetrance analysis of the BRCA1 and BRCA2 genes in breast cancer families. The Breast Cancer Linkage Consortium. *Am J Hum Genet.* 1998;62:676–689.
18. Foulkes WD, Smith IE, Reis-Filho JS. Triple-negative breast cancer. *N Engl J Med.* 2010;363:1938–1948.
19. Frank TS, Deffenbaugh AM, Reid JE, et al. Clinical characteristics of individuals with germline mutations in BRCA1 and BRCA2: analysis of 10,000 individuals. *J Clin Oncol.* 2002;20:1480–1490.
20. Genetic/Familial High-Risk Assessment: Breast and Ovarian. NCCN; 2016. Accessed October 9, 2016.
21. Geurts-Giele WR, Leenen CH, Dubbink HJ, et al. Somatic aberrations of mismatch repair genes as a cause of microsatellite-unstable cancers. *J Pathol.* 2014;234:548–559.
22. Giardiello FM, Allen JI, Axilbund JE, et al. Guidelines on genetic evaluation and management of Lynch syndrome: a consensus statement by the US Multi-Society Task Force on colorectal cancer. *Gastroenterology.* 2014;147:502–526.
23. Giardiello FM, Brensinger JD, Tersmette AC, et al. Very high risk of cancer in familial Peutz-Jeghers syndrome. *Gastroenterology.* 2000;119:1447–1453.
24. Giardiello FM, Trimbath JD. Peutz-Jeghers syndrome and management recommendations. *Clin Gastroenterol Hepatol.* 2006;4:408–415.
25. Gismondi V, Meta M, Bonelli L, et al. Prevalence of the Y165C, G382D and 1395delGGA germline mutations of the MYH gene in Italian patients with adenomatous polyposis coli and colorectal adenomas. *Int J Cancer.* 2004;109:680–684.
26. Grover S, Kastrinos F, Steyerberg EW, et al. Prevalence and phenotypes of APC and MUTYH mutations in patients with multiple colorectal adenomas. *JAMA.* 2012;308:485–492.
27. Hall MJ, Forman AD, Pilarski R, Wiesner G, Giri VN. Gene panel testing for inherited cancer risk. *J Natl Compr Canc Netw.* 2014;12:1339–1346.
28. Hansford S, Kaurah P, Li-Chang H, et al. Hereditary diffuse gastric cancer syndrome: CDH1 mutations and beyond. *JAMA Oncol.* 2015;1:23–32.
29. Haraldsdottir S, Hampel H, Tomsic J, et al. Colon and endometrial cancers with mismatch repair deficiency can arise from somatic, rather than germline, mutations. *Gastroenterology.* 2014;147:1308–1316 e1.
30. Heald B, Mester J, Rybicki L, Orloff MS, Burke CA, Eng C. Frequent gastrointestinal polyps and colorectal adenocarcinomas in a prospective series of PTEN mutation carriers. *Gastroenterology.* 2010;139:1927–1933.
31. Heald B, Rigelsky C, Moran R, et al. Prevalence of thoracic aortopathy in patients with juvenile Polyposis Syndrome-Hereditary Hemorrhagic Telangiectasia due to SMAD4. *Am J Med Genet A.* 2015;167A:1758–1762.
32. Herrmann LJ, Heinze B, Fassnacht M, et al. TP53 germline mutations in adult patients with adrenocortical carcinoma. *J Clin Andocrinol Metab.* 2012;97:E476–E485.
33. Howe JR, Mitros FA, Summers RW. The risk of gastrointestinal carcinoma in familial juvenile polyposis. *Ann Surg Oncol.* 1998;5:751–756.
34. Howe JR, Sayed MG, Ahmed AF, et al. The prevalence of MADH4 and BMPR1A mutations in juvenile polyposis and absence of BMPR2, BMPR1B, and ACVR1 mutations. *J Med Genet.* 2004;41:484–491.
35. Jenkins MA, Croitoru ME, Monga N, et al. Risk of colorectal cancer in monoallelic and biallelic carriers of MYH mutations: a population-based case-family study. *Cancer Epidemiol Biomarkers Prev.* 2006;15:312–314.
36. Jones N, Vogt S, Nielsen M, et al. Increased colorectal cancer incidence in obligate carriers of heterozygous mutations in MUTYH. *Gastroenterology.* 2009;137:489–494, 94 e1; quiz 725–726.
37. Kadmon M, Tandara A, Herfarth C. Duodenal adenomatosis in familial adenomatous polyposis coli. A review of the literature and results from the Heidelberg Polyposis Register. *Int J Colorectal Dis.* 2001;16:63–75.
38. Kauff ND, Satagopan JM, Robson ME, et al. Risk-reducing salpingo-oophorectomy in women with a BRCA1 or BRCA2 mutation. *N Engl J Med.* 2002;346:1609–1615.
39. King MC, Marks JH, Mandell JB. New York Breast Cancer Study G. Breast and ovarian cancer risks due to inherited mutations in BRCA1 and BRCA2. *Science.* 2003;302:643–646.
40. King MC, Wieand S, Hale K, et al. Tamoxifen and breast cancer incidence among women with inherited mutations in BRCA1 and BRCA2: National Surgical Adjuvant Breast and Bowel Project (NSABP-P1) Breast Cancer Prevention Trial. *JAMA.* 2001;286:2251–2256.
41. Kravochuck SE, Kalady MF, Burke CA, Heald B, Church JM. Defining HNPCC and Lynch syndrome: what's in a name? *Gut.* 2014;63:1525–1526.
42. Li FP, Fraumeni JF, Jr., Mulvihill JJ, et al. A cancer family syndrome in twenty-four kindreds. *Cancer Res.* 1988;48:5358–5362.
43. Lubbe SJ, Di Bernardo MC, Chandler IP, Houlston RS. Clinical implications of the colorectal cancer risk associated with MUTYH mutation. *J Clin Oncol.* 2009;27:3975–3980.
44. Mensenkamp AR, Vogelaar IP, van Zelst-Stams WA, et al. Somatic mutations in MLH1 and MSH2 are a frequent cause of mismatch-repair deficiency in Lynch syndrome-like tumors. *Gastroenterology.* 2014;146:643–646 e8.
45. Mester JL, Schreiber AH, Moran RT. Genetic counselors: your partners in clinical practice. *Cleve Clin J Med.* 2012;79:560–568.
46. Narod SA, Brunet JS, Ghadirian P, et al. Tamoxifen and risk of contralateral breast cancer in BRCA1 and BRCA2 mutation carriers: a case-control study. Hereditary Breast Cancer Clinical Study Group. *Lancet.* 2000;356:1876–1881.
47. NCCN. Genetic/Familial High-Risk Assessment: Colorectal, Version 2.2016. 2016.

48. NCCN. NCCN Clinical Practice Guidelines in Oncology Genetic/Familial High-Risk Assessment: Breast and Ovarian, Version 1.2018. 2016.

49. Nelen MR, Kremer H, Konings IB, et al. Novel PTEN mutations in patients with Cowden disease: absence of clear genotype-phenotype correlations. *Eur J Hum Genet.* 1999;7:267–273.

50. Nielsen M, Poley JW, Verhoef S, et al. Duodenal carcinoma in MUTYH-associated polyposis. *J Clin Pathol.* 2006;59:1212–1215.

51. O'Malley M, LaGuardia L, Kalady MF, et al. The prevalence of hereditary hemorrhagic telangiectasia in juvenile polyposis syndrome. *Dis Colon Rectum.* 2012;55:886–892.

52. Pederson HJ, Padia SA, May M, Grobmyer S. Managing patients at genetic risk of breast cancer. *Cleve Clin J Med.* 2016;83:199–206.

53. Rebbeck TR, Friebel T, Wagner T, et al. Effect of short-term hormone replacement therapy on breast cancer risk reduction after bilateral prophylactic oophorectomy in BRCA1 and BRCA2 mutation carriers: the PROSE Study Group. *J Clin Oncol.* 2005;23:7804–7810.

54. Rebbeck TR, Kauff ND, Domchek SM. Meta-analysis of risk reduction estimates associated with risk-reducing salpingo-oophorectomy in BRCA1 or BRCA2 mutation carriers. *J Natl Cancer Inst.* 2009;101:80–87.

55. Robson M, Dabney MK, Rosenthal G, et al. Prevalence of recurring BRCA mutations among Ashkenazi Jewish women with breast cancer. *Genet Test.* 1997;1:47–51.

56. Robson ME, Bradbury AR, Arun B, et al. American Society of Clinical Oncology policy statement update: genetic and genomic testing for cancer susceptibility. *J Clin Oncol.* 2015;33:3660–3667.

57. Rubin SC, Benjamin I, Behbakht K, et al. Clinical and pathological features of ovarian cancer in women with germ-line mutations of BRCA1. *N Engl J Med.* 1996;335:1413–1416.

58. Sampson JR, Dolwani S, Jones S, et al. Autosomal recessive colorectal adenomatous polyposis due to inherited mutations of MYH. *Lancet.* 2003;362:39–41.

59. Sayed MG, Ahmed AF, Ringold JR, et al. Germline SMAD4 or BMPR1A mutations and phenotype of juvenile polyposis. *Ann Surg Oncol.* 2002;9:901–906.

60. Sieber OM, Lipton L, Crabtree M, et al. Multiple colorectal adenomas, classic adenomatous polyposis, and germ-line mutations in MYH. *N Engl J Med.* 2003;348:791–799.

61. Smith M, Mester J, Eng C. How to spot heritable breast cancer: a primary care physician's guide. *Cleve Clin J Med.* 2014;81:31–40.

62. Sourrouille I, Coulet F, Lefevre JH, et al. Somatic mosaicism and double somatic hits can lead to MSI colorectal tumors. *Fam Cancer.* 2013;12:27–33.

63. Spigelman AD, Thomson JP, Phillips RK. Towards decreasing the relaparotomy rate in the Peutz-Jeghers syndrome: the role of peroperative small bowel endoscopy. *Br J Surg.* 1990;77:301–302.

64. Tai YC, Domchek S, Parmigiani G, Chen S. Breast cancer risk among male BRCA1 and BRCA2 mutation carriers. *J Natl Cancer Inst.* 2007;99:1811–1814.

65. Tan MH, Eng C. RE: Cowden syndrome and PTEN hamartoma tumor syndrome: systematic review and revised diagnostic criteria. *J Natl Cancer Inst.* 2014;106:dju130.

66. Tan MH, Mester JL, Ngeow J, Rybicki LA, Orloff MS, Eng C. Lifetime cancer risks in individuals with germline PTEN mutations. *Clin Cancer Res.* 2012;18:400–407.

67. Thompson ER, Rowley SM, Li N, et al. Panel testing for familial breast cancer: calibrating the tension between research and clinical care. *J Clin Oncol.* 2016;34:1455–1459.

68. Tovar JA, Eizaguirre I, Albert A, Jimenez J. Peutz-Jeghers syndrome in children: report of two cases and review of the literature. *J Pediatr Surg.* 1983;18:1–6.

69. Tung N, Battelli C, Allen B, et al. Frequency of mutations in individuals with breast cancer referred for BRCA1 and BRCA2 testing using next-generation sequencing with a 25-gene panel. *Cancer.* 2015;121:25–33.

70. Tung N, Lin NU, Kidd J, et al. Frequency of germline mutations in 25 cancer susceptibility genes in a sequential series of patients with breast cancer. *J Clin Oncol.* 2016;34:1460–1468.

71. Tutt A, Robson M, Garber JE, et al. Oral poly(ADP-ribose) polymerase inhibitor olaparib in patients with BRCA1 or BRCA2 mutations and advanced breast cancer: a proof-of-concept trial. *Lancet.* 2010;376:235–244.

72. Umar A, Boland CR, Terdiman JP, et al. Revised Bethesda Guidelines for hereditary nonpolyposis colorectal cancer (Lynch syndrome) and microsatellite instability. *J Natl Cancer Inst.* 2004;96:261–268.

73. van der Post RS, Vogelaar IP, Carneiro F, et al. Hereditary diffuse gastric cancer: updated clinical guidelines with an emphasis on germline CDH1 mutation carriers. *J Med Genet.* 2015;52:361–374.

74. van der Post RS, Vogelaar IP, Manders P, et al. Accuracy of hereditary diffuse gastric cancer testing criteria and outcomes in patients with a germline mutation in CDH1. *Gastroenterology.* 2015;149:897–906 e19.

75. Vasen HF, Mecklin JP, Khan PM, Lynch HT. The International Collaborative Group on Hereditary Non-Polyposis Colorectal Cancer (ICG-HNPCC). *Dis Colon Rectum.* 1991;34:424–425.

76. Vasen HF, Watson P, Mecklin JP, Lynch HT. New clinical criteria for hereditary nonpolyposis colorectal cancer (HNPCC, Lynch syndrome) proposed by the International Collaborative group on HNPCC. *Gastroenterology.* 1999;116:1453–1456.

77. Vogt S, Jones N, Christian D, et al. Expanded extracolonic tumor spectrum in MUTYH-associated polyposis. *Gastroenterology*. 2009;137:1976–1985 e1–10.
78. von Minckwitz G, Schneeweiss A, Loibl S, et al. Neoadjuvant carboplatin in patients with triple-negative and HER2-positive early breast cancer (GeparSixto; GBG 66): a randomised phase 2 trial. *Lancet Oncol*. 2014;15:747–756.
79. Warner E, Plewes DB, Hill KA, et al. Surveillance of BRCA1 and BRCA2 mutation carriers with magnetic resonance imaging, ultrasound, mammography, and clinical breast examination. *JAMA*. 2004;292:1317–1325.
80. Whittemore AS, Gong G, Itnyre J. Prevalence and contribution of BRCA1 mutations in breast cancer and ovarian cancer: results from three U.S. population-based case-control studies of ovarian cancer. *Am J Hum Genet*. 1997;60:496–504.
81. Win AK, Dowty JG, Cleary SP, et al. Risk of colorectal cancer for carriers of mutations in MUTYH, with and without a family history of cancer. *Gastroenterology*. 2014;146:1208–12211 e1–5.
82. Win AK, Parry S, Parry B, et al. Risk of metachronous colon cancer following surgery for rectal cancer in mismatch repair gene mutation carriers. *Ann Surg Oncol*. 2013;20:1829–1836.

Jason M. Redman, Julius Strauss, and Ravi A. Madan

FDA-APPROVED IMMUNOTHERAPIES

Cytokine Therapies

Interferon Alpha 2b

- FDA approved for the adjuvant treatment of melanoma with microscopic or gross nodal involvement within 84 days of definitive surgical resection, including complete lymphadenectomy (see Table 45.1).
- This approval is based upon a phase III study, which randomized 1,256 patients with surgically resected Stage III melanoma to pegylated interferon alpha 2b or observation. Based on 696 relapse-free survival (RFS) events, an improvement in RFS was seen for those receiving interferon (HR 0.82; 95% CI 0.71 to 0.96; $P = 0.011$). The estimated median RFS was 34.8 months with interferon as compared to 25.5 months with observation. Of note, no difference in overall survival (OS) between interferon and observation was appreciated (HR 0.98; 95% CI 0.82 to 1.16).
- For adjuvant treatment of melanoma interferon alpha 2b is administered subcutaneously at a dose of 6 mcg/kg per week for eight doses followed by 3 mcg/kg per week for up to 5 years.
- Reported common adverse reactions (>60%) include fatigue, increased ALT, increased AST, pyrexia, headache, anorexia, myalgia, nausea, chills, and injection site reaction. There is also a black box warning for the risk of worsening depression, suicidal ideation or other serious neuropsychiatric disorders.
- FDA approved in combination with bevacizumab for metastatic renal cell carcinoma.
- This approval is based upon a phase III trial which randomized 649 patients with previously untreated, metastatic clear cell RCC to receive IFN-α (9 million units subcutaneously three times weekly) with or without bevacizumab (10 mg/kg intravenously every 2 weeks). Median PFS was significantly longer in the bevacizumab plus interferon alfa group (10.2 vs. 5.4 months; HR 0.63; 95% CI, 0.52 to 0.75; $P = 0.0001$).
- Of note the addition of bevacizumab to interferon was found to significantly increase the rates of grade 3 and 4 hypertension, anorexia, fatigue, and proteinuria as compared to IFN-α alone.
- Although the combination of interferon alpha 2b and bevacizumab is FDA approved for metastatic renal cell carcinoma, it is rarely used in clinical practice due to the more recent FDA approval of multiple tyrosine kinase inhibitors (sunitinib, pazopanib, etc.) for the same indication.

Aldesleukin (Proleukin; IL-2)

- Aldesleukin is a recombinant analog of the endogenous cytokine interleukin-2 (IL-2).
- FDA approved for the treatment of patients with metastatic melanoma as well as metastatic renal cell carcinoma.
- The same treatment dose and schedule was employed in all studies demonstrating efficacy for both metastatic melanoma and metastatic RCC. Aldesleukin was given at a dose of 600,000 International

TABLE 45.1 FDA-Approved Immunotherapies

Agent	Indications
Inteferon alpha 2b	▪ Adjuvant treatment of melanoma with microscopic or gross nodal involvement within 84 days of definitive surgical resection including complete lymphadenectomy ▪ In combination with bevacizumab for metastatic renal cell carcinoma
Aldesleukin	▪ Metastatic melanoma ▪ Metastatic renal cell carcinoma (RCC)
Sipuleucel-T	▪ Asymptomatic or minimally symptomatic metastatic castration-resistant prostate cancer (mCRPC)
Talimogene laherparepvec (T-VEC)	▪ Local treatment of unresectable cutaneous, subcutaneous, and nodal lesions in patients with melanoma who have recurrent disease after initial surgery
Ipilimumab	▪ Unresectable or metastatic melanoma ▪ Adjuvant therapy in patients who have cutaneous melanoma with pathologic involvement of regional lymph nodes of more than 1 mm and who have undergone complete resection, including total lymphadenectomy
Nivolumab	▪ As single agent or in combination with ipilimumab for unresectable or metastatic melanoma (BRAF V600 mutant or BRAF wild type) ▪ Metastatic NSCLC following previous platinum based chemotherapy and where EGFR or ALK sensitizing genomic alterations exist following EGFR or ALK TKI therapy ▪ Advanced renal cell carcinoma following previous anti-angiogenic therapy ▪ Classical Hodgkin's lymphoma following autologous HSCT and post-transplant brentuximab vendotin ▪ Recurrent or metastatic squamous cell carcinoma of the head and neck with disease progression on or after a platinum-based therapy ▪ Locally advanced or metastatic urothelial carcinoma progressing on or following platinum-containing chemotherapy or progressing within 12 months of neoadjuvant or adjuvant treatment with a platinum-containing chemotherapy
Pembrolizumab	▪ As treatment in patients with unresectable or metastatic melanoma (BRAF V600 mutant or BRAF wild type) ▪ Recurrent or metastatic head and neck squamous cell carcinoma (HNSCC) following platinum based chemotherapy ▪ Metastatic NSCLC with high tumor expression of PD-L1 (>50%) with no prior chemotherapy treatment in the absence of EGFR or ALK sensitizing genomic alterations ▪ Metastatic NSCLC with positive tumor expression of PD-L1 (>1%) following platinum based chemotherapy and where EGFR or ALK sensitizing genomic alterations exist following treatment with EGFR or ALK TKI therapy
Atezolizumab	▪ Locally advanced or metastatic urothelial carcinoma who have progressed following platinum based chemotherapy or have disease progression within 12 months of neoadjuvant or adjuvant treatment with platinum based chemotherapy ▪ Metastatic NSCLC following platinum based chemotherapy and where EGFR or ALK sensitizing genomic alterations exist following treatment with EGFR or ALK TKI therapy
Durvalumab	▪ Locally advanced or metastatic urothelial carcinoma who have progressed following platinum based chemotherapy or have disease progression within 12 months of neoadjuvant or adjuvant treatment with platinum based chemotherapy
Avelumab	▪ Locally advanced or metastatic urothelial carcinoma who have progressed following platinum based chemotherapy or have disease progression within 12 months of neoadjuvant or adjuvant treatment with platinum based chemotherapy ▪ Metastatic Merkel cell carcinoma in adults or childen 12 years of age

Units/kg (0.037 mg/kg) by 15 minutes intravenous infusion every 8 hours for up to 5 days (maximum of 14 doses). No treatment was given on days 6 to 14 and then dosing was repeated for up to 5 days on days 15 to 19 (maximum of 14 doses). These two cycles constituted one course of therapy. Patients could receive a maximum of 28 doses during a course of therapy. Although up to 28 doses were allowed, the vast majority of patients had doses withheld due to toxicity. For metastatic RCC patients treated with this schedule a median of 20 doses were given. For metastatic melanoma patients a median of 18 doses were received.

▪ In eight clinical trials, 270 patients with metastatic melanoma were treated with single agent aldesleukin. Of the 270 patients, 43 (16%) had an objective response, with 17 (6%) having a complete response and 26 (10%) having a partial response. In addition, in seven clinical trials, 255 patients with metastatic renal cell cancer (RCC) were treated with single agent aldesleukin. Of the 255 patients, 37 (15%) had an objective response with 17 (7%) having a complete response and 20 (8%) having a partial response. It should also be noted that patients achieving a complete response with this therapy have a near 90% ten year disease-free survival.

▪ Because of the potential for high-dose aldesleukin to cause capillary leak syndrome, hypotension, and reduced organ perfusion, it is recommended that aldesleukin be administered under the supervision of an experienced physician and in a hospital containing an intensive care unit. In addition, because of the potential for aldesleukin to cause cardiac arrhythmias, angina, myocardial infarction, and respiratory insufficiency, it is recommended that use of aldesleukin be limited to patients with normal cardiac and pulmonary function tests and without a history of cardiac or pulmonary disease. Aldesleukin may also cause gastrointestinal bleeding or infarction, renal insufficiency, edema, mental status changes, as well as an increased risk of sepsis due to impaired neutrophil function (reduced chemotaxis). Aldesleukin should be withheld in patients developing moderate to severe lethargy or somnolence as conti

▪ nued administration may result in coma.

Vaccines

Sipuleucel-T

▪ Sipuleucel-T is an autologous dendritic cell-based vaccine platform.
▪ FDA approved for the treatment of patients with minimally symptomatic metastatic castration-resistant prostate cancer (mCRPC).
▪ This approval is based on results of the IMPACT trial, a phase III double-blind placebo-controlled trial in which 512 patients with minimally symptomatic mCRPC were randomized to receive sipuleucel-T every 2 weeks for a total of three doses, or placebo. Patients receiving sipuleucel-T had a 4.1-month improvement in median OS (25.8 vs. 21.7 months; HR 0.78; 95% CI, 0.61 to 0.98; P = 0.03).
▪ Based on this trial the approved dosing is every 2 weeks for a total of three doses.
▪ Patients receiving sipuleucel-T should be premedicated with acetaminophen and an antihistamine such as diphenhydramine. Infusion reactions have been observed with sipuleucel-T. In the event of an acute infusion reaction, the infusion rate may be decreased or the infusion stopped, depending on the severity of reaction. The most common adverse reactions (incidence ≥ 15%) reported with sipuleucel-T are chills, fatigue, fever, back pain, nausea, joint ache, and headache. Most of these adverse events have been reported to occur within one day of the infusion and typically resolve within 1 to 2 days with supportive care.
▪ Retrospective analysis suggests patients with relatively lower PSA values (likely a marker for less tumor volume) benefit most from the vaccine.

Oncolytic Viruses

Talimogene Laherparepvec (T-VEC)

▪ T-VEC is a genetically modified oncolytic viral therapy derived from HSV-1.
▪ FDA approved for the local treatment of unresectable cutaneous, subcutaneous, and nodal lesions in patients with melanoma who have recurrent disease after initial surgery.

- The recommended starting dose is up to a maximum of 4 mL at a concentration of 10^6 (1 million) plaque-forming units (PFU) per mL. Subsequent doses should be administered up to 4 mL at a concentration of 10^8 (100 million) PFU per mL.
- FDA approval was based on a phase III trial, which randomized 436 patients with unresected stage IIIB, IIIC, or IV melanoma 2:1 to receive T-VEC or control therapy with GM-CSF. The objective response rate for T-VEC was 26% with 11% CR, versus 6% with 1% CR in those receiving GM-CSF. The durable response rate (lasting more > 6 months) for T-VEC was 16% versus 2% with GM-CSF (P < 0.0001). In addition, a final planned survival analysis showed a trend in favor of T-VEC. Median OS for T-VEC was 23.3 months versus 18.9 months for GM-CSF (HR 0.80; 95% CI 0.62 to 1.01; P = 0.06).
- The most commonly reported adverse drug reactions (≥25%) in patients treated with T-VEC are fatigue, chills, pyrexia, nausea, influenza-like illness, and injection site pain. It is recommended that healthcare providers and close contacts should avoid direct contact with injected lesions, dressings or body fluids of patients to minimize the risk of transmission of T-VEC and herpetic infection. Healthcare providers who are immunocompromised and pregnant women are recommended against administering T-VEC.

Immune Checkpoint Inhibitors

Ipilimumab

- Ipilimumab is a monoclonal antibody and inhibitor of CTLA-4.
- The first immune checkpoint inhibitor approved by the FDA.
- FDA approved for use in unresectable or metastatic melanoma at a dose of 3 mg/kg administered intravenously every 3 weeks for a total of four doses.
- This approval is based upon a phase III trial of 676 patients with unresectable stage III or IV melanoma who were randomized 3:1:1 to receive ipilimumab plus gp100 (a peptide-based vaccine against glycoprotein 100), ipilimumab alone, or gp100 alone. Median overall survival (OS) of ipilimumab was significantly improved when compared to gp100 alone (10.1 vs. 6.4 months; HR 0.66; P = 0.003). The combination of gp100 and ipilimumab did not show any added survival benefit compared to ipilimumab alone (10 vs. 10.1 months; HR 1.04; P = 0.76).
- Ipilimumab is also approved as adjuvant therapy in patients who have cutaneous melanoma with pathologic involvement of regional lymph nodes of more than 1 mm and who have undergone complete resection, including total lymphadenectomy.
- The approved dose for adjuvant treatment is 10 mg/kg administered intravenously over 90 minutes every 3 weeks for four doses, followed by 10 mg/kg every 12 weeks for up to 3 years or until documented disease recurrence or unacceptable toxicity.
- This approval was based on results from the phase III EORTC 18071 trial, in which 951 patients with stage 3 resected cutaneous melanoma were randomized to receive adjuvant ipilimumab versus placebo. At a median follow up of 2.74 years, the median recurrence-free survival for adjuvant ipiluimumab was 26.1 months as compared to 17.1 months with placebo (HR 0.75; 95% CI 0.64 to 0.90; P = 0.0013).
- The most common adverse reactions at the 3 mg/kg dose (≥5%) are fatigue, diarrhea, pruritus, rash, and colitis. Additional common adverse reactions at the 10 mg/kg dose (≥5%) include nausea, vomiting, headache, weight loss, pyrexia, decreased appetite, and insomnia.

Nivolumab

- Nivolumab is a monoclonal antibody and inhibitor of PD-1.
- FDA approved for several indications, including
  - As single agent or in combination with ipilimumab for unresectable or metastatic melanoma (BRAF V600 mutant or BRAF wild type).
  - Metastatic NSCLC following previous platinum based chemotherapy and following EGFR or ALK-targeted therapy when EGFR or ALK sensitizing genomic alterations exist.
  - Advanced renal cell carcinoma following previous antiangiogenic therapy.

- • Classical Hodgkin's lymphoma following autologous HSCT and post-transplant brentuximab vendotin.
- • Recurrent or metastatic squamous cell carcinoma of the head and neck with disease progression on or after a platinum-based therapy.
- • Locally advanced or metastatic urothelial carcinoma progressing on or following platinum-containing chemotherapy or progressing within 12 months of neoadjuvant or adjuvant treatment with a platinum-containing chemotherapy.
- ▪ Nivolumab gained FDA approval for metastatic melanoma based on several trials.
  - • In a randomized phase III trial, nivolumab was compared to dacarbazine or carboplatin, standard second-line chemotherapy options, in patients with metastatic melanoma that had been previously treated with ipilimumab and if BRAF V600 mutant a BRAF inhibitor as well. After 167 patients were followed for at least 6 months, the median overall response rate (ORR) was 32% for nivolumab compared to 11% for chemotherapy. After a median 8.4 months of follow up, the median duration of response for nivolumab was not reached, with 95% of nivolumab-treated patients still in response, compared to 80% in the chemotherapy-treated group.
  - • A phase III trial in patients with previously untreated BRAF-negative melanoma showed that nivolumab produced an ORR of 40% versus 13.9% for dacarbazine (HR 4.06; $P < 0.001$). At one year of follow-up, OS was 72.9% in the nivolumab group versus 42.1% in the dacarbazine group (HR 0.42; 99.8% CI 0.25 to 0.73; $P < 0.001$).
  - • The approval of nivolumab in combination with ipilimumab was based upon a phase III trial in previously untreated advanced melanoma (CheckMate 067), which randomized 945 patients to receive ipilimumab, nivolumab, or the combination. PFS was 11.5 months (95% CI, 8.9 to 16.7) for the combination compared to 2.9 months (95% CI, 2.8 to 3.4; $P < 0.001$) for ipilimumab alone and 6.9 months (95% CI, 4.3 to 9.5; $P < 0.001$) for nivolumab alone.
- ▪ FDA approval for Nivolumab in NSCLC is based on two key trials, one in squamous NSCLC and one in nonsquamous NSCLC.
  - • A phase III trial comparing nivolumab to standard dosing of docetaxel in patients with metastatic squamous non–small cell lung cancer (NSCLC who had failed at least two prior regimens showed a median OS of 9.2 months for nivolumab versus 6.0 months for docetaxel (HR 0.59; 95% CI, 0.44 to 0.79; $P = 0.00025$). The ORR in the nivolumab group was a modest 20%, but, notably, these patients developed durable responses, with a median duration of response still not reached after a median 11 months of follow-up.
  - • A similar phase III trial evaluated nivolumab versus docetaxel in patients with non-squamous NSCLC who had failed standard platinum-based doublet chemotherapy. In this study, nivolumab produced a median OS of 12.2 months versus 9.4 months with docetaxel (HR 0.73; 96% CI, 0.59 to 0.89; $P = 0.00155$).
- ▪ Nivolumab was granted FDA approval for advanced renal cell carcinoma (RCC) after progression on antiangiogenic therapy based on a phase III trial, which found that such patients treated with nivolumab had a median OS of 25.0 months compared to a median 19.6 months with standard second-line everolimus (HR 0.73; 98.5% CI, 0.57 to 0.93; $P = 0.002$).
- ▪ Nivolumab was granted FDA approval for recurrent or metastatic squamous cell carcinoma of the head and neck (SCCHN) with disease progression on or after a platinum-based therapy based on a randomized phase III trial ($n = 361$), which found that such patients treated with nivolumab had a median OS of 7.5 months compared to a median 5.1 months with standard second line therapy (HR 0.70; 97.73% CI, 0.51 to 0.96; $P = 0.01$).
- ▪ Nivolumab was granted FDA approval for locally advanced or metastatic urothelial carcinoma progressing on or following platinum-containing chemotherapy or progressing within 12 months of neoadjuvant or adjuvant treatment with a platinum-containing chemotherapy based on a phase II trial ($n = 270$) which found that such patients treated with nivolumab had an objective response rate of 19.6%.
- ▪ Finally, nivolumab received FDA approval for the treatment of refractory classical Hodgkin's lymphoma, based on data in a small cohort of 23 patients showing an ORR of 87%, including 17% with a complete response and 70% with a partial response.

- When nivolumab is given as a single agent, the same dosing and administration schedule is used for metastatic melanoma, NSCLC, RCC, urothelial carcinoma, SCCHN, or refractory classical Hodgkin's lymphoma. It is given by intravenous infusion over 60 minutes at a dose of 3 mg/kg every 2 weeks. When nivolumab is given in combination with ipilimumab for metastatic melanoma, the FDA approved dose is 1 mg/kg, followed by ipilimumab 3 mg/kg on the same day, every 3 weeks for four doses, then nivolumab 3 mg/kg as monotherapy every 2 weeks thereafter.
- Although the combination of ipilimumab and nivolumab is not yet FDA approved for advanced RCC, it is worth noting that CheckMate 016 which evaluated varying doses of ipilimumab plus nivolumab in RCC suggested that nivolumab 3 mg/kg in combination with ipilimumab 1 mg/kg was just as efficacious as nivolumab 1 mg/kg in combination with ipilimumab 3 mg/kg (ORR 38.3% vs. 40.4%) but with significantly reduced grade 3 to 4 toxicity (34% vs. 64%).
- The most common adverse reactions (≥20%) in patients with melanoma being treated with nivolumab are fatigue, rash, musculoskeletal pain, pruritus, and diarrhea. When combined with ipilimumab for advanced melanoma nausea, vomiting, pyrexia, and dyspnea are also common. In addition, data from CheckMate 067 in metastatic melanoma strongly suggests that the overall risk of grade 3 to 4 toxicity increases with the combination of ipilimumab and nivolumab compared to each agent alone (55% as compared to 16.3% with nivolumab or 27.3% with ipilimumab).
- In patients with metastatic NSCLC the most common adverse reactions (≥20%) are fatigue, musculoskeletal pain, decreased appetite, cough, and constipation.
- In those with advanced RCC, the most common adverse reactions (≥20%) are asthenic conditions, cough, nausea, rash, dyspnea, diarrhea, constipation, decreased appetite, back pain, and arthralgia.
- In those with urothelial carcinoma, the most common adverse reactions (>20%) were fatigue, musculoskeletal pain, nausea, and decreased appetite.
- In those with SCCHN, the most common adverse reactions (>10%) were cough and dyspnea.
- Finally, in patients with classical Hodgkin's the most common (>20%) adverse reactions are fatigue, upper respiratory tract infection, pyrexia, diarrhea, and cough.

Pembrolizumab

- Pembrolizumab is also an anti-PD-1 antibody.
- FDA approved for several indications including:
  - As treatment in patients with unresectable or metastatic melanoma (BRAF V600 mutant or BRAF wild type).
  - Recurrent or metastatic HNSCC following platinum based chemotherapy.
  - Metastatic NSCLC with no prior systemic chemotherapy treatment in the absence of EGFR or ALK sensitizing genomic alterations.
    - First line treatment of metastatic NSCLC in patients with >50% PD-L1 tumor expression, as measured by an FDA-approved.
  - Metastatic NSCLC following platinum-based chemotherapy and where EGFR or ALK sensitizing genomic alterations exist following treatment with EGFR or ALK TKI therapy.
    - Metastatic NSCLC with positive tumor expression of PD-L1 (>1%) measured by an FDA-approved assay.
- Pembrolizumab gained FDA approval for metastatic melanoma based on two trials, one evaluating pembrolizumab in ipilimumab naïve melanoma and one evaluating pembrolizumab in ipilimumab refractory melanoma.
  - In an open label, multicenter, active controlled trial, 834 patients with ipilimumab naïve metastatic melanoma were randomized 1:1:1 to pembrolizumab at 10 mg/kg every 2 weeks or 10 mg/kg every 3 weeks or ipilimumab 3 mg/kg every 3 weeks for a total of four doses. Patients with BRAF V600E mutated melanoma were not required to receive prior BRAF inhibitor therapy. Objective responses were found in 34% and 33% of those treated with pembrolizumab at 2 weeks and 3 weeks, respectively, as compared to 12% in those treated with ipilimumab. In addition, OS was significantly longer in patients treated with pembrolizumab at 2 weeks (HR 0.69;

95% CI, 0.52 to 0.90; $P = 0.004$) and 3 weeks (HR 0.63; 95% CI, 0.47 to 0.83; $P < 0.001$) compared to those treated with ipilimumab.
- A multicenter, active controlled trial randomized 540 patients with ipilimumab refractory metastatic melanoma 1:1:1 to pembrolizumab 2 mg/kg or 10 mg/kg every 3 weeks or investigator's choice chemotherapy. Objective responses were found in 21% and 25% of those treated with pembrolizumab at 2 mg/kg and 10 mg/kg, respectively, as compared to 4% in those treated with chemotherapy. In addition, PFS was significantly longer in patients treated with pembrolizumab at 2 mg/kg (HR 0.57; 95% CI 0.45 to 0.73; $P < 0.001$) and 10 mg/kg (HR 0.50; 95% CI 0.39 to 0.64; $P < 0.001$) as compared to those treated with chemotherapy.

- FDA approval for pembrolizumab in NSCLC as first-line therapy is based upon a phase III trial which randomized 305 patients with previously untreated advanced NSCLC with PD-L1 expression on at least 50% of tumor cells to pembrolizumab 200 mg every 3 weeks or platinum-based chemotherapy. PFS was significantly longer for pembrolizumab as compared to platinum-based chemotherapy (10.3 vs. 6.0 months; HR 0.50; 95% CI 0.37 to 0.68; $P < 0.001$).

- FDA approval for pembrolizumab in NSCLC as second-line therapy is based upon an open-label, phase 2/3 study, which randomized 1,034 patients with previously treated advanced NSCLC with PD-L1 expression on at least 1% of tumor cells 1:1:1 to pembrolizumab 2 mg/kg, pembrolizumab 10 mg/kg, or docetaxel 75 mg/m^2 every 3 weeks. OS was significantly longer for pembrolizumab 10 mg/kg versus docetaxel (12.7 vs. 8.5 months; HR 0.71; 95% CI 0.58 to 0.88; $P = 0.0008$) and for pembrolizumab 2 mg/kg versus docetaxel (10.4 vs. 8.5; HR 0.61; 95% CI 0.49 to 0.75; $P < 0.0001$).

- Pembrolizumab received FDA approval for HNSCC based upon a multicenter, nonrandomized, open-label phase 1b trial that enrolled 192 patients with recurrent or metastatic HNSCC with disease progression following platinum-containing chemotherapy. Patients received pembrolizumab at 10 mg/kg every 2 weeks ($n = 53$) or 200 mg every 3 weeks ($n = 121$). The ORR was 17.7%. Among responding patients, the median duration of response had not been reached after a median 12.5 months of follow-up. ORR was 21.9% in HPV$^+$ patients and 15.9% in HPV$^-$ patients.

- Pembrolizumab is administered as an intravenous infusion over 30 minutes at a dose of 2 mg/kg every 3 weeks for melanoma or as a flat dose of 200 mg every 3 weeks for HNSCC and NSCLC.

- The most common adverse reactions ($\geq$20%) seen with pembrolizumab in clinical trials were fatigue, decreased appetite, and dyspnea. Cough was common in patients with NSCLC, and in patients with melanoma, pruritus, rash, constipation, diarrhea, and nausea were also common.

Atezolizumab

- Atezolizumab is an anti-PD-L1 antibody.
- FDA approved for two indications:
  - Locally advanced or metastatic urothelial carcinoma with progression following platinum-based chemotherapy or progression within 12 months of neoadjuvant or adjuvant treatment with platinum-based chemotherapy.
- Metastatic NSCLC following platinum-based chemotherapy and where EGFR or ALK sensitizing genomic alterations exist following treatment with EGFR or ALK TKI therapy. The approval for locally advanced or metastatic urothelial carcinoma was based on a phase II study, where 316 patients with metastatic urothelial carcinoma who had disease progression on platinum-based chemotherapy were given atezolizumab 1,200 mg every 3 weeks. The ORR was 15%, with 91% of responses still ongoing after 24 weeks of follow-up.
- The approval for metastatic NSCLC was based on a phase III trial, where 850 patients with previously treated metastatic NSCLC were randomized to atezolizumab 1,200 mg or docetaxel 75 mg/m^2 every 3 weeks. Median OS was improved with atezolizumab as compared with docetaxel (13.8 vs. 9.6 months; HR 0.73; 95% CI, 0.62 to 0.87; $P = 0.0003$).
- Atezolizumab is administered by intravenous infusion over 60 minutes at a flat dose of 1,200 mg every 3 weeks for both NSCLC and urothelial carcinoma.
- The most common adverse reactions ($\geq$20% of patients) seen with atezolizumab in patients with urothelial carcinomas are fatigue, decreased appetite, nausea, urinary tract infection, pyrexia, and constipation.

- The most common adverse reactions (≥20% of patients) seen with atezolizumab in patients with NSCLC are fatigue, decreased appetite, dyspnea, cough, nausea, musculoskeletal pain, and constipation.

Durvalumab

- Durvalumab is an anti-PD-L1 antibody
- The FDA granted accelerated approved in May 2017 for locally advanced or metastatic urothelial carcinoma that has progressed on or following platinum-based chemotherapy or has progressed within 12 months of adjuvant/neoadjuvant platinum-based therapy.
- The approvals were based on findings from a single arm trial in patients with locally advanced or metastatic urothelial carcinoma with progression following platinum-based chemotherapy (n = 182). The ORR by RECIST 1.1 was 17.0% (95% CI: 11.9, 23.3). At the time of analysis, median response duration was not reached (range: 0.9+ to 19.9+ months). The VENTANA PD-L1 (SP263) assay was used for evaluation of PD-L1 status. For 95 patients who were PD-L1high, ORR was 26.3% (95% CI: 17.8, 36.4). The ORR was 4.1% (95% CI: 0.9, 11.5) for the 73 patients who were PD-L1low or PD-L1-. The VENTANA PD-L1 assay is also FDA approved as a companion diagnostic (package insert, data not published).
  - The manufacturer must complete a currently ongoing trial to confirm clinical benefit, as a condition of the accelerated approval.
- The recommended durvalumab dosing, based on the 182 patient study, 10 mg/kg i.v. every 2 weeks until disease progression or unacceptable toxicity.
- Commonly reported adverse reactions included fatigue, nausea, decreased appetite, constipation, musculoskeletal pain, peripheral edema, and urinary tract infections, with 43% of patients experiencing grade 3-4 toxicities.
  - Immune-related pneumonitis, hepatitis, colitis, thyroid disease, adrenal insufficiency, and diabetes have been observed with durvalumab.

Avelumab

- Avelumab is an anti-PD-L1 antibody
- FDA approvals:
  - Avelumab was granted accelerated approval by FDA for treatment of metastatic Merkel cell carcinoma in children over 12 years old and adults in March 2017.
  - In May 2017, Avelumab received approval for locally advanced or metastatic urothelial carcinoma that has progressed on or following platinum-based chemotherapy or has progressed within 12 months of adjuvant/neoadjuvant platinum-based therapy.
- Approval of avelumab for Merkel cell carcinoma was based upon data from the phase I multicenter JAVELIN Merkel 200 trial, demonstrating an ORR of 33% (95% CI: 23.3, 43.8). The complete response rate was 22% and partial response rate was 11%, with 86% of responses durable 6 months. No correlation between tumor PD-L1 status and responses was observed.
- Approval for urothelial carcinoma was based upon findings from the urothelial cohorts (n = 242) in the multicenter JAVELIN phase I, single arm trial in solid tumors.
  - Data reported in March 2016 from 153 patients with 6 months follow-up demonstrated an ORR of 17.7% (95% CI: 12.0, 24.6) with 9 completes responses and 18 partial responses. The 24-week duration of response rate was 92% (95% CI: 71.6,97.9), and the median was not reached. The median OS was 7 months (95% CI: 5.6,11.2). Of evaluable tumors, 56 patients' tumors were PD-L1+ (based on 5% PD-L1 staining) and 75 were PD-L1-. ORR was 25% (95% CI: 14.4, 38.4) and 14.7% (95% CI: 7.6, 24.7; p = 0.178, respectively, suggesting that PD-L1 tumor status by this method is not a predictor of response.
- Dosing of Avelumab for both Merkel cell and urothelial carcinoma is 10 mg/kg i.v. every 2 weeks until disease progression.
- Premedication with acetaminophen and an anti-histamine is recommended for at least the first 4 doses of avelumab to prevent infusion reactions.

- The most commonly reported adverse reactions in Merkel cell carcinoma patients (≥ 20%) were fatigue, musculoskeletal pain, diarrhea, nausea, infusion-related reaction, rash, decreased appetite, and peripheral edema.
- The most common adverse events in patients with urothelial carcinoma (at least 20%) of were fatigue, infusion-related reaction, musculoskeletal pain, nausea, decreased appetite, and urinary tract infection.
  - Serious adverse reactions occurred in 41% of urothelial carcinoma patients (41%). The most common (≥ 2%) were urinary tract infection/urosepsis, hematuria/urinary tract hemorrhage, small bowel obstruction, abdominal pain, musculoskeletal pain, renal function decrease, dehydration, and pyrexia.
  - Death due to an adverse reaction occurred in 6% of urothelial carcinoma patients who received avelumab.
- Avelumab can cause immune-mediated pneumonitis, colitis, hepatitis, endocrinopathy and nephritis.

MANAGING IMMUNE-RELATED ADVERSE EVENTS DUE TO IMMUNE CHECKPOINT INHIBITORS

- Although occurring rarely, a number of serious immune-related adverse events (irAEs) have been reported with immune checkpoint inhibitors (i.e., ipilimumab, nivolumab, pembrolizumab, atezolizumab) including colitis, nephritis, pneumonitis, endocrinopathies (hypothyroidism, Type 1 DM, adrenal insufficiency, hypopituitarism), myasthenia gravis, Guillain-Barré, meningoencephalitis, pericarditis, uveitis, iritis, nerve palsies, hemolytic anemia, pancreatitis, hepatitis leading to hepatotoxicity and hyperacute GVHD following allogeneic stem cell transplant.
- Because of these risks it is recommended that in addition to routine bloodwork including CBC and chemistries that include liver function tests, ACTH and thyroid function also be routinely monitored.
- In the event of a severe immune-mediated adverse reaction, permanently discontinue treatment and administer systemic high-dose corticosteroids (prednisone 1 to 2 mg/kg/day or equivalent). Patients should continue corticosteroids until symptoms improve at which time a steroid taper lasting over a month should be initiated (see Fig. 45.1).

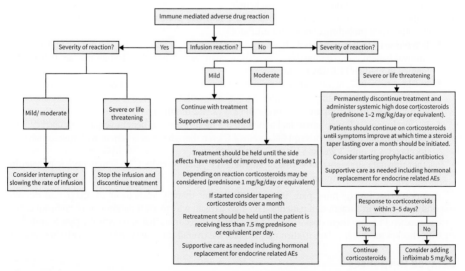

FIGURE 45.1 Recommendations for managing immune-related adverse events due to immune checkpoint inhibitors.

- While patients may be concerned about corticosteroids abrogating the effects of checkpoint inhibitor therapy, at least one small trial evaluating ipilimumab in 139 patients with advanced melanoma, suggested that corticosteroids given for irAEs do not affect the duration of objective responses ($P = 0.23$).
- If patients do not respond to corticosteroids within 3 to 5 days (occurs rarely), then treatment with infliximab 5 mg/kg with or without the continuation of steroids should be considered after ruling out bowel perforation or sepsis. A second dose of infliximab 5 mg/kg may be given 2 weeks after the first dose if severe symptoms persist.
- For moderate immune-mediated adverse reactions, it is recommended that treatment be held until the side effects have resolved or improved to at least grade 1. For ipilimumab it is recommended that treatment be held until the patient is receiving less than 7.5 mg prednisone or equivalent per day.
- Prophylactic antibiotics should be administered to patients on long-term immune suppression, particularly to pneumocystis pneumonia.
- Infusion reactions have also been described. For severe and life-threatening infusion reactions stop the infusion and discontinue treatment. For mild or moderate reactions consider interrupting or slowing the rate of infusion.
- Special attention should be paid to patients with diarrhea or dyspnea as colitis and pneumonis, respectively, can be lethal toxicities if not addressed in an appropriate time frame.

RESPONSE TO IMMUNOTHERAPY

Assessing Clinical Benefit

- A number of immunotherapies have been found to significantly improve overall survival even when no or minimal benefit is seen in short term outcomes (e.g., TTP, PFS, decline in tumor markers).
  - In the IMPACT trial, Sipuleucel-T was found to provide a median OS benefit of 4.1 months over placebo (25.8 vs. 21.7 months) in men with mCRPC. Yet no significant difference in TTP was observed between sipuleucel-T and the control arm. In addition, only 2.6% of patients receiving sipuleucel-T were observed to have confirmed PSA declines (>50%).
  - A lack of improvement in short term outcomes (e.g. lack of PSA decline) should not be misinterpreted as a lack of potential long-term benefit.
- This phenomenon is not unique to sipulecuel-T and has been reported with a number of other immunotherapies including checkpoint inhibitors.
  - In a phase III trial in patients with advanced melanoma, ipilimumab showed a median 3.7 month survival benefit compared gp100 vaccination (10.1 vs. 6.4 months) despite the fact that no difference in median PFS was found.
  - In Checkmate 057, nivolumab had a median 2.8 month survival benefit as compared to docetaxel (12.2 vs. 9.4 months) in patients with non-squamous NSCLC. However, PFS was not improved with nivolumab as compared to docetaxel (2.3 vs. 4.2 months).
  - In Checkmate 017, nivolumab had a median 3.2 month survival benefit versus docetaxel (9.2 vs. 6.0 months) in patients with squamous NSCLC even though the PFS benefit with nivolumab over docetaxel was only 3 weeks (3.5 vs. 2.8 months).
- Together this data suggests that surrogate markers (i.e., change in PSA, PFS) may underestimate the clinical impact of many immunotherapies.

It appears that for the most part, immune checkpoint therapy leads to rapid, deep, and durable responses, but only in a fraction of patients. That may explain why many trials show no significant difference in median PFS, but there does appear to be a tail on PFS curves that is statistically significantly better with checkpoint therapy. This in turn may explain the overall survival benefit seen with these agents.

Delayed Responses

- Effective anti-tumor immune activation by immunotherapy may take weeks to months to occur, leading to delayed responses. This is more commonly seen with vaccine and oncolytic virus–based therapies but may occasionally also occur with immune checkpoint inhibitors.

- In the phase III trial of T-VEC in locally advanced and metastatic melanoma, the median time to response was 4.1 months ranging from 1.2 to as long as 16.7 months.
- In the phase III trial of nivolumab versus dacarbazine in patients with previously untreated advanced melanoma, the median time to response with nivolumab was 2.1 months ranging from 1.6 to up to 7.6 months.
- In the phase III trial of nivolumab versus docetaxel in non-squamous NSCLC the median time to response was also 2.1 months and ranged from 1.2 to up to 8.6 months. In the phase Ib trial of pembrolizumab in patients with HNSCC, the median time to response was two months but ranged from two to as many as 17 months.
- Specifically, with regard to checkpoint inhibitors, a median of 2 months until response likely reflects the time point of first restaging in clinical trials suggesting that these therapies for the most part lead to relatively rapid responses although occasionally delayed responses may occur.

Durable Responses

- Once an objective response with immunotherapy is achieved, the response is usually durable.
  - In the phase III T-VEC trial in locally advanced and metastatic melanoma, after a median 44.4 months of follow up, the median duration of response was still not reached.
  - In the phase III trial of ipilimumab with or without gp100 versus gp100 alone in advanced melanoma, after a median follow up of 8.9 months, the median duration of response to ipilimumab was also not reached.
  - In the phase III trials of nivolumab in previously treated advanced melanoma and squamous NSCLC, the median durations of response were again not reached after a median of 8.9 and minimum of 11 months of follow-up, respectively.

In the phase III trial of nivolumab in advanced non-squamous NSCLC, the median duration of response was 17.2 months after a minimum 13.2 months of follow-up.

Pseudo-progression

- Pseudo-progression is a phenomenon where tumors appear to progress radiographically following treatment, but the apparent increase in tumor size on scans is due to other factors such as edema rather than tumor growth. Before the use of immune checkpoint inhibitors, this phenomenon was best described in glioblastoma following radiotherapy.
- With respect to immune checkpoint inhibitors, the term pseudo-progression is usually used to refer to the observation of apparent tumor progression radiographically after treatment followed by tumor regression and objective response.
- In the case of immune checkpoint inhibition, the initial increase in size is hypothesized to be due to tumor immune cell infiltration.
- The finding that certain tumors seem to have pseudo-progression following immune checkpoint inhibition has led to the development of newer immune-related response criteria, which have been developed to limit the number of patients cutting treatment short for pseudo-progression. Among other changes to traditional response criteria (i.e., RECIST), these newer criteria introduce the concept of confirmation of progression on follow-up scans. Based on this, it is generally recommended that patients who are receiving immune checkpoint inhibition have confirmatory scans about 4 weeks after first radiographic progression to confirm disease progression.
- However, while this is the general rule it should be noted that pseudo-progression is relatively rare following immune checkpoint inhibition.
  - A recent study retrospectively looked at 356 patients with a variety of cancers (i.e., melanoma, lung, breast) receiving immune checkpoint inhibitors and found that only 6% of patients developed pseudo progression by immune-related response criteria.
- In every day practice the decision to continue with treatment and wait for confirmation of disease progression should not be made automatically because pseudo progression occurs in a substantial minority (less than 10%) of patients. Factors such as patient preference, their symptoms, and rate of tumor growth and velocity of tumor markers may be used to help make an educated clinical decision about continuing versus switching treatment.

PD-L1 Staining

- Data from studies in melanoma, head and neck, lung, and bladder cancers all suggest that response rates to anti-PD-1/PD-L1 treatment are substantially higher in patients who have biopsy proven PD-L1 expression in the tumor microenvironment (TME).
  - Head and neck tumors (PD-L1-positive: 46% vs. PD-L1 negative: 11%).
  - Bladder cancer (PD-L1-positive: 43% vs. PD-L1-negative: 11%).
  - Lung cancer (PD-L1-positive: 46% vs. PD-L1-negative: 15%).
  - Melanoma (PD-L1-positive: 49% vs. PD-L1-negative: 13%).
    - In addition, a recent meta-analysis of patients with metastatic melanoma, NSCLC, and renal cell carcinoma showed a significant correlation between response to anti PD-1/PDL-1 therapy and PDL-1 expression in the TME.

  Interestingly, many studies have associated increased PD-L1 expression in the TME with an underlying baseline tumor immune response (e.g., T cell infiltration in tumors). Tumors with a preexisting, underlying immune response are often referred to as "hot" tumors whereas their counterparts without an underlying immune response are often referred to as "cold" tumors. Immune checkpoint inhibitors, especially anti PD-1/PD-L1 therapies, do not create a tumor specific immune response de novo but allow a baseline immune response to proceed unchecked. This may explain why "hot" tumors, which are associated with increased PD-L1 expression, seem to respond better to anti PD-1/PD-L1 therapy. Although beyond the scope of this chapter, a massive research effort is underway to turn "cold" tumors into "hot" tumors and thereby increase the percentage of patients who may benefit from immune checkpoint therapy.

Mismatch Repair Deficiency and Microsatellite Instability

- Growing clinical data suggest that patients harboring mismatch repair deficient tumors (bearing microsatellite instability) have a significant chance of responding to immune checkpoint inhibition.
- In a phase II study of pembrolizumab in patients with progressive metastatic carcinoma, four of ten (40%) patients with mismatch repair deficient colorectal cancers had an objective response compared with 0 of 18 (0%) patients with mismatch repair proficient colorectal cancers.
- In addition, objective responses were observed in five of seven (71%) patients with mismatch repair deficient noncolorectal cancers.
- It has been hypothesized that mismatch repair deficiency results in a high somatic mutational and antigenic burden, which predisposes to response with immune checkpoint inhibitors. In the preceding trial, whole exome sequencing of tumors showed significantly more mutations tumor in mismatch repair deficient versus mismatch repair proficient tumors (mean of 1,782 vs. 73; $P = 0.007$). A high somatic mutational burden was also found to be significantly associated with longer-free survival (PFS) ($P = 0.02$).

Suggested Readings

1. Andtbacka RHI, Collichio FA, Amatruda T, et al. Final planned overall survival (OS) from OPTiM, a randomized phase III trial of talimogene laherparepvec (T-VEC) versus GM-CSF for the treatment of unresected stage IIIB/C/IV melanoma (NCT00769704). *J Immunother Cancer.* 2014;2(suppl 3):P263.
2. Andtbacka RHI, Kauffman HL, Collichio FA, et al. Talimogene laherparepvec improves durable response rate in patients with advanced melanoma. *J Clin Oncol.* 2015 Sep 1;33(25):2780–2788.
3. Ansell SM, Lesokhin AM, Borrello I, et al. PD-1 blockade with nivolumab in relapsed or refractory Hodgkin's lymphoma. *N Engl J Med.* 2015;372:311–319.
4. Atkins MB, Lotze MT, Dutcher JP, et al. High-dose recombinant interleukin 2 therapy for patients with metastatic melanoma: analysis of 270 patients treated between 1985 and 1993. *JCO.* 1999 July;17(7):2105.
5. Brahmer J, Reckamp KL, Baas P, et al. Nivolumab versus docetaxel in advanced squamous-cell non–small-cell lung cancer. *N Engl J Med.* 2015;373:123–135. (This trial led to FDA approval of nivolumab for advanced squamous NSCLC.)
6. Downey SG, Klapper JA, Smith FO, et al. Prognostic factors related to clinical response in patients with metastatic melanoma treated by CTL-associated antigen-4 blockade. *Cancer Res.* 2007 Nov 15;13(22 Pt 1):6681–6688.
7. Eggermont AM, Chiarion-Sileni V, Grob JJ, et al. Adjuvant ipilimumab versus placebo after complete resection of high-risk stage III melanoma (EORTC 18071): a randomised, double-blind, phase 3 trial. *Lancet Oncol.* 2015 May;16(5):522–530.

8. Eggermont AM, Suciu S, Testori A, et al. Long-term results of the randomized phase III trial EORTC 18991 of adjuvant therapy with pegylated interferon alfa-2b versus observation in resected stage III melanoma. *J Clin Oncol.* 2012 Nov 1;30(31):3810.

9. Escudier B, Pluzanska A, Koralewski P, et al. Bevacizumab plus interferon alfa-2a for treatment of metastatic renal cell carcinoma: a randomised, double-blind phase III trial. *Lancet.* 2007 Dec 22;370(9605):2103–2111.

10. Ferris RL, Blumenschein G, Fayette J, et al. Nivolumab for recurrent squamous-cell carcinoma of the head and neck. *N Engl J Med.* 2016;375:1856–1867.

11. Fisher RI, Rosenberg SA, Sznol M, et al. High-dose aldesleukin in renal cell carcinoma: long-term survival update. *Cancer J Sci Am.* 1997 Dec;3(suppl 1):S70–S72.

12. Fu J, Malm IJ, Kadayakkara DK, et al. Preclinical evidence that PD1 blockade cooperates with cancer vaccine TEGVAX to elicit regression of established tumors. *Cancer Res.* 2014;74:4042–4052.

13. Gandini S, Massi D, Mandalà M. PD-L1 expression in cancer patients receiving anti PD-1/PD-L1 antibodies: a systematic review and meta-analysis. *Crit Rev Oncol Hematol.* 2016;100:88–98.

14. Hammers H, Plimack E, Infante J, et al. Expanded cohort results from CheckMate 016: a phase I study of nivolumab in combination with ipilimumab in metastatic renal cell carcinoma (mRCC). *J Clin Oncol.* 2015;33(suppl):abstr 4516.

15. Herbst RS, Baas P, Kim DW, et al. Pembrolizumab versus docetaxel for previously treated, PD-L1-positive, advanced non-small-cell lung cancer (KEYNOTE-010): a randomised controlled trial. *Lancet.* 2016 April 9;387(10027):1540–1550.

16. Hodi FS, O'Day SJ, McDermott DF, et al. Improved survival with ipilimumab in patients with metastatic melanoma. *N Engl J Med.* 2010;363:711–723.

17. Hoffman-Censits J, Grivas P, Van Der Heijden M, et al. IMvigor 210, a phase II trial of atezolizumab (MPDL3280A) in platinum-treated locally advanced or metastatic urothelial carcinoma (mUC). *J Clin Oncol.* 2016;34(suppl 2S):abstr 355.

18. Kantoff PW, Higano CS, Shore ND, et al. Sipuleucel-T immunotherapy for castration-resistant prostate cancer. *N Engl J Med.* 2010;363:411–422.

19. Kaufman HL, Russell L, Hamid O, et al. Avelumab in patients with chemotherapy-refractory metastatic Merkel cell carcinoma: a multicentre, single-group, open-label, phase 2 trial. *Lancet Oncol.* 2016;17:1374–1385.

20. Kurra V, Sullivan RJ, Gaino JF, et al. Pseudoprogression in cancer immunotherapy: rates, time course and patient outcomes. *J Clin Oncol.* 2016;34(suppl):abstr 6580.

21. Larkin J, Chiarion-Sileni V, Gonzalez R, et al. Combined nivolumab and ipilimumab or monotherapy in untreated melanoma. *N Engl J Med.* 2015;373:23–34.

22. Le DT, Uram JN, Wang H, et al. PD-1 blockade in tumors with mismatch-repair deficiency. *N Engl J Med.* 2015;372:2509–2520.

23. Mehra R, Seiwert TY, Mahipal A, et al. Efficacy and safety of pembrolizumab in recurrent/metastatic head and neck squamous cell carcinoma (R/M HNSCC): pooled analyses after long-term follow-up in KEYNOTE-012. *J Clin Oncol.* 2016;34(suppl):abstr 6012.

24. Motzer RJ, Escudier B, McDermott DF, et al. Nivolumab versus everolimus in advanced renal-cell carcinoma. *N Engl J Med.* 2015;373:1803–1813.

25. Pages C, Gornet JM, Monsel G, et al. Ipilimumab-induced acute severe colitis treated by infliximab. *Melanoma Res.* 2013;23:227–230.

26. Pardoll DM. The blockade of immune checkpoints in cancer immunotherapy. *Nat Rev Cancer.* 2012 April;12(4):252–264.

27. Patel MR, Ellerton JA, Infante JR, et al. Avelumab in patients with metastatic urothelial carcinoma: pooled results from two cohorts of the phase 1b JAVELIN Solid Tumor trial. *J Clin Oncol.* 2017;35(6_suppl):330–330.

28. Paz-Ares L, Horn L, Borghaei H, et al. Phase III, randomized trial (CheckMate 057) of nivolumab (NIVO) versus docetaxel (DOC) in advanced non-squamous cell (non-SQ) non-small cell lung cancer (NSCLC). *J Clin Oncol.* 2015;33(suppl):abstr LBA109.

29. Powles T, Eder JP, Fine GD, et al. MPDL3280A (anti-PD-L1) treatment leads to clinical activity in metastatic bladder cancer. *Nature* 2014;515:558–562.

30. Reck M, Rodríguez-Abreu D, Robinson AG, et al. Pembrolizumab versus chemotherapy for PD-L1–positive non–small-cell lung cancer. *N Engl J Med.* 2016 Nov 10;375:1823–1833.

31. Ribas A, Hodi F, Kefford R, et al. Efficacy and safety of the anti-PD-1 monoclonal antibody MK-3475 in 411 patients (pts) with melanoma (MEL). *J Clin Oncol.* 2014;32(5s):abstr LBA9000.

32. Ribas A, Puzanov I, Dummer R, et al. Pembrolizumab versus investigator-choice chemotherapy for ipilimumab-refractory melanoma (KEYNOTE-002): a randomised, controlled, phase 2 trial. *Lancet Oncol.* 2015 Aug;16(8):908–918.

33. Rittmeyer A, Barlesi F, Waterkamp D, et al. Atezolizumab versus docetaxel in patients with previously treated non-small-cell lung cancer (OAK): a phase 3, open-label, multicentre randomised controlled trial. *Lancet.* 2017 Jan 21;389(10066):255–265.

34. Rizvi N, Chow L, Dirix L, et al. Clinical trials of MPDL3280A (anti-PDL1) in patients (pts) with non-small cell lung cancer (NSCLC). *J Clin Oncol.* 2014;32(5s):abstr TPS8123.

35. Robert C, Long GV, Brady B, et al. Nivolumab in previously untreated melanoma without BRAF mutation. *N Engl J Med.* 2015;372:320–330.

36. Robert C, Schachter J, Long GV, et al. Pembrolizumab versus ipilimumab in advanced melanoma. *N Engl J Med.* 2015 Jun 25;372(26):2521–232.

37. Seiwert T, Burtness B, Weiss J, et al. A phase Ib study of MK-3475 in patients with human papillomavirus (HPV)-associated and non-HPV–associated head and neck (H/N) cancer. *J Clin Oncol.* 2014;32(5s):abstr 6011.

38. Sharma P, Retz M, Siefker-Radtke A, et al. Nivolumab in metastatic urothelial carcinoma after platinum therapy (CheckMate 275): a multicentre, single-arm, phase 2 trial. *Lancet Oncol.* 2017 Jan 25:pii: S1470-2045(17)30065-7.

39. Thompson ED, Zahurak M, Murphy A. Patterns of PD-L1 expression and CD8 T cell infiltration in gastric adenocarcinomas and associated immune stroma. *Gut.* 2016 Jan 22:pii: gutjnl-2015-310839.

40. Webb JR, Milne K, Kroeger DR, et al. PD-L1 expression is associated with tumor-infiltrating T cells and favorable prognosis in high-grade serous ovarian cancer. *Gynecol Oncol.* 2016 May;141(2):293–302.

41. Weber J, Minor D, D'Angelo S, et al. A phase 3 randomized, open-label study of nivolumab (anti-PD-1; BMS-936558; ONO-4538) versus investigator's choice chemotherapy (ICC) in patients with advanced melanoma after prior anti-CTLA-4 therapy. *Ann Oncol.* 2014;25(suppl 4):abstr LBA3-PR.

42. YERVOY™ (ipilimumab) US Prescribing Information: Risk Evaluation and Mitigation Strategy (REMS). Princeton, NJ: Bristol-Myers Squibb Company; 2011. https://www.hcp.yervoy.com/pages/rems.aspx. Accessed April 2015.

Anticancer Agents 46

Erin F. Damery and Thomas E. Hughes

INTRODUCTION

Please note that all information has been obtained from current product labeling as of January 31, 2017. Doses listed are those from the package insert and apply when the agent is given alone, unless otherwise noted. Doses are expressed in accordance with nomenclature guidelines from Kohler et al.

ADVERSE REACTIONS

Adverse reactions to anticancer agents involve the following:

- Cardiovascular system (CV)
- Skin and integument system (DERM)
- Electrolyte abnormalities (ELECTRO)
- Endocrine system (ENDO)
- Gastrointestinal system (GI)
- Genitourinary system (GU)
- Hematopoietic system (HEMAT)
- Hepatic system (HEPAT)
- Infusion-related reactions (INFUS)
- Neurologic system, central and peripheral (NEURO)
- Ocular system
- Pulmonary system (PULM)
- Liver function
- Serum creatinine (Cr)
- Creatinine clearance (CrCl)
- Nausea and vomiting (N/V): Classified on a four-level system. Emetogenic potential is based on the incidence of acute emesis in product labeling and/or based on classification by national chemotherapy-induced nausea and vomiting (CINV) guidelines—minimal, <10%; low, 10% to 30%; moderate, 30% to 90%; and high, >90% (see Chapter 38).

ABIRATERONE (ZYTIGA)

Mechanism of Action

- Androgen biosynthesis inhibitor of 17 α-hydroxylase/C17, 20-lyase (CYP17). This enzyme is expressed in testicular, adrenal, and prostatic tumor tissues and is required for androgen biosynthesis.

FDA-Approved Indications

- In combination with prednisone for the treatment of metastatic castration-resistant prostate cancer.

FDA-Approved Dosage

- 1,000 mg (four 250 mg tablets) PO once daily in combination with prednisone 5 mg administered PO twice daily. Abiraterone must be taken on an empty stomach, swallowed whole with water. No food should be consumed for at least 2 hours before the dose and for at least 1 hour after the dose of abiraterone.

Dose Modification Criteria

- Renal: no
- Hepatic (moderate, Child–Pugh class B): yes
- Hepatic (severe, Child–Pugh class C): avoid use

Adverse Reactions

- CV: hypertension
- ELECTRO: hypokalemia, hypernatremia, and hypophosphatemia
- ENDO: adrenal insufficiency, hypercholesterolemia, hyperglycemia, and hypertriglyceridemia
- GI: constipation, diarrhea, and dyspepsia
- GU: hematuria and urinary tract infection
- HEMAT: anemia and lymphopenia
- HEPAT: elevated alkaline phosphatase, elevated bilirubin, and elevated LFTs
- PULM: cough, dyspnea, nasopharyngitis, and upper respiratory tract infection
- OTHER: confusion, edema, fatigue, hot flush, insomnia, joint swelling/discomfort, and muscle discomfort

Comments

- Use abiraterone with caution in patients with a history of CV disease. The safety of abiraterone in patients with LVEF <50% or New York Heart Association (NYHA) class II to IV heart failure was not established in clinical studies. Control hypertension and correct hypokalemia before treatment. Monitor blood pressure, serum potassium, and symptoms of fluid retention at least monthly.
- Monitor for signs and symptoms of adrenocortical insufficiency. Increased dosage of corticosteroids may be indicated before, during, and after stressful situations.
- Hepatotoxicity can be severe and fatal. Monitor liver function and modify, interrupt, or discontinue based on the recommendations outlined in product labeling.
- Abiraterone is an inhibitor of CYP2D6. Avoid coadministration of abiraterone with substrates of CYP2D6 with a narrow therapeutic index (e.g., thioridazine). Based on in vitro data, avoid or use with caution with strong CYP3A4 inhibitors or inducers.
- Abiraterone peak concentration (Cmax) and area under the concentration–time curve (AUC) exposure were increased up to 17- and 10-fold higher, respectively, when a single dose of abiraterone was administered with a meal compared to a fasted state. Patients must be counseled to take abiraterone on an empty stomach.
- Abiraterone is not indicated for use in women. Embryo-fetal toxicity: abiraterone can cause fetal harm when administered to a pregnant woman.

ADO-TRASTUZUMAB EMTANSINE (KADCYLA)

Mechanism of Action

- Human epidermal growth factor receptor protein (HER2) targeted antibody-drug conjugate composed of the humanized anti-HER2 IgG1 antibody trastuzumab, and the small molecule cytotoxin DM1, which is a microtubule inhibitor. Once ado-trastuzumab emtansine binds to the HER2 receptor, receptor-mediated internalization occurs, leading to intracellular release of DM1.

FDA-Approved Indications

- HER2-positive metastatic breast cancer in patients who have previously received trastuzumab and a taxane, separately or in combination. Patient should have either received prior therapy for metastatic disease or developed disease recurrence during or within 6 months of completing adjuvant therapy.

FDA-Approved Dosage

- 3.6 mg/kg IV infusion every 3 weeks until disease progression or unacceptable toxicity.

Dose Modification Criteria

- Renal (mild to moderate, CrCl ≥30 mL/min): no
- Renal (severe, CrCl <30 mL/min): limited data available
- Hepatic (mild to moderate): no
- Hepatic (severe): not studied, use with caution
- Myelosuppression: yes
- Nonhematologic toxicity: yes

Adverse Reactions

- CV: left ventricular dysfunction
- GI: diarrhea, constipation, and N/V (low)
- HEMAT: hemorrhage, thrombocytopenia, and anemia
- HEPAT: increased transaminases
- INFUS: flushing, chills, pyrexia, dyspnea, hypotension, wheezing, bronchospasm, and tachycardia
- NEURO: peripheral neuropathy and headache
- PULM: dyspnea, cough, pulmonary infiltrates, and pneumonitis
- OTHER: arthralgia, myalgia, and fatigue

Comments

- Do not substitute ado-trastuzumab emtansine for or with trastuzumab.
- Do not administer as an intravenous push or bolus. Do not use Dextrose 5% (D5W) solution.
- Hepatotoxicity and liver failure have occurred in patients treated with ado-trastuzumab emtansine. Monitor hepatic function prior to initiation of therapy and prior to each dose. Dose withholding or dose modification may be necessary.
- Ado-trastuzumab emtansine may lead to reductions in left ventricular ejection fraction (LVEF). Assess LVEF prior to initiation and at regular intervals during treatment and monitor for signs or symptoms of cardiac toxicity.
- Interstitial lung disease has been reported. Monitor and withhold for acute onset or worsening of pulmonary symptoms.
- Monitor for signs or symptoms of neurotoxicity. Temporarily discontinue for grade 3 or 4 peripheral neuropathy.
- Embryo-fetal toxicity: Ado-trastuzumab may cause fetal harm when administered to a pregnant woman.

AFATINIB (GILOTRIF)

Mechanism of Action

- Covalently binds to the kinase domains of epidermal growth factor receptor (EGFR), HER2, and HER4 and irreversibly inhibits tyrosine kinase autophosphorylation, resulting in down regulation of ErbB signaling.

FDA-Approved Indications

- First-line treatment of metastatic non-small cell lung cancer (NSCLC) tumors that have EGFR exon 19 deletions or exon 21 (L858R) substitution mutations as detected by an FDA-approved test
- Metastatic, squamous NSCLC progressing after platinum-based chemotherapy

FDA-Approved Dosage

- 40 mg orally, once daily. Take at least 1 hour before or 2 hours after a meal.

Dose Modification Criteria

- Renal (mild or moderate, CrCl > 30ml/min): no
- Renal (severe, CrCl 15–29 mL/min): yes
- Hepatic (mild or moderate): no
- Hepatic (severe, Child–Pugh C): no data available, use with caution
- Nonhematologic toxicity: yes

Adverse Reactions

- DERM: bullous and exfoliative skin disorders, rash/acneiform dermatitis, dry skin, pruritus, and paronychia
- ELECTRO: decreased potassium
- GI: diarrhea, stomatitis, and N/V (low)
- GU: decreased CrCl, cystitis
- HEMAT: decreased lymphocytes
- HEPAT: increased ALT/AST, increased alkaline phosphate, and increased bilirubin
- PULM: interstitial lung disease
- Ocular System: keratitis and conjunctivitis
- OTHER: pyrexia

Comments

- Diarrhea may result in dehydration and renal failure. Withhold afatinib for severe or prolonged diarrhea not responsive to antidiarrheal agents.
- Withhold afatinib for severe or prolonged cutaneous reactions.
- Afatinib may cause interstitial lung disease. Withhold afatinib for acute onset or worsening of pulmonary symptoms.
- Monitor liver function tests (LFTs) periodically during therapy. Withhold afatinib for severe or worsening liver tests.
- Afatinib may cause ulcerative keratitis. Withhold and evaluate for new symptoms of keratitis.
- Embryo-fetal toxicity: Afatinib may cause fetal harm when administered to a pregnant woman.
- Co-administration of afatinib and p-glycoprotein inhibitors or inducers can lead to changes in afatinib exposure and may require dose modification. See product labeling for recommendations on dose modifications.

ALDESLEUKIN (PROLEUKIN)

Mechanism of Action

- Cellular immunity activation

FDA-Approved Indications

- Metastatic renal cell carcinoma (RCC)
- Metastatic melanoma

FDA-Approved Dosage

- 600,000 international units/kg IV over 15 minutes every 8 hours for a maximum of 14 doses
- May be repeated after 9 days of rest for a maximum of 28 doses per course

Dose Modification Criteria

- Withhold or interrupt a dose for toxicity

Adverse Reactions

- CV: hypotension, tachycardia, and arrhythmia
- DERM: rash and pruritis
- GI: diarrhea, N/V (moderate), mucositis, and anorexia
- GU: oliguria and acute renal failure
- HEMAT: myelosuppression
- NEURO: confusion, somnolence, anxiety, and dizziness
- PULM: dyspnea and pulmonary edema
- OTHER: pain, fever, chills, and malaise

Comments

- Restrict use to patients with normal cardiac and pulmonary function.
- Monitor for capillary leak syndrome.
- Associated with impaired neutrophil function; consider antibiotic prophylaxis for patients with indwelling central lines.
- Withhold in patients developing moderate-to-severe lethargy or somnolence; continued administration may result in coma.

ALECTINIB (ALECENSA)

Mechanism of Action

- Inhibitor of tyrosine kinases, including anaplastic lymphoma kinase (ALK) and re-arranged during transfection (RET) kinase

FDA-Approved Indications

- ALK-positive, metastatic NSCLC patients who have progressed on or are intolerant to crizotinib

FDA-Approved Dosage

- 600 mg orally twice daily with food until disease progression or unacceptable toxicity

Dose Modification Criteria

- Renal (mild to moderate, CrCl >30 ml/min): no
- Renal (severe, CrCl < 30 ml/min): no data, use with caution
- Hepatic (mild): no
- Hepatic (moderate to severe): no data, use with caution
- Nonhematologic toxicity: yes

Adverse Reactions

- CV: bradycardia
- DERM: rash
- ELECTRO: hypocalcemia, hypokalemia, hypophosphatemia, and hyponatremia
- ENDO: hyperglycemia
- GI: constipation, N/V (low), and diarrhea
- GU: increased creatinine
- HEMAT: anemia and lymphopenia
- HEPAT: ALT/AST elevations, elevated bilirubin, and increased bilirubin
- NEURO: headache
- PULM: interstitial lung disease, pneumonitis, cough, and dyspnea
- OTHER: myalgia, creatine phosphokinase (CPK) elevation, fatigue, edema (peripheral, generalized, eyelid, and periorbital)

Comments

- Hepatotoxicity: Monitor liver function tests every 2 weeks during the first 3 months of treatment, then once monthly and as clinically indicated.
- Alectinib may cause interstitial lung disease. Withhold alectinib for acute onset or worsening of pulmonary symptoms.
- Bradycardia: Monitor heart rate and blood pressure regularly and withhold and modify therapy if a patient becomes symptomatic from bradycardia.
- Myalgia and musculoskeletal pain are common toxicities. Monitor CPK every 2 weeks during the first month of treatment and in patients reporting musculoskeletal pain. Withholding therapy and dose modifications may be necessary.
- Embryo-fetal toxicity: Alectinib may cause fetal harm when administered to a pregnant woman.

ALEMTUZUMAB (CAMPATH)

Mechanism of Action

- Humanized monoclonal antibody directed against the cell surface protein CD52. The CD52 antigen is expressed on the surface of normal and malignant B and T lymphocytes, NK cells, monocytes, macrophages, and a subpopulation of granulocytes. The proposed mechanism of action is antibody-dependent lysis of leukemic cells following cell-surface binding.

FDA-Approved Indication

- B-cell chronic lymphocytic leukemia (CLL)

FDA-Approved Dosage

- Alemtuzumab is dose escalated in a stepwise format to a maintenance dose of 30 mg.
- The initial recommended dose is 3 mg IV over 2 hours daily. When this dose is tolerated (infusion-related toxicities ≤ grade 2), the daily dose should be escalated to 10 mg IV over 2 hours daily and continued until tolerated. When the 10 mg dose is tolerated, the maintenance dose of 30 mg may be initiated. The maintenance dose is 30 mg IV over 2 hours administered three times per week (i.e., Monday, Wednesday, and Friday) for up to 12 weeks. In most patients, escalation to 30 mg can be accomplished in 3 to 7 days. If therapy is interrupted for 7 or more days, alemtuzumab should be reinitiated with gradual dose escalation.
- Single doses of Campath >30 mg or cumulative doses >90 mg per week should not be administered because these doses are associated with a higher incidence of pancytopenia.
- Premedicate patients with an antihistamine (e.g., diphenhydramine 50 mg oral or IV) and acetaminophen (650 mg oral) 30 minutes prior to alemtuzumab to ameliorate or avoid infusion-related toxicity. Antiemetics, meperidine, and corticosteroids have also been used to prevent or treat infusion-related toxicities.

Dose Modification Criteria

- Myelosuppression: yes

Adverse Reactions

- CV: hypotension and edema/peripheral edema
- DERM: rash, urticaria, and pruritus
- GI: N/V (minimal), diarrhea, anorexia, and mucositis/stomatitis
- HEMAT: myelosuppression and lymphopenia
- INFUS: rigors, fever, chills, N/V, hypotension, dyspnea, bronchospasm, headache, rash, and urticaria
- NEURO: headache, dysthesias, and dizziness

▪ PULM: dyspnea, cough, bronchitis, pneumonia, and bronchospasm
▪ OTHER: opportunistic infections, sepsis, fatigue, asthenia, and pain

Comments

▪ Alemtuzumab (Campath) was removed from the commercial market in September 2012. The Campath Distribution Program was developed to ensure continued access to alemtuzumab for appropriate patients. Drug supplies are provided free of charge, but in order to receive drug, the healthcare provider is required to document and comply with certain requirements. For additional information, refer to www.campath.com or contact the Campath Distribution Program (1-877-422-6728).
▪ Alemtuzumab-treated patients are at risk for opportunistic infections due to profound lymphopenia. Anti-infective prophylaxis is recommended upon initiation of therapy and for a minimum of 2 months following the last dose of alemtuzumab or until the CD4 count is ≥200 cells/μL. Prophylaxis directed against *Pneumocystis* pneumonia (PJP) (e.g., trimethoprim/sulfamethoxazole) and herpesvirus infections (e.g., famciclovir or equivalent) should be utilized.
▪ Do not administer as an intravenous push or bolus.
▪ Careful monitoring of blood pressure and hypotension is recommended especially in patients with ischemic heart disease and in patients on antihypertensive medications.
▪ Patients who have recently received alemtuzumab should not be immunized with live viral vaccines.

ALTRETAMINE (HEXALEN)

Mechanism of Action

▪ Unknown, but like an alkylating agent in structure

FDA-Approved Indications

▪ Ovarian cancer: second-line, palliative treatment of persistent or recurrent ovarian cancer

FDA-Approved Dosage

▪ 65 mg/m^2 orally four times daily; total daily dose: 260 mg/m^2 for 14 or 21 consecutive days every 28 days

Dose Modification Criteria

▪ Myelosuppression: yes
▪ Nonhematologic toxicity (GI intolerance and progressive neurotoxicity): yes

Adverse Reactions

▪ GI: N/V (moderate)
▪ HEMAT: myelosuppression (WBC, RBC, and platelets)
▪ NEURO: peripheral sensory neuropathy, mood disorders, ataxia, and dizziness

Comments

▪ Monitor for neurologic toxicity

ANASTROZOLE (ARIMIDEX)

Mechanism of Action

▪ Selective, nonsteroidal aromatase inhibitor

FDA-Approved Indications

- Breast cancer
- Adjuvant treatment: postmenopausal women with hormone receptor-positive early breast cancer
- First-line therapy: postmenopausal women with hormone receptor-positive or hormone receptor unknown locally advanced or metastatic breast cancer
- Second-line therapy (after tamoxifen) in postmenopausal women with advanced breast cancer

FDA-Approved Dosage

- 1 mg orally daily (no requirement for glucocorticoid or mineralocorticoid replacement)

Dose Modification Criteria

- Renal: no
- Hepatic (mild-to-moderate impairment): no
- Hepatic (severe impairment): unknown

Adverse Reactions

- CV: hot flashes/flushing
- GI: N/V (low) and diarrhea
- HEPAT: LFTs (in patients with liver metastases)
- NEURO: headache
- PULM: dyspnea
- OTHER: asthenia, pain, back pain, and vaginal bleeding

Comments

- Patients with estrogen receptor (ER)-negative disease and patients who do not respond to tamoxifen rarely respond to anastrozole.
- In women with pre-existing ischemic heart disease, an increased incidence of ischemic cardiovascular events associated with anastrozole use compared to tamoxifen use has been demonstrated.
- Decreases in bone mineral density and increases in total cholesterol may occur. Consider monitoring.

ARSENIC TRIOXIDE (TRISENOX)

Mechanism of Action

- The mechanism is not completely defined.
- Induces apoptosis in NB4 human promyelocytic leukemia cells in vitro and causes damage or degradation of the fusion protein PML/RAR-α.

FDA-Approved Indications

- Acute promyelocytic leukemia (APL): Second-line treatment for the induction of remission and consolidation of APL patients who are refractory to, or have relapsed from, retinoid and anthracycline chemotherapy.

FDA-Approved Dosage

- APL induction: 0.15 mg/kg IV over 1 to 2 hours daily until bone marrow remission. Total induction dose should not exceed 60 doses.
- APL consolidation: 0.15 mg/kg IV over 1 to 2 hours daily × 25 doses over a period up to 5 weeks. Consolidation treatment should begin 3 to 6 weeks after completion of induction therapy.

Dose Modification Criteria

▪ Renal: no data, use with caution
▪ Hepatic: no data

Adverse Reactions

▪ CV: QT interval prolongation, complete atrioventricular block, torsades de pointes-type ventricular arrhythmia, atrial dysrhythmias, tachycardia, hypotension, and edema
▪ DERM: rash, dermatitis, dry skin, and pruritus
▪ ENDO: hyperglycemia, hypokalemia, and hypomagnesemia
▪ GI: N/V (moderate), diarrhea, abdominal pain, anorexia, and constipation
▪ HEMAT: leukocytosis and myelosuppression
▪ HEPAT: elevated LFTs
▪ NEURO: headache, dizziness, and paresthesias
▪ PULM: dyspnea and cough
▪ OTHER: fatigue, arthralgia, myalgia, pain, and APL differentiation (RA-APL) syndrome (RA-APL syndrome—fever, dyspnea, weight gain, radiographic pulmonary infiltrates, and pleural or pericardial effusion)

Comments

▪ The APL differentiation syndrome (RA-APL syndrome) has occurred in some patients treated with arsenic trioxide. Early recognition and high-dose corticosteroids (dexamethasone 10 mg IV every 12 hours × 3 days or until the resolution of symptoms) have been used for management.
▪ Prior to stating arsenic trioxide, a 12-lead ECG should be performed and serum electrolytes (potassium, calcium, and magnesium) and creatinine should be assessed; preexisting electrolyte abnormalities should be corrected. Avoid concomitant drugs that may prolong the QT interval. During therapy with arsenic trioxide, monitor and maintain normal potassium and magnesium concentrations (see package insert).
▪ Risk factors for QT prolongation and subsequent arrhythmias include other QT prolonging drugs, a history of torsades de pointes, preexisting QT prolongation, congestive heart failure (CHF), administration of potassium wasting diuretics, or other drugs or conditions that result in hypokalemia or hypomagnesemia.

ASPARAGINASE (ERWINAZE)

Mechanism of Action

▪ Asparaginase depletes asparagine, an amino acid required by some leukemic cells

FDA-Approved Indications

▪ Erwinaze (asparaginase derived from *Erwinia chrysanthemi*): Acute lymphoblastic leukemia (ALL) induction therapy for patients who have developed hypersensitivity to *Escherichia coli*–derived asparaginase

FDA-Approved Dosage

▪ Consult current literature for doses.
▪ Erwinaze: ALL induction therapy—25,000 international units/m² intramuscularly or intravenously substituting for each planned dose of either pegaspargase or *E. coli*–derived asparaginase.

Dose Modification Criteria

▪ None available

Adverse Reactions

- DERM: skin rash
- ENDO: hyperglycemia
- GI: N/V (minimal) and pancreatitis
- GU: prerenal azotemia
- HEMAT: coagulopathy (thrombosis or hemorrhage)
- HEPAT: increased LFTs, hyperbilirubinemia, and decreased serum albumin
- NEURO: variety of mental status changes
- OTHER: hypersensitivity, anaphylactic reactions, and hyperthermia

Comments

- Contraindicated in patients with active pancreatitis or history of pancreatitis. Discontinue asparaginase should severe or hemorrhagic pancreatitis develops while on therapy. Hypersensitivity and anaphylactic reactions can occur. Discontinue with serious reactions.
- Glucose intolerance may be irreversible. Monitor and treat accordingly.
- Serious thrombotic or hemorrhagic events may occur and should lead to discontinuation of therapy.
- Intramuscular administration has a lower incidence of hypersensitivity reactions compared to intravenous administration.
- Intravenous infusions of Erwinaze should be over 1 to 2 hours.
- The asparaginase formulation derived from *E.coli* (Elspar) was discontinued in December 2012.

ATEZOLIZUMAB (TECENTRIQ)

Mechanism of Action

- Humanized monoclonal antibody that binds to programmed death-ligand 1 (PD-L1) and blocks interactions with the programmed death 1 (PD-1) and B7.1 receptors

FDA-Approved Indications

- Locally advanced or metastatic urothelial carcinoma that has progressed during or following platinum-containing chemotherapy, or progressed within 12 months of neoadjuvant or adjuvant treatment with platinum-containing chemotherapy.
- Metastatic non-small cell lung cancer who have disease progression during or following platinum-containing chemotherapy. Patients with EGFR or ALK genomic tumor aberrations should have disease progression on FDA-approved therapy for these aberrations prior to receiving atezolizumab.

FDA-Approved Dosage

- 1200 mg IV every 3 weeks until disease progression or unacceptable toxicity

Dose Modification Criteria

- Renal: no.
- Hepatic (mild): no.
- Hepatic (moderate to severe): no data.
- Nonhematologic toxicity: Doses should be held, not reduced due to toxicities. See package insert for specific recommendations regarding holding doses and starting corticosteroids.

Adverse Reactions

- DERM: rash and pruritus
- ELECTRO: hyponatremia

- ENDO: immune-related hypophysitis, thyroid disorders, adrenal insufficiency, and diabetes mellitus
- GI: immune-related colitis, immune-related pancreatitis, decreased appetite, constipation, diarrhea, and N/V (low)
- GU: urinary tract infection
- HEMAT: lymphopenia
- HEPAT: immune-related hepatitis
- INFUS: infusion reactions
- NEURO: immune-related myasthenic syndrome/myasthenia gravis, Guillain-Barré, and meningoencephalitis
- OCULAR: ocular inflammatory toxicity
- PULM: immune-related pneumonitis or interstitial lung disease, dyspnea, and cough
- OTHER: fatigue, pyrexia, arthralgia, peripheral edema, and back/neck pain

Comments

- Interrupt or flow the rate of infusion for mild or moderate infusion reactions and discontinue for severe or life-threatening reactions.
- Withholding parameters for immune-related toxicities are provided in the product labeling.
- Embryo-fetal toxicity: Atezolizumab may cause fetal harm when administered to a pregnant woman.

AXITINIB (INLYTA)

Mechanism of Action

- Inhibits receptor tyrosine kinases including vascular endothelial growth factor receptors (VEGFR)-1, VEGFR-2, and VEGFR-3

FDA-Approved Indications

- Advanced Renal Cell Carcinoma (RCC) after failure of one prior systemic therapy

FDA-Approved Dosage

- 5 mg orally twice daily. Swallow whole with a glass of water. Administer axitinib doses approximately 12 hours apart with or without food.

Dose Modification Criteria

- Renal (mild, moderate, and severe): no
- Renal (end-stage renal disease) (CrCl <15 mL/minute): use caution
- Hepatic (mild, Child–Pugh class A): no
- Hepatic (moderate, Child–Pugh class B): yes
- Hepatic (severe, Child–Pugh class C): not studied
- Nonhematologic toxicity: yes

Adverse Reactions

- Cr: creatinine increased
- CV: hypertension and cardiac failure
- DERM: dry skin, palmar-plantar erythrodysesthesia, and rash
- ELECTRO: decreased bicarbonate, hyperkalemia, hypernatremia, hypocalcemia, hyponatremia, and hypophosphatemia
- ENDO: hyperglycemia, hypoglycemia, and hypothyroidism
- GI: abdominal pain, anorexia, constipation, diarrhea, N/V (minimal to low), and stomatitis
- GU: proteinuria
- HEMAT: anemia, leukopenia, lymphopenia, and thrombocytopenia

- HEPAT: hypoalbuminemia, hyperbilirubinemia, increased alkaline phosphatase, and increased LFTs
- NEURO: headache and dysgeusia
- PULM: cough and dyspnea
- OTHER: asthenia, arterial and venous thromboembolic events, dysphonia, fatigue, hemorrhage, pain in extremity, and weight decreased

Comments

- Blood pressure should be well controlled prior to starting axitinib, and should be monitored regularly during treatment.
- Cardiac failure has been observed and can be fatal. Monitor for signs of symptoms of cardiac failure.
- Use with caution in patients who are at an increased risk for arterial and venous thrombotic events, as these events have been observed.
- Hemorrhagic events have been reported. Axitinib has not been studied in patients with evidence of untreated brain metastasis or recent active gastrointestinal bleeding and should not be used in these patients.
- Gastrointestinal perforation and fistula have occurred.
- Hypothyroidism requiring thyroid hormone replacement has been reported. Thyroid function should be monitored prior to and throughout treatment.
- Stop axitinib at least 24 hours prior to scheduled surgery. The decision to resume axitinib after surgery should be based on clinical judgment of adequate wound healing.
- Reversible posterior leukoencephalopathy syndrome (RPLS) has been observed. Permanently discontinue axitinib if signs or symptoms of RPLS, such as headache, seizure, lethargy, confusion, blindness, and other visual and neurologic disturbances, occur.
- Monitor for proteinuria before initiation of, and periodically throughout, treatment with axitinib.
- Concomitant use of strong CYP3A4/5 inhibitors should be avoided. If coadministration is necessary, decrease the axitinib dose by half.
- Embryo-fetal toxicity: Axitinib may cause fetal harm when administered to a pregnant woman.

AZACITIDINE (VIDAZA)

Mechanism of Action

- Antimetabolite. A pyrimidine nucleoside analog of cytidine. Azacitidine causes hypomethylation of DNA and direct cytotoxicity on abnormal hematopoietic cells in the bone marrow.

FDA-Approved Indications

- Myelodysplastic syndrome (MDS): The specific subtypes of MDS for which azacitidine is indicated include refractory anemia or refractory anemia with ringed sideroblasts (if accompanied by neutropenia or thrombocytopenia or requiring transfusions), refractory anemia with excess blasts, refractory anemia with excess blasts in transformation, and chronic myelomonocytic leukemia (CML).

FDA-Approved Dosage

- First treatment cycle: The recommended starting dose for all patients regardless of baseline hematology laboratory values is 75 mg/m^2 SC or IV, daily for 7 days.
- Subsequent treatment cycles: A cycle should be repeated every 4 weeks. The dose may be increased to 100 mg/m^2 if no beneficial effect is seen after two treatment cycles and if no toxicity other than N/V has occurred.
- Duration: Minimum duration of four treatment cycles is recommended; complete or partial response may take more than four treatment cycles; may be continued as long as the patient continues to benefit.

Dose Modification Criteria

- Renal: no data, use with caution (dose modify for renal toxicity)
- Hepatic: no data (use with caution)
- Myelosuppression: yes
- Nonhematologic toxicity (renal tubular acidosis, renal toxicity): yes

Adverse Reactions

- DERM: injection site erythema or pain, ecchymosis, rash, and pruritus
- ELECTRO: renal tubular acidosis (alkaline urine, fall in serum bicarbonate, and hypokalemia)
- GI: N/V (moderate), diarrhea, constipation, anorexia, abdominal pain, and hepatotoxicity
- GU: increased Cr and BUN, renal failure, and renal tubular acidosis
- HEMAT: anemia, neutropenia, and thrombocytopenia
- NEURO: headache and dizziness
- PULM: cough and dyspnea
- OTHER: fever, rigors, fatigue, weakness, peripheral edema, and tumor lysis syndrome

Comments

- Embryo-fetal toxicity: Teratogenic, women of childbearing potential should be advised to avoid becoming pregnant while receiving azacitidine. Men should be advised to not father a child while receiving azacitidine.
- Use caution in patients with liver disease. Azacitidine is potentially hepatotoxic in patients with preexisting hepatic impairment.
- Azacitidine is contraindicated in patients with advanced malignant hepatic tumors.
- Azacitidine and its metabolites are primarily cleared renally. Patients with renal impairment should be closely monitored for toxicity. Renal toxicity has been reported rarely with intravenous azacitidine in combination with other chemotherapeutic agents for non-MDS conditions.

BCG LIVE (INTRAVESICAL) [THERACYS, TICE BCG]

Mechanism of Action

- Local inflammatory and immune response

FDA-Approved Indications

- Treatment and prophylaxis of carcinoma in situ of the urinary bladder and for the prophylaxis of primary or recurrent-stage Ta and/or T1 papillary tumors following transurethral resection (TUR)

FDA-Approved Dosage

- TheraCys: Vial contains 81 mg (dry weight) or $10.5 \pm 8.7 \times 10^8$ colony-forming units with accompanying 3 mL diluent vial.
  - One reconstituted vial (81 mg/3 mL), diluted in 50 mL sterile, preservative-free normal saline (0.9% sodium chloride injection, USP), instilled into bladder for as long as possible (up to 2 hours) once weekly for 6 weeks (induction therapy) followed by one treatment at 3, 6, 12, 18, and 24 months after initial treatment (maintenance therapy)
- TICE Bacillus Calmette-Guérin (BCG): Vial contains 50 mg (wet weight) or 1 to 8×10^8 colony-forming units.
  - One reconstituted vial (50 mg/1 mL), diluted in a total volume of 50 mL preservative-free normal saline (0.9% sodium chloride injection, USP), instilled into bladder for as long as possible (up to 2 hours) once weekly for 6 weeks followed by once monthly for 6 to 12 months

Dose Modification Criteria

- Withhold on any suspicion of systemic infection

Adverse Reactions

- GU: irritative bladder symptoms (e.g., dysuria, typically beginning 4 to 6 hours after instillation and lasting for 24 to 72 hours).
- OTHER: malaise, fever, and chills; infectious complications (uncommon)

Comments

- TheraCys and TICE BCG are not bioequivalent products and may not be used interchangeably.
- May complicate tuberculin skin test interpretation.
- BCG live products contain live, attenuated mycobacteria. Because of the potential risk of transmission, it should be prepared, handled, and disposed of as a biohazard material.
- BCG live products are contraindicated in immunosuppressed patients or those with congenital or acquired immune deficiencies.

BELINOSTAT (BELEODAQ)

Mechanism of Action

- Histone deacetylase (HDAC) inhibitor

FDA-Approved Indications

- Relapsed or refractory peripheral T-cell lymphoma (PTCL)

FDA-Approved Dosage

- 1,000 mg/m^2 IV on days 1 to 2 of a 21-day cycle until disease progression or unacceptable toxicity

Dose Modification Criteria

- Renal (mild to moderate, CrCl >39 ml/min): no
- Renal (severe, CrCl ≤39): no data available
- Hepatic: moderate to severe (total bilirubin >1.5 X ULN): no data available
- Myelosuppression: yes
- Nonhematologic toxicity: yes
- Reduced UGT1A1 activity (homozygous for UGT1A1*28 allele): yes

Adverse Reactions

- CV: prolonged QT
- DERM: rash, pruritus
- GI: N/V (low), diarrhea, constipation
- HEMAT: thrombocytopenia, neutropenia, lymphopenia, and anemia
- HEPAT: liver function test abnormalities
- INFUS: infusion site pain and phlebitis
- NEURO: headache
- PULM: dyspnea and cough
- OTHER: infection, fatigue, pyrexia, peripheral edema, and chills

Comments

- Monitor liver function tests before treatment and before each cycle. Interrupting therapy or dose modification may be necessary for hepatic toxicity.

- Monitor patients for tumor lysis syndrome particularly in patients with advanced stage disease and/ or high tumor burden.
- Avoid concomitant administration of strong UGT1A1 inhibitors.
- Embryo-fetal toxicity: Belinostat may cause fetal harm when administered to a pregnant woman.

BENDAMUSTINE HYDROCHLORIDE (TREANDA)

Mechanism of Action

- Alkylating agent

FDA-Approved Indications

- CLL
- Indolent B-cell non-Hodgkin Lymphoma (NHL): Disease progression during or within 6 months of treatment with rituximab or a rituximab-containing regimen

FDA-Approved Dosage

- CLL: 100 mg/m² IV over 30 minutes on days 1 and 2 of a 28-day cycle, up to six cycles
- NHL: 120 mg/m² IV over 60 minutes on days 1 and 2 of a 21-day cycle, up to eight cycles

Dose Modification Criteria

- Renal: no data; use with caution in patients with mild-to-moderate renal impairment, avoid in patients with CrCL <40 mL per minute.
- Hepatic: no data; use with caution in patients with mild hepatic impairment, avoid in patients with moderate to severe hepatic impairment.
- Myelosuppression: yes
- Nonhematologic toxicity: yes

Adverse Reactions

- DERM: rash, pruritis, toxic skin reactions, and bullous exanthema
- GI: N/V (moderate), diarrhea, and mucositis
- HEMAT: myelosuppression
- INFUS: fever, chills, pruritis, rash, anaphylaxis, or anaphylactoid reactions
- PULM: cough
- OTHER: tumor lysis syndrome, asthenia, and infections

Comments

- Infusion reactions occurred commonly in clinical trials. Monitor clinically and discontinue drug for severe reactions (grade 3 or worse). Measures to prevent severe reactions (e.g., antihistamines, antipyretics, and corticosteroids) should be considered in subsequent cycles in patients who have previously experienced grade 1 or 2 infusion reactions.
- Monitor for tumor lysis syndrome, particularly with the first treatment cycle, and utilize allopurinol during the first 1 to 2 weeks of therapy in patients at high risk.
- Severe skin reactions have been reported necessitating drug therapy to be withheld or discontinued.
- Bendamustine hydrochloride is primarily metabolized via hydrolysis to metabolites with low cytotoxic activity. Some metabolism via cytochrome P450 1A2 (CYP1A2) occurs forming active metabolites; thus, potential drug interactions with CYP1A2 inhibitors or inducers should be considered.
- Embryo-fetal toxicity: Bendamustine may cause fetal harm when administered to a pregnant woman.

- Do not use bendamustine solution for injection with devices that contain polycarbonate or acrylo-nitrile-butadiene-styrene including most closed system transfer devices (CSTDs).
- Concomitant CYP1A2 inducers or inhibitors have the potential to alter the exposure of bendamustine.

BEVACIZUMAB (AVASTIN)

Mechanism of Action

- Recombinant humanized monoclonal IgG1 antibody that binds to and inhibits the biologic activity of human vascular endothelial growth factor (VEGF).

FDA-Approved Indications

- Metastatic colorectal cancer: First- or second-line treatment of patients with metastatic carcinoma of the colon or rectum; in combination with intravenous 5-fluorouracil (5-FU)-based chemotherapy. Second-line treatment of metastatic colorectal carcinoma (in combination with fluoropyrimidine–irinotecan-based or fluoropyrimidine–oxaliplatin-based therapy) in patients who have progressed on a first-line bevacizumab-containing regimen.
- Nonsquamous, NSCLC: First-line treatment of patients with unresectable, locally advanced, recurrent, or metastatic nonsquamous NSCLC, in combination with carboplatin and paclitaxel.
- Glioblastoma: Second-line single-agent therapy in patients with progressive disease following prior therapy.
- Metastatic RCC: In combination with interferon-α.
- Cervical cancer: persistent, recurrent, or metastatic disease in combination with paclitaxel and cisplatin or paclitaxel and topotecan.
- Recurrent epithelial ovarian, fallopian tube or primary peritoneal cancer that is
  - platinum-resistant in combination with paclitaxel, pegylated liposomal doxorubicin, or topotecan.
  - platinum-sensitive in combination with carboplatin and paclitaxel or in combination with carboplatin and gemcitabine, followed by bevacizumab as a single agent.

FDA-Approved Dosage

- Metastatic colorectal cancer: Administered as an intravenous infusion (5 mg/kg or 10 mg/kg) every 2 weeks when used in combination with intravenous fluorouracil-based chemotherapy.
  - 5 mg/kg IV every 2 weeks when used in combination with bolus-IFL
  - 10 mg/kg IV every 2 weeks when used in combination with FOLFOX4
  - 5 mg/kg IV every 14 days or 7.5 mg/kg IV every 3 weeks when used in combination with a fluoropyrimidine-irinotecan-based or fluoropyrimidine-oxaliplatin-based chemotherapy regimen in patients who have progressed on a first-line bevacizumab-containing regimen
  - Nonsquamous NSCLC: 15 mg/kg intravenous infusion every 3 weeks in combination with carboplatin and paclitaxel
- Glioblastoma: 10 mg/kg intravenous infusion every 2 weeks.
- Metastatic RCC: 10 mg/kg intravenous infusion every 2 weeks in combination with interferon-α.
- Cervical cancer: 15 mg/kg IV every 3 weeks with paclitaxel/cisplatin or paclitaxel/topotecan.
- Platinum-resistant recurrent epithelial ovarian, fallopian tube, or primary peritoneal cancer:
  - 10 mg/kg IV every 2 weeks with paclitaxel, pegylated liposomal doxorubicin, or weekly topotecan.
  - 15 mg/kg IV every 3 weeks with topotecan given every 3 weeks.
- Platinum-sensitive recurrent epithelial ovarian, fallopian tube, or primary peritoneal cancer:
  - 15 mg/kg IV every 3 weeks in combination with carboplatin/paclitaxel for 6 to 8 cycles, followed by 15 mg/kg IV every 3 weeks as a single agent
  - 15 mg/kg IV every 3 weeks in combination with carboplatin/gemcitabine for 6 to 10 cycles, followed by 15 mg/kg IV every 3 weeks as a single agent
- Do not administer as an intravenous push or bolus. The initial bevacizumab dose should be delivered over 90 minutes as an IV infusion following chemotherapy. If the first infusion is well tolerated, the

second infusion may be administered over 60 minutes. If the 60-minute infusion is well tolerated, all subsequent infusions may be administered over 30 minutes.

Dose Modification Criteria

- Renal: no
- Hepatic: no
- Myelosuppression: no
- Nonhematologic toxicity: yes

Adverse Reactions

- CV: hypertension, hypertensive crisis, and CHF
- DERM: dry skin, exfoliative dermatitis
- GI: N/V (minimal), taste alteration, diarrhea, abdominal pain, gastrointestinal perforation, and wound dehiscence
- GU: proteinuria and nephrotic syndrome
- INFUS: fever, chills, wheezing, and stridor
- NEURO: headache
- PULM: dyspnea and wheezing stridor
- OTHER: rhinitis, back pain, epistaxis, and other mild-to-moderate hemorrhagic events; serious hemorrhagic events; wound healing complications; deep vein thrombosis or other thromboembolic events; and asthenia

Comments

- Bevacizumab can result in the development of gastrointestinal perforation and wound dehiscence and other wound healing complications. The appropriate interval between termination of bevacizumab and subsequent elective surgery required to avoid the risks of wound healing/wound dehiscence has not been determined. Product labeling suggests that bevacizumab should not be initiated for at least 28 days following major surgery and the surgical incision should be fully healed.
- Bleeding complications secondary to bevacizumab occur in two distinct patterns: minor hemorrhage (most commonly grade 1 epistaxis) and serious, and in some cases, fatal hemorrhagic events. Patients with squamous cell NSCLC appear to be at higher risk for serious hemorrhagic events. There is a risk of CNS bleeding in patients with CNS metastases based on limited data (refer to product labeling).
- Blood pressure monitoring should be conducted every 2 to 3 weeks during therapy and more frequently in patients who develop hypertension.
- Arterial and venous thromboembolic events have been associated with bevacizumab. Discontinue bevacizumab for severe or life-threatening thromboembolic events.
- Posterior reversible encephalopathy syndrome associated with bevacizumab use has been reported rarely (<0.5%).
- Monitor urinalysis serially for proteinuria; patients with a 2+ or greater urine dipstick reading should undergo further assessment (e.g., a 24-hour urine collection).
- Bevacizumab may increase the risk of ovarian failure in premenopausal females.
- Embryo-fetal toxicity: Angiogenesis is critical to fetal development and bevacizumab has been shown to be teratogenic in rabbits.

BEXAROTENE (TARGRETIN)

Mechanism of Action

- A retinoid that selectively binds and activates retinoid X receptor subtypes (RXRs).
- Once activated, these receptors function as transcription factors that regulate the expression of genes that control cellular differentiation and proliferation.

FDA-Approved Indications

- Cutaneous T-cell lymphoma (CTCL): second-line treatment of the cutaneous manifestations of CTCL in patients who are refractory to at least one prior systemic therapy

FDA-Approved Dosage

- 300 mg/m^2 orally daily with a meal

Dose Modification Criteria

- Renal: no (caution due to possible protein binding alterations)
- Hepatic: use with caution
- Nonhematologic toxicity: yes

Adverse Reactions

- CV: peripheral edema
- DERM: dry skin, photosensitivity, rash, and pruritus
- ENDO: hypothyroidism and hypoglycemia (diabetic patients)
- GI: nausea, pancreatitis, and abdominal pain
- HEMAT: leukopenia and anemia
- HEPAT: elevated LFTs
- NEURO: headache
- Ocular: cataracts
- OTHER: lipid abnormalities (elevated triglycerides, elevated total and LDL cholesterol, and decreased HDL cholesterol), asthenia, and infection

Comments

- Monitor fasting blood lipid tests prior to initiation of bexarotene and weekly until the lipid response is established (usually occurs within 2 to 4 weeks) and then at 8-week intervals thereafter.
- Monitor LFTs prior to initiation of bexarotene and then after 1, 2, and 4 weeks of treatment, and if stable, at least every 8 weeks thereafter during treatment.
- Monitor complete blood count (CBC) and thyroid function tests at baseline and periodically thereafter.
- Pancreatitis: interrupt bexarotene and evaluate if suspected.
- Minimize exposure to sunlight and artificial ultraviolet light during treatment with bexarotene.
- Embryo-fetal toxicity: Bexarotene is a teratogen and may cause fetal harm when administered to a pregnant woman. Bexarotene must not be given to a pregnant woman or a woman who intends to become pregnant. A negative pregnancy test in female patients of childbearing potential should be obtained within 1 week prior to starting bexarotene therapy and then repeated at monthly intervals while the patient remains on therapy. Effective contraception (two reliable forms used simultaneously) must be used for 1 month prior to initiation of therapy, during therapy, and for at least 1 month following discontinuation of therapy. Bexarotene may induce the metabolism of hormonal contraceptives and reduce their effectiveness; thus one form of contraception should be nonhormonal.

BICALUTAMIDE (CASODEX)

Mechanism of Action

- Antiandrogen

FDA-Approved Indications

- Prostate cancer: palliation of advanced prostate cancer (stage D2) in combination therapy with a luteinizing hormone-releasing hormone (LHRH) agonist

FDA-Approved Dosage

▪ 50 mg orally daily

Dose Modification Criteria

▪ Renal: no
▪ Hepatic (mild-to-moderate impairment): no
▪ Hepatic (severe impairment): use with caution

Adverse Reactions

▪ ENDO: loss of libido, hot flashes, and gynecomastia
▪ GI: N/V, diarrhea, and constipation
▪ GU: impotence
▪ HEPAT: hepatitis

Comments

▪ Monitor LFTs prior to treatment, at regular intervals for the first 4 months, and periodically thereafter. Severe hepatic injury including fatalaties have been observed.
▪ R-bicalutamide is an inhibitor of CYP 3A4; use caution when bicalutamide is used concurrently with CYP 3A4 substrates.

BLEOMYCIN (BLENOXANE)

Mechanism of Action

▪ Unknown, but may inhibit DNA and RNA synthesis

FDA-Approved Indications

▪ Squamous cell cancers, NHL, testicular cancer, Hodgkin disease, and malignant pleural effusions

FDA-Approved Dosage

▪ The product labeling recommends a test dose (2 units or less) for the first two doses in lymphoma patients.
▪ From 0.25 to 0.50 units/kg (10 to 20 units/m²) IV or IM or SC weekly or twice weekly.
▪ Malignant pleural effusions: 60 units as single intrapleural bolus dose.

Dose Modification Criteria

▪ Renal: yes

Adverse Reactions

▪ DERM: erythema, rash, striae, vesiculation, hyperpigmentation, skin tenderness, alopecia, nail changes, pruritus, and stomatitis
▪ PULM: pulmonary fibrosis (increases at cumulative doses >400 units, but can happen at lower total doses), and pneumonitis
▪ OTHER: fever and chills; idiosyncratic reaction consisting of hypotension, mental confusion, fever, chills, and wheezing has been reported in 1% of lymphoma patients; local pain with intrapleural administration

Comments

▪ Risk factors for bleomycin-induced pulmonary toxicity include age (>70 years old), underlying emphysema, prior thoracic radiotherapy, high cumulative doses (e.g., >450 units), and high single doses (>30 units).

■ Patients who have received bleomycin may be at increased risk of respiratory failure during the post-operative recovery period after surgery. Use the minimal tolerated concentration of inspired oxygen and modest fluid replacement to prevent pulmonary edema.

BLINATUMOMAB (BLINCYTO)

Mechanism of Action

■ CD19-directed CD3 T-cell engager that binds to CD19 expressed on the surface of cells of B-lineage origin and CD3 expressed on the surface of T cells. Blinatumomab activates endogenous T cells by connecting CD3 in the T-cell receptor complex with CD19 on benign and malignant B cells, leading to lysis of CD19+ cells.

FDA-Approved Indications

■ Philadelphia chromosome-negative relapsed or refractory B-cell precursor ALL

FDA-Approved Dosage

■ Premedicate with dexamethasone 20 mg IV 1 hour prior to the first dose of each cycle, prior to an increase in dose (ex. cycle 1 day 8), and when restarting an infusion after an interruption ≥4 hours.
■ For patients ≥45 kg:
  ● During cycle 1 administer 9 mcg/day via continuous infusion on days 1 to 7 and 28 mcg/day via continuous infusion on days 8 to 28.Days 29 to 42 are treatment-free days.During subsequent cycles administer 28 mcg/day via continuous infusion on days 1 to 28.
■ For patients <45 kg:
  ● During cycle 1 administer 5 mcg/m^2/day (not to exceed 9mcg/day) via continuous infusion on days 1 to 7 and 15 mcg/m^2/day (not to exceed 28 mcg/day) on days 8 to 28.Days 29 to 42 are treatment-free days.During subsequent cycles administer 15 mcg/m^2/day (not to exceed 28 mcg/day) on days 8 to 28.

Dose Modification Criteria

■ Renal (mild to moderate, CrCl >30 ml/min): no (limited data)
■ Renal: (CrCl <30 mL/min) no information available
■ Hepatic: no information available
■ Nonhematologic toxicity: yes

Adverse Reactions

■ DERM: rash
■ ELECTRO: hypokalemia
■ GI: N/V (low), constipation, diarrhea, pancreatitis, and abdominal pain
■ HEMAT: anemia, neutropenia, and thrombocytopenia
■ HEPAT: increased ALT/AST
■ INFUS: infusion reactions
■ NEURO: encephalopathy, convulsions, speech disorders, disturbances in consciousness, confusion and disorientation, coordination and balance, seizures, headache, tremor
■ PULM: pneumonia, cough, and dyspnea
■ OTHER: Cytokine release syndrome, febrile neutropenia, pyrexia, peripheral edema, fatigue, and chills

Comments

■ Cytokine release syndrome and neurologic toxicity may be life threatening or fatal. Patients should be closely monitored for signs and symptoms of these events. Guidance on criteria for interruption or discontinuation of blinatumomab is provided in the product labeling.

- Prepare according to the package insert to minimize errors.
- Do not flush infusion lines when changing bags or at the completion of infusion.
- Hospitalization is recommended for the first 9 days of the first cycle and the first 2 days of the second cycle.
- Advise patient to refrain from driving and engaging in hazardous occupations while blinatumomab is being administered due to the potential for neurologic events.

BORTEZOMIB (VELCADE)

Mechanism of Action

- Bortezomib is a reversible inhibitor of the 26S proteosome, a large protein complex that degrades ubiquinated proteins. Inhibition of the 26S proteosome prevents targeted proteolysis, which can effect multiple signaling cascades within the cell. This disruption of normal homeostatic mechanisms can lead to cell death.

FDA-Approved Indications

- Multiple myeloma
- Mantle cell lymphoma

FDA-Approved Dosage

- General dosing guidelines: The recommended starting dose for bortezomib is 1.3 mg/m². Bortezomib may be administered intravenously at a concentration of 1 mg/mL or subcutaneously at a concentration of 2.5 mg/mL. When administered intravenously, bortezomib is administered as a 3- to 5-second bolus intravenous injection.
- Multiple myeloma (first-line therapy in combination with melphalan and prednisone): 1.3 mg/m² IV or SC twice weekly on a 6-week treatment cycle on days 1, 4, 8, 11, 22, 25, 29, and 32 for cycles 1 to 4. In cycles 5 to 9, bortezomib is administered once weekly on days 1, 8, 22, and 29 of a 6-week treatment cycle (note that week 3 and week 6 of cycle are rest periods).
- Mantle cell lymphoma (first-line therapy in combination with rituximab, cyclophosphamide, doxorubicin, and prednisone [VcR-CAP]): 1.3 mg/m² IV twice weekly for two weeks (Days 1, 4, 8 and 11) followed by a 10-day rest period on days 12 to 21.
- Multiple myeloma (relapsed disease) and mantle cell lymphoma (relapsed disease): 1.3 mg/m² IV or SC administered twice weekly for 2 weeks (days 1, 4, 8, and 11) followed by a 10-day rest period (days 12 to 21). For extended therapy of more than eight cycles, bortezomib may be administered on the standard schedule or on a maintenance schedule of once weekly for 4 weeks (days 1, 8, 15, and 22) followed by a 13-day rest period (days 23 to 35). At least 72 hours should elapse between consecutive doses of bortezomib.
- Retreatment for multiple myeloma may be considered in patients who had previously responded to treatment and who have relapsed at least 6 months after completing prior therapy. Treatment may be started at the last tolerated dose.

Dose Modification Criteria

- Renal: no data (use caution)
- Hepatic (moderate or severe hepatic impairment): yes
- Myelosuppression: yes
- Nonhematologic toxicity (e.g., neuropathy and neuropathic pain): yes

Adverse Reactions

- CV: hypotension (including orthostatic hypotension and syncope), edema, and heart failure
- DERM: rash

- GI: N/V (low), diarrhea, anorexia, and constipation
- HEMAT: myelosuppression (thrombocytopenia > anemia > neutropenia)
- HEPAT: hepatotoxicity
- NEURO: peripheral neuropathy, neuropathic pain, dizziness, headache, and posterior reversible encephalopathy syndrome (PRES)
- Ocular: diplopia and blurred vision
- PULM: dyspnea, acute respiratory syndromes
- OTHER: asthenia, fatigue, fever, insomnia, arthralgia, and tumor lysis syndrome

Comments

- The reconstitution volume/concentration is different for the intravenous and subcutaneous routes. Use caution when calculating the volume to be administered.
- The incidence of peripheral neuropathy is lower when bortezomib is administered by the subcutaneous route of administration compared to the intravenous route. Starting bortezomib subcutaneously may be considered for patients with preexisting or at high risk of peripheral neuropathy.
- Use caution in treating patients with a history of syncope, who are on medications associated with hypotension, and in patients who are dehydrated.
- Embryo-fetal toxicity: bortezomib may cause fetal harm when administered to a pregnant woman.
- Bortezomib is a substrate of CYP 3A4. Use caution in patients who are concomitantly receiving medications that are strong inhibitors or inducers of CYP 3A4.

BOSUTINIB (BOSULIF)

Mechanism of Action

- Tyrosine kinase inhibitor (TKI) that inhibits the Bcr–Abl kinase that promotes CML); also an inhibitor of Src-family kinases including Src, Lyn, and Hck.

FDA-Approved Indications

- Chronic, accelerated, or blast-phase Philadelphia chromosome-positive (Ph+) CML with resistance or intolerance to prior therapy.

FDA-Approved Dosage

- 500 mg orally once daily with food.
- Consider dose escalation to 600 mg orally once daily in patients who have not reached a complete hematologic response by week 8 or a complete cytogenetic response by week 12.

Dose Modification Criteria

- Renal (CrCL <50 mL/minute): yes
- Hepatic (mild, moderate, and severe): yes
- Myelosuppression: yes
- Nonhematologic toxicity: yes

Adverse Reactions

- DERM: pruritus and rash
- GI: abdominal pain, anorexia, diarrhea, and N/V (low)
- GU: renal toxicity (decline in GFR)
- HEMAT: anemia, neutropenia, and thrombocytopenia
- HEPAT: elevated LFTs
- NEURO: dizziness and headache

- PULM: cough, nasopharnygitis, and respiratory tract infection
- OTHER: arthralgia, asthenia, back pain, fatigue, fluid retention, and pyrexia

Comments

- Avoid the concomitant use of strong or moderate CYP3A and/or P-glycoprotein (P-gp) inhibitors and inducers.
- Bosutinib may increase the plasma concentrations of drugs that are P-gp substrates, such as digoxin.
- Proton pump inhibitors (PPIs) may decrease bosutinib drug levels. Consider short-acting antacids or H_2-blockers in place of PPIs, and separate antacid or H_2-blocker dosing from bosutinib by more than 2 hours.
- Bosutinib did not inhibit the T315I and V299L mutant cells in mice.
- Monitor hepatic enzymes at least monthly for the first 3 months and as needed.
- Embryo-fetal toxicity: Bosutinib may cause fetal harm when administered to a pregnant woman.

BRENTUXIMAB VEDOTIN (ADCETRIS)

Mechanism of Action

- Antibody–drug conjugate (ADC) consisting of a chimeric IgG1 directed against CD30 and mono-methyl auristatin E (MMAE), a microtubule disrupting agent that is covalently attached to the anti-body via a linker. The ADC binds to CD30-expressing cells, is internalized and, subsequently, MMAE is released via proteolytic cleavage. Binding of MMAE to tubulin disrupts the microtubule network within the cell, subsequently inducing cell cycle arrest and apoptosis.

FDA-Approved Indications

- Hodgkin lymphoma (HL) after failure of autologous stem cell transplant (ASCT) or after failure of at least two prior multiagent chemotherapy regimens in patients who are not ASCT candidates.
- Classical Hodgkin Lymphoma (cHL) at high risk of relapse or progression as post-auto-HSCT consolidation.
- Systemic anaplastic large cell lymphoma after failure of at least one prior multiagent chemotherapy regimen.

FDA-Approved Dosage

- 1.8 mg/kg as an intravenous infusion over 30 minutes every 3 weeks.
- Do not administer as an intravenous push or bolus.
- Continue treatment until a maximum of 16 cycles, disease progression, or unacceptable toxicity.
- The dose for patients weighing greater than 100 kg should be calculated based on a weight of 100 kg (max dose 180 mg).

Dose Modification Criteria

- Renal (mild to moderate, CrCl 30 to 80 ml/min): no
- Renal (severe, CrCl <30 ml/min): avoid use
- Hepatic (mild, Child–Pugh A): yes
- Hepatic (moderate to severe, Child–Pugh B or C): avoid use
- Myelosuppression: yes
- Nonhematologic toxicity: yes

Adverse Effects

- DERM: alopecia, night sweats, pruritus, rash, serious dermatologic reactions (e.g., Stevens-Johnson syndrome or toxic epidermal necrolysis)
- GI: abdominal pain, constipation, diarrhea, N/V (low), oropharyngeal pain, serious gastrointestinal complications (e.g., perforation)

- HEMAT: anemia, neutropenia, lymphadenopathy, and thrombocytopenia
- HEPAT: hepatotoxicity
- INFUS: anaphylaxis, breathing problems, chills, fever, and rash
- NEURO: dizziness, headache, and motor and sensory peripheral neuropathy
- PULM: cough, dyspnea, upper respiratory tract infection, and noninfectious pulmonary toxicity
- OTHER: arthralgia, back pain, chills, fatigue, insomnia, myalgia, pain in extremity, pyrexia, and tumor lysis syndrome

Comments

- JC virus infection resulting in progressive multifocal leukoencephalopathy (PML) and death can occur. Consider the diagnosis of PML in any patient presenting with new-onset signs and symptoms of central nervous system abnormalities.
- Concomitant use of brentuximab vedotin and bleomycin is contraindicated due to pulmonary toxicity.
- Brentuximab vedotin-induced peripheral neuropathy is predominantly sensory, and is cumulative.
- A higher incidence of infusion-related reactions was observed in patients who developed persistently positive antibodies.
- MMAE is primarily metabolized by CYP3A. Patients who are receiving strong CYP3A4 inhibitors concomitantly with brentuximab vedotin should be closely monitored for adverse reactions. Coadministration of brentuximab vedotin with strong CYP3A4 inducers should be avoided.
- Embryo-fetal toxicity: Brentuximab vedotin may cause fetal harm when administered to a pregnant woman.

BUSULFAN (MYLERAN); BUSULFAN INJECTION (BUSULFEX)

Mechanism of Action

- Alkylating agent

FDA-Approved Indications

- Oral busulfan: palliative treatment of CML
- Parenteral busulfan: conditioning regimen (in combination with cyclophosphamide) prior to allogeneic hematopoietic progenitor cell transplantation for CML

FDA-Approved Dosage

- Oral busulfan: induction, 4 to 8 mg orally daily; Weight or BSA based: 60 mcg/kg or 1.8 mg/m² orally daily; maintenance, 1 to 3 mg orally daily
- Parenteral busulfan
- Patients should receive phenytoin or an alternative antiseizure regimen prior to starting busulfan and continuing through the busulfan regimen
- For nonobese patients, use ideal body weight (IBW) or actual body weight, whichever is lower
- For obese or severely obese patients, use adjusted IBW. Adjusted IBW (AIBW) should be calculated as follows: AIBW = IBW + 0.25 × (actual weight − IBW).
- 0.8 mg/kg IV over 2 hours every 6 hours × 16 doses (total course dose: 12.8 mg/kg) with cyclophosphamide.

Dose Modification Criteria

- Myelosuppression: yes

Adverse Reactions

- DERM: hyperpigmentation
- GI: N/V oral (<4 mg/kg/day): low, intravenous: moderate
- HEMAT: severe myelosuppression

- HEPAT: hepatic veno-occlusive disease
- NEURO: seizures
- PULM: pulmonary fibrosis

Comments

- Therapeutic drug monitoring to determine area under the curve (AUC) with the first administered dose is frequently done with high-dose parenteral busulfan.
- Alternative high-dose once daily parenteral dose regimens and multiple dose oral regimens have been utilized for conditioning regimens in the allogeneic blood and marrow transplant setting. Consult current literature for dosing regimens.
- Phenytoin reduces busulfan plasma AUC by 15%. Use of other anticonvulsants may result in higher busulfan plasma AUCs, and potentially increased toxicity. Consult current literature in regard to the antiseizure regimen utilized within a regimen.
- Embryo-fetal toxicity: busulfan may cause fetal harm when administered to a pregnant woman.

CABAZITAXEL (JEVTANA)

Mechanism of Action

- Microtubule inhibitor that binds to tubulin and promotes its assembly into microtubules while simultaneously inhibiting disassembly. This leads to stabilization of microtubules, which results in inhibition of mitotic and interphase cellular functions.

FDA-Approved Indication

- In combination with prednisone for the treatment of hormone-refractory metastatic prostate cancer previously treated with a docetaxel-containing treatment regimen

FDA-Approved Dosage

- 25 mg/m^2 as a 1-hour intravenous infusion every 3 weeks in combination with oral prednisone 10 mg administered daily throughout cabazitaxel treatment

Dose Modification Criteria

- Renal (CrCL >15 mL/min/1.73 m^2): no
- Renal (CrCL <15 mL/min/1.73 m^2): use caution
- Hepatic (mild to moderate): yes
- Hepatic (severe): avoid use
- Myelosuppression: yes
- Nonhematologic toxicity: yes

Adverse Effects

- DERM: alopecia
- GI: abdominal pain, anorexia, constipation, diarrhea, dyspepsia, and N/V (low)
- GU: hematuria and renal toxicity
- HEMAT: anemia, leukopenia, neutropenia, and thrombocytopenia
- INFUS: hypersensitivity reactions
- NEURO: peripheral neuropathy and dysgeusia
- PULM: cough and dyspnea and severe noninfectious respiratory disorders
- OTHER: arthralgia, asthenia, back pain, fatigue, and pyrexia

Comments

- Cabazitaxel should not be used in patients with neutrophil counts of ≤1,500/mm^3.
- Primary prophylaxis with G-CSF should be considered in patients with high-risk clinical features (age >65 years, poor performance status, previous episodes of febrile neutropenia, extensive prior

radiation ports, poor nutritional status, or other serious comorbidities) that predispose them to increased complications from prolonged neutropenia. Monitoring of CBCs is essential on a weekly basis during cycle 1 and before each treatment cycle thereafter so that the dose can be adjusted, if needed.

- Elderly patients (≥65 years of age) may be more likely to experience certain adverse reactions. The incidence of neutropenia, fatigue, asthenia, pyrexia, dizziness, urinary tract infection, and dehydration occurred at rates ≥5% higher in patients who were aged ≥65 years compared to younger patients.
- Since cabazitaxel is extensively metabolized in the liver, it should be dose modified in patients with mild to moderate impairement and not given to patients with severe hepatic impairment (see product labeling for definitions).
- Cabazitaxel is contraindicated in patients who have a history of severe hypersensitivity reactions to other drugs formulated with polysorbate 80.
- Cabazitaxel requires two dilutions prior to administration, one with the supplied diluent (contains 5.7 mL of 13% w/w ethanol in water), followed by dilution in either 0.9% sodium chloride or 5% dextrose solution.
- Do not use PVC infusion containers and polyurethane infusion sets for preparation and administration. Use an in-line filter of 0.22 μm nominal pore size during administration.
- Cabazitaxel requires premedication with an antihistamine, corticosteroid, and H_2 antagonist, and patients should be observed closely for hypersensitivity reactions.
- Diarrhea and electrolyte abnormalities may be severe, and require intensive measures.
- Since cabazitaxel is primarily metabolized through CYP3A, concomitant administration of strong CYP3A inhibitors and inducers should be avoided. Patients should refrain from taking St. John's Wort.
- Embryo-fetal toxicity: Cabazitaxel may cause fetal harm when administered to a pregnant woman.

CABOZANTINIB (COMETRIQ, CABOMETYX)

Mechanism of Action

- Inhibits tyrosine activity of RET; MET; VEGFR-1, -2, and -3; KIT; TRKB; FLT-3; AXL; and TIE-2

FDA-Approved Indications

- Progressive, metastatic medullary thyroid cancer (Cometriq)
- Advanced RCC who have received prior antiangiogenic therapy (Cabometyx)

FDA-Approved Dosage

- Thyroid cancer: 140 mg orally once daily. (Cometriq)
- RCC: 60 mg orally once daily. (Cabometyx)
- Do not eat for at least 2 hours before and at least 1 hour after taking cabozantinib.

Dose Modification Criteria

- Renal (mild or moderate): no
- Renal (severe): unknown
- Hepatic: mild or moderate: yes
- Hepatic (severe): use not recommended
- Myelosuppression: yes
- Nonhematologic toxicity: yes

Adverse Effects

- CV: hypertension
- DERM: palmar-plantar erythrodysesthesia and wound complications

- ELECTRO: hypocalcemia and hypophosphatemia
- GI: N/V (low), abdominal pain, constipation, decreased appetite, diarrhea, oral pain, and stomatitis
- GU: proteinuria
- HEMAT: lymphopenia, neutropenia, and thrombocytopenia
- HEPAT: hyperbilirubinemia and transaminitis
- OTHER: decreased weight, dysgeusia, fatigue, hair color changes, hemorrhage, and thrombosis

Comments

- Gastrointestinal perforations and fistula formation have been reported. Severe, sometimes fatal, hemorrhage including hemoptysis and gastrointestinal hemorrhage have been reported. Monitor patients for signs and symptoms of bleeding, and do not administer cabozantinib to patients with a recent history of hemorrhage or hemoptysis.
- Cabozantinib treatment results in an increased incidence of thrombotic events.
- Withhold cabozantinib for wound dehiscence or complications requiring medical intervention. Stop treatment with cabozantinib at least 28 days prior to scheduled surgery.
- Monitor blood pressure and discontinue for hypertensive crisis.
- Treatment with cabozantinib can cause osteonecrosis of the jaw. Oral examination should be performed prior to initiation of cabozantinib and periodically during therapy. Patients should maintain good oral hygiene practices. For invasive dental procedures, therapy should be withheld for at least 28 days prior to scheduled surgery, if possible.
- Perform an evaluation for RPLS in any patient presenting with seizures, headache, visual disturbances, confusion, or altered mental function.
- Cabozantinib is a substrate of CYP 3A4. For patients who require concomitant treatment with a strong CYP3A4 inhibitor or inducer, a dose modification of cabozantinib is necessary. Refer to product labeling for recommendations.
- Embryo-fetal toxicity: Cabozantinib may cause fetal harm when administered to a pregnant woman. Effective contraception during treatment with cabozantinib and up to 4 months after completion of therapy is recommended.

CAPECITABINE (XELODA)

Mechanism of Action

- Antimetabolite that is enzymatically converted to fluorouracil in tumors

FDA-Approved Indications

- Colorectal cancer
  - Adjuvant therapy: Indicated as a single agent for adjuvant treatment in patients with Dukes C colon cancer who have undergone complete resection of the primary tumor when treatment with fluoropyrimidine therapy alone is preferred.
  - Metastatic disease: First-line treatment of patients with metastatic colorectal carcinoma when treatment with fluoropyrimidine therapy alone is preferred.
- Breast cancer
  - Combination therapy: Capecitabine combined with docetaxel is indicated for the treatment of patients with metastatic breast cancer after failure with prior anthracycline-containing chemotherapy.
  - Breast cancer monotherapy: Third-line therapy for metastatic breast cancer (after paclitaxel and an anthracycline-containing chemotherapy regimen) or second-line (after paclitaxel) if anthracycline is not indicated.

FDA-Approved Dosage

- Give 1,250 mg/m^2 orally twice daily (total daily dose: 2,500 mg/m^2) at the end of a meal for 2 weeks, followed by a 1-week rest period, given as 3-week cycles. See product labeling for a dosing chart.

Dose Modification Criteria

- Renal (mild impairment, CrCl 51 to 80 mL per minute): no
- Renal (moderate impairment, CrCl 30 to 50 mL per minute): yes
- Hepatic (mild-to-moderate impairment due to liver metastases): no
- Toxicity (grade 2 toxicity or higher): yes
- See product labeling for dose modification guidelines

Adverse Reactions

- DERM: hand and foot syndrome (palmar-plantar erythrodysesthesia) and dermatitis
- GI: N/V (low), diarrhea, mucositis, abdominal pain, anorexia
- HEMAT: myelosuppression
- HEPAT: hyperbilirubinemia
- NEURO: fatigue/weakness, paresthesia, and peripheral sensory neuropathy

Comments

- Altered coagulation parameters and/or bleeding have been reported in patients receiving concomitant capecitabine and oral coumarin-derivative anticoagulation therapy. Anticoagulant response (INR and prothrombin time [PT]) should be monitored frequently to adjust anticoagulant dose accordingly.
- Cardiotoxicity has been observed with capecitabine and is more common in patients with a history of coronary artery disease.
- Severe mucocutaneous reactions, Steven Johnson syndrome, toxic epidermal necrolysis have been reported with capecitabine. Discontinue therapy for severe mucocutaneous reactions or dermatologic toxicity.
- Patients with low or absent dihydropyridine dehydrogenase (DPD) activity are at increased risk of severe or fatal adverse reactions. In patients with evidence of acute early onset or unusually severe toxicity, withhold or permanently discontinue capecitabine as this might indicate low or absent DPD activity.
- Dehydration may occur secondary to gastrointestinal toxicities and this has been observed to cause acute renal failure. Interrupt capecitabine therapy for grade 2 dehydration or greater until dehydration is corrected.
- Embryo-fetal toxicity: Capecitabine may cause fetal harm when administered to a pregnant woman.
- Severe mucocutaneous dermatologic toxicity (e.g., Stevens Johnson syndrome or toxic epidermal necrolysis have been observed in patients treated with capecitabine.
- Geriatric patients (greater than 80 years old) may experience a greater incidence of grade 3 and 4 adverse events.

CARBOPLATIN (PARAPLATIN)

Mechanism of Action

- Alkylating-like agent producing interstrand DNA cross-links

FDA-Approved Indications

- Advanced ovarian cancer
  - First-line therapy (in combination with other agents)
  - Second-line therapy (including patients who have previously received cisplatin)

FDA-Approved Dosage

- With cyclophosphamide: 300 mg/m^2 IV × one dose on day 1 of the cycle; repeat cycles every 4 weeks × six cycles.
- Single agent: 360 mg/m^2 IV × one dose every 4 weeks.

- Formula dosing may be used as an alternative to body surface area (BSA)-based dosing.
- Calvert formula for carboplatin dosing:
  Total dose in milligrams = (target AUC) × [glomerular filtration rate (GFR) + 25].
- The target AUC of 4 to 6 mg/mL/minute using single-agent carboplatin appears to provide the most appropriate dose range in previously treated patients.
- The Calvert formula was based on studies where GFR was measured by ^{51}Cr-EDTA clearance. Alternatively, many clinicians commonly use estimated CrCl equations to determine GFR.

Dose Modification Criteria

- Renal: yes
- Myelosuppression: yes

Adverse Reactions

- GI: N/V (moderate to high)
- ELECTRO: Mg, Na, Ca, and K alterations
- GU: Inc. Cr and BUN
- HEMAT: myelosuppression (thrombocytopenia > leukopenia and anemia)
- HEPAT: increased LFTs
- NEURO: neuropathy
- OTHER: anaphylactic reactions, pain, and asthenia

Comments

- Do not confuse with cisplatin for dosing or during preparation.
- Use caution when estimating CrCl for use in formula (e.g., Calvert equation) dosing. The current isotope dilution mass spectrometry (IDMS) method to measure serum creatinine appears to underestimate serum creatinine values compared to older methods when the serum creatinine values are relatively low (e.g., 0.7 mg/dL). Overestimating the GFR may result when using a serum creatinine measured by the IDMS method. The FDA recommends that physicians consider capping the dose of carboplatin for desired exposure (AUC) to avoid potential toxicity due to overdosing. The maximum dose recommended by the FDA is based on a GFR estimate that is capped at 125 mL to minute for patients with normal renal function.

CARFILZOMIB (KYPROLIS)

Mechanism of Action

- Tetrapeptide epoxyketone proteasome inhibitor that irreversibly binds to the N-terminal threonine-containing active sites of the 20S proteasome, the proteolytic core particle within the 26S proteasome

FDA-Approved Indications

- Multiple myeloma
  - In combination with dexamethasone or with lenalidomide plus dexamethasone in patients with relapsed or refractory disease who have received one to three lines of therapy.
  - As a single agent in patients with relapsed or refractory disease who have received one or more lines of therapy.

FDA-Approved Dosage

- 20/27 mg/m^2 regimen by 10 minute infusion: used in combination therapy with lenalidomide and dexamethasone or as monotherapy
  - Recommended cycle 1 dose is 20 mg/m^2/day on days 1 and 2. If tolerated, increase on day 8 of cycle 1 dose and subsequent cycle doses to 27 mg/m^2/day.

- For cycles 1 to 12, carfilzomib is administered intravenously over 10 minutes, on 2 consecutive days each week for 3 weeks (days 1, 2, 8, 9, 15, and 16), followed by a 12-day rest period (days 17 to 28). Each 28-day period is considered one treatment cycle. With cycle 13 and beyond, omit carfilzomib doses on days 8 and 9.
- 20/56 mg/m^2 regimen by 30 minute infusion: used in combination with dexamethasone or as monotherapy
  - Recommended cycle 1 dose is 20 mg/m^2 on days 1 and 2. If tolerated, increase on day 8 of cycle 1 dose and subsequent cycle doses to 56 mg/m^2/day.
  - For cycles 1 to 12, carfilzomib is administered intravenously over 30 minutes on 2 consecutive days each week for 3 weeks (days 1, 2, 8, 9, 15, and 16) followed by a 12-day rest period (days 17 to 28). Each 28-day period is considered one treatment cycle. With cycle 13 and beyond, omit carfilzomib doses on days 8 and 9.

Dose Modification Criteria

- Renal (for baseline impairment): no
- Hepatic (for baseline impairment): not studied
- Hematologic toxicity: yes
- Nonhematologic toxicity: yes

Adverse Reactions

- CV: cardiac toxicity, CHF, hypertension
- ELECTRO: hypokalemia
- GI: diarrhea and nausea (low)
- GU: acute renal failure and increased serum creatinine
- HEMAT: anemia, neutropenia, and thrombocytopenia
- HEPAT: increased bilirubin and increased LFTs
- INFUS: angina, arthralgia, chest tightness, chills, facial edema, facial flushing, fever, hypotension, myalgia, shortness of breath, syncope, vomiting, and weakness
- NEURO: headache and peripheral neuropathy
- PULM: cough, dyspnea, upper respiratory tract infection, pulmonary arterial hypertension (PAH)
- OTHER: back pain, edema, fatigue, pyrexia, muscle spasm, insomnia, and tumor lysis syndrome

Comments

- Dosing is capped at a BSA of 2.2 m^2. Dose adjustments do not need to be made for weight changes of less than or equal to 20%.
- Hydrate patients prior to and following administration of carfilzomib to prevent tumor lysis syndrome and renal toxicity. Prior to each dose in cycle 1, give 250 to 500 mL of IV normal saline or other appropriate IV fluid. Give an additional 250 mL to 500 mL of IV fluids as needed following carfilzomib administration. Continue IV hydration as needed in subsequent cycles.
- Premedicate with the recommended dose of dexamethasone for carfilzomib monotherapy (4 mg for 10 minute carfilzomib infusion regimen and 8 mg for 30 minute carfilzomib infusion regimen) or the recommended dexamethasone dose for combination therapy orally or intravenously prior to all cycle 1 doses, during the first cycle of dose escalation, and if infusion reaction symptoms develop or reappear. Administer at least 30 minutes and no more than 4 hours prior to carfilzomib. Infusion reactions can develop up to 24 hours after administration of carfilzomib.
- Monitor platelet counts frequently during treatment.
- Monitor serum potassium levels regularly during treatment.
- New onset or worsening of preexisting CHF with decreased left ventricular function or myocardial ischemia has occurred following administration of carfilzomib. Monitor for cardiac complications. Patients with NYHA class III and IV heart failure, myocardial infarction in the preceding 6 months, and conduction abnormalities uncontrolled by medications were not eligible for the clinical trials; these patients may be at greater risk for cardiac complications.

- Monitor for and manage dyspnea immediately. Severe pulmonary toxicity, and pulmonary hypertension have been observed.
- Venous thromboembolic events have been observed with carfilzomib. Thromboprophylaxis is recommended for patients treated with the combination of carfilzomib with dexamethasone or lenalidomide plus dexamethasone.
- Cases of hepatic failure have been reported. Monitor liver enzymes and bilirubin frequently during treatment.
- Serious of fatal cases of hemorrhage have been observed. Promptly evaluate signs and symptoms of bleeding or blood loss.
- Cases of thrombotic microangiopathy have been observed in patients receiving carfilzomib including thrombotic thrombocytopenic purpura/hemolytic uremic syndrome (TTP/HUS). Monitor and discontinue drug therapy if suspected.
- Cases of posterior reversible encephalopathy syndrome (PRES) have been observed in patients receiving carfilzomib. Consider neuro-radiological imaging and discontinue drug therapy if suspected.
- Consider antiviral prophylaxis for patients who have a history of herpes zoster infection.
- Embryo-fetal toxicity: Carfilzomib can cause fetal harm if administered to a pregnant woman.

CARMUSTINE (BICNU)

Mechanism of Action

- Alkylating agent

FDA-Approved Indications

- Indicated as palliative therapy as a single agent or in established combination therapy with other approved chemotherapeutic agents in the following: brain tumors, multiple myeloma, Hodgkin lymphoma, and NHL.

FDA-Approved Dosage

- Single agent in previously untreated patients: 150 to 200 mg/m^2 IV × one dose every 6 weeks *or* 75 to 100 mg/m^2 IV daily × two doses every 6 weeks

Dose Modification Criteria

- Myelosuppression: yes

Adverse Reactions

- GI: N/V >250 mg/m^2 (high), ≤250 mg/m^2 (moderate)
- GU: nephrotoxicity with large cumulative doses
- HEMAT: myelosuppression (can be delayed)
- HEPAT: increased LFTs
- Ocular: retinal hemorrhages
- PULM: pulmonary fibrosis (acute and delayed)

Comments

- Risk of pulmonary toxicity increases with cumulative total doses >1,400 mg/m^2 and in patients with a history of lung disease, radiation therapy, or concomitant bleomycin.
- Myelosuppression is delayed and blood counts should be monitored weekly for at least 6 weeks after a dose. Bone marrow toxicity is cumulative and dose adjustment must be considered based on nadir blood counts from the prior dose.

CERITINIB (ZYKADIA)

Mechanism of Action

- Tyrosine kinase inhibitor of anaplastic lymphoma kinase (ALK)

FDA-Approved Indications

- ALK+ metastatic NSCLC who have progressed or are intolerant to crizotinib

FDA-Approved Dosage

- 750 mg orally once daily on an empty stomach until disease progression or unacceptable toxicity

Dose Modification Criteria

- Renal (mild to moderate, CrCl >30 mL/min): no
- Renal (severe, CrCl <30ml/min): no information
- Hepatic (mild): no
- Hepatic (moderate to severe): no information
- Nonhematologic toxicity: yes

Adverse Reactions

- CV: QT prolongation, bradycardia
- DERM: rash
- ENDO: hyperglycemia
- GI: diarrhea, N/V (moderate), abdominal pain, constipation, decreased appetite, pancreatitis
- GU: creatinine increase
- HEMAT: decreased hemoglobin
- HEPAT: elevated ALT/AST, elevated total bilirubin
- PULM: interstitial lung disease/pneumonitis
- OTHER: fatigue

Comments

- Severe or persistent gastrointestinal toxicity may require withholding therapy and subsequent dose reduction of ceritinib.
- Ceritinib is a substrate of CYP3A4 and p-glycoprotein. Strong inhibitors of CYP3A4 or p-glycoprotein will increase ceritinib drug exposure and should be avoided or may require ceritinib dose reduction. Strong inducers of CYP3A4 should be avoided. Ceritinib may also effect the metabolism of other concomitant drugs; screen for potential drug interactions.
- Embryo-fetal toxicity: Ceritinib may cause fetal harm when administered to a pregnant woman.

CETUXIMAB (ERBITUX)

Mechanism of Action

- Recombinant chimeric monoclonal antibody that binds to the extracellular domain of the human EGFR on both normal and tumor cells, and competitively inhibits the binding of epidermal growth factor (EGF) and other ligands, thus blocking phosphorylation and activation of receptor-associated kinases.

FDA-Approved Indications

- Head and neck cancer
  - Locally or regionally advanced squamous cell carcinoma of the head and neck in combination with radiation therapy

- Recurrent locoregional disease or metastatic squamous cell carcinoma of the head and neck in combination with platinum-based therapy with 5-FU
- Recurrent or metastatic squamous cell carcinoma of the head and neck progressing after platinum-based therapy as single-agent therapy
▪ Metastatic colorectal carcinoma (*K-Ras* mutation-negative [wild-type], EGFR-expressing metastatic disease)
    - Monotherapy: single-agent therapy in patients who have failed irinotecan- and oxaliplatin-based regimens or in patients who are intolerant of irinotecan-based chemotherapy
    - Combination therapy: in combination therapy with FOLFIRI (irinotecan, 5-FU, leucovorin) for first-line treatment OR in combination with irinotecan in patients who are refractory to irinotecan-based chemotherapy

FDA-Approved Dosage

▪ Squamous cell carcinoma of the head and neck: 400 mg/m^2 intravenous infusion over 120 minutes administered 1 week prior to the first course of radiation therapy or on the day of initiation of platinum-based therapy with 5-FU followed by subsequent weekly doses of 250 mg/m^2 intravenous infusion over 60 minutes for the duration of radiation therapy (6 to 7 weeks) or until disease progression or unacceptable toxicity when administered in combination with platinum-based therapy with 5-FU. Complete cetuximab administration 1 hour prior to radiation therapy or platinum-based therapy with 5-FU.
▪ Squamous cell carcinoma of the head and neck (monotherapy): The recommended initial dose is 400 mg/m^2 intravenous infusion over 120 minutes followed by subsequent weekly doses of 250 mg/m^2 intravenous infusion over 60 minutes until disease progression or unacceptable toxicity.
▪ Metastatic colorectal carcinoma (monotherapy or in combination with irinotecan or FOLFIRI [irinotecan, 5-FU, leucovorin]): 400 mg/m^2 intravenous infusion over 120 minutes as an initial loading dose (first infusion) followed by a weekly maintenance dose of 250 mg/m^2 IV infusion over 60 minutes. Therapy is continued until disease progression or unacceptable toxicity. Complete cetuximab administration 1 hour prior to FOLFIRI.
▪ Premedication with an H$_1$ antagonist (e.g., 50 mg of diphenhydramine intravenously 30 to 60 minutes prior to the first dose) is recommended. Premedication should be administered for subsequent doses based upon clinical judgment and presence/severity of prior infusion reactions.

Dose Modification Criteria

▪ Renal: no
▪ Hepatic: no
▪ Nonhematologic toxicity (dermatologic toxicity): yes

Adverse Reactions

▪ DERM: acneiform rash, skin drying and fissuring, and nail toxicity
▪ ELECTRO: Mg, Ca, and K alterations
▪ GI: nausea, constipation, and diarrhea
▪ INFUS: chills, fever, dyspnea, airway obstruction (bronchospasm, stridor, and hoarseness), urticaria, and hypotension
▪ PULM: interstitial lung disease
▪ OTHER: asthenia, malaise, and fever

Comments

▪ *K-Ras* mutation predicts for a lack of response to cetuximab. Determine *K-Ras* mutation and EGFR-expression status using FDA-approved tests prior to initiating treatment.
▪ Grade 1 and 2 infusion reactions (chills, fever, and dyspnea) are common (16% to 23%) usually on the first day of initial dosing. Severe infusion reactions have been observed in approximately 2% to 5% of patients and are characterized by a rapid onset of airway obstruction, urticaria, and/or

hypotension. Severe infusion reactions require immediate interruption of the cetuximab infusion and permanent discontinuation from further treatment.

- Cardiopulmonary arrest and/or sudden death have been reported in patients with squamous cell carcinoma of the head and neck treated with radiation therapy and cetuximab.
- An acneiform rash is common (approximately 76% to 88% overall, 1% to 17% severe) with cetuximab therapy and is most commonly observed on the face, upper chest, and back. Skin drying and fissuring were common and can be associated with inflammatory or infections sequelae. Interruption of therapy and dose modification are recommended for severe dermatologic toxicity (see product labeling).
- Interstitial lung disease has been reported with cetuximab therapy rarely. In the event of acute onset or worsening pulmonary symptoms, interrupt cetuximab therapy and promptly investigate symptoms.
- Hypomagnesemia and other electrolyte abnormalities are common and patients should be monitored closely during therapy and for at least 8 weeks following the completion of cetuximab.
- Embryo-fetal toxicity: No animal reproduction studies have been conducted and effects in pregnant women are unknown. However, EGFR has been implicated in the control of prenatal development and human IgG1 is known to cross the placental barrier.
- Do not administer as an intravenous push or bolus.

CHLORAMBUCIL (LEUKERAN)

Mechanism of Action

- Alkylating agent

FDA-Approved Indications

- Palliation of chronic lymphocytic leukemia (CLL), Hodgkin lymphoma, and NHL

FDA-Approved Dosage

- Initial and short courses of therapy: 0.1 to 0.2 mg/kg orally daily for 3 to 6 weeks as required. Usually the 0.1 mg/kg/day dose is used except for Hodgkin lymphoma, in which 0.2 mg/kg/day is used.
- Alternate regimen in CLL (intermittent, biweekly, or once monthly pulses). Initial single dose of 0.4 mg/kg orally × one dose. Increase dose by 0.1 mg/kg until control of lymphocytosis.
- Maintenance: not to exceed 0.1 mg/kg/day.

Dose Modification Criteria

- Myelosuppression: yes

Adverse Reactions

- DERM: rash and rare reports of progressive skin hypersensitivity reactions
- GI: N/V (minimal)
- HEMAT: myelosuppression and lymphopenia
- HEPAT: increased LFTs
- NEURO: seizures, confusion, twitching, and hallucinations
- PULM: pulmonary fibrosis
- OTHER: allergic reactions, secondary acute myelomonocytic leukemia (AML) (long-term therapy), and sterility

Comments

- Radiation and cytotoxic drugs render the bone marrow more vulnerable to damage; chlorambucil should be used with caution within 4 weeks of a full course of radiation therapy or chemotherapy.

CISPLATIN (PLATINOL)

Mechanism of Action

- Alkylating-like agent producing interstrand DNA cross-links

FDA-Approved Indications

- Metastatic testicular tumors (in combination with other agents) in patients who have already received appropriate surgical and/or radiotherapeutic procedures.
- Metastatic ovarian tumors (in combination with other agents) in patients who have already received appropriate surgical and/or radiotherapeutic procedures.
- Metastatic ovarian tumors (as a single agent) as secondary therapy in patients who are refractory to standard chemotherapy and who have not previously received cisplatin.
- Advanced transitional cell bladder cancer, which is no longer amenable to local treatments such as surgery and/or radiotherapy.

FDA-Approved Dosage

- Metastatic testicular tumors: 20 mg/m^2 IV daily × 5 days every 4 weeks (in combination with other agents).
- Metastatic ovarian tumors: 75 to 100 mg/m^2 IV × one dose (in combination with cyclophosphamide) every 4 weeks, OR as single-agent therapy: 100 mg/m^2 IV × one dose every 4 weeks.
- Advanced bladder cancer: 50 to 70 mg/m^2 IV × one dose every 3 to 4 weeks (single-agent therapy).

Dose Modification Criteria

- Renal: no (consider delay in therapy for toxicity)
- Myelosuppression: no (consider delay in therapy based on nadir blood counts)

Adverse Reactions

- ELECTRO: Mg, Na, Ca, and K alterations
- GI: N/V (≥50 mg/m^2: high, <50 mg/m^2: moderate
- GU: increased Cr and BUN (cumulative)
- HEMAT: myelosuppression and anemia
- HEPAT: increased LFTs (especially AST and bilirubin)
- NEURO: neuropathy, paresthesia, and ototoxicity
- Ocular: optic neuritis, papilledema, and cerebral blindness infrequently reported
- OTHER: anaphylactic reactions and rare vascular toxicities

Comments

- Check auditory acuity.
- Vigorous hydration recommended before and after cisplatin administration.
- Use other nephrotoxic agents (e.g., aminoglycosides) concomitantly with caution.
- Exercise precaution to prevent inadvertent cisplatin overdose and confusion with carboplatin.

CLADRIBINE (LEUSTATIN)

Mechanism of Action

- Antimetabolite

FDA-Approved Indications

- Hairy cell leukemia (HCL)
- Chronic Lymphocytic Leukemia (CLL)—second line therapy in patients refractory to alkylating agents

FDA-Approved Dosage

- HCL: 0.09 mg/kg intravenously by continuous infusion over 24 hours daily × 7 days (a single course of therapy)
- CLL: 0.12 mg/kg (or 4.8 mg/m²) intravenous infusion over 2 hours once daily x 5 days and repeated every 28 days up to a maximum of 6 cycles

Dose Modification Criteria

- Renal: no data
- Hepatic: no data

Adverse Reactions

- CV: edema
- DERM: rash, pruritis, and diaphoresis
- GI: N/V (minimal), decreased appetite, diarrhea, constipation, and abdominal pain
- HEMAT: myelosuppression and lymphopenia
- NEURO: fatigue, headache, dizziness, and peripheral neuropathy
- PULM: cough
- OTHER: fever, chills, fatigue, asthenia, administration site reactions, infections, and tumor lysis syndrome

Comments

- Immunosuppression (lymphopenia) is prolonged after cladribine therapy
- Embryo-fetal toxicity: cladribine may cause fetal harm if administered to a pregnant woman.

CLOFARABINE (CLOLAR)

Mechanism of Action

- Antimetabolite

FDA-Approved Indications

- ALL: pediatric patients (age 1 to 21 years) with relapsed or refractory ALL after at least two prior regimens

FDA-Approved Dosage

- 52 mg/m² by intravenous infusion over 2 hours daily for 5 consecutive days.
- Treatment cycles are repeated following recovery or return to baseline organ function, approximately every 2 to 6 weeks.

Dose Modification Criteria

- Renal: yes
- Hepatic: no data, use with caution
- Myelosuppression: yes
- Nonhematologic toxicity: yes

Adverse Reactions

- CV: tachycardia and hypotension
- DERM: dermatitis and palmar-plantar erythrodysesthesia syndrome
- GI: N/V (moderate), abdominal pain, diarrhea, gingival bleeding, and anorexia

- GU: elevated Cr
- HEMAT: myelosuppression
- HEPATIC: elevated LFTs, hyperbilirubinemia, hepatomegaly, and hepatic veno-occlusive disease
- INFUS: fever, chills, and rigors
- NEURO: headache and dizziness
- PULM: dyspnea, respiratory distress, and pleural effusion
- OTHER: tumor lysis syndrome; infections, fatigue, and asthenia

Comments

- Prophylaxis for tumor lysis syndrome (hydration, allopurinol) should be considered and patients should be closely monitored during therapy.
- Capillary leak syndrome or systemic inflammatory response syndrome (SIRS) has been reported and patients should be closely monitored. The use of prophylactic corticosteroids (e.g., 100 mg/m² hydrocortisone on days 1 through 3) may be of benefit in preventing SIRS or capillary leak.
- Myelosuppression may be severe and prolonged. Severe hemorrhagic events have been observed often associated with thrombocytopenia.
- Hepatobiliary toxicities were frequently observed in clinical trials.
- Severe and fatal cases of enterocolitis have been observed with clofarabine therapy.
- Severe mucocutaneous dermatologic toxicity (e.g., Stevens Johnson syndrome or toxic epidermal necrolysis) has been observed in patients treated with clofarabine.
- Dose adjustment is required in patients with renal impairment. Clofarabine may also cause nephrotoxicity; avoid concomitant nephrotoxic agents during therapy.
- Embryo-fetal toxicity: Clofarabine may cause fetal harm when administered to a pregnant woman.

COBIMETINIB (COTELLIC)

Mechanism of Action

- Reversible inhibitor of mitogen-activated protein kinase (MAPK)/extracellular signal regulated kinase 1 (MEK1) and MEK2. BRAF V600E and K mutations result in constitutive activation of the BRAF pathway, which includes MEK1 and MEK2.

FDA-Approved Indications

- Unresectable or metastatic melanoma with a BRAF V600E or V600K mutation, in combination with vemurafenib

FDA-Approved Dosage

- 60 mg orally once daily for the first 21 days of a 28 day cycle until disease progression or unacceptable toxicity

Dose Modification Criteria

- Renal (mild to moderate, CrCl ≥30 mL/min): no
- Renal (severe, CrCl <30 mL/min): no established recommendation
- Hepatic (mild to severe, Child–Pugh A-C): no
- Nonhematologic toxicty: yes

Adverse Reactions

- CV: cardiomyopathy
- DERM: new primary malignancies (cutaneous squamous cell carcinoma, keratoacanthoma, basal cell carcinoma, and second primary melanoma), severe rash, and severe photosensitivity
- ELECTRO: hyponatremia and hypophosphatemia

- GI: diarrhea, N/V (low)
- GU: increased creatinine
- HEMAT: anemia, lymphopenia, thrombocytopenia, and hemorrhage
- HEPAT: increased ALT/AST and increased alkaline phosphatase
- Ocular System: retinopathy and retinal vein occlusion
- OTHER: rhabdomyolysis, CPK elevations, and pyrexia

Comments

- Cobimetinib is a substrate of CYP3A4. Avoid concomitant moderate or strong inhibitors or inducers of CYP3A4.
- New primary malignancies may occur following cobimetinib. Monitor prior to initiation of therapy, while on therapy, and for 6 months following the last dose of cobimetinib.
- Cardiomyopathy: Evaluate LVEF prior to initiation of therapy, one month after initiation and then every 3 months during therapy with cobimetinib.
- Monitor for severe skin rashes and interrupt, reduce, or discontinue cobimetinib if necessary. Have patients avoid sun exposure due to photosensitivity.
- Ocular toxicity: Perform an ophthalmological exam at regular intervals and for any visual disturbances.
- Embryo-fetal toxicity: Cobimetinib may cause fetal harm when administered to a pregnant woman.

CRIZOTINIB (XALKORI)

Mechanism of Action

- Inhibitor of receptor tyrosine kinases including anaplastic lymphoma kinase (ALK), hepatocyte growth factor receptor (HGFR, c-Met), ROS1 (c-ros), and recepteur d'origine nantais (RON).

FDA-Approved Indications

- Metastatic NSCLC that is ALK-positive as detected by an FDA-approved test or ROS1-positive.

FDA-Approved Dosage

- 250 mg orally twice daily with or without food.

Dose Modification Criteria

- Renal (mild, moderate): no
- Renal (severe, end-stage renal disease): yes
- Hepatic: not studied, use caution
- Myelosuppression: yes (except lymphopenia, unless associated with clinical events)
- Nonhematologic toxicity/tolerability: yes

Adverse Reactions

- CV: QT interval prolongation
- GI: abdominal pain, anorexia, constipation, diarrhea, esophageal disorder, N/V (moderate), and stomatitis
- HEMAT: lymphopenia
- HEPAT: increased LFTs
- NEURO: dizziness, headache, dysgeusia, and neuropathy
- Ocular: vision disorder
- PULM: cough, dyspnea, pneumonitis, and upper respiratory infection
- OTHER: arthralgia, back pain, chest pain, edema, fatigue, insomnia, and pyrexia

Comments

- Detection of ALK-positive NSCLC using an FDA-approved test or ROS-1 positive is necessary for selection of patients for treatment with crizotinib.
- Advise patients to keep crizotinib in the original container. Do not crush, dissolve, or open capsules.
- The aqueous solubility of crizotinib is pH dependent, with higher pH resulting in lower solubility. Drugs that elevate the gastric pH may decrease the solubility of crizotinib and subsequently reduce its bioavailability.
- Avoid concurrent use of crizotinib with strong CYP3A inhibitors or inducers. Avoid grapefruit or grapefruit juice. Dose reduction may be needed for coadministered drugs that are predominantly metabolized by CYP3A. Avoid concurrent use of crizotinib with CYP3A substrates with narrow therapeutic indices.
- Monitor patients for pulmonary symptoms indicative of pneumonitis.
- Avoid crizotinib in patients with congenital long QT syndrome. Consider periodic monitoring with ECGs and electrolytes in patients with CHF, bradyarrhythmias, and electrolyte abnormalities, or who are taking medications that are known to prolong the QT interval. Permanently discontinue crizotinib in patients who develop grade 4 QTc prolongation, and in those who have recurrent grade 3 QTc prolongation.
- Severe and fatal cases of hepatotoxicity have been observed with crizotinib. Monitor LFTs every 2 weeks during the first 2 months of therapy then once a month and as clinically indicated.
- Visual disorders generally start within 2 weeks of drug administration. Ophthalmologic evaluation should be considered, particularly if patients experience photopsia or experience new or increased vitreous floaters. Severe or worsening vitreous floaters and/or photopsia could be signs of a retinal hole or pending retinal detachment. Advise patients to exercise caution when driving or operating machinery due to the risk of developing a vision disorder.
- Embryo-fetal toxicity: Crizotinib may cause fetal harm when administered to a pregnant woman. Patients of childbearing potential should use adequate contraceptive methods during therapy and for at least 90 days after completing therapy.

CYCLOPHOSPHAMIDE (CYTOXAN)

Mechanism of Action

- Activated by liver to alkylating agent

FDA-Approved Indications

- Lymphomas, leukemias, multiple myeloma, mycosis fungoides (advanced disease), neuroblastoma (disseminated disease), adenocarcinoma of the ovary, retinoblastoma, and breast cancer

FDA-Approved Dosage

- Parenteral (intravenous): many dosing regimens reported; consult current literature
- Oral: 1 to 5 mg/kg/day (many other regimens reported; consult current literature)

Dose Modification Criteria

- Myelosuppression: yes

Adverse Reactions

- DERM: rash, skin and nail pigmentation, and alopecia
- GI: N/V ($\geq$1,500 mg/m^2: high, <1,500 mg/m^2: moderate), anorexia, and diarrhea
- GU: hemorrhagic cystitis and renal tubular necrosis
- HEMAT: myelosuppression (leukopenia > thrombocytopenia and anemia)

- NEURO: syndrome of inappropriate antidiuretic hormone (SIADH)
- PULM: pulmonary fibrosis
- OTHER: secondary malignancies; sterility, amenorrhea; anaphylactic reactions; cardiac toxicity with high-dose regimens

Comments

- Encourage forced fluid intake and frequent voiding to reduce the risk of hemorrhagic cystitis. Consider using vigorous intravenous hydration and MESNA therapy with high-dose cyclophosphamide.

CYTARABINE (CYTOSAR AND OTHERS)

Mechanism of Action

- Antimetabolite

FDA-Approved Indications

- In combination with other agents for induction therapy of ANLL, ALL, blast-phase CML, intrathecal prophylaxis, and treatment of meningeal leukemia

FDA-Approved Dosage

- ALL: consult current literature for doses.
- ANLL induction (in combination with other agents): 100 mg/m^2 IV by continuous infusion over 24 hours × 7 days *or* 100 mg/m^2 IV every 12 hours × 7 days. Consult current literature for alternative dosing regimens (e.g., high-dose regimens such as ≥1 gm/m^2/dose).
- Intrathecally: (use preservative-free diluents) 30 mg/m^2 intrathecally every 4 days until cerebrospinal fluid (CSF) clear, and then one additional dose. Other doses and frequency of administration have been utilized.

Dose Modification Criteria

- Hepatic/renal: Use with caution and at possibly reduced dose in patients with poor hepatic or renal function (no specific criteria).
- Nonhematologic toxicity (neurotoxicity): Yes.

Adverse Reactions

- DERM: rash and alopecia
- GI: N/V (>1 g/m^2: moderate; ≤200 mg/m^2: low), anorexia, diarrhea, mucositis, and pancreatitis (in patients who have previously received asparaginase)
- HEMAT: myelosuppression
- HEPAT: increased LFTs
- NEURO: cerebellar dysfunction, somnolence, coma (generally seen with high-dose regimens), and chemical arachnoiditis (intrathecal administration)
- Ocular: conjunctivitis (generally seen with high-dose regimens)
- OTHER: cytarabine (Ara-C) syndrome (includes fever, myalgia, bone pain, rash, conjunctivitis, and malaise); acute respiratory distress syndrome reported with high-dose regimens

Comments

- Consider appropriate prophylaxis for tumor lysis syndrome when treating acute leukemias.
- Consider local corticosteroid eye drops to provide prophylaxis for conjunctivitis when employing high-dose regimens of cytarabine.
- Withhold therapy if acute CNS toxicity occurs with high-dose regimens.

CYTARABINE LIPOSOME INJECTION (DEPOCYT)

Mechanism of Action

▪ Antimetabolite

FDA-Approved Indications

▪ Intrathecal treatment of lymphomatous meningitis

FDA-Approved Dosage

▪ Given only by intrathecal route either via an intraventricular reservoir or directly into the lumbar sac over a period of 1 to 5 minutes.
▪ Patients should be started on dexamethasone, 4 mg PO or IV twice daily × 5 days beginning on the day of the cytarabine liposome injection.
▪ Induction: 50 mg intrathecally every 14 days × two doses (weeks 1 and 3).
▪ Consolidation: 50 mg intrathecally every 14 days × three doses (weeks 5, 7, and 9) followed by an additional dose at week 13.
▪ Maintenance: 50 mg intrathecally every 28 days × four doses (weeks 17, 21, 25, and 29).

Dose Modification Criteria

▪ Nonhematologic toxicity (neurotoxicity): yes

Adverse Reactions

▪ NEURO: Chemical arachnoiditis, headache, asthenia, confusion, and somnolence

DABRAFENIB (TAFINLAR)

Mechanism of Action

▪ Inhibitor of the mutated BRAF kinases V600E, V600K, and V600D

FDA-Approved Indications

▪ As a single agent for the treatment of unresectable or metastatic melanoma with BRAF V600E mutation as detected by an FDA-approved test
▪ In combination with trametinib for the treatment of unresectable or metastatic melanoma with BRAF V600E or V600K mutation as detected by an FDA-approved test

FDA-Approved Dosage

▪ 150 mg orally twice daily as a single or combination agent until disease progression or unacceptable toxicity. Take at least 1 hour before or 2 hours after a meal.

Dose Modification Criteria

▪ Renal (severe impairment): no data available
▪ Hepatic (moderate-to-severe impairment): no data available
▪ Nonhematologic toxicity: yes

Adverse Reactions

▪ CV: cardiomyopathy
▪ DERM: new primary malignancies (cutaneous squamous cell carcinoma, keratoacanthoma, and second primary melanoma), hyperkeratosis, palmar-plantar erythrodysesthesia syndrome, papilloma, alopecia, and rash

- ENDO: hyperglycemia
- HEMAT: hemorrhage
- NEURO: headache
- Ocular System: uveitis
- OTHER: pyrexia, chills, and arthralgia

Comments

- Screen for drug interactions. Dabrafenib is metabolized through CYP3A4 and CYP2C8. Strong inhibitors or inducers of these enzymes will effect drug concentrations of dabrafenib. Dabrafenib is an inducer of CYP3A4 and CYP2C9, which may decrease the systemic exposure of other concomitant medications that are substrates of these enzymes.
- New primary malignancies may occur following dabrafenib. Monitor prior to initiation of therapy, while on therapy, and for 6 months following the last dose of dabrafenib.
- Cardiomyopathy: Evaluate LVEF prior to initiation of therapy, one month after initiation and then every 2 to 3 months during therapy with dabrafenib.
- Monitor for severe skin toxicity and interrupt or discontinue dabrafenib if necessary.
- Uveitis: Monitor for visual signs or symptoms of uveitis (e.g., change in vision, photophobia, and eye pain). Uveitis may require ocular therapy and interruption of discontinuation of dabrafenib.
- Serious febrile reactions may occur. The incidence of febrile reactions is higher when dabrafenib is used in combination with trametinib.
- Dabrafenib may cause hemolytic anemia in patients with G6PD deficiency.
- Embryo-fetal toxicity: Dabrafenib may cause fetal harm when administered to a pregnant woman.

DACARBAZINE (DTIC-DOME)

Mechanism of Action

- Methylation of nucleic acids, direct DNA damage, and inhibition of purine synthesis

FDA-Approved Indications

- Metastatic malignant melanoma
- Hodgkin disease (second-line therapy)

FDA-Approved Dosage

- Malignant melanoma: 2 to 4.5 mg/kg IV daily × 10 days; repeat every 4 weeks, OR 250 mg/m² IV daily × 5 days; repeat every 3 weeks
- Hodgkin disease: 150 mg/m² IV daily × 5 days, repeat every 4 weeks (in combination with other agents), OR 375 mg/m² IV on day 1, repeat every 15 days (in combination with other agents)

Adverse Reactions

- DERM: alopecia, rash, facial flushing, and facial paresthesia
- GI: N/V (high), anorexia, and diarrhea
- HEPAT: increased LFTs and hepatic necrosis
- OTHER: pain and burning at infusion, anaphylaxis, fever, myalgias, and malaise

DACTINOMYCIN (COSMEGEN)

Mechanism of Action

- Intercalating agent

FDA-Approved Indications

- Indicated as part of a combination chemotherapy or multimodality treatment regimen for the following malignancies:
  - Wilms tumor
  - Childhood rhabdomyosarcoma
  - Ewing sarcoma
  - Metastatic, nonseminomatous testicular cancer
  - Indicated as a single agent or as part of a combination regimen for gestational trophoblastic neoplasia
  - Indicated as a component of regional perfusion in the treatment of locally recurrent or locoregional solid malignancies

FDA-Approved Dosage

- For obese or edematous patients, dose should be based on BSA.
- Dose intensity should not exceed 15 μg/kg IV daily × 5 days *OR* 400 to 600 μg/m² IV daily × 5 days, repeated every 3 to 6 weeks.
- Consult with current literature for dosage regimens and guidelines.

Dose Modification Criteria

- Myelosuppression: yes

Adverse Reactions

- DERM: alopecia, erythema, skin eruptions, radiation recall, and tissue damage/necrosis with extravasation
- ELECTRO: hypocalcemia
- GI: N/V (moderate), mucositis, anorexia, and dysphagia
- HEMAT: myelosuppression
- HEPAT: increased LFTs and hepatotoxicity
- OTHER: fever, fatigue, myalgia, and secondary malignancies

Comments

- Vesicant

DARATUMUMAB (DARZALEX)

Mechanism of Action

- An immunoglobulin G1 kappa human monoclonal antibody that binds to CD38 and inhibits the growth of CD38 expressing tumor cells

FDA-Approved Indications

- Multiple myeloma
  - Combination therapy with lenalidomide and dexamethasone or bortezomib and dexamethasone in patients who have received one prior therapy
  - Monotherapy after at least 3 prior lines of therapy including a proteasome inhibitor (PI) and an immunomodulatory agent or who are double-refractory to a PI and an immunomodulatory agent

FDA-Approved Dosage

- 16 mg/kg IV infusion according to the following schedule:

- Monotherapy and in combination with lenalidomide and dexamethasone: weekly during weeks 1 to 8, every two weeks during weeks 9 to 24 and then every 4 weeks until disease progression
- In combination with bortezomib and dexamethasone: weekly during weeks 1 to 9, every three weeks during weeks 10 to 24 and then every 4 weeks until disease progression
- See chart below for specific dilutions and infusion rates

	Dilution volume	Initial rate (first hour)	Rate increment	Maximum rate
First infusion	1000 mL	50 mL/hour	50 mL/hour	200 mL/hr
Second infusion	500 mL	50 mL/hour	every hour	
Subsequent infusions	500 mL	100 mL/hour		

- premedicate with an IV corticosteroid (see product labeling for recommendation), oral antipyretics, and an oral or IV antihistamine
- Infusion should be completed within 15 hours
- Postinfusion medications: oral corticosteroid (see product labeling for recommendation) on the first and second day after all infusions for monotherapy and may be considered for combination therapy

Dose Modification Criteria

- Renal (CrCl > 15 ml/min): no
- Hepatic (mild to moderate) no
- Hepatic (severe): no data
- Myelosuppression: no (dose delays may be needed)

Adverse Reactions

- GI: N/V (low), diarrhea, constipation, and decreased appetite
- HEMAT: anemia, thrombocytopenia, neutropenia, and lymphopenia
- INFUS: Infusion reactions (e.g., bronchospasm, hypoxia, dyspnea, hypertension, laryngeal edema, pulmonary edema, respiratory symptoms, chills, and N.V)
- PULM: cough, nasal congestion, dyspnea, upper respiratory tract infection, and nasopharyngitis
- OTHER: fatigue, pyrexia, back pain, and arthralgia

Comments

- Daratumumab may cause severe infusion reactions. Approximately half of all patients experience a reaction, most during the first infusion. Administer in a setting with immediate access to emergency equipment and appropriate medical support to manage infusion reactions.
- Initiate antiviral prophylaxis to prevent herpes zoster reactivation within 1 week of starting daratumumab and continue for 3 months following treatment.
- Daratumumab binds to CD38 on red blood cells, resulting in a positive indirect antiglobulin test (Coombs test).
- Daratumumab may be detected on serum protein electrophoresis (SPE) and immunofixation (IFE) assays and interfere with clinical monitoring of endogenous M-protein.

DASATINIB (SPRYCEL)

Mechanism of Action

- Tyrosine kinase inhibitor (BCR–ABL, SRC family, c-KIT, EPHA-2, and PDGFRβ)

FDA-Approved Indications

- CML

- Initial therapy in newly diagnosed adults with Ph+ CML in chronic phase.
- Chronic, accelerated, or myeloid or lymphoid blast-phase CML with resistance or intolerance to prior therapy including imatinib.
- ALL: adults with Ph+ ALL with resistance or intolerance to prior therapy

FDA-Approved Dosage

- CML, chronic phase: 100 mg orally once daily
- CML, accelerated phase or myeloid or lymphoid blast phase: 140 mg orally once daily
- ALL (Ph+): 140 mg orally once daily

Dose Modification Criteria

- Renal: no data
- Hepatic: no (use with caution)
- Myelosuppression: yes
- Nonhematologic toxicity: yes

Adverse Reactions

- CV: CHF, QT prolongation, left ventricular dysfunction, and myocardial infarction
- DERM: skin rash
- GI: N/V (minimal) and diarrhea
- HEMAT: myelosuppression and hemorrhage
- NEURO: headache
- PULM: pleural effusion, pulmonary edema, pericardial effusion, dyspnea, and PAH
- OTHER: fluid retention (e.g., edema), fatigue, musculoskeletal pain, and tumor lysis syndrome

Comments

- Myelosuppression may require dose interruption or reduction. Monitor closely.
- Severe bleeding-related events, mostly related to thrombocytopenia, have been reported. Use with caution in patients requiring medications that inhibit platelet function or anticoagulants.
- Dasatinib is metabolized through cytochrome P450 3A4 isoenzyme. Screen for drug interactions with CYP 3A4 inhibitors or inducers.
- Use with caution in patients who have or may develop QT prolongation. Correct hypokalemia or hypomagnesemia prior to starting therapy.
- Dasatinib may increase the risk of developing PAH, which may occur any time after initiation and is reversible upon discontinuation.
- Severe mucocutaneous dermatologic toxicity (e.g., Stevens Johnson syndrome or toxic epidermal necrolysis have been observed in patients treated with dasatinib.
- The bioavailability of dasatinib is pH dependent. Long-term suppression of gastric acid secretion by H_2 antagonists or PPIs is likely to reduce dasatinib exposure. Administration of antacids should be separated from dasatinib by a minimum of 2 hours.
- Embryo-fetal toxicity: Dasatinib may cause fetal harm when administered to a pregnant woman.

DAUNORUBICIN (CERUBIDINE)

Mechanism of Action

- Intercalating agent; topoisomerase II inhibition

FDA-Approved Indications

- In combination with other agents for remission induction in adult ANLL or ALL, children, and adults

FDA-Approved Dosage

- ANLL: in combination with cytarabine
  - Age <60 years: (first course) 45 mg/m² IV daily × 3 days (days 1, 2, and 3); (subsequent course) 45 mg/m² IV daily × 2 days (days 1 and 2)
  - Age ≥ 60 years: (first course) 30 mg/m² IV daily × 3 days (days 1, 2, and 3); (subsequent course) 30 mg/m² IV daily × 2 days (days 1 and 2)
- ALL: (combined with vincristine, prednisone, L-asparaginase) 45 mg/m² IV daily × 3 days (days 1, 2, and 3).
- Pediatric ALL: (combined with vincristine, prednisone) 25 mg/m² IV × one dose weekly × 4 weeks initially. In children aged <2 years or below 0.5 m² BSA, dosage should be based on weight (1 mg/kg) instead of BSA.

Dose Modification Criteria

- Renal: yes
- Hepatic: yes

Adverse Reactions

- CV: congestive heart failure (CHF) (risk of cardiotoxicity increases rapidly with total lifetime cumulative doses >400 to 550 mg/m² in adults or >300 mg/m² in children), arrhythmias
- DERM: nail hyperpigmentation, rash, alopecia, tissue damage/necrosis with extravasation
- GI: N/V (moderate) and mucositis
- HEMAT: myelosuppression
- OTHER: red-tinged urine, fever, chills, and secondary malignancies

Comments

- Consult current literature for dosing information. High-dose daunorubicin regimens (e.g., 90 mg/m²/dose) have been evaluated and shown to be superior to standard doses in younger patient populations.
- Vesicant.
- Consider appropriate prophylaxis for tumor lysis syndrome when treating acute leukemias.

DECITABINE (DACOGEN)

Mechanism of Action

- Decitabine is an analog of the natural nucleoside 2′-deoxycytidine. Decitabine's mechanism of action is as a hypomethylating agent of DNA and also via direct incorporation into DNA.

FDA-Approved Indications

- Myelodysplastic Syndromes (MDS): Previously treated and untreated de novo and secondary MDS of all FAB subtypes and intermediate-1, intermediate-2, and high-risk International Prognostic Scoring System groups

FDA-Approved Dosage

There are two dosing regimens for decitabine. For either regimen, it is recommended that patients be treated for a minimum of four cycles; however, a complete or partial response may take longer than four cycles.

- 15 mg/m² by intravenous infusion over 3 hours repeated every 8 hours for 3 days. Cycles may be repeated every 6 weeks.
- 20 mg/m² by intravenous infusion over 1 hour once daily for 5 days. Repeat cycle every 4 weeks.

Dose Modification Criteria

- Renal: not studied (use with caution)
- Hepatic: not studied (use with caution)
- Myelosuppression: yes
- Nonhematologic toxicity: yes

Adverse Reactions

- CV: edema and peripheral edema
- DERM: rash, erythema, and ecchymosis
- ELECTRO: hypomagnesemia, hypokalemia, and hyponatremia
- ENDO: hyperglycemia
- GI: N/V (low), diarrhea, constipation, abdominal pain, stomatitis, and dyspepsia
- HEMAT: myelosuppression
- HEPAT: hyperbilirubinemia and increased LFTs
- NEURO: headache, dizziness, insomnia, and confusion
- PULM: cough and pharyngitis
- OTHER: fatigue, fever, rigors, arthralgis, and limb or back pain

Comments

- Embryo-fetal toxicity: Decitabine may cause fetal harm if administered to a pregnant woman. Men should not father a child while receiving treatment with decitabine or for 2 months afterward.

DEGARELIX (FIRMAGON)

Mechanism of Action

- Gonadotropin-releasing hormone (GnRH) antagonist that binds reversibly to the pituitary GnRH receptors, thereby reducing the release of gonadotropins and consequently testosterone

FDA-Approved Indications

- Treatment of advanced prostate cancer

FDA-Approved Dosage

- Treatment is started with a dose of 240 mg given subcutaneously as two injections of 120 mg each.
- The starting dose is followed by maintenance doses of 80 mg administered as a single injection every 28 days. The first maintenance dose should be given 28 days after the starting dose.

Dose Modification Criteria

- Renal (CrCL 50 to 80 mL per minute): No
- Renal (CrCL <50 mL per minute): Use with caution.
- Hepatic (mild, moderate): No testosterone concentrations should be monitored monthly until medical castration is achieved since hepatic impairment can lower degarelix exposure.
- Hepatic (severe): Use with caution.

Adverse Reactions

- CV: hypertension and prolonged QT interval
- DERM: injection site reactions, including erythema, induration and nodule, pain, and swelling
- ENDO: hot flashes
- HEPAT: elevated LFTs and elevated γ-glutamyltransferase (GGT)
- OTHER: back pain, chills, fatigue, and increased weight

Comments

- Long-term androgen deprivation therapy prolongs the QT interval. The benefits of androgen deprivation therapy should be weighed against the potential risks in patients with congenital long QT syndrome, electrolyte abnormalities, or CHF and in patients taking class IA (e.g., quinidine, procainamide) or class III (e.g., amiodarone, sotalol) antiarrhythmic medications.
- Degarelix is administered as a subcutaneous injection in the abdominal region to areas that will not be exposed to pressure. The injection site should vary periodically. To minimize the risk of dermal exposure, impervious gloves should be worn when handling degarelix. If degarelix solution contacts the skin, immediately wash it thoroughly with soap and water. If degarelix contacts mucous membranes, the membranes should be flushed immediately and thoroughly with water.
- Following subcutaneous administration of 240 mg degarelix at a concentration of 40 mg/mL to prostate cancer patients, degarelix is eliminated in a biphasic fashion, with a median terminal half-life of approximately 53 days. The long half-life after subcutaneous administration is a consequence of a very slow release of degarelix from depot formed at the injection site.
- The therapeutic effect of degarelix should be monitored by measuring serum concentrations of prostate-specific antigen (PSA) periodically. If PSA increases, serum concentrations of testosterone should be measured.
- Embryo-fetal toxicity: Degarelix is not indicated for use in women. Degarelix can cause fetal harm when administered to a pregnant woman.

DINUTUXIMAB (UNITUXIN)

Mechanism of action

- Binds to the glycolipid GD2, which is expressed on neuroblastoma cells and normal cells of neuroectodermal origin. The binding of dinutuximab to cell surface GD2 induces cell lysis through antibody-dependent cell-mediated cytotoxicity (ADCC) and complement-dependent cytotoxicity (CDC).

FDA-Approved Indications

- High-risk neuroblastoma in combination with GM-CSF, interleukin-2 (IL-2) and 13-cis-retinoic acid (RA) in pediatric patients who achieved at least a partial response to prior first-line multiagent, multimodalilty therapy.

FDA-Approved Dosage

- Prehydration: 0.9% sodium chloride 10 mL/kg IV over 1 hour just prior to initiating dinutuximab infusion
- Premedications
  - Antihistamine IV 20 minutes prior to infusion and as tolerated every 4 to 6 hours during the infusion
  - Acetaminophen 20 minutes prior to each infusion and every 4 to 6 hours as needed for fever or pain. Administer ibuprofen every 6 hours as needed for control of persistent fever or pain
  - Morphine sulfate (50 mcg/kg) IV immediately prior to initiation of dinutuximab followed by a morphine sulfate drip 20 to 50 mcg/kg/hour during and for two hours following completion of dinutuximab infusion
- 17.5 mg/m^2/day as an IV infusion over 10 to 20 hours for 4 consecutive days
- Initiate at an infusion rate of 0.875 mg/m^2/hour for 30 minutes then increase as tolerated to a maximum rate of 1.75 mg/m^2/hour
- Administer on days 4 to 7 of a 24-day cycle during cycles 1, 3, and 5 and on days 8 to 11 of a 32 day cycle during cycles 2 and 4.

Dose Modification Criteria

- Renal: no data available
- Hepatic: no data available
- Nonhematologic toxicity: yes

Adverse Reactions

- CV: capillary leak syndrome and hypotension
- DERM: urticaria
- ELECTRO: hyponatremia, hypokalemia, and hypocalcemia
- GI: N/V (moderate) and diarrhea
- HEMAT: thrombocytopenia, anemia, neutropenia, and lymphopenia
- HEPAT: increased ALT/AST
- INFUS: facial and upper airway edema, dyspnea, bronchospasm, stridor, urticarial, and hypotension
- NEURO: pain during infusion (generalized pain, extremity pain, back pain, musculoskeletal chest pain, and arthralgia)
- Ocular system: neurological disorders of the eye
- OTHER: capillary leak syndrome, pyrexia, hypoalbuminemia, atypical hemolytic uremic syndrome

Comments

- Infusion reactions: Life-threatening infusion adverse reactions occur with dinutuximab infusions. Immediately interrupt for severe infusion reactions and permanently discontinue for anaphylaxis.
- Dinutuximab causes severe neuropathic pain. Administer intravenous opioid prior to, during and for 2 hours following completion of the dinutuximab infusion. If morphine is not tolerated as a premedication, consider using fentanyl or hydromorphone.
- If pain is inadequately managed with opioids, consider use of gabapentin or lidocaine in conjunction with intravenous morphine.
- Capillary leak syndrome and hypotension may require interruption, infusion rate reduction, or permanent discontinuation.
- Neurological disorders of the eye: Evaluate patients for visual disturbances. Dinutuximab has been reported to cause eye disorders characterized by blurred vision, photophobia, mydriasis, fixed or unequal pupils, optic nerve disorder, eyelid ptosis, and papilledema.
- Embryo-fetal toxicity: Dinutuximab may cause fetal harm if administered to a pregnant woman.

DOCETAXEL (TAXOTERE)

Mechanism of Action

- Microtubule assembly stabilization

FDA-Approved Indications

- NSCLC
  - First-line therapy in combination with cisplatin for unresectable, locally advanced, or metastatic NSCLC
  - Second-line therapy as single agent after failure of prior platinum-based chemotherapy
- Breast cancer
  - Locally advanced or metastatic breast cancer (after failure of prior chemotherapy)
  - For the adjuvant treatment of patients with operable node-positive breast cancer (in combination with doxorubicin and cyclophosphamide)

- Prostate cancer: androgen-independent (hormone refractory) metastatic-prostate cancer (in combination with prednisone)
- Gastric cancer: advanced gastric adenocarcinoma, including adenocarcinoma of the gastroesophageal junction (in combination with cisplatin and fluorouracil), first-line therapy in advanced disease
- Head and neck cancer: induction treatment of locally advanced squamous cell carcinoma of the head and neck (in combination with cisplatin and fluorouracil)

FDA-Approved Dosage

- Premedication for hypersensitivity reactions and fluid retention: dexamethasone, 8 mg PO twice daily for 3 days starting 1 day before docetaxel administration.
- NSCLC
  - First-line therapy (combined with cisplatin): 75 mg/m^2 IV over 1 hour × one dose every 3 weeks (administered immediately prior to cisplatin)
  - Second-line therapy (single agent): 75 mg/m^2 IV over 1 hour × one dose every 3 weeks
- Breast cancer
  - Locally advanced or metastatic breast cancer: 60 to 100 mg/m^2 IV over 1 hour × one dose every 3 weeks.
  - In the adjuvant treatment setting: 75 mg/m^2 IV over 1 hour after doxorubicin 50 mg/m^2 and cyclophosphamide 500 mg/m^2 every 3 weeks for six cycles. Prophylactic filgrastim may be used.
- Prostate cancer: 75 mg/m^2 IV over 1 hour × one dose every 3 weeks; prednisone 5 mg orally twice daily is administered continuously.
- Gastric adenocarcinoma: 75 mg/m^2 IV over 1 hour on day 1 only every 3 weeks (in a combination regimen with cisplatin and fluorouracil).
- Head and neck cancer
  - Induction chemotherapy followed by radiotherapy (TAX323): 75 mg/m^2 IV over 1 hour on day 1 only (in a combination regimen with cisplatin and fluorouracil), repeat cycle every 3 weeks for four cycles.
  - Induction chemotherapy followed by chemoradiotherapy (TAX324): 75 mg/m^2 IV over 1 hour on day 1 only (in a combination regimen with cisplatin and fluorouracil), repeat cycle every 3 weeks for three cycles.
  - All patients in the TAX323 and TAX324 docetaxel study arms received prophylactic antibiotics.

Dose Modification Criteria

- Hepatic: yes
- Myelosuppression: yes
- Nonhematologic toxicity: yes (consult with package labeling for dose modification guidelines)

Adverse Reactions

- DERM: rash with localized skin eruptions, erythema and pruritis, nail changes (pigmentation, onycholysis, and pain), and alopecia
- GI: N/V (low), diarrhea, and mucositis
- HEMAT: myelosuppression
- HEPAT: increased LFTs
- INFUS: acute hypersensitivity-type reactions consist of hypotension and/or bronchospasm or generalized rash/erythema
- NEURO: peripheral neurosensory toxicity (paresthesia, dysesthesia, and pain)
- OTHER: severe fluid retention, myalgia, fever, and asthenia

Comments

- Patients with preexisting hepatic dysfunction are at increased risk of severe toxicity.
- Patients with preexisting effusions should be closely monitored from the first dose for the possible exacerbation of the effusions.
- Cystoid macular edema has been reported in patients treated with docetaxel. Patients who develop impaired vision should be evaluated promptly.

- Alcohol content: Cases of intoxication have been reported with some formulations of docetaxel due to the alcohol content. Patients should be counseled on the potential CNS effects and avoidance of driving or operating machinery. Lower dose, weekly dosage regimens are commonly utilized. Consult current literature for dose guidelines.
- Use non-di(2-ethyylhexyl)phthalate (non-DEHP) plasticized solution containers and administration sets.
- Embryo-fetal toxicity: Docetaxel may cause fetal harm when administered to a pregnant woman.

DOXORUBICIN (ADRIAMYCIN AND OTHERS)

Mechanism of Action

- Intercalating agent; topoisomerase II inhibition

FDA-Approved Indications

- Breast cancer: as a component of multiagent adjuvant chemotherapy for treatment of women with axillary lymph node involvement following resection of primary breast cancer
- Acute lymphoblastic leukemia, acute myeloblastic leukemia, Wilms tumor, neuroblastoma, soft tissue and bone sarcoma, breast, ovarian, thyroid, bronchiogenic, gastric cancer, transitional cell bladder cancer, Hodgkin disease, and malignant lymphoma

FDA-Approved Dosage

- Many dosing regimens reported; consult current literature; common dose regimens listed below
- Single agent: 60 to 75 mg/m² IV × one dose repeated every 21 days
- In combination with other agents: 40 to 75 mg/m² IV × one dose, repeated every 21 to 28 days

Dose Modification Criteria

- Hepatic: yes
- Myelosuppression: yes

Adverse Reactions

- CV: CHF (risk of cardiotoxicity increases rapidly with total lifetime cumulative doses >450 mg/m²) and arrhythmias
- DERM: nail hyperpigmentation, onycholysis, alopecia, radiation recall, and tissue damage/necrosis with extravasation
- GI: N/V (moderate) and mucositis
- HEMAT: myelosuppression
- OTHER: red-tinged urine, fever, chills, and secondary malignancies

Comments

- Secondary malignancies: secondary acute myelogenous leukemia and myelodysplastic syndrome occur at a higher incidence in patients treated with anthracyclines.
- Radiation-induced toxicity can be increased by the administration of doxorubicin. Radiation recall can occur in patients who receive doxorubicin after prior radiotherapy.
- Embryo-fetal toxicity: doxorubicin may cause fetal harm when administered to a pregnant woman.
- Vesicant

DOXORUBICIN HCL LIPOSOME INJECTION (DOXIL)

Mechanism of Action

- Intercalating agent; topoisomerase II inhibition

FDA-Approved Indications

- AIDS-related Kaposi sarcoma (progressive disease after prior combination chemotherapy or in patients intolerant to such therapy)
- Ovarian cancer (progressive or recurrent disease after platinum-based chemotherapy)
- Multiple myeloma: in combination with bortezomib for patients who have not received bortezomib and have received at least one prior therapy

FDA-Approved Dosage

- AIDS-related Kaposi sarcoma: 20 mg/m^2 IV over 30 minutes × one dose, repeated every 3 weeks
- Ovarian cancer: 50 mg/m^2 IV over 60 minutes × one dose, repeated every 4 weeks
- Multiple myeloma: 30 mg/m^2 IV over 60 minutes on day 4 only following bortezomib (bortezomib dose is 1.3 mg/m^2 IV bolus on days 1, 4, 8, and 11), every 3 weeks for up to eight cycles until disease progression or unacceptable toxicity
- Note: Infusion should start at an initial rate of 1 mg per minute to minimize the risk of infusion reactions. If no infusion-related adverse events are observed, the rate of infusion can be increased to complete administration of the drug over 1 hour

Dose Modification Criteria

- Hepatic: yes
- Myelosuppression: yes
- Nonhematologic toxicity (palmar-plantar erythrodysesthesia, stomatitis): yes

Adverse Reactions

- CV: CHF and arrhythmias
- DERM: palmar-plantar erythrodysesthesia, alopecia, and rash
- GI: N/V (low) and mucositis/stomatitis
- HEMAT: myelosuppression
- INFUS: flushing, shortness of breath, facial swelling, headache, chills, chest pain, back pain, tightness in chest or throat, fever, tachycardia, pruritis, rash, cyanosis, syncope, bronchospasm, asthma, apnea, and/or hypotension
- OTHER: asthenia and red-tinged urine

Comments

- Do not confuse with nonliposomal forms of doxorubicin.
- Liposomal formulations of the same drug may not be equivalent.
- Irritant.
- Mix only with D5W; do not use in-line filters.
- The majority of infusion-related events occur during the first infusion.
- Experience with large cumulative doses of doxorubicin HCl liposome injection is limited and cumulative dose limits based on cardiotoxicity risk have not been established. It is recommended by the manufacturer that cumulative dose limits established for conventional doxorubicin be followed for the liposomal product (e.g., cumulative doses ≥400 to 550 mg/m^2 depending on risk factors).
- Embryo-fetal toxicity: doxorubicin HCl liposome may cause fetal harm when administered to a pregnant woman.

ELOTUZUMAB (EMPLICITI)

Mechanism of Action

- Humanized IgG1 monoclonal antibody that targets the signaling lymphocytic activation molecule family member 7 (SLAMF7) protein expressed on myeloma cells and natural killer cells. The binding of elotuzumab to SLAMF7 facilitates the interaction between activated natural killer cells and myeloma cells leading to antibody dependent cellular cytotoxicity (ADCC).

FDA-Approved Indications

▪ Multiple myeloma in combination with lenalidomide and dexamethasone for patients who have received 1 to 3 prior therapies.

FDA-Approved Dosage

▪ Premedicate with dexamethasone 28 mg orally 3 to 24 hours before administration, and dexamethasone 8 mg IV, an H_1 antagonist, an H_2 antagonist and acetaminophen 45 to 90 minutes before administration.
▪ 10 mg/kg administered IV every week for the first two cycles and every 2 weeks thereafter in combination with lenalidomide and dexamethasone. Cycles are 28 days.
▪ Initiate cycle 1 dose 1 at 0.5 mL/min. Rate may be doubled in 30 minute intervals to a maximum rate of 2 mL/min. Cycle 1 dose 2 may be initiated at 1 mL/min and increased to 2 mL/min after 30 minutes. Subsequent doses may start at 2 mL/min.

Dose Modification Criteria

▪ Renal: no
▪ Hepatic (mild): no
▪ Hepatic (moderate to severe): no data

Adverse Reactions

▪ GI: diarrhea, constipation
▪ HEMAT: thrombocytopenia
▪ HEPAT: elevated ALT/AST
▪ INFUS: fever, chills, and hypertension
▪ NEURO: peripheral neuropathy, headache
▪ PULM: pneumonia, cough, and nasopharyngitis
▪ OTHER: fatigue, pyrexia

Comments

▪ Elotuzumab can cause infusion reactions, which may be severe. Premedication is required and severe reactions may require dose interruption and rate reduction.
▪ A higher incidence of second primary malignancies has been observed in patients treated with elotuzumab and patients should be monitored.
▪ Elotuzumab may be detected in the serum protein electrophoresis (SPEP) and serum immunofixation assays of myeloma patients, interfering with correct response classification.

ENZALUTAMIDE (XTANDI)

Mechanism of Action

▪ Inhibits androgen binding to androgen receptors and inhibits androgen receptor nuclear translocation and interaction with DNA.

FDA-Approved Indications

▪ Prostate cancer; Patients with metastatic castration-resistant prostate cancer

FDA-Approved Dosage

▪ 160 mg orally once daily with or without food

Dose Modification Criteria

- Hepatic (Child–Pugh class A, B, or C): no
- Renal (CrCL 30 to 89 mL per minute): no
- Renal (<30 mL per minute, end-stage renal disease): unknown
- Nonhematologic toxicity: yes

ADVERSE EFFECTS

- CV: hypertension
- ENDO: hot flashes
- GI: diarrhea
- GU: hematuria
- HEMAT: neutropenia
- HEPAT: elevated LFTs
- PULM: lower respiratory infection
- NEURO: cauda equina syndrome, hallucinations, headache, paresthesia, seizure, and spinal cord compression
- OTHER: anxiety, arthralgia, asthenia, back pain, fatigue, muscular weakness, musculoskeletal pain, and peripheral edema

Comments

- The half-life of enzalutamide is 5.8 days. With daily dosing, enzalutamide steady state is achieved by day 28.
- Avoid strong CYP2C8 inhibitors (e.g., gemfibrozil, ritonavir, and sorafenib). If coadministration is necessary, reduce the dose of enzalutamide to 80 mg once daily. If coadministration of the strong inhibitor is discontinued, restart the original dose.
- Avoid moderate and strong CYP3A4 inducers or CYP2C8 inducers as they can alter the plasma exposure of enzalutamide.
- Avoid CYP3A4, CYP2C9, and CYP2C19 substrates with a narrow therapeutic index, as enzalutamide may decrease the plasma exposure of these drugs.
- If enzalutamide is coadministered with warfarin, conduct additional INR monitoring.
- In the clinical trial, 0.9% patients treated with enzalutamide experienced a seizure. Seizures occurred from 31 to 603 days after initiation of therapy. The safety of enzalutamide in patients with predisposing factors for seizure is not known.
- Neuro-toxicity: seizures and posterior reversible encephalopathy syndrome have been reported with enzalutamide.
- Embryo-fetal toxicity: enzalutamide is not indicated for use in women: enzalutamide can cause fetal harm when administered to a pregnant woman.

EPIRUBICIN (ELLENCE)

Mechanism of Action

- Intercalating agent; topoisomerase II inhibition

FDA-Approved Indications

- Breast cancer: Adjuvant therapy of axillary node-positive breast cancer

FDA-Approved Dosage

- The following dosage regimens were used in the trials supporting use of epirubicin as a component of adjuvant therapy in patients with axillary-node-positive breast cancer.
- CEF 120: 60 mg/m² IV × one dose on days 1 and 8 (120 mg/m² total dose each cycle), repeated every 28 days for six cycles (combined with cyclophosphamide and fluorouracil)

- FEC 100: 100 mg/m² IV × one dose on day 1 only, repeated every 21 days for six cycles (combined with cyclophosphamide and fluorouracil)

Dose Modification Criteria

- Renal: yes
- Hepatic: yes
- Myelosuppression: yes

Adverse Reactions

- CV: CHF (risk of cardiotoxicity increases rapidly with total lifetime cumulative doses >900 mg/m²) and arrhythmias
- DERM: alopecia, rash, pruritus, radiation recall, and tissue damage/necrosis with extravasation
- GI: N/V (moderate), mucositis, and diarrhea
- HEMAT: myelosuppression
- Ocular: conjunctivitis, keratitis
- OTHER: facial flushing, amenorrhea, lethargy, and secondary malignancies

Comments

- Embryo-fetal toxicity: epirubicin may cause fetal harm when administered to a pregnant woman.
- Vesicant.

ERIBULIN (HALAVEN)

Mechanism of Action

- Inhibits the growth phase of microtubules without affecting the shortening phase and sequesters tubulin into nonproductive aggregates. Eribulin is a nontaxane microtubule dynamics inhibitor.

FDA-Approved Indications

- Breast cancer: Metastatic breast cancer in patients who have previously received at least two chemotherapeutic regimens for the treatment of metastatic disease. Prior therapy should have included an anthracycline and a taxane in either the adjuvant or metastatic setting.
- Liposarcoma: Unresectable or metastatic liposarcoma who have received a prior anthracycline-containing regimen.

FDA-Approved Dosage

- 1.4 mg/m² IV over 2 to 5 minutes on days 1 and 8 of a 21-day cycle.

Dose Modification Criteria

- Renal (mild): no
- Renal (CrCL 15 to 49 mL per minute): yes
- Renal (CrCL <15 mL per minute): not studied
- Hepatic (mild impairment, Child–Pugh class A): no
- Hepatic (moderate impairment, Child–Pugh class B): yes
- Hepatic (Child–Pugh class C): not studied
- Hematologic toxicity: yes
- Nonhematologic toxicity: yes

Adverse Effects

- DERM: alopecia
- CV: QT prolongation
- ELECTRO: hypokalemia, hypocalcemia, hypophosphatemia
- GI: anorexia, constipation, diarrhea, abdominal pain, and N/V (low)
- GU: urinary tract infection
- HEMAT: anemia and neutropenia
- HEPAT: elevated LFTs
- NEURO: headache, peripheral motor, and sensory neuropathy
- PULM: cough and dyspnea
- OTHER: alopecia, arthralgia/myalgia, asthenia, back pain, bone pain, decreased weight, fatigue, pain in extremity, and pyrexia

Comments

- Do not mix with other drugs or administer with dextrose-containing solutions.
- Monitor for prolonged QT intervals in patients with CHF, bradyarrhythmias, drugs known to prolong the QT interval, including classes Ia and III antiarrhythmics, and electrolyte abnormalities. Avoid in patients with congenital long QT syndrome. Correct hypokalemia or hypomagnesemia prior to initiating eribulin and monitor electrolytes periodically during therapy.
- Patients should be monitored closely for signs of peripheral motor and sensory neuropathy.
- Embryo-fetal toxicity: Eribulin is expected to cause fetal harm when administered to a pregnant woman. Women should use effective contraception during treatment.

ERLOTINIB (TARCEVA)

Mechanism of Action

- Tyrosine kinase inhibitor (EGFR type I [EGFR/HER1])

FDA-Approved Indications

- NSCLC
  - First-line treatment of patients with metastatic disease whose tumors have EGFR exon 19 deletions or exon 21 (L858R) substitution mutations as detected by an FDA-approved test
  - Maintenance therapy in patients with locally advanced or metastatic disease whose disease has not progressed after four cycles of platinum-based first-line chemotherapy
  - Locally advanced or metastatic disease after failure of at least one prior chemotherapy regimen
- Pancreatic cancer: first-line treatment in combination with gemcitabine in patients with locally advanced, unresectable, or metastatic pancreatic cancer

FDA-Approved Dosage

- NSCLC: 150 mg orally daily (administer at least 1 hour before or 2 hours after the ingestion of food)
- Pancreatic cancer: 100 mg orally daily (administer at least 1 hour before or 2 hours after the ingestion of food) in combination with gemcitabine

Dose Modification Criteria

- Renal: no
- Hepatic: use with caution
- Myelosuppression: no
- Nonhematologic toxicity: yes

Adverse Reactions

- DERM: rash, pruritis, dry skin, bullous, and exfoliative skin disorders
- GI: N/V (minimal), diarrhea, anorexia, and gastrointestinal perforation
- GU: renal insufficiency, acute renal failure, and hepatorenal syndrome
- HEPAT: elevated LFTs, hepatic failure, and hepatorenal syndrome
- Ocular: conjunctivitis, keratoconjunctivitis sicca, corneal perforation, or ulceration
- PULM: dyspnea, cough, and interstitial lung disease
- OTHER: fatigue

Comments

- KRAS mutation predicts for a lack of response to anti-EGFR agents like erlotinib. Consider evaluating for the KRAS mutation prior to initiating therapy.
- Interrupt therapy in patients who develop an acute onset of new or progressive pulmonary symptoms (e.g., dyspnea, cough, or fever) for diagnostic evaluation. If interstitial lung disease is diagnosed, erlotinib should be discontinued.
- Diarrhea can usually be managed with loperamide. Interruption of therapy or dose reduction may be necessary in patients with severe diarrhea who are unresponsive to loperamide or who become dehydrated.
- Monitor liver transaminases, bilirubin, and alkaline phosphatase during therapy with erlotinib. Therapy with erlotinib should be interrupted if changes in liver function are severe.
- The risk of myocardial infarction, cerebrovascular accidents, and microangiopathic hemolytic anemia is increased in patients with pancreatic cancer treated with erlotinib.
- Erlotinib is metabolized through cytochrome P450 3A4 and 1A2 isoenzymes. Screen for drug interactions with CYP 3A4 and 1A2 inhibitors or inducers. Other interactions include cigarette smoking (reduced erlotinib exposure), coumarin-derived anticoagulants (increased INR and bleeding events), and agents which reduced gastric pH (PPIs, H_2 antagonists, and antacids).
- Embryo-fetal toxicity: Erlotinib may cause fetal harm when administered to a pregnant woman.

ESTRAMUSTINE (EMCYT)

Mechanism of Action

- Alkylating agent, estrogen, and microtubule instability

FDA-Approved Indications

- Prostate cancer: palliative treatment of metastatic and/or progressive carcinoma of the prostate

FDA-Approved Dosage

- 4.67 mg/kg orally three times daily OR 3.5 mg/kg orally four times daily (QID); total daily dose: 14 mg/kg.
- Administer with water 1 hour before or 2 hours after meals. Avoid the simultaneous administration of milk, milk products, and calcium-rich foods or drugs.

Dose Modification Criteria

- Hepatic: administer with caution, no specific dose modifications

Adverse Reactions

- CV: edema, fluid retention, venous thromboembolism, and hypertension
- ENDO: hyperglycemia, gynecomastia, and impotence
- GI: diarrhea and nausea
- HEPAT: elevated LFTs (especially AST or LDH)
- PULM: dyspnea

ETOPOSIDE (VEPESID)

Mechanism of Action

- Topoisomerase II inhibition

FDA-Approved Indications

- Testicular cancer: in combination therapy for refractory disease
- Small cell lung cancer (SCLC), first-line therapy in combination with other agents

FDA-Approved Dosage

- Testicular cancer: 50 to100 mg/m^2 IV over 30 to 60 minutes daily × 5 days (days 1 to 5), repeated every 3 to 4 weeks OR 100 mg/m^2 IV over 30 to 60 minutes on days 1, 3, and 5, repeated every 3 to 4 weeks (in combination with other approved agents). Consult current literature for dose recommendations.
- SCLC: 35 to 50 mg/m^2 IV over 30 to 60 minutes daily × 4 to 5 days, repeated every 3 to 4 weeks (in combination with other agents). Consult current literature for dose recommendations.
- Oral capsules: In SCLC, the recommended dose of etoposide capsules is two times the intravenous dose rounded to the nearest 50 mg.

Dose Modification Criteria

- Renal: yes

Adverse Reactions

- DERM: alopecia, rash, urticaria, and pruritis
- GI: N/V (low), mucositis, and anorexia
- HEMAT: myelosuppression
- INFUS: hypotension (infusion rate–related), anaphylactic-like reactions (characterized by chills, fever, tachycardia, bronchospasm, dyspnea, and/or hypotension)
- OTHER: secondary malignancies

ETOPOSIDE PHOSPHATE (ETOPHOS)

Mechanism of Action

- Rapidly and completely converted to etoposide in plasma, leading to topoisomerase II inhibition

FDA-Approved Indications

- Testicular cancer: in combination therapy for refractory disease
- SCLC, first-line therapy in combination with other agents

FDA-Approved Dosage

- Testicular cancer: 50 to 100 mg/m^2 IV daily × 5 days (days 1 to 5), repeated every 3 to 4 weeks OR 100 mg/m^2 IV on days 1, 3, and 5, repeated every 3 to 4 weeks (in combination with other approved agents). Consult current literature for dose recommendations.
- SCLC: 35 to 50 mg/m^2 IV daily × 4 to 5 days, repeated every 3 to 4 weeks (in combination with other agents). Consult current literature for dose recommendations.
- Higher rates of intravenous administration have been utilized and tolerated by patients with etoposide phosphate compared to etoposide. Etoposide phosphate can be administered at infusion rates from 5 to 210 minutes (generally infusion durations of 5 to 30 minutes have been utilized).

Dose Modification Criteria

■ Renal: yes

Adverse Reactions

■ DERM: alopecia, rash, urticaria, and pruritis
■ GI: N/V (low), mucositis, and anorexia
■ HEMAT: myelosuppression
■ INFUS: hypotension (infusion rate–related) and anaphylactic-like reactions (characterized by chills, fever, tachycardia, bronchospasm, dyspnea, and/or hypotension)
■ OTHER: secondary malignancies

Comments

■ Etoposide phosphate is a water soluble ester of etoposide. The water solubility of etoposide phosphate lessens the potential for precipitation following dilution and during intravenous administration. Enhanced water solubility also allows for lower dilution volumes and more rapid intravenous administration compared to conventional etoposide.

EVEROLIMUS (AFINITOR, AFINITOR DISPERZ)

Mechanism of Action

■ Inhibits mammalian target of rapamycin (mTOR), a serine–threonine kinase, downstream of the PI3K/AKT pathway. Everolimus binds to an intracellular protein, FKBP-12, resulting in an inhibitory complex formation with mTOR complex 1 (mTORC1) and thus inhibition of mTOR kinase activity.

FDA-Approved Indications

■ Postmenopausal women with advanced hormone receptor-positive, HER2-negative breast cancer (advanced HR+ BC) in combination with exemestane after failure of treatment with letrozole or anastrozole.
■ Progressive neuroendocrine tumors (PNETs) of pancreatic origin and progressive, well-differentiated, nonfunctional neuroendocrine tumors of gastrointestinal or lung origin that are unresectable, locally advanced, or metastatic.
■ Advanced RCC after failure of treatment with sunitinib or sorafenib.
■ Renal angiomyolipoma and tuberous sclerosis complex (TSC), not requiring immediate surgery.
■ Pediatric and adult patients with TSC who have subependymal giant cell astrocytoma (SEGA) that requires therapeutic intervention but cannot be curatively resected.

FDA-Approved Dosage

■ Advanced HR+ BC, advanced NET, advanced RCC, or renal angiomyolipoma with TSC: 10 mg orally once daily with or without food.
■ SEGA with TSC: 4.5 mg/m² orally once daily.

Dose Modification Criteria

■ Renal: no
■ Hepatic (Child–Pugh class A, B, or C): yes
■ Nonhematologic toxicity: yes

Adverse Reactions

■ Cr: increased creatinine and renal failure
■ CV: edema

- DERM: mouth ulcers and rash
- ELECTRO: hypophosphatemia
- ENDO: hypercholesterolemia, hyperglycemia, and hypertriglyceridemia
- GI: abdominal pain, decreased appetite, diarrhea, mucositis, nausea (minimal to low), and stomatitis
- GU: proteinuria
- HEMAT: anemia, lymphopenia, neutropenia, and thrombocytopenia
- NEURO: headache
- PULM: cough, pneumonitis, and respiratory tract infection
- OTHER: asthenia, fatigue, fever, impaired wound healing, and infections

Comments

- Contraindicated in patients with hypersensitivity to everolimus, other rapamycin derivatives or to any of the excipients. Afinitor Disperz® contains mannitol.
- Available as tablets and tablets for oral suspension (Afinitor Disperz®). Afinitor Disperz® is recommended only for the treatment of patients with SEGA and TSC in conjunction with therapeutic drug monitoring. Maintain trough concentrations of 5 to15 ng/mL.
- Avoid the use of live vaccines and avoid close contact with individuals who have received live vaccines.
- Avoid the use of alcohol-, peroxide-, iodine-, or thyme-containing mouthwashes, since they may exacerbate mouth ulcers, oral mucositis, and stomatitis.
- Everolimus is a substrate of CYP3A4, and a substrate and moderate inhibitor of P-gp. Avoid the concomitant use of strong inhibitors or inducers of CYP3A4. Dose modifications are recommended when everolimus is used concomitantly with moderate inhibitors of CYP3A4 and/or P-gp or strong inducers of CYP3A4.
- Everolimus has immunosuppressive properties and may predispose patients to bacterial, fungal, protozoal, or viral infections, including reactivation of hepatitis B.
- Noninfectious pneumonitis is a class effect of rapamycin derivatives. Patients should be monitored for hypoxia, pleural effusion, cough, or dyspnea.
- Embryo-fetal toxicity: Everolimus can cause fetal harm when administered to a pregnant woman.

EXEMESTANE (AROMASIN)

Mechanism of Action

- Irreversible steroidal aromatase inactivator

FDA-Approved Indications

- Breast cancer
    - Adjuvant treatment of ER-positive early breast cancer in postmenopausal women who have received 2 to 3 years of tamoxifen and are switched to exemestane for completion of a total of 5 consecutive years of adjuvant hormonal therapy.
    - Advanced breast cancer after tamoxifen failure in postmenopausal women.

FDA-Approved Dosage

- 25 mg orally, daily after a meal

Dose Modification Criteria

- Renal: no
- Hepatic: no (note: drug exposure is increased with hepatic and/or renal insufficiency. The safety of chronic dosing in these settings has not been studied. Based on experience with exemestane at repeated doses up to 200 mg daily that demonstrated a moderate increase in nonlife-threatening adverse effects, dosage adjustment does not appear to be necessary.)

Adverse Reactions

- CV: hot flashes and edema
- GI: nausea and increased appetite
- HEMAT: lymphocytopenia
- NEURO: headache, depression, insomnia, and anxiety
- OTHER: tumor site pain, asthenia, fatigue, increased sweating, and fever

Comments

- Reductions in bone mineral density (BMD) over time are seen with exemestane use. Women with osteoporosis or at risk for osteoporosis should have BMD assessed and monitored. Assessment of vitamin D levels should be performed prior to start of therapy and replacement of vitamin D should provided if deficiency is identified.
- Concomitant use of strong CYP 3A4 inducers (e.g. rifampin, phenytoin) with exemestane decreases exemestane exposure and require dose modification to 50 mg once daily.

FLOXURIDINE

Mechanism of Action

- Antimetabolite (catabolized to fluorouracil)

FDA-Approved Indications

- Palliative management of gastrointestinal adenocarcinoma metastatic to the liver when given by continuous regional intra-arterial infusion in carefully selected patients who are considered incurable by surgery or other means.

FDA-Approved Dosage

- 0.1 to 0.6 mg/kg/day by continuous arterial infusion. The higher dose ranges (0.4 to 0.6 mg/kg/day) are usually employed for hepatic artery infusion because the liver metabolizes the drug, thus reducing the potential for systemic toxicity. Therapy may be given until adverse reactions appear; when toxicities have subsided, therapy may be resumed. Patients may be maintained on therapy as long as response to floxuridine continues.

Dose Modification Criteria

- Renal: no
- Hepatic: no, use with caution
- Myelosuppression: yes
- Nonhematologic toxicity: yes

Adverse Reactions

- CV: myocardial ischemia
- DERM: alopecia, dermatitis, and rash
- GI: N/V, stomatitis, diarrhea, enteritis, gastrointestinal ulceration, and bleeding
- HEMAT: myelosuppression
- HEPAT: elevated LFTs
- INFUS: procedural complications of regional arterial infusion—arterial aneurysm, arterial ischemia, arterial thrombosis, embolism, fibromyositis, thrombophlebitis, hepatic necrosis, abscesses, infection at catheter site, bleeding at catheter site, catheter blocked, displaced, or leaking
- OTHER: fever, lethargy, malaise, and weakness

FLUDARABINE (FLUDARA)

Mechanism of Action

- Antimetabolite

FDA-Approved Indications

- B-cell Chronic lymphocytic leukemia (CLL): second-line after alkylating agent therapy

FDA-Approved Dosage

- CLL: 25 mg/m^2 IV over 30 minutes daily × 5 days, repeated every 28 days

Dose Modification Criteria

- Renal: yes

Adverse Reactions

- CV: edema
- DERM: rash
- GI: N/V (minimal), diarrhea, and anorexia
- HEMAT: myelosuppression, autoimmune hemolytic anemia, and lymphopenia
- NEURO: weakness, agitation, confusion, visual disturbances, coma (severe neurotoxicity generally seen with high-dose regimens but have been reported rarely at recommended doses), and peripheral neuropathy
- PULM: pneumonitis and cases of severe pulmonary toxicity have been reported
- OTHER: myalgia, tumor lysis syndrome, and fatigue

Comments

- Monitor for hemolytic anemia.
- A high incidence of fatal pulmonary toxicity was seen in a trial investigating the combination of fludarabine with pentostatin. The combined use of fludarabine and pentostatin is not recommended.
- Transfusion-associated graft-versus-host disease has been observed rarely after transfusion of nonirradiated blood in fludarabine-treated patients. Consideration should be given to using only irradiated blood products if transfusions are necessary in patients undergoing treatment with fludarabine.
- Monitor for tumor lysis syndrome and consider prophylaxis in CLL patients with a large tumor burden initiated on fludarabine.
- Embryo-fetal toxicity: fludarabine may cause fetal toxicity when given to a pregnant woman.

FLUOROURACIL (ADRUCIL AND OTHERS)

Mechanism of Action

- Antimetabolite

FDA-Approved Indications

- Palliative management of colon, rectal, breast, stomach, and pancreatic cancer

FDA-Approved Dosage

- Consult current literature

Adverse Reactions

- CV: angina, ischemia
- DERM: dry skin, photosensitivity, hand–foot syndrome (palmar-plantar erythrodysesthesia), alopecia, dermatitis, and thrombophlebitis
- GI: N/V (low), mucositis, diarrhea, anorexia, gastrointestinal ulceration, and bleeding
- HEMAT: myelosuppression
- NEURO: acute cerebellar syndrome, nystagmus, headache, visual changes, and photophobia
- OTHER: anaphylaxis and generalized allergic reactions

Comments

- Fluorouracil may be given as continuous intravenous infusion or by rapid intravenous administration (intravenous bolus or push). The method of administration will change the toxicity profile of fluorouracil (e.g., greater potential for GI toxicities such as mucositis and diarrhea with continuous intravenous infusions and more hematologic toxicity with bolus administration).

FLUTAMIDE (EULEXIN)

Mechanism of Action

- Antiandrogen

FDA-Approved Indications

- Prostate cancer: Stage D2 metastatic prostate carcinoma (in combination with LHRH agonists) or locally confined stage B2-C prostate carcinoma (in combination with LHRH agonists and radiation therapy)

FDA-Approved Dosage

- Stage D2 metastatic prostate carcinoma: 250 mg orally three times daily (every 8 hours)
- Stage B2-C prostate cancer: 250 mg orally three times daily (every 8 hours) beginning 8 weeks before and continuing through radiation

Adverse Reactions

- DERM: rash
- GI: N/V, diarrhea, and constipation
- GU: impotence
- ENDO: loss of libido, hot flashes, and gynecomastia
- HEPAT: increased LFTs (monitor LFTs periodically because of rare associations with cholestatic jaundice, hepatic necrosis, and encephalopathy)

Comments

- Interacts with warfarin; monitor international normalized ratio (INR) closely

FULVESTRANT (FASLODEX)

Mechanism of Action

- Estrogen receptor antagonist

FDA-Approved Indications

- Breast cancer

- Treatment of hormone receptor (HR)-positive metastatic breast cancer in postmenopausal women with disease progression following antiestrogen therapy.
- Treatment of HR-positive, human epidermal growth factor receptor 2 (HER2)-negative advanced or metastatic breast cancer in combination with palbociclib in women with disease progression after endocrine therapy.

FDA-Approved Dosage

- 500 mg intramuscular injection (two 5 mL injections, one in each buttock) on days 1, 15, and 29 and once monthly thereafter

Dose Modification Criteria

- Renal: no
- Hepatic (mild impairment): no
- Hepatic (moderate impairment): yes
- Hepatic (severe impairment): not tested

Adverse Reactions

- CV: peripheral edema
- ENDO: hot flashes
- GI: N/V, constipation, diarrhea, abdominal pain, and anorexia
- HEPAT: increased LFTs
- NEURO: headache
- PULM: cough, dyspnea
- OTHER: pain, fatigue, pharyngitis, injection site reactions, and asthenia

Comments

- Use with caution in patients with bleeding diathesis, thrombocytopenia, or anticoagulant use.
- Embryo-fetal toxicity: fulvestrant may cause fetal harm when used in pregnant women.

GEFITINIB (IRESSA)

Mechanism of Actions

- Tyrosine kinase inhibitor (primarily EGFR)

FDA-Approved Indications

- NSCLC: first-line treatment of patients with metastatic NSCLC whose tumors have epidermal growth factor receptor (EGFR) exon 19 deletions or exon 21 (L858R) substitution mutations as detected by an FDA approved test.

FDA-Approved Dosage

- 250 mg orally once daily

Dose Modification Criteria

- Renal: not evaluated in severe impairment, use with caution
- Hepatic: no; monitor for adverse effects in moderate or severe impairment

Adverse Reactions

- DERM: rash, acne, dry skin, and pruritus
- GI: N/V (minimal), diarrhea, anorexia
- HEPAT: elevated LFTs

- Ocular: conjunctivitis, blepharitis, keratitis, dry eye, eye pain, and corneal erosion/ulcer (sometimes in association with aberrant eyelash growth)
- PULM: interstitial lung disease (interstitial pneumonia, pneumonitis, and alveolitis)
- OTHER: asthenia and weight loss

Comments

- In a patient who presents with acute onset or worsening of pulmonary symptoms (dyspnea, cough, and fever), gefitinib therapy should be interrupted and a prompt investigation of these symptoms should occur. Fatalities related to interstitial lung disease have been reported.
- Diarrhea can be severe; withhold gefitinib for severe or persistent diarrhea.
- Bullous or exfoliative skin disorders have been reported. Interrupt or discontinue gefitinib for severe bullous, blistering or exfoliative skin disorders.
- Embryo-fetal toxicity: gefitinib may cause fetal toxicity when given to a pregnant woman.
- Gefitinib is extensively hepatically metabolized, predominantly by cytochrome (CYP) 3A4. Be aware of potential drug interactions with either potent inhibitors or inducers of CYP 3A4. A dose increase of gefitinib to 500 mg per day may be considered when given concomitantly with a potent CYP 3A4 enzyme inducer such as phenytoin or rifampin.
- Gefitinib may potentially interact with warfarin leading to an elevated PT and INR and bleeding events; monitor PT/INR regularly with concomitant use.

GEMCITABINE (GEMZAR)

Mechanism of Action

- Antimetabolite

FDA-Approved Indications

- Pancreatic cancer: first-line treatment for patients with locally advanced (nonresectable stage II or stage III) or metastatic (stage IV) adenocarcinoma of the pancreas and in pancreatic cancer patients previously treated with fluorouracil.
- NSCLC: first-line treatment (in combination with cisplatin) for patients with inoperable, locally advanced (stage IIIa or IIIb) or metastatic (stage IV) NSCLC.
- Metastatic breast cancer: first-line treatment (in combination with paclitaxel) for patients with metastatic breast cancer after failure of prior anthracycline-containing adjuvant chemotherapy, unless anthracyclines were clinically contraindicated.
- Ovarian cancer: in combination with carboplatin for advanced ovarian cancer that has relapsed at least 6 months after completion of platinum-based therapy.

FDA-Approved Dosage

- Pancreatic cancer (single-agent use): 1,000 mg/m^2 IV over 30 minutes once weekly for up to 7 weeks, followed by 1 week of rest from treatment. Subsequent cycles should consist of 1,000 mg/m^2 IV over 30 minutes once weekly for 3 consecutive weeks out of every 4 weeks.
- NSCLC (combination therapy with cisplatin)
  - 4-week schedule: 1,000 mg/m^2 IV over 30 minutes on days 1, 8, and 15 of each 28-day cycle. Cisplatin (100 mg/m^2 IV × one dose) should be administered after gemcitabine only on day 1, OR
  - 3-week schedule: 1,250 mg/m^2 IV over 30 minutes on days 1 and 8 of each 21-day cycle. Cisplatin (100 mg/m^2 IV × one dose) should be administered after gemcitabine only on day 1
- Metastatic breast cancer (combination therapy with paclitaxel): 1,250 mg/m^2 IV over 30 minutes on days 1 and 8 of each 21-day cycle. Paclitaxel should be administered at 175 mg/m^2 IV over 3 hours × one dose (day 1 only) before gemcitabine administration.
- Ovarian cancer: 1,000 mg/m^2 IV over 30 minutes on days 1 and 8 of each 21-day cycle. Carboplatin AUC 4 IV should be administered on day 1 after gemcitabine administration.

Dose Modification Criteria

- Renal: use with caution
- Hepatic: use with caution
- Myelosuppression: yes
- Nonhematologic toxicity: yes

Adverse Reactions

- DERM: rash and alopecia
- GI: N/V (low), constipation, diarrhea, and mucositis
- GU: proteinuria, hematuria, and hemolytic-uremic syndrome
- HEMAT: myelosuppression
- HEPAT: increased LFTs and bilirubin, and rare reports of severe hepatotoxicity
- PULM: dyspnea and rare reports of severe pulmonary toxicity (pneumonitis, pulmonary fibrosis, pulmonary edema, and acute respiratory distress syndrome)
- OTHER: fever, pain, and rare reports of vascular toxicity (vasculitis)

Comments

- Intravenous administration rate has been shown to influence both efficacy and toxicity. Refer to the published literature for the appropriate rate of administration for a specific regimen.
- Pulmonary toxicity: discontinue gemcitabine for unexplained new or worsening dyspnea or evidence of severe pulmonary toxicity.
- Hemolytic uremic syndrome (HUS) has been reported in patients treated with gemcitabine. Assess renal function prior to initiating therapy and periodically during treatment. Discontinue gemcitabine in patients with HUS or severe renal impairment.
- Exacerbation of radiation therapy toxicity: may cause severe or life-threatening toxicity when administered during or within 7 days of radiation therapy.
- Capillary leak syndrome has been reported in patients treated with gemcitabine.
- Posterior reversible encephalopathy syndrome (PRES) has been reported in patients treated with gemcitabine. Discontinue gemcitabine if PRES develops during therapy.
- Embryo-fetal toxicity: gemcitabine may cause fetal toxicity when given to a pregnant woman.

GOSERELIN ACETATE IMPLANT (ZOLADEX)

Mechanism of Action

- LHRH agonist; chronic administration leads to sustained suppression of pituitary gonadotropins and subsequent suppression of serum testosterone in men and serum estradiol in women.

FDA-Approved Indications

- Prostate cancer.
  - Palliative treatment of advanced carcinoma of the prostate.
  - Stage B2-C prostatic carcinoma: in combination with flutamide and radiation therapy. Goserelin acetate and flutamide treatment should start 8 weeks prior to initiating radiation therapy.
- Breast cancer: palliative treatment of advanced breast cancer in pre- and perimenopausal women.
- Other indications: endometriosis and endometrial thinning.

FDA-Approved Dosage

- Advanced carcinoma of the prostate: 3.6 mg subcutaneous depot monthly, OR 10.8 mg subcutaneous depot every 12 weeks.
- Stage B2-C prostatic carcinoma: Start 8 weeks prior to initiating radiotherapy and continue through radiation. A treatment regimen of 3.6 mg subcutaneous depot, followed in 28 days by 10.8 mg

subcutaneous depot. Alternatively, four injections of 3.6 mg subcutaneous depot can be administered at 28-day intervals, two depots preceding and two during radiotherapy.
▪ Breast cancer: 3.6 mg subcutaneous depot every 4 weeks.

Dose Modification Criteria

▪ Renal: no
▪ Hepatic: no

Adverse Reactions

▪ CV: transient changes in blood pressure (hypo- or hypertension)
▪ ENDO: men—hot flashes, gynecomastia, sexual dysfunction, and decreased erections; women—hot flashes, headache, vaginal dryness, vaginitis, emotional lability, change in libido, depression, increased sweating, and change in breast size
▪ GU: erectile dysfunction and lower urinary tract symptoms
▪ NEURO: pain
▪ OTHER: tumor flare in the first few weeks of therapy, loss of bone mineral density, osteoporosis, bone fracture, and asthenia

Comments

▪ Use with caution in patients at risk of developing ureteral obstruction or spinal cord compression.

HISTRELIN ACETATE IMPLANT (VANTAS)

Mechanism of Action

▪ LHRH agonist; chronic administration leads to sustained suppression of pituitary gonadotropins and subsequent suppression of serum testosterone in men and serum estradiol in women.

FDA-Approved Indications

▪ Prostate cancer: palliative treatment of advanced carcinoma of the prostate
▪ Other indications: central precocious puberty (alternative product: supprelin LA)

FDA-Approved Dosage

▪ Advanced carcinoma of the prostate: 50 mg subcutaneous depot every 12 months. The once yearly implant is inserted subcutaneously in the inner aspect of the upper arm. The implant must be removed after 12 months of therapy prior to a new implant insertion for continuation of therapy. Implant insertion is a surgical procedure.

Dose Modification Criteria

▪ Renal: no
▪ Hepatic: not studied

Adverse Reactions

▪ ENDO: men—hot flashes, gynecomastia, sexual dysfunction, decreased erections
▪ DERM: implant site reactions (pain, soreness, tenderness, erythema)
▪ GU: erectile dysfunction and renal impairment
▪ OTHER: tumor flare in the first few weeks of therapy, loss of bone mineral density, osteoporosis, bone fracture, and fatigue

Comments

▪ Use with caution in patients at risk of developing ureteral obstruction or spinal cord compression.

HYDROXYUREA (HYDREA, DROXIA)

Mechanism of Action

- Antimetabolite; inhibits DNA synthesis; radiation sensitizer

FDA-Approved Indications

- CML: resistant CML
- Locally advanced squamous cell carcinomas of the head and neck (excluding the lip) in combination with chemoradiation therapy
- Sickle cell anemia with recurrent moderate-to-severe painful crises

FDA-Approved Dosage

- Dose based on actual or ideal body weight, whichever is less
- Individualize treatment based on tumor type, disease state, and response to treatment, patient risk factors, and current clinical practice standards. Sickle cell anemia: Initial starting dose of 15 mg/kg orally daily

Dose Modification Criteria

- Renal: yes
- Hepatic: use with caution
- Myelosuppression: yes

Adverse Reactions

- DERM: rash, peripheral and facial erythema, skin ulceration, dermatomyositis-like skin changes, hyperpigmentation, and cutaneous vasculitic toxicities
- GI: N/V (minimal), diarrhea, anorexia, mucositis, and constipation
- HEMAT: myelosuppression (leukopenia, anemia > thrombocytopenia)
- NEURO: drowsiness (large doses)

Comments

- Cutaneous vasculitic toxicities, including vasculitic ulcerations and gangrene have occurred in patients with myeloproliferative disorders receiving hydroxyurea. If cutaneous vasculitic ulcers occur, discontinue hydroxyurea.
- Radiation recall may occur. Monitor for skin erythema in patients who have previously received radiation therapy.
- Embryo-fetal toxicity: hydroxyurea may cause fetal toxicity when given to a pregnant woman.
- Avoid live vaccines and concomitant antiretroviral agents with hydroxyurea.
- Hydoxyurea may cause a self-limiting macrocytosis early in the course of therapy; Prophylactic administration of folic acid is recommended.

IBRUTINIB (IMBRUVICA)

Mechanism of Action

- Small-molecule inhibitor of Bruton's tyrosine kinase (BTK)

FDA-Approved Indications

- Mantle Cell Lymphoma (MCL) patients who have received at least one prior therapy
- Chronic Lymphocytic Leukemia (CLL)/Small Lymphocytic Lymphoma (SLL)
- CLL/SLL with 17p deletion
- Waldenstrom's Macroglobulinemia (WM)

FDA-Approved Dosage

- MCL: 560 mg orally once daily until disease progression or unacceptable toxicity
- CLL/SLL and WM: 420 mg orally once daily until disease progression or unacceptable toxicity
- CLL/SLL when used in combination with bendamustine and rituximab: 420 mg orally once daily

Dose Modification Criteria

- Renal (CrCl > 25 mL/min): no dose adjustment necessary
- Renal (CrCl < 25 mL/min): no data available
- Hepatic (mild, Child–Pugh class A): yes
- Hepatic (moderate to severe, Child–Pugh class B and C): use not recommended
- Myelosuppression: yes
- Nonhematologic toxicity: yes

Adverse Reactions

- CV: Atrial fibrillation, hypertension
- DERM: rash
- GI: diarrhea, N/V (low), constipation, abdominal pain, decreased appetite
- HEMAT: hemorrhage, neutropenia, thrombocytopenia, anemia
- PULM: upper respiratory tract infection
- OTHER: fatigue, peripheral edema, musculoskeletal pain, pyrexia, tumor lysis syndrome

Comments

- Ibrutinib is a substrate of CYP3A4. Avoid concomitant use of moderate or strong 3A4 inhibitors and strong inducers of CYP3A4. If a moderate CYP3A4 must be used concomitantly with ibrutinib, a dose reduction of ibrutinib is recommended.
- Second primary malignancies have been observed in patients treated with ibrutinib including skin cancer and other carcinomas.
- Embryo-fetal toxicity: Ibrutinib may cause fetal harm if administered to a pregnant woman.

IDARUBICIN (IDAMYCIN)

Mechanism of Action

- Intercalating agent; topoisomerase II inhibition

FDA-Approved Indications

- In combination with other agents for adult AML (FAB M1 to M7)

FDA-Approved Dosage

- AML induction in combination with cytarabine: 12 mg/m^2 slow intravenous injection (over 10 to 15 minutes) daily for 3 days

Dose Modification Criteria

- Renal: use with caution
- Hepatic: yes
- Nonhematologic toxicity (mucositis): yes

Adverse Reactions

- CV: CHF and arrhythmia
- DERM: alopecia, radiation recall, and rash

- GI: N/V (moderate), mucositis, abdominal cramps, and diarrhea
- HEMAT: myelosuppression

Comments

- Vesicant.
- Myocardial toxicity is increased in patients with prior anthracycline therapy or heart disease. Cumulative dose limit not established within package literature.
- Consider appropriate prophylaxis for tumor lysis syndrome when treating acute leukemias.
- Embryo-fetal toxicity: Idarubicin may cause fetal toxicity when given to a pregnant woman.

IDELALISIB (ZYDELIG)

Mechanism of Action

- Inhibitor of PI3Kδ kinase, which is expressed in normal and malignant B-cells.

FDA-Approved Indications

- Relapsed chronic lymphocytic leukemia (CLL) in combination with rituximab in patients for whom rituximab alone would be considered appropriate therapy due to other co-morbidities
- Relapsed follicular B-cell non-Hodgkin lymphoma (FL) patients who have received at least 2 prior systemic therapies
- Relapsed small lymphocytic lymphoma (SLL) patients who have received at least 2 prior systemic therapies

FDA-Approved Dosage

- 150 mg orally twice daily until disease progression or unacceptable toxicity

Dose Modification Criteria

- Renal (≥ 15 mL/min): no
- Hepatic (ALT/AST > 2.5 X ULN or bilirubin > 1.5 X ULN): no data available
- Myelosuppression: yes
- Nonhematologic toxicity: yes

Adverse Reactions

- DERM: rash, severe cutaneous reactions
- GI: diarrhea or colitis, intestinal perforation, N/V (low), abdominal pain
- HEMAT: neutropenia
- HEPAT: ALT/AST elevations
- PULM: cough, pneumonia, and pneumonitis
- OTHER: severe allergic reactions, including anaphylaxis, pyrexia, chills, and fatigue

Comments

- Idelalisib is a substrate of CYP3A4. Avoid concomitant administration with strong CYP3A inducers. Monitor for signs of toxicity if used concurrently with a strong CYP3A inhibitor. Idelalisib is also a strong CYP3A inhibitor and increase drug exposure of other CYP3A substrates. Screen for potential drug interactions.
- Hepatotoxicity: Fatal or serious hepatotoxicity has been reported. Monitor hepatic function prior to and during treatment. Interruption of discontinuation of idelalisib may be necessary.
- Severe diarrhea or colitis may occur and require interruption of discontinuation of therapy.
- Pneumonitis may occur. Monitor for pulmonary symptoms and bilateral interstitial infiltrates. Interruption of discontinuation of therapy may be necessary.

- Severe cutaneous reactions have been reported, which may require interruption of discontinuation of therapy.
- Monitor for signs or symptoms of infection, which can be serious and/or fatal.
- Embryo-fetal toxicity: Idelalisib may cause fetal harm if administered to a pregnant woman.

IFOSFAMIDE (IFEX)

Mechanism of Action

- Alkylating agent

FDA-Approved Indications

- Germ cell testicular cancer (third-line therapy in combination with other agents)

FDA-Approved Dosage

- 1.2 g/m^2 IV daily for 5 days, repeated every 3 weeks. Extensive hydration and mesna should be used to reduce the incidence of hemorrhagic cystitis. Mesna is given either as 3 IV bolus doses or as an IV dose followed by 2 oral doses. When administered as 3 IV bolus injections, give mesna 20% (wt/wt; 240 mg/m^2 per dose for a 1.2 g/m^2 ifosfamide dose) at time of ifosfamide, and then 4 and 8 hours after ifosfamide. Alternatively, give 20% of the ifosfamide dose as an IV bolus injection at time of ifosfamide, and then 40% of the ifosfamide dose orally at 2 and 6 hours after ifosfamide.

Dose Modification Criteria

- Renal: unknown
- Hepatic: unknown
- Myelosuppression: yes
- Nonhematologic toxicity (neurotoxicity): yes

Adverse Reactions

- DERM: alopecia
- GI: N/V (moderate)
- GU: hemorrhagic cystitis, Fanconi syndrome (proximal tubular impairment), and glomerular or tubular toxicity
- HEMAT: myelosuppression
- HEPAT: increased LFTs
- NEURO: encephalopathy, somnolence, confusion, depressive psychosis, hallucinations, and dizziness

Comments

- Ensure adequate hydration (at least 2 liters or oral or intravenous hydration per day); administer MESNA concurrently; monitor for microscopic hematuria.
- Nephrotoxicity can be severe and result in renal failure.
- Discontinue therapy with the occurrence of neurologic toxicity. The incidence of CNS toxicity may be higher in patients with impaired renal function and/or low serum albumin.
- Cardiotoxicity including arrhythmias and cardiomyopathy has been associated with ifosfamide. Use with caution in patients with cardiac risk factors or preexisting cardiac disease.
- Interstitial pneumonitis, pulmonary fibrosis, and other forms of pulmonary toxicity with fatal outcomes can occur. Monitor for signs and symptoms of pulmonary toxicity.
- Ifosfamide is a substrate of CYP3A4 and CYP2B6. Inhibitors or inducers of CYP3A4 will alter the metabolism of ifosfamide and impact efficacy or increase risk of toxicity.
- Embryo-fetal toxicity: Ifosfamide may cause fetal toxicity when given to a pregnant woman.

IMATINIB MESYLATE (GLEEVEC)

Mechanism of Action

- Inhibitor of multiple tyrosine kinases including the Bcr–Abl tyrosine kinase, which is created by the Philadelphia chromosome abnormality in CML. Imatinib is also an inhibitor of the receptor tyrosine kinases for platelet-derived growth factor (PDGF) and stem cell factor (SCF), c-kit, and inhibits PDGF- and SCF—mediated cellular events.

FDA-Approved Indications

- CML:
  - First-line therapy for newly diagnosed adult and pediatric patients with Ph+ CML in chronic phase
  - Second-line therapy for patients in blast crisis, accelerated phase, or in chronic phase after failure of interferon-α therapy
- ALL:
  - Adult patients with relapsed or refractory Ph+ ALL
  - Pediatric patients with newly diagnosed Ph+ ALL in combination with chemotherapy
- Myelodysplastic/myeloproliferative disease (MDS/MPD): adult patients with MDS/MPD associated with PDGFR gene rearrangement
- Adult patients with aggressive systemic mastocytosis (ASM) without the D816V c-Kit mutation or with c-Kit mutational status unknown
- Hypereosinophilic syndrome (HES) and/or chronic eosinophilic leukemia (CEL): adult patients who have FIP1L1–PDGFR α-fusion kinase and patients who are FIP1L1-PDGFR α-infusion kinase negative or unknown
- Dermatofibrosarcoma protuberans (DFSP): adult patients with unresectable, recurrent, and/or metastatic DFSP
- Gastrointestinal stromal tumors (GISTs)
  - Treatment of patients with Kit (CD117)–positive unresectable and/or metastatic malignant GIST
  - Adjuvant treatment of adult patients following resection of Kit (CD17)-positive GIST

FDA-Approved Dosage

- CML
  - Adult patients, chronic phase: 400 mg orally daily. Doses may be escalated to 600 mg per day as clinically indicated (see package insert for criteria).
  - Adult patients, accelerated phase: 600 mg orally daily. Doses may be escalated to 800 mg per day (400 mg orally twice daily) as clinically indicated (see package insert for criteria).
  - Pediatric patients: 340 mg/m^2 orally daily (NTE 600 mg per day).
- ALL
  - Adult patients: 600 mg orally daily
  - Pediatric patients: 340 mg/m^2 orally daily (NTE 600 mg per day)
- MDS/MDP: 400 mg orally daily for adult patients
- ASM—adult patients with
  - ASM without the D816V c-Kit mutation: 400 mg orally daily.
  - Unknown c-Kit mutation status: 400 mg orally daily may be considered for patients not responding to satisfactorily to other therapies.
  - ASM associated with eosinophilia: starting dose of 100 mg per day is recommended, consider increasing dose from 100 to 400 mg per day in the absence of adverse drug reactions and insufficient response to therapy.
- HES and/or CEL: 400 mg orally daily (adults). For HES/CEL with demonstrated FIP1L1–PDGFR α-fusion kinase start with 100 mg per day, may consider increasing dose from 100 to 400 mg per day in the absence of adverse drug reactions and insufficient response to therapy.
- DFSP: 800 mg per day (400 mg orally twice daily).
- GIST—metastatic or unresectable disease: 400 mg orally daily; adjuvant therapy: 400 mg orally daily.

▪ The prescribed dose should be administered orally, with a meal and a large glass of water. Doses of 400 or 600 mg should be administered once daily, whereas a dose of 800 mg should be administered as 400 mg twice a day. In children, imatinib can be given as a once-daily dose or divided into two doses (bid).

Dose Modification Criteria

▪ Renal: yes
▪ Hepatic: yes
▪ Myelosuppression: yes
▪ Nonhematologic toxicity: yes

Adverse Reactions

▪ CV: superficial edema (periorbital, lower limb), severe fluid retention (pleural effusion, ascites, pulmonary edema, and rapid weight gain), CHF, and left ventricular dysfunction
▪ DERM: rash and bullous exfoliative dermatologic reactions
▪ GI: N/V, diarrhea, GI irritation, and dyspepsia
▪ HEMAT: myelosuppression and hemorrhage
▪ HEPAT: elevated LFTs and severe hepatotoxicity
▪ NEURO: headache and dizziness
▪ PULM: cough
▪ OTHER: muscle cramps, pain (musculoskeletal, joint, abdominal), myalgia, arthralgia, nasopharyngitis, fatigue, and fever

Comments

▪ The cytochrome p450 (CYP) 3A4 enzyme is the major enzyme responsible for the metabolism of imatinib. Be aware of potential drug interactions with either potent inhibitors or inducers of CYP 3A4. Dosage of imatinib should be increased at least 50% and clinical response carefully monitored, in patients receiving imatinib with a potent CYP3A4 inducer such as rifampin or phenytoin.
▪ Monitor regularly for weight gain and signs and symptoms of fluid retention. An unexpected rapid weight gain should be carefully investigated and appropriate treatment provided. The probability of edema is increased with higher doses of imatinib and age >65 years.
▪ Monitor LFTs prior to initiation of imatinib therapy and monthly thereafter or as clinically indicated.
▪ Monitor CBCs prior to initiation of imatinib therapy, weekly for the first month, biweekly for the second month, and periodically thereafter as clinically indicated (e.g., every 2 to 3 months).
▪ Embryo-fetal toxicity: Imatinib may cause fetal harm when administered to a pregnant woman.

INGENOL MEBUTATE (PICATO)

Mechanism of Action

▪ The mechanism by which ingenol mebutate induces cell death in actinic keratosis lesions is unknown.

FDA-Approved Indications

▪ Topical treatment of actinic keratosis.

FDA-Approved Dosage

▪ Actinic keratosis on the face and scalp: Apply 0.015% gel to the affected area once daily for 3 consecutive days.
▪ Actinic keratosis on the trunk and extremities: apply 0.05% gel to the affected area once daily for 2 consecutive days.
▪ Not for oral, ophthalmic, or intravaginal use.

Dose Modification Criteria

- None

Adverse Reactions

- DERM: Application site infection, irritation, and pruritus, crusting, erosion/ulceration, erythema, flaking/scaling, swelling, and vesculation/postulation
- NEURO: headache
- Ocular: periorbital edema
- OTHER: nasopharyngitis

Comments

- Ingenol mebutate may be applied to the affected area, up to one contiguous skin area of approximately 25 cm^2 using one unit dose tube. After spreading evenly over the treatment area, the gel should be allowed to dry for 15 minutes, and patients should avoid washing and touching the treated area for a period of 6 hours. Following this time, patients may wash the area with a mild soap.
- Administration of ingenol mebutate is not recommended until skin is healed from any previous drug or surgical treatment.
- Eye disorders, including severe eye pain, eyelid edema, eyelid ptosis, and periorbital edema, can occur after exposure. Patients should wash their hands well after applying ingenol mebutate gel, and avoid transfer of the drug to the periocular area during and after application. If accidental exposure occurs, the area should be flushed with water and the patient should seek medical care as soon as possible.
- Local skin reactions typically occurred within 1 day of treatment initiation, peaked in intensity up to 1 week following completion of treatment, and resolved within 2 weeks for areas treated on the face and scalp, and within 4 weeks for areas treated on the trunk and extremities.

INTERFERON A-2B (INTRON A)

Mechanism of Action

- Cell proliferation suppression, macrophage phagocytic activity enhancement, lymphocyte cytotoxicity enhancement

FDA-Approved Indications

- Oncology indications (adults, ≥18 years of age): hairy cell leukemia, malignant melanoma (adjuvant therapy to surgical treatment), AIDS-related Kaposi sarcoma, follicular lymphoma (clinically aggressive disease in conjunction with anthracycline-containing combination chemotherapy)
- Other indications: condyloma acuminata, chronic hepatitis C, and chronic hepatitis B

FDA-Approved Dosage

- Hairy cell leukemia: 2 million international units/m^2 IM or SC three times a week for up to 6 months.
- Malignant melanoma—Induction: 20 million international units/m^2 IV for 5 consecutive days per week for 4 weeks. Maintenance: 10 million international units/m^2 SC three times per week for 48 weeks.
- Kaposi sarcoma: 30 million international units/m^2 SC or IM three times a week until disease progression or maximal response has been achieved after 16 weeks of treatment.
- Follicular lymphoma (in combination with an anthracycline-containing chemotherapy regimen): 5 million international units SC three times a week for up to 18 months.

Dose Modification Criteria

- Serious adverse events: yes

Adverse Reactions

- DERM: skin rash and alopecia
- ENDO: thyroid abnormalities
- GI: diarrhea, N/V, anorexia, taste alteration, and abdominal pain
- HEMAT: myelosuppression
- HEPAT: increased LFTs
- NEURO: dizziness, depression, suicidal ideation, and paresthesias
- PULM: dyspnea, pulmonary infiltrates, pneumonitis, and pneumonia
- OTHER: flu like symptoms (fever, chills, headache, fatigue, malaise, and myalgia), hypersensitivity reactions, ophthalmologic disorders, and autoimmune disorders

Comments

- Patients with a preexisting psychiatric condition, especially depression, should not be treated.
- Use with caution in patients with pulmonary disease, diabetes mellitus, coagulopathies, cardiac disorders, autoimmune diseases, or ophthalmologic disorders.
- Recommended laboratory monitoring includes CBCs, blood chemistries, LFTs, and thyroid-stimulating hormone (TSH) prior to beginning treatment and then periodically thereafter.
- Other recommended baseline studies include a chest x-ray and an ophthalmologic exam.

IPILIMUMAB (YERVOY)

Mechanism of Action

- Human cytotoxic T-lymphocyte antigen 4 (CTLA-4) antibody that binds to CTLA-4 and blocks the interaction of CTLA-4 with its ligands, CD80/CD86. Blockade of CTLA-4 has been shown to augment T-cell activation and proliferation.

FDA-Approved Indications

- Malignant Melanoma
  - Treatment of unresectable or metastatic melanoma
  - Adjuvant treatment of cutaneous melanoma with pathologic involvement of regional lymph nodes of more than 1 mm who have undergone complete resection, including total lymphadenectomy.

FDA-Approved Dosage

- Unresectable or metastatic melanoma: 3 mg/kg administered IV over 90 minutes every 3 weeks for a total of four doses
- Adjuvant melanoma: 10 mg/kg administered IV over 90 minutes every 3 weeks for 4 doses, followed by 10 mg/kg IV every 12 weeks for up to 3 years or until documented recurrence or unacceptable toxicity

Dose Modification Criteria

- Renal: no
- Hepatic (mild): none
- Hepatic (moderate, severe): not studied
- Immune-mediated toxicity: yes
- Nonhematologic toxicity: yes

Adverse Reactions

- DERM: dermatitis, rash, and pruritus
- ENDO: adrenal insufficiency, hypogonadism, hypophysitis, hypopituitarism, hyperthyroidism, and hypothyroidism

- GI: N/V (low at 10 mg/kg dose), enterocolitis, and diarrhea
- HEPAT: elevated LFTs, hyperbilirubinemia, and immune-mediated hepatitis
- NEURO: motor or sensory neuropathy and headache
- OTHER: fatigue, weight loss, and pyrexia

Comments

- Ipilimumab can cause severe and fatal immune-mediated adverse reactions due to T-cell activation and proliferation. These immune-mediated reactions may involve any organ system; however, the most common severe immune-mediated adverse reactions are enterocolitis, hepatitis, dermatitis (including toxic epidermal necrolysis), neuropathy, and endocrinopathy. The majority of these reactions manifest during treatment; however, a minority can occur weeks to months after discontinuation of therapy.
- Permanently discontinue ipilimumab for severe immune-mediated adverse reactions and administer systemic high-dose corticosteroids for severe, persistent, or recurring immune-mediated reactions.
- Assess patients for signs and symptoms of enterocolitis, dermatitis, neuropathy, and endocrinopathy and evaluate clinical chemistries including LFTs and thyroid function tests at baseline and before each dose.
- Do not shake ipilimumab. Administer the diluted solution through a nonpyrogenic, low-protein-binding in-line filter.
- Embryo-fetal toxicity: Use during pregnancy only if potential benefit justifies risk to fetus. Human IgG1 is known to cross the placental barrier and ipilimumab is an IgG1; therefore, ipilimumab has the potential to be transmitted from the mother to the developing fetus.

IRINOTECAN (CAMPTOSAR)

Mechanism of Action

- Topoisomerase I inhibitor

FDA-Approved Indications

- Metastatic colon or rectal cancer
  - First-line therapy in combination with fluorouracil and leucovorin
  - Second-line therapy (single agent) after fluorouracil-based therapy

FDA-Approved Dosage

- First-line combination-agent dosing: See product labeling for fluorouracil/leucovorin dosing.
  - Regimen 1: 125 mg/m^2 IV over 90 minutes weekly × four doses (days 1, 8, 15, 22) followed by 2 weeks of rest. Repeat every 6 weeks.
  - Regimen 2: 180 mg/m^2 IV over 90 minutes every 2 weeks (days 1, 15, 29) for each cycle. Each cycle is 6 weeks in duration.
- Second-line single-agent dosing.
  - Weekly regimen: 125 mg/m^2 IV over 90 minutes weekly for four doses (days 1, 8, 15, 22) followed by 2 weeks rest. Repeat every 6 weeks, OR
  - Once-every-3-weeks regimen: 350 mg/m^2 IV over 90 minutes every 3 weeks.

Dose Modification Criteria

- Renal: no data, use with caution
- Hepatic: yes
- Pelvic/abdominal irradiation: yes
- Myelosuppression: yes
- Nonhematologic toxicity: yes (see package labeling for dose modifications)

Adverse Reactions

- CV: vasodilation
- DERM: alopecia, sweating, and rash
- GI: N/V (moderate), diarrhea (early and late), abdominal pain, mucositis, and anorexia, flatulence
- HEMAT: myelosuppression
- HEPAT: increased bilirubin and LFTs
- NEURO: insomnia and dizziness
- PULM: dyspnea, coughing, and rhinitis
- OTHER: asthenia, fever, and hypersensitivity reactions

Comments

- Can induce both early (within 24 hours of administration) and late forms of diarrhea. The early-onset diarrhea is cholinergic in nature and may be accompanied by symptoms of rhinitis, increased salivation, miosis, lacrimation, diaphoresis, flushing, and abdominal cramping. These early cholinergic symptoms can be treated by administration of atropine. Late-onset diarrhea (generally after 24 hours) should be treated aggressively with high-dose loperamide. Each patient should be instructed to have loperamide readily available so that treatment can be initiated at the earliest onset of diarrhea. See package labeling for dosage recommendations for atropine and loperamide.
- Patients with reduced UGT1A1 activity (homozygous for the UGT1A1*28 allele) are at increased risk of neutropenia with irinotecan.
- Interstitial pulmonary disease-like events, including fatalities, have occurred with irinotecan. Interrupt therapy for new or progressive dyspnea, cough, and fever pending evaluation.
- Embryo-fetal toxicity: irinotecan may cause fetal toxicity when given to a pregnant woman.
- Irinotecan and the active metabolite SN-38 are metabolized through CYP3A4 and UGT1A1. Screen for drug interactions with inhibitors or inducers of CYP3A4 and inhibitors of UGT1A1.

IRINOTECAN LIPOSOME INJECTION (ONIVYDE)

Mechanism of Action

- Topoisomerase 1 inhibitor encapsulated in a lipid bilayer vesicle or liposome.

FDA-Approved Indications

- Metastatic adenocarcinoma of the pancreas in combination with fluorouracil and leucovorin after progression following gemcitabine-based therapy

FDA-Approved Dosage

- Administer a corticosteroid and an anti-emetic 30 minutes prior to infusion
- 70 mg/m^2 infused over 90 minutes every 2 weeks

Dose Modification Criteria

- Renal (mild to moderate, CrCl > 30 ml/min): no
- Renal (severe, CrCl <30 mL/min): no data available
- Hepatic: limited data, use with caution
- Hematologic or nonhematologic toxicity: yes

Adverse Reactions

- ENDO: hypomagnesemia and hypokalemia
- GI: diarrhea, N/V (moderate), stomatitis, and decreased appetite

- HEMAT: neutropenia, anemia, lymphopenia, and thrombocytopenia
- HEPAT: elevated ALT
- INFUS: hypersensitivity reaction
- PULM: interstitial lung disease
- OTHER: fatigue/asthenia, pyrexia, and cholinergic reactions

Comments

- Do not substitute for other drugs containing irinotecan.
- Protect diluted solution from light.
- Patients with reduced UGT1A1 activity (homozygous for the UGT1A1*28 allele) are at increased risk of neutropenia with irinotecan liposome and require dose reduction.
- Avoid the use of strong CYP3A4 inducers and strong CYP3A4 or UGT1A1 inhibitors if possible
- Severe or life-threatening neutropenia and neutropenic sepsis can occur. Monitor blood cell counts during treatment.
- Severe diarrhea (early and late) may occur as with nonliposomal irinotecan. See comments above with nonliposomal irinotecan regarding diarrhea management.
- Embryo-fetal toxicity: Irinotecan liposome may cause fetal harm when administered to a pregnant woman.

IXABEPILONE (IXEMPRA)

Mechanism of Action

- Microtubule inhibitor

FDA-Approved Indications

- Breast cancer
  - In combination with capecitabine in patients with metastatic or locally advanced breast cancer after failure of an anthracycline and a taxane.
  - Monotherapy in patients with metastatic or locally advanced breast cancer after failure of an anthracycline, a taxane, and a capecitabine.

FDA-Approved Dosage

- 40 mg/m^2 IV over 3 hours every 3 weeks

Dose Modification Criteria

- Renal: no
- Hepatic: yes
- Myelosuppression: yes
- Nonhematologic toxicity: yes

Adverse Reactions

- DERM: alopecia
- GI: N/V (low), stomatitis/mucositis, and diarrhea
- HEMAT: myelosuppression
- HEPAT: elevated LFTs
- INFUS: hypersensitivity reactions (e.g., flushing, rash, dyspnea, and bronchospasm)
- NEURO: peripheral neuropathy
- OTHER: fatigue, asthenia, myalgia/arthralgia, and alopecia

Comments

- Patients should be premedicated approximately 1 hour before the infusion of ixabepilone with an H$_1$ antagonist (e.g., diphenhydramine) and an H$_2$ antagonist (ranitidine).

- Monitor for peripheral neuropathy. Neuropathy is cumulative, generally reversible, and should be managed by dose adjustment and delays.
- Ixabepilone is metabolized through CYP 3A4 isoenzyme. Screen for drug interactions with CYP 3A4 inhibitors or inducers. A dose modification is suggested if concomitantly used with a potent CYP 3A4 inhibitor.
- Embryo-fetal toxicity: Ixabepilone may cause fetal harm when administered to a pregnant woman.

IXAZOMIB (NINLARO)

Mechanism of Action

- Reversible proteasome inhibitor

FDA-Approved Indications

- Multiple myeloma in combination with lenalidomide and dexamethasone for patients who have received at least 1 prior therapy

FDA-Approved Dosage

- 4 mg orally once a week on days 1, 8, and 15 of a 28 day cycle in combination with lenalidomide and dexamethasone.

Dose Modification Criteria

- Renal (severe, CrCl < 30 mL/min or dialysis): yes
- Hepatic (moderate to severe, total bilirubin > 1.5 X ULN): yes
- Hematologic toxicity: yes
- Nonhematologic toxicity: yes

Adverse Reactions

- DERM: rash
- GI: diarrhea, constipation, N/V (low)
- HEMAT: thrombocytopenia, neutropenia
- HEPAT: increased LFTs, hepatotoxicity
- NEURO: peripheral neuropathy
- OTHER: peripheral edema, back pain

Comments

- Avoid concomitant administration with strong CYP3A inducers.
- Embryo-fetal toxicity: Ixazomib may cause fetal harm when administered to a pregnant woman.

LAPATINIB (TYKERB)

Mechanism of Action

- Tyrosine kinase inhibitor of EGFR Type I (EGFR/HER1) and human epidermal receptor type II (HER2/ErbB2)

FDA-Approved Indications

- Breast cancer
  - In combination with capecitabine for the treatment of patients with advanced or metastatic breast cancer who overexpress HER2 and who have received prior therapy, including an anthracycline, a taxane, and trastuzumab.

- In combination with letrozole for the treatment of postmenopausal women with hormone receptor-positive metastatic breast cancer that overexpresses the HER2 receptor for whom hormonal therapy is indicated.

FDA-Approved Dosage

- Breast cancer
  - HER2-positive metastatic breast cancer: 1,250 mg orally once daily on days 1 to 21 continuously in combination with capecitabine (dosed on days 1 to 14) in a repeating 21-day cycle.
  - Hormone receptor-positive, HER2-positive metastatic breast cancer: 1,500 mg orally once daily continuously in combination with letrozole.
  - Lapatinib should be administered once daily (not in divided doses) at least 1 hour before or 1 hour after the ingestion of food.

Dose Modification Criteria

- Renal: no
- Hepatic: yes
- Myelosuppression: no
- Nonhematologic toxicity: yes

Adverse Reactions

- CV: reduced LVEF and QT prolongation
- DERM: palmar-plantar erythrodysesthesia and rash
- GI: N/V (low), diarrhea, and stomatitis
- HEMAT: myelosuppression
- HEPAT: elevated LFTs
- PULM: interstitial lung disease and pneumonitis
- OTHER: fatigue

Comments

- Product labeling suggests monitoring LVEF at baseline and during therapy. Interrupt therapy for grade 2 or greater reductions in LVEF. Upon recovery, restart at lower dose.
- Monitor patients for interstitial lung disease or pneumonitis. Lapatinib should be discontinued in patients who experience pulmonary symptoms indicative of ≥grade 3 toxicity.
- Severe cutaneous reactions have been reported. Discontinue lapatinib if life-threatening reactions are suspected.
- Lapatinib is metabolized through CYP 3A4 isoenzyme. Screen for drug interactions with CYP 3A4 inhibitors or inducers. Dose modifications may be necessary if concomitant use is unavoidable with potent inhibitors or inducers.
- Embryo-fetal toxicity: Lapatinib may cause fetal harm when administered to a pregnant woman.

LENALIDOMIDE (REVLIMID)

Mechanism of Action

- Immunomodulatory agent with antineoplastic and antiangiogenic properties

FDA-Approved Indications

- Myelodysplastic Syndrome (MDS): treatment of patients with transfusion-dependent anemia due to low- or intermediate-1 risk MDSs associated with a deletion 5q cytogenetic abnormality with or without additional cytogenetic abnormalities
- Multiple myeloma: in combination with dexamethasone
- Mantle Cell Lymphoma (MCL): treatment of relapsed or progressive disease after two prior therapies, one of which included bortezomib

FDA-Approved Dosage

- MDS: 10 mg orally daily
- Multiple myeloma: 25 mg orally daily on days 1 to 21 of a 28-day treatment cycle in combination with dexamethasone
- MCL: 25 mg orally once daily on days 1 to 21 of a 28-day treatment cycle

Dose Modification Criteria

- Renal: yes
- Hepatic: no data
- Myelosuppression: yes
- Nonhematologic toxicity: yes

Adverse Reactions

- CV: edema
- DERM: rash, pruritis, and dry skin
- ELECTRO: hypokalemia
- GI: diarrhea, constipation, N/V (minimal to low), abdominal pain, and anorexia
- HEMAT: myelosuppression
- HEPAT: hepatotoxicity
- NEURO: dizziness, headache, insomnia, and tremor
- PULM: dyspnea, cough, and nasopharyngitis
- OTHER: thromboembolic events, fatigue, fever, arthralgia, back or limb pain, muscle cramps, asthenia, hypersensitivity reactions, and tumor lysis syndrome

Comments

- Lenalidomide is only available through a restricted distribution program (Revlimed REMS program). Only prescribers and pharmacists registered with the program are allowed to prescribe and dispense lenalidomide.
- Embryo-fetal toxicity. Lenalidomide is an analog of thalidomide, which is a known teratogen. Lenalidomide may cause severe birth defects or death to an unborn baby. Refer to the product labeling for information regarding requirements for patient consent, pregnancy testing, and patient consent as part of the Revlimid REMS program.
- Myelosuppression (particularly neutropenia and thrombocytopenia) is a common and dose-limiting toxicity. Monitor blood counts closely as indicated in the product labeling.
- Lenalidomide may cause venous thromboembolic events. There is an increased risk of thrombotic events when lenalidomide is combined with standard chemotherapeutic agents, including dexamethasone. Consider concurrent prophylactic anticoagulation or aspirin treatment.
- Lenalidomide is not indicated or recommended for the treatment of chronic lymphocytic leukemia per product labeling. Serious and fatal cardiac adverse events occurred in CLL patients treated with lenalidomide.
- A higher incidence of second primary malignancies have been observed in multiple myeloma patients treated with lenalidomide.
- Tumor flare reactions have been observed in clinical trials of lenalidomide in CLL and lymphoma.
- Impaired stem cell mobilization: A decrease in the number of CD34+ cells collected after treatment (>4 cycles) with lenalidomide has been reported.

LENVATINIB (LENVIMA)

Mechanism of Action

- Receptor tyrosine kinase (RTK) inhibitor that inhibits the kinase activity of VEGFR-1, -2, and -3 fibroblast growth factor receptors (FGFR) -1, -2, -3, and -4, platelet-derived growth factor receptor alpha (PDGFRα), KIT, and RET.

FDA-Approved Indications

- Differentiated thyroid cancer (DTC): single agent for patients with locally recurrent or metastatic, progressive, radioactive iodine-refractory DTC
- Renal cell cancer (RCC): in combination with everolimus, for patients with advanced RCC following one prior antiangiogenic therapy

FDA-Approved Dosage

- DTC: 24 mg orally, once daily until disease progression or unacceptable toxicity
- RCC: 18 mg orally, once daily in combination with everolimus 5 mg once daily until progression or unacceptable toxicity

Dose Modification Criteria

- Renal (severe, CrCl <30 mL/min): yes; ESRD not studied
- Hepatic (severe, Child–Pugh C): yes
- Nonhematologic toxicity: yes

Adverse Reactions

- CV: hypertension, cardiac dysfunction, arterial thromboembolic events, QT interval prolongation
- DERM: palmar-plantar erythrodysesthesia, rash
- ELECTRO: hypcalcemia
- ENDO: hypothyroidism
- GI: diarrhea, gastrointestinal perforation, fistula formation, N/V (moderate), stomatitis, constipation, abdominal pain, oral pain, decreased appetite, dyseusia
- GU: proteinuria, renal failure/impairment
- HEMAT: hemorrhagic events
- HEPAT: increased LFTs, hepatotoxicity
- NEURO: headache, dizziness
- PULM: dysphonia, cough
- OTHER: fatigue, peripheral edema, arthralgia/myalgia, pyrexia

Comments

- Hypertension: Control blood pressure before starting lenvatinib. Monitor blood pressure after 1 week, then every 2 weeks for the first 2 months, then at least monthly thereafter. Hypertension may require withholding therapy or discontinuation.
- Hepatotoxicity: Monitor LFTs before starting lenvatinib. Monitor LFTs every 2 weeks for the first 2 months, then at least monthly thereafter.
- Proteinuria: Monitor for proteinuria before starting lenvatinib and periodically throughout therapy.
- Diarrhea may be severe and recurrent. Promptly initiate standard antidiarrheal therapy if needed. Monitor for dehydration and withhold therapy for grade 3 or 4 diarrhea.
- Reversible posterior leukoencephalopathy syndrome (RPLS) has been reported with lenvatinib.
- Patients who cannot swallow capsules whole may dissolve capsules in 1 tablespoon of water or apple juice.
- Embryo-fetal toxicity: Lenvatinib may cause fetal harm when administered to a pregnant woman.

LETROZOLE (FEMARA)

Mechanism of Action

- Selective, nonsteroidal aromatase inhibitor

FDA-Approved Indications

- Breast cancer
    - For adjuvant treatment of postmenopausal women with hormone receptor-positive early breast cancer

- For the extended adjuvant treatment of early breast cancer in postmenopausal women who have received 5 years of adjuvant tamoxifen therapy
- First-line and second-line treatment of postmenopausal women with hormone receptor-positive or hormone receptor unknown locally advanced or metastatic breast cancer

FDA-Approved Dosage

- 2.5 mg orally daily

Dose Modification Criteria

- Renal (CrCl ≥10 mL per minute): no
- Hepatic (mild-to-moderate impairment): no
- Hepatic (severe impairment): yes

Adverse Reactions

- GI: nausea (minimal), constipation, and diarrhea
- NEURO: headache, dizziness
- OTHER: hot flashes, fatigue, somnolence, musculoskeletal pain, arthralgia, increased sweating, hypercholesterolemia, and peripheral edema

Comments

- Femara may cause a decrease in bone mineral density and an increase in total cholesterol. Consider monitoring for both parameters.

LEUPROLIDE ACETATE (LUPRON, ELIGARD, VIADUR)

Mechanism of Action

- Gonadotropin-releasing hormone (GnRH or LHRH) agonist; chronic administration leads to sustained suppression of pituitary gonadotropins and subsequent suppression of serum testosterone in men and serum estradiol in women.

FDA-Approved Indications

- Palliative treatment of advanced prostate cancer
- Other indications: endometriosis, uterine leiomyomata (fibroids), central precocious puberty

FDA-Approved Dosage

- Prostate cancer: Lupron—1 mg SC daily; Lupron and Eligard depot injections—7.5 mg IM monthly; 22.5 mg IM every 3 months; 30 mg IM every 4 months; 45 mg IM every 6 months; Viadur implant— one implant (contains 72 mg of leuprolide acetate) every 12 months

Adverse Reactions

- CV: transient changes in blood pressure (hypo- or hypertension), QT interval prolongation
- ENDO: hot flashes, gynecomastia, sexual dysfunction, and decreased erections
- GU: erectile dysfunction, lower urinary tract symptoms, and testicular atrophy
- OTHER: tumor flare in the first few weeks of therapy, bone pain, injection site reactions, loss of bone mineral density, osteoporosis, bone fracture, convulsions, and asthenia

Comments

- Use with caution in patients at risk of developing ureteral obstruction or spinal cord compression.
- Hyperglycemia and an increased risk of developing diabetes have been reported in men receiving GnRH analogs such as leuprolide. Monitor blood glucose.

- An increased risk of cardiovascular disease (myocardial infarction, sudden cardiac death, stroke) has been associated in men receiving GnRH analogs such as leuprolide.
- Because of different release characteristics, a fractional dose of the 3-month or 4-month lupron depot formulation is not equivalent to the same dose of the monthly formulation and should not be given.

LOMUSTINE, CCNU (CEENU)

Mechanism of Action

- Alkylating agent

FDA-Approved Indications

- Primary and metastatic brain tumors; Hodgkin disease (second-line therapy in combination with other agents)

FDA-Approved Dosage

- Single-agent therapy: 100 to 130 mg/m² as a single oral dose every 6 weeks

Dose Modification Criteria

- Myelosuppression: yes

Adverse Reactions

- GI: N/V (>60 mg/m²–high, ≤ 60 mg/m²–moderate) and mucositis
- GU: increased BUN and Cr
- HEMAT: severe delayed myelosuppression and cumulative myelosuppression
- HEPAT: increased LFTs
- PULM: pulmonary infiltrates and/or fibrosis (cumulative and usually occurs after 6 months of therapy or a cumulative lifetime dose of 1,100 mg/m², although it has been reported with total lifetime doses as low as 600 mg)
- OTHER: secondary malignancies

Comments

- A single dose is given every 6 weeks.
- Monitor blood counts at least weekly for 6 weeks after a dose.
- Embryo-fetal toxicity: lomustine may cause fetal harm when administered to a pregnant woman.

MECHLORETHAMINE (MUSTARGEN)

Mechanism of Action

- Alkylating agent

FDA-Approved Indications

- Systemic (intravenous) palliative treatment of bronchogenic carcinoma, chronic lymphocytic leukemia (CLL), CML, Hodgkin disease (stages III and IV), lymphosarcoma, malignant effusions, mycosis fungoides, and polycythemia vera
- Palliative treatment of malignant effusions from metastatic carcinoma administered intrapleurally, intraperitoneally, or intrapericardially

FDA-Approved Dosage

■ Intravenous administration: Consult current literature for dose recommendations. A total dose of 0.4 mg/kg IV × one dose per course OR in divided doses of 0.1 to 0.2 mg/kg per day. Dosage should be based on ideal dry body weight.
■ MOPP regimen (Hodgkin disease): Mechlorethamine 6 mg/m² IV × 1 dose administered on days 1 and 8 of a 28-day cycle (combined with vincristine, prednisone, and procarbazine).
■ Intracavitary administration: 0.2 to 0.4 mg/kg for intracavitary injection. Consult current literature for dose and administration technique. The technique and the dose used for the various intracavitary routes (intrapleural, intraperitoneal, and intrapericardial) vary.

Dose Modification Criteria

■ Myelosuppression: yes

Adverse Reactions

■ DERM: alopecia, phlebitis, tissue damage/necrosis with extravasation, and rash
■ GI: N/V (high), metallic taste in mouth, and diarrhea
■ HEMAT: myelosuppression
■ NEURO: vertigo, tinnitus, and diminished hearing
■ OTHER: hyperuricemia, secondary malignancies, infertility, and azospermia

Comments

■ Vesicant
■ Embryo-fetal toxicity: Mechlorethamine may cause fetal harm when administered to a pregnant woman.

MEDROXYPROGESTERONE ACETATE (DEPO-PROVERA)

Mechanism of Action

■ Derivative of progesterone

FDA-Approved Indications

■ Adjunctive therapy and palliative treatment of inoperable, recurrent, and metastatic endometrial or renal cancer.

FDA-Approved Dosage

■ 400 to 1,000 mg intramuscular injection × one dose. Doses may be repeated weekly initially; if improvement is noted, the dose may be reduced to maintenance doses as low as 400 mg IM monthly.

Adverse Reactions

■ CV: edema, weight gain, and thromboembolic events
■ DERM: urticaria, pruritus, rash, acne, alopecia, and hirsutism
■ ENDO: breast tenderness and galactorrhea
■ GI: nausea and cholestatic jaundice
■ GU: breakthrough bleeding, spotting, change in menstrual flow, amenorrhea, changes in cervical erosion, and secretions
■ NEURO: headache, nervousness, dizziness, and depression
■ Ocular: neuro-ocular lesions (retinal thrombosis, optic neuritis)
■ OTHER: hypersensitivity reactions, fever, fatigue, insomnia, somnolence, and injection site reactions

Comments

- The oncology indications only apply to the 400 mg/mL formulation for intramuscular administration.

MEGESTROL (MEGACE AND OTHERS)

Mechanism of Action

- Progestational agent

FDA-Approved Indications

- Palliative therapy of advanced breast cancer and endometrial cancer

FDA-Approved Dosage

- Breast cancer: 40 mg PO QID (four times daily; total daily dose: 160 mg per day)
- Endometrial cancer: 10 mg PO QID to 80 mg PO QID (four times daily; total daily dose: 40 to 320 mg per day)

Adverse Reactions

- CV: deep vein thrombosis
- DERM: alopecia
- ENDO: Cushing-like syndrome, hyperglycemia, glucose intolerance, weight gain, and hot flashes
- GU: vaginal bleeding
- NEURO: mood changes
- OTHER: carpal tunnel syndrome and tumor flare

Comments

- Other indications include cancer and AIDS-related anorexia and cachexia as an appetite stimulant and to promote weight gain. Usual dose range is 160 to 800 mg per day (consult current literature).

MELPHALAN (ALKERAN, EVOMELA)

Mechanism of Action

- Alkylating agent

FDA-Approved Indications

- Multiple myeloma
  - Palliative treatment of multiple myeloma (oral tablets and injection)
  - For use as a high-dose conditioning treatment prior to hematopoietic progenitor (stem) cell transplantation in patients with multiple myeloma.
- Ovarian cancer: palliative treatment of nonresectable epithelial carcinoma of the ovary (oral tablets)

FDA-Approved Dosage

- Multiple myeloma.
  - Oral administration: 6 mg orally daily × 2 to 3 weeks. Wait up to 4 weeks for count recovery, and then a maintenance dose of 2 mg orally daily may be initiated to achieve mild myelosuppression. Refer to package insert and current literature for other dosing regimens.
  - Intravenous administration (if oral therapy not appropriate)—16 mg/m^2 IV over 15 to 20 minutes every 2 weeks × four doses, and then after adequate recovery from toxicity, repeat administration at 4-week intervals. Refer to current literature for other dosing regimens.

- For conditioning treatment, the recommended dose of melphalan is 100 mg/m²/day IV over 30 minutes once daily for 2 consecutive days (Day -3 and -2) prior to autologous stem cell transplantation (ASCT, Day 0).
- Ovarian cancer: 0.2 mg/kg orally daily × 5 days, repeated every 4 to 5 weeks depending on hematologic tolerance. Refer to current literature for other dosing regimens.

Dose Modification Criteria

- Renal: yes
- Myelosuppression: yes

Adverse Reactions

- DERM: vasculitis, alopecia, and skin ulceration/necrosis at injection site (rare)
- HEMAT: myelosuppression and hemolytic anemia
- GI: N/V (oral: minimal; high dose intravenous: moderate); diarrhea, mucositis, and anorexia
- HEPAT: increased LFTs
- PULM: pulmonary toxicity (pulmonary fibrosis and interstitial pneumonitis)
- OTHER: hypersensitivity reactions, secondary malignancies, and infertility

Comments

- Oral absorption is highly variable with considerable patient-to-patient variability in systemic availability. Oral dosages may be adjusted based on the basis of blood counts to achieve some level of myelosuppression to assure that potentially therapeutic levels of the drug have been reached.
- High-dose intravenous regimens of melphalan are utilized in preparative regimens prior to autologous and allogeneic blood and marrow stem cell transplants. Consult current literature for dosing regimens.
- Embryo-fetal toxicity: melphalan may cause fetal harm when administered to a pregnant woman.

MERCAPTOPURINE (PURINETHOL)

Mechanism of Action

- Antimetabolite

FDA-Approved Indications

ALL: indicated in the maintenance therapy of ALL as part of a combination regimen

FDA-Approved Dosage

- ALL maintenance therapy: 1.5 to 2.5 mg/kg orally once daily

Dose Modification Criteria

- Renal: yes (consider dose reduction)
- Hepatic: yes (consider dose reduction)
- Myelosuppression: yes

Adverse Reactions

- DERM: rash, alopecia;
- GI: anorexia, N/V (minimal), mucositis
- HEMAT: myelosuppression

- HEPAT: hepatotoxicity
- OTHER: tumor lysis syndrome

Comments

- Monitor LFTs and bilirubin at weekly intervals initially and then at monthly intervals.
- Usually there is complete cross-resistance with thioguanine.
- Oral mercaptopurine dose should be reduced to 25% to 33% of usual daily dose in patients receiving allopurinol concomitantly.
- Variability in mercaptopurine metabolism may occur in patients due to genetic polymorphisms in the gene for the enzyme thiopurine S-methyltransferase (TMPT). TMPT genotyping or phenotyping can identify patients who are homozygous deficient or who have low or intermediate TMPT activity and who would need dose reduction to avoid mercaptopurine toxicity.
- Embryo-fetal toxicity: mercaptopurine may cause fetal harm when administered to a pregnant woman.

METHOTREXATE

Mechanism of Action

- Antimetabolite

FDA-Approved Indications

- Neoplastic disease indications: gestational tumors (choriocarcinoma, chorioadenoma destruens, hydatidiform mole), (ALL-maintenance therapy in combination with other agents and in the prophylaxis of meningeal leukemia), treatment of meningeal leukemia, breast cancer, epidermoid cancers of the head or neck, advanced mycosis fungoides, lung cancers (particularly squamous cell and small cell types), advanced-stage NHL, and nonmetastatic osteosarcoma (high-dose therapy followed by leucovorin rescue)
- Other indications: psoriasis (severe, recalcitrant, disabling); rheumatoid arthritis (severe)

FDA-Approved Dosage

- Choriocarcinoma and similar trophoblastic diseases: 15 to 30 mg orally or intramuscularly daily × 5 days. Treatment courses are repeated three to five times with rest periods of 1 or more weeks between courses to allow for toxic symptoms to subside. Refer to current literature.
- ALL maintenance therapy (following induction): 15 mg/m² orally or intramuscularly twice weekly (total weekly dose of 30 mg/m²) OR 2.5 mg/kg IV every 14 days (in combination with other agents). Refer to current literature for combination regimens for both induction and maintenance regimens in ALL.
- Meningeal leukemia (intrathecal administration): Younger than 1 year: 6 mg intrathecally; 1 to younger than 2 years: 8 mg intrathecally; 2 to younger than 3 years: 10 mg intrathecally; older than 3 years: 12 mg intrathecally. Refer to current literature.
- Nonmetastatic osteosarcoma: 12 g/m² IV over 4 hours × one dose (with leucovorin rescue, vigorous hydration, and urinary alkalinization) given weekly (weeks 4, 5, 6, 7 after surgery), and then weeks 11, 12, 15, 16, 29, 30, 44, and 45. Leucovorin doses should be adjusted based on methotrexate concentrations. Methotrexate is generally given with other agents. Refer to current literature.
- Other indications: Refer to current literature.

Dose Modification Criteria

- Renal: yes

Adverse Reactions

- DERM: alopecia, rash, urticaria, telangiectasia, acne, photosensitivity, and severe dermatologic reactions
- GI: N/V (≤50 mg/m²: minimal, >50 to <250 mg/m²: low, ≥250 mg/m²: moderate), mucositis/stomatitis, and diarrhea
- GU: renal failure (high-dose therapy) and cystitis

- HEMAT: myelosuppression
- HEPAT: increased LFTs and acute and chronic hepatotoxicity
- NEURO: acute chemical arachnoiditis (intrathecal), subacute myelopathy (intrathecal), chronic leuko-encephalopathy (intrathecal), acute neurotoxicity, or encephalopathy (high-dose intravenous therapy)
- PULM: interstitial pneumonitis
- OTHER: fever, malaise, chills, fatigue, teratogenic, and tumor lysis syndrome

Comments

- Clearance reduced in patients with impaired renal function or third space fluid accumulations (e.g., ascites and pleural effusions). Methotrexate distributes to third space fluid accumulations with subsequent slow and delayed clearance leading to prolonged terminal plasma half-life and toxicity.
- Nonsteroidal anti-inflammatory drugs and acidic drugs inhibit methotrexate clearance. Multiple potential drug interactions; review current literature.
- Use vigorous hydration, urinary alkalinization, and leucovorin rescue with high-dose therapy.
- Use preservative-free product and diluents when administering intrathecally or with high-dose intravenous regimens.
- Embryo-fetal toxicity: methotrexate is teratogenic and may cause fetal harm when administered to a pregnant woman.

MITOMYCIN

Mechanism of Action

- Induces DNA cross-links through alkylation; inhibits DNA and RNA synthesis.

FDA-Approved Indications

- Disseminated gastric cancer or pancreatic cancer (in combination with other agents and as palliative treatment when other modalities have failed)

FDA-Approved Dosage

- Single-agent therapy: 20 mg/m^2 IV × 1 dose repeated every 6 to 8 weeks.
- Refer to current literature for alternative dosing regimens and combination regimens.

Dose Modification Criteria

- Renal: yes
- Myelosuppression: yes

Adverse Reactions

- CV: congestive heart failure (patients with prior doxorubicin exposure)
- DERM: alopecia, pruritus, and tissue damage/necrosis with extravasation
- GI: anorexia, N/V (low), mucositis, and diarrhea
- GU: hemolytic-uremic syndrome and increased Cr
- HEMAT: myelosuppression (may be cumulative)
- PULM: nonproductive cough, dyspnea, and interstitial pneumonia
- OTHER: fever, malaise, and weakness

Comments

- Vesicant
- Alternative routes of administration for mitomycin include intravesical instillation (bladder cancer), intra-cavitary administration for malignant pleural or pericardial administration, and topical application (adjunct for glaucoma filtration surgery). See primary literature for more information.

MITOTANE (LYSODREN)

Mechanism of Action

- Adrenal cytotoxic agent

FDA-Approved Indications

- Inoperable, functional, and nonfunctional adrenal cortical carcinoma

FDA-Approved Dosage

- Initial dose: 2 to 6 g orally per day in three to four divided doses. Increase dose incrementally to achieve a blood concentration of 14 to 20 mg/L, or as tolerated.

Adverse Reactions

- DERM: transient skin rashes
- GI: anorexia, N/V, and diarrhea
- NEURO: vertigo, depression, lethargy, somnolence, and dizziness
- OTHER: adrenal insufficiency

Comments

- Institute adrenal insufficiency precautions. In patients taking mitotane, adrenal crisis occurs in the setting of shock or severe trauma and response to shock is impaired.
- Patients should be counseled regarding the common CNS side effects and ambulatory patients should be cautioned about driving, operating machinery, and other hazardous pursuits requiring mental and physical alertness. Plasma concentrations greater than 20 mg/L (mcg/mL) are associated with a greater incidence of CNS toxicity.
- Mitotane is a strong inducer of cytochrome p450 3A4 (CYP3A4). Screen patients for potential drug interactions with medications that are substrates of CYP3A4.
- Embryo-fetal toxicity: mitotane may cause fetal harm when administered to a pregnant woman.

MITOXANTRONE (NOVANTRONE)

Mechanism of Action

- Interacts with DNA; intercalating agent; topoisomerase II inhibition

FDA-Approved Indications

- Acute nonlymphocytic leukemia (ANLL: myelogenous, promyelocytic, monocytic, erythroid acute leukemia) in adults (initial therapy in combination with other agents)
- Advanced hormone-refractory prostate cancer (in combination with corticosteroids)
- Other indications: multiple sclerosis

FDA-Approved Dosage

- ANLL: induction, 12 mg/m^2 IV daily × 3 days (days 1, 2, and 3) in combination with cytarabine; consolidation, 12 mg/m^2 IV daily × 2 days (days 1 and 2) in combination with cytarabine
- Prostate cancer: 12 to 14 mg/m^2 IV × one dose every 21 days with prednisone or hydrocortisone

Dose Modification Criteria

- Renal: no data, unknown
- Hepatic: yes (use with caution; consider dose adjustment)

Adverse Reactions

- CV: CHF (clinical risk increases after a lifetime cumulative dose of 140 mg/m^2), tachycardia, ECG changes, and chest pain

- DERM: rash, alopecia, urticaria, and nail-bed changes
- GI: N/V (low to moderate), mucositis, constipation, and anorexia
- HEMAT: myelosuppression
- HEPAT: increased LFTs
- PULM: dyspnea
- OTHER: bluish-green urine, sclera may turn bluish, phlebitis (irritant), fatigue, secondary leukemias, and tumor lysis syndrome

Comments

- Consider appropriate prophylaxis for tumor lysis syndrome when treating acute leukemias.
- Mitoxantrone may increase the risk of secondary malignancies such as leukemias.
- Embryo-fetal toxicity: mitoxantrone may cause fetal harm when administered to a pregnant woman.

NECITUMUMAB (PORTRAZZA)

Mechanism of Action

- Recombinant human IgG1 monoclonal antibody that binds to human epidermal growth factor receptor (EGFR) and blocks the binding of EGFR to its ligand.

FDA-Approved Indications

- First-line treatment of metastatic squamous NSCLC in combination with gemcitabine and cisplatin

FDA-Approved Dosage

- 800 mg by IV infusion over 60 minutes on Days 1 and 8 of a 21 day cycle until disease progression or unacceptable toxicity

Dose Modification Criteria

- Renal: no
- Hepatic (mild to moderate): no
- Hepatic (severe): no data available
- Nonhematologic toxicity (dermatologic): yes

Adverse Reactions

- DERM: rash, dermatitis acneiform, acne, dry skin, pruritis
- ELECTRO: hypomagnesemia, hypokalemia, hypocalcemia, hypophosphatemia
- INFUS: infusion-related reactions (usually occurs during first or second infusion)

Comments

- Necitumumab is not indicated for the treatment of nonsquamous NSCLC.
- Infusion-related reactions may require rate reductions or interruptions in infusion. Patients who experience a grade 1 or 2 infusion-related reaction should receive diphenhydramine prior to subsequent infusions. Patients who experience a second infusion reaction should receive diphenhydramine, acetaminophen, and dexamethasone prior to future infusions.
- Cardiopulmonary arrest and/or sudden death has been reported in patients treated with necitumumab in combination with gemcitabine and cisplatin. Closely monitor serum electrolytes including serum magnesium, potassium, and calcium with aggressive replacement when warranted.
- Venous and arterial thromboembolic events may occur while on therapy.
- Embryo-fetal toxicity: Necitumumab may cause fetal harm when administered to a pregnant woman.

NELARABINE (ARRANON)

Mechanism of Action

- Antimetabolite

FDA-Approved Indications

- T-cell ALL and T-cell lymphoblastic lymphoma: in patients whose disease has not responded to or has relapsed following treatment with at least two chemotherapy regimens

FDA-Approved Dosage

- Adult: 1,500 mg/m^2 intravenous infusion over 2 hours on days 1, 3, and 5 repeated every 21 days
- Pediatric: 650 mg/m^2 IV infusion over 1 hour daily for 5 consecutive days repeated every 21 days

Dose Modification Criteria

- Renal: unknown, use with caution in patients with moderate or severe renal impairment
- Hepatic: unknown, use with caution in patients with severe hepatic impairment
- Myelosuppression: no
- Nonhematologic toxicity: yes

Adverse Reactions

- GI: N/V (low), diarrhea, and constipation
- HEMAT: myelosuppression
- HEPAT: increased LFTs
- NEURO: neurotoxicity (see comments), somnolence, dizziness, headache, and peripheral neuropathy
- PULM: cough, dyspnea, and pleural effusion
- OTHER: tumor lysis syndrome, fever, asthenia, fatigue, edema, and myalgia/arthralgia

Comments

- Neurotoxicity is the dose-limiting toxicity of nelarabine. Common signs of nelarabine-induced neurotoxicity include somnolence, confusion, convulsions, ataxia, paresthesias, and hypoesthesia. Severe neurologic toxicity can manifest as coma, status epilepticus, craniospinal demyelination, or ascending neuropathy similar in presentation to Guillain–Barré syndrome. Patients treated previously or concurrently with intrathecal chemotherapy or previously with craniospinal irradiation may be at increased risk for neurologic adverse events.
- Appropriate prevention measures for tumor lysis syndrome (e.g., intravenous hydration, urinary alkalization, and allopurinol) should be initiated prior to nelarabine therapy for patients considered to be at risk.
- Embryo-fetal toxicity: Nelarabine may cause fetal harm when administered to a pregnant woman.

NILOTINIB (TASIGNA)

Mechanism of Action

- Tyrosine kinase inhibitor (Bcr–Abl, PDGFR, and c-KIT)

FDA-Approved Indications

- CML
    - Initial therapy in newly diagnosed adults with Ph+ CML in chronic phase
    - Chronic-phase and accelerated-phase Ph+ CML in adult patients resistant to or intolerant to prior therapy that included imatinib

FDA-Approved Dosage

▪ CML—Newly diagnosed Ph+ CML-chronic phase: 300 mg orally twice daily; resistant or intolerant Ph (+) CML-chronic phase or accelerative phase: 400 mg orally twice daily. Nilotinib should be taken approximately 12 hours apart on an empty stomach (no food 2 hours before and 1 hour after taking dose)

Dose Modification Criteria

▪ Renal: no
▪ Hepatic: yes
▪ Myelosuppression: yes
▪ Nonhematologic toxicity: yes

Adverse Reactions

▪ CV: QT prolongation
▪ DERM: rash, pruritis
▪ ELECTRO: hypophosphatemia, hypokalemia, hyperkalemia, hypocalcemia, and hyponatremia
▪ GI: N/V (minimal), constipation, and diarrhea
▪ HEMAT: myelosuppression
▪ HEPAT: elevated LFTs
▪ NEURO: headache
▪ PULM: cough and dyspnea
▪ OTHER: fatigue, pancreatitis and elevated lipase, fever, asthenia, peripheral edema, fluid retention (e.g. pleural or pericardial effusions), arthralgia/mylagia, nasopharyngitis, pyrexia, night sweats, and tumor lysis syndrome

Comments

▪ Myelosuppression common. Monitor CBC every 2 weeks for the first 2 months of therapy and at least monthly thereafter, or as clinically indicated.
▪ Correct electrolyte abnormalities (e.g., hypokalemia and hypomagnesemia) prior to initiating therapy and monitor periodically during therapy. Obtain an ECG at baseline, 7 days after initiation, and periodically as clinically indicated. Do not use nilotinib concomitantly with other agents that cause QT prolongation. Sudden deaths have been reported on patients treated with nilotinib.
▪ Nilotinib is metabolized through the CYP 3A4 isoenzyme. Screen for potential drug interactions with CYP 3A4 inhibitors or inducers. Dose modification may be necessary if concomitant use with a potent CYP 3A4 inducer or inhibitor cannot be avoided. In addition, nilotinib is a competitive inhibitor and inducer of multiple CYP isoenzymes and P-gp, and subsequently may either increase or decrease concentrations of concomitant medications. Refer to product labeling for additional information.
▪ Embryo-fetal toxicity: Nilotinib may cause fetal harm when administered to a pregnant woman.

NILUTAMIDE (NILANDRON)

Mechanism of Action

▪ Antiandrogen

FDA-Approved Indications

▪ Metastatic prostate cancer (stage D2; in combination therapy with surgical castration). Dosing should begin on same day or day after surgical castration.

FDA-Approved Dosage

- Give 300 mg orally daily × 30 days, and then 150 mg orally daily (with or without food)

Adverse Reactions

- CV: hypertension and angina
- ENDO: hot flashes, impotence, and decreased libido
- GI: nausea, anorexia, and constipation
- HEPAT: increased LFTs (monitor LFTs periodically because of rare associations with cholestatic jaundice, hepatic necrosis, and encephalopathy)
- NEURO: dizziness
- Ocular: visual disturbances and impaired adaptation to dark
- PULM: interstitial pneumonitis and dyspnea

Comments

- Obtain baseline chest x-ray prior to initiating therapy (with consideration of baseline pulmonary function tests). Patients should be instructed to report any new or worsening shortness of breath and if symptoms occur, nilutamide should be immediately discontinued.
- Monitor LFTs at baseline and at regular intervals × 4 months and then periodically thereafter.

NIVOLUMAB (OPDIVO)

Mechanism of Action

- Human monoclonal antibody that binds to programmed death 1 (PD-1) receptors, blocking the binding of PD-1 ligands

FDA-Approved Indications

- Unresectable or metastatic melanoma as a single agent or in combination with ipilimumab
- Metastatic NSCLC with progression on or after platinum-based chemotherapy. Patients with EGFR or ALK genomic tumor aberrations should have progressed FDA-approved therapy for these aberrations
- Advanced RCC patients that have received prior antiangiogenic therapy
- cHL that has relapsed or progressed after autologous hematopoietic stem cell transplantation and post-transplantant brentuximab vedotin
- Recurrent or metastatic squamous cell carcinoma of the head and neck with disease progression on or after a platinum-based therapy
- Locally advanced or metastatic urothelial carcinoma who have disease progression during or following platinum-containing chemotherapy or within 12 months of neoadjuvant or adjuvant treatment with platinum-containing chemotherapy

FDA-Approved Dosage

- Melanoma (single agent), NSCLC, RCC, Urothelial carcinoma: 240 mg IV every 2 weeks
- Melanoma: 1 mg/kg infused over 60 minutes every 3 weeks in combination with ipilimumab for 4 doses, followed by single agent nivolumab 240 mg every 2 weeks
- Hodgkin lymphoma, head and neck squamous cell carcinoma: 3 mg/kg IV every 2 weeks

Dose Modification Criteria

- Renal: no.
- Hepatic (mild): no.
- Hepatic (moderate or severe): has not been studied.
- Doses should be held, not reduced due to toxicities. See package insert for specific recommendations regarding holding doses and starting corticosteroids.

Adverse Reactions

- DERM: rash, pruritus, and immune-mediated dermatologic toxi
- ELECTRO: hyponatremia and hyperkalemia
- ENDO: immune-mediated endocrinopathies (hypophysitis, adrenal insufficiency, hypo/hyperthyroidism, and type I diabetes mellitus)
- GI: immune-mediated colitis, nausea, diarrhea, and constipation
- GU: immune-mediated nephritis and renal dysfunction
- HEPAT: immune-mediated hepatitis, increased LFTs
- INFUS: infusion-related reactions
- NEURO: immune-mediated encephalitis
- PULM: immune-mediated pneumonitis, cough, and dyspnea
- OTHER: arthralgia, musculoskeletal pain, fatigue, asthenia, and pyrexia

Comments

- Severe transplant-related complications, including fatal events, have occurred in patients who have received an allogeneic hematopoietic stem cell transplant after having received nivolumab. Follow patients closely for early evidence of transplant-related complications such as graft-versus-host disease (GVHD), febrile syndromes, hepatic veno-occlusive disease (VOD), and other immune-mediated adverse reactions.
- Embryo-fetal toxicity: Nivolumab may cause fetal harm when administered to a pregnant woman.

OBINUTUZUMAB (GAZYVA)

Mechanism of Action

- Monoclonal antibody that targets the CD20 antigen expressed on the surface of preB- and mature B-lymphocytes

FDA-Approved Indications

- Previously untreated chronic lymphocytic leukemia (CLL) in combination with chlorambucil
- Follicular lymphoma (FL) in combination with bendamustine followed by obinutuzumab monotherapy in patients that have relapsed or are refractory to a rituximab containing regimen

FDA-Approved Dosage

- CLL
  - Cycle 1, day 1: 100 mg infused over 4 hours
  - Cycle 1 day 2: 900 mg initiated at a rate of 50 mg/hr and increased by 50 mg/hr every 30 minutes to a maximum rate of 400 mg/hr
  - Cycle 1 days 8 and 15, and cycles 2 to 6 day 1: 1000 mg initiated at a rate of 100 mg/hr if the previous infusion was well tolerated, and increased by 100 mg/hr every 30 minutes to a maximum rate of 400 mg/hr. Each cycle is 28 days
- FL
  - 1000 mg on cycle 1 days 1, 8, and 15, and cycles 2 to 6 on day 1. Each cycle is 28 days. Initiate the first dose at 50 mg/hr and increase by 50 mg/hr every 30 minutes at maximum of 400 mg/hr. If the previous infusion was well tolerated, subsequent infusions may be initiated at 100 mg/hr and increased by 100 mg/hr every 30 minutes to a maximum of 400 mg/hr.
  - After cycle 6 administer 1000 mg every 2 months for 2 years

Dose Modification Criteria

- Renal (mild to moderate, CrCl > 30 mL/min): no
- Rental (severe, CrCl < 30 ml/min): no data

- Hepatic: no data
- Hematologic and nonhematologic toxicity: Doses should be held, not reduced due to toxicities. See package insert for specific recommendations regarding holding parameters.

Adverse Reactions

- ELECTRO: hypocalcemia, hyponatremia, and tumor lysis syndrome
- GI: N/V (low), diarrhea, and constipation
- HEMAT: neutropenia, thrombocytopenia, lymphopenia, and anemia
- INFUS: hypotension, tachycardia, dyspnea, respiratory symptoms, nausea, fatigue, dizziness, diarrhea, hypertension, flushing, headache, pyrexia and chills. May occur in 38% to 65% of patients during first infusion.
- OTHER: Hepatitis B virus reactivation, fatigue, asthenia, arthralgia, tumor lysis syndrome

Comments

- Assess risk for tumor lysis syndrome prior to initiation of treatment.
- Premedicate with an IV glucocorticoid, acetaminophen and anti-histamine prior to first infusion. Subsequent premedication recommendations are based on the patient's disease state and tolerability of previous infusions.
- Screen all patients for hepatitis B virus (HBV) infection before initiating therapy. For patients who show evidence of HBV infection, consult physicians with expertise in managing HBV regarding monitoring and consideration for HBV antiviral therapy.
- Progressive Multifocal Leukoencephalopathy (PML) has been observed in patients treated with obinutuzumab.
- Immunization with live virus vaccines is not recommended during treatment and until B-cell recovery.

OFATUMUMAB (ARZERRA)

Mechanism of Action

- Cytolytic monoclonal antibody that targets CD20, which is expressed on normal B lymphocytes and on B-cell CLL.

FDA-Approved Indications

- Chronic lymphocytic leukemia (CLL)
  - Treatment of previously untreated patients with CLL in combination with chlorambucil in patients for whom therapy with fludarabine is considered inappropriate.
  - Treatment of patients with relapsed CLL in combination with fludarabine and cyclophosphamide.
  - Extended treatment of patients with recurrent or progressive CLL who are in complete or partial response after at least two lines of therapy.
  - Treatment of CLL patients refractory to fludarabine and alemtuzumab

FDA-Approved Dosage

- Previously untreated CLL in combination with chlorambucil:
  - 300 mg IV infusion on Day 1 followed by 1,000 mg IV infusion on day 8 (Cycle 1) followed by:
  - 1,000 mg IV infusion on Day 1 of 28 day cycles for a minimum of 3 cycles until best response or a maximum of 12 cycles
- Relapsed CLL in combination with fludarabine and cyclophosphamide
  - 300 mg IV infusion on Day1 followed by 1,000 mg IV infusion on day 8 (Cycle 1) followed by:
  - 1,000 mg IV infusion on Day 1 of 28 day cycles for a maximum of 6 cycles
- Extended treatment in CLL
  - 300 mg IV infusion on Day 1 followed by 1,000 mg IV infusion on Day 8 (Cycle 1) followed by:

- 1,000 mg IV infusion 7 weeks later and every 8 weeks thereafter for up to a maximum of 2 years
▪ Refractory CLL
  - 300 mg IV infusion on Day 1 followed 1 week later by
  - 2,000 mg IV infusion weekly x 7 doses, followed 4 weeks later with:
  - 2,000 mg IV infusion every 4 weeks x 4 doses
▪ Do not administer as an intravenous push or bolus.
▪ Premedicate with acetaminophen, antihistamine, and corticosteroid.

Dose Modification Criteria

▪ Infusion reactions: modify rate
▪ Renal (> 30 mL per minute): no
▪ Hepatic: unknown

Adverse Reactions

▪ DERM: rash
▪ GI: diarrhea and nausea (minimal)
▪ HEMAT: anemia, neutropenia and thrombocytopenia
▪ INFUS: abdominal pain, angioedema, back pain, bronchospasm, cardiac ischemia/infarction, dyspnea, laryngeal edema, pulmonary edema, flushing, hypertension, hypotension, pyrexia, rash, syncope, and urticaria
▪ PULM: bronchitis, cough, dyspnea, pneumonia, and upper respiratory tract infections
▪ OTHER: pyrexia, fatigue, and tumor lysis syndrome

Comments

▪ Serious infusion reactions can occur. Premedicate prior to each dose with oral acetaminophen, oral or intravenous antihistamine, and intravenous corticosteroid. Refer to product labeling for recommendations on premedication agents and doses and corticosteroid dose modifications. Infusion reactions occur more frequently with the first two infusions.
▪ Anticipate and provide prophylaxis for tumor lysis syndrome in high-risk patients.
▪ Severe cytopenias may occur. Late onset (>42 days after last treatment) and prolonged neutropenia (not resolved between 24 and 42 days after last treatment) has been reported. Monitor complete blood counts at regular intervals during and after conclusion of therapy.
▪ Progressive multifocal leukoencephalopathy (PML) can occur. Monitor for neurologic signs or symptoms.
▪ Screen patients at high risk of hepatitis B virus (HBV) infection before initiation of ofatumumab. Reactivation of HBV can occur following treatment.
▪ Obstruction of the small intestine can occur.
▪ Do not administer live viral vaccines to patients who have recently received ofatumumab.
▪ Embryo-fetal toxicity: There are no adequate or well-controlled studies of ofatumumab in pregnant women.

OLAPARIB (LYNPARZA)

Mechanism of Action

▪ Inhibitor of poly (ADP-ribose) polymerase (PARP) enzymes, including PARP1, PARP2, and PARP3 which play a role in DNA repair.

FDA-Approved Indications

▪ Ovarian cancer patients with confirmed or suspected BRCA mutation that have received 3 or more prior lines of chemotherapy

FDA-Approved Dosage

- 400 mg orally, twice daily until disease progression or unacceptable toxicity

Dose Modification Criteria

- Renal (mild, CrCl 51 to 80 mL/min): no
- Renal (moderate, CrCl 31 to 50 ml/min): yes
- Renal (severe, CrCl < 30 ml/min): no data
- Hepatic (mild, Child–Pugh A): no
- Hepatic (moderate to severe): no data available
- Myelosuppression: yes
- Nonhematologic toxicity: yes

Adverse Reactions

- DERM: rash and dermatitis
- GI: abdominal pain/discomfort, decreased appetite, N/V (moderate), diarrhea, and dyspepsia
- HEMAT: anemia, neutropenia, thrombocytopenia, and lymphopenia
- NEURO: headache and dysgeusia
- PULM: cough, upper respiratory infection/nasopharyngitis, and pneumonitis
- OTHER: fatigue/asthenia, arthralgia/musculoskeletal pain, and myalgia

Comments

- Myelodysplastic syndrome / acute myeloid leukemia has been reported in patients who have received olaparib. Monitor patients for hematologic toxicity at baseline and monthly thereafter.
- Pneumonitis, including fatal cases, has been reported in patients receiving olaparib. Interrupt therapy and evaluate if patients present with new or worsening pulmonary symptoms.
- Olaparib is a substrate of CYP3A4. Avoid concomitant use of CYP3A inducers and strong or moderate CYP3A4 inhibitors. Dose reduction of olaparib is recommended if a moderate or strong CYP3A4 inhibitor must be used concomitantly.
- Embryo-fetal toxicity: Olaparib may cause fetal harm when administered to a pregnant woman.

OLARATUMAB (LARTRUVO)

Mechanism of Action

- Human IgG1 antibody that binds platelet-derived growth factor receptor alpha (PDGFR-α), which prevents binding of the receptor with PDGF ligands, receptor activation, and downstream PDGF-α pathway signaling.

FDA-Approved Indications

- Soft tissue sarcoma (STS): adults with STS with a histologic subtype for which an anthracycline-containing regimen is appropriate and which is not amenable to curative treatment with radiotherapy or surgery.

FDA-Approved Dosage

- 15 mg/kg IV infusion over 60 minutes on days 1 and 8 of each 21-day cycle until disease progression or unacceptable toxicity. For the first 8 cycles, olaratumab is administered with doxorubicin.
- Premedicate with diphenhydramine and dexamethasone intravenously prior to the first infusion of olaratumab on day 1 of cycle 1.

Dose Modification Criteria

- Renal (mild to moderate, CrCl > 30 ml/min): no
- Renal (severe, CrCl < 30ml/min): no data

■ Hepatic (mild to moderate, total bilirubin < 3 x ULN): no
■ Hepatic (severe): no data
■ Myelosuppression: yes

Adverse Reactions

■ DERM: alopecia
■ ELECTRO: hypokalemia, hypophosphatemia, and hypomagnesemia
■ ENDO: hyperglycemia
■ INFUS: fever, chills, flushing, shortness of breath, and bronchospasm
■ GI: N/V (moderate), mucositis, diarrhea, decreased appetite, and abdominal pain
■ HEMAT: neutropenia, lymphopenia, and thrombocytopenia
■ NEURO: neuropathy and headache
■ OTHER: fatigue, asthenia, and musculoskeletal pain

Comments

■ Infusion-related reactions: Monitor for signs and symptoms during and following infusion. For grade 1 or 2 reactions, interrupt infusion and reduce rate by 50% following resolution of symptoms. Permanently discontinue for grade 3 or 4 infusion-related reactions.
■ Embryo-fetal toxicity: Olaratumab may cause fetal harm when administered to a pregnant woman. Advise females of reproductive potential to use effective contraception during treatment with olaratumab and for 3 months after the last dose.

OMACETAXINE MEPESUCCINATE (SYNRIBO)

Mechanism of Action

■ Inhibits protein synthesis and is independent of direct Bcr–Abl binding.

FDA-Approved Indications

■ Chronic or accelerated-phase CML with resistance and/or intolerance to two or more TKIs.

FDA-Approved Dosage

■ CML induction dose: 1.25 mg/m^2 administered by subcutaneous injection twice daily for 14 consecutive days of a 28-day cycle.
■ CML maintenance dose: 1.25 mg/m^2 administered by subcutaneous injection twice daily for 7 consecutive days of a 28-day cycle.
■ Cycles should be repeated every 28 days until patients achieve a hematologic response. Treatment should continue as long as patients are clinically benefiting from therapy.

Dose Modification Criteria

■ Renal: no data
■ Hepatic: no data
■ Myelosuppression: yes

Adverse Reactions

■ Cr: increased serum creatinine
■ DERM: alopecia and rash
■ ELECTRO: increased uric acid
■ ENDO: hyperglycemia and hypoglycemia
■ GI: abdominal pain, constipation, diarrhea, N/V, and upper abdominal pain
■ HEMAT: anemia, leukocytopenia, neutropenia, and thrombocytopenia

- INFUS: injection site reaction
- PULM: cough
- OTHER: arthralgia, asthenia, edema, epistaxis, fatigue, hemorrhage, infection, pain in extremity, and pyrexia

Comments

- Monitor CBCs weekly during induction and initial maintenance cycles and every 2 weeks during maintenance cycles, as clinically indicated. A high incidence of grade 3/4 thrombocytopenia, neutropenia, and anemia was seen in trials with omacetaxine mepesuccinate.
- Fatalities from cerebral hemorrhage and severe, nonfatal, gastrointestinal hemorrhage occurred in 2% of patients treated with omacetaxine mepesuccinate in the clinical trials that evaluated for safety.
- Monitor blood glucose levels frequently, especially in patients with diabetes or risk factors for diabetes.
- Embryo-fetal toxicity: Omacetaxine mepesuccinate may cause fetal harm when administered to a pregnant woman. Omacetaxine mepesuccinate may impair male fertility.

OSIMERTINIB (TAGRISSO)

Mechanism of Action

- Kinase inhibitor of epidermal growth factor receptor (EGFR) that binds irreversibly to the T790M, L858R, and exon 19 deletion mutant forms of EGFR at 9-fold lower concentrations than wild-type

FDA-Approved Indications

- NSCLC with the EGFR T790M mutation that has progressed on or after EGFR tyrosine kinase inhibitor therapy

FDA-Approved Dosage

- 80 mg orally, once daily

Dose Modification Criteria

- Renal (mild to moderate, CrCl >30 ml/min): no
- Renal (severe, CrCl <30 mL/min): no data
- Hepatic (mild): no
- Hepatic (moderate or severe): no data
- Nonhematologic toxicity: yes

Adverse Reactions

- CV: QTc prolongation and cardiomyopathy
- DERM: rash, dry skin, and nail toxicity
- ELECTRO: hyponatremia and hypermagnesemia
- GI: diarrhea and N/V (low)
- HEMAT: lymphopenia, thrombocytopenia, anemia, and neutropenia
- PULM: pneumonitis

Comments

- Patients who have difficulty swallowing may dissolve the tablet in 4 tablespoons (50 mL) of water
- Cardiomyopathy: Assess LVEF prior to initiation, then every 3 months thereafter.
- Interstitial lung disease/pneumonitis has been reported with osimertinib. Withhold therapy and evaluate for new or worsening pulmonary symptoms.

- Osimertinib is a substrate of CYP3A4. Avoid concomitant use with strong CYP3A4 inducers or consider dose modification if concomitant administration is necessary. Osimertinib is an inhibitor of BCRP and will impact the drug exposure of BCRP substrates. Screen for drug interactions.
- Embyro-fetal toxicity: osimertinib may cause fetal harm when administered to a pregnant woman.

OXALIPLATIN (ELOXATIN)

Mechanism of Action

- Alkylating-like agent producing interstrand DNA cross-links

FDA-Approved Indications

- Colorectal cancer
  - Adjuvant treatment of stage III colon cancer in patients who have undergone complete resection of the primary tumor in combination with infusional fluorouracil and leucovorin.
  - Treatment of advanced colorectal cancer in combination with infusional fluorouracil and leucovorin.

FDA-Approved Dosage

- Combined therapy with infusional fluorouracil and leucovorin (FOLFOX regimen)
- **Day 1**: Oxaliplatin 85 mg/m^2 IV infusion over 120 minutes × 1 dose given concurrently with leucovorin 200 mg/m^2 IV infusion over 120 minutes × 1 dose *followed by* fluorouracil 400 mg/m^2 intravenous bolus over 2 to 4 minutes × 1 dose *followed by* fluorouracil 600 mg/m^2 intravenous continuous infusion over 22 hours.
- **Day 2**: Leucovorin 200 mg/m^2 IV infusion over 120 minutes × 1 dose *followed by* fluorouracil 400 mg/m^2 intravenous bolus over 2 to 4 minutes × 1 dose *followed by* fluorouracil 600 mg/m^2 intravenous continuous infusion over 22 hours.
- Cycles are repeated every 2 weeks. For adjuvant use, treatment is recommended for a total of 6 months (12 cycles). For advanced disease, treatment is recommended until disease progression or unacceptable toxicity.

Dose Modification Criteria

- Renal (mild to moderate, CrCl > 30 ml/min): no
- Renal (severe, CrCl < 30 ml/min): yes
- Myelosuppression: yes
- Nonhematologic toxicity: yes

Adverse Reactions

- CNS: peripheral sensory neuropathies (see comments below) and headache
- CV: edema, thromboembolic events, and QT prolongation
- DERM: injection site reactions
- GI: N/V (moderate), diarrhea, mucositis/stomatitis, abdominal pain, anorexia, and taste perversion
- GU: elevated serum creatinine
- HEMAT: myelosuppression
- HEPAT: elevated LFTs
- PULM: cough, dyspnea, and interstitial lung disease
- OTHER: fatigue, fever, back pain, pain, rhabdomyolysis, and hypersensitivity reaction.

Comments

- Anaphylactic reactions have been reported, and may occur within minutes of oxaliplatin administration. Epinephrine, corticosteroids, and antihistamines have been used to alleviate symptoms of anaphylaxis.
- Embryo-fetal toxicity: oxaliplatin may cause fetal harm when administered to a pregnant woman.
- Oxaliplatin is associated with two types of peripheral neuropathy

1. An acute, reversible, primarily peripheral, and sensory neuropathy that is of early onset (within hours to 1 to 2 days of dosing), that resolves within 14 days, and that frequently recurs with further dosing. The symptoms include transient paresthesia, dysesthesia, and hypoesthesia in the hands, feet, perioral area, or throat. Symptoms may be precipitated or exacerbated by exposure to cold temperature or cold objects. Patients should be instructed to avoid cold drinks, use of ice, and should cover exposed skin prior to exposure to cold temperature or cold objects.
2. A persistent (>14 days), primarily peripheral, sensory neuropathy usually characterized by paresthesias, dysesthesias, hypoesthesias, but may also include deficits in proprioception that can interfere with daily activities. Dose modifications are recommended for persistent grade 2 neurotoxicity and discontinuation of therapy is recommended for persistent grade 3 neurotoxicity.

PACLITAXEL (TAXOL)

Mechanism of Action

- Microtubule assembly stabilization.

FDA-Approved Indications

- Advanced ovarian cancer (first-line and subsequent therapy). As first-line therapy, paclitaxel is indicated in combination with cisplatin.
- Breast cancer.
- Adjuvant treatment of node-positive breast cancer (administered sequentially to standard doxorubicin-containing combination chemotherapy).
- Second-line therapy for breast cancer (after failure of combination chemotherapy for metastatic disease or relapse within 6 months of adjuvant therapy).
- NSCLC: First-line therapy in combination with cisplatin in patients who are not candidates for potentially curative surgery and/or radiation therapy.
- AIDS-related Kaposi sarcoma (second-line treatment).

FDA-Approved Dosage

- Premedicate patients with dexamethasone, diphenhydramine (or its equivalent), and H_2 antagonists (e.g., cimetidine or ranitidine) to prevent severe hypersensitivity reactions. Suggested package literature premedication regimen: dexamethasone 20 mg orally × two doses administered approximately 12 and 6 hours before paclitaxel; diphenhydramine 50 mg IV 30 to 60 minutes before paclitaxel; and cimetidine 300 mg IV OR ranitidine 50 mg IV 30 to 60 minutes before paclitaxel. Consult current literature for alternative premedication regimens.
- First-line ovarian cancer: 135 mg/m^2 IV continuous infusion over 24 hours OR 175 mg/m^2 IV infusion over 3 hours (followed by cisplatin 75 mg/m^2 IV) every 3 weeks.
- Second-line ovarian cancer: 135 mg/m^2 OR 175 mg/m^2 IV infusion over 3 hours every 3 weeks. Consult current literature for alternative regimens.
- Adjuvant therapy of node-positive breast cancer: 175 mg/m^2 IV infusion over 3 hours every 3 weeks × four cycles (administered sequentially with doxorubicin-containing chemotherapy).
- Second-line breast cancer: 175 mg/m^2 IV over 3 hours every 3 weeks.
- NSCLC: 135 mg/m^2 IV continuous infusion over 24 hours (followed by cisplatin 75 mg/m^2 IV) every 3 weeks.
- AIDS-related Kaposi sarcoma: 135 mg/m^2 IV infusion over 3 hours every 3 weeks or 100 mg/m^2 IV infusion over 3 hours every 2 weeks (note: reduce the dose of dexamethasone premedication dose to 10 mg orally) per dose (instead of the suggested 20 mg oral dose).

Dose Modification Criteria

- Hepatic: yes
- Myelosuppression: yes
- Nonhematologic toxicity (neuropathy): yes

Adverse Reactions

- CV: hypotension, bradycardia, and ECG changes
- DERM: alopecia, onycholysis (more common with weekly dosing), and injection site reactions
- GI: N/V (low), diarrhea, and mucositis
- HEMAT: myelosuppression
- INFUS: acute hypersensitivity-type reactions
- NEURO: peripheral neurosensory toxicity (paresthesia, dysesthesia, and pain)
- OTHER: arthralgia and myalgia.

Comments

- Use non-DEHP plasticized solution containers and administration sets.
- In-line filtration (0.22 μm filter) required during administration.
- Lower dose, weekly dosage regimens are commonly utilized. Consult current literature for dose guidelines.
- Embryo-fetal toxicity: paclitaxel may cause fetal harm when administered to a pregnant woman.

PACLITAXEL PROTEIN-BOUND (ABRAXANE)

Mechanism of Action

- Microtubule inhibitor that promotes the assembly of microtubules from tubulin dimers and stabilizes microtubules by preventing depolymerization.

FDA-Approved Indications

- Breast cancer: after failure of combination chemotherapy for metastatic disease or relapse within 6 months of adjuvant chemotherapy. Prior therapy should have included an anthracycline unless clinically contraindicated.
- NSCLC: locally advanced or metastatic disease as first-line treatment in combination with carboplatin, in patients who are not candidates for curative surgery or radiation therapy.
- Pancreatic cancer: metastatic adenocarcinoma of the pancreas as first-line treatment in combination with gemcitabine.

FDA-Approved Dosage

- Metastatic breast cancer: 260 mg/m^2 IV infusion over 30 minutes every 3 weeks.
- NSCLC: 100 mg/m^2 IV over 30 minutes on days 1, 8, and 15 of each 21-day cycle; carboplatin AUC 6 mg·min/mL is given intravenously on day 1 of each 21-day cycle immediately after protein-bound paclitaxel administration.
- Pancreatic cancer: 125 mg/m^2 IV infusion over 30 to 40 minutes on days 1, 8, and 15 of each 28 day cycle; administer gemcitabine immediately after protein-bound paclitaxel on days 1, 8, and 15 of each 28 day cycle.

Dose Modification Criteria

- Renal (mild to moderate): no
- Renal (severe): no data
- Hepatic (mild): no
- Hepatic (moderate, severe): yes
- Myelosuppression: yes
- Nonhematologic toxicity: yes

Adverse Effects

- Cr: increased serum creatinine
- CV: abnormal ECG

- DERM: alopecia and rash
- GI: diarrhea, nausea/vomiting (low), and decreased appetite
- HEMAT: anemia, neutropenia, and thrombocytopenia
- HEPAT: alkaline phosphatase elevation and increased LFTs
- INFECT: infections
- INFUS: anaphylaxis, arrhythmia, chest pain, dyspnea, flushing, and hypotension
- NEURO: sensory neuropathy
- Ocular: blurred vision, keratitis, and ocular/visual disturbances
- PULM: pneumonitis
- OTHER: arthralgia, asthenia, edema, fatigue, pyrexia, myalgia, and nail changes

Comments

- Contraindicated if neutrophil count is <1,500 cells/mm^3.
- Do not substitute for or with other paclitaxel formulations.
- Protein-bound paclitaxel contains albumin (human). Based on effective donor screening and product manufacturing processes, it carries a remote risk for transmission of viral diseases.
- No premedication is required prior to administration, but premedication may be needed in patients who have had prior hypersensitivity reactions.
- Severe hypersensitivity reactions with fatal outcome have been reported. Do not rechallenge.
- The use of an in-line filter is not recommended.
- Embryo-fetal toxicity: Protein-bound paclitaxel may cause fetal harm when administered to a pregnant woman. Men should be advised not to father a child while receiving protein-bound paclitaxel.

PALBOCICLIB (IBRANCE)

Mechanism of Action

- Inhibitor of cyclin-dependent kinase (CDK) 4 and 6, which is downstream of signaling pathways that lead to cellular proliferation.

FDA-Approved Indications

- Breast Cancer: Hormone receptor (HR)-positive, HER2-negative advanced or metastatic breast cancer in combination with letrozole as initial endocrine-based therapy in postmenopausal women, or with fulvestrant in women with disease progression following endocrine therapy

FDA-Approved Dosage

- 125 mg once daily with food on days 1 to 21 of a 28 day cycle in combination with letrozole or fulvestrant.

Dose Modification Criteria

- Renal (mild to moderate, CrCl > 30 ml/min): no
- Renal (severe, CrCl < 30 ml/min): no data
- Hepatic (mild): no
- Hepatic (moderate to severe, total bilirubin >1.5 X ULN): no data
- Myelosuppression: yes
- Nonhematologic toxicity: yes

Adverse Reactions

- DERM: alopecia and rash
- GI: decreased appetite, stomatitis, N/V (low), diarrhea, and constipation
- HEMAT: neutropenia, leukopenia, anemia, and thrombocytopenia

- NEURO: headache
- PULM: upper respiratory tract infection, and pulmonary embolism
- OTHER: fatigue

Comments

- Pulmonary embolism has been reported at a higher rate in patients treated with palbociclib. Monitor for signs and symptoms of pulmonary embolism and treat as medically appropriate.
- Embryo-fetal toxicity: Palbociclib may cause fetal harm when administered to a pregnant woman.

PANITUMUMAB (VECTIBIX)

Mechanism of Action

- Monoclonal antibody to the human EGFR.

FDA-Approved Indications

- Colorectal cancer: wild-type*KRAS* (exon 2) metastatic disease determined by an FDA-approved test as follows:
  - First-line treatment in combination with FOLFOX combination chemotherapy
  - Monotherapy for the treatment metastatic colorectal carcinoma with disease progression on or following fluoropyrimidine-, oxaliplatin-, and irinotecan-containing chemotherapy regimens.

FDA-Approved Dosage

- 6 mg/kg intravenous infusion over 60 minutes every 14 days. Doses higher than 1,000 mg should be administered over 90 minutes.

Dose Modification Criteria

- Renal (mild to moderate): no
- Renal (severe): no data
- Hepatic (mild to moderate): no
- Hepatic (severe): no data
- Myelosuppression: no
- Nonhematologic toxicity: yes

Adverse Reactions

- DERM: dermatitis acneiform, pruritis, erythema, rash, skin exfoliation, paronychia, dry skin, skin fissures, and photosensitivity
- ELECTRO: hypomagnesemia and hypocalcemia
- GI: N/V (low), abdominal pain, diarrhea, and stomatitis/mucositis
- INFUS: infusion reactions may include fever, chills, dyspnea, bronchospasm, and hypotension
- Ocular: conjunctivitis, ocular hyperemia, and increased lacrimation
- PULM: interstitial lung disease and pulmonary fibrosis (rare)
- OTHER: fatigue

Comments

- KRAS mutation predicts for a lack of response to anti-EGFR agents like panitumumab. Panitumumab is not indicated for the treatment of patients with KRAS mutation-positive metastatic colorectal cancer or for whom KRAS status is unknown.
- Patients enrolled in the colorectal cancer clinical studies were required to have immunohistochemical evidence of EGFR expression; these are the only patients studied and for whom benefit has been shown.

- Reduce infusion rate by 50% in patients experiencing a mild or moderate (grade 1 or 2) infusion reaction for the duration of that infusion. Immediately and permanently discontinue panitumumab in patients experiencing a severe (grade 3 or 4) infusion reaction. The use of premedication was not standardized in the clinical trials and thus the utility of premedication is not known.
- Withhold panitumumab for dermatologic toxicities that are grade 3 or higher or considered intolerable. If toxicity does not improve to ≤grade 2 within 1 month, permanently discontinue panitumumab. If dermatologic toxicity does improve to ≤grade 2 after withholding no more than two doses, treatment may be resumed at 50% of the original dose. See product labeling for further information on dose adjustments.

PANOBINOSTAT (FARYDAK)

Mechanism of Action

- Histone deacetylase (HDAC) inhibitor

FDA-Approved Indications

- Multiple myeloma in combination with bortezomib and dexamethasone after receiving at least 2 prior regimens, including bortezomib and an immunomodulatory agent

FDA-Approved Dosage

- 20 mg orally once every other day for 3 doses per week (on days 1, 3, 5, 8, 10, and 12) during weeks 1 and 2 of a 3 week cycle for 8 cycles. Extended therapy may be considered for another 8 cycles if there is clinical benefit.

Dose Modification Criteria

- Renal (mild to severe): no (not studied in end stage renal disease)
- Hepatic (mild to moderate): yes
- Hepatic (severe impairment): avoid use
- Myelosuppression: yes
- Nonhematologic toxicity: yes

Adverse Reactions

- CV: cardiac ischemic events, severe arrhythmias, and electrocardiogram changes
- ELECTRO: hypokalemia, hypophosphatemia, and hyponatremia
- GI: diarrhea, N/V (low), and decreased appetite
- HEMAT: thrombocytopenia, neutropenia, anemia, and hemorrhage
- HEPAT: elevated ALT/AST and elevated total bilirubin
- OTHER: fatigue, peripheral edema, and pyrexia

Comments

- Panobinostat is a substrate of CYP3A4 and P-glycoprotein. Avoid strong inhibitors or inducers of CYP3A4. Dose reductions of panobinostat may be considered if strong CYP3A4 inhibitors must be used concomitantly. Panobinostat is an inhibitor of CYP2D6. Screen for drug interactions.
- Diarrhea may be severe. Promptly initiate antidiarrheal medication at the onset of diarrhea. Monitor hydration status and electrolytes. Interrupt panobinostat for moderate diarrhea (4 to 6 stools per day) and evaluate for consideration of dose reduction or discontinuation.
- Severe and fatal ischemic events, severe arrhythmias, and ECG changes have occurred in patients treated with panobinostat. Obtain ECG and electrolytes at baseline and periodically during treatment as clinically indicated. Concomitant use with anti-arrhythmics and medications that prolong the QT interval is not recommended.
- Embryo-fetal toxicity: Panobinostat may cause fetal harm when administered to a pregnant woman.

PAZOPANIB (VOTRIENT)

Mechanism of Action

- Multityrosine kinase inhibitor of VEGF receptor (VEGFR)-1, VEGFR-2, and VEGFR-3, PDGFR-α and -β, fibroblast growth factor receptor (FGFR)-1 and -3, cytokine receptor (Kit), IL-2 receptor inducible T-cell kinase (Itk), leukocyte-specific protein tyrosine kinase (Lck), and transmembrane glycoprotein receptor tyrosine kinase (c-Fms).

FDA-Approved Indications

- Advanced RCC.
- Advanced soft tissue sarcoma (STS) who have received prior chemotherapy.
- Limitations of use: the efficacy of pazopanib for adipocytic STS or GISTs has not been demonstrated.

FDA-Approved Dosage

- 800 mg orally once daily without food, at least 1 hour before or 2 hours after a meal

Dose Modification Criteria

- Renal (mild to severe): no (not studied in end stage renal disease)
- Hepatic (mild): no
- Hepatic (moderate): yes
- Hepatic (severe): not recommended

Adverse Effects

- CV: cardiac dysfunction, hypertension, and QT prolongation
- DERM: hair color changes, skin hypopigmentation, and wound healing complications
- ELECTRO: hypomagnesemia, hyponatremia, and hypophosphatemia
- ENDO: hyperglycemia and hypothyroidism
- GI: diarrhea, N/V (minimal to low)
- GU: proteinuria
- HEMAT: leucopenia, lymphocytopenia, neutropenia, and thrombocytopenia
- HEPAT: increased bilirubin and increased LFTs
- NEURO: headache and dysgeusia
- PULM: dyspnea and interstitial lung disease
- OTHER: fatigue, decreased appetite, decreased weight, hemorrhage, infection, musculoskeletal pain, thrombosis, tumor pain, and increased lipase

Comments

- Severe and fetal hepatotoxicity has occurred. Measure liver chemistries before the initiation of treatment and regularly during treatment.
- Pazopanib is not indicated for use in combination with other cancer therapy.
- CYP3A4 inhibitors: Avoid use of strong inhibitors. If concomitant administration is necessary, reduce the dose of pazopanib. Avoid grapefruit and grapefruit juice.
- CYP3A4 inducers: Consider an alternate concomitant medication with no or minimal enzyme induction potential, or avoid pazopanib.
- CYP Substrates: Concomitant use of pazopanib with agents with narrow therapeutic windows that are metabolized by CYP3A4, CYP2D6, or CYP2C8 is not recommended.
- Concomitant use of pazopanib and simvastatin increases the risk of ALT elevations and should be undertaken with caution and close monitoring.
- Use with caution in patients at higher risk of developing QT interval prolongation. Monitoring electrocardiograms and electrolytes should be considered.
- CHF and decreased LVEF have occurred. Monitor blood pressure and manage hypertension promptly. Baseline and period evaluation of LVEF is recommended in patients at risk of cardiac dysfunction.

- Pazopanib has not been studied in patients who have a history of hemoptysis, cerebral, or clinically significant gastrointestinal hemorrhage in the past 6 months and should not be used in those patients.
- Use with caution in patients who are at an increased risk for arterial and venous thrombotic events. Monitor for signs and symptoms of venous thromboembolism (VTE) and pulmonary embolism (PE).
- Use with caution in patients at risk for gastrointestinal perforation or fistula.
- Permanently discontinue pazopanib if signs or symptoms of RPLS occur.
- Blood pressure should be well controlled prior to initiating pazopanib. Monitor blood pressure within 1 week after starting pazopanib and frequently thereafter.
- Interruption of therapy with pazopanib is recommended in patients undergoing surgical procedures. Pazopanib should be stopped at least 7 days prior to scheduled surgery.
- Interrupt pazopanib for 24-hour urine protein ≥3 g and discontinue for repeat episodes despite dose reductions.
- Serious infections (with or without neutropenia), some with fatal outcome, have been reported. Monitor for signs and symptoms and treat active infection promptly.
- Embryo-fetal toxicity: Pazopanib may cause fetal harm when administered to a pregnant woman.

PEMBROLIZUMAB (KEYTRUDA)

Mechanism of Action

- Humanized monoclonal antibody that blocks the interaction between programmed death 1 (PD-1) and its ligands, programmed death-ligand 1 (PD-L1) and PD-L2

FDA-Approved Indications

- Unresectable or metastatic melanoma
- Metastatic NSCLC that expresses PD-L1 as determined by an FDA-approved test, and
  - No EGFR or ALK mutations and no prior systemic chemotherapy OR
  - Disease progression on or after platinum-containing chemotherapy. Patients with EGFR or ALK genomic tumor aberrations should have disease progression on FDA-approved therapy for these mutations prior to receiving pembrolizumab.
  - Recurrent or metastatic head and neck squamous cell carcinoma (HNSCC) with disease progression on or after platinum-containing chemotherapy.

FDA-Approved Dosage

- Melanoma: 2 mg/kg IV infusion over 30 minutes every 3 weeks until disease progression or unacceptable toxicity.
- NSCLC and HNSCC: 200 mg IV infusion over 30 minutes every 3 weeks until disease progression, unacceptable toxicity, or up to 24 months in patients without disease progression.

Dose Modification Criteria

- Renal: no (initial dosing).
- Hepatic: (mild): no (initial dosing).
- Hepatic (moderate to severe): no data.
- Doses should be held, not reduced due to toxicities. See package insert for specific recommendations regarding holding doses and starting corticosteroids.

Adverse Reactions

- DERM: rash, pruritus
- ELECTRO: hyponatremia
- ENDO: immune-mediated endocrinopathies (hypophysitis, hypo/hyperthyroidism, type 1 diabetes mellitus)
- GI: immune-mediated colitis, nausea, diarrhea, constipation, decreased appetite

- GU: immune-mediated nephritis and renal dysfunction
- HEMAT: anemia and lymphopenia
- HEPAT: immune-mediated hepatitis
- INFUS: infusion-related reactions
- PULM: immune-mediated pneumonitis and, dyspnea
- OTHER: fatigue and arthralgia

Comments

- Embryo-fetal toxicity: Pembrolizumab may cause fetal harm when administered to a pregnant woman.

PEGASPARGASE (ONCASPAR)

Mechanism of Action

- A modified (pegylated) version of the enzyme L-asparaginase. L-Asparaginase depletes asparagine, an amino acid required by some leukemic cells.

FDA-Approved Indications

- ALL
  - First-line therapy as a component of a multiagent chemotherapeutic regimen.
  - ALL and hypersensitivity to native forms of L-asparaginase.

FDA-Approved Dosage

- ALL: 2,500 international units/m² IM or IV infusion over 1 to 2 hours × one dose every 14 days.

Adverse Reactions

- CV: chest pain, hypertension, and hypotension
- DERM: alopecia, itching, and injection site reactions
- ENDO: hyperglycemia
- GI: anorexia; N/V (minimal), and pancreatitis
- GU: increased BUN and Cr
- HEMAT: hypofibrinogenemia and coagulopathy (thrombosis or hemorrhage)
- HEPAT: hepatotoxicity and increased LFTs
- NEURO: malaise, confusion, lethargy, and depression
- PULM: respiratory distress, cough, and epistaxis
- OTHER: hypersensitivity reaction, fever, arthralgia, musculoskeletal pain, and tumor lysis syndrome.

Comments

- Contraindications: history of pancreatitis with prior L-asparaginase therapy, history of serious hemorrhagic event or thrombosis with prior L-asparaginase therapy, and history of serious allergic reactions to pegasparagase

PEGINTERFERON A-2B (SYLATRON)

Mechanism of Action

- Pleiotropic cytokine; the mechanism by which it exerts its effects in patients with melanoma is unknown.

FDA-Approved Indications

- Adjuvant treatment of melanoma with microscopic or gross nodal involvement within 84 days of definitive surgical resection including complete lymphadenectomy

FDA-Approved Dosage

- 6 mcg/kg SC weekly for eight doses followed by,
- 3 mcg/kg SC weekly for up to 5 years.

Dose Modification Criteria

- Renal (moderate to severe): yes
- Hepatic: not studied (contraindicated in moderate to severe impairment for viral hepatitis)
- Hematologic toxicity: yes
- Nonhematologic toxicity: yes
- Performance status, tolerability: yes

Adverse Effects

- CV: angina pectoris, arrhythmias, cardiomyopathy, hypotension, and tachycardia
- DERM: alopecia, injection site reactions, and rash
- ENDO: diabetes mellitus, hyperthyroidism, and hypothyroidism
- GI: anorexia, diarrhea, and N/V (minimal)
- HEPAT: hyperbilirubinemia, increased alkaline phosphatase, and increased LFTs
- NEURO: dysgeusia, aggressive behavior, bipolar disorders, depression, encephalopathy, hallucinations, headache, increased risk of relapse in recovering drug addicts, mania, psychoses, and suicidal and homicidal ideation
- Ocular: retinopathy
- OTHER: chills, decreased weight, dizziness, fatigue, myalgia, olfactory nerve disorder, and pyrexia

Comments

- Peginterferon α-2b is contraindicated if the patient has a known hypersensitivity reaction to interferon α-2b or peginterferon α-2b, autoimmune hepatitis, or hepatic decompensation (Child–Pugh classes B and C).
- Premedicate with acetaminophen 500 to 1,000 mg PO 30 minutes prior to the first dose of peginterferon α-2b and as needed for subsequent doses.
- Use caution with concomitant medications that are metabolized by CYP2C9 or CYP2D6.
- Advise patients and their caregivers to immediately report any symptoms of depression or suicidal ideation to their healthcare provider. Monitor patients frequently during treatment and for at least 6 months after the last dose.
- Hepatic function should be monitored at 2 and 8 weeks, and 2 and 3 months following initiation of peginterferon α-2b, then every 6 months while receiving peginterferon α-2b.
- TSH levels should be obtained within 4 weeks prior to initiation of peginterferon α-2b, and at 3 and 6 months following initiation, then every 6 months thereafter while receiving peginterferon α-2b.
- Embryo-fetal toxicity: Use peginterferon α-2b only if the potential benefit justifies the potential risk to the fetus.

PEMETREXED (ALIMTA)

Mechanism of Action

- Antimetabolite. An antifolate that disrupts folate-dependent metabolic process essential for cell replication.

FDA-Approved Indications

- Malignant pleural mesothelioma: in combination with cisplatin in patients whose disease is unresectable or who are otherwise not candidates for curative surgery
- Nonsquamous NSCLC

- First-line therapy in patients with locally advanced or metastatic nonsquamous NSCLC in combination with cisplatin
- Maintenance therapy in patients with locally advanced or metastatic nonsquamous NSCLC whose disease has not progressed after four cycles of platinum-based first-line chemotherapy
- Second-line therapy as a single agent in patients with locally advanced or metastatic nonsquamous NSCLC after prior chemotherapy

FDA-Approved Dosage

- Malignant pleural mesothelioma: 500 mg/m^2 IV infusion over 10 minutes on day 1 of each 21-day cycle.
- NSCLC: 500 mg/m^2 IV infusion over 10 minutes on day 1 of each 21-day cycle.
- When pemetrexed is combined with cisplatin for malignant pleural mesothelioma or in first-line therapy for NSCLC, the recommended dose of cisplatin (in combination with pemetrexed) is 75 mg/m^2 IV over 2 hours beginning approximately 30 minutes after the end of pemetrexed.
- See comments below regarding premedication regimen for pemetrexed.

Dose Modification Criteria

- Renal (CrCl >45 mL per minute): no
- Renal (CrCl <45 mL per minute): yes—administration is not recommended
- Hepatic: no data
- Myelosuppression: yes
- Nonhematologic toxicity: yes

Adverse Reactions

- DERM: rash and desquamation
- GI: N/V (low), mucositis, pharyngitis, diarrhea, and anorexia
- HEMAT: neutropenia, thrombocytopenia, and anemia
- HEPAT: increased LFTs
- OTHER: fatigue and fever

Comments

- Vitamin supplementation: Patients treated with pemetrexed must be instructed to take folic acid and vitamin B$_{12}$ as a prophylactic measure to reduce treatment-related hematologic and GI toxicity. Patients should receive at least five daily doses of folic acid (most common daily dose: 400 μg) during the 7-day period prior to the first dose of pemetrexed and dosing should continue during the full course of therapy and for 21 days after the last dose. Patients must also receive one intramuscular dose of vitamin B$_{12}$ (1,000 μg) during the week prior to the first dose of pemetrexed and every three cycles (9 weeks) thereafter.
- Corticosteroid premedication: Pretreatment with dexamethasone (or equivalent) reduces the incidence and severity of cutaneous reactions. Recommended regimen (product labeling): dexamethasone 4 mg orally twice daily × 3 days (six doses) beginning the day prior to each dose of pemetrexed (the day before, the day of, and the day after pemetrexed).
- Embryo-fetal toxicity: pemetrexed may cause fetal harm when administered to a pregnant woman. Pemetrexed is fetotoxic and teratogenic in mice; there are no studies of pemetrexed in pregnant women.

PENTOSTATIN (NIPENT)

Mechanism of Action

- Antimetabolite (adenosine deaminase inhibitor).

FDA-Approved Indications

- Hairy cell leukemia (first-line and in α-interferon-refractory disease).

FDA-Approved Dosage

- 4 mg/m^2 IV every other week. Pentostatin may be given as a bolus injection or diluted in a larger volume and infused over 20 to 30 minutes. The optimal treatment duration has not been determined. The package insert suggests continued treatment until a complete response has been achieved followed by two additional doses.

Dose Modification Criteria

- Renal: yes
- Myelosuppression: yes

Adverse Reactions

- DERM: rash;
- GI: N/V (moderate)
- GU: elevated serum creatinine (generally mild and reversible but mild-to-moderate renal toxicity may occur)
- HEMAT: leukopenia, anemia, and thrombocytopenia
- HEPAT: elevated LFTs
- OTHER: fever, infection, and fatigue

Comments

- A high incidence of fatal pulmonary toxicity was seen in a trial investigating the combination of fludarabine with pentostatin. The combined use of fludarabine and pentostatin is not recommended.
- Patients should receive intravenous hydration (500 to 1,000 mL) before and after each pentostatin dose to reduce the risk of nephrotoxicity.
- Embryo-fetal toxicity: pentostatin may cause fetal harm when administered to a pregnant woman.

PERTUZUMAB (PERJETA)

Mechanism of Action

- Recombinant humanized monoclonal antibody that targets the extracellular dimerization domain (subdomain II) of the human epidermal growth factor receptor 2 protein (HER2) and, thereby, blocks ligand-dependent heterodimerization of HER2 with other HER family members, including EGFR, HER3, and HER4.

FDA-Approved Indications

- Breast cancer
  - HER2-positive metastatic breast cancer in combination with trastuzumab and docetaxel in patients who have not received prior anti-HER2 therapy or chemotherapy for metastatic disease.
  - Neoadjuvant treatment in combination with trastuzumab and docetaxel for patients with HER-2-positive, locally advanced, inflammatory, or early-stage breast cancer (either greater than 2 cm in diameter or node positive) as part of a complete treatment regimen for early breast cancer.

FDA-Approved Dosage

- Initial dose is 840 mg administered as a 60-minute intravenous infusion.
- Followed every 3 weeks thereafter by 420 mg administered as a 30 to 60 minute intravenous infusion.

Dose Modification Criteria

- Renal (mild to moderate): no
- Renal (severe <30 mL per minute): unknown

■ Hepatic: no data
■ Nonhematologic toxicity: yes

Adverse Reactions

■ CV: Left ventricular dysfunction
■ DERM: alopecia, mucosal inflammation, paronychia, and rash
■ GI: diarrhea and nausea (mild)
■ HEMAT: anemia, leucopenia, and neutropenia
■ INFUS: chills, dysgeusia, fatigue, headache, hypersensitivity, myalgia, pyrexia, and vomiting
■ NEURO: headache and peripheral neuropathy
■ PULM: upper respiratory tract infection
■ OTHER: asthenia and fatigue

Comments

■ Detection of HER2 protein overexpression is necessary for appropriate patient selection.
■ If a significant infusion reaction occurs, slow or interrupt the infusion.
■ For delayed or missed doses, if the time between two sequential infusions is less than 6 weeks, administer 420 mg IV. If the time between two sequential infusions is 6 weeks or more, the initial dose of 840 mg should be re-administered as a 60-minute infusion followed by the normal dosing schedule.
■ When administered with pertuzumab, the recommended initial dose of docetaxel is 75 mg/m^2, which can be escalated to 100 mg/m^2 every 3 weeks if the initial dose is well tolerated.
■ Left ventricular dysfunction, which includes symptomatic left ventricular systolic dysfunction and decreases in LVEF, may occur. Assess LVEF prior to initiation and at regular intervals during treatment. Withhold pertuzumab and trastuzumab and repeat LVEF assessment within 3 weeks in patients with significant decrease in LVEF (i.e., a drop in LVEF to <45% or LVEF of 45% to 49% with a 10% or greater absolute decrease below pretreatment values); discontinue if the LVEF has not improved or has declined further after 3 week unless the benefits for the patient outweigh the risks.
■ Pertuzumab should be withheld or discontinued if trastuzumab is withheld or discontinued. If docetaxel is discontinued, treatment with pertuzumab and trastuzumab may continue.
■ Dose reductions are not recommended for pertuzumab.
■ Embryo-fetal toxicity: pertuzumab may cause fetal harm when administered to a pregnant woman. Studies in animals have resulted in oligohydramnios, delayed renal development, and death.

POLIFEPROSAN 20 WITH CARMUSTINE IMPLANT (GLIADEL WAFER)

Mechanism of Action

■ The polifeprosan 20 with carmustine implant is designed to deliver carmustine directly into the surgical cavity created when a brain tumor is resected. On exposure to the aqueous environment of the resection cavity, carmustine is released from the copolymer and diffuses into the surrounding brain tissue. Carmustine is an alkylating agent.

FDA-Approved Indications

■ High-grade malignant glioma (first-line treatment in newly diagnosed patients as an adjunct to surgery and radiation.
■ Recurrent glioblastoma multiforme (GBM) as an adjunct to surgery.

FDA-Approved Dosage

■ Each wafer contains 7.7 mg of carmustine. Up to eight wafers should be implanted at time of surgery (eight wafers results in a dose of 61.6 mg).

Adverse Reactions

- GI: N/V (low)
- NEURO: meningitis, abscess, and brain edema
- OTHER: abnormal wound healing, pain, asthenia and fever

Comments

- Wafers can be broken in half. Proper handling and disposal precautions should be observed.

POMALIDOMIDE (POMALYST)

Mechanism of Action

- Immunomodulatory agent with antineoplastic activity

FDA-Approved Indications

- Multiple myeloma in combination with dexamethasone after at least two prior therapies including lenalidomide and a proteasome inhibitor and have demonstrated disease progression on or within 60 days of completion of last therapy

FDA-Approved Dosage

- 4 mg orally, once daily on days 1 to 21 of a 28 day cycle in combination with dexamethasone

Dose Modification Criteria

- Renal: (mild to severe, not requiring dialysis): no
- Renal (severe impairment requiring dialysis: yes
- Hepatic (mild to severe, Child–Pugh classes A, B, C): yes
- Hematologic toxicity: yes
- Nonhematologic toxicity: yes

Adverse Reactions

- CV: venous and arterial thromboembolism
- DERM: rash
- GI: N/V (low), constipation, diarrhea, and decreased appetite
- HEMAT: neutropenia, anemia, and thrombocytopenia
- HEPAT: elevated ALT and bilirubin and hepatic failure
- NEURO: neuropathy, fatigue, and dizziness
- PULM: upper respiratory tract infection and dyspnea
- OTHER: hypersensitivity reactions (angioedema, severe dermatologic reactions), peripheral edema, pyrexia, back pain, muscle spasms, arthralgia, fatigue, asthenia, and tumor lysis syndrome

Comments

- Pomalidomide is only available through a restricted distribution program (Pomalyst REMS program). Only prescribers and pharmacists registered with the program are allowed to prescribe and dispense pomalidomide.
- Embryo-fetal toxicity. Pomalidomide is an analog of thalidomide which is a known teratogen. Pomalidomide may cause severe birth defects or death to an unborn baby. Refer to the product labeling for information regarding requirements for patient consent, pregnancy testing, and patient consent as part of the Pomalyst REMS program.
- Myelosuppression (particularly neutropenia and thrombocytopenia) is a common and dose-limiting toxicity. Monitor blood counts closely as indicated in the product labeling.

- Pomalidomide may cause venous and arterial thromboembolic event. Prophylactic anticoagulation treatment is recommended.
- Pomalidomide is a substrate of CYP1A2. Avoid concomitant use with strong CYP1A2 inhibitors. If concomitant use with a CYP1A2 inhibitor is unavoidable, a dose reduction of pomalidomide is recommended.
- Smoking reduces pomalidomide AUC by 32% due to CYP1A2 induction. Advise patients that smoking may reduce efficacy.

PONATINIB (ICLUSIG)

Mechanism of Action

- Tyrosine kinase inhibitor of BCR–ABL and T315I mutant ABL, and additional kinases including members of the VEGFR, PDGFR, FGFR, and EPH receptors and SRC families of kinase, and KIT, RET, TIE2, and FLT-3

FDA-Approved Indications

- CML: treatment of adults with chronic-phase, accelerated-phase, or blast-phase CML for whom no other tyrosine kinase inhibitor is indicated or with T315I-positive disease.
- Acute lymphoblastic leukemia (Ph+ ALL): adults for whom no other tyrosine kinase inhibitor is indicated or with T315I-positive disease

FDA-Approved Dosage

- 45 mg orally once daily with or without food. Continue treatment as long as the patient does not show evidence of disease progression or unacceptable toxicity.

Dose Modification Criteria

- Renal: not studied
- Hepatic (mild to severe): yes
- Hematologic toxicity: yes
- Nonhematologic toxicity: yes

Adverse Effects

- CV: cardiac arrhythmias, CHF, hypertension, left ventricular dysfunction, myocardial infarction, and worsening coronary artery disease
- DERM: dry skin and rash
- ELECTRO: decreased bicarbonate, hyperglycemia, hyperkalemia, hypernatremia, hyperphosphatemia, hypocalcemia, hypoglycemia, hypokalemia, and hyponatremia
- GI: abdominal pain, constipation, mucositis, N/V (low), and pancreatitis
- HEMAT: anemia, lymphopenia, neutropenia, and thrombocytopenia
- HEPAT: elevated LFTs
- NEURO: headache, peripheral neuropathy, and stroke
- Ocular: retinal and other ocular toxicities
- PULM: cough, dyspnea, nasopharyngitis, pneumonia, and upper respiratory tract infection
- OTHER: arterial thrombosis, arthralgia, asthenia, back pain, fatigue, fluid retention, hemorrhage, impaired wound healing, infections, muscle spasms, myalgia, pain in extremity, pyrexia, tumor lysis syndrome, venous thromboembolism, and increased lipase

Comments

- Patients with CV risk factors are at increased risk for arterial thrombosis with ponatinib.
- Monitor LFTs as baseline, at least monthly, or as clinically indicated.
- Monitor patients for signs or symptoms consistent with CHF.
- Monitor and manage blood pressure elevations.

- Check serum lipase every 2 weeks for the first 2 months and then monthly thereafter or as clinically indicated. Consider additional serum lipase monitoring in patients with a history of pancreatitis or alcohol abuse.
- Interrupt ponatinib for at least 1 week prior to major surgery. The decision when to resume ponatinib after surgery should be based on clinical judgment of adequate wound healing.
- Conduct a comprehensive eye exam at baseline and periodically during treatment to monitor for ocular toxicity.
- Patients taking strong inhibitors of CYP3A require a dose reduction of ponatinib. Concomitant strong inhibitors may increase risk for adverse reactions.
- Coadministration of strong CYP3A inducers should be avoided.
- Elevated gastric pH may reduce bioavailability and exposure of ponatinib. Coadministration of ponatinib with PPIs, H_2 blockers, or antacids should be avoided unless the benefit outweighs the possible risk of ponatinib underexposure.
- Patients aged ≥65 years may be more likely to experience adverse reactions including decreased platelet count, peripheral edema, increased lipase, dyspnea, asthenia, muscle spasms, and decreased appetite. Dose selection for an elderly patient should be cautious.
- Reversible posterior leukoencephalopathy syndrome (RPLS) has been reported in ponatinib-treated patients. Interrupt therapy for signs and symptoms consistent with RPLS.
- Embryo-fetal toxicity: Ponatinib can cause fetal harm when administered to a pregnant woman.

PORFIMER (PHOTOFRIN)

Mechanism of Action

- Photosensitizing agent

FDA-Approved Indications

- Esophageal cancer (palliation of complete or partial obstruction)
- Endobronchial NSCLC
  - For reduction of obstruction and palliation of symptoms in patients with completely or partially obstructed endobronchial NSCLC.
  - For treatment of microinvasive endobronchial NSCLC in patients for whom surgery and radiotherapy are not indicated.
- High-grade dysplasia in Barrett esophagus (ablation of high-grade dysplasia in patients who do not undergo esophagectomy).

FDA-Approved Dosage

- 2 mg/kg intravenous injection over 3 to 5 minutes × one dose followed by photodynamic therapy. For the treatment of esophageal and endobronchial cancer, patients may receive up to three additional courses; each course should be administered no sooner than 30 days after the prior course. For the ablation of high-grade dysplasia in Barrett esophagus, patients may receive up to three additional courses; each course should be administered no sooner than 90 days after the prior course.

Adverse Reactions

- CV: hypertension, hypotension, heart failure, chest pain, atrial fibrillation, and tachycardia
- DERM: photosensitivity
- HEMAT: anemia
- GI: N/V, abdominal pain, anorexia, constipation, dysphagia, esophageal edema, and esophageal stricture
- NEURO: anxiety, confusion, and insomnia
- PULM: pleural effusion, dyspnea, pneumonia, pharyngitis, cough, respiratory insufficiency, and tracheoesophageal fistula
- OTHER: fever

Comments

■ Patients are photosensitive (including eyes) for at least 30 days after administration.

PRALATREXATE (FOLOTYN)

Mechanism of Action

■ Folate analog metabolic inhibitor that competitively inhibits dihydrofolate reductase. It is also a competitive inhibitor for polyglutamylation by the enzyme folylpolyglutamyl synthetase. This inhibition results in the depletion of thymidine and other biologic molecules, the synthesis of which depends on single carbon transfer.

FDA-Approved Indications

■ Treatment of relapsed or refractory peripheral T-cell lymphoma (PTCL)

FDA-Approved Dosage

■ 30 mg/m^2 administered as an intravenous push over 3 to 5 minutes once weekly for 6 weeks in 7-week cycles

Dose Modification Criteria

■ Renal (mild to moderate): no; monitor for toxicity
■ Renal (severe 15 to 30 ml/min/1.73 m^2): yes and monitor for toxicity
■ Renal (end stage renal disease and/or dialysis): avoid use
■ Hepatic: not evaluated
■ Hematologic toxicity: yes
■ Nonhematologic toxicity: yes

Adverse Effects

■ Cr: increased serum creatinine
■ CV: tachycardia
■ DERM: bullous exfoliative skin reactions including toxic epidermal necrolysis and Stevens–Johnson, pruritus, and rash
■ ELECTRO: hypokalemia
■ GI: abdominal pain, constipation, diarrhea, mucositis, and N/V (low)
■ HEMAT: anemia, neutropenia, and thrombocytopenia
■ HEPAT: elevated LFTs
■ PULM: cough, dyspnea, and upper respiratory tract infection
■ OTHER: asthenia, back pain, dehydration, edema, epistaxis, fatigue, night sweats, pain in extremity, pharyngolaryngeal pain, pyrexia, sepsis, and tumor lysis syndrome

Comments

■ Prior to initiating pralatrexate, patients should be supplemented with vitamin B$_{12}$ 1 mg IM every 8 to 10 weeks and folic acid 1.0 to1.25 mg orally on a daily basis.
■ Monitor for mucositis weekly and if ≥ grade 2 mucositis is observed omit or reduce dose as recommended in product labeling.
■ Pralatrexate should not be diluted. It is a clear, yellow solution.
■ Coadministration with probenecid or other drugs that may affect relevant transporter systems (e.g., NSAIDs) require close monitoring for signs of systemic toxicity.
■ Embryo-fetal toxicity: Pralatrexate can cause fetal harm when administered to a pregnant woman. Women should be advised against breastfeeding while being treated with pralatrexate.

PROCARBAZINE (MATULANE)

Mechanism of Action

- The mechanism is unknown. There is evidence that the drug may act by inhibition of protein, and RNA and DNA synthesis.

FDA-Approved Indications

- Stage III and IV Hodgkin lymphoma: first-line treatment in combination with other anticancer drugs. (Procarbazine is used as part of the MOPP [mechlorethamine, vincristine, procarbazine, and prednisone] chemotherapy regimen.)

FDA-Approved Dosage

- All doses based on actual body weight unless the patient is obese or there has been a spurious weight increase, in which case lean body weight (dry weight) should be used.
- Doses may be given as a single daily dose or divided throughout the day.
- MOPP regimen for Hodgkin lymphoma: 100 mg/m^2 orally daily × 14 days (in combination with mechlorethamine, vincristine, and prednisone).
- Adult single-agent therapy: 2 to 4 mg/kg orally daily × 7 days, and then 4 to 6 mg/kg orally daily until maximal response is obtained. Maintenance dose: 1 to 2 mg/kg orally daily.
- Pediatric single-agent therapy: 50 mg/m^2 orally daily × 7 days, and then 100 mg/m^2 orally daily until maximum response is obtained. Maintenance dose: 50 mg/m^2 orally daily.

Adverse Reactions

- DERM: pruritus, hyperpigmentation, and alopecia
- GI: anorexia, N/V (moderate), stomatitis, xerostomia, diarrhea, and constipation
- HEMAT: myelosuppression
- NEURO: paresthesias, confusion, lethargy, and mental depression
- OTHER: fever and myalgia.

Comments

- Disulfiram-like (Antabuse) reaction can occur; avoid alcoholic beverages while taking procarbazine.
- Procarbazine is a weak monoamine oxidase (MAO) inhibitor; avoid tyramine-rich foods, sympathomimetic drugs, antidepressant agents (e.g., tricyclic or SSRIs). Screen for other potential drug–drug interactions.

RALOXIFENE (EVISTA)

Mechanism of Action

- Estrogen agonist/antagonist (selective ER modulator)

FDA-Approved Indications

- Reduction in risk of invasive breast cancer in postmenopausal women with osteoporosis
- Reduction in risk of invasive breast cancer in postmenopausal women at high risk of invasive breast cancer
- Treatment and prevention of osteoporosis in postmenopausal women

FDA-Approved Dosage

- 60 mg orally once daily

Dose Modification Criteria

- Renal: no (use with caution in patients with moderate or severe impairment)
- Hepatic: no (use with caution in patients with impairment)

■ Myelosuppression: no
■ Nonhematologic toxicity: no

Adverse Reactions

■ CV: peripheral edema
■ GI: N/V (minimal)
■ OTHER: hot flashes, leg cramps, flu syndrome, arthralgia, sweating, and venous thromboembolic events (deep venous thrombosis, PE, retinal vein thrombosis, and superficial thrombophlebitis)

Comments

■ Women with active or past history of VTE should not take raloxifene. Raloxifene should be discontinued at least 72 hours prior to and during prolonged immobilization (e.g., postsurgical recovery and prolonged bed rest), and raloxifene should be resumed only after the patient is fully ambulatory. Women should be advised to move about periodically during prolonged travel.
■ In a clinical trial of postmenopausal women with documented coronary heart disease or at increased risk of coronary events, an increased risk of death due to stroke was observed after treatment with raloxifene. However, there was no statistically significant difference between treatment groups in the incidence of stroke.
■ Cholestyramine (and other anion exchange resins) should not be used concurrently with raloxifene.
■ If used concomitantly with warfarin, monitor PT when starting or stopping raloxifene.
■ Raloxifene is highly protein bound (95%); use with caution with other highly protein-bound drugs.
■ Embryo-fetal toxicity: raloxifene may cause fetal harm when administered to a pregnant woman.

RAMUCIRUMAB (CYRAMZA)

Mechanism of Action

■ Recombinant human IgG1 monoclonal antibody that binds to VEGF receptor 2.

FDA-Approved Indications

■ Advanced gastric or gastro-esophageal junction adenocarcinoma that has progressed on or after prior fluoropyrimidine or platinum containing chemotherapy. May be used as a single agent or in combination with paclitaxel.
■ In combination with docetaxel for treatment of metastatic NSCLC with disease progression on or after platinum-based therapy. Patients with EGFR or ALK mutations should have disease progression on FDA-approved therapy specific for these mutations.
■ In combinations with FOLFIRI for the treatment of metastatic colorectal cancer with disease progression on or after prior therapy with bevacizumab, oxaliplatin, and a fluoropyrimidine.

FDA-Approved Dosage

■ Gastric Cancer: 8 mg/kg IV over 60 minutes every 2 weeks as either a single agent or in combination with weekly paclitaxel
■ NSCLC: 10 mg/kg IV over 60 minutes on day 1 of a 21 day cycle prior to docetaxel infusion
■ Colorectal Cancer: 8 mg/kg IV over 60 minutes every 2 weeks prior to FOLFIRI administration
■ All indications: continue until disease progression or unacceptable toxicity

Dose Modification Criteria

■ Renal: no
■ Hepatic (mild to moderate (total bilirubin < 3 X ULN): no; clinical deterioration was reported in patients with Child–Pugh B or C cirrhosis who received single-agent ramucirumab
■ Nonhematologic toxicity: yes

Adverse Reactions

- CV: hypertension and arterial thromboembolic events
- ENDO: hypothyroidism
- GI: gastrointestinal perforations, diarrhea, and stomatitis
- GU: proteinuria
- HEMAT: hemorrhage, neutropenia, and thrombocytopenia
- INFUS: rigors/tremors, back pain/spasms, chest pain, chills, flushing, dyspnea, wheezing, and hypoxia
- OTHER: impaired wound healing, fatigue, asthenia

Comments

- Premedicate with an IV histamine H_1 antagonist prior to each infusion. Patients who have experienced a grade 1 or 2 infusion-related reaction should also receive dexamethasone and acetaminophen as premedication.
- Hemorrhage: Ramucirumab increased the risk of hemorrhage and gastrointestinal hemorrhage, including severe and sometimes fatal hemorrhagic events. Discontinue therapy in patients who experience severe bleeding.
- Ramucirumab is an antiangiogenic therapy, which can lead to complications such as gastrointestinal (GI) perforation and impaired wound healing. Discontinue ramucirumab prior to surgery and in patients who develop GI perforation or develop wound healing complications.
- Hypertension: Control hypertension prior to initiating therapy and monitor blood pressure every 2 weeks or more frequently as indicated during therapy.
- Reversible posterior leukoencephalopathy syndrome (RPLS) has been reported rarely with ramucirumab.
- Embryo-fetal toxicity: Ramucirumab may cause fetal harm when administered to a pregnant woman.

REGORAFENIB (STIVARGA)

Mechanism of Action

- Kinase inhibitor of multiple membrane-bound and intracellular kinases

FDA-Approved Indications

- Colorectal cancer: metastatic colorectal cancer in patients who have been previously treated with fluoropyrimidine-, oxaliplatin- and irinotecan-based chemotherapy, an anti-VEGF therapy, and, if KRAS wild type, an anti-EGFR therapy.
- Gastrointestinal stromal tumor (GIST): locally advanced, unresectable, or metastatic GIST who have been previously treated with imatinib mesylate and sunitinib malate.

FDA-Approved Dosage

- 160 mg orally once daily with a low-fat breakfast for the first 21 days of each 28-day cycle

Dose Modification Criteria

- Renal (mild to severe): no
- Renal (end stage renal disease or dialysis): no data
- Hepatic (mild to moderate, Child–Pugh class A or B): no
- Hepatic (severe, Child–Pugh class C): not studied
- Nonhematologic toxicity: yes

Adverse Effects

- CV: cardiac ischemia, cardiac infarction, and hypertension
- DERM: Hand–foot skin reaction, rash,
- ELECTRO: hypocalcemia, hypokalemia, hyponatremia, and hypophosphatemia

- GI: decreased appetite, diarrhea, mucositis, abdominal pain, and N/V (minimal to low)
- GU: proteinuria
- HEMAT: anemia, lymphopenia, and thrombocytopenia
- HEPAT: increased bilirubin and increased LFTs
- OTHER: asthenia, dysphonia, fatigue, hemorrhage, infection, weight loss, wound healing complications, fever, increased amylase, and/or lipase

Comments

- Severe and sometimes fatal hepatotoxicity has been observed in clinical trials. Obtain LFTs before initiation of regorafenib and monitor at least every 2 weeks during the first 2 months of treatment. Thereafter, monitor monthly or more frequently as clinically indicated. Monitor LFTs weekly in patients experiencing elevated LFTs until improvement to <3 times the ULN or baseline. Temporarily hold and then reduce or permanently discontinue regorafenib depending on the severity and persistence of hepatotoxicity as manifested by elevated LFTs or hepatocellular necrosis.
- For dermatologic toxicity, withhold regorafenib, reduce dose, or permanently discontinue therapy depending on the severity and persistence of toxicity.
- Regorafenib caused an increased incidence of hemorrhage. Permanently discontinue regorafenib in patients with severe or life-threatening hemorrhage. Monitor INR levels more frequently in patients receiving warfarin.
- Regorafenib increased the incidence of myocardial ischemia and infarction. Withhold regorafenib in patients who develop new or acute onset cardiac ischemia or infarction.
- Monitor blood pressure weekly for the first 6 weeks of treatment and then every cycle, or more frequently, as clinically indicated. Temporarily or permanently withhold regorafenib for severe or uncontrolled hypertension.
- Gastrointestinal perforation or fistula can occur. Permanently discontinue regorafenib in these patients.
- Treatment with regorafenib should be stopped at least 2 weeks prior to scheduled surgery.
- Regorafenib should be discontinued in patients with wound dehiscence.
- Monitor for RPLS. Confirm the diagnosis of RPLS with MRI and discontinue regorafenib in patients who develop RPLS.
- Strong CYP3A4 inhibitors and inducers should be avoided with regorafenib. Regorafenib and its metabolites competitively inhibit uridine diphosphate glucuronsyltransferases (UGT) 1A9 and 1A1, which may increase the exposure of UGT1A1 substrates (e.g., irinotecan). Regorafenib may also increase the exposure to breast cancer resistance protein (BCRP) substrates (e.g., methotrexate, rosuvastatin).
- Embryo-fetal toxicity: regorafenib may cause fetal harm when administered to a pregnant woman. Results from animal studies indicate that regorafenib can impair male and female infertility.

RITUXIMAB (RITUXAN)

Mechanism of Action

- Chimeric (murine, human) monoclonal antibody directed at the CD20 antigen found on the surface of normal and malignant B lymphocytes.

FDA-Approved Indications

- Non-Hodgkin's Lymphoma (NHL)
  - Relapsed or refractory low-grade or follicular, CD20-positive, B-cell, NHL as a single agent.
  - Previously untreated follicular, CD20-positive, B-cell NHL in combination with first-line chemotherapy and, in patients achieving a complete or partial response to rituximab in combination with chemotherapy, as single-agent maintenance therapy.
  - Nonprogressive (including stable disease), low-grade, CD20-positive, B-cell NHL, as a single agent, after first-line CVP chemotherapy.
  - Previously untreated diffuse large B-cell, CD20-positive NHL in combination with CHOP or other anthracycline-based chemotherapy regimens.

- Chronic Lymphocytic Leukemia (CLL): In combination with fludarabine and cyclophosphamide (FC) in previously untreated and previously treated CD20-positive CLL.
- Other: Rheumatoid arthritis, granulomatosis with polyangiitis (GPA) (Wegener's granulomatosis) and microscopic polyangiitis (MPA).

FDA-Approved Dosage

- Premedication with acetaminophen and an antihistamine (e.g., diphenhydramine) should be considered before each infusion.
- If a patient experiences an infusion-related reaction, the infusion should be stopped, the patient managed symptomatically, and then the infusion should be restarted at half the rate once the symptoms have resolved.
- NHL—375 mg/m^2/ dose IV infusion according to the following schedules:
  - Relapsed or refractory, low-grade or follicular, CD20-positive, B-cell NHL: Administer once weekly for four or eight doses
  - Retreatment for relapsed or refractory, low-grade or follicular, CD20-positive B-cell NHL: Administer once weekly for four doses
  - Previously untreated, follicular, CD20-positive, B-cell NHL: Administer on day 1 of each cycle of chemotherapy, for up to eight doses. For maintenance therapy in patients who obtain a complete or partial response, administer as a single-agent every 8 weeks for 12 doses.
  - Nonprogressing, low-grade, CD20-positive, B-cell NHL, after first-line CVP chemotherapy: Administer once weekly for four doses at 6-month intervals to a maximum of 16 doses.
  - Diffuse large B-cell NHL: Administer on day 1 of each cycle of chemotherapy for up to eight infusions.
- CLL: 375 mg/m^2 IV infusion × 1 dose the day prior to initiation of FC chemotherapy, followed by 500 mg/m^2 IV infusion on day 1 of cycles 2 to 6 (every 28 days).
- Rate titration: For the first infusion start at 50 mg per hour, and then may increase by 50 mg per hour every 30 minutes up to a maximum of 400 mg per hour. If the initial infusion is tolerated, subsequent infusions can be administered at an advanced rate either in a standard infusion rate titration or a more rapid 90 minute titration format for certain patient populations.
  - Standard infusion titration: Start at 100 mg per hour, and then may increase by 100 mg per hour every 30 minutes up to a maximum of 400 mg per hour.
  - Advanced rate 90 minute infusion (evaluated in previously untreated follicular NHL and DLBCL patients with a glucocorticoid-containing chemotherapy regimen): Start at a rate of 20% of the total dose given in the first 30 minutes and the remaining 80% of the total dose given over the next 60 minutes.

Adverse Reactions

- CV: hypotension, arrhythmias, and peripheral edema
- DERM: rash, pruritis, urticaria, and severe mucocutaneous reactions
- GI: N/V (minimal) and abdominal pain
- HEMAT: leukopenia, thrombocytopenia, and neutropenia
- INFUS: fever, chills, rigors, hypoxia, pulmonary infiltrates, adult respiratory distress syndrome, angioedema, myocardial infarction, ventricular fibrillation, or cardiogenic shock
- NEURO: headache and dizziness
- OTHER: throat irritation, rhinitis, bronchospasm, hypersensitivity reaction, myalgia, back pain, tumor lysis syndrome, asthenia, and infections

Comments

- Tumor lysis syndrome has been reported within 12 to 24 hours after the infusion (high-risk: high numbers of circulating malignant cells).
- Mild-to-moderate infusion reactions consisting of fever, chills, and rigors occur in the majority of patients during the first infusion. The reactions resolve with slowing or interruption of the infusion and with supportive care measures. The incidence of infusion reactions declines with subsequent infusions.

- A more severe infusion-related complex, usually reported with the first infusion (hypoxia, pulmonary infiltrates, adult respiratory distress syndrome, myocardial infarction, ventricular fibrillation, or cardiogenic shock), has resulted in fatalities.
- Severe mucocutaneous reactions, some with fatal outcome, have been reported in association with rituximab treatment.
- Serious infections including bacterial, fungal, and new or reactivated viral infections can occur during and following the completion of rituximab-based therapy. Reported infectious complications include PML secondary to the JC virus, and hepatitis B virus (HBV) reactivation resulting in fulminant hepatitis, hepatic failure, and death.
- Hepatitis B virus reactivation: Screen all patients for HBV infection by measuring HBsAg and anti-HBc before initiating rituximab therapy. For patients who show evidence of prior hepatitis B infection (HBsAg positive or HBsAg negative but anti-HBc positive), monitor for reactivation during and for several months after rituximab therapy. Consult with physicians with expertise in managing hepatitis B in regards to monitoring and consideration of antiviral prophylaxis.
- Rituximab is commonly combined with cytotoxic chemotherapy agents in various subtypes of B-cell NHL. Consult current literature for dosing regimens.

ROMIDEPSIN (ISTODAX)

Mechanism of Action

- Histone deacetylase inhibitor

FDA-Approved Indications

- Cutaneous T-cell Lymphoma (CTCL) in patients who have received at least one prior systemic therapy
- Peripheral T-cell lymphoma (PTCL) in patients who have received at least one prior therapy

FDA-Approved Dosage

- 14 mg/m^2 administered intravenously over a 4-hour period on days 1, 8, and 15 of a 28-day cycle. Repeat cycles every 28 days provided that the patient continues to benefit from and tolerates the drug.

Dose Modification Criteria

- Renal (mild to severe): no
- Renal (end-stage renal disease): no data, use with caution
- Hepatic (mild): no
- Hepatic (moderate to severe): no data, use with caution
- Myelosuppression: yes
- Nonhematologic toxicity: yes

Adverse Reactions

- CV: ECG T-wave and ST-segment changes, hypotension, and tachycardia
- DERM: dermatitis, exfoliative dermatitis, and pruritus
- ELECTRO: hypermagnesemia, hyperuricemia, hypocalcemia, hypokalemia, hypomagnesemia, hyponatremia, and hypophosphatemia
- ENDO: hyperglycemia
- GI: abdominal pain, anorexia, constipation, diarrhea, N/V (low), and stomatitis
- HEMAT: anemia, lymphopenia, neutropenia, and thrombocytopenia
- HEPAT: elevated LFTs and hypoalbuminemia
- NEURO: dysgeusia

- PULM: cough and dyspnea
- OTHER: asthenia, chills, decreased weight, fatigue, infections, peripheral edema, pyrexia, and tumor lysis syndrome

Comments

- Serious and sometimes fatal infections have been reported during treatment and within 30 days after treatment with romidepsin. Viral reactivation, including Epstein Barr and hepatitis B have been reported in clinical trials. In patients with evidence of prior hepatitis B infection, consider monitoring for reactivation and antiviral prophylaxis.
- Carefully monitor PT and INR in patients concurrently administered romidepsin and warfarin derivatives.
- Strong CYP3A4 inhibitors and inducers should be avoided with romidepsin.
- In patients with congenital long QT syndrome, those with a history of significant CV disease, and in those taking antiarrhythmic medicine that lead to significant QT prolongation, appropriate CV monitoring precautions should be considered, such as the monitoring of electrolytes and ECGs at baseline and periodically during treatment. Potassium and magnesium should be within the normal range before administration of romidepsin.
- Embryo-fetal toxicity: Based on its mechanism of action and findings in animals, romidepsin may cause fetal harm when administered to a pregnant woman.

RUCAPARIB (RUBRACA)

Mechanism of Action

- Inhibitor of poly (ADP-ribose) polymerase (PARP) enzymes, including PARP1, PARP2, and PARP3 which play a role in DNA repair.

FDA-Approved Indications

- Ovarian cancer: monotherapy for the treatment of patients with advanced disease and deleterious BRCA mutation (germline and/or somatic) who have been treated with 2 or more prior lines of chemotherapy.

FDA-Approved Dosage

- 600 mg orally, twice daily until disease progression or unacceptable toxicity

Dose Modification Criteria

- Renal (mild to moderate, CrCl > 30 mL/min): no
- Renal (severe, CrCl < 30 ml/min): no data
- Hepatic (mild): no
- Hepatic (moderate to severe): no data
- Myelosuppression: yes
- Nonhematologic toxicity: yes

Adverse Reaction

- GI: abdominal pain, decreased appetite, N/V (moderate), diarrhea, and constipation
- GU: increased serum creatinine
- HEMAT: anemia, neutropenia, thrombocytopenia, and lymphopenia
- HEPAT: increased AST/ALT
- NEURO: dysgeusia
- PULM: dyspnea
- OTHER: fatigue/asthenia and hypercholesterolemia

Comments

■ Myelodysplastic syndrome / acute myeloid leukemia has been reported in patients who have received rucaparib. Monitor patients for hematologic toxicity at baseline and monthly thereafter.
■ Embryo-fetal toxicity: Rucaparib may cause fetal harm when administered to a pregnant woman.

RUXOLITINIB (JAKAFI)

Mechanism of Action

■ Inhibits Janus-associated kinases (JAKs) JAK1 and JAK2, which mediate the signaling of cytokines and growth factors that are important for hematopoiesis and immune function. JAK signaling involves recruitment of signal transducers and activators of transcription (STATs) to cytokine receptors, activation, and subsequent localization of STATs to the nucleus leading to modulation of gene expression.

FDA-Approved Indications

■ Myelofibrosis: intermediate or high-risk myelofibrosis, including primary myelofibrosis, postpolycythemia vera myelofibrosis, and postessential thrombocythemia myelofibrosis.
■ Polycythemia vera: patients who have had an inadequate response to or intolerant of hydroxyurea.

FDA-Approved Dosage

■ Myelofibrosis:
  ● Starting dose is based on patient's baseline platelet count:
  ● 20 mg orally twice daily for patients with a platelet count greater than $200 \times 10^9/L$
  ● 15 mg orally twice daily for patients with a platelet count between $100 \times 10^9/L$ and $200 \times 10^9/L$
  ● 5 mg orally twice daily for patients with a platelet count between $50 \times 10^9/L$ to less than $100 \times 10^9/L$
  ● Increase dose based on response to a maximum of 25 mg orally twice daily
  ● Discontinue after 6 months if no spleen reduction or symptom improvement
■ Polycythemia vera:
  ● Starting dose is 10 mg orally twice daily. Doses may be titrated based on safety and efficacy.

Dose Modification Criteria

■ Renal (mild): no
■ Renal (moderate, severe, end-stage renal disease): use and dose modification depend on platelet count
■ Hepatic impairment: use and dose modification depend on platelet count
■ Hematologic toxicity: yes

Adverse Reactions

■ DERM: bruising
■ GI: flatulence
■ GU: urinary tract infection
■ HEME: anemia, neutropenia, and thrombocytopenia
■ NEURO: dizziness and headache
■ OTHER: infection and weight gain

Comments

■ Can be administered through a nasogastric tube (≥8 Fr). Suspend one tablet in 40 mL of water with stirring for approximately 10 minutes. Within 6 hours after the tablet hast dispersed, the suspension can be administered through a nasogastric (NG) tube using an appropriate syringe. Flush NG tube with 75 mL of water.

- Active serious infections should have resolved before starting therapy.
- May cause lipid elevations. Monitor lipid levels 8 to 12 weeks after starting therapy.
- Screen for drug interactions. Concomitant use with strong CYP3A4 inhibitors or fluconazole may require dose interruption, reduction, or discontinuation.
- Ruxolitinib may increase the risk of nonmelanoma skin cancer; perform periodic skin examinations.
- Embryo-fetal toxicity: There are no adequate and well-controlled studies of ruxolitinib in pregnant women.

SIPULEUCEL-T (PROVENGE)

Mechanism of Action

- Autologous cellular immunotherapy designed to induce an immune response targeted against prostatic acid phosphatase (PAP), an antigen expressed in most prostate cancers. Sipuleucel-T consists of autologous peripheral blood mononuclear cells that have been activated with a recombinant human protein consisting of PAP linked to granulocyte macrophage colony-stimulating factor.

FDA-Approved Indications

- Asymptomatic or minimally symptomatic metastatic castrate-resistant (hormone refractory) prostate cancer

FDA-Approved Dosage

- Administer three doses at approximately 2-week intervals.
- Each dose of sipuleucel-T contains a minimum of 50 million autologous CD54+ cells activated with PAP-GM-CSF.

Dose Modification Criteria

- Infusion reactions: slow rate

ADVERSE REACTIONS

- INFU: fever, chills, fatigue, syncope, hypotension, hypertension, nausea, joint ache, back pain, respiratory events (dyspnea, hypoxia, bronchospasm), and tachycardia

Comments

- Thromboembolic events, including deep venous thrombosis and pulmonary embolism, can occur following infusion of sipuleucel-T. Use with caution in patients with risk factors for thromboembolic events.
- The patient's peripheral blood mononuclear cells are obtained via a standard leukapheresis procedure 3 days prior to the infusion date. The cellular composition of sipuleucel-T depends on the composition of cells obtained from the patient's leukapheresis. In addition to antigen-presenting cells, the final product contains T cells, B cells, natural killer cells, and other cells.
- Sipuleucel-T is not routinely tested for transmissible infectious diseases; thus universal precautions should be employed when handling sipuleucel-T or leukapheresis material.
- For autologous use only. For intravenous use only. Do not use a cell filter. Do not infuse expired product. The sipuleucel-T infusion bag must remain within the insulated polyurethane container until the time of administration.
- If the infusion must be interrupted, it should not be resumed if the sipuleucel-T infusion bag will be held at room temperature for more than 3 hours.
- Premedicate with acetaminophen and an oral antihistamine 30 minutes prior to infusion of sipuleucel-T.
- If the patient is unable to receive a scheduled infusion of sipuleucel-T, the patient will need to undergo an additional leukapheresis procedure.
- Concomitant use of chemotherapy and immunosuppressive medications with sipuleucel-T has not been studied.

SONIDEGIB (ODOMZO)

Mechanism of Action

- Inhibits the Hedgehog pathway

FDA-Approved Indications

- Locally advanced basal cell carcinoma (BCC) that has recurred following surgery or radiation therapy, or BCC patients who are not candidates for surgery or radiation therapy

FDA-Approved Dosage

- 200 mg orally once daily until disease progression or unacceptable toxicity. Take on an empty stomach, at least 1 hour before or 2 hours after a meal

Dose Modification Criteria

- Renal (mild to moderate, CrCl ≥30 mL/min): no
- Hepatic (mild to severe, Child–Pugh A, B, C): no
- Nonhematologic toxicity (musculoskeletal and elevated CK): yes

Adverse Reactions

- DERM: alopecia and pruritis
- GI: N/V (low), diarrhea, decreased appetite, and abdominal pain
- NEURO: headache and dysgeusia
- OTHER: serum creatine kinase elevations, muscle spasms, musculoskeletal pain, myalgia, and fatigue

Comments

- Embryo-fetal toxicity: Verify pregnancy status of females of reproductive potential prior to initiating sonidegib. Sonidegib can cause embryo-fetal death or severe birth defects when administered to a pregnant woman.
- Musculoskeletal toxicity: Obtain serum creatine kinase (CK) levels prior to initiating sonidegib and periodically during treatment and as clinically indicated.
- Blood donation: Advise patients not to donate blood or blood products during therapy with sonidegib and for at least 20 months after the last dose.
- Sonidegib is a substrate of CYP3A4. Avoid concomitant administration with strong or moderate CYP3A4 inhibitors or inducers.

SORAFENIB (NEXAVAR)

Mechanism of Action

- Tyrosine kinase inhibitor (Raf kinases, VEGFR-2, -3, FLT-3, KIT, PDGFR-β)

FDA-Approved Indications

- Advanced RCC
- Unresectable hepatocellular carcinoma
- Differentiated thyroid carcinoma: locally recurrent or metastatic, progressive, differentiated thyroid carcinoma refractory to radioactive iodine treatment

FDA-Approved Dosage

- 400 mg orally twice daily without food (1 hour before or 2 hours after eating)

Dose Modification Criteria

- Renal: no (not studied in patients who are on dialysis)
- Hepatic: no (not studied in patients with severe hepatic impairment)
- Myelosuppression: no
- Nonhematologic toxicity: yes

Adverse Reactions

- CV: hypertension, cardiac ischemia/infarction (see comments), QT prolongation
- DERM: palmar-plantar erythrodysesthesia, rash, alopecia, pruritis, dry skin, erythema, severe bullous, and exfoliative skin reactions
- ELECTRO: hypophosphatemia
- GI: N/V (minimal), diarrhea, anorexia, abdominal pain, and gastrointestinal perforation (rare)
- HEMAT: myelosuppression
- HEPAT: elevated LFTs and drug-induced hepatitis
- NEURO: peripheral neuropathy (sensory)
- OTHER: bleeding/hemorrhage, fatigue, asthenia, weight loss, and increased lipase/amylase

Comments

- Hand–foot skin reaction (palmar-plantar erythrodysesthesia) and rash are the most common adverse events with sorafenib. Monitor closely, provide supportive care, and evaluate for dose interruption of modification for severe toxicity (see product labeling).
- Monitor blood pressure weekly during the first 6 weeks of therapy and thereafter monitor and treat according to standard medical practice.
- Sorafenib may impair wound healing. Temporary interruption of sorafenib is recommended in patients undergoing major surgical procedures.
- In placebo controlled trials for the FDA-approved indications, the incidence of cardiac ischemia/infarction was higher in the sorafenib-treated patients compared to the placebo group. Temporary or permanent discontinuation of sorafenib should be considered in patients who develop cardiac ischemia and/or infarction.
- Sorafenib impairs exogenous thyroid suppression. In patients with differentiated thyroid carcinoma, monitor TSH levels monthly and adjust thyroid replacement medication as needed.
- Sorafenib is hepatically metabolized undergoing oxidative metabolism through CYP isoenzyme 3A4 as well as glucuronidation mediated by UGT1A9 and thus drug exposure may be influenced by inhibitors or inducers of CYP3A4 or UGT1A9. Sorafenib is also a competitive inhibitor of multiple cytochrome enzymes (e.g., CYP2B6, CYP2C8) and of glucuronidation by the UGT1A1 and UGT1A9 pathways. Refer to product labeling and other appropriate references to screen for potential drug interactions.
- Embryo-fetal toxicity sorafenib may cause fetal harm when administered to a pregnant woman.

STREPTOZOTOCIN (ZANOSAR)

Mechanism of Action

- Alkylating agent

FDA-Approved Indications

- Metastatic islet cell carcinoma of the pancreas (functional and nonfunctional carcinomas)

FDA-Approved Dosage

- Daily schedule
  - 500 mg/m^2 IV daily × 5 days every 6 weeks until maximum benefit or treatment limiting toxicity is observed, OR

▪ Weekly schedule
  ● Initial dose: 1 g/m² IV weekly for the first two courses (weeks). In subsequent courses, drug doses may be escalated in patients who have not achieved a therapeutic response and who have not experienced significant toxicity with the previous course of treatment. However, a single dose should not exceed 1,500 mg/m².

Dose Modification Criteria
▪ Renal: use with caution, consider dose reduction

Adverse Reactions
▪ DERM: injection site reactions (irritant)
▪ ELECTRO: hypophosphatemia
▪ ENDO: dysglycemia, may lead to insulin-dependent diabetes
▪ GI: N/V (high) and diarrhea
▪ GU: azotemia, anuria, renal tubular acidosis, increased BUN and serum creatinine, glycosuria
▪ HEMAT: myelosuppression
▪ HEPAT: increased LFTs

Comments
▪ Renal complications are dose related and cumulative. Mild proteinuria is usually an early sign of impending renal dysfunction. Serial urinalysis is important for the early detection of proteinuria and should be quantified with a 24-hour collection when proteinuria is detected. Adequate hydration may help reduce the risk of nephrotoxicity. Avoid other nephrotoxic agents.

SUNITINIB MALATE (SUTENT)

Mechanism of Action
▪ Tyrosine kinase inhibitor (VEGFR-1, -2, -3, FLT-3, KIT, PDGFR-α, β, CSF-1R, RET)

FDA-Approved Indications
▪ Gastrointestinal stromal tumor (GIST): after disease progression on or intolerance to imatinib mesylate
▪ Advanced RCC
▪ Advanced pancreatic neuroendocrine tumors (pNET)—progressive, well-differentiated pNET in patients with unresectable locally advanced or metastatic disease

FDA-Approved Dosage
▪ GIST and RCC: 50 mg orally once daily on a schedule of 4 weeks on treatment followed by 2 weeks off. Sunitinib may be taken with or without food.
▪ pNET: 37.5 mg orally once daily continuously without a scheduled off-treatment period.

Dose Modification Criteria
▪ Renal: no
▪ Hepatic: no (not studied in patients with severe hepatic impairment)
▪ Myelosuppression: no
▪ Nonhematologic toxicity: yes

Adverse Reactions
▪ CV: hypertension, left ventricular dysfunction, and QT interval prolongation
▪ DERM: palmar-plantar erythrodysesthesia, rash, skin discoloration (yellow), and dry skin
▪ ENDO: hypothyroidism and hypoglycemia

- GI: N/V (low), diarrhea, mucositis/stomatitis, dyspepsia, abdominal pain, constipation, altered taste, and anorexia
- GU: proteinuria and nephrotic syndrome
- HEMAT: myelosuppression
- HEPAT: increased LFTs and hepatotoxicity
- NEURO: peripheral neuropathy (sensory)
- OTHER: bleeding/hemorrhage, fatigue, asthenia, myalgia/limb pain, increased amylase/lipase, osteonecrosis of the jaw, and tumor lysis syndrome

Comments

- Hepatotoxicity, including liver failure, has been observed. Monitor LFTs before initiation of sunitinib, during each cycle, and as clinically indicated. Interrupt therapy for grade 3 or 4 drug-related hepatic adverse events and discontinue therapy if there is no resolution.
- Hypertension may occur. Monitor blood pressure and treat as needed.
- Proteinuria and nephrotic syndrome have been reported with sunitinib. Monitor for the development or worsening of proteinuria.
- Severe cutaneous reactions have been reported such as erythema multiforme, Stevens-Johnson syndrome, toxic epidermal necrolysis, and necrotizing fasciitis. Discontinue sunitinib if severe cutaneous reactions are observed or suspected.Thombotic microangiopathy (TMA) has been associated with sunitinib therapy. Discontinue sunitinib if TMA occurs during therapy.
- Left ventricular ejection declines have occurred. Monitor patients for signs or symptoms of CHF.
- Prolonged QT intervals and torsades de pointes have been observed. Use with cation in patients at higher risk. Consider baseline and on-treatment electrocardiograms and monitor electrolytes.
- Hemorrhagic events including tumor-related hemorrhage have occurred. Perform serial CBCs and physical examination.
- Hypothyroidism may occur. Patients with signs or symptoms suggestive of hypothyroidism should have laboratory monitoring of thyroid function and be treated as per standard medical practice.
- Adrenal hemorrhage was observed in animal studies. Monitor adrenal function in case of stress such as surgery, trauma, or severe infection.
- Temporary interruption of sunitinib is recommended in patients undergoing major surgical procedures.
- Sunitinib is hepatically metabolized undergoing oxidative metabolism through CYP isoenzyme 3A4 and thus drug exposure may be influenced by potent inhibitors or inducers of CYP3A4. Refer to product labeling and other appropriate references to screen for potential drug interactions.
- Embryo-fetal toxicity: Sunitinib may cause fetal harm when administered to a pregnant woman.

TALIMOGENE LAHERPAREPVEC (IMLYGIC)

Mechanism of Action

- Talimogene laherparepvec is a live, attenuated HSV-1 genetically modified to replicate within tumors and produce the immune stimulatory protein GM-CSF, which leads to lysis of tumors and is followed by release of tumor-derived antigens, promoting an antitumor immune response.

FDA-Approved Indications

- Local treatment of unresectable cutaneous, subcutaneous, and nodal lesions of melanoma that is recurrent after initial surgery

FDA-Approved Dosage

- 10^6 plaque-forming units (PFU) per mL—for initial dose only
- 10^8 PFU per mL—for all subsequent doses

▪ Second treatment should be 3 weeks after initial injection. All subsequent injections should be every 2 weeks.
▪ Maximum injection volume per visit is 4 mL. See product labeling for injection volume based on lesion size. Continue for at least 6 months or until there are no injectable lesions to treat.

Dose Modification Criteria

▪ Renal: not studied
▪ Hepatic: not studied

Adverse Reactions

▪ DERM: injection site pain and complications (e.g., necrosis or ulceration of tumor tissue)
▪ GI: N/V (low) and diarrhea
▪ NEURO: headache
▪ OTHER: herpetic infection (including cold sores and herpetic keratitis), fatigue, chills, pyrexia, influenza-like illness

Comments

▪ Immune-mediated events: In clinical studies, immune-mediated events including glomerulonephritis, vasculitis, pneumonitis, worsening psoriasis, and vitiligo have been reported in patients treated with talimogene laherparepvec. Consider the risks and benefits before initiating therapy in patients who have underlying autoimmune disease or before continuing therapy in patients who have developed immune-mediated events.
▪ For intralesional injection only. Do not administer intravenously.
▪ Do not administer to immunocompromised patients.
▪ Healthcare providers who are immunocompromised or pregnant should not prepare or administer talimogene laherparepvec or come into contact with injection sites, dressings, or body fluids of treated patients
▪ Do not administer to pregnant patients.
▪ Talimogene laherparepvec is sensitive to acyclovir and other antiviral agents and thus concurrent use of antiviral agents may compromise efficacy of therapy.
▪ Follow universal biohazard precautions for preparation, administration, and handling.

TAMOXIFEN (NOLVADEX)

Mechanism of Action

▪ Nonsteroidal antiestrogen

FDA-Approved Indications

▪ Breast cancer treatment
  • Treatment of metastatic breast cancer
  • Adjuvant treatment of node-positive and node-negative breast cancer following breast surgery and breast irradiation
  • Reduction in breast cancer incidence
    • Ductal carcinoma in situ (DCIS): to reduce the risk of invasive breast cancer following breast surgery and radiation
    • High-risk women, at least 35 years of age with a 5-year predicted risk of breast cancer ≥1.67% as calculated by the Gail model (see package insert).

FDA-Approved Dosage

▪ Breast cancer treatment: 20 mg orally daily or 10 to 20 mg PO twice daily (20 to 40 mg per day). Adjuvant therapy should be continued × 5 years. Doses >20 mg per day should be given in divided doses (morning and evening).
▪ Breast cancer incidence reduction (DCIS and in high risk women): 20 mg orally daily × 5 years.

Adverse Reactions

- CV: thromboembolism, stroke, pulmonary embolism
- DERM: skin rash
- ENDO: hot flashes
- GI: N/V (minimal) and anorexia
- GU: menstrual irregularities, pruritis vulvae, vaginal discharge, or bleeding
- HEMAT: bone marrow depression
- Ocular: vision disturbances and cataracts
- PULM: dyspnea, chest pain, and hemoptysis
- OTHER: dizziness, headaches, tumor or bone pain, pelvic pain, and uterine malignancies

Comments

- High risk is defined as women at least 35 years old with a 5-year predicted risk of breast cancer of 1.67%, as predicted by the Gail model. Healthcare professionals can access a breast cancer risk assessment tool on the NCI website (www.cancer.gov/bcrisktool/).
- Serious and life-threatening events associated with tamoxifen in the risk reduction setting include uterine malignancies, stroke, and PE. Consult package insert for additional information.

TEMOZOLOMIDE (TEMODAR)

Mechanism of Action

- Alkylating agent

FDA-Approved Indications

- Glioblastoma Multiforme (GBM): Newly diagnosed patients used concomitantly with radiotherapy and then as maintenance treatment in adults.
- Anaplastic astrocytoma: Second-line treatment in adults with progressive disease after a regimen-containing nitrosourea and procarbazine.

FDA-Approved Dosage

- Newly diagnosed GBM: 75 mg/m^2 orally or IV daily × 42 days concomitant with focal radiotherapy followed by maintenance temozolomide for six cycles. The temozolomide dose should be continued throughout the 42-day concomitant period up to 49 days to achieve acceptable hematologic and nonhematologic parameters (see package insert). *Pneumocystis jiroveci* prophylaxis is required during the concomitant administration of temozolomide and radiotherapy and should be continued in patients who develop lymphocytopenia.
- Maintenance phase
  - Cycle 1: 150 mg/m^2 orally or IV daily × 5 followed by 23 days without treatment starting 4 weeks after the temozolomide + RT phase.
  - Cycles 2 to 6: Dose is escalated to 200 mg/m^2 if the nonhematologic and hematologic parameters are met (see package insert). The dose remains at 200 mg/m^2 per day for the first 5 days of each subsequent cycle except if toxicity occurs.
- Refractory anaplastic astrocytoma—initial dose: 150 mg/m^2 orally or IV daily × 5 consecutive days every 28 days. If the initial dose leads to acceptable hematologic parameters at the nadir and on day of dosing (see criteria in package insert), the temozolomide dose may be increased to 200 mg/m^2 orally or IV daily × 5 consecutive days per 28-day treatment cycle.
- Bioequivalence between the oral and intravenous formulations has only been established when the intravenous infusion is administered over 90 minutes. Infusion over a shorter or longer period may lead to suboptimal dosing.

Dose Modification Criteria

- Renal (severe impairment): use with caution
- Hepatic (severe impairment): use with caution
- Myelosuppression: yes

Adverse Reactions

- HEMAT: myelosuppression
- GI: N/V (moderate—reduced by taking on an empty stomach), constipation, and anorexia
- HEPAT: increased LFTs and hepatotoxicity
- NEURO: headache
- OTHER: asthenia, fatigue, and alopecia. Myelodysplastic syndrome (MDS) and secondary malignancies have been reported

Comments

- Capsules should be taken with water. Administer consistently with respect to food and to reduce the risk of N/V it is recommended that temozolomide be taken on an empty stomach. Bedtime administration may be advised.
- Myelosuppression occurs late in the treatment cycle. The median nadirs in a study of 158 patients with anaplastic astrocytoma occurred at 26 days for platelets (range 21 to 40 days) and 28 days for neutrophils (range 1 to 44 days). The package insert recommends obtaining a CBC on day 22 (21 days after the first dose) and then weekly until the ANC is above $1.5 \times 10^9/L$ and the platelet count exceeds $100 \times 10^9/L$. The next cycle of temozolomide should not be started until the ANC and platelet count exceed these levels. See the package insert for dose modification guidelines.
- Fatal and severe hepatotoxicity has been reported with temozolomide. Monitor LFTs at baseline, midway through the first cycle, prior to each subsequent cycle, and 2 to 4 weeks after the last dose.
- Embryo-fetal toxicity: temozolomide can cause fetal harm when administered to a pregnant woman.

TEMSIROLIMUS (TORISEL)

Mechanism of Action

- Inhibitor of mammalian target of rapamycin (mTOR)

FDA-Approved Indications

- Advanced RCC

FDA-Approved Dosage

- 25 mg infused IV over 30 to 60 minutes once a week. Treat until disease progression or unacceptable toxicity. Antihistamine pretreatment is recommended.

Dose Modification Criteria

- Renal: no
- Hepatic: yes
- Myelosuppression: yes
- Nonhematologic toxicity: no

Adverse Reactions

- DERM: rash, pruritis, nail disorder, and dry skin
- ENDO: hyperglycemia/glucose intolerance
- ELECTRO: hypophosphatemia and hypokalemia
- GI: N/V (low); mucositis, anorexia, weight loss, diarrhea, constipation, taste loss/perversion, and bowel perforation (rare)
- GU: elevated serum creatinine and renal failure
- HEMAT: myelosuppression
- HEPAT: elevated LFTs (AST, alkaline phosphatase)
- INFUS: hypersensitivity reactions (anaphylaxis, dyspnea, flushing, and chest pain)
- NEURO: headache and insomnia
- PULM: interstitial lung disease
- OTHER: asthenia, fever, immunosuppression; hyperlipidemia, hypertriglyceridemia, impaired wound healing, bleeding/hemorrhage, edema, and back pain/arthralgias

Comments

- To reduce the risk of hypersensitivity reactions, premedicate patients with an H_1 antihistamine prior to the administration of temsirolimus. Interrupt the infusion if a patient develops an infusion reaction for patient observation. At the discretion of the physician, the infusion may be resumed after administration of additional antihistamine therapy (H_1 and/or H_2 receptor antagonists) and with a slower rate of infusion for the temsirolimus.
- Serum glucose should be tested before and during treatment with temsirolimus. Patients may require an increase in the dose of, or initiation of, insulin and/or oral hypoglycemic agent therapy.
- Elevations in triglycerides and/or lipids are common side effects and may require treatment. Monitor lipid profiles.
- Monitor for symptoms or radiographic changes of interstitial lung disease. Therapy with temsirolimus should be discontinued if toxicity occurs and corticosteroid therapy should be considered.
- Bowel perforation may occur. Evaluate fever, abdominal pain, bloody stools, and/or acute abdomen promptly.
- Renal failure has occurred; monitor renal function at baseline and while on therapy.
- Due to abnormal wound healing, use temsirolimus with caution in the perioperative period.
- Live vaccinations and close contact with those who received live vaccines should be avoided.
- Temsirolimus is hepatically metabolized undergoing oxidative metabolism through CYP isoenzyme 3A4 and thus drug exposure may be influenced by potent inhibitors or inducers of CYP3A4. Refer to product labeling and other appropriate references to screen for potential drug interactions.
- Embryo-fetal toxicity: temsirolimus may cause fetal harm when administered to a pregnant woman.

TENIPOSIDE (VUMON)

Mechanism of Action

- Topoisomerase II inhibitor

FDA-Approved Indications

- Refractory childhood ALL: induction therapy as a second-line treatment (in combination with other agents)

FDA-Approved Dosage

- Refer to current literature for dosing regimens. The package insert cites two dosage regimens based on two different studies:

- In combination with cytarabine: 165 mg/m² IV over 30 to 60 minutes twice weekly × eight to nine doses
- In combination with vincristine and prednisone: 250 mg/m² IV over 30 to 60 minutes weekly × four to eight doses

Dose Modification Criteria

- Renal: use with caution, no guidelines available
- Hepatic: use with caution, no guidelines available

Adverse Reactions

- CV: hypotension with rapid infusion
- DERM: alopecia, thrombophlebitis, and tissue damage secondary to drug extravasation
- GI: diarrhea, N/V (low), and mucositis
- HEMAT: myelosuppression
- INFUS: anaphylaxis and hypersensitivity reactions (fever, chills, urticarial, tachycardia, bronchospasm, dyspnea, hypertension, hypotension, rash, and facial flushing)

Comments

- Hypersensitivity reactions may occur with the first dose of teniposide. The reactions may be due to the presence of cremaphor EL (polyoxyethylated castor oil) in the vehicle or to teniposide itself. Observe the patient for at least 60 minutes after dose.
- Consider premedication with antihistamines and/or corticosteroids for retreatment (if indicated) after a hypersensitivity reaction.
- Use non-DEHP plasticized solution containers and administration sets.
- Embryo-fetal toxicity: teniposide may cause fetal harm when administered to a pregnant woman.

THALIDOMIDE (THALOMID)

Mechanism of Action

- Immunomodulatory agent with antineoplastic and antiangiogenic properties

FDA-Approved Indications

- Multiple myeloma: first-line therapy of newly diagnosed multiple myeloma in combination with dexamethasone
- Other indications: erythema nodosum leprosum

FDA-Approved Dosage

- Multiple myeloma: 200 mg orally once daily, preferably at bedtime and at least 1 hour after the evening meal. Thalidomide is administered in combination with dexamethasone in 28-day treatment cycles. Dexamethasone is dosed at 40 mg orally once daily on days 1 to 4, 9 to 12, and 17 to 20 every 28 days. Refer to current literature for alternative dosing recommendations.

Dose Modification Criteria

- Renal: no (not studied except in patients on dialysis)
- Hepatic: no data
- Myelosuppression: yes
- Nonhematologic toxicity: yes

Adverse Reactions

- CV: edema, orthostatic hypotension, and bradycardia
- DERM: rash, desquamation, dry skin, and bullous exfoliative skin reactions
- ELECTRO: hypocalcemia
- GI: constipation and N/V (minimal to low)
- HEMAT: myelosuppression
- NEURO: peripheral neuropathy (sensory and motor), drowsiness, somnolence, dizziness, confusion, tremor, and seizures
- PULM: dyspnea
- OTHER: thromboembolic events, hypersensitivity reactions, fatigue, and tumor lysis syndrome

Comments

- Thalidomide is only available through a restricted distribution program (Thalomid REMS). Only prescribers and pharmacists registered with the program are allowed to prescribe and dispense thalidomide.
- Embryo-fetal toxicity. Thalidomide is a known teratogen and can cause severe birth defects or death to an unborn baby. Refer to the product labeling for information regarding requirements for patient consent, pregnancy testing, and patient consent as part of the Thalomid REMS program.
- Thalidomide may cause venous thromboembolic events. There is an increased risk of thrombotic events when thalidomide is combined with standard chemotherapeutic agents, including dexamethasone. Ischemic heart disease and stroke have also occurred in patients treated with thalidomide and dexamethasone. Consider concurrent prophylactic anticoagulation or aspirin treatment.
- Peripheral neuropathy is a common, potentially severe toxicity that may be irreversible. Consideration should be given to electrophysiologic testing at baseline and periodically thereafter.
- Serious dermatologic reactions (e.g., Stevens-Johnson syndrome, toxic epidermal necrolysis) have been reported with thalidomide. Discontinue if a dermatological reaction is suspected.

THIOGUANINE (TABLOID)

Mechanism of Action

- Antimetabolite

FDA-Approved Indications

- Acute nonlymphocytic leukemias (ANLL): remission induction, remission consolidation. Thioguanine is not recommended for use during maintenance therapy or similar long-term continuous treatments due to high risk of liver toxicity.

FDA-Approved Dosage

- Combination therapy: Refer to current literature.
- Single-agent therapy: 2 mg/kg orally daily as a single daily dose. May increase to 3 mg/kg orally daily as a single daily dose after 4 weeks if no clinical improvement.

Adverse Reactions

- GI: anorexia, stomatitis, and N/V (minimal)
- HEMAT: myelosuppression
- HEPAT: increased LFTs and increased bilirubin (cases of veno-occlusive hepatic disease have been reported in patients receiving combination chemotherapy for leukemia)
- OTHER: hyperuricemia and tumor lysis syndrome

Comments

- Variability in thioguanine metabolism may occur in patients due to genetic polymorphisms in the gene for the enzyme thiopurine S-methyltransferase (TMPT). TMPT genotyping or phenotyping can identify patients who are homozygous deficient or who have low or intermediate TMPT activity and who would need dose reduction to avoid thioguanine toxicity.
- Cross-resistance with mercaptopurine.
- Consider appropriate prophylaxis for tumor lysis syndrome when treating acute leukemias.
- Embryo-fetal toxicity: thioguanine may cause fetal harm when administered to a pregnant woman.

THIOTEPA (THIOPLEX, TEPADINA)

Mechanism of Action

- Alkylating agent

FDA-Approved Indications

- Superficial papillary carcinoma of the bladder
- Controlling intracavitary effusions secondary to diffuse or localized neoplastic diseases of various serosal cavities
- Adenocarcinoma of the breast
- Adenocarcinoma of the ovary
- To reduce the risk of graft rejection when used in conjunction with high-dose busulfan and cyclophosphamide as a preparative regimen for allogeneic hematopoietic progenitor (stem) cell transplantation for pediatric patients with class-3 beta thalassemia (Tepadina)

Dose Modification Criteria

- Renal (moderate to severe): use caution and monitor for toxicity
- Hepatic (moderate to severe): use caution and monitor for toxicity

FDA-Approved Dosage

- Adenocarcinoma of the breast or ovary: 0.3 to 0.4 mg/kg IV × one dose repeated at 1- to 4-week intervals. Consult current literature for alternative dosing regimens.
- Superficial papillary carcinoma of the bladder: Intravesical administration: Patients are dehydrated for 8 to 12 hours before procedure. Then 60 mg of thiotepa in 30 to 60 mL of sodium chloride injection is instilled into the bladder. For maximum effect, the solution should be retained in the bladder for 2 hours. If desired, reposition the patient every 15 minutes to maximize contact. Repeat administration weekly × 4 weeks. A course of treatment (four doses) may be repeated for up to two more courses if necessary, but with caution secondary to bone marrow depression.
- Intracavitary administration: 0.6 to 0.8 mg/kg × one dose through tubing used to remove fluid from cavity.
- Preparative regimen for class-3 beta thalassemia: 5 mg/kg IV infusion over 3 hours administered every 12 hours for 2 doses on Day -6 before allogeneic HSCT in conjunction with high-dose busulfan and cyclophosphamide.

Adverse Reactions

- CNS: dizziness, headache, blurred vision, conjunctivitis, encephalopathy (high dose)
- DERM: alopecia and pain at the injection site, rash, cutaneous toxicity (high dose)
- GI: anorexia, N/V (low to moderate), diarrhea, and mucositis at high doses
- GU: amenorrhea, reduced spermatogenesis, dysuria, and chemical or hemorrhagic cystitis (intravesical)
- HEMAT: myelosuppression and hemorrhage
- HEPAT: increased LFTs (AST, ALT, bilirubin), hepatic veno-occlusive disease (high dose)
- OTHER: fever, hypersensitivity reactions, fatigue, weakness, and anaphylaxis

Comments

- Cutaneous toxicity: In high doses thiotepa and/or its active metabolites may be excreted in part via skin, which may cause skin discoloration, pruritis, blistering, desquamation, and peeling. Patients should be instructed to shower or bathe with water at least twice daily through 48 hours post administration and bed sheets should be changed daily.
- Embryo-fetal toxicity: Thiotepa may cause fetal harm when administered to a pregnant woman.

TOPOTECAN (HYCAMTIN)

Mechanism of Action

- Topoisomerase I inhibitor

FDA-Approved Indications

- Metastatic ovarian cancer: second-line therapy after failure of initial or subsequent chemotherapy (topotecan injection)
- Small cell lung cancer (SCLC): second-line therapy in sensitive disease after failure of first-line chemotherapy (topotecan injection and oral capsules)
- Cervical cancer: combination therapy with cisplatin for stage IV-B, recurrent, or persistent carcinoma of the cervix, which is not amenable to curative treatment with surgery and/or radiation therapy

FDA-Approved Dosage

- Ovarian cancer: 1.5 mg/m^2 IV over 30 minutes daily × 5 days, starting on day 1 of a 21-day course
- SCLC
  - Injection: 1.5 mg/m^2 IV over 30 minutes daily × 5 days, repeated every 21 days
  - Oral capsules: 2.3 mg/m^2 orally once daily × 5 days, repeated every 21 days
- Cervical cancer: 0.75 mg/m^2 IV over 30 minutes daily × 3 days (days 1, 2, and 3), followed by cisplatin 50 mg/m^2 by intravenous infusion on day 1 only; repeated every 21 days (21-day cycle)

Dose Modification Criteria

- Renal (mild impairment, CrCl 40 to 60 mL per minute): no
- Renal (moderate impairment, CrCl 20 to 39 mL per minute): yes
- Renal (severe impairment, <20 mL per minute): unknown
- Hepatic (bilirubin, mild-to-moderate elevation): no
- Myelosuppression: yes
- Nonhematologic toxicity: yes

Adverse Reactions

- DERM: alopecia, rash, and injection site reactions
- HEMAT: myelosuppression
- GI: N/V (low), diarrhea, constipation, abdominal pain, stomatitis, and anorexia
- NEURO: headache and pain
- PULM: dyspnea, coughing, and interstitial lung disease
- OTHER: fatigue, asthenia, and fever

Comments

- Bone marrow suppression (primarily neutropenia) is a dose-limiting toxicity of topotecan. Topotecan should be administered only to patients with baseline neutrophil counts of ≥1,500 cells/mm^3 and a platelet count ≥100,000 cells/mm^3.

■ Topotecan-induced neutropenia can lead to neutropenic colitis.
■ Severe diarrhea requiring hospitalization has been reported with oral topotecan capsules. Dose may need to be adjusted.
■ Concomitant filgrastim may worsen neutropenia. If used, start filgrastim at least 24 hours after last topotecan dose.
■ P-gp inhibitors (e.g., cyclosporine, elacridar, ketoconazole, ritonavir, saquinavir) can cause significant increases in topotecan exposure.
■ Embryo-fetal toxicity: Topotecan may cause fetal harm if administered to a pregnant woman.

TOREMIFENE (FARESTON)

Mechanism of Action

■ Nonsteroidal antiestrogen

FDA-Approved Indications

■ Metastatic breast cancer in postmenopausal women with ER-positive or unknown tumors

FDA-Approved Dosage

■ 60 mg orally once daily

Adverse Reactions

■ CV: thromboembolism, stroke, PE, and QT prolongation
■ DERM: skin discoloration and dermatitis
■ ELECTRO: hypercalcemia
■ ENDO: hot flashes
■ GI: N/V (minimal), constipation, and elevated LFTs
■ GU: vaginal discharge and vaginal bleeding
■ NEURO: dizziness and depression
■ Ocular: dry eyes, ocular changes, and cataracts
■ OTHER: sweating and tumor flare

Comments

■ Do not use in patients with a history of thromboembolic disease or endometrial hyperplasia.
■ Toremifene has been shown to prolong the QTc interval in a dose- and concentration-related manner. Avoid in patients with long QT syndrome. Use with caution in patients with CHF, hepatic impairment, and electrolyte abnormalities. Concomitant use with other drugs that may prolong the QT interval should be avoided. Monitor ECG in patients at increased risk.
■ Toremifene is extensively metabolized principally by CYP enzyme 3A4 (CYP3A4). Coadministration with strong inhibitors or inducers of CYP3A4 will significantly impact serum concentrations of toremifene and should be avoided or used with caution. Toremifene is a weak inhibitor of CYP2C9 and may interact with CYP2C9 substrates (e.g., wafarin and phenytoin).
■ Embryo-fetal toxicity: Toremifene may cause fetal harm when administered to a pregnant woman.

TRABECTEDIN (YONDELIS)

Mechanism of Action

■ An alkylating agent that binds guanine residues in the minor groove of DNA, forming adducts and resulting in a bending of the DNA helix toward the major groove

FDA-Approved Indications

- Unresectable or metastatic liposarcoma or leiomyosarcoma after prior anthracycline-containing regimen

FDA-Approved Dosage

- 1.5mg/m² as an IV infusion over 24 hours through a central venous line every 21 days until disease progression or unacceptable toxicity
- Administer dexamethasone 20 mg IV 30 minutes prior to each dose

Dose Modification Criteria

- Renal (mild to moderate, CrCl > 30 ml/min): no
- Renal (severe, CrCl < 30 ml/min): no data
- Hepatic (moderate): yes
- Hepatic (severe): avoid use
- Myelosuppression: yes
- Nonhematologic toxicity: yes

Adverse Reactions

- CV: cardiomyopathy
- DERM: tissue damage/necrosis with extravasation
- GI: N/V (moderate), constipation, diarrhea, and decreased appetite
- GU: increased creatinine
- HEMAT: neutropenia, anemia, and thrombocytopenia
- HEPAT: elevated AST/ALT and increased alkaline phosphatase
- NEURO: headache and insomnia
- PULM: dyspnea
- OTHER: rhabdomyolysis/musculoskeletal toxicity, arthralgia, myalgia, elevated creatine phosphokinase (CPK), fatigue, and peripheral edema

Comments

- Vesicant
- Rhabdomyolysis: Trabectedin has been associated with rhabdomyolysis and musculoskeletal toxicity. Assess CPK levels prior to each dose of trabectadin and withhold therapy if serum CPK levels exceed 2.5 x the upper level of normal.
- Cardiomyopathy: Assess left ventricular ejection fraction prior to starting therapy and at 2 to 3 month intervals during therapy.
- Trabectedin is a substrate of CYP3A4. Avoid coadministration with strong CYP3A inhibitors or inducers.
- Embryo-fetal toxicity: Trabectedin may cause fetal harm when administered to a pregnant woman.

TRAMETINIB (MEKINIST)

Mechanism of Action

- A reversible inhibitor of mitogen-activated extracellular signal-regulated kinase 1 (MEK1) and MEK2 activation, and MEK1 and MEK2 kinase activity. MEK proteins are upstream regulators of the extracellular signal-related kinase (ERK) pathway, which promotes cellular proliferation. BRAF V600E mutations result in constitutive activation of the BRAF pathway, which includes MEK1 and MEK2.

FDA-Approved Indications

- Unresectable or metastatic melanoma with BRAF V600E or V600K mutations, given as a single agent or in combination with dabrafenib

FDA-Approved Dosage

▪ 2 mg orally once daily until disease progression or unacceptable toxicity. Take at least 1 hour before or 2 hours after a meal.

Dose Modification Criteria

▪ Renal (mild to moderate): no
▪ Renal (severe): no data
▪ Hepatic (mild): no
▪ Hepatic (moderate or severe): no data
▪ Nonhematologic toxicity: yes

Adverse Reactions

▪ CV: cardiomyopathy and hypertension
▪ DERM: new primary malignancies (cutaneous squamous cell carcinoma, keratoacanthoma, basal cell carcinoma, and second primary melanoma), rash, acneiform dermatitis, palmar-plantar erythrodysesthesia, erythema, pruritus
▪ ELECTRO: hyponatremia
▪ ENDO: hyperglycemia
▪ GI: diarrhea, stomatitis, and N/V (low)
▪ HEMAT: hemorrhage, venous thromboembolism, anemia, neutropenia, lymphopenia, and thrombocytopenia
▪ HEPAT: increased AST/ALT, increased alkaline phosphatase
▪ Ocular System: retinal vein occlusion
▪ PULM: interstitial lung disease
▪ OTHER: serious febrile reactions (when administered with dabrafenib), chills, lymphedema, hypoalbuminemia

Comments

▪ New primary malignancies (cutaneous and noncutaneous) may occur following trametinib. Monitor prior to initiation of therapy, while on therapy, and for 6 months following the last dose of trametinib.
▪ Cardiomyopathy: Evaluate LVEF prior to initiation of therapy, one month after initiation and then every 2 to 3 months during therapy with trametinib.
▪ Monitor for severe skin rashes and interrupt, reduce, or discontinue trametinib if necessary.
▪ Ocular toxicity: Perform an ophthalmological exam at regular intervals and for any visual disturbances.
▪ Embryo-fetal toxicity: Trametinib may cause fetal harm when administered to a pregnant woman.

TRASTUZUMAB (HERCEPTIN)

Mechanism of Action

▪ Humanized monoclonal antibody directed at the human epidermal growth factor receptor 2 protein (HER2)

FDA-Approved Indications

▪ Adjuvant breast cancer
  • For the adjuvant treatment of HER2-overexpressing node-positive or node-negative (ER/PR-negative or with one high-risk feature) breast cancer as part of a regimen containing doxorubicin, cyclophosphamide, and either paclitaxel or docetaxel OR with docetaxel and carboplatin OR as a single agent following multimodality anthracycline-based therapy.
▪ Metastatic breast cancer in patients in which tumor overexpresses the HER2 protein including
  • First-line treatment in combination with paclitaxel.

- Single-agent therapy in patients who have received one or more chemotherapy regimens for metastatic disease.
■ Metastatic gastric cancer: First-line therapy in patients with HER2 overexpressing metastatic gastric or gastroesophageal junction adenocarcinoma in combination with cisplatin and capecitabine or 5-fluorouracil.

FDA-Approved Dosage

■ Adjuvant breast cancer—administer according to one of the following doses and schedules for a total of 52 weeks of therapy
   - During and following paclitaxel, docetaxel, or docetaxel/carboplatin
   - Initial dose of 4 mg/kg by intravenous infusion over 90 minutes followed by subsequent once weekly doses of 2 mg/kg by intravenous infusion over 30 minutes for the first 12 weeks (paclitaxel or docetaxel) or 18 weeks (docetaxel/carboplatin). One week following the last weekly dose, administer trastuzumab at 6 mg/kg as an intravenous infusion over 30 to 90 minutes every 3 weeks.
   - As a single agent within 3 weeks following completion of multimodality, anthracycline-based chemotherapy regimens
   - Initial dose of 8 mg/kg as an intravenous infusion over 90 minutes followed by subsequent doses of 6 mg/kg as an intravenous infusion over 30 to 90 minutes every 3 weeks.
■ Metastatic breast cancer—administered alone or in combination with paclitaxel: Initial dose of 4 mg/kg by intravenous infusion over 90 minutes followed by subsequent once weekly doses of 2 mg/kg by intravenous infusion over 30 minutes until disease progression.
■ Metastatic gastric cancer: Initial dose of 8 mg/kg as an intravenous infusion over 90 minutes followed by subsequent doses of 6 mg/kg as an intravenous infusion over 30 to 90 minutes every 3 weeks until disease progression.

Adverse Reactions

■ CV: cardiomyopathy, ventricular dysfunction, CHF (incidence higher in patients receiving concurrent chemotherapy), and hypotension (infusion reactions)
■ DERM: rash
■ HEMAT: myelosuppression (anemia and leukopenia with concurrent chemotherapy)
■ GI: diarrhea, nausea, vomiting, and anorexia
■ INFUS: (first infusion) chills, fever, nausea, vomiting, pain (at tumor sites), rigors, headache, dizziness, dyspnea, rash, hypotension, and asthenia
■ NEURO: headache, dizziness (see infusion reactions)
■ PULM: cough, dyspnea, rhinitis, adult respiratory distress syndrome, bronchospasm, angioedema, wheezing, pleural effusions, pulmonary infiltrates, noncardiogenic pulmonary edema, pulmonary insufficiency, and hypoxia (some severe pulmonary reactions required supplemental oxygen or ventilatory support)
■ OTHER: infection (higher incidence of mild upper respiratory infections and catheter infections observed in one randomized trial), asthenia, allergic reactions, and anaphylaxis

Comments

■ Death within 24 hours of a trastuzumab infusion has been reported. The most severe reactions seem to occur in patients with significant preexisting pulmonary compromise secondary to intrinsic lung disease and/or malignant pulmonary involvement.
■ Do not administer by intravenous push or bolus.
■ May use sterile water for injection for reconstitution if patient is allergic to benzyl alcohol (supplied diluent is bacteriostatic water for injection); product should be used immediately and unused portion discarded.
■ Alternative dosing regimens have been studied including dosing at longer dosing intervals; consult current literature.
■ Embryo-fetal toxicity: Trastuzumab can cause fetal harm when administered to a pregnant woman.

TRETINOIN (VESANOID)

Mechanism of Action

- Induces maturation, cytodifferentiation, and decreased proliferation of acute promyelocytic leukemia cells.

FDA-Approved Indications

- Acute promyelocytic leukemia (APL): Induction of remission in patients with APL FAB M3 (including the M3 variant), characterized by the t(15:17) translocation and/or the presence of the PML/RAR α gene, who are refractory to or relapsed after anthracycline chemotherapy or for whom anthracycline therapy is contraindicated.

FDA-Approved Dosage

- 22.5 mg/m² orally twice daily (total daily dose: 45 mg/m²) until complete remission is documented. Therapy should be discontinued 30 days after complete remission is obtained or after 90 days of treatment, whichever comes first.

Adverse Reactions

- CV: hypertension, arrhythmias, and flushing
- DERM: dry skin/mucous membranes, rash, pruritis, alopecia, and mucositis
- GI: N/V, diarrhea, constipation, and dyspepsia
- HEMAT: leukocytosis
- HEPAT: elevated LFTs
- NEURO: dizziness, anxiety, insomnia, headache, depression, confusion, intracranial hypertension, agitation, earaches, hearing loss, and pseudotumor cerebri
- Ocular: visual changes
- OTHER: dyspnea, fever, shivering, retinoic acid–APL syndrome (RA-APL syndrome: fever, dyspnea, weight gain, radiographic pulmonary infiltrates, and pleural or pericardial effusion), and hyperlipidemia

Comments

- Teratogenic; women must use effective contraception during and for 1 month after therapy.
- RA-APL syndrome occurs in up to 25% of patients usually within the first month. Early recognition and high-dose corticosteroids (dexamethasone 10 mg IV every 12 hours × 3 days or until the resolution of symptoms) have been used for management.
- During tretinoin treatment about 40% of patients will develop rapidly evolving leukocytosis, which is associated with a higher risk of life-threatening complications. If signs and symptoms of the RA-APL syndrome are present together with leukocytosis, high-dose corticosteroids should be initiated immediately. Chemotherapy is often combined with tretinoin in patients who present with leukocytosis (WBC count of >5 × 10⁹/L) or with rapidly evolving leukocytosis.
- Consult current literature for APL treatment regimens.

TRIFLURIDINE/TIPIRACIL (LONSURF)

Mechanism of Action

- Trifluridine is a thymidine-based nucleoside analog and tipiracil is a thymidine phosphorylase inhibitor. Tipiracil increases exposure to trifluridine by inhibiting its metabolism by thymidine phosphorylase.

FDA-Approved Indications

- Metastatic colorectal cancer that has previously been treated with fluoropyrimidine-, oxaliplatin- and irinotecan-based chemotherapy, an anti-VEGF biological therapy, and if RAS wild-type, an anti-EGFR therapy

FDA-Approved Dosage

- 35 mg/m^2 up to a maximum of 80 mg per dose (based on the trifluridine component) orally twice daily on days 1 to 5 and 8 to 12 of a 28-day cycle until disease progression or unacceptable toxicity. Take within one hour of morning and evening meals.

Dose Modification Criteria

- Renal (mild to moderate, CrCl ≥ 30 mL/min): no (monitor for toxicity)
- Renal (severe, CrCl < 30 mL/min): no data
- Hepatic (mild): no
- Hepatic (moderate to severe): no data
- Myelosuppression: yes
- Nonhematologic toxicity: yes

Adverse Reactions

- GI: N/V (low), diarrhea, abdominal pain, decreased appetite
- HEMAT: anemia, neutropenia, thrombocytopenia (myelosuppression may be severe)
- OTHER: asthenia/fatigue, pyrexia

Comments

- Embryo-fetal toxicity: Trifluridine/tipiracil may cause fetal harm when administered to a pregnant woman.

TRIPTORELIN (TRELSTAR)

Mechanism of Action

- Gonadotropin-releasing hormone (GnRH or LHRH) agonist; chronic administration leads to sustained suppression of pituitary gonadotropins and subsequent suppression of serum testosterone in men and serum estradiol in women.

FDA-Approved Indications

- Palliative treatment of advanced prostate cancer

FDA-Approved Dosage

- Trelstar 3.75 mg intramuscular injection every 4 weeks
- Trelstar 11.25 mg intramuscular injection every 12 weeks
- Trelstar 22.5 mg intramuscular injection every 24 weeks

Adverse Reactions

- CV: hypertension, peripheral edema, QT interval prolongation
- ENDO: hot flashes, gynecomastia, breast pain, sexual dysfunction, decreased erections, and hyperglycemia
- GU: erectile dysfunction, lower urinary tract symptoms, and testicular atrophy
- OTHER: tumor flare in the first few weeks of therapy, bone pain, injection site reactions, loss of bone mineral density, osteoporosis, bone fracture, and asthenia

Comments

- Use with caution in patients at risk of developing ureteral obstruction or spinal cord compression.

VALRUBICIN (VALSTAR)

Mechanism of Action

▪ Intercalating agent; topoisomerase II inhibition

FDA-Approved Indications

▪ Carcinoma in situ of the urinary bladder: Second-line intravesical treatment after BCG therapy in patients for whom immediate cystectomy would be associated with unacceptable morbidity or mortality.

FDA-Approved Dosage

▪ 800 mg intravesically weekly × 6 weeks. For each instillation, 800 mg of valrubicin is diluted with 0.9% sodium chloride to a total volume of 75 mL. Once instilled into the bladder, the patient should retain drug in bladder for 2 hours before voiding.

Adverse Reactions

▪ GU: Irritable bladder symptoms: urinary frequency, dysuria, urinary urgency, hematuria, bladder spasm, bladder pain, urinary incontinence, cystitis, local burning symptoms related to the procedure, and red-tinged urine

Comments

▪ Patients should maintain adequate hydration after treatment.
▪ Irritable bladder symptoms may occur during instillation and retention of valrubicin and for a limited period following voiding. For the first 24 hours following administration, red-tinged urine is typical. Patients should report prolonged irritable bladder symptoms or prolonged passage of red-colored urine immediately to their physician.
▪ Use non-DEHP plasticized solution containers and administration sets.

VANDETANIB (CAPRELSA)

Mechanism of Action

▪ Kinase inhibitor. In vitro studies have shown that vandetanib inhibits the activity of EGFR, VEGF, rearranged during transfection (RET), protein tyrosine kinase 6 (BRK), TIE2, members of the EPH receptors kinase family, and members of the Src family of tyrosine kinases.

FDA-Approved Indications

▪ Symptomatic or progressive medullary thyroid cancer in patients with unresectable locally advanced or metastatic disease

FDA-Approved Dosage

▪ 300 mg orally once daily with or without food

Dose Modification Criteria

▪ Renal (mild): no
▪ Renal (CrCL <30 to 49 mL per minute): yes
▪ Hepatic (mild): no
▪ Hepatic (moderate, severe): use is not recommended
▪ Nonhematologic toxicities: yes

Adverse Reactions

- CV: heart failure, hypertension, and QT prolongation
- DERM: acne, dermatitis acneiform, dry skin, pruritis, rash, photosensitivity, palmar-plantar erythrodysesthesia, and severe bullous/exfoliative skin reactions (including Stevens–Johnson syndrome)
- ELECTRO: hypocalcemia, hypoglycemia, hypokalemia, and hyperkalemia
- ENDO: hypothyroidism
- GI: abdominal pain, anorexia, diarrhea, dyspepsia, and nausea (minimal to low)
- GU: proteinuria
- HEPAT: increased ALT
- NEURO: headache and ischemic cerebrovascular events
- PULM: interstitial lung disease and upper respiratory tract infection
- OTHER: asthenia, fatigue, and hemorrhage

Comments

- Only prescribers and pharmacies certified with the restricted distribution program (Caprelsa® REMS Program) are able to prescribe and dispense vandetanib.
- Vandetanib should not be used in patients with hypocalcemia, hypokalemia, hypomagnesemia, or long QT syndrome. Electrolyte abnormalities should be corrected before drug administration. Drugs known to prolong the QT interval should be avoided. Given the half-life of 19 days, ECGs should be obtained to monitor the QT at baseline, at 2 to 4 weeks and 8 to 12 weeks after starting treatment with vandetanib, and every 3 months thereafter. Following any dose reduction for QT prolongation, or any dose interruptions greater than weeks, QT assessment should be conducted.
- Use of vandetanib in patients with indolent, asymptomatic, or slowly progressing disease should be carefully considered because of the treatment-related risks of vandetanib.
- Interrupt vandetanib and investigate unexplained dyspnea, cough, and fever. Advise patients to report promptly any new or worsening respiratory symptoms.
- Do not administer vandetanib to patients with recent history of hemoptysis of ≥1/2 teaspoon of red blood.
- Consider RPLS in any patient presenting with seizures, headache, visual disturbances, confusion, or altered mental function.
- Routine antidiarrheal agents are recommended. If severe diarrhea develops, vandetanib treatment should be stopped until diarrhea improves, and upon improvement, treatment should be resumed at a reduced dose.
- Avoid the concomitant use of strong CYP3A4 inducers, and with agents that may prolong the QT interval.
- Mild-to-moderate skin reactions have been treated with topical and systemic corticosteroids, oral antihistamines, and topical and systemic antibiotics. If CTCAE grade 3 or greater skin reactions occur, vandetanib should be stopped until improved, and upon improvement, consideration should be given to continuing treatment at a reduced dose or permanent discontinuation of vandetanib.
- Patients should be advised to wear sunscreen and protective clothing when exposed to the sun. Due to the long half-life of vandetanib, protective clothing and sunscreen should continue for 4 months after discontinuation of treatment.
- Vandetanib tablets should not be crushed. If patients have difficulty swallowing tablets, the tablets can be dispersed in a glass containing two ounces of noncarbonated water and stirred for approximately 10 minutes until the tablet is dispersed (it will not completely dissolve). See product labeling for additional information.
- Embryo-fetal toxicity: Vandetanib may cause fetal harm when administered to a pregnant woman.

VEMURAFENIB (ZELBORAF)

Mechanism of Action

- Inhibits some mutated forms of BRAF serine–threonine kinase, including BRAF^{v600E}. Some mutations in the *BRAF* gene including V600E result in constitutively activated BRAF proteins, which can cause cell proliferation in the absence of growth factors that would normally be required for proliferation.

FDA-Approved Indications

▪ Unresectable or metastatic melanoma with BRAF^{V600E} mutation as detected by an FDA-approved test.

FDA-Approved Dosage

▪ 960 mg orally twice daily.

Dose Modification Criteria

▪ Renal (mild to moderate): no
▪ Renal (severe): exercise caution
▪ Hepatic (mild to moderate): no
▪ Hepatic (severe): exercise caution
▪ Nonhematologic toxicity: yes

Adverse Reactions

▪ CV: QT prolongation
▪ DERM: alopecia, cutaneous squamous cell carcinoma, dry skin, erythema, hyperkeratosis, hypersensitivity reaction (generalized rash, erythema, bullous exfoliative skin reactions [e.g., Stevens–Johnson, toxic epidermal necrolysis]), new primary malignant melanoma, photosensitivity, pruritus, rash, and skin papilloma
▪ GI: decreased appetite, constipation, diarrhea, and N/V (minimal to low)
▪ GU: increased serum creatinine, interstitial nephritis, acute tubular necrosis
▪ HEPAT: increased alkaline phosphatase, increased bilirubin, and increased LFTs
▪ NEURO: headache
▪ Ocular: blurry vision, iritis, photophobia, retinal vein occlusion, and uveitis
▪ OTHER: arthralgia, edema, fatigue, myalgia, and pain in extremity

Comments

▪ Vemurafenib is not recommended for use in patients with wild-type BRAF melanoma. An FDA-approved test must be used to detect the BRAF^{V600E} mutation.
▪ Vemurafenib increases photosensitivity to UVA light, which can penetrate glass. Patients should be advised to apply broad spectrum UVA/UVB sunscreen and lip balm (SPF ≥30) when outdoors and when driving.
▪ Cutaneous squamous cell carcinomas occurred in 24% of patients. Perform dermatologic evaluations prior to initiation of therapy and every 2 months while on therapy. Manage with excision and continue treatment without dose adjustment. Dose modifications or interruptions are not recommended. Vemurafenib may also promote new noncutaneous squamous cell carcinoma and other malignancies.
▪ Radiation sensitization and recall involving cutaneous and visceral organs have been reported in patients treated with radition therapy prior to, during or subsequent to vemurafenib treatment. Concomitant use of vemurafenib with drugs with narrow therapeutic windows that are metabolized by CYP3A4, CYP1A2, or CYP2D6 is not recommended.
▪ Vemurafenib may increase exposure to concomitantly administered warfarin. Exercise caution and consider additional INR monitoring.
▪ Vemurafenib is not recommended in patients with uncorrectable electrolyte abnormalities, with long QT syndrome, or who are taking QT-prolonging drugs.
▪ Embryo-fetal toxicity: Vemurafenib may cause fetal harm when administered to a pregnant woman.

VENETOCLAX (VENCLEXTA)

Mechanism of Action

- Selective inhibitor of the anti-apoptotic protein BCL-2.

FDA-Approved Indications

- CLL with 17p deletion, as detected by an FDA approved test, who have received at least one prior therapy

FDA-Approved Dosage

- Dose is increased from 20 to 400 mg using the following 5 week ramp-up schedule: 20 mg daily X 1 week, 50 mg daily X 1 week, 100 mg daily X 1 week, 200 mg daily X 1 week, 400 mg daily during week 5 and beyond.
- Venetoclax tablets should be taken orally once daily with a meal and water.

Dose Modification Criteria

- Renal (mild to moderate): no
- Renal (severe, CrCl <30 mL/min): no data
- Hepatic (mild to moderate): no (monitor for toxicity)
- Hepatic (severe, total bilirubin > 3 X ULN): no data
- Myelosuppression: yes
- Nonhematologic toxicity: yes

Adverse Reactions

- GI: diarrhea, N/V (low)
- HEMAT: neutropenia, anemia, and thrombocytopenia
- NEURO: headache
- PULM: upper respiratory tract infection
- OTHER: fatigue, pyrexia, and tumor lysis syndrome

Comments

- Anticipate and assess risk for tumor lysis syndrome (TLS) and provide prophylaxis as appropriate. Labs may suggest TLS as early as 6 to 8 hours following the first dose. The slow ramp up of dosing is to reduce the potential for TLS.
- Venetoclax is a substrate of CYP3A4/5, P-glycoprotein, and BCRP. Concomitant use of strong CYP3A inhibitors during the ramp-up phase is contraindicated. When possible, avoid moderate or strong CYP3A4 inhibitors, strong CYP3A4 inducers, and P-glycoprotein inhibitors. Venetoclax dose reductions may be employed when moderate or strong inhibitors must be used concurrently. Screen for drug interactions.
- Do not administer live attenuated vaccines prior to, during or after treatment with venetoclax until B-cell recovery.
- Embryo-fetal toxicity: Venetoclax may cause fetal harm when administered to a pregnant woman.

VINBLASTINE (VELBAN)

Mechanism of Action

- Inhibits microtubule formation

FDA-Approved Indications

- Palliative treatment of the following malignancies:
  - Frequently responsive malignancies: testicular cancer, Hodgkin disease, NHL, mycosis fungoides, Kaposi sarcoma, histiocytic lymphoma, Letterer–Siwe disease (histiocytosis X)
  - Less frequently responsive malignancies: breast cancer and resistant choriocarcinoma

FDA-Approved Dosage

- Initial (adults): 3.7 mg/m^2 IV weekly. May increase weekly dose in a step wise format up to a maximum dose of 18.5 mg/m^2 to maintain WBC >3,000 cells/mm^3 (see package insert for schema).
- Pediatric: Consult current literature for dose regimens.
- Consult current literature for alternative dosing regimens.

Dose Modification Criteria

- Renal: no
- Hepatic: yes
- Myelosuppression: yes

Adverse Reactions

- CV: hypertension
- DERM: alopecia and tissue damage/necrosis with extravasation
- GI: N/V (minimal), stomatitis, constipation, and ileus
- GU: urinary retention and polyuria
- HEMAT: myelosuppression
- NEURO: peripheral neuropathy, paresthesias, loss of deep tendon reflexes, and SIADH
- OTHER: bone pain, jaw pain, tumor pain, weakness, malaise, and Raynaud phenomenon

Comments

- Vesicant.
- Administer only by the intravenous route. Fatalities have been reported when other vinca alkaloids have been given intrathecally.
- Label syringe: Administer only intravenously; fatal if given intrathecally. Label outerwrap (if used): "Do not remove covering until moment of injection. Fatal if given intrathecally. For intravenous use only." Alternatively, administration of vinblastine via an IV minibag as a short infusion may be used and can potentially help to prevent errors in administration. Refer to recommendations provided by the Institute of Safe Medication Practices (www.ismp.org).
- Embryo-fetal toxicity: vinblastine may cause fetal harm when administered to a pregnant woman.

VINCRISTINE (ONCOVIN AND OTHERS)

Mechanism of Action

- Inhibits microtubule formation

FDA-Approved Indications

- Acute leukemia.
- Vincristine has shown to be useful in combination with other agents for Hodgkin disease, NHL, neuroblastoma, Wilms tumor, and rhabdomyosarcoma.

FDA-Approved Dosage

- Adults: 1.4 mg/m^2 IV × one dose. Doses may be repeated at weekly intervals. Some clinicians will limit ("cap") individual doses to a maximum of 2 mg.
- Pediatrics: 1.5 to 2 mg/m^2 IV × one dose. For pediatric patients weighing 10 kg or less: 0.05 mg/kg IV × one dose. Doses may be repeated at weekly intervals. Some clinicians will limit ("cap") individual doses to a maximum of 2 mg.

Dose Modification Criteria

- Renal: no
- Hepatic: yes

Adverse Reactions

- DERM: alopecia and tissue damage/necrosis with extravasation
- GI: N/V (minimal), stomatitis, anorexia, diarrhea, constipation, and ileus
- GU: urinary retention
- NEURO: peripheral neuropathy, paresthesias, numbness, loss of deep tendon reflexes, and SIADH
- Ocular: ophthalmoplegia and extraocular muscle paresis
- PULM: pharyngitis
- OTHER: jaw pain

Comments

- Vesicant.
- Administer only by the intravenous route. Fatalities have been reported when vinca alkaloids have been given intrathecally.
- Label syringe: Administer only intravenously; fatal if given intrathecally. Label outerwrap (if used): "Do not remove covering until moment of injection. Fatal if given intrathecally. For intravenous use only." Alternatively, administration of vincristine via an IV minibag as a short infusion may be used and can potentially help to prevent errors in administration. Refer to recommendations provided by the Institute of Safe Medication Practices (www.ismp.org).
- Medications that are inhibitors of cytochrome 3A4 will increase vincristine drug exposure and increase the risk of neurotoxicity.
- Embryo-fetal toxicity: vincristine may cause fetal harm when administered to a pregnant woman.
- A routine prophylactic regimen against constipation is recommended for all patients receiving vincristine.

VINCRISTINE SULFATE LIPOSOME (MARQIBO)

Mechanism of Action

- Binds to tubulin, altering the tubulin polymerization equilibrium, resulting in altered microtubule structure and function, and stabilizes the spindle apparatus, preventing chromosome segregation, triggering metaphase arrest, and inhibition of mitosis.

FDA-Approved Indications

- ALL: Philadelphia chromosome-negative ALL in second or greater relapse or whose disease has progressed following two or more antileukemia therapies.

FDA-Approved Dosages

- 2.25 mg/m² IV over 1 hour once every 7 days
- For intravenous use only; fatal if given by other routes

Dose Modification Criteria

- Renal: no data
- Hepatic (mild, moderate): no
- Hepatic (severe): no data
- Myelosuppression: yes
- Nonhematologic toxicity: yes

Adverse Effects

- CV: hypotension
- GI: bowel obstruction, constipation, diarrhea, ileus, and nausea (minimal)
- HEMAT: anemia, febrile neutropenia, neutropenia, and thrombocytopenia
- HEPAT: elevated LFTs

- NEURO: motor and sensory peripheral neuropathy
- OTHER: fatigue, insomnia, pain, pyrexia, and tumor lysis syndrome

Comments

- Fatal if given intrathecally.
- Vincristine sulfate liposome has different dosage recommendations than vincristine sulfate injection.
- Vincristine sulfate liposome requires extensive preparation time (60 to 90 minutes to prepare).
- Vincristine sulfate liposome is contraindicated in patients with demyelinating conditions including Charcot–Marie–Tooth syndrome.
- Vincristine sulfate liposome is a vesicant. If extravasation is suspected, discontinue infusion immediately and consider local treatment measures.
- Monitor patients for peripheral motor and sensory, central and autonomic neuropathy, and reduce, interrupt, or discontinue dosing. Sensory and motor neuropathies are cumulative.
- Institute a prophylactic bowel regimen to prevent potential constipation, bowel obstruction, and/or paralytic ileus.
- Vincristine sulfate liposome is expected to interact with drugs known to interact with nonliposomal vincristine sulfate. The concomitant use of strong CYP3A inhibitors and inducers should be avoided, as well as P-glycoprotein inhibitors or inducers.
- Embryo-fetal toxicity: Vincristine sulfate liposome may cause fetal harm when administered to a pregnant woman.

VINORELBINE (NAVELBINE)

Mechanism of Action

- Inhibits microtubule formation

FDA-Approved Indications

- NSCLC: First-line treatment as a single agent (stage IV) or in combination with cisplatin (stage III or IV) for ambulatory patients with unresectable, advanced NSCLC.

FDA-Approved Dosage

- Single agent: 30 mg/m^2 IV over 6 to 10 minutes weekly.
- Vinorelbine in combination with cisplatin:
  - Vinorelbine 25 mg/m^2 IV over 6 to 10 minutes weekly, *plus*
  - Cisplatin 100 mg/m^2 IV every 4 weeksOR
  - Vinorelbine 30 mg/m^2 IV over 6 to 10 minutes weekly, *plus*
  - Cisplatin 120 mg/m^2 IV × one dose on day 1 and 29, then every 6 weeks
- Flush line with 75 to 125 mL of fluid (e.g., 0.9% sodium chloride) after administration of vinorelbine.

Dose Modification Criteria

- Renal: no
- Hepatic: yes
- Myelosuppession: yes
- Nonhematologic toxicity (neurotoxicity): yes

Adverse Reactions

- CV: thromboembolic events and chest pain
- DERM: alopecia, vein discoloration, venous pain, chemical phlebitis, and tissue damage/necrosis with extravasation
- GI: N/V (minimal), stomatitis, anorexia, constipation, and ileus

- HEMAT: myelosuppression (granulocytopenia > thrombocytopenia or anemia)
- HEPAT: elevated LFTs
- NEURO: peripheral neuropathy and loss of deep tendon reflexes
- PULM: interstitial pulmonary changes and shortness of breath
- OTHER: jaw pain, tumor pain, fatigue, and anaphylaxis

Comments

- Vesicant.
- Administer only by the intravenous route. Fatalities have been reported when other vinca alkaloids have been given intrathecally.
- Embryo-fetal toxicity: vinorelbine may cause fetal harm when administered to a pregnant woman.

VISMODEGIB (ERIVEDGE)

Mechanism of Action

- Hedgehog pathway inhibitor that binds to and inhibits smoothened, a transmembrane protein involved in Hedgehog signal transduction.

FDA-Approved Indications

- Metastatic basal cell carcinoma.
- Locally advanced basal cell carcinoma that has recurred following surgery or in patients who are not candidates for surgery, and who are not candidates for radiation.

FDA-Approved Dosage

- 150 mg orally once daily

Dose Modification Criteria

- Renal: no
- Hepatic: no

Adverse Reactions

- DERM: alopecia
- ELECTRO: azotemia, hypokalemia, and hyponatremia
- GI: anorexia, constipation, diarrhea, and N/V (low)
- NEURO: taste disorders (ageusia and dysgeusia)
- OTHER: amenorrhea, decreased appetite, fatigue, muscle spasms, and arthralgias

Comments

- Embryo-fetal toxicity: Vismodegib can result in embryo-fetal death or severe birth defects. Verify pregnancy status prior to initiation. Advise females of the need for contraception during and for 7 months after treatment, and advise males of the potential risk of vismodegib exposure through semen. Male patients should use condoms with spermicide, even after a vasectomy, during sexual intercourse with female partners during treatment and for 2 months after the last dose. Report immediate exposure during pregnancy to the Genentech Adverse Event Line at 1-888-835-2555. Encourage patient participation in the vismodegib pregnancy pharmacovigilance program.
- Advise patients not to donate blood or blood products while receiving vismodegib and for at least 7 months after the last dose.

VORINOSTAT (ZOLINZA)

Mechanism of Action

- Histone deacetylase inhibitor

FDA-Approved Indications

- Cutaneous T cell lymphoma (CTCL): treatment of cutaneous manifestations in patients with CTCL who have progressive, persistent, or recurrent disease on or following two systemic therapies.

FDA-Approved Dosage

- 400 mg orally once daily with food

Dose Modification Criteria

- Renal: no (use with caution)
- Hepatic: yes (mild-to-moderate impairment, limited data with severe impairment)
- Myelosuppression: yes
- Nonhematologic toxicity: yes

Adverse Reactions

- CV: QTc prolongation
- DERM: alopecia
- ENDO: hyperglycemia
- GI: N/V (low), diarrhea, anorexia, weight loss, constipation, and dry mouth
- GU: increased Cr and proteinuria
- HEMAT: myelosuppression (thrombocytopenia and anemia)
- NEURO: taste disorders (dysgeusia)
- OTHER: constitutional symptoms (fatigue and chills), thromboembolic events (including PE), dehydration, and muscle spasms

Comments

- Deep venous thrombosis and PE have been reported. Monitor for pertinent signs and symptoms.
- Patients may require antiemetics, antidiarrheals, and fluid and electrolyte replacement to prevent dehydration.
- Hyperglycemia has been commonly reported. Adjustment of diet and/or therapy for increased glucose may be necessary.
- QTc prolongation has been observed. Monitor electrolytes and ECGs at baseline and periodically during treatment.
- Monitor blood counts and chemistry tests every 2 weeks during the first 2 months of therapy and monthly thereafter.
- Severe thrombocytopenia and gastrointestinal bleeding have been reported with concomitant use of vorinostat and other HDAC inhibitors (e.g., valproic acid).
- Embryo-fetal toxicity: vorinostat may cause fetal harm when administered to a pregnant woman.

ZIV-AFLIBERCEPT (ZALTRAP)

Mechanism of Action

- Ziv-aflibercept acts as a soluble receptor that binds to VEGF-A, VEGF-B, and PIGF. By binding to these endogenous ligands, ziv-aflibercept can inhibit the binding and activation of their cognate receptors. This inhibition can result in decreased neovascularization and decreased vascular permeability.

FDA-Approved Indications

- Metastatic colorectal cancer that is resistant to or has progressed following an oxaliplatin-containing regimen: Ziv-aflibercept is used in combination with 5-fluorouracil, leucovorin, and irinotecan (FOLFIRI).

FDA-Approved Dosage

- 4 mg/kg IV over 1 hour every 2 weeks

Dose Modification Criteria

- Renal: no
- Hepatic (mild to moderate): no
- Hepatic (severe): no data
- Nonhematologic toxicity: yes

Adverse Reactions

- CV: hypertension and arterial thromboembolic events
- GI: diarrhea, stomatitis, weight loss, decreased appetite, abdominal pain, gastrointestinal fistula, perforation, or hemorrhage
- GU: increased serum creatinine and proteinuria
- HEMAT: myelosuppression (leukopenia, neutropenia, and thrombocytopenia)
- HEPAT: increased LFTs
- NEURO: headache, RPLS
- OTHER: fatigue, epistaxis, dysphonia, and compromised wound healing

Comments

- Ziv-aflibercept/FOLFIRI should not be administered until the neutrophil count is $\geq 1.5 \times 10^9$/L.
- Ziv-aflibercept should be held for at least 4 weeks prior to elective surgery, and for at least 4 weeks following major surgery. Do not resume ziv-aflibercept until the surgical wound has fully healed. Monitor blood pressure at least every 2 weeks. Suspend ziv-aflibercept for recurrent or severe hypertension. Once hypertension is controlled, reduce the dose of ziv-aflibercept upon restarting treatment.
- Ziv-aflibercept should be suspended for proteinuria of 2 g per 24 hours. Reduce the dose of ziv-aflibercept for recurrent proteinuria.
- Elderly patients may be at a higher risk for diarrhea and dehydration with ziv-aflibercept/FOLFIRI, and should be monitored closely.
- Ziv-aflibercept should be administered through a 0.2 μm polyethersulfone filter. Polyvinylidene fluoride or nylon filters should not be used.
- Embryo-fetal toxicity: there are no adequate and well-controlled studies with ziv-aflibercept in pregnant women. Male and female contraception should be used during treatment and for at least 3 months following the last dose of ziv-aflibercept.

Suggested Readings

1. Kohler DR, Montello MJ, Green L, et al. Standardizing the expression and nomenclature of cancer treatment regimens. *Am J Health Syst Pharm.* 1998;55:137–144.

1 PERFORMANCE STATUS SCALES/SCORES: PERFORMANCE STATUS CRITERIA

TABLE 1

ECOG (Zubrod)		Karnofsky		Lansky[a]	
Score	Description	Score	Description	Score	Description
0	Fully active, able to carry on all predisease performance without restriction	100	Normal, no complaints, no evidence of disease	100	Fully active, normal
1	Restricted in physically strenuous activity but ambulatory and able to carry out work of a light or sedentary nature, for example, light housework/office work	90	Able to carry on normal activity; minor signs or symptoms of disease	90	Minor restrictions in physically strenuous activity
2	Ambulatory and capable of all self-care but unable to carry out any activities related to work. Up and about more than 50% of waking hours	80	Normal activity with effort; some signs or symptoms of disease	80	Active, but tires faster than in previous phase
3	Capable of only limited self-care, confined to bed or chair more than 50% of waking hours	70	Cares for self, unable to carry on normal activity or do active work	70	Both greater restriction of play activity and less time spent in such activity than in previous phase
4	Completely disabled. Cannot carry on any self-care; totally confined to bed or chair	60	Requires occasional assistance, but is able to care for most of his/her needs	60	Up and around, but minimally active in play; keeps busy with quieter activities than in previous phase
		50	Requires considerable assistance and frequent medical care	50	Gets dressed, but lies around much of the day; no active play; able to participate in quiet play and activities
		40	Disabled, requires special care and assistance	40	Mostly in bed; participates in quiet activities
		30	Severely disabled, hospitalization indicated; death not imminent	30	In bed; needs assistance even for quiet play
		20	Very sick, hospitalization indicated; death not imminent	20	Often sleeping; play entirely limited to very passive activities
		10	Moribund, fatal processes progressing rapidly	10	No play; does not even get out of bed

[a] The conversion of the Lansky to ECOG scales is intended for National Cancer Institute reporting purposes only.

ECOG, Eastern Cooperative Oncology Group.

Karnofsky and Lansky performance scores are intended to be multiples of 10.

Index